THE INTERNATIONAL SYSTEM OF UNITS
(Continued)

Selected Typical Reference Intervals

SOME TYPICAL CLINICAL CHEMISTRY REFERENCE INTERVALS IN CONVENTIONAL AND SI UNITS

Component	System	Typical Reference Intervals		
		in Conventional Units	Factor*	in SI Units*†
Albumin	Serum	3.8–5.0 gm/dl	10	38–50 g/l
Bicarbonate	Plasma	21–28 mM	1	21–28 mmol/l
Bilirubin	Serum			
direct		<0.3 mg/dl	17.1	<5.1 μmol/l
indirect		0.1–1.0 mg/dl		1.7–17.1 μmol/l
total		0.1–1.2 mg/dl		1.7–20.5 μmol/l
Calcium	Serum	9.2–11.0 mg/dl	0.25	2.3–2.8 mmol/l
		4.6–5.5 mEq/l	0.5	
Chloride	Serum	95–103 mEq/l	1	95–103 mmol/l
Cholesterol	Serum	150–250 mg/dl	0.026	3.90–6.50 mmol/l
Creatinine	Serum	0.6–1.2 mg/dl	88.4	53–106 μmol/l
Globulins	Serum	2.3–3.5 gm/dl	10	23–35 g/l
Glucose	Serum	70–110 mg/dl	0.055	3.85–6.05 mmol/l
Iron	Serum	60–150 μg/dl	0.179	11–27 μmol/l
Lactate dehydrogenase	Serum	80–129 units at 25°C. (lactate→pyruvate)	0.48	38–62 U/l at 25°C.
		185–640 units at 30°C. (pyruvate→lactate)	0.48	90–310 U/l at 30°C.
Phosphatase, alkaline	Serum	20–90 IU/l at 30°C. (p-nitro phenylphosphate)	1	20–90 U/l at 30°C.
Phosphorus	Serum	2.3–4.7 mg/dl	0.323	0.78–1.52 mmol/l
Potassium	Plasma	3.8–5.0 mEq/l	1	3.8–5.0 mmol/l
Protein, total	Serum	6.0–7.8 gm/dl	10	60–78 g/l
Sodium	Plasma	136–142 mEq/l	1	136–142 mmol/l
Thyroxine	Serum	5.0–11.0 μg/dl	13.0	65–143 nmol/l
Transferases:	Serum			
aspartate amino-		16–60 U/ml (Karmen) at 30°C.	0.48	8–29 U/l at 30°C.
alanine amino-		8–50 U/ml (Karmen) at 30°C.	0.48	4–24 U/l at 30°C.
Triglyceride	Serum	10–190 mg/dl	0.011	0.11–2.09 mmol/l
Urea nitrogen	Serum	8–23 mg/dl	0.357	2.9–8.2 mmol/l
Uric acid	Serum			
male		4.0–8.5 mg/dl	0.059	0.24–0.5 mmol/l
female		2.7–7.3 mg/dl		0.16 mmol/l

*Factor = Number factor (the units are not presented).
†Value in SI units = Value in conventional units × factor.

SOME TYPICAL HEMATOLOGY REFERENCE INTERVALS IN CONVENTIONAL AND SI UNITS

Component	Typical Reference Intervals		
	in Conventional Units	Factor	in SI Units*
Complete Blood Count (CBC)			
Hematocrit			
male	40–54%	0.01	0.40–0.54
female	38–47%		0.38–0.47
Hemoglobin			
male	13.5–18.0 gm/dl	0.155	2.09–2.79 mmol/l
female	12.0–16.0 gm/dl		1.86–2.48 mmol/l
Erythrocyte count			
male	$4.6–6.2 \times 10^6/\mu l$	10^6	$4.6–6.2 \times 10^{12}/l$
female	$4.2–5.4 \times 16^6/\mu l$		$4.2–5.4 \times 10^{12}/l$
Leukocyte count	$4.5–11.0 \times 10^3/\mu l$	10^6	$4.5–11.0 \times 10^9/l$
Erythrocyte indices			
mean corpuscular volume	80–96 cu. microns	1	80–96 fl
mean corpuscular hemoglobin	27–31 pg.	1	27–31 pg
Platelet Count	$150–440 \times 10^3/\mu l$	10^6	$0.15–0.4 \times 10^{12}/l$
Reticulocytes	0.5–1.5% of erythrocytes	0.01	0.005–0.015
	$25,000–75,000$ cells/μl	10^6	$25–75 \times 10^9/l$

*Value in SI units = Value in conventional units × factor.

(Tables continue on back cover)

Volume II

Todd • Sanford • Davidsohn

CLINICAL DIAGNOSIS *and* MANAGEMENT by LABORATORY METHODS

Sixteenth Edition

JOHN BERNARD HENRY, M.D.

Professor of Pathology, College of Medicine, and Director of Clinical Pathology, University Hospital, State University of New York, Upstate Medical Center, Syracuse

1979

W. B. SAUNDERS COMPANY
Philadelphia   London   Toronto

W. B. Saunders Company: West Washington Square
Philadelphia, PA 19105

1 St. Anne's Road
Eastbourne, East Sussex BN 21 3UN, England

1 Goldthorne Avenue
Toronto, Ontario M8Z 5T9, Canada

Clinical Diagnosis and Management by Laboratory Methods

Volume 1	0-7216-4652-2
Volume 2	0-7216-4653-0
Single Volume	0-7216-4654-9
Set ISBN	0-7216-4639-5

Last digit is the print number: 9   8   7   6   5   4   3   2   1

To my wife Georgette and
our children
Maureen, Julie, Bill, Paul, John, and David
who accepted patiently the inconvenience
associated with my long preoccupation
with this work

CONTRIBUTORS

BERTIE F. ARGYRIS, Ph.D.
*Professor of Microbiology, State
University of New York, Upstate
Medical Center College of Medicine,
Syracuse, New York.*
THE IMMUNE RESPONSE AND
IMMUNOBIOLOGY

MYRTON FREEMAN BEELER, M.D.
*Professor, Department of Pathology,
Louisiana State University School of
Medicine in New Orleans; Director,
Clinical Chemistry Section, Pathology
Department, Charity Hospital of
Louisiana, Consultant in Clinical
Pathology, Veterans Administration
Hospital and United States Public
Health Service Hospital, New Orleans,
Louisiana.*
EXAMINATION OF EXOCRINE PANCREATIC
FUNCTION; MALABSORPTION, DIARRHEA,
AND EXAMINATION OF FECES

MARY BRADLEY, M.D.
*Associate Professor, Department of
Laboratory Medicine and Pathology,
University of Minnesota Medical
School, Minneapolis, Minnesota.*
EXAMINATION OF URINE

M. DESMOND BURKE, M.D.
*Associate Professor, Department of
Laboratory Medicine and Pathology,
University of Minnesota Medical
School; Associate Pathologist, Mt. Sinai
Hospital, Minneapolis, Minnesota.*
QUANTITATIVE EVALUATION OF
LABORATORY MEASUREMENTS

WILLIAM G. CANNADY
*Director of Phoresis and Assistant
Director of HLA, American Red Cross
Blood Services—Northeast Region,
Boston, Massachusetts.*
HLA: THE MAJOR HISTOCOMPATIBILITY
COMPLEX

DONALD C. CANNON, M.D., Ph.D.
*Professor and Chairman, Department
of Pathology and Laboratory Medicine,
University of Texas Health Science
Center at Houston Medical School;
Chief, Department of Pathology and
Laboratory Medicine, Hermann
Hospital, Houston, Texas.*
METABOLIC INTERMEDIATES AND
INORGANIC IONS; EXAMINATION OF
SEMINAL FLUID; EXAMINATION OF
GASTRIC AND DUODENAL CONTENTS.

MARY E. CHANDLER, Ph.D.
*Postdoctoral Fellow, Medical Genetics
Division, Department of Laboratory
Medicine and Pathology, University of
Minnesota Medical School,
Minneapolis, Minnesota.*
CYTOGENETICS

RONALD P. DANIELE, M.D.
*Associate Professor of Medicine and
Pathology, University of Pennsylvania
School of Medicine; Chief, Pulmonary
Clinic, Hospital of the University of
Pennsylvania, Philadelphia,
Pennsylvania.*
LYMPHOCYTES

FREDERICK R. DAVEY, M.D.
*Associate Professor of Pathology and
Medicine and Associate Director of
Clinical Pathology, State University of
New York, Upstate Medical Center
College of Medicine, Syracuse, New
York.*
BLOOD VESSELS AND HEMOSTASIS;
PLATELETS AND PLATELET DISORDERS;
BLOOD COAGULATION AND ITS DISORDERS

WILLIAM C. DeWOLF, M.D.
*Research Associate, Sidney Farber
Cancer Institute, Boston,
Massachusetts.*
HLA: THE MAJOR HISTOCOMPATIBILITY
COMPLEX

MERLE A. EVENSON, Ph.D.
*Professor, Department of Medicine,
University of Wisconsin Medical
School Center for the Health Sciences;
Director, Toxicology Laboratories,
University of Wisconsin Hospitals,
Madison, Wisconsin.*
PRINCIPLES OF INSTRUMENTATION

JOHN R. FEEGEL, M.D., J.D.
*Associate Professor of Pathology,
Emory University; Associate
Pathologist, Grady Memorial Hospital,
Atlanta, Georgia.*
LEGAL ASPECTS OF LABORATORY
MEDICINE

HJORDIS M. FOY, M.D., Ph.D.
*Professor, Department of Epidemiology,
School of Public Health and
Community Medicine, University of
Washington School of Medicine, Seattle,
Washington.*
MYCOPLASMAL INFECTION

MICHAEL M. FRANK, M.D.
*Clinical Director and Chief,
Laboratory of Clinical Investigation,
National Institutes of Allergy and
Infectious Diseases, Bethesda,
Maryland.*
COMPLEMENT

THELMA A. GAITHER, B.S.
*Research Biologist, National Institutes
of Allergy and Infectious Diseases,
Bethesda, Maryland.*
COMPLEMENT

ROBERT S. GALEN, M.D., M.P.H.
*Assistant Professor of Clinical
Pathology, Columbia University College
of Physicians and Surgeons, New
York, New York; Associate Director of
Laboratories, Overlook Hospitals,
Summit, New Jersey.*
QUANTITATIVE EVALUATION OF
LABORATORY MEASUREMENTS

THOMAS L. GAVAN, M.D.
*Head, Department of Microbiology, The
Cleveland Clinic Foundation,
Cleveland, Ohio.*
SPACE, EQUIPMENT, MATERIALS, AND
TECHNIQUES; QUALITY CONTROL

ROBERT GILBERT, M.D.
*Professor of Medicine, State University
of New York, Upstate Medical Center
College of Medicine, Syracuse;
Attending Physician, University
Hospital of Upstate Medical Center,
Syracuse, New York.*
SPIROMETRY, BLOOD GASES, ACID-BASE,
AND PULMONARY FUNCTION SPIROMETRY

MILTON GOLDEN, Ph.D.
*Associate Professor, Microbiology, Rush
Medical College, Chicago; Director,
Microbiology, Mt. Sinai Hospital
Medical Center, Chicago, Illinois*
MONITORING THE QUALITY OF
LABORATORY MEASUREMENTS

GEORGE F. GRANNIS, Ph.D.
*Department of Pathology, Ohio State
University College of Medicine,
Columbus, Ohio.*
MONITORING THE QUALITY OF
LABORATORY MEASUREMENTS

YEZID GUTIERREZ, M.D., Ph.D.
*Assistant Professor of Pathology, Case
Western Reserve University School of
Medicine, Cleveland, Ohio.*
MEDICAL PARASITOLOGY

JOHN BERNARD HENRY, M.D.
*Professor of Pathology, State
University of New York, Upstate
Medical Center College of Medicine,
Syracuse; Director of Clinical
Pathology, University Hospital of
Upstate Medical Center, Syracuse,
New York.*
THEORY AND PRACTICE OF LABORATORY
TECHNIQUE; EVALUATION OF RENAL
FUNCTION, AND WATER, ELECTROLYTE,
AND ACID-BASE BALANCE; CLINICAL
ENZYMOLOGY; THERAPEUTIC DRUG
MONITORING AND TOXICOLOGY; AMNIOTIC
FLUID AND ANTENATAL DIAGNOSIS;
IMMUNOHEMATOLOGY, BLOOD BANKING,
AND HEMOTHERAPY; LABORATORY
EVALUATION OF DISPUTED PARENTAGE;
EFFECTIVE UTILIZATION OF CLINICAL
LABORATORIES

MARY JANE HICKS, M.D.
*Assistant Professor of Pathology,
University of Arizona College of
Medicine; Attending Physician in
Pathology, Arizona Health Science
Center, Tucson, Arizona.*
LABORATORY DIAGNOSIS OF VIRUSES,
RICKETTSIA, AND CHLAMYDIA

JOAN HOLOHAN HOWANITZ, M.D.
*Assistant Professor of Pathology, State
University of New York, Upstate
Medical Center College of Medicine,
Syracuse; Assistant Director of
Clinical Pathology, University
Hospital of Upstate Medical Center,
Syracuse, New York.*
CARBOHYDRATES; RADIOIMMUNOASSAY;
EVALUATION OF ENDOCRINE FUNCTION;
THERAPEUTIC DRUG MONITORING AND
TOXICOLOGY

PETER JOHN HOWANITZ, M.D.
Assistant Professor of Pathology, State University of New York, Upstate Medical Center College of Medicine, Syracuse; Assistant Director of Clinical Pathology, University Hospital of Upstate Medical Center, Syracuse, New York.
CARBOHYDRATES; RADIOIMMUNOASSAY; EVALUATION OF ENDOCRINE FUNCTION; THERAPEUTIC DRUG MONITORING AND TOXICOLOGY

YUAN S. KAO, M.D.
Associate Professor of Pathology, Louisiana State University School of Medicine in New Orleans; Visiting Pathologist, Charity Hospital of Louisiana, New Orleans, Louisiana.
EXAMINATION OF EXOCRINE PANCREATIC FUNCTION; MALABSORPTION, DIARRHEA, AND EXAMINATION OF FECES

RICHARD T. KELLY, M.D.
Associate Professor, Department of Pathology and Microbiology, University of Tennessee College of Medicine, Memphis; Pathologist in Microbiology/Serology, Baptist Memorial Hospital, Nashville, Tennessee.
SPIROCHETES AND SPIRAL BACTERIA

GEORGE E. KENNY, Ph.D.
Professor and Chairman, Department of Pathobiology, School of Public Health and Community Medicine, University of Washington School of Medicine, Seattle, Washington.
MYCOPLASMAL INFECTION

THOMAS F. KEYS, M.D.
Assistant Professor of Medicine, Mayo Medical School, Rochester; Consultant, Division of Infectious Diseases and Internal Medicine, Mayo Clinic-Foundation, Rochester, Minnesota.
HOSPITAL INFECTION CONTROL

ELMER W. KONEMAN, M.D.
Executive Director, Colorado Association for Continuing Medical Laboratory Education (CACMLE), Denver, Colorado.
DIAGNOSIS OF MYCOTIC DISEASE

ARTHUR F. KRIEG, M.D.
Professor of Pathology, Pennsylvania State University College of Medicine, Hershey; Director of Clinical Laboratories, The Milton S. Hershey
Medical Center, Hershey, Pennsylvania.
CEREBROSPINAL FLUIDS AND OTHER BODY FLUIDS; PREGNANCY TESTS AND EVALUATION OF PLACENTAL FUNCTION

MICHAEL W. LAPINSKI, M.D.
Pathologist, Woman's Christian Association Hospital, Jamestown, New York, and Warren General Hospital, Warren, Pennsylvania.
BLOOD GASES

CHANG LING LEE, M.D.
Professor of Medicine and Pathology, Rush Medical College, Chicago; Director, Charles Hymen Blood Center of Mount Sinai Hospital Medical Center of Chicago; Scientific Director, American Red Cross Blood Services Mid-America Region, Chicago, Illinois.
IMMUNOHEMATOLOGY, BLOOD BANKING, AND HEMOTHERAPY; LABORATORY EVALUATION OF DISPUTED PARENTAGE

H. PETER LEHMANN, Ph.D.
Assistant Professor, Department of Pathology, Louisiana State University School of Medicine in New Orleans, Louisiana.
SI UNITS

ROBERT I. LEVY, M.D.
Director, National Heart, Lung, and Blood Institute, National Institutes of Health, Bethesda, Maryland.
MEASUREMENT OF LIPIDS AND EVALUATION OF LIPID DISORDERS

ERNEST GEORGE LINKE, Ph.D.
Clinical Chemist, Pathology Associates, Gadsden, Alabama.
THEORY AND PRACTICE OF LABORATORY TECHNIQUE

ROBERT P. LISAK, M.D.
Associate Professor of Neurology, University of Pennsylvania School of Medicine; Associate Neurologist, Hospital of the University of Pennsylvania; Consultant Neurologist, Veterans Administration Hospital, Philadelphia; Director, Multiple Sclerosis Clinic, Hospital of the University of Pennsylvania, Philadelphia, Pennsylvania.
AUTOIMMUNITY AND AUTOIMMUNE DISEASE

EUFRONIO G. MADERAZO, M.D.
Assistant Professor, Department of Pathology, University of Connecticut School of Medicine, Farmington; Director, Medical Research Laboratory, and Assistant Director, Infectious Disease Division, Department of Medicine, Hartford Hospital, Hartford, Connecticut.
PHAGOCYTIC CELLS

JOHN M. MATSEN, M.D.
Professor of Pathology, University of Utah College of Medicine, Salt Lake City, Utah.
ANTIMICROBIAL SUSCEPTIBILITY TESTS

WILLIAM W. McLENDON, M.D.
Professor of Pathology, University of North Carolina School of Medicine; Chairman, Department of Hospital Laboratories, North Carolina Memorial Hospital, Chapel Hill, North Carolina.
ORGANIZATION AND MANAGEMENT OF THE CLINICAL LABORATORY; FISCAL MANAGEMENT; COMMUNICATIONS AND DATA PROCESSING

JOHN E. MURPHY, M.D.
Assistant Clinical Professor of Pathology, Southern Illinois University School of Medicine; Associate Pathologist, Department of Laboratory Medicine, Memorial Medical Center, Springfield, Illinois.
EVALUATION OF RENAL FUNCTION, AND WATER, ELECTROLYTE, AND ACID-BASE BALANCE; EFFECTIVE UTILIZATION OF CLINICAL LABORATORIES

ROBERT M. NAKAMURA, M.D.
Adjunct Professor of Pathology, University of California, San Diego, School of Medicine, La Jolla; Chairman, Department of Pathology, Green Hospital of Scripps Clinic, La Jolla, California.
ANTIBODY AS REAGENT

DOUGLAS A. NELSON, M.D.
Professor of Pathology, State University of New York, Upstate Medical Center College of Medicine, Syracuse; Deputy Director of Clinical Pathology and Attending Pathologist, University Hospital of Upstate Medical Center, Syracuse, New York.
BASIC METHODOLOGY (OF HEMATOLOGY); HEMATOPOIESIS; ERYTHROCYTIC DISORDERS; LEUKOCYTIC DISORDERS

DANIEL C. NIEJADLIK, M.D.
Assistant Professor of Laboratory Medicine, University of Connecticut School of Medicine, Farmington; Pathologist, Middlesex Memorial Hospital, Middletown, Connecticut.
SPUTUM

ALLEN L. PUSCH, M.D.
Associate Professor of Pathology, Rush Medical College, Chicago; Pathologist, Christ Hospital, Oak Lawn, Illinois.
SERODIAGNOSTIC TESTS

C. GEORGE RAY, M.D.
Professor of Pathology and Pediatrics, University of Arizona College of Medicine, Tucson; Attending Physician in Pathology and Pediatrics, Arizona Medical Center, and Attending Physician in Pediatrics, Tucson Medical Center, Tucson, Arizona.
LABORATORY DIAGNOSIS OF VIRUSES, RICKETTSIA, AND CHLAMYDIA

MICHAEL D. REICH
Assistant Director, Professional Support Services, North Carolina Memorial Hospital, Chapel Hill, North Carolina.
ORGANIZATION AND MANAGEMENT OF THE CLINICAL LABORATORY; FISCAL MANAGEMENT

MANUEL J. RICARDO, JR., Ph.D.
Assistant Professor of Microbiology, University of Tennessee College of Medicine, Memphis, Tennessee.
THE IMMUNOGLOBULINS

BASIL M. RIFKIND, M.D.
Chief, Lipid Metabolism Branch, National Heart, Lung, and Blood Institute of the National Institutes of Health, Bethesda, Maryland.
MEASUREMENTS OF LIPIDS AND EVALUATION OF LIPID DISORDERS

ROBERT F. RITCHIE, M.D.
Associate Professor of Medicine, Tufts University School of Medicine, Boston, Massachusetts; Medical Director, Foundation for Blood Research, Scarborough, and Attending Physician, Maine Medical Center, Portland, Maine.
SPECIFIC PROTEINS

GLENN D. ROBERTS, Ph.D.
Assistant Professor of Microbiology and of Laboratory Medicine, Mayo Medical School, Rochester; Director, Mycology Laboratory, Section of Clinical Microbiology, Department of

Laboratory Medicine, Mayo Clinic-Foundation, Rochester, Minnesota.
CLINICAL AND LABORATORY DIAGNOSIS OF MYCOTIC DISEASE

JERALD M. ROSENBAUM, M.D.
Instructor in Pathology, University of Massachusetts Medical School, Worcester; Attending Pathologist, Baystate Medical Center, Springfield, Massachusetts.
AMNIOTIC FLUID AND ANTENATAL DIAGNOSIS

DAVID T. ROWLANDS, JR., M.D.
Professor of Pathology, University of Pennsylvania School of Medicine; Pathologist, Hospital of the University of Pennsylvania, Philadelphia, Pennsylvania.
LYMPHOCYTES

THOMAS A. RUMA, M.D.
Chief Resident, Clinical Pathology, University Hospital of Upstate Medical Center, Syracuse, New York
THERAPEUTIC PHERESIS AND PLASMA EXCHANGE

WILLIAM DOUGLAS SCHEER, Ph.D.
Instructor, Department of Pathology, Louisiana State University School of Medicine in New Orleans; Clinical Chemist, Charity Hospital of Louisiana, New Orleans, Louisiana.
MALABSORPTION, DIARRHEA, AND EXAMINATION OF FECES

G. BERRY SCHUMANN, M.D.
Assistant Professor of Pathology, University of Cincinnati College of Medicine; Director of Cytopathology, University of Cincinnati Medical Center, Cincinnati, Ohio.
EXAMINATION OF URINE

JAMES WARREN SMITH, M.D.
Professor of Clinical Pathology, Indiana University School of Medicine; Director, Division of Clinical Microbiology, Indiana University Hospitals, Wishard Memorial Hospital, and Veterans Administration Hospital, Indianapolis, Indiana.
MEDICAL PARASITOLOGY

HERBERT M. SOMMERS, M.D.
Professor of Pathology, Northwestern University Medical School, Chicago; Attending Pathologist and Director, Clinical Microbiology Laboratory, Northwestern Memorial Hospital;

Consultant Pathologist, Lakeside Veterans Hospital, Chicago, Illinois.
MYCOBACTERIAL DISEASE

BERNARD EUGENE STATLAND, M.D., Ph.D.
Associate Professor of Pathology, University of California, Davis, School of Medicine; Director of Clinical Chemistry, Sacramento Medical Center, Sacramento, California.
SOURCES OF VARIATION IN LABORATORY MEASUREMENTS; REFERENCE VALUES; THEORY AND PRACTICE OF LABORATORY TECHNIQUE; QUANTITATIVE EVALUATION OF LABORATORY MEASUREMENTS; MONITORING THE QUALITY OF LABORATORY MEASUREMENTS

ISRAEL TAMIR, M.D.
Associate Professor, Department of Pediatrics, Sackler School of Medicine, University of Tel-Aviv, Israel.
MEASUREMENTS OF LIPIDS AND EVALUATION OF LIPID DISORDERS

RUSSELL H. TOMAR, M.D.
Associate Professor of Pathology and Assistant Professor of Medicine, State University of New York, Upstate Medical Center College of Medicine, Syracuse; Associate Director of Clinical Pathology, University Hospital of Upstate Medical Center, Syracuse, New York.
LABORATORY APPROACHES TO IMMUNOLOGICALLY RELATED DISORDERS

JOHN J. TREUTING, Ph.D.
Assistant Professor, Department of Pathology and Laboratory Medicine, University of Texas Health Science Center at Houston Medical School; Assistant Director, Clinical Chemistry, Hermann Hospital, Houston, Texas.
METABOLIC INTERMEDIATES AND INORGANIC IONS

ERNEST S. TUCKER, III, M.D.
Clinical Associate Professor of Pathology and Pediatrics, University of California, San Diego, School of Medicine, La Jolla; Head, Section of Immunology—Department of Pathology, Green Hospital of Scripps Clinic, La Jolla, California.
ANTIBODY AS REAGENT

PATRICK C. J. WARD, M.D.
Associate Professor, Department of Laboratory Medicine and Pathology, University of Minnesota Medical School, Minneapolis; Director of

Laboratories, *Mount Sinai Hospital, Minneapolis, Minnesota.*
EXAMINATION OF URINE

PETER A. WARD, M.D.
Professor and Chairman, Department of Pathology, University of Connecticut School of Medicine, Farmington; Chief Pathologist, University of Connecticut Health Center, Farmington, Connecticut.
PHAGOCYTIC CELLS

JOHN A. WASHINGTON, II, M.D.
Professor, Microbiology and Laboratory Medicine, Mayo Medical School, Rochester; Head, Section of Clinical Microbiology, Mayo Clinic-Foundation, Rochester, Minnesota.
INTRODUCTION TO MEDICAL MICROBIOLOGY; MEDICAL BACTERIOLOGY

ROBERT EDMUND WENK, M.D.
Assistant Professor, Johns Hopkins University School of Medicine, Baltimore; Attending Pathologist and Head, Division of Clinical Pathology, Sinai Hospital, Baltimore, Maryland.
AMNIOTIC FLUID AND ANTENATAL DIAGNOSIS

THERESA L. WHITESIDE, Ph.D.
Assistant Professor of Pathology, University of Pittsburgh School of Medicine; Associate Director, Clinical Immunopathology Laboratory, University Health Center of Pittsburgh, Pennsylvania.
LYMPHOCYTES

PER WINKEL, M.D., Doc. Sci. Med.
Visiting Professor, Department of Pathology, University of North Carolina School of Medicine, Chapel Hill; Co-Director, Department of Clinical Chemistry, Finseninstitutet, Copenhagen, Denmark.
SOURCES OF VARIATION IN LABORATORY MEASUREMENTS; REFERENCE VALUES; QUANTITATIVE EVALUATION OF LABORATORY MEASUREMENTS

JANNIE WOO, Ph.D.
Assistant Professor, Department of Pathology and Laboratory Medicine, University of Texas Health Science Center at Houston Medical School; Assistant Director, Clinical Chemistry, Hermann Hospital, Houston, Texas.
METABOLIC INTERMEDIATES AND INORGANIC IONS

WEI TING WU, Ph.D.
Assistant Professor, Department of Pathology, Louisiana State University School of Medicine in New Orleans; Senior Clinical Chemist, Pathology, Charity Hospital of Louisiana, New Orleans, Consultant in Clinical Chemistry, West Jefferson Hospital, Merrero, Louisiana.
EXAMINATION OF EXOCRINE PANCREATIC FUNCTION

EDMOND J. YUNIS, M.D.
Professor of Pathology, Harvard Medical School, Boston; Chief, Division of Immunogenetics, Sidney Farber Cancer Institute, Boston, Massachusetts.
HLA: THE MAJOR HISTOCOMPATIBILITY COMPLEX

JORGE J. YUNIS, M.D.
Professor and Director, Medical Genetics Division, University of Minnesota Medical School, Minneapolis, Minnesota.
CYTOGENETICS

HYMAN J. ZIMMERMAN, M.D.
Professor of Medicine, George Washington University School of Medicine and Health Sciences; Chief, Medical Service, Veterans Administration Hospital, Washington, D.C.
EVALUATION OF THE FUNCTION AND INTEGRITY OF THE LIVER; CLINICAL ENZYMOLOGY

BURTON ZWEIMAN, M.D.
Professor of Medicine and Neurology, University of Pennsylvania School of Medicine; Chief, Section of Allergy and Immunology, Hospital of the University of Pennsylvania; Attending Physician, Veterans Administration Hospital, Philadelphia, Pennsylvania.
AUTOIMMUNITY AND AUTOIMMUNE DISEASE

PREFACE

With this sixteenth edition, Todd and Sanford reaches the mature age of 70 years of service to at least three generations of clinical pathologists and medical laboratory personnel (especially technologists and medical technicians), medical students, and physicians in training and in practice, i.e., family physicians, internists, surgeons, and pediatricians, in particular.

Our goals in this edition include the following:

1. Identify appropriate measurements and examinations for diagnosis, confirmation of a clinical impression, therapeutic or management guideline data, prognosis, and screening or detection of disease.
2. Indicate the order in which such measurements and examinations should be requested.
3. Interpret and translate laboratory measurements and examinations.
4. Recognize pitfalls, problems, and limitations of laboratory data, including discussion of quality control and drug interaction as well as relative merits in terms of methodology, patient preparation, communication, and cost effectiveness.
5. Understand pathophysiology or sequence of disease as reflected by clinical pathology data.
6. Appreciate and understand the importance of laboratory organization and management for efficient and cost-effective medical care delivery.

The content of this edition has been reorganized to represent more closely the working structure of the modern clinical pathology laboratory and to be more useful in solving medical problems.

It is significant that this edition begins with a discussion of bias and random variation in laboratory measurements and concludes with material on monitoring the quality of laboratory measurements. These two subjects identify a basic approach and understanding of laboratory medicine and currently play vital roles in effective utilization of the laboratory.

In terms of the six parts, with their constituent chapters, the organization of the laboratory is reflected in a functional manner:

1. Chemical Pathology and Clinical Chemistry
2. Medical Microscopy and Examination of Other Body Fluids
3. Hematology and Coagulation
4. Immunology and Immunopathology
5. Medical Microbiology
6. Administration of the Clinical Laboratory

The thrust of special competence in clinical pathology and subspecialization in medicine is consistent with the restructuring of this edition.

The sixty-three chapters in this edition represent a virtual doubling of the number of chapters from the previous edition and also reflect the comprehensive and intensive development of laboratory medicine and its application to medical care in recent years.

Not only is the massive technology of clinical pathology expanded as well as delineated, but also the role of the physician in terms of laboratory medicine is emphasized. Among these six parts, Immunology and Immunopathology represents a recent thrust in laboratory medicine which, by virtue of its technology as well as scientific and clinical applications, could for all practical purposes embrace most other areas of the laboratory. Cellular as well as humoral aspects of the immune response and laboratory applications are emphasized throughout this part. These range from a consideration of the immune response and discussion of the antibody as reagent to immunogenetics, immunohematology, and hemotherapy.

The second greatest impact in laboratory medicine since the previous edition is reflected in Chemical Pathology and Clinical Chemistry. What was embraced in the previous edition in terms of a chapter on Clinical Chemistry, as well as several other chapters, has been extensively revised. This includes blood gases, carbohydrates, lipids, proteins, water, electrolytes and renal function, metabolites and inorganic ions, liver function and clinical enzymology, and the sophisticated and substantial developments in evaluation of endocrine function, including radioimmunoassay and also therapeutic drug monitoring. Radioisotopic pathology in terms of *in vitro* assays or radioimmunoassays replaces nuclear medicine in the previous edition.

The final chapter of this part underscores quantitative approaches used in evaluating laboratory measurements and other types of data emphasizing the likelihood of values, e.g., probability that the patient is a member of a clinical class or probability of one outcome occurring. This important approach embraces probabilistic reasoning, which makes even greater demands on the clinician, necessitating a keen awareness of the various assumptions and conditions intrinsic in an approach embracing values of multiple variates and discriminate analysis.

Cytogenetics, as well as various topics ranging from urinalysis, cerebrospinal fluid, amniotic fluid, semen, and sputum to pancreatic function, gastric analysis, malabsorption, diarrhea, and examination of feces, is reviewed in the Medical Microscopy part of this edition.

Hematology and Coagulation, which were considered in two chapters in the previous edition, here constitute seven chapters: basic hematology, including a section on physiologic variations; hematopoiesis, including revised concepts of blood cell production; erythrocyte disorders and leukocyte disorders, each occupying an extensively revised chapter; the role of blood vessels in hemostasis, and normal and disordered platelet function, each discussed in a new chapter; and a new chapter on coagulation, which incorporates many of the extensive advances in this area.

In Medical Microbiology not only are all the elements of this broad discipline reviewed in 14 chapters, but special attention is given to antimicrobial susceptibility testing, mycoplasmal, viral, and chlamydial infections, and spirochetes, as well as quality control and hospital infection control. The important subject of hospital infection control pertains not only to the laboratory but to the entire hospital and thus has been expanded and updated.

Finally, in a part entitled Administration of the Clinical Laboratory—which embraces the organization and operation of the clinical laboratory, including fiscal—communication and data processing, personnel administration, and effective utilization are reviewed at length.

In summary, the sixteenth edition embraces a complete as well as thorough revision that is consistent with the new title of this text, as well as the role of the laboratory through its professional staff in not only translating this information into patient care, but also facilitating and amplifying the effectiveness of medical care delivery through sophisticated medical technology coupled with medical and scientific skills and knowledge.

Even the appendices provide information which is useful to the clinician and laboratorian, in terms of reference (normal) values and intervals. An introduction to SI units has been added not only on the inside cover but also in Appendix 4. New terminology has been incorporated not only with the reference intervals, but also throughout the text whenever feasible and consistent with optimal medical care.

My own special interest in effective utilization of the laboratory is reflected on the inside cover, which outlines an alternative strategy for ordering blood in elective surgery.

After working with Israel Davidsohn, M.D., on the two previous editions, I have enthusiastically assumed the burden of responsibility for this effort. Although I have missed my former association with Israel Davidsohn in this role, to some extent this has been replaced by the opportunity to work closely with several new colleagues in this endeavor. In addition to my associates at the Upstate Medical Center who have participated in this edition, Douglas Nelson, M.D., and Russell Tomar, M.D., I have enjoyed working with and appreciate the tremendous contribution of John Washington, M.D., as well as William McLendon, M.D., and Bernard E. Statland, M.D., Ph.D. Chosen for their extensive knowledge and current activity in their respective disciplines, distinguished scientists and physicians have been attracted as additional contributors to this edition.

I am grateful to my associate and assistant editors as well as contributors, who have been faithful to their task and gracious in cooperation.

I accept full responsibility for any errors of omission or commission and welcome any comments or reactions to this edition.

JOHN BERNARD HENRY, M.D.

ACKNOWLEDGMENT

It is with great pleasure and deep satisfaction that I acknowledge the collaboration of my esteemed colleagues and friends as associate editors, Douglas A. Nelson, M.D., and John A. Washington II, M.D., and assistant editors, William McLendon, M.D., Bernard E. Statland, M.D., Ph.D., and Russell H. Tomar, M.D. Each has been most gracious, diligent, and resourceful in his efforts. A work of multiple authors requires the willingness of the contributors to accept the guidance of the editors. I am delighted to acknowledge that our collaborators have been responsible and responsive in this respect.

Several individuals have been particularly helpful with suggestions and critical review of selected manuscripts, galley proofs, page proofs, and chapter outlines. Among these are: Drs. Peter Boyd, Robert A. Calhoun, Frederick R. Davey, Joan Howanitz, Peter Howanitz, Harold V. Lamberson, Frances Lapinski, Michael Lapinski, Leonard Madoff, Erik Mitchell, Vernon Pilon, Niles Rosen, Thomas A. Ruma, James Terzian, and Russell H. Tomar, and Ms. Nadine Bartholoma, Ms. Shirley Boyd, Mr. Samir ELSamahy, Mr. Lawrence Fiske, Ms. Charlene Hubbell, Ms. Shirley Irving, Ms. JoAnne Iwanski, Mr. Reginaldo Lauzon, Mr. Harry Ludke, Ms. Bettina Martin, Mr. Richard Martin, Ms. Jane MacCallum, Ms. Mildred McDermott, Ms. Frances Morgenstern, Mr. Michael Morris, Mr. Ricardo Narvaez, Mr. David Pettit, Ms. Celeste Schreck, Ms. Kathleen Sheedy, Ms. Joanne Shovan, Ms. Karen Strouse, and Mr. Robert Sunheimer, all of Clinical Pathology; Dr. George Collins, Department of Pathology; Drs. Lytt Gardner, Frank Oski, and Margaret Williams, Department of Pediatrics; Dr. Raja Abdul-Karim, Department of Obstetrics and Gynecology; Dr. Robert Levine, Department of Medicine; Dr. Richard Oates, Department of Preventive Medicine; Upstate Medical Center in Syracuse; Dr. Paul Granato, Veterans Administration Hospital, Syracuse; Mr. Thomas Grimshaw, Administration, Upstate Medical Center, Syracuse; Dr. Ritchard Cable, Regional Red Cross Blood Services, Syracuse; Ms. Margaret Over, Nurse-Epidemiologist, Upstate Medical Center, Syracuse; Dr. Vernie A. Stembridge, Southwestern Medical School, Dallas, Texas. Thanks are also due to Ms. Janet Bungay for editorial assistance and to Ms. Karen Wishnow for manuscript preparation of the lipid chapter. Ms. Joanne Beaudoin and Drs. Charles Alper, Myron Johnson, and James Haddow deserve special thanks for assistance in the preparation of the protein chapter. Dr. Laurence M. Demers and Ms. Lucille K. Shearer provided assistance in the preparation of the cerebrospinal fluid and pregnancy test chapters.

I also acknowledge the stimulus of former residents, medical students, and colleagues who have helped in so many ways.

For sustained devotion and meticulous attention to detail I express my deepest gratitude and appreciation to Ms. Sharon Putney, who has not only supported me throughout this entire effort but has simultaneously been devoted and dedicated to this edition. Our association for 15 years has made it possible for me to be involved with this undertaking as well as to participate in so many other activities that have enhanced this effort.

In addition, I am grateful to the excellent clerical support which has been rendered in a superb manner by others, including Ms. Deborah Body, Ms. Melody Doxtater, Ms. Patricia Fiorello, Ms. Ruth Jackson, and Ms. Ivy West, Upstate Medical Center, Syracuse; Ms. Karen Prescott, LaJolla, California; Ms. Karen Russell and Ms. Mary Buchanan, Chapel Hill, North Carolina; Ms. Lola Jaeger, Rochester, Minnesota; Ms. Sharon Kitagawa and Ms. Nancy Wolf, Mt. Sinai Hospital Medical Center, Chicago.

Acknowledgment is also due to Fred H. Allen, Jr., M.D., of the New York Blood Center, Herbert Polesky, Minneapolis War Memorial Blood Bank, Leon Sussman, Beth Israel Medical Center, New York, and Richard Walker, William Beaumont Hospital, Royal Oak, Michigan, for their review and valuable suggestions on Chapter 44.

I am grateful to Dr. John H. Thompson of the Mayo Clinic for review and comments on the parasitology chapter.

For Part 6 I am especially grateful to Ms. Bettina Martin, my administrative assistant, whose critical comments and review were invaluable.

Special thanks are due to Dorothea Nelson, Maaja Washington, Ann McLendon, Alexandra Statland, and Karen Tomar. Without their understanding and faithful support, the contributions of my associate and assistant editors would not have been possible.

Dr. William McLendon and the University of North Carolina should be recognized for their support of Dr. Bernard Statland, who made his contributions to this edition while serving on the faculty there.

To Dr. James N. Patterson goes my sincere thanks for bringing Doctor Israel Davidsohn and me together.

My deep appreciation and gratitude are due to Dr. Israel Davidsohn, who for 15 years shared with me the satisfaction as well as the joys, rigors, and pleasure of writing.

I want to express my sincere appreciation for the cooperation and guidance of Albert Meier, Herb Powell, and Donna Musser, as well as the entire staff of W. B. Saunders Company, who shared and supported this effort. Thanks are also due to Mr. Robert Rowan, whose availability and support over the past 15 years have been invaluable as well as delightful, and to Mr. John Hanley, whose involvement in this edition, although early and brief, was nevertheless significant.

JOHN BERNARD HENRY, M.D.

CONTENTS

Part 4

IMMUNOLOGY AND IMMUNOPATHOLOGY

Edited by John Bernard Henry, M.D.,
and Russell H. Tomar, M.D.

THE IMMUNE RESPONSE
AND IMMUNOBIOLOGY

Bertie F. Argyris, Ph.D.

4

Immunologic responses are commonly divided into two types—humoral and cell-mediated. In humoral immunity, a specific circulating antibody is induced, which rids the body of the antigen. Humoral immunity includes the response to simple chemicals and microorganisms. Hypersensitivity resulting in tissue injury may also be mediated by circulating antibodies and has been subdivided by Gell (1975) into immediate, anaphylactic (I), cytotoxic (II), and complex-mediated (III) hypersensitivity.

In cell-mediated immunity (CMI), the immunocompetent cells are activated, leading to the destruction of a foreign target. Histocompatibility antigens are involved in this process. Cell-mediated immunity includes the rejection of foreign organ transplants, delayed type hypersensitivity, graft-vs-host reactions, and tumor immunity. Delayed type hypersensitivity may also result in tissue injury and has been termed Type IV hypersensitivity (Gell, 1975). In selected cases, cell-mediated immunity may be accompanied by the production of circulating antibodies.

Both cell-mediated and humoral immune responses are induced by antigens. In addition to these *induced* responses, the body contains a natural resistance. This natural resistance, which may be our first line of defense, appears to be mediated by a special population of cells, called natural killer (NK) cells (Perlmann, 1976).

This chapter focuses primarily on the cellular basis of the immune response, i.e., the nature of the immunocompetent cells (T cells, B cells, null cells, NK cells, and macrophages), and their interaction during humoral and cell-mediated immunity. This is followed by a short section on the experimental techniques which can be used to detect and/or remove a specific population of immunocompetent cells from the circulation, discussed in further detail in Chapter 39.

After discussing the nature and interaction of cells involved in the immune response, we will briefly consider genetic factors.

The remainder of the chapter is devoted to selected aspects of cell-mediated immunity. In the discussion on organ transplantation, the concepts of host-vs-graft and graft-vs-host reactions, tissue typing, and immunosuppression will be introduced.

Many tumors possess surface tumor-specific transplantation antigens (TSTA) which evoke cell-mediated immune responses. A short section in this chapter will suggest how tumors may grow despite these immune responses and some current rationale for tumor immunotherapy.

A fetus can also be viewed as a "foreign transplant." We will therefore present a possible mechanism which may explain the survival of this immunologically "foreign object" during gestation.

Some recipients of kidneys can be withdrawn from their immunosuppressive therapy without jeopardizing the fate of their organ transplants. These individuals appear to have become immunologically tolerant to the foreign antigens on the kidney graft. Immunological tolerance can also be induced experimentally by introducing foreign antigens into an immunologically immature animal. The discussion on immunologic tolerance will show that it may have important implications for the establishment of "self-tolerance" and how a breakdown of this self-tolerance can lead to autoimmunity.

There has been a rapid accumulation of information about the immune response in general but in particular about the cellular interactions and the regulation by gene products. Much of this knowledge has been gained through the study of genetically well-defined animal models, especially mice. Thus far mouse and man have generally been quite similar in their immune behavior. Insights gained from studying the mouse are rapidly tested in the human. Therefore, to understand the directions of new information for man, we have tried to include relevant non-human data.

CELLS INVOLVED IN THE IMMUNE RESPONSE

There are currently four major populations of mononuclear cells believed to be involved in the immune response. Some of these populations have subpopulations, and their interactions are complex.

Monocytes and macrophages

These are large mononuclear phagocytic cells which originate in the bone marrow as monocytes and settle as fixed macrophages or histiocytes in various organs or migrate as ameboid-like cells throughout the body. The exact function of macrophages has been in dispute for some time. One of their functions—and it may be the function of a subpopulation—is waste disposal. The cells phagocytize and digest debris that results from tissue damage. In addition, macrophages ingest and "process" foreign antigens and transfer these antigens into more immunogenic molecules. This may be done via an informational RNA molecule (i-RNA) produced

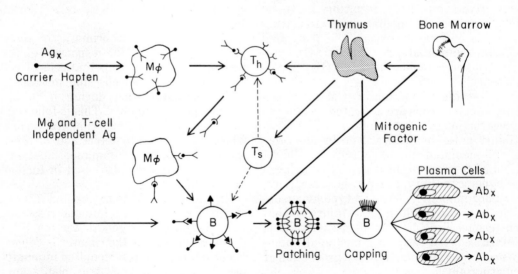

Figure 34–1. Humoral antibody production. Ag, antigen; Ab, antibody; B, B lymphocyte; Mφ, macrophage; T_h, helper T-cell; T_s, suppressor T-cell.

by the macrophage, by attaching an RNA molecule onto the antigen, or by retaining part of the ingested antigen near or on the surface of the macrophage, thereby becoming the functional "immunogen" (Unanue, 1975). While macrophages are required for antibody production to most antigens, there are exceptions. The macrophage-independent antigens can convert an antibody-producing precursor B-lymphocyte into an antibody-forming cell through direct contact (Fig. 34-1).

Macrophages also play a role in cell-mediated immunity (CMI). Optimal stimulation in mixed lymphocyte cultures, an *in vitro* correlate of CMI (Bach, 1976), requires the presence of macrophages or supernatant fluids from macrophage cultures. Macrophages can become non-specifically activated by agents like Bacillus Calmette-Guerin (BCG) or *Corynebacterium parvum*, to kill tumor cells or bacteria (Bast, 1974). These cells can also become specifically activated ("armed") through contact with sensitized T-lymphocytes; macrophages armed by sensitized T-lymphocytes will kill, specifically, the target cell to which the T-lymphocytes are sensitized (Fig. 34-2).

Lastly, macrophages can function as suppressor cells. These suppressor macrophages can inhibit immunocompetent cells and function as regulators of the immune response. Suppressor macrophages appear to have an important role in the regulation of tumor growth and immunoglobulin production (Waldmann, 1977). Functional assays of macrophages are discussed on page 1347.

T Cells

Thymus-derived lymphocytes, or T cells, originate in the bone marrow and mature in the thymus, where they obtain some of their T cell characteristics. They then home to the lymph node and spleen via the lymphatics and blood stream. Some of the maturation steps are under the influence of a thymic hormone, thymosin, which is produced by the reticuloendothelial cells of the thymus. Thymosin, a protein of small molecular weight, can be isolated from bovine thymus and has been used in several instances for the treatment of thymic deficiencies (Goldstein, 1975).

There are a number of subpopulations of T cells (Cantor, 1977). These include helper T (T_h) cells, which are required for the production of antibody to most antigens. The T_h cells are believed to concentrate the antigen via specific receptor molecules on the cell surface. These receptors bind the carrier part of the antigen molecule. The antigen-receptor complex is next picked up by a macrophage and presented to the potential antibody-forming cells. Previously we mentioned that there are macrophage-independent antigens. These antigens are also thymus-independent and do not require the cooperation of T_h cells (Fig. 34-1).

T_h cells also play a role in the cell-mediated immune response. In a graft-vs-host reaction (GVHR), for instance, T_h ("amplifier") cells cooperate with the GVH-reactive T cell. In mixed lymphocyte cultures, the proliferation of T cells, or the generation of cytotoxic T cells, requires interaction with a T_h cell. It is not certain that the T_h cell involved in humoral antibody synthesis is the same cell required for CMI. In addition, there may be other T cells required for full expression of helper functions (Fig. 34-2).

In addition to T_h cells, there are cytotoxic T-lymphocytes (T_{cx}) which are involved in cell-mediated immunity (Cerottini, 1974). The T_{cx} cells are activated by tissue or tumor antigens and can kill specifically, without the help of antibody, target cells which have this antigen on their surfaces. T_{cx} cells may also render macrophages specifically cytotoxic to tumor target cells.

A third subpopulation of T cells functions as suppressor cells (T_s) (Gershon, 1975). These T_s cells can be activated during humoral immunity or in cell-mediated immunity. The mechanism by which T_s cells suppress the immune response is not clear but it may be via a soluble factor produced by T_s cells.

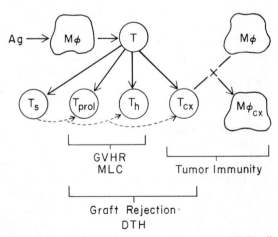

Figure 34–2. Cell-mediated immunity. Ag, antigen; T, T-cell; T_s, suppressor T-cell; T_{prol}, proliferating T-cell; T_h, helper T-cell; T_{cx}, cytotoxic T-lymphocytes; Mϕ, macrophage; Mϕ_{cx}, cytotoxic macrophage; GVHR, graft-vs. host reaction; MLC, mixed lymphocyte culture; DTH, delayed-type hypersensitivity.

B Cells

Bone marrow-derived lymphocytes, or B cells, are the antibody-forming precursor cells. They migrate from the bone marrow to the germinal centers of lymphoid tissues where they accept the antigen/T cell receptor complexes from macrophages. The B cell accepts the antigen/T cell receptor complex via hapten-specific receptor molecules. After shedding the T cell receptor, the antigen molecules distribute themselves in patches over the surface of the B cell ("patching") and subsequently migrate to the polar cap of the cell ("capping"), where they are ingested. At this time the B cells divide (possibly under the influence of a soluble factor secreted by thymic cells) and differentiate into antibody-forming plasma cells (Fig. 34-1).

Upon initial contact with most antigens, plasma cells produce IgM, an immunoglobulin of high molecular weight. On further exposure the cells switch and produce an antibody of smaller molecular weight which may be of IgG, IgA, IgD, or IgE isotype (p. 1216). Some antigens, especially the bacterial polysaccharides, evoke only IgM. Antibody production, after first exposure to an antigen, is called a primary antibody response. After restimulation with a similar antigen, the body responds with a secondary or anamnestic response, which generally results in the more rapid production of an increased quantity of antibody. During an anamnestic response the cells usually avoid the IgM phase and immediately produce the antibody of lower molecular weight. In addition, antibodies produced during a secondary response are usually more avid. A detailed discussion on the nature and function of the various antibodies is presented in Chapter 36 (p. 1215).

Null cells

During selected "cell-mediated" immune responses, cytotoxic cells are found to be neither macrophages nor T or B cells. These lymphocytes are called null cells. They possess Fc-receptors for IgG (p. 140) and are capable of killing antibody-coated target cells *in vitro* (antibody-dependent cytotoxic cells—ADCC). Null cells are also called killer, or *K*, cells (Perlmann, 1976). The precise role of these cells in CMI is currently under active investigation, but it is thought that they may play a role in autoimmune disorders (Allison, 1976).

NK Cells

The peripheral lymphocytes from non-immunized individuals or the spleen of non-sensitized mice may also contain a population of cells which are cytotoxic for several targets. These natural killer, or NK, cells are non-phagocytic and do not have markers for T- or B-lymphocytes. They are therefore also "null cells." NK cells may represent our first line of defense in "natural resistance" and may be responsible for immunosurveillance against tumor cells. The origin of NK cells and their mechanism of action are uncertain.

SPECIFIC REMOVAL OR DEPLETION OF SUBPOPULATIONS OF MONONUCLEAR CELLS

Macrophages

Macrophages can be removed from a cell population by incubation on a glass or plastic surface. The non-adherent cells can be poured off and the adherent macrophages collected by gently scraping with a rubber policeman, or by treatment with EDTA or lidocaine (Rabinovitch, 1975). Macrophages can also be removed by filtration through columns of glass wool or glass beads.

In addition to their ability to adhere to glass, macrophages phagocytize foreign substances. To deplete macrophages from a mixed population of cells, one can incubate the cells with iron particles. The macrophages ingest the iron and can subsequently be passed through a strong magnetic field, attracting the iron-laden macrophages. The resultant cell population is free of phagocytic cells. There are substances such as carrageenan and silica which can destroy macrophages of several species. Treatment of a mixed cell population with anti-macrophage serum and complement can also eliminate macrophage activity.

Detection, separation, and removal of T and B cells

Mitogens are plant lectins which stimulate the proliferation of lymphocytes in culture and, in certain instances, promote the non-specific generation of cytotoxic cells. Mitogens, like phytohemagglutinin (PHA) and concanavalin A (Con A), are more stimulatory for T cells and may, therefore, be used to detect the presence of these cells. Human peripheral T cells respond better to PHA than to Con A. Lipopolysaccharide (LPS) is a mitogen specific for mouse B cells. Pokeweed mitogen (PWM) has been used to assay for B-lymphocytes in man, but its specificity is in question.

Nylon wool columns can be used to separate B and T cells. If one removes macrophages from a lymphoid cell population and then filters the remaining cells through a nylon wool column, the effluent cells are predominantly T cells, whereas the column-adherent cells are predominantly B cells. The purity of these separated cell populations can be determined by using mitogens and/or specific surface markers.

Rosette formation occurs when lymphoid cells are incubated with sheep red blood cells (SRBC): T-lymphocytes bind SRBC and form rosette-like structures. The number of rosette-forming cells (RFC) can be counted under the microscope. To deplete T cells from a mixed population of cells, one can induce rosette formation and then centrifuge the cells on a density gradient. Under these conditions the RFC settle out at the bottom of the gradient.

B cells can also form rosettes, but only with SRBC which have been pretreated with an anti-SRBC antibody and sublytic doses of complement. The complement receptors on the B-cell bind the red cell-antibody-complement complex, and the number of B cells which have formed such rosettes can be counted microscopically (EAC rosettes).

Studies in the mouse have demonstrated the presence of *specific T and B cell surface antigens*. There is no compelling reason to doubt that equivalent antigens exist on human lymphocytes.

Specific B cell antigens have been described and heterologous anti-B cell antisera prepared. Rabbit anti-mouse B cell will, in the presence of complement, deplete a mouse lymphoid cell population of B cells. The absence of B cells can be monitored by a loss of LPS-responsiveness or by a failure of fluorescence-labeled anti-immunoglobulin serum to tag any cells in a previously mixed lymphocyte population. Anti-immunoglobulin specifically attaches to B cells because of the immunoglobulin molecules present on B cells and absent (or masked) on T cells. There are also reports on the preparation of anti-human B cell serum (Geier, 1977).

T cells have a number of specific antigens to which antisera can be raised. The first one,

which was described by Reif (1964), is the theta antigen of the mouse, also called Thy 1. Investigators have cleverly exploited mice which differ genetically only in some relatively small, well-defined manner (congenic). Thus, mouse strains lacking Thy 1 have produced anti-Thy 1 after immunization with the appropriate thymocytes. This anti-Thy 1 or anti-theta serum, in the presence of complement, will kill those T cells with the appropriate surface Thy 1 antigen.

Other specific T cell antigens are called Ly antigens and have been described by Boyse and Cantor (Cantor, 1977). At the moment there are three known Ly antigens (Ly_1, Ly_2, and Ly_3) on T cells. Like theta, the Ly antigens are genetically determined. Subpopulations of T cells have different Ly phenotypes—for example T_h cells are $Ly_1^+{}_2^-{}_3^-$; T_{cx} cells are $Ly_1^-{}_2^+{}_3^+$, and T_s cells are $Ly_1^-{}_2^+{}_3^+$. By producing a specific anti-Ly serum one can therefore, with the help of complement, eliminate a specific subpopulation of T cells from a mixed population. Interestingly enough, the genes coding for Ly_1 and $Ly_{2,3}$ are located on different chromosomes.

The fluorescence-activated cell sorter can also help in the separation of T and B cells. One can, for instance, allow B cells to combine with a fluorescent-labeled anti-immunoglobulin. The cell sorter can then isolate these fluorescent cells from a mixed cell population.

Further discussion of cell separation can be found on p. 1318.

GENETIC CONTROL OF THE IMMUNE RESPONSE

The immune response is controlled by a small region on chromosome 6 in man and chromosome 17 in the mouse. The major histocompatibility complex (MHC) in the mouse (also called H-2 complex) is subdivided into 5 regions: K, I, S, G, and D (see Fig. 41–1, p. 1354). The K and D regions, which are located on each side of the MHC, regulate the production of serologically defined (SD) antigens. In addition to SD antigens, there are antigens called lymphocyte-activating determinants (LaD; also referred to as LD) which control the proliferation of lymphocytes. These LD antigens are regulated by genes located in the I region, which is just to the right of the K region. The I region also controls the strength of the immune response, i.e., whether the animal will be a high or a low responder to antigens. To the right of the I region is the S locus, which controls the concentration of some serum proteins, including complement. To the right of this, and bordering the D region on the far right, is the G region, which determines some of the antigens expressed on red blood cells.

The MHC in man, also called HLA, was redefined in 1975 by a committee organized by the World Health Organization. The MHC consists of loci A, B, and C whose alleles control the production of SD antigens. A fourth locus, D, controls the production of LaD antigens (Bach, 1976).

There is some indication that the susceptibility to some diseases is under control of the MHC. In mice, for instance, the genes which influence the development of virally induced leukemia map at the K-end of the H-2 complex. In man, association has been found between HLA-SD antigens and some lymphomas or leukemias and some types of autoimmune and infectious diseases (Albert, 1977). The MHC is discussed in Chapter 41.

ORGAN TRANSPLANTATION

The exchange of tissue between two individuals with different genetic constitution leads to the immunologic phenomenon of graft rejection. Table 34-1 defines the various types of grafts which can be exchanged. *Syngeneic* and *autologous grafts* are acceptable to a recipient on a permanent basis. When one transplants *allogeneic* or *xenogeneic* grafts, the histocompatibility antigens, which are glycoprotein molecules located on the surface of the grafted cells, provoke the proliferation of host lymphocytes (the result of stimulation by LaD antigens) and promote the generation of cyto-

toxic cells (the result of stimulation by SD antigens). This leads to the rejection of the foreign tissue. When the transplant itself contains immunocompetent cells, the grafted cells can react immunologically against the foreign transplantation antigens of the host. This *graft-vs-host reaction* can result in major problems in the transplantation of immunocompetent tissues like bone marrow, spleen, or thymus.

There are certain sites in the body, called *immunologically privileged sites*, where allogeneic and xenogeneic grafts are protected from the rejection process. Some examples are the brain and the anterior chamber of the eye. The mechanism by which the transplanted tissue is protected in the privileged site is not clear, but it is probably due to a physical and/or chemical barrier which prevents the histocompatibility antigens from reaching the host lymphoid system and/or the activated host lymphocytes from reaching the transplanted tissue.

When a graft is placed in a healthy recipient, the signs of graft rejection are usually not overt until 7 to 10 days later. After about one week, however, the graft will begin to show signs of deterioration and will be infiltrated with host immunocompetent cells (*first set* or *acute rejection*). If an individual has been sensitized to tissue antigens prior to transplantation, rejection will occur more rapidly, within 5 to 6 days (*second set rejection*). Upon repeated grafting with foreign transplants, an individual may develop, in addition to cytotoxic cells, cytotoxic antibodies. Such individuals are hypersensitized and often will reject a transplant in a matter of hours. This phenomenon is called *hyperacute rejection*. In most instances the recipient of a foreign transplant is not in perfect health and/or is partially immunosuppressed. If graft rejection does occur in such individuals it can be a very slow and gradual process (*chronic rejection*).

To determine whether a particular individual is a suitable donor for a potential organ transplant recipient, the blood and tissue types of both are determined. Compatibility with respect to red blood cell antigens is of prime importance. Next the type of SD antigens on the potential donor and recipient peripheral white blood cells (WBC) are determined by incubating them in a microcytotoxicity test, with a panel of relatively monospecific anti-HLA sera. The killing of WBC by a particular antiserum indicates

Table 34-1. TERMINOLOGY OF TYPES OF GRAFTS USED IN TRANSPLANTATION

NAME OF GRAFT	GRAFTS EXCHANGED BETWEEN INDIVIDUALS OF
Syngeneic	genetically identical nature
Allogeneic (allograft)	genetically dissimilar nature within same species
Xenogeneic (xenograft)	genetically dissimilar nature of different species
Autologous (autograft)	grafts relocated within same individual

Table 34–2. CRITERIA FOR SELECTING SUITABLE DONOR/HOST TRANSPLANT COMBINATIONS

TEST FOR	TEST	TO PREVENT
Blood group antigens	ABO blood cell typing	Blood cell incompatibility
SD (serologically defined) antigen	Microcytotoxicity (HLA typing)	Generation of cytotoxic cells
LaD (Lymphocyte-activating determinant) antigen	Mixed lymphocyte culture (MLC)	Generation of proliferating cells
Circulating antibodies	Crossmatch	Hyperacute rejection

the presence of a specific SD antigen. The number of incompatibilities (i.e., the number of SD antigens present on the cells from the donor but absent in the recipient) and the locus (e.g., locus A, B, or C) where the incompatibilities are located are taken into consideration when a suitable combination of donor/recipient is selected for transplantation.

For the selection of a bone marrow transplant donor it is also important to take into consideration the presence of SD antigens in the recipient which are absent in the donor, since the immunocompetent donor cells may recognize the host antigens, leading to a graft-vs-host (GVH) reaction.

To avoid hyperacute rejection, a potential recipient is tested for the presence of circulating antibodies to the SD antigens on the donor cells. In this test the prospective donor's WBC are incubated with the serum of the potential recipient (crossmatch). The presence of circulating antibodies is indicated by destruction of the WBC (positive crossmatch).

In addition to comparing the profile of SD antigens on the cells from the prospective donor and recipient, the LaD antigenic difference is measured by incubating host and donor peripheral WBC in a mixed lymphocyte culture (MLC). The lymphocytes respond to the allogeneic LaD antigens by proliferating, which is measured by the incorporation of tritiated thymidine into cellular DNA. To determine the response of host lymphocytes to the LaD antigens on the donor cells, the latter are treated with mitotic inhibitors such as mitomycin-C (one-way MLC). When a bone marrow transplant needs to be performed, the MLC culture should be carried out in both directions, to predict the severity of the rejection of the graft by the host (HVG) as well as the rejection of the host by the graft (GVH). This can be done with an MLC using the host lymphocytes treated with mitomycin.

Immunologic selection of a potential donor is based on ABO compatibility, a low number of SD incompatibilities, a negative crossmatch, and, if time permits an MLC, low mixed lymphocyte reactivity (Table 34–2).

Despite a larger pool of cadaver donor transplants, owing to regional centers and more sophisticated techniques for donor selection of live transplants, the likelihood of a "perfect" match between two genetically dissimilar individuals is slim. For this reason, immunosuppressive treatment is almost always necessary. The most commonly used immunosuppressive drugs are azathioprine, a purine analog, and prednisone. Both of these are anti-inflammatory agents and inhibit the function of lymphocytes. It is apparent that these non-specific immunosuppressive agents can be deleterious to the general health of the individual and need to be administered with great caution. The above-mentioned treatment is occasionally accompanied by the use of anti-lymphocyte (ALS) or anti-thymocyte (ATS) serum. ALS and ATS are produced in horses, monkeys, goats, or rabbits against human lymphocytes or thymocytes, and can inactivate human lymphocytes. ALS or ATS cannot be used over a long period of time, however, since many individuals eventually develop serum sickness. A more detailed discussion on immunogenetics, organ transplantation, tissue typing, and immunosuppression can be found in Chapter 41.

TUMOR IMMUNITY

There is strong evidence that tumor cells have specific antigens, called tumor-specific transplantation antigens (TSTA), on their cell surfaces (Klein, 1968). These TSTA, which may be modified histocompatibility antigens, can elicit an immune response in the tumor-bearing host (Table 34–3). Indeed, it is believed by many immunologists that tumor cells continually arise in our body but are rejected by the immunocompetent cells activated by the

Table 34-3. ACTIVATION OF IMMUNE RESPONSE BY TUMOR-SPECIFIC TRANSPLANTATION ANTIGEN (TSTA)

TSTA ACTIVATE	EFFECT
Cytotoxic T cells	Kill tumor target by contact
Cytotoxic macrophages	Kill tumor target by contact(?)
B cells producing cytotoxic antibody	Kill tumor target by complement-dependent lysis
Null cells	Kill antibody-coated tumor target cells

TSTA. This concept is called *"immunologic surveillance."* If immunologic surveillance does exist, one must find an explanation for the fact that tumors grow, in spite of the immune response they provoke. A number of possible explanations have been offered. First, it is possible that a delicate balance exists between tumor growth and rejection, with the fate of the tumor depending on this tug of war. Second, there is the possibility that the presence of the tumor elicits the production of a tumor-enhancing factor. Indeed there is evidence for a factor in the serum of tumor-bearing individuals which actually inhibits the immunologic function of host lymphocytes. This substance, called *blocking factor,* appears to consist of an antigen-antibody complex (Hellström, 1974). Third, it is possible that a tumor activates suppressor cells which inhibit the immunologic response of host lymphocytes. The presence of suppressor cells in tumor-bearing mice has indeed been demonstrated. It has also been observed that low levels of an immune response can occasionally stimulate tumor growth, whereas high levels inhibit it. The mechanism of this dual response is not clear.

T cells, null cells, and macrophages all may be cytotoxic for tumors. The cytotoxic T cells develop through cooperation with another subpopulation of T cells, the amplifier or helper T cells. This interaction appears to be mediated by a soluble factor. Cytotoxic T cells eradicate tumor cells by direct contact.

Macrophages become cytotoxic ("armed") by interacting with cytotoxic T cells. This arming takes place through the action of a soluble factor. It is not clear how macrophages destroy tumor cells.

Null cells kill antibody-coated target cells via the Fc receptors on their surfaces (ADCC).

However, null cells are also effective in the absence of detectable antibody. This mechanism of action is not known. Both T cells and macrophages have been found to function as suppressor cells in tumor immunity. The precise role of suppressor cells in regulating tumor growth is under active investigation.

Several biochemical markers for the early detection of cancer are available. One is the *carcinoembryonic antigen (CEA),* a cell surface glycoprotein, which appears in the bloodstream of many patients with tumors. Originally it was thought that CEA was a specific marker for colonic cancer, but it is now apparent that CEA can also appear in the bloodstream of many groups of individuals, including heavy smokers. Monitoring CEA levels in patients is useful in detecting tumor recurrence after therapy.

A second biochemical marker for the detection of cancer is *alpha-fetoprotein (AFP).* This fetal serum protein, also a glycoprotein molecule, disappears in the adult but may reappear in patients with certain tumors. These proteins are discussed on page 326.

A number of approaches for the *immunotherapy* of cancer are available. The most common one is to stimulate immunocompetent cells, especially macrophages, non-specifically. This can be done, for instance, by injections of BCG (Bacillus Calmette-Guerin), an attenuated strain of the bacterium that causes bovine tuberculosis. It has been reported that the use of BCG can successfully contribute to the control of cancer, especially leukemia (Mathé, 1973). Immunostimulatory drugs such as Levamisole are also currently being explored for non-specific stimulation of the immune system (Symoens, 1977).

Another way to boost the immune system is by the injection of transfer factor. Transfer factor, discovered by H. S. Lawrence some 20 years ago, is a small molecule which can be prepared from human leukocytes and can confer immunity to normal non-sensitized individuals. Transfer factor has been used, clinically, in the treatment of several groups of patients, including some with osteogenic sarcoma and breast cancer (Levin, 1973).

Specific stimulation of the immune system in the tumor-bearing patient can, theoretically, be done in a number of ways. One way is to boost the immune reactivity of the cytotoxic T cells by injecting the patients with small numbers of their own tumor cells which previously had been surgically removed.

These tumor cells may be pretreated so that they are still immunogenic but are unable to proliferate. This approach, however, can also lead to enhanced growth of the residual tumor cells, possibly by stimulating blocking factor or activating suppressor cells.

Another possibility is to extract "immune" RNA (I-RNA) from sensitized lymphocytes. Pilch (1973) has reported that he was able to extract RNA from the lymphocytes of patients who had recovered from melanoma. This I-RNA was able to transform normal human lymphocytes into cells which were cytotoxic to cultured melanoma cells. Immune RNA could possibly be used to specifically boost the immune response of tumor patients.

Another approach is to sensitize lymphocytes *in vitro* to the tumor antigen. All these approaches show potential but are still in the experimental stage.

FETAL-MATERNAL INTERACTION

We have noted that allografts evoke an immune response in their host, which in most cases leads to graft rejection. The question arises why a fetus, which possesses one half of the histocompatibility antigens of the father and therefore represents an allograft, is not rejected during pregnancy. Indeed, alloantigens are expressed in the fetal tissue at a very early stage of development. It has been established that pregnant females are immunologically competent and capable of rejecting normal allografts. The survival of the fetus is therefore not the result of an immunodeficiency on the part of the mother. The uterus is not an immunologically privileged site because normal allografts transplanted experimentally in the uterus of normal or pseudopregnant mice are rejected (Beer, 1974).

The survival of the immunologically foreign fetus is probably due to a number of factors. One is the presence of a placental barrier, the trophoblast. This is a single layer of cells of fetal origin which forms a protective wall between fetus and mother. The trophoblast layer prevents the exchange of fetal and maternal histocompatibility antigens.

In addition to the placental barrier, the survival of the fetus may be assured by the presence of blocking factors and/or suppressor cells. Blocking factors, presumably similar to those found in individuals with progressive tumors, have been detected in the bloodstream of pregnant mice. The activation of suppressor cells during pregnancy has also been reported.

When an Rh-negative woman bears an Rh-positive child, some of the Rh-positive antigens may enter the maternal bloodstream during late pregnancy and delivery. When such an individual has a second Rh-positive child, an anamnestic response occurs. The maternal IgG antibody penetrates the placenta and injures the fetal erythrocytes (erythroblastosis fetalis). To prevent this, anti-Rh antibody is administered to the mother shortly after the birth of the first child. The antibody inhibits the immune response of the mother, possibly by "mopping up" the Rh antigen, and reduces the chances for sensitization during a second pregnancy (see Chap. 43).

During gestation, the fetus is protected immunologically by the passive transfer of maternal IgG. After birth, the fetus may receive maternal IgA antibody and other protective molecules through colostrum and breast milk. IgA antibody seems to be particularly important at a time when immunocompetence is low, perhaps to help prevent overgrowth of microorganisms in the gastrointestinal tract. A neonate is relatively immunodeficient, partly owing to a lack of functional T-helper, T-cytotoxic, antibody-forming precursor B cells and macrophages, and partly to an overabundance of suppressor cells. The possible significance of high suppressor cell activity at birth will be discussed below.

Soon after birth the human infant begins to produce antibodies and develop cell-mediated immune responses.

IMMUNOLOGIC TOLERANCE AND AUTOIMMUNITY

Immunologic tolerance is defined as specific immunologic unresponsiveness. It is most easily induced in the neonatal animal at a time when immunocompetence is low. Unresponsiveness to tissue antigens can be evoked by the injection of living cells; the resulting tolerant animal is a chimera of host and donor cells. When tolerance is induced by injection of immunocompetent cells, such as spleen, the chances for a graft-vs-host reaction are high, resulting in fatal "runt" disease. Long-lasting tolerance to a non-replicating antigen can be induced only by repeated injection of the neonate; unresponsiveness disappears when the antigen is finally eliminated.

Even though the induction of immunologic tolerance in the human newborn is not yet practical, an understanding of its mechanism has important implications in the development of autoimmunity and the prevention of transplant rejection. It is, for instance, apparent that in some organ transplant patients, the foreign transplant survives, even though immunosuppressive therapy has been discontinued. Such patients are immunologically tolerant and we may conclude that the antigens on the foreign transplant provided the tolerance-inducing stimulus at a time when immunocompetence was suppressed. Gradual decrease of immunosuppressive drugs allows a gradual return of immunocompetence, just as in the newborn, and establishment of a chimera state between the patient and the foreign transplant.

High susceptibility to tolerance during early development has important implications for the establishment of self-tolerance. During fetal and early postnatal development many tissue-specific as well as organ-specific antigens develop, and a failure to induce self-tolerance can lead to autoantibodies and/or autoreactive cells, i.e., autoimmunity.

Most tissue-specific and organ-specific antigens arise when the individual is immunologically immature and susceptible to the induction of self-tolerance. Some organ-specific antigens, however, do not arise until after immunologic immaturity has been established. These antigens, however, are thought to be shielded by a protective barrier from contact with the immune system. When a "leak" in this protective barrier occurs, the immune system responds to the "foreign" antigen, and an autoimmune response takes place. One example is the development of antigens on spermatozoa, which are present inside the testicular follicles, and are normally protected from the immune system. When the testes are damaged, sperm antigens may get into the bloodstream and induce an immune response, which may lead to further destruction of the testis. Other events can also lead to the breakdown of self-tolerance and autoimmunity. One example is damage to a particular organ, altering the antigens usually presented to the immune system and eliciting an autoimmune response.

The mechanism of tolerance is still under investigation. Burnet's classic theory of immunologic tolerance involves deletion of a clone of immunologically specific cells. This clonal deletion theory evolved from Burnet's clonal selection theory (Burnet, 1959) which postulated that in the immunologically mature individual, antigens select out a specific cell. This cell proliferates into a clone of immunocompetent cells, all with a specific function, i.e., reacting to that specific antigen. Tolerance occurs when the individual is immunologically immature and the cell which is selected by the antigen does not divide to form a clone but is destroyed. Continued presence of the foreign antigen keeps eliminating newly arising cells with specificity for that antigen, and permanent tolerance can be established. Clonal selection has received experimental support from the discovery of specific receptors on lymphocytes which could be responsible for the antigenic selection of cells. The relationship between antigen receptors on cell surfaces and susceptibility to tolerance-inducing stimuli is receiving close scrutiny.

Another explanation for immunologic tolerance is based on immunologic paralysis. This theory suggests that tolerance is due to an exhaustion of lymphocyte function by an antigen overload. Paralysis is likely to be a contributing factor, especially in cases where immunologic tolerance is induced with high doses of antigen (high zone tolerance). It should, however, be pointed out that in some instances tolerance can also be induced with low doses of antigen (low zone tolerance).

Finally, it is possible that immunologic tolerance is due to an increased suppressor cell activity. Indeed, the recent literature contains a number of reports demonstrating increased suppressor cell activity during immunologic tolerance (Waldmann, 1977).

At this time it is obvious that induction of specific immunologic tolerance is still in the experimental stage.

REFERENCES

Albert, E. D.: The HLA system: Serologically defined antigens. Clin. Immunobiol., *3*:237, 1977.

Allison, A. S.: Self-tolerance and autoimmunity in the thyroid. N. Engl. J. Med., *295*:821, 1976.

Bach, F. H.: Mixed leukocyte cultures: A cellular approach to histocompatibility testing. Clin. Immunobiol., *3*:273, 1976.

Bach, F. H., and Van Rood, J. J.: The major histocompatibility complex—genetics and biology. N. Engl. J. Med., *295*:806, 872, and 927, 1976.

Bast, R. C., Zbar, B., Borsos, T., and Rapp, H. J.: BCG and cancer. N. Engl. J. Med., *290*:1413, 1974.

Beer, A. E., and Billingham, R. E.: The embryo as a transplant. Sci. Am., *230*:36, 1974.

Burnet, F. M.: The clonal selection theory of acquired immunity. Cambridge, Cambridge University Press, 1959.

Cantor, H., and Boyse, E. A.: Lymphocytes as models for the study of mammalian cellular differentiation. Immunol. Rev., *33*:105, 1977.

Cerottini, J. C., and Brunner, K. T.: Cell-mediated cytotoxicity, allograft rejection, and tumor immunity. Adv. Immunol., *18*:67, 1974.

Geier, S. S., and Cresswell, P.: Rabbit antisera to human B cell alloantigens. Cell. Immunol., *28*:341, 1977.

Gell, P. G. H., Coombs, R. A., and Lachmann, P. (eds): Clinical Aspects of Immunology, 3rd ed. Oxford, Blackwell Scientific Publications, 1975.

Gershon, R. K.: Immunoregulations by T cells. Miami Winter Symposium, *9*:267, 1975.

Goldstein, A. L., Thurman, G. B., Cohen, G. H., and Hooper, J. A.: The role of thymosin and the endocrine thymus on the ontogenesis and function of T cells. Miami Winter Symposium, *9*:243, 1975.

Hellström, K. E., and Hellström, I.: The role of cell-mediated immunity in control and growth of tumors. Clin. Immunobiol., *2*:233, 1974.

Klein, G.: Tumor-specific transplantation antigens. Cancer Res., *4*:625, 1968.

Levin, A. S., Spitler, L. E., and Fudenberg, H.: Transfer factor therapy in immune deficiency states. Ann. Rev. Med., *24*:175, 1973.

Mathé, G., Weiner, R., Pouillart, P., Schwarzenberg, L., Jasmen, C., Schneider, M., Hayat, M., Amiel, J. L., DeVarral, F., and Rosenfeld, C.: BCG in cancer immunotherapy. Natl. Cancer Inst. Monogr., *39*:165, 1973.

Perlmann, P.: Cellular immunity: Antibody dependent cytotoxicity (K cell activity). Clin. Immunobiol., *3*:107, 1976.

Pilch, Y. H., Ramming, K. P., and Deckers, P. J.: Induction of anti-cancer immunity with RNA. Ann. N.Y. Acad. Sci., *207*:409, 1973.

Rabinovitch, M., and DeStefano, N. J.: Use of local anesthetic lidocaine for cell harvesting and subcultivation. In Vitro, *11*:379, 1975.

Reif, A. E., and Allen, J. M. V.: The AKR thymic antigen and its distribution in leukemias and nervous tissues. J. Exp. Med., *120*:413, 1964.

Symoens, J., and Rosenthal, M.: Levamisole in the modulation of the immune response: The current experimental and clinical state. Reticuloendothel. Soc., *21*:176, 1977.

Unanue, E. R., and Calderon, J.: Evaluation of the role of macrophages in immune induction. Fed. Proc., *34*:1737, 1975.

Waldmann, T. A., and Broder, S.: Suppressor cells in the regulation of the immune response. Prog. Clin. Immunol., *3*:155, 1977.

4

35

ANTIBODY AS REAGENT

Robert M. Nakamura, M.D.
Ernest S. Tucker, III, M.D.

GENERAL NATURE AND CHARACTERISTICS OF ANTIBODIES

NATURE OF ANTIBODIES

All antibodies are globulins that are made up of heavy and light polypeptide chains. They are distinct from other globulins by their capability of complexing with antigenic determinants of complementary combining sites. The immunologic specificity of the antibody refers to its ability to combine with substances bearing a unique physicochemical feature, the corresponding antigenic determinant.

Certain generalizations can be made about antibodies:

1. They are produced in response to antigenic stimulation.

2. There are five classes (isotypes) of immunoglobulins. IgG immunoglobulins are further divided into four subgroups and the IgA and IgM into two subgroups. All known antibody molecules have either kappa or lambda light chains.

3. Antibodies are heterogeneous in structure, in affinity with corresponding antigenic sites, and in their function *in vivo* and *in vitro*.

4. All antibodies have the capacity to bind with their respective antigens.

Antibodies may be classified according to their origin, their host specificity, or the characteristics of the immunologic reactions in which they are involved. Most antibodies are found free and circulating in plasma, but some specific immunoglobulins such as IgE occur as cell-associated or cytophilic antibodies which after being synthesized become associated with other cells through the Fc part of the molecule.

The term *natural antibody* is customarily applied to isohemagglutinins which are hereditary and may reflect bacterial antibodies and which sometimes occur in low concentrations in human and animal sera. The term natural antibodies probably should be limited to those immunoglobulins which, like the isohemagglutinins, are inherited and appear in the serum at certain times in the life of the individual.

IMMUNOLOGIC REACTION
(Weir, 1973)

The binding reaction between antigen and antibody may be represented by the following equation:

$$Ag + Ab \underset{Kd}{\overset{Ka}{\rightleftharpoons}} Ag \cdot Ab$$

Ag represents one of the often multiple antigenic sites on a given molecule, and Ab represents one or two or more antigenic binding sites on a given antibody molecule. Similar to a chemical reaction, there is an association and dissociation constant and the summated effect of the two yields an equilibrium constant. The total concentration of antibody in the sample is the sum of the free and bound antibody sites, and the concentration of the free antibody sites under any given circumstance is governed by the law of mass action, according to the following equation:

$$K = \frac{Ag \cdot Ab}{(Ag) \times (Ab)}$$

The antibody populations with high avidity or affinity are those with high K values, and the antibody populations with relatively low avidity have low K values (Hudson, 1976).

TYPES OF IMMUNOLOGIC REACTION

Antigen-antibody tests may be classified according to whether the test is dependent upon a primary interaction between the antibody and antigen or is based on a secondary manifestation such as precipitation, flocculation, agglutination, complement fixation, etc., following the primary interaction. The tertiary manifestations of antigen-antibody reactions are those that occur as biologic reactions which follow primary and secondary levels of antigen-antibody reactions. The tertiary reactions include many of the biologic effects of

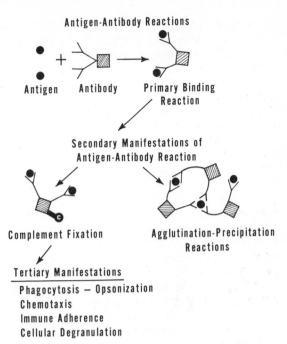

Antigen-Antibody Reactions

Antigen   Antibody   Primary Binding Reaction

Secondary Manifestations of Antigen-Antibody Reaction

Complement Fixation   Agglutination-Precipitation Reactions

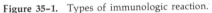

Tertiary Manifestations

Phagocytosis — Opsonization
Chemotaxis
Immune Adherence
Cellular Degranulation

Figure 35–1. Types of immunologic reaction.

complement activation, such as opsonization, phagocytosis, chemotaxis, etc. (Fig. 35–1).

The primary interaction between antigen and antibody is the first step in a series of reactions and biochemical processes which may or may not proceed to a secondary or tertiary reaction discussed below. The primary interaction is the specific recognition and combination of an antigenic determinant with the binding site of its corresponding antibody.

Quantitative tests dependent entirely on primary interaction between antigen and antibody include immunofluorescence, radioimmunoassay, and immunoenzymatic assays. The *primary tests* are more sensitive than the secondary or tertiary tests and are not dependent upon variables which control secondary or tertiary reactions. The primary tests require the following: (1) Either a purified antigen or an antibody preparation for the reaction. (2) A technique to quantitate the antigen or antibody with use of a radioisotope, enzyme, or fluorescent label. (3) A method to separate the antigen-antibody reaction complex from free antigen or antibody in solution. *Secondary manifestations* of antigen-antibody reactions include precipitation in solution or in gel, direct agglutination or agglutination of erythrocyte or other particles coated with antigen or antibody, and complement fixation.

Tertiary manifestations of antigen-antibody reactions include phagocytosis-opsonization, chemotaxis, immune adherence, and cellular degranulation.

Antibody molecules are capable of recognizing binding and complexing with specific antigen. In the case of reaction of specific IgG with a hapten antigen, the complexes are usually $(hapten)_2 - (antibody)_1$. In the case of multivalent protein antigens, complexes of varying size may be formed proportional to the concentrations of the antibody and antigen. Immune complexes of varying size have different degrees of solubility; their ability to localize along vascular basement membrane and fix complement *in vivo* is responsible for a wide range of immune complex-mediated hypersensitivity diseases. Thus, a full understanding of antigen-antibody interaction involves a knowledge first of type, specificity, affinity, and concentration of antibody, then of antigen concentration, and finally of biologic activity.

SENSITIVITY AND SPECIFICITY OF IMMUNOLOGIC TESTS

A wide spectrum of different immunologic methods is currently available. Antibodies differ widely in their specificity and sensitivity. Primary antigen-antibody binding assays can be sensitive in the nanogram to picogram per milliliter range. Variation in standardization and specificity of immunologic methods is a common problem. Antibodies which have a high affinity and are potent may give unwanted cross-reactions while weak antisera may be specific but not sensitive. Cross-reaction refers to immunologic reactivity of two or more antigens with the same antiserum or to the reactivity of two or more sera with one antigen.

Varying levels of sensitivity are well illustrated by the numerous tests available for the detection of hepatitis B associated surface antigen (HBsAg). The agar gel diffusion test may be considered to be a precipitin test with the sensitivity value of one. The cross electrophoretic or electroimmunodiffusion method increases the sensitivity 10 times, whereas the radioimmunoassay procedure for HBsAg will increase the sensitivity 10,000 times.

The sensitivity of the agar gel test for alpha-1-fetoprotein is in the range of 3000 ng/ml. Most of the positive determinations are significant and may be diagnostic for

Table 35–1. RELATIVE SENSITIVITY OF IMMUNOLOGIC TESTS INVOLVING SECONDARY MANIFESTATIONS OF ANTIGEN-ANTIBODY REACTIONS*

IMMUNOLOGIC TEST	MINIMUM OF ANTIBODY N (μg) DETECTABLE OR NEEDED FOR REACTION
Precipitation	
Tube precipitation	0.1
Immunodiffusion	0.1–0.3
Agglutination	
Qualitative	0.05
Quantitative	0.02–0.1
Hemagglutination, passive	0.001
Hemagglutination-inhibition	0.001
Coombs' reaction	0.01
Complement fixation	0.05

*Modified from Kwapinski, J.B.G.: Methodology of Immunochemical and Immunological Research. New York, Wiley-Interscience, Inc., 1972.

hepatocellular carcinoma or embryonal cell carcinoma. A current radioimmunoassay procedure, however, has a sensitivity to 1 ng/ml but will reveal many more "positive" specimens. The former method will have more false negatives, the latter more false positives.

Relative sensitivity of immunologic tests involving secondary manifestations of antigen-antibody reactions is listed below in Table 35-1.

PRECIPITIN REACTIONS

The precipitin reaction occupies an important position in immunology and occurs when serum from a sensitized animal is mixed with the immunizing antigen. The precipitate that forms represents large complexes of antigen and antibody that have combined to form an insoluble lattice. The first observation of the reaction was reported by Kraus in 1897 when he observed a precipitin reaction on mixing antisera to typhoid bacillus with cell-free filtrates of cultures from typhoid organisms. Many investigators since then have used the precipitin reaction to identify and quantitate immunologic reactions. Some major investigators who have contributed to our knowledge of the precipitin reaction include such prominent individuals as Ehrlich, Heidelberger, Kendall, Pauling, Boyd, Nuttal, and Landsteiner.

The modern refinements of the quantitative precipitin technique as an analytical tool for measurement of antibody were extensively developed by Heidelberger and Kendall. Much of their work, which was carried out during the early 1930's, stands today as a major contribution to the science of immunology and immunochemistry.

Varied applications of the precipitin reaction will be discussed as an important tool in immunochemistry for the identification and quantification of a wide range of antigenic substances. Each of the modes of application of the precipitin technique has a differing advantage of sensitivity, specificity, and simplicity. Immunoprecipitin techniques will no doubt enjoy a continually broadening application in the clinical laboratory. The disadvantages of these techniques are relatively minor compared with other more cumbersome, less direct, and complex techniques for macromolecular analysis. A diversity of specific antisera is critical in the continued growth and application of these techniques. Currently such antisera are available from only a limited number of commercial or research sources and for only a limited number of antigenic substances. Another major problem is availability of stable and well-defined standards. Also lacking are control sera of sufficient stability to compare favorably with those used in other areas of clinical laboratory analysis.

The limitation of the sensitivity of these assays is a major consideration. Even under the best conditions of enhanced sensitivity afforded by the newer light-scattering techniques, the accuracy and sensitivity of immunoprecipitin assays are not satisfactory below a range of 0.1 to 0.5 mg/dl. This limits certain applications of immunoprecipitin assays, but the techniques appear quite sufficient for quantification of many major serum proteins and a wide range of other biologic molecules of importance in clinical medicine. Some important trace proteins, polypeptides, and endocrine factors cannot be accurately measured by the current methods of immunoprecipitin assay. Their measurement by the more sensitive techniques of radioimmunoassay, enzyme-linked immunoassay, and immunofluorescence will be discussed in other sections of this text.

PRINCIPLES

The quantitative precipitin reaction, as it is known today, provides a systematic approach to determining the amount of either antibody or antigen by defining the optimal proportions of each reactant in the formation of the immune precipitate. The approach usually followed is to prepare a series of test tubes, each containing a fixed amount of antisera; to each tube in sequence an increasing quantity of the antigen used for immunization is added. Following addition of antigen, an appropriate period of time is allowed for the reaction to occur and precipitate to form. The amount of nitrogen or protein in the precipitate is then determined by measuring the nitrogen, often by the micro Kjeldahl method. In appropriate proportions, all the antigen is precipitated; therefore, the nitrogen of the precipitate due to antigen can be subtracted and a direct determination of antibody nitrogen in the immune sera can be made. As will be noted subsequently, the precipitin reaction forms the basis for many quantitative and qualitative immunochemical techniques now used in the clinical laboratory (Kabat, 1961).

Investigation of factors affecting the precipitin reaction was extensively pursued by Heidelberger and Kendall, who found that, in addition to the relative proportions of reactants, conditions of temperature, pH, ionic strength of the medium, and certain characteristics of antibody known as avidity and affinity are important in formation of the immune precipitate. A graphic illustration of the pattern of precipitin formation when there is sequential addition of increasing quantities of antigen to a fixed quantity of antiserum is shown in Figure 35-2. It can be noted that there occurs a point of maximum, or optimal, precipitation designated as the *point of equivalence*. Continued addition of antigen following the equivalence point results in a solubilizing effect on the precipitate. This is thought to occur because of the formation of small complexes with the excess antigen. These small complexes do not lead to the formation of the lattice structure. In such conditions, it can be seen that the small soluble complexes may have a ratio of two molecules of antigen to a single molecule of antibody. Indeed, antigen excess may sometimes be adjusted to a point where the precipitate completely redissolves, leaving no visible evidence of an antigen/antibody reaction. This zone of solubility in antigen excess is referred to as the *post-zone* phenomenon. By contrast, inspection of Figure 35-2 also shows that early in the course of adding antigen a condition of marked antibody excess exists and there is also a lack of

4

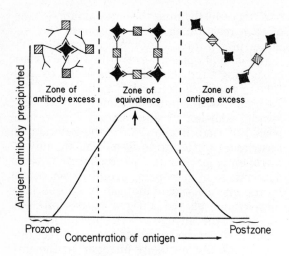

THE QUANTITATIVE PRECIPITIN CURVE

Plot obtained by adding increasing amounts of a soluble antigen to fixed volumes of monospecific antiserum. Maximum precipitate (↑) is formed at optimal ratio of antigen to antibody called the equivalence point.

Figure 35-2.

precipitate formation. This is presumably due to formation of highly soluble complexes with abundant antibody so that antibody molecules may exceed six to seven for each molecule of antigen. This area of the precipitin curve in antibody excess where no precipitate is observed is known as the *pro-zone*.

Inspection of the contour of the precipitin curve in Figure 35-2 also reveals that the equivalence point, or point of maximum precipitate, generally occurs over a narrow range of antibody/antigen ratios. The ratios commonly found are in the range of three or four molecules of antibody to one molecule of antigen. It should be emphasized that this relatively narrow zone of equivalence occurs largely with those antigens which are easily soluble and which contain a minimum number of antigen reactive sites in each molecule. By contrast, the precipitin curves for large poorly soluble or particulate antigens exhibit a very broad zone of precipitate and, in such instances, the precipitin reaction does not offer the degree of quantitation that can be obtained with a smaller soluble antigen (Kabat, 1961).

Another circumstance which alters the narrow zone of equivalence in the precipitin curve occurs when a mixture of antibodies is present

in the immune serum, and these react with the differing antigens in the immunizing material. Such a multicomponent reactant system will also give a broader zone of equivalence than the singular reactive systems. The zone of equivalence in multicomponent reactions tends to be somewhat rounded in contrast to a sharply narrow zone with the single reactant. The explanation for this is that in the multicomponent system each subgroup of antigen/antibody reactants forms a precipitate with varied ratios of antigen to antibody. Consequently, some begin to precipitate early on addition of the antigen mixture, while increasing additions of antigen precipitate with other antibody populations. As will be noted later, the individual antigen/antibody reactants in such a multicomponent precipitin system can best be separated by using a semisolid supporting medium such as agar gel rather than a liquid medium for the reaction (see Fig. 35-5).

The chemical structure of the precipitate is important in further understanding the nature of the precipitin reaction. As shown in Figure 35-3, the immune complexes formed throughout the range of any precipitin reaction will vary in the composition ratio of antibody to antigen. As discussed elsewhere (p. 1232), we know much about the structure and combining sites of various classes of antibody in vertebrates and other animals. These data clearly reveal that each molecule of antibody has a minimum of at least two combining sites for antigen. Classically, two combining sites are described for immunoglobulins of the classes IgG, IgA, and IgE. IgM is known to be composed of multiple subunits which resemble the 7-S structure of IgG and generally will possess from 5 to 6 combining sites for antigens. IgA may also occur in the form of a dimer or trimer and exhibit additional combining sites. Antigens, on the other hand, usually exhibit extensive variation in chemical structure and reactive antigenic sites. Knowledge of and characterization of all the possible ranges of antigen configurations are beyond our current scope. However, it can be assumed that, since antigen as well as antibody link together to form a three-dimensional lattice structure, antigen must provide the key link in the lattice. Based on this assumption, antigen sites would of necessity occur in clusters of at least 4 to 5 per molecule in order to link up the bivalent combining antibody in a lattice configuration. As the foregoing discussion indi-

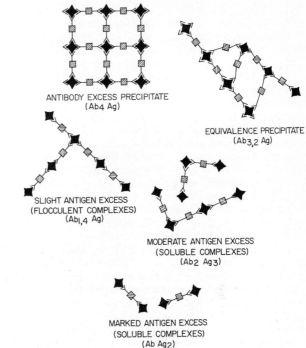

Figure 35-3. Schematic representation of lattice structures of immune complexes formed at various ratios of antibody to antigen. (Stoichiometry of complexes indicated below each structure.)

cates, the point of equivalence is taken to represent the maximum linkage between antigen and antibody, and this configuration gives rise to the greatest amount of precipitate. The drawings in Figure 35-3 diagrammatically show the variability in antigen/antibody structure which is presumed to exist at different parts of the precipitin curve. At the point of equivalence the regular lattice structure as shown is expected, while in the conditions of high solubility of an immune complex in antigen excess an increase of antigen could give a ratio of antibody to antigen as low as 0.5. In those circumstances in which the antigen possesses only a single reactive site, linkage and lattice formation would not occur and a precipitate would not be formed (Kabat, 1961).

FACTORS AND CONDITIONS AFFECTING THE PRECIPITIN REACTION

Brief mention has been made of the conditions of temperature, pH, and antibody reactivity which affect the precipitin reaction. In some reactant conditions the precipitate may form equally well at 0°C. and at 37°C. However, many antisera will be found which exhibit higher specific reactivity at some temperatures than at others. Commonly the conditions of wide ranges of temperature are met

by initially allowing incubation to proceed at 37°C. for a few hours, then followed by a period of incubation at 0 to 4°C. The relative amount of precipitate which forms under the different conditions is then determined. pH appears to have an effect in that immune complexes appear to form most abundantly in the neutral range between 6 and 7.5, while higher and lower pH extremes may dissociate or prevent the formation of the complexes (Kabat, 1961).

Salt concentration of the reactant medium, usually as sodium chloride concentration, exhibits a substantial effect on immune complex formation in the precipitin reaction. In general, high quantities of salt appear to increase solubility of the complexes and cause a shift in equilibrium between the reactants so that dissociation occurs in those complexes which have formed, and formation of new complexes is prevented. The increase in salt concentration above 0.15 M brings a striking decrease in the amount of precipitate. However, it has been observed that antisera from birds and other avian species may exhibit increased precipitin reaction in the presence of higher salt concentrations.

Certain characteristics of the antibody itself will have an effect on the precipitin reaction. The specificity and affinity of the antibody for antigenic sites affect the velocity of the reaction. The specificity of an antibody is measured by determining affinity of the antisera for a group of closely related antigens. Usually, when there is high specificity and strong affinity for the antigens, precipitin reaction will readily result with both the immunizing and closely related antigens. In contrast, antibodies with low affinity, even if highly specific, tend to react only with the immunizing antigen and not to any extent with related antigens and to give weak precipitin reactions.

The avidity of the antibody is also important in the precipitin reaction. This characteristic of the antibody determines the degree of stability of the antigen/antibody complex at the antigen binding site. The tendency of complexes to dissociate and dissolve decreases substantially as the avidity of the antiserum increases. Avidity also affects the amount of antibody in the precipitate as well as the contour of the zone of equivalence. With increased avidity there is an increase in the combining stability of the antibody with the antigen.

In addition to the known characteristics of antibodies there are other less well understood factors of molecular structure which affect the ability of antibody to form precipitates that remain stable combined with antigen. Other factors affect the rate of formation and solubilization of the complexes. In general, as was indicated earlier, the precipitates will dissolve or become solubilized with increasing additions of antigen or in the presence of excess antibody. However, instances have been observed in which certain antigen/antibody precipitates do not exhibit this easily reversible solubility. They remain as precipitates for long periods and often appear to undergo reversible solubility at a very slow rate or not at all. Such a phenomenon was described by Danysz in 1902 and the term Danysz phenomenon is now used to designate insolubility of some immune precipitates. In contrast to the poorly soluble precipitates, there also are populations of antibody which are so poorly reactive with antigen that they are non-precipitating. Such non-precipitating antibody can only be detected by special techniques. One technique is known as co-precipitation, in which known precipitating reactants are added to a suspension of non-precipitating antibody to produce a carrier, or co-precipitation, effect on the otherwise non-reacting antibody (Kabat, 1961; Campbell, 1970).

CLINICAL LABORATORY APPLICATIONS OF THE PRECIPITIN REACTION

The sensitivity, simplicity, and specificity of the precipitin reaction have provided the basis for its importance as an analytical technique in the clinical laboratory. Adaptation of the precipitin reaction to semisolid media such as agar gel and agarose greatly simplified the routine applications of the technique. Investigators such as Preer, Oakley-Fulthorpe, and Oudin refined the use of precipitin reaction in gel diffusion systems for the quantitative es-

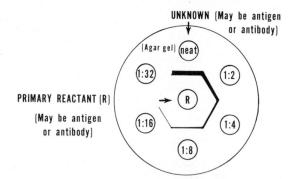

Figure 35–4. Estimate of antigen (or antibody) content using serial dilution of unknown against primary reactant. (Double immunodiffusion Ouchterlony technique.) Note decreasing thickness of precipitin line which disappears at fivefold dilution of unknown.

timate of antibody content of immune sera. These investigators emphasized the quantitative significance of the thickness of the precipitin line formed in gels at the point of equivalence (Fig. 35-4). In the early 1960's, investigators such as Mancini, Carbonara, and Heremans, as well as Fahey and McKelvey, adapted the immunoprecipitin reaction in gels to a highly sensitive and specifically quantitative technique of single radial immunodiffusion which is now in common use. This technique will be covered in detail later in this section. Grabar and Williams combined the techniques of electrophoresis and immunodiffusion in gel media to introduce yet another dimension to identification and quantification of complex macromolecules. All of these techniques are now used in determinations of specific antibody concentration and in the determination of the identity and concentration of a wide variety of antigenic macromolecules. These antigens include a wide range of serum proteins and tissue proteins, as well as complex polysaccharides, nucleic acids, and a variety of synthetic chemical compounds (Crowle, 1961; Mancini, 1965; Fahey, 1965).

In the following sections there will be discussion of particular applications of the immunodiffusion reaction in gels. Many of these applications relate to specific design of the gel chamber and the points of application of antigen and antibody.

Single immunodiffusion involves incorporation of antibody into the agar gel at a temperature sufficiently low to prevent denaturation and yet allow subsequent filling of an appropriate chamber—either small test tubes, Petri dishes, or glass slide surfaces (Fig. 35-5). Direct application of the test antigen is then

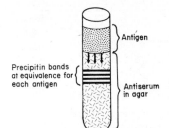

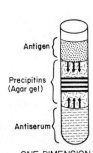

Figure 35-5. Single and double immunodiffusion reactions: Use of immunoprecipitin reactions in gel to determine presence of multiple reactants in antigen and antibody preparations.

ONE DIMENSION-SINGLE IMMUNODIFFUSION(OUDIN TUBE)(Antigen diffuses from overlay into agar containing antiserum where precipitin lines form at the equivalence points for each separate antigen)

ONE DIMENSION-DOUBLE IMMUNODIFFUSION (Antigen diffuses into agar from overlay while antibody diffuses from below. Precipitin bands form at equivalence points for each separate antigen)

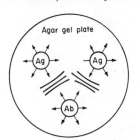

TWO DIMENSION-DOUBLE IMMUNODIFFUSION OUCHTERLONY (Antigens and antibody diffuse radially into agar. Precipitin bands form at equivalence points for each separate antigen. Location and arrangement of wells in agar can vary to compare a variety of antigens and antibodies)

made either as an overlay in the test tube or by diffusion from a well punched in the agar plates. After a period of time to allow for diffusion and equilibrium, there occurs formation of precipitin bands in the agar. Visual observation by inspection confirms the presence of a precipitin line in the agar. This line is formed at the point of optimum antigen/antibody ratio, which is the same as the equivalence point earlier described in the precipitin reaction. The distance of the precipitin line from the point of application of antigen has been shown to be directly proportional to the concentration of antigen when using a defined quantity of antiserum in the agar. By a graphic comparison with preparations of antigen standards, the quantity of the unknown antigen can be determined. The principle of the technique is that antigen diffuses through the agar-containing antibody until the point of equivalence is reached and a precipitin line forms (Williams, 1970).

Double immunodiffusion incorporates an agar gel to act as a supporting medium which separates the antigen and antibody (Figs. 35-5 and 35-6). The type of chamber selected for the study can be a test tube, a Petri dish, or a glass slide containing agar. The antigen and antibody are applied at separate points by punching wells in the agar or placing antibody at the base of the test tube separating it from the antigen by a layer of agar gel. After diffusion of the reactants into the agar over a suitable period, usually 18 to 48 hours, the reactants will contact at the interface of diffusion, and at the equivalence point there will be formation of a precipitin line. This method can be used in a semi-quantitative way by inspecting the thickness of the precipitin line and determining the distance of migration from the reactant wells. Comparison is made with a standard antigen of known concentration which has reacted in a companion set-up.

The double immunodiffusion reaction also affords a rapid and simple method of determining relative concentrations of antigen and antibody in different preparations. As shown in Figure 35-6, the diffusion of antigen and

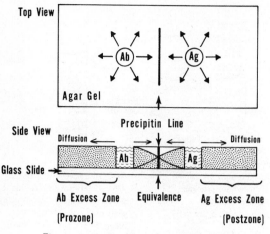

Figure 35-6. Double immunodiffusion.

antibody from application sites in the wells leads to formation of a precipitin line at some point between the two wells. The precipitin line forms at the point of equivalence. In those situations in which the line forms equidistant from antigen and antibody wells, this finding is direct evidence that the amount of antibody and antigen in each preparation is balanced at the optimal ratio. When a precipitin band forms close to the antigen well, this indicates an excess of antibody over that of antigen. By contrast, when the precipitin band develops

near the antibody well, excess antigen is indicated. In some instances a precipitin band may not form. In such a case, the cause could be either antibody excess (pro-zone phenomenon) or antigen excess (post-zone phenomenon). In such instances, alternate serial dilution of each one of the reactants with repeat of the assay will eventually give precipitin formation. The dilutions required and position of the precipitin line reveal the presence of antigen or antibody excess (Campbell, 1970).

Double immunodiffusion in two dimensions is a method described by Ouchterlony which represents a variation of the double immunodiffusion technique. This procedure is usually carried out in a gel medium in a Petri dish or on a glass slide and it is used for comparing different antigens or different antibodies. Figure 35-7 illustrates the appearance of precipitin patterns that may be encountered in this analysis. Molecules that share an identical antigenic structure exhibit a pattern of complete coalescence of the precipitin lines, while those with partial antigenic differences exhibit a spur pattern. Those of complete antigenic difference show crossing of the precipitin bands (Williams, 1970; Campbell, 1970).

The *electroimmunodiffusion reaction* (counter immunoelectrophoresis) is a variation of the double immunodiffusion reaction created by augmenting the diffusion of the reactants

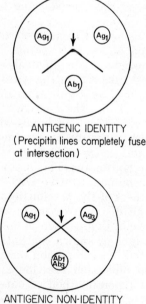

ANTIGENIC IDENTITY
(Precipitin lines completely fuse at intersection)

ANTIGENIC NON-IDENTITY
(Precipitin lines cross at intersection indicative of no shared antigens)

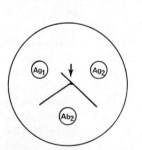

PARTIAL ANTIGENIC IDENTITY
(Precipitin line of Ag_1 fuses completely with Ag_2; Ag_2 exibits a precipitin spur beyond intersection with Ag_1 indicative of non-shared antigens)

Figure 35-7. Precipitin patterns observed in double immunodiffusion reactions by the Ouchterlony technique.

Ag_1 = Antigen 1 Ab_1 = Antibody to Ag_1
Ag_2 = Antigen 2 Ab_2 = Antibody to Ag_2
Ag_3 = Antigen 3 Ab_3 = Antibody to Ag_3

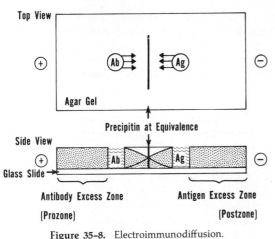

Figure 35-8. Electroimmunodiffusion.

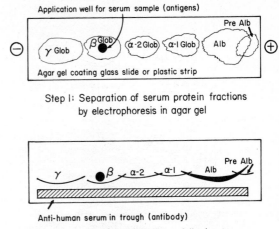

Step 1: Separation of serum protein fractions by electrophoresis in agar gel

Step 2: Precipitin lines form following two dimensional immunodiffusion reaction in agar after application of specific antiserum in trough. (Incubate in moist chamber overnight)

Figure 35-9. Steps involved in precipitin analysis by the technique of immunoelectrophoresis.

in agar gel by use of an electric current. The schematic for this technique is illustrated in Figure 35-8 and is similar to that followed in the usual double immunodiffusion reaction. Antibody is placed in the well favoring its migration in the direction of the cathode, while antigens that tend to be more negatively charged are placed in the well favoring migration to the anode. The electrophoretic effect enhances mobility of the reactants and speeds up their movement toward each other. A precipitin line which occurs at a point of equivalence thus requires a much shorter time for development owing to the augmentation by electrophoresis. The size and position of the precipitin band provides the same type of information regarding equivalence or antigen/antibody excess as in the simple double immunodiffusion system (Ritzmann, 1975).

Immunoelectrophoresis couples electrophoretic separation with the two-dimensional immunodiffusion reaction and is now used extensively for specific identification and semiquantitative estimation of a wide range of antigens. The steps of the technique are outlined diagrammatically in Figure 35-9. The first step involves application of a macromolecular sample such as human serum for electrophoresis in agar gel on a plastic or glass support. On completion of the electrophoresis, a trough is prepared along one margin of the slide and specific antiserum is applied in the trough. Diffusion is then allowed to proceed. In the diagram of Step 2 in Figure 35-9 there is shown a representative pattern of precipitin lines which form with human serum using a multispecific antiserum to human serum proteins. Notice that the relative thickness of

individual bands is proportional to their relative concentrations. Their respective positions in the electrophoretic migration also aid in their identity. By using this method homogeneous populations of macromolecules such as those which occur in monoclonal gammopathies of multiple myeloma or Waldenstrom's macroglobulinemia exhibit narrow localized areas of thickening of the precipitin bands. Indeed, this approach is the definitive method for identifying such monoclonal immunoglobulins. By using monospecific antisera to different components of immunoglobulins, a differential immunoelectrophoretic study of monoclonal proteins can give a definite identification as to light and heavy chain composition. This technique also finds wide application in other areas of immunologic investigation where separation and identification of different macromolecules are required. It is also quite useful in the study of cleavage or proteolytic breakdown of macromolecules such as those of the serum complement and properdin systems, which will be discussed later in this chapter (Rose, 1973; Ritzmann, 1975).

QUANTITATIVE TECHNIQUES
UTILIZING IMMUNOPRECIPITIN
REACTIONS IN GELS

Brief mention has already been made of using precipitin reactions in gel to quantify

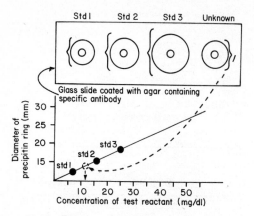

Figure 35–10. Diagram of immunoquantitation by method of single radial immunodiffusion (Techniques of Mancini, Carbonara, and Heremans; and of Fahey and McKelvey).

both antigens and antibody. The *radial immunodiffusion* (RID) technique has proved to be a most useful method for immunoglobulin and serum protein quantitation in the clinical laboratory during the past few years. The essential elements of the technique are diagrammed in Figure 35–10. This illustration shows that the RID technique indeed has advantages of operational simplicity as well as sensitivity and specificity. The approach basically represents a variation of the single immunodiffusion technique where antibody has been incorporated into the agar which is poured into a plate or onto a glass slide. Wells are then cut in the agar and test material is placed in the wells. Antigen standards of known amount are placed in some wells along with unknown test material in others. After allowing an adequate time for diffusion and formation of precipitin rings about the wells, a standard curve is graphically drawn by measuring the diameters (or areas) of the precipitin rings for the different concentration standards. These are plotted on orthographic

or semilog paper. The diameters of precipitin rings of the unknown (or areas) are then measured and plotted on the standard curve. By direct inspection a determination of the concentration of the unknown test material can be made. The specificity of this reaction quite obviously depends on the quality and monospecificity of the antiserum used as the reagent in the gel. Antisera which lack sharp specificity may give rise to more than one precipitin ring. In some instances deterioration of the unknown test material may result in breakdown fragments that also give rise to artifactual double or triple precipitin ring formation. However, such problems are only infrequently encountered and, in general, the method is the simplest and most direct for quantitation of complex macromolecules (Mancini, 1965; Fahey, 1965).

Single dimension electroimmunodiffusion, developed by Laurell in the 1960's, represents an important variation of the single immunodiffusion reaction. The method involves the use of agar gel with antibody incorporated into the agar as in RID. Sample application is made at one margin of the gel plate into wells followed by electrophoresis of the test samples into the agar. The elements of this technique are diagrammed in Figure 35–11. The effect of electrophoresis is to enhance migration into the agar of the test specimens, which form precipitin lines with the intrinsic antibody in a configuration that resembles a rocket. Indeed, the technique has often been referred to as the "rocket technique" because of the conical shape of the precipitin lines exhibiting an apex at the far point of migration from the application well. The height of the "rocket" or length of the precipitin arc from the application well to the apex has been shown to be directly proportional to the amount of applied antigen. Antigen standards are applied along with the unknown test material in the assay.

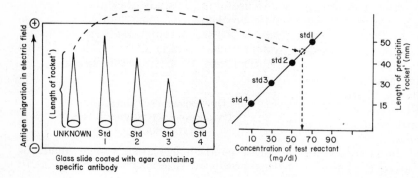

Figure 35–11. Diagram of immunoquantitation by method of single one-dimensional electroimmunodiffusion (Laurell technique of "rocket" electrophoresis).

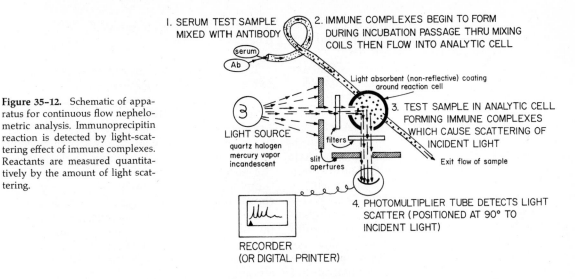

1. SERUM TEST SAMPLE MIXED WITH ANTIBODY

serum
Ab

2. IMMUNE COMPLEXES BEGIN TO FORM DURING INCUBATION PASSAGE THRU MIXING COILS THEN FLOW INTO ANALYTIC CELL

Light absorbent (non-reflective) coating around reaction cell

LIGHT SOURCE
quartz halogen
mercury vapor
incandescent

filters

slit apertures

3. TEST SAMPLE IN ANALYTIC CELL FORMING IMMUNE COMPLEXES WHICH CAUSE SCATTERING OF INCIDENT LIGHT

Exit flow of sample

4. PHOTOMULTIPLIER TUBE DETECTS LIGHT SCATTER (POSITIONED AT 90° TO INCIDENT LIGHT)

RECORDER
(OR DIGITAL PRINTER)

Figure 35–12. Schematic of apparatus for continuous flow nephelometric analysis. Immunoprecipitin reaction is detected by light-scattering effect of immune complexes. Reactants are measured quantitatively by the amount of light scattering.

The heights of the precipitin "rockets" of each standard are plotted graphically to establish a standard curve. The concentration of the unknown is then determined by locating the height of the precipitin "rocket" of the unknown on the standard plot. This method closely parallels that of radial immunodiffusion (RID). It offers the advantage of more rapid completion of the assay owing to the enhanced migration achieved by use of electrophoresis. Commonly, this procedure can be completed in a few hours, whereas the radial immunodiffusion (RID) techniques require from 18 to 48 hours to complete precipitin ring formation. One important limitation of the "rocket" technique is that the relative net charge of macromolecules at the pH used in the test must be accurately estimated. This charge on the molecules will determine the direction of migration to either anode or cathode. Those antigens with positive net charges will migrate to the cathode, while those with negative charge will exhibit anodal migration. This point is of importance to determine actual positioning of the positive and negative electrodes in the electrophoretic assembly. The use of chemical cross-linking of antigens to carriers such as albumin by formaldehyde or glutaraldehyde can be employed to alter the electrophoretic migration of many antigens (Axelsen, 1975).

During the past decade, a number of investigators have developed techniques for *immunoprecipitin analysis by the use of light scattering* devices. The occurrence of immune complex formation has been related to the amount of such light scattering and used as a basis for antigen quantitation. This approach has been accompanied by the development of sophisticated instruments specifically designed to rapidly measure light scattering, a technique known as nephelometry. The technique of nephelometry, as contrasted to turbidimetric absorbance or emission spectroscopy, is based on scatter reflectance of the transmitted light, which is detected by a photomultiplier tube and not on absorbance of transmitted light as in turbidimetric assays. This approach has proved useful because of its sensitivity and specificity for rapidly detecting immune complex formation. The technique is diagrammed in Figure 35-12. It can be observed in the diagram that filtered light of a certain wavelength enters the analytical cell containing a suspension of reactant material and on striking the immune complexes scatters randomly. The photomultiplier tube located at an angle of 30 to 90 degrees from incident light collects the light scatter as it is reflected from the small particles of the immune complex formations in the test material. The sensitivity of the reflectance system has been further enhanced by using a fluorescent light source. Also, use of enhancing reagents such as polyethylene glycol (PEG) has improved the assay by increasing the speed and sensitivity of immune complex formation so that measurements can be made within seconds to minutes after antigen-antibody mixing, thus affording an extremely rapid approach to immunoquantitation. Within the last few years, improved instruments utilizing laser and other light sources along with microprocessors to determine rate reactions of precipitin formation have appeared. Such devices offer the promise of even more rapid and sensitive precipitin assays (Larson, 1970).

One limitation of this technique is that the antisera and test specimens must have low levels of intrinsic light scattering activity. The antiserum must have high affinity and monospecificity for the assay antigen. Antiserum exhibiting these properties is referred to as "nephelometric grade." Those nephelometric systems which employ "steady state" conditions require that optimum antigen-antibody ratios be established for use in the assays. This is necessary in order to determine those dilutions of antigen and antibody which are sufficient to produce a light scattering by developing immune complex formation but avoid rapid development of large particulates that cause an uneven distortion of the light-scattering response. Once the ratios have been determined, the antiserum is mixed to the diluted test specimen either individually, in a continuous flow system, or under conditions of constant mixing as in a rotary chemical analyzer. Once "steady state" conditions have developed, light-scattering measurements are made. The peak height of response from the photomultiplier tube is recorded by a recorder on a graphic plot or on a digital print-out. Standards that contain known concentrations of the antigen are recorded in order to plot a standard curve using the height of the response that is proportional to the concentration. By plotting the peak response of the test unknown, the concentration can then be determined by direct inspection of the plot of the standards. Alternative methods for determining the unknown concentration are based on use of a microprocessor or programmable calculator. These devices are now commonly employed with the analytical instruments and simplify the reduction of data in an analytical program to determine the amount of the unknown in a given specimen (Larson, 1970).

AGGLUTINATION TESTS

Agglutination is a classic serologic reaction that involves clumping of a cell suspension by specific antibody. This phenomenon may be observed when particulate antigens such as blood cells or bacteria are exposed to specific antibody under appropriate conditions. Reactions of soluble antigens can be adapted to agglutination tests by the coated or covalent linking of the antigen or specific antibody to a particulate carrier, e.g., red cells, latex particles.

The agglutination reaction takes place in two stages: the antibody first unites with antigen, and then the agglutination occurs. When a given antibody to red cells causes agglutination, the antibody is called "complete." If the antibody unites with specific antigen on the red cells without agglutination, the antibody is called "incomplete." An "incomplete" antibody can be demonstrated by the antiglobulin test. Certain incomplete antibodies do not cause agglutination of red cells in saline, but only when the reaction mixture has a 20 to 30 per cent albumin concentration or the red cells are treated with certain proteolytic enzymes.

The agglutination test is semi-quantitative and the agglutination of either insoluble native antigens or antigen-coated particles can be assessed visually with or without a microscope. Advantages of the agglutination reactions are the high degree of sensitivity and the wide variety of antigens that may be detected with the use of antigen or antibody-coated particles. The simplicity of the reaction is deceiving, since correct interpretation of the reaction requires a strict quality control program with use of well-characterized reagents and knowledge of causes of false positive and false negative results. Major requirements in the agglutination tests are the availability of stable cell or particle suspension, the presence of one or more antigens close to the surface, and the knowledge that the incomplete or non-agglutinating antibodies are not detectable without modification. The IgM antibody is about 750 times

Table 35–2. AGGLUTINATION TESTS

Direct Agglutination Tests
  Simple
  High viscosity
  Enzyme treated cells
Indirect (Passive) Agglutination
  Antigen coated or covalently linked to particles
    Red cells
    Inert particles such as latex, bentonite
  Antibody-coated or covalently linked to particles
    (reverse passive)
Antiglobulin Tests
  Direct Coombs' (red cells)
  Indirect Coombs' (red cells)
  General antiglobulin tests
  Rose Waaler
  Rheumatoid factor

more efficient than IgG in agglutinations and the presence of IgM antibody will definitely influence the test results.

Agglutination reactions may generally be classified as either *direct, indirect* (*passive*), or *antiglobulin,* as shown in the Table 35-2 (Kwapinski, 1972; Singer, 1973-74).

DIRECT AGGLUTINATION ASSAY

The simple direct agglutination assay is a classic reaction which involves clumping of a cell or insoluble particulate suspension, as bacteria, fungi, and other microbial organisms, by specific antibody. The aggregation is brought about by antibody molecules with two or more combining receptors linking the cells or particles. A reaction is possible with antigens at or close to the cell surface. Special modifications are required to demonstrate incomplete antibodies that may fail to produce agglutination. For example, with Rh blood group antibodies and human bacilli antibodies, the agglutinins are IgM, while the incomplete antibodies are smaller IgG and IgA molecular species. Tests for detection of specific antibody are performed by determination of the dilution of serum that will agglutinate a constant amount of antigen. Because of the inherent variability of the test, a titer of a given serum is not considered significantly different from that of another serum sample value unless there is a four-fold difference.

In many cases, incomplete antibodies may fail to produce agglutination of red cells in saline or dilutions of serum and saline, whereas if this medium is replaced by one with a *higher viscosity,* such as 5 to 30 per cent bovine serum albumin, dextran, or polyvinyl pyrolidine, agglutination may be visible and a more sensitive assay established.

Treatment of human red cells with certain *enzymes* renders them directly agglutinable by some incomplete antibodies such as Rh_0. Many enzymes, such as trypsin, papain, ficin, and bromelin, have been investigated and found to be effective. This procedure has become standard in blood grouping laboratories for detection of many of the incomplete antibodies and is discussed on p. 1449.

PASSIVE OR INDIRECT AGGLUTINATION

This technique has wide and versatile application in the clinical laboratory and involves

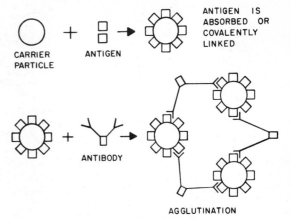

Figure 35-13. Passive agglutination.

the agglutination of cells or inert particles coated with soluble antigen or antibody. The cells or inert particles are passive carriers and the antigens may be physically absorbed or covalently coupled to the surface (Fig. 35-13). In the development of passive agglutination tests, cells or particles are needed to which antigens of different chemical nature may be firmly adsorbed or chemically linked. The cell or particle should also form stable and agglutinable suspensions.

Human red cells are often used as agglutinable carriers, but cells of other species may also be used. When erythrocytes are used as the inert particles, the serum samples must first be absorbed with uncoated cells to remove heterophile and other non-specific antibodies that may cause non-specific agglutination. The cells are usually readily available and can often be fixed with formalin, glutaraldehyde, or pyruvic aldehyde and stored for prolonged periods.

Many antigens will spontaneously adsorb to red blood cells and form good reagents for antibody detection. Examples are bacterial lipopolysaccharides, purified protein derivative (PPD), penicillin, and many microbial antigens. Since many proteins adsorb poorly to cells, mild treatment of erythrocytes with *tannic acid* or similar reagent may increase the amount of cell-bound antigen or antibody. This test has wide diagnostic application.

Protein antigen may be *chemically coupled* by covalent bonds to the red cell membrane. One common procedure involves cross-linking with bidiazotized benzidine (BDB). The BDB method has had similar applications to the tanned red cell technique. Other coupling

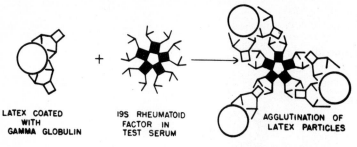

Figure 35-14. Latex agglutination test for rheumatoid factor. (Reproduced with permission from Nakamura, R. M.: Immunopathology: Clinical Laboratory Concepts and Methods. Boston, Little, Brown & Co., 1974.)

LATEX COATED WITH GAMMA GLOBULIN

19S RHEUMATOID FACTOR IN TEST SERUM

AGGLUTINATION OF LATEX PARTICLES

agents, such as chromic chloride, glutaraldehyde, cyanuric chloride, and a water-soluble carbodiimide have also found use.

Inert particles such as bentonite, latex, colloidion, and charcoal have been used to adsorb many classes of antigens, including proteins, carbohydrates, and DNA. Latex is a suspension of spherical polystyrene polymer particles. Proteins or polysaccharides adsorb to the surface and will encourage particles to be clumped by specific antibody. Latex particles with carboxyl group can be covalently linked to various protein antigens. Examples are latex fixation for detection of rheumatoid factor (Fig. 35-14), and agglutination of DNA-coated red cells for detection of anti-DNA antibody (Singer, 1973-74).

ANTIGLOBULIN TESTS (COOMBS' TEST)

This ingenious test was first described in 1908 by Moreschi and was rediscovered by

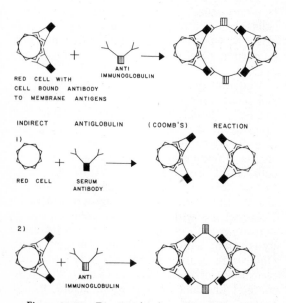

RED CELL WITH CELL BOUND ANTIBODY TO MEMBRANE ANTIGENS

ANTI IMMUNOGLOBULIN

INDIRECT   ANTIGLOBULIN   (COOMB'S)   REACTION

1)

RED CELL   SERUM ANTIBODY

2)

ANTI IMMUNOGLOBULIN

Figure 35-15. Direct and indirect Coombs' reaction.

Coombs and co-workers in 1945 to demonstrate incomplete antibodies to red cell antigens. "Incomplete" antibodies such as anti-Rh IgG, fail to produce agglutination of a saline suspension of homologous red cells, but nevertheless combine firmly with antigens on the erythrocyte. After washing away other serum proteins, the anti-Rh IgG remains on the cell surface. The erythrocytes may then be agglutinated by the addition of rabbit anti-human IgG (Fig. 35-15). The antiglobulin test is a simple serologic method of showing globulins firmly attached to the cell. The *indirect test* assays serum for antibody by allowing it to react with reference cells. The *direct test* assays for antibody already on the patient's erythrocytes. These determinations are discussed on p. 1450.

The reaction between the antiglobulin serum and red cells sensitized with Rh(D) incomplete antibody may be *inhibited* by gamma globulin in solution. The specific nature of this inhibition has been utilized in determining the species specificities of gamma globulin in unknown samples of serum, blood stains, etc. This technique is much more sensitive than the direct precipitin method.

The *Rose-Waaler test* is an antiglobulin test using sheep red cells sensitized with a sub-agglutinating dose of rabbit anti-sheep erythrocyte IgG. Rheumatoid factor, 19S IgM, will combine with the fixed 7S IgG and produce agglutination.

FLUORESCENT ANTIBODY TECHNIQUES

Fluorescent-labeled antibody was first used by Coons and associates in 1941 for studying localization of antigens in tissues. The fluorescent dye was used as a chemically linked marker on the specific antibody and did not alter its immunologic reactivity. The two fluorochromes most widely used today are fluorescein and rhodamine or their stable derivative. Fluorescein has a yellowish green fluorescence with a maximum at about 520 nm and rhodamine has a reddish orange fluorescence with a maximum at about 620 nm. These compounds have been the fluorochromes of choice because of intensity or efficiency of fluorescence.

The green fluorescence of fluorescein offers two important advantages over the red fluorescence of rhodamine: (a) The human eye is more sensitive to the apple-green color than to the reddish orange color, and (b) red autofluorescence is more common in nature than green autofluorescence. The most popular conjugate used in the clinical laboratory is the fluorescein isothiocyanate conjugated antiserum. The isothiocyanate derivative is stable and is coupled to the free amino groups of the protein to form a carbamido linkage. Tetramethylrhodamine isothiocyanate can be conjugated in a similar manner as fluorescein isothiocyanate for the reddish orange fluorescent reagent (Nakamura, 1974).

IMMUNOHISTOCHEMICAL METHODS FOR USE OF FLUORESCENT ANTIBODY

In the use of fluorescent-labeled antibody, there are various methods that can be used to detect the presence both of unknown antigens and tissues or smears and of unknown antibodies in the patient's serum. The common

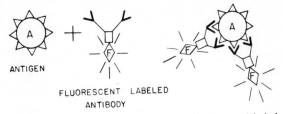
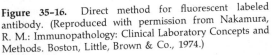

Figure 35–16.   Direct method for fluorescent labeled antibody. (Reproduced with permission from Nakamura, R. M.: Immunopathology: Clinical Laboratory Concepts and Methods. Boston, Little, Brown & Co., 1974.)

methods are the direct, indirect, inhibition, and complement staining methods (Kawamura, 1977).

In the *direct method*, the antibody is labeled with fluorescent compound and is used to detect the presence of antigen in tissue fixed to a slide. The fluorescent-labeled antibodies are added to the antigen in its optimal dilution and allowed to react for at least 30 minutes at room temperature or at 37° C. (Fig. 35-16). The preparation is next washed to remove the labeled gamma globulins, which do not react with the antigen. The smear tissue sections are blotted and the preparation mounted with buffered glycerol for examination with the fluorescent microscope.

The *indirect method* is utilized for detection of either unknown antigen in tissue sections or unknown antibody in the patient's serum (Fig. 35-17). The specific antigen-antibody—both unlabeled—reaction may be visualized by addition of labeled antibody directed against the antibody in the primary reaction. The an-

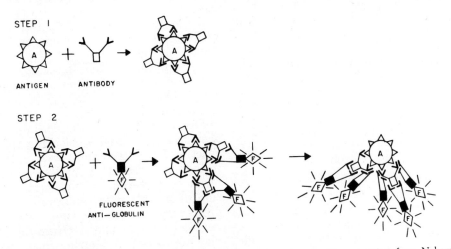

Figure 35–17.   Indirect method for fluorescent labeled antibody. (Reproduced with permission from Nakamura, R. M.: Immunopathology: Clinical Laboratory Concepts and Methods. Boston, Little, Brown & Co., 1974.)

tigen plus antibody globulin plus labeled anti-antibody complex results in fluorescence of the coated antigen. The indirect method has the advantage of utilizing a single-labeled anti-antibody globulin to detect many different specific antigen-antibody reactions occurring within a given species. For example, fluoresceinated rabbit or goat anti-human globulin may be used to detect a wide variety of human antibody-antigen reactions. In the detection of the unknown antigen or antibody the tissue sections or smear is reacted with unlabeled antiserum and allowed to react for 30 to 60 minutes at room temperature or at 37°C. The preparation is thoroughly washed to remove unlabeled antibody unattached to the antigen. Labeled anti-antibody globulin is then incubated with the preparation as in the direct technique.

The *inhibition method* is often employed as a control for testing the specificity of the antibodies in the direct fluorescent procedure. It has also been applied for detection of certain microorganisms such as *Toxoplasma gondii*. Antigen becomes saturated when treated with unlabeled specific antibody. Therefore, upon subsequent exposure to specific labeled antibody, no antigen fluorescence can be detected. Optimal concentrations of both labeled and unlabeled antibodies must be determined.

The *complement staining method* is similar to the indirect technique except that the labeled antibody is directed against complement components, often of guinea pig origin. The method is useful to detect either unknown antigen or antibody in patient's serum. For example, tissue is treated with serum which may contain the antibody in question. This antibody must be able to fix complement. A source of complement is added and finally the antigen-antibody complex is reacted with labeled anticomplement. This results in fluorescence of the complement-binding complexes.

APPLICATIONS OF FLUORESCENT ANTIBODY METHODS
(Cherry, 1974)

Fluorescent-labeled antibody methods are primarily used as a histochemical or cytochemical tool for detection and localization of antigen and antibody reactions. The procedure has been used for the detection of specific antibodies in patients' sera; localization of antigen, antibody, complement, and immune complexes on various cells and tissue sections; localization and fate of injected foreign antigens; localization and site of multiplication of infectious agents for use in the rapid diagnosis of microbial infections; and localization of various hormones and enzymes in cells and tissue sections.

More recently, fluorescent-labeled antibody methods are being used to quantitate antigen and antibodies similar to radioimmunoassay methods with comparable levels of sensitivity. The procedures require extensive purification and characterizations of the fluorescent reagents, as well as special instrumentation to decrease non-specific background while increasing specificity and sensitivity.

The immunofluorescent methods may in many instances be replaced by enzyme-labeled antibody methods. The fluorescent antibody methods have been used for a longer period of time and have the advantages of greater availability of well-characterized, standardized reagents and procedures.

QUALITY CONTROL

Controls in the staining with labeled antibodies, as in any standard laboratory procedure, are a necessary part of the procedure. Control procedures include:

1. Absorption of the antibody from the labeled antiserum by the specific antigen before staining the preparation.

2. Comparison of the fluorescence of the experimentally positive slide with similar tissue material known to be non-reacting, e.g., a tissue exhibiting a different pathologic process.

3. The use of unrelated fluorescent antisera or fluorescent normal globulin on the experimental tissue.

4. Inhibition or the "blocking" of fluorescence by prior application of unlabeled antibody. This method may yield only partial inhibition.

The specificity of the staining reaction should be monitored by blocking the staining reaction by pretreatment with unlabeled homologous antiserum. Complete inhibition can often be achieved by appropriate manipulation of pretreatment and staining times. A pretreatment: staining time ratio of 8:1 is generally recommended. Often the inhibition may not be complete owing to the continuous exchange of conjugate with unlabeled antibody. The specificity may also be checked by

Table 35-3. FACTORS IN
NON-SPECIFIC IMMUNOFLUORESCENT
STAINING REACTIONS

1. Quality of conjugate dye
2. Fraction of antiserum conjugated, i.e., IgG or
   gamma globulin fraction
3. Titer of specific antibody
4. Specificity of antiserum conjugation procedure
5. Presence of free dye
6. Dye:protein ratio
7. Procedures to remove high dye:protein conjugates
   a. DEAE cellulose chromatography
   b. Tissue powder absorption
8. Counterstains
9. Tissue preparation

blocking the reaction by absorbing the labeled antibody with specific antigen. The antigen should be coupled to a solid phase carrier to avoid formation of soluble immune complexes. Lastly, the labeled antibody may be displaced with unlabeled antibody.

Several causes of non-specific staining are listed in Table 35-3. A common cause is a high dye:protein ratio of the conjugate which is more negatively charged and produces artificial staining reactions. The more highly negatively charged conjugates may be selectively removed by DEAE-cellulose chromatography or by precipitation and after dialysis with buffers in a pH range of 6.0 to 6.2. The non-specific staining may be reduced by means of the classic procedure of absorption of conjugates with tissue homogenates.

Several procedures are required to control fluorescein-labeled conjugates. They may be checked by dialysis for absence of unbound fluorescein and may be separated from unbound fluorescein by gel filtration. Protein concentrations may be determined by the biuret reaction with readings at 560 nm instead of the usual 540 nm to avoid interference from fluorescein absorbency. An alternative method for determination of the protein concentration is measuring absorbance at 280 nm and 495 nm and using the following formula:

Protein (mg/ml)
$$= \frac{\text{O.D. } 280 \text{ nm} - 0.35 \text{ (O.D. } 495 \text{ nm)}}{1.4}$$

Cellulose acetate or gel electrophoresis may be used to evaluate for the presence of unbound fluorescent material and of protein added to previously conjugated protein. After electrophoresis the strip is examined under a Woods' light (366 nm) for fluorescence of separated proteins. The location and brightness of each band should be noted and sketched. The strip is then stained with an appropriate protein stain such as Ponceau S and scanned by a densitometer. The Ponceau S-stained strip is compared with the sketch of fluorescence made

before protein staining. A fluorescent band beyond the albumin position indicates the presence of unreacted fluorescein. A strong fluorescence in the gamma globulin region with no fluorescence in the beta area denotes a high concentration of labeled gamma globulin and indicates that the gamma globulin fraction alone was labeled with fluorescein. The absence of fluorescein in bands stained by Ponceau S as alpha one, alpha two, or albumin indicates that protein has been added to FITC-(fluorescent conjugate) labeled protein.

Immunoelectrophoresis is performed in which the fluoresceinated antisera are reacted against normal whole human sera. A heavy line of precipitation in the IgG region should be obtained. Additional lines with antibodies to serum proteins other than immunoglobulins are often seen in commercial antisera. The extraneous antibodies may not necessarily interfere with the specificity of the immunofluorescent test; however, they contribute to increased non-specific staining. Also, the presence of contaminant antibodies casts doubt on the purity of the antigen used for immunization. Spurs from the IgG line produced by cross-reaction of the anti-IgG conjugate with IgM or IgA in the electrophoresed normal human serum may be expected in the presence of antibodies to the light chain of IgG. The light-chain antibodies may be specifically removed by absorption with purified human IgM or IgA preparations. Cross-reactions of antibodies to the light chain in antisera to IgG with light-chain antibodies of IgM and IgA do not usually occur in immunofluorescent staining, provided that the immunization is carried out with purified IgG and the conjugate is diluted to $\frac{1}{4}$ unit/ml. Thus at $\frac{1}{4}$ unit/ml of anti-IgG, no visible immunofluorescent staining occurs with IgA or IgM immunoglobulins in indirect immunofluorescent staining reactions. If a concentration of 1 unit/ml of labeled anti-IgG is used and there are anti-light chain antibodies present, then the IgG antiserum will detect the presence of IgA and IgM immunoglobulins.

The gel diffusion precipitin test is performed with reference antiserum to IgG; and the test conjugate against normal human serum should give precipitin lines of complete identity. Cross-reactions of anti-human IgG conjugate with human IgM and IgA may be detected by the precipitin tests.

Determination of immunologic sensitivity of the conjugate is accomplished by measuring the level of specific precipitating antibodies which can be expressed in units/ml. The units of conjugate are based on the titer of antiglobulin determined in the standard gel diffusion precipitin test using 1 mg IgG/ml antigen and twofold dilutions of the conjugate. The conjugate is more specific for purified IgG than for normal human serum. However, the units of antibody may be determined with normal human serum diluted to contain 1 mg/ml IgG (normal serum diluted 1:12). An agar gel template, recommended for determining the units of antibodies, is a horizontally placed line of wells 2.8 mm in diameter, placed 7.5 mm apart in a gel with a depth of 1.5 mm. Titration is performed by serial two-fold dilutions of the conjugates, which are placed opposite the wells containing the antigen test in a concentration of 1 mg/ml. Pipets are changed with each dilution and plates are incubated at room temperature for 24 hours and read for the highest dilution which gives a visible line of precipitation. This titer is the unitage. A linear pattern agar gel template for gel diffusion should be used instead of one with a circular pattern. Acceptable conjugates should have at least 4 units/1% protein when the unitage assay is employed. This is approximately equivalent to 1 mg precipitating antibody/10 mg protein. Conjugates with lower antibody levels are not recommended for use.

Expressing a fluorescein:protein (F:P) ratio as the ratio of absorbance at 495 nm to that at 280 nm can be recommended only for screening purposes, since the absolute levels of FITC, as well as the F:P ratio, influence non-specific staining. Also, aromatic compounds having a high absorbance at 280 nm are sometimes added to commercial conjugates as preservatives. F:P ratios may be expressed as micrograms of bound FITC per milligram of protein.

To obtain F:P molar ratios, the weight ratios are multiplied by a factor of 0.411. The conversion formula is derived as follows:

$$\frac{160,000}{389 \times 10^3} = 0.411$$

The average molecular weight of immunoglobulin is 160,000 and 389 is the molecular weight of FITC; 10^3 converts milligrams to micrograms. The F:P ratio must be determined before the conjugate is diluted with a protein carrier such as albumin. In an indirect antinuclear antibody test utilizing mouse liver, a molar F:P ratio of approximately 3:1 was found to be optimal for conjugates with 4 units antibody/ml. However, a different molar F:P ratio may be optimal for other systems.

DETERMINATION OF WORKING DILUTION OF CONJUGATES

Fluoresceinated immunoglobulin can be evaluated in the indirect antinuclear antibody tests with substrate. Chessboard titrations should be carried out with different unit dilutions of fluoresceinated antisera against different high and lower titered sera known to contain antinuclear antibodies. With good fluoresceinated antisera, a plateau end point of $\frac{1}{6}$ or $\frac{1}{64}$ units may be seen when reacted against high-titered sera. A working dilution of the fluorescein conjugate should be $\frac{1}{4}$ to $\frac{1}{8}$ unit/ml. In the antinuclear antibody test, a working dilution of $\frac{1}{4}$ unit/ml is recommended, provided the F:P ratio is approximately 3 to 5. This provides for a satisfactory background and will insure detection of the low-titered sera containing antinuclear antibodies. Also, reproducible titers can be obtained on the same serum containing antinuclear antibodies when tested with a different source of conjugated antisera.

Usually the working dilutions of the anti-IgA and anti-IgM conjugate used should be at least 1 unit/ml. Polyvalent anti-immunoglobulin conjugate should be used at the dilution of 1 unit/ml. In fluorescent kidney biopsy studies, anti-IgM and anti-IgA are recommended for use at a concentration of 1 unit/ml.

When conjugated anti-β_{1C} is used, a working dilution of $\frac{1}{2}$ unit/ml is satisfactory for kidney biopsies. A chessboard titration may be performed in a test system and if a plateau end point of $\frac{1}{16}$ unit/ml is seen, then a working dilution of $\frac{1}{4}$ unit may be used. Criteria for evaluation of anti-β_{1C} conjugates are the same as above. The conjugates should also have 4 units antibody/1% protein/ml.

Conjugates should be stored sterile after membrane filtration, and precautions should be taken to avoid aggregation. Protein concentration for storage should be 2 mg/ml or greater (other proteins such as albumin may be helpful). The conjugates should be divided into small aliquots and thawed only once before use. They should be ultracentrifuged (150,000 g for 30 minutes) before storage and subjected to high-speed centrifugation before use.

TISSUE PROCESSING

In tissue immunofluorescence work, it is essential that the tissue be processed so as to preserve antigenic reactivity and general structural morphology. Many antigens are rendered inactive after treatment with the usual fixatives employed for non-immunologic studies.

Substrate and biopsy tissue specimens should be "snap" frozen in liquid nitrogen, liquid nitrogen-isopentane, or dry ice-acetone mixture. The tissue is kept frozen in a non-frost-free freezer, preferably at −70°C, in a sealed container to prevent drying by evaporation. The material can be shipped in dry ice to a reference laboratory if necessary.

Fresh substrate tissue to be frozen is cut into small cubes approximately 3 mm in dimension. The blocks are placed on aluminum foil and covered with optimal cutting temperature compound (OCT, Ames Co., Elkhart, Indiana) and snap frozen by immersion in liquid nitrogen or dry ice and acetone. Then they are wrapped in aluminum foil and placed in a precooled screw cap bottle for storage in a −70°C. freezer. Composite blocks containing several tissues are prepared by placing small folds and pieces of tissue close together on one plate. The frozen section wrapped in aluminum foil is best stored in a tightly sealed bottle with a screw cap at

−70°C. The chuck and tissue sections can be carried from the freezer to the cryostat in pressed polystyrene boxes containing solid carbon dioxide. The tissue should not be allowed to thaw before sectioning, since the slightest degree of thawing would allow sections to become unrecognizable. Alternatively, the tissue may be placed in a test tube or small bottle containing isopentane and frozen by immersion into liquid nitrogen or dry ice and acetone. A few minutes should be sufficient for freezing. The tissue should not be left in the solvent for a long period of time, as it dries out and becomes very difficult to section. After the tissue is completely frozen it is removed from the test tube with forceps and placed in another test tube, sealed, and stored in a freezer, preferably at −70°C. Tissue may be stored in a regular freezer at −20°C. or below but should not be stored in an automatic frost-free freezer.

Preparation of needle biopsy tissue

Small needle biopsies of kidney, thyroid, or other excisional biopsies of the skin can be collected directly from the operation and carried to the laboratory and mounted upon a section of tongue blade or small sponge (Onkosponge No. 1, Histo-Med, Inc., Paterson, N.J.) with the optimal cutting temperature compound (OCT) and quickly frozen by immersion in liquid nitrogen. The OCT has not been found to interfere with the immunochemical studies.

The sections are cut from 4 to 6 μ on a standard cryostat. The optimum temperature for cutting most tissues depends on the amount of fatty tissue and may vary from −22°C. to lower than −30°C. for tissue with a large amount of lipids. Cleaned microscopic slides should be used. The sections are placed on the slide after drying and may be stored in a −70°C. cabinet.

In order to prevent the loss of water-soluble antigens or antibodies, the tissue or other material on the microscope slide is placed in a mild fixative. One may employ an equal mixture of absolute ethyl alcohol and ethyl ether at room temperature for 10 minutes, followed by 95 per cent ethyl alcohol at room temperature for 10 minutes. However, other agents such as acetone and methyl alcohol have been used. In certain studies, fixatives are not used, as they may destroy the immunologic reactivity of the antigen.

EQUIPMENT FOR FLUORESCENT
MICROSCOPY

The fluorescence microscope can be designed in many ways, and in choosing the type

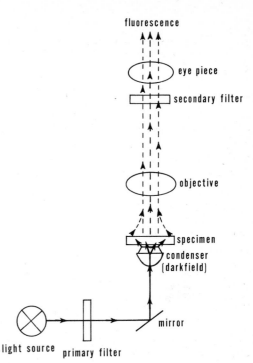

Figure 35–18. Transmitted Darkfield immunofluorescence.

of equipment desired the various factors described below should be considered. Two principles are used in the construction of fluorescence microscopes: transmitted illumination and incident or epi-illumination.

For *transmitted illumination* (Fig. 35–18) two condenser systems are available: the brightfield condenser used in ordinary light microscopy and the darkfield condenser. The brightfield condenser will produce a satisfactory excitation, i.e., a good signal, but the problem of filtering away light of unwanted wavelengths, i.e., optical noise, has not been satisfactorily solved, and brightfield condensers are not recommended for routine fluorescent work. *Darkfield condensers* (oil immersion) are to be preferred. They will give an optimal signal by concentrating the excitation light in a narrow area, but at the same time most of the excitation light will be directed away from the objective front lens, so that the optical noise is significantly decreased.

For *incident or epi-illumination* (Fig. 35–19) no condenser problems exist, in that the microscope objective itself functions as a condenser. The excitation light is admitted to the microscope tube at a right angle, reflected to the fluorescent specimen by means of a di-

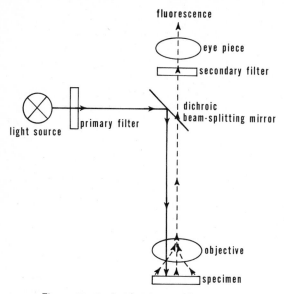

Figure 35–19. Incident immunofluorescence.

chroic mirror (i.e., an interference filter), and the fluorescence observed through the dichroic mirror.

The two most effective systems for fluorescence microscopy are transmitted light illumination with a darkfield condenser system and the brightfield incident or epi-illumination.

A conventional microscope can be usually converted to a fluorescence microscope by adding a darkfield condenser and suitable filter systems with a low voltage tungsten or halogen light source. The level of fluorescence produced is suitable for most procedures in the clinical laboratory.

The Ploem type vertical illuminator can be attached to a research type microscope stand. The illuminator is equipped with an interference dividing plate (dichroic mirror) which is mounted above the objective at an angle of 45 degrees to the illuminating beam. The dichroic mirror is matched for excitation and transmission to the fluorochrome. The objective acts as the condenser. A major advantage of epi-illumination is that a narrow band excitation beam may be employed with interchangeable filter systems to detect the two different fluorochromes. Another advantage of epi-illumination is that it can be combined with transmitted illumination, such as phase contrast or polarized light microscopy.

The *light source* must give ample energy in the wavelength range corresponding to the absorption maximum of the fluorochrome used.

High-pressure arc lamps (mercury, xenon, cesium) are traditional light sources for fluorescence microscopy. Their wavelength spectrum extends from the ultraviolet through the visible to the infrared part, consisting of a light continuum and a line spectrum. Subsequent primary filtration is necessary. The ultraviolet component may give rise to fluorescence of tissue proteins and nucleoproteins, the so-called *autofluorescence*, unless suitable filtration is provided.

Halogen lamps (e.g., iodine-quartz lamps) can be operated at very high temperatures, thanks to the quartz bulb and the halogen filling of the bulb. They are cheap, easy to run, and will provide enough excitation energy for most purposes when used in connection with a suitable primary filter system.

Lasers such as the argon ion laser, helium-cadmium laser, and pulsed organic dye laser are ideal light sources that can provide a very high energy excitation of the two fluorochromes most commonly used: FITC and TRITC. Laser excitation studies have given extremely promising results, but so far laser excitation has been used only in highly specialized laboratories. The availability of relatively cheap, reliable lasers will lead to more widespread use in the future. No filtration of the laser light is needed because of the monochromatic nature of the laser light.

There are generally two types of *primary filters*: (1) the absorption filter, which absorbs light of a certain wavelength and allows light of another wavelength to pass, and (2) the interference filter, which selects the desired band of light by reflection and dispersion of the undesired light. The advantage of the interference filter is that the light passed has a higher intensity than the light passed by the absorption filters.

The primary absorption filters traditionally used were glass or gelatin filters. Their transmission curves must be characterized as far from ideal in most cases, but still such filters have given excellent results when used in combination with high-energy light sources, e.g., high-pressure mercury arc lamps or xenon lamps.

When fluorescein is used as the fluorescent label the common absorption filters used are the Schott BG-12 (2 to 4 mm thick) or No. 5040 Corning filter. The transmission maximum for these filters is frequently in the 366 nm region near ultraviolet. Another set of primary absorption filters looks dark blue and is used for a blue light excitation. Their transmission includes the blue portion of the visible spectrum from 420 to 450 nm. Blue light excitation filters are used in conjunction with secondary filters of a yellow-orange color.

A UG-1 filter with a mercury arc vapor lamp will pass light from 300 to 400 nm and utilizes a moderate absorption band of FITC found between 300 and 400 nm. With use of a UG-1 filter, there is good contrast although the intensity is reduced. The UG-1 filter is useful for immunofluorescence work with liver biopsies for hepatitis B antigen localization. The liver tissue has many autofluorescent tissue substances.

Special fluorescein isothiocyanate (FITC) primary interference filters are now available and recommended for most of the fluorescent work using FITC.

In addition to the above primary exciter filters and heat absorbing filter, one can use a skyblue Schott BG-38 filter. The BG-38 suppresses the transmission in the far red spectrum given by many primary filters. The purpose of the BG-38 is to make the background in the field of view completely black.

A 480 nm yellow filter can be used to reduce tissue autofluorescence associated with excitation by primary BG-12 or FITC interference filters.

The purpose of the *secondary filter* is to transmit all the fluorescence wavelengths and stop all the excitation wavelengths. The secondary filters are inserted in the body of the tube or the eye pieces, or a variety of filters can be utilized in the rotating device in the body of the microscope. The secondary filters serve to remove remnants of exciting light so that only the fluorescent light reaches the observer's eyes. They are inserted between the objective and the observer's eyes, either above the nose piece or in the rotating disc in the stands. Various filters are complementary to the primary filters. For use with FITC labeled compounds, the secondary filter can be a Zeiss 53, which has a peak cut-off point near the maximal emission peak of FITC at 525 nm.

In general, high numerical aperture objectives are to be recommended to increase the *optical signal* at this level also. Fluorite objectives give very satisfactory results in fluorescence microscopy. Dry lenses are easier to handle than oil immersion lenses. For very high aperture objectives an objective diaphragm may be necessary to exclude optical noise.

ENZYME-LINKED IMMUNOASSAY (ELISA)

A number of approaches may be used to identify specific antibody. Immunofluorescence (p. 1199) and radioimmunoassay (p. 385) are two such techniques. Ferritin-labeled proteins have been quite useful in identifying such materials in tissue electron microscopy. However, this technique has limited applications for the clinical laboratory. Enzyme-linked immunoassays (Elisa) are rapidly supplementing and at times replacing RIA and immunofluorescence. The principle of Elisa is similar to that of immunofluorescences, i.e., a purified enzyme is linked in a stable manner to a specific antibody. The activity of the enzyme should be easily detectable either by a cytochemical method or by a change in absorbance at a specified wavelength. For cytochemical uses, the enzyme-substrate should not be readily diffusible. In fact, it is preferable if a precipitate results from the reaction. It is useful especially in tissue work if the optimal pH of the enzyme is at, or nearly, neutral. Of course, the enzyme should not affect tissue structure.

The active enzyme should be available in pure form. Otherwise, immunoglobulins could be labeled with "inactive" materials and could decrease the sensitivity and specificity of the reaction. Binding enzymes to antibodies often decreases the enzymic activity somewhat, but obviously it must not abolish it. The enzyme must be stable for storage purposes. A small enzyme is less likely to interfere with antigen-antibody reactions by steric hindrance and more likely to penetrate tissue. There should be no natural substrates in tissue or the clinical specimen to be examined. Horseradish peroxidase and alkaline phosphatase are two commonly used enzymes. The enzyme-conjugate method is probably less sensitive than radioimmunoassay or immunofluorescence. Sensitivity is lost by preparation of the conjugate and competition from unlabeled immunoglobulins. The so-called unlabeled-antibody-enzyme method, which usually utilizes soluble enzyme-anti-enzyme complexes, may be more specific and is more sensitive. Its sensitivity is gained by saturation of all of the tissue antigen sites with specific antibody and by allowing little excess enzyme or anti-enzyme in the mixture (Sternberger, 1974). These techniques have been used for toxicology, viral antibody studies, electron microscopy, and light microscopy for identification of antigens and immunoglobulins. Elisa methods can be automated and are stable and do not carry the potential hazards of radioisotopes. Tissue preparations do not fade as with fluorescent work, and light microscopy may be used. Elisa is also discussed on page 1242.

CELL SURFACE MARKERS IN TISSUE PREPARATIONS

Mononuclear cell surface markers may be identified in frozen sections of tissue. This is accomplished by indicator materials, such as sheep erythrocytes or zymosan, coated with IgG, IgM, and/or complement reacting with unfixed tissue. Thymic-derived lymphocytes are not easily defined in such tissue, since they form only a loose association with sheep erythrocytes and are readily washed away (Dukor, 1970). This technique is discussed on p. 1322.

QUALITY CONTROL AND STANDARDS

The same types of quality control programs described in Chapter 63 may be implemented in the immunopathology laboratory. For example, high and low stable control samples should be examined with each set of determinations. Some laboratories have used aliquots of normal sera, either quick frozen and stored at $-70°$C. or lyophilized for such a purpose. Assaying aliquots of the same sample on one day provides not only within-day variation, but also a mean and standard deviation with which all future results may be compared. Of course, new reagents must always be compared with existing ones and adjusted if necessary. Several states require unknown identification for continued certification or licensure. Unknowns may also be obtained from other laboratories—often on a reciprocal basis—or from national groups such as the College of American Pathologists. It is vital to establish good rapport with clinicians who utilize the laboratory results for diagnosis and management. A result which "doesn't fit" the clinical appraisal may be a clue to a problem in that procedure; for example, a negative ANA in someone with clinical SLE. If possible, it is helpful, and usually reassuring, to obtain the clinical histories of patients with "abnormal" determinations.

The *precision* of a test refers to its reproducibility or repeatability; it is the degree to which results from repeated assays from the same specimen agree with one another. The precision of the test is measured by the magnitude of the difference between quantitative results obtained with repeated assays on the same specimen without particular reference to the true value of the substance measured.

On the other hand, *accuracy* refers to the amount of the discrepancy between the quantitative test results and the true quantity of the substance measured. The accuracy of an immunologic procedure can only be estimated, since absolute values in immunopathology are seldom established.

There are immunochemical and clinical definitions of sensitivity. Immunochemically, *sensitivity* is measured by the lowest level at which the antigen-antibody reaction can be detected reliably. Clinically, the sensitivity is measured by the incidence of true positive test results found among all patients known to have a particular disease.

Specificity may also be defined immunochemically and clinically. Immunochemically, the specificity of the test is measured by its ability to react with all subsets of the prescribed antigenic determinants and with no other. Clinically, the specificity is measured by the incidence of true negative test results among patients known to be free from a particular disease. In the clinical definition of specificity, it is assumed that any false positive specimen does not contain the component being assayed.

Precision, accuracy, and specificity are discussed further on p. 17 (Rose, 1976).

Reference preparations are absolutely necessary to any quality control program. There are several types of standards available (Table 35-4). Currently available standards are listed below:

Immunoglobulin Quantitation. A WHO International Reference Preparation for human

Table 35-4. WORLD HEALTH ORGANIZATION (WHO) NOMENCLATURE OF STANDARDS*

1. *WHO International Standards*
   Biologic substances which official organizations have agreed to subject to national control of quality and to express the values in international units or equivalents.

2. *WHO International Reference Preparations*
   Biologic substances provided as a service but for which national control of quality has not been considered obligatory.

3. *WHO International Reference Reagents*
   Reagents for qualitative use in identification.

4. *National Standards*
   Preparations which have designated unitage calibrated in terms of WHO International Standards or International Reference Preparations.

5. *WHO Reference Laboratories Working Standards*
   Preparations often of the same material as the WHO International or National Standards with directly related unitage values.

6. *Other Standards*
   Preparations provided by the manufacturers and other organizations, including research laboratories.

*Modified from Batty, I.: Standards and quality control in clinical immunology. *In* Thompson, R.A. (ed.): Techniques in Clinical Immunology. Oxford, Blackwell Scientific Publications, 1977.

serum immunoglobulins IgG, IgA and IgM was established in 1970 (Batty, 1977). It is a freeze-dried, slightly diluted, pooled human serum. It is designated 67/86 and by definition there are 100 units of activity of IgG, IgM, and IgA per ampule. There are two other lots of the same source material processed in similar ways but freeze-dried at different times. These are designated 67/95 and 67/97 and are generally available to immunologists for the calibration of their internal standards. They are all suitable for use in single radial diffusion and are not suitable for the nephelometric procedures.

Each laboratory should make or have available a standard antigen pool of human sera which has been calibrated against the International Reference Preparation either directly or through one of the substandards 67/95 or 67/97.

An International Reference Preparation of human immunoglobulin IgE is available. The standard is suitable for a modified single radial immunodiffusion technique where the technique is rendered more sensitive by the use of either ^{131}I-labeled anti-sheep immunoglobulin serum or ^{125}I-labeled IgE. Recently, the reference preparation has been found to contain hepatitis B antigen and should be used only with the necessary precautions.

Rheumatoid Factor. Many reported surveys have shown a wide variation in interlaboratory reproducibility of both the Rose-Waaler and the latex agglutination tests.

Division of Biological Standards, National Institute for Medical Research, London, England, on behalf of the WHO Expert Committee on Biological Standardization, arranged a collaborative study of a possible reference preparation of a pool of serum from 197 patients with rheumatoid arthritis. The aim was to see whether a greater uniformity of results could be obtained if samples were assayed in comparison with a standard.

The participants used the Rose-Waaler method and the same batch of rabbit amboceptor was provided to each laboratory. The study demonstrated that a reference standard was useful in markedly reducing the within-laboratory variation to fourteen-fold.

Each standard ampule of the International Reference Preparation of Rheumatoid Arthritis Serum by definition contains 100 International Units of Rheumatoid Factor. A local pool of serum should be calibrated in terms of this reference preparation, the appropriate value assigned, and unknown sera calibrated on this basis.

It has been demonstrated that the latex test can be made more reproducible and precise if the laboratory standard is calibrated against the International Reference Preparation.

Antinuclear and Other Autoantibody Assays. A research standard for fluorochrome-labeled antihuman immunoglobulin 68/45 was established by the Immunology Committee of the British Research Council. More recently the International Union of Immunological Societies submitted a batch of lyophilized FITC-labeled antihuman immunoglobulin to WHO. The accepted International Standard immunoglobulin conjugate reacts strongly with IgG, IgM, and IgA immunoglobulins.

An International Research Standard for antinuclear factor is available to workers in autoimmune disease. The Research Standard A for antinuclear factor (homogeneous) 66/223 was made available by the Division of Biological Standards, National Institute for Medical Research, London, England. There are also National Reference preparations of anti-thyroid microsome serum and anti-thyroglobulin serum held by the same National Institute.

The International Union of Immunological Societies, in collaboration with WHO, the Communicable Disease Center, USPHS, and other organizations, is developing standards for various serum proteins, complement components, and other immunologic-related substances. Certain data should be available for all antisera used in diagnostic studies (Table 35-5).

SPECIAL APPLICATIONS OF IMMUNOASSAYS

EVALUATION OF COMPLEMENT ACTIVATION

There are a number of diseases and disorders in which activation of the complement

Table 35-5. INFORMATION DESIRED ON LABEL OF ANTISERA*

1. Name and address of the manufacturer.
2. Proper name of the product and its batch or lot number and date of manufacture.
3. Manufacturer's recommended expiration date.
4. Species of animals used in preparing the batch and whether the batch contains a single serum or pooled sera.
5. Source of antigen—individual donor or pool of donors (state minimum number in pool)—general method of preparation.
6. Immunization schedule—single or repeated injection; adjuvant or not; route.
7. Absorption procedures, with description of absorbant and description of evidence of specificity (immunoelectrophoretic or other) before and after absorption.
8. Immunoglobulin separation process or other chemical treatment, and preservative used.
9. Potency, with reference to a standard in a functional test (for instance, direct or reversed single diffusion test) of antibody content.

Other desirable information is specific evidence and manner of specificity evaluation, i.e., precipitin methods, passive hemagglutination, radioimmunoassay, etc. Besides the potency of the antibody, the affinity and avidity values would be helpful in the use of the antibody for sensitive radioimmunoassay procedures.

*Information from MRC Working Party: Immunology, *20*:3, 1971.

system is important. These include both immune and non-immune processes. The immune disorders which are complement-dependent involve antigen/antibody reactions where the antibody is of the IgG or IgM class. Complement activation in non-immunologic disorders may be found in disseminated intravascular coagulation, various forms of cardiovascular shock including both endotoxic and hemorrhagic shock, myocardial infarcts, acute hypocomplementemic glomerulonephritis, and a variety of other inflammatory and infectious diseases. There are also some situations in which acute tissue injury causes release of proteolytic enzymes from the damaged tissues. These enzymes can produce a local or systemic activation of certain complement components (Lachman, 1973; Tucker, 1974; Müller-Eberhard, 1975).

The determination of complement activation can aid in the etiologic diagnosis of the clinical disorder. By using specific antisera for complement components C3 and C4 and antisera for the properdin Factor B, also known as C3 Pro-Activator, activation can be detected by employing the technique of immunoelectrophoresis. Such studies are performed using either fresh serum or fresh serum that has been stored at −40°C. or preferably EDTA

plasma. The sample serum or plasma is applied directly to a multi-well electrophoretic plate of agar or agarose as in a study for routine immunoelectrophoresis. After completion of the electrophoresis, the specific antisera for C3, C4, and properdin Factor B are placed in individual troughs on the electrophoretic plate. Time is then allowed for immunodiffusion to occur with formation of precipitin lines. Test samples are always run with a normal control serum (Alper, 1975; Ruddy, 1975).

After precipitin lines have formed, the position of migration of the complement components and properdin Factor B can be visually determined and compared with the control. Figure 35-20 is a diagrammatic illustration of the changes in mobility of each of the components which occurs as a result of activation. Activation follows a proteolytic cleavage of the individual components. It can be observed that intact C3 migrates in the β1C position, while the split product C3c shows a precipitin line in the β1A position. The shift in mobility is clear evidence of cleavage activation of C3. Also, intact C4, which normally migrates in the β1E position, shifts to a faster migrating β1D position as a result of cleavage activation. Properdin Factor B, also known as C3 Pro-Activator, likewise exhibits a major change in

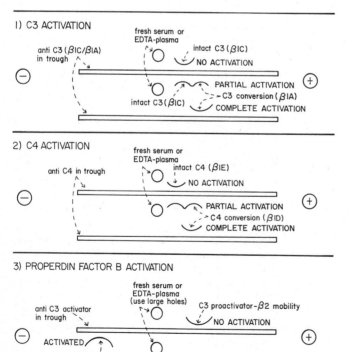

Figure 35-20. Patterns of change in electrophoretic mobility on activation of complement components C3, C4, and properdin factor B (C3 proactivator).

Table 35–6 INTERPRETATION OF IMMUNOELECTROPHORETIC PATTERNS OF COMPLEMENT ACTIVATION

CLINICAL DISORDER	MOBILITY PATTERN		
	C3	C4	Properdin B
Immunologic injury	$\beta 1C \rightarrow \beta 1A$	$\beta 1E \rightarrow \beta 1D$	No change
Alternative pathway mediated	$\beta 1C \rightarrow \beta 1A$	No change	$\beta 2 \rightarrow \gamma$
Proteolytic enzymes from traumatic or inflammatory injury	$\beta 1C \rightarrow \beta 1A$	No change	No change

mobility on cleavage activation, with conversion to C3 Activator. Factor B in the proactivator state normally migrates in a β_2 position and on activation shifts its mobility pattern to the gamma region. This shift can easily be detected by immunoelectrophoresis with specific antisera.

Studies of cleavage activation by immunoelectrophoresis provide a rapid means of determining different patterns of complement activation. Table 35–6 provides a summary for interpreting the different activation patterns. It can be seen that C3 cleavage indicates general complement activation and can be used as a screening test. The cleavage activation of C4 is found in those instances of immunologic activation of the complement system. A shift in mobility of C3 ProActivator, or Factor B, is indicative of activation of the alternative pathway (properdin pathway) of complement activation. In those conditions where only C3 activation is found without change in C4 or Factor B, one can surmise that endogenous release of proteolytic enzymes from injured tissue or other causes have brought about the change in C3 mobility.

Further discussion of the complement system and other tests to determine complement activity are discussed on pp. 1245–1261.

LABORATORY TESTS FOR DETECTION OF AUTOANTIBODIES

Many of the techniques discussed in this chapter have been applied to the measurement of autoantibodies in body fluids or on tissue. A summary of *organ-directed autoantibodies* is provided in Table 35–7.

Autoantibodies to nuclear antigens can now be classified according to their immunologic specificities. They include antibodies which react with DNA, deoxyribonucleoprotein, nuclear histones, and nuclear acidic protein antigens. It has been established that there are several antinuclear antibodies which react with nuclear acidic proteins, including antibodies to Sm antigen, nuclear ribonucleoprotein, and SS-A and SS-B antigens.

Recent developments have demonstrated that it is important not only to detect the presence and quantity of the ANA but also to identify the immunologic specificities of the ANA in a given patient. It has also been established that certain systemic rheumatic diseases such as systemic lupus erythematosus, Sjögren's syndrome, and scleroderma are characterized by antibodies of some specificities and not of others. Certain of these antibodies, such as antibody to Sm antigen and scleroderma-1 (Scl-1) antigen are specific "marker" antibodies for systemic lupus erythematosus and progressive systemic sclerosis, respectively. The identification of immunologic specificity of the ANA helps in the diagnosis, management, and treatment of rheumatic disease patients. Immunologic specificity of ANA with characteristic clinical and laboratory features is shown in Table 35–8.

Low levels of DS-DNA (double-strand DNA) antibodies are usually found in diseases such as rheumatoid arthritis, Sjögren's syndrome, progressive systemic sclerosis, dermatomyositis, discoid lupus erythematosus, and mixed connective tissue disease (MCTD) (Fernandez-Madrid, 1976).

Recently, an immunofluorescent method capable of detecting antibodies to DS-DNA with use of the kinetoplast of the hemoflagellate *Crithidia luciliae* method for detection of antibodies for DS-DNA was supported by studies with known specificity for DS-DNA and SS-DNA, respectively. The immunofluorescent method was positive in subjects with SLE and drug-induced antinuclear factors. The immunofluorescent technique is easy to perform and allows a check on immunoglobulin character of the DNA-binding activity and is not liable to interference from antibodies to SS-DNA. The disadvantages of the *Crithidia luciliae* method are that the test is less sensitive and not as quantitative as the standard radioimmunoassay methods.

It is currently believed that antibodies with specificity for insoluble *deoxyribonucleoprotein*

4

Table 35-7. ANTIBODIES IN ORGAN-SPECIFIC AUTOIMMUNE DISEASES*

DISEASES	ANTIGEN INVOLVED	METHODS FOR DETECTION OF ANTIBODY
Organ-Specific, Endocrine		
Autoimmune thyroiditis, primary myxedema, thyrotoxicosis	Thyroglobulin	Immunofluorescence test (IFT) (indirect)—methanol-fixed human thyroid Passive hemagglutination Latex agglutination
	Cytoplasmic microsome	IFT (indirect)—unfixed human hyperplastic thyroid tissue Passive hemagglutination Complement fixation
Thyrotoxicosis	Thyroid cell surface antigen	Bioassay—mouse thyroid stimulation *in vivo* Radioimmunoassay with inhibition of *TSH-tissue receptor
Addison's disease	Adrenal cell cytoplasm	IFT (indirect)—unfixed human adrenal cortex
Parathyroid	Parathyroid cytoplasmic antigen	IFT (indirect)—human parathyroid gland
Early onset diabetes	Islet cell	IFT on human or guinea pig pancreas
Alimentary Tract Diseases		
Atrophic gastritis	Parietal cell microsomes	IFT (indirect)—human or mouse gastric mucosa substrate
Pernicious anemia	Intrinsic factor	Radioactive vitamin B_{12} binding assay
Sjögren's syndrome	Salivary duct cells	IFT (indirect)—unfixed human salivary gland
Ulcerative colitis	Colon, lipopolysaccharide	IFT (indirect)—human or rat colon
Celiac disease	Reticulin	IFT (indirect)—rat kidney and liver
Crohn's disease	Reticulin	IFT (indirect)—rat kidney and liver
Liver Diseases		
Chronic aggressive hepatitis	Smooth muscle (actin)	IFT (indirect)—rat gastric mucosa, human cervical tissue
	Liver/kidney microsomal	IFT (indirect)—rat kidney and liver
Primary biliary cirrhosis	Mitochondrial	IFT (indirect)—rat kidney, unfixed
Neuromuscular Diseases		
Myasthenia gravis	Skeletal or heart muscle	IFT (indirect)—rat skeletal muscle and calf thymus
	Acetylcholine receptor	Radioimmunoassay
Demyelinating diseases (i.e., multiple sclerosis)	Myelin	IFT (indirect)—mammalian spinal cord
Dermatologic Diseases		
Pemphigus vulgaris	Prickle cell desmosomes	IFT (direct and indirect)—human skin Peroxidase-labeled antibody
Bullous pemphigoid	Epithelial basement membrane	IFT (direct and indirect)—human skin Peroxidase-labeled antibody
Cicatricial pemphigoid	Epithelial basement membrane	IFT (direct) on biopsy of mucous membrane—indirect on human skin
Dermatitis herpetiformis	Reticulin	IFT (indirect)—rat kidney and liver
Others		
Autoimmune hemolytic anemia	Red cell	Coombs' antiglobulin test (direct and indirect)
Goodpasture's syndrome	Glomerular and lung basement membrane	IFT (direct)—biopsy of patient's kidney IFT (indirect)—patient's serum on human kidney substrate Radioimmunoassay on serum

*Modified from Nakamura, R. M., Chisari, F. V., and Edgington, T. S.: Laboratory tests for diagnosis of autoimmune diseases. *In* Stefannini, M. (ed.): Progress in Clinical Pathology. New York, Grune & Stratton, Inc., 1975.

Table 35–8. IMMUNOLOGIC SPECIFICITY OF ANTINUCLEAR ANTIBODIES (ANA)*

TYPES OF ANTIBODIES	DISEASES IN WHICH ANTIBODIES SEEN	CHARACTERISTICS OF ANTIGENIC DETERMINANTS	PATTERN OBSERVED BY INDIRECT IMMUNOFLUORESCENT TEST USING ACETONE-FIXED MOUSE KIDNEY SUBSTRATE	OTHER TESTS USED TO DETECT SPECIFIC ANTIBODY†
Antibodies to DNA				
1. React *only* with double-stranded DNA	Characteristic of SLE; few cases reported	Double-strandedness of DNA essential	Rim and/or homogeneous	RIA, ID, CIE, HA, CF, special IF
2. React with both double- and single-stranded DNA	High levels in SLE, lower levels in other rheumatic diseases	Relate to deoxyribose, purines, and pyrimidines but not dependent on double helix	Same	Same as above
3. React only with single-stranded DNA	Rheumatic and non-rheumatic diseases	Relates to purines and pyrimidines with ribose or deoxyribose equally reactive	Not detected on routine screen. Special treatment necessary.	RIA, ID, CIE, HA, CF
Deoxynucleoprotein soluble form (sNP)	LE cell antibody in SLE; drug-induced LE	DNA-histone complex necessary. Dissociated components are nonreactive	Rim and/or homogeneous	RIA, ID, LATEX, HA, Bentonite, LE cell
Histone	Infrequent and present in low titer in SLE	Different classes of histones may have different determinants	Homogeneous	CF or special IF test
Sm	Highly diagnostic of SLE	Glycoprotein	Speckled	ID, CIE, HA, CF using either calf or rabbit thymus extract
RNP	High levels in mixed connective tissue disease (MCTD); lower levels in other rheumatic diseases	RNA-protein complex	Speckled	ID, CIE, HA, CF with thymus extract
Scl-1	Highly diagnostic of scleroderma	An extractable antigen. Chemical nature unknown	Atypical speckled	ID using rabbit thymus and prototype sera
SS-A	High prevalence in Sjögren's syndrome sicca complex and lower prevalence in other rheumatic diseases	Chemical nature unknown	Negative	ID, CIE using Wil₂ extract and prototype serum
SS-B	High prevalence in Sjögren's syndrome sicca complex and lower prevalence in other rheumatic diseases	An extractable antigen. Chemical nature unknown	Speckled	ID, CIE using rabbit thymus or Wil₂ extract and prototype serum
RAP	Present in rheumatoid arthritis (RA) and Sjögren's syndrome with RA	Chemical nature unknown	Negative	ID using Wil₂ extract and prototype serum
PM-1	High prevalence in patients with polymyositis	Chemical nature unknown	Variable, speckled	ID using calf thymus extract and prototype serum
Nucleolar	High prevalence in progressive systemic sclerosis; Sjögren's syndrome	4-6S RNA	Nucleolar	—

4

* From Greenwald, C., Peebles, C., and Nakamura, R. M.: Current status of laboratory tests for antinuclear antibody (ANA) in the evaluation of rheumatic disease. Lab. Med., *9*:19, 1978.

†RIA = radioimmunoassay

ID = agar gel double immunodiffusion

CIE = counterimmunoelectrophoresis in agar gel

HA = passive hemagglutination

IF = immunofluorescence

CF = complement fixation

are responsible for the LE cell phenomenon. The LE cell test is positive in 60 to 70 per cent of cases of acutely ill patients with SLE.

Deoxyribonucleoprotein has been extracted from calf thymus nuclei in soluble form (sNP), and a sensitive radioimmunoassay procedure has been developed to detect antibodies to (^{125}I) sNP. The sera of SLE patients showed (^{125}I) sNP binding in 21 of 36 cases (58 per cent). The majority of SLE patients have antibodies to sNP and DS-DNA (native DNA) present simultaneously. In contrast, individuals with other systemic rheumatic diseases rarely showed binding to (^{125}I) sNP. Thus, it appears that the presence of antibody to sNP is relatively specific for SLE (Notman, 1975).

Sm and ribonucleoprotein antigens are non-histone acidic "nuclear proteins" (see p. 1269).

The passive red cell agglutination test for Sm and RNP antibodies may not detect the presence of low titers of anti-RNP in the presence of a high level of anti-Sm antibodies. The test determines the agglutination titers of antigen-coated red cells before and after the cells are digested with RNAse. Thus, if the serum contains antibody to nuclear RNP in higher titer than antibody to Sm, the agglutination titer of untreated cells will be higher than that of RNAse-treated cells. In contrast, if antibody to Sm is present in higher titer than antibody to nuclear RNP, the agglutination titer of untreated cells and of RNAse-treated cells will be the same.

In order to detect low levels of anti-RNP antibodies in the presence of high titers of anti-Sm antibodies, one should routinely test the sera with either the immunodiffusion or the counterimmuno-electrophoresis procedure. In the gel procedures, both the Sm and RNP antibodies can be detected in the same serum samples by specific precipitin lines of identity with known prototype sera.

Autoantibodies to other nuclear acidic proteins (Nakamura, 1978)

In recent years, there has been much work directed at elucidating the nature of autoantibodies to other nuclear acidic protein antigens. These include antibodies to SS-A and SS-B antigens, and those antigens which are reactive with rheumatoid arthritis sera and scleroderma sera (Scl-1). An antibody to nuclear acidic protein antigen can be identified by immunodiffusion methods in which immunologic identity has been demonstrated with a standard reference serum.

The nuclear acidic protein antigens such as the SS-A antigen and the RAP antigen appear to be present in significant concentration only in lymphoid tissue culture cells. With the use of lymphoid tissue culture cell lines such as Wil$_2$ and Raji, extracts of these cell lines can be shown to contain nuclear antigens that precipitate immunologically with antibodies in the sera of patients with Sjögren's syndrome (SS-A antibody) and rheumatoid arthritis (RA precipitin-RAP).

Many of these new studies, particularly antibodies of the SS-A and SS-B system, have been of great help in the diagnosis of Sjögren's syndrome. The availability of these serologic tests to aid in diagnosis has helped in expanding our understanding of Sjögren's syndrome. In many instances, the diagnosis of

Table 35-9. FREQUENCIES OF ANA IN RHEUMATIC DISEASES*

DISEASE†	\multicolumn{7}{c}{TYPES OF ANTIBODIES}						
	DNA	sNP	Sm	RNP	SS-A	SS-B	RAP
SLE	70%	52%	28%	26%	0%	0%	7%
RA	40%‡	3%	0%	10%	0%	0%	65%
SS-sicca syndrome	29%‡	3%	0%	3%	70%	48%	5%
SS-RA					9%	3%	76%
PSS	55%‡	0%	0%	22%	0%	1%	0%
Dermatomyositis	25%‡	0%	0%	0%	–	–	–
DLE	50%‡	0%	0%	25%	0%	0%	0%
MCTD	50%‡	8%	8%	100%	0%	0%	0%
Controls	4%‡	4%	0%	0%	0%	0%	1%

*Percentage of patients with abnormal results compared to 95th percentile for control groups for antibodies to DNA, sNP, Sm, and RNP antigens. (From Greenwald, C., Peebles, C., and Nakamura, R. M.: Current status of laboratory tests for antinuclear antibody (ANA) in the evaluation of rheumatic diseases. Lab. Med., 9:19, 1978.)

†SS = Sjögren's syndrome; control groups included 42 sera negative for IF-ANA with mouse kidney substrate, 29 non-rheumatic disease patients, and 25 normal healthy patients.

‡Generally present in significantly lower titer compared to SLE.

Sjögren's syndrome is overlooked by the physician because of the predominance of rheumatic symptoms and the relative insignificance of sicca symptoms. In a recent study, it was demonstrated that the serologic tests for Sjögren's syndrome helped to establish the diagnosis in approximately 40 per cent of patients with Sjögren's syndrome (Table 35-9).

The differentiation of ANA into antibodies with different immunologic specificities will help in the diagnosis of patients with systemic rheumatic diseases and aid in the management of patients, as has been demonstrated in SLE in cases of antibodies to native DNA. The occurrence of antibodies of such diverse specificities and the selective restriction of specific "marker" antibodies in certain diseases would suggest that different systemic rheumatic diseases are induced by different etiologic mechanisms.

A more extensive discussion of autoimmune disease is presented in Chapter 38.

REFERENCES

Alper, C. A., and Rosen, F. S.: Complement in laboratory medicine. *In* Vyas, G. N., Stites, D. P., and Brecher, G. (eds.): Laboratory Diagnosis of Immunologic Disorders. New York, Grune & Stratton, Inc., 1975.

Axelsen, N. H. (ed.): Quantitative immunoelectrophoresis: New developments and applications. Scand. J. Immunol. (Suppl. 2), 1975.

Batty, I.: Standards and quality control in clinical immunology. *In* Thompson, R. A. (ed.): Techniques in Clinical Immunology. Oxford, Blackwell Scientific Publications, 1977.

Campbell, D. H., Garvey, J. S., Cremer, N. E., and Sussdorf, D. H. (eds.): Methods in Immunology, 2nd ed. New York, W. A. Benjamin, Inc., 1970, pp. 235-267.

Cherry, W. B.: Immunofluorescence techniques. *In* Lennette, E. H., Spaulding, E. H., and Truant, J. P. (eds.): Manual of Clinical Microbiology, 2nd ed. Washington, D.C., American Society of Microbiology, 1974.

Crowle, A. J.: Immunodiffusion. New York, Academic Press, 1961.

Dukor, P., Bianco, C., and Nussenzweig, V.: Cell surface markers in tissue preparations. Proc. Natl. Acad. Sci., *67*:991, 1970.

Fahey, J. L., and McKelvey, E. M.: Quantitative determination of serum immunoglobulins in antibody-agar plates. J. Immunol., *94*:84, 1965.

Fernandez-Madrid, F., and Mattioli, M: Antinuclear antibodies (ANA): Immunologic and clinical significance. *In* Talbott, J. (ed.): Seminars in Arthritis and Rheumatism, vol. VI. New York, Grune & Stratton, Inc., 1976, pp. 83-124.

Greenwald, C., Peebles, C., and Nakamura, R. M.: Current status of laboratory tests for antinuclear antibody (ANA) in the evaluation of rheumatic diseases. Lab. Med., *9*:19, 1978.

Hudson, L., and Hay, F. C.: Practical Immunology. London, Blackwell Scientific Publications, 1976.

Kabat, E. A.: Kabat and Mayer's Experimental Immunochemistry, 2nd ed. Springfield, Ill., Charles C Thomas, Publisher, 1961.

Kawamura, A., Jr.: Fluorescent Antibody Techniques and Their Applications. Baltimore, University Park Press, 1977.

Kwapinski, J. B. G.: Methodology of Immunochemical and Immunological Research. New York, Wiley-Interscience, Inc., 1972.

Lachmann, P. J., Hobart, M. J., and Aston, W. P.: Complement. *In* Weir, D. M. (ed.): Handbook of Experimental Immunology, 2nd ed. Oxford, Blackwell Scientific Publications, 1973.

Larson, C., Orenstein, B., and Ritchie, R. F.: An automated method for quantitation of proteins in body fluids. *In* Advances in Automated Analysis. vol. 1. Technicon International Congress. Miami, Thurman Associates, 1970, pp. 101-104.

Müller-Eberhard, H. J.: Complement. Ann. Rev. Biochem., *44*:697, 1975.

Nakamura, R. M.: Immunopathology: Clinical Laboratory Concepts and Methods. Boston, Little, Brown and Co., 1974.

Nakamura, R. M., and Tan, E. M.: Recent progress in autoantibodies to nuclear antigens (ANA). Hum. Pathol., *9*:85-91, 1978.

Nakamura, R. M., Chisari, F. V., and Edgington, T. S.: Laboratory tests for diagnosis of autoimmune diseases. *In* Stefannini, M. (ed.): Progress in Clinical Pathology, vol. VI. New York, Grune & Stratton, Inc., 1975.

Notman, D., Kurata, N., and Tan, E. M.: Profiles of antinuclear antibodies in systemic rheumatic diseases. Ann. Intern. Med., *83*:464, 1975.

Ritzmann, S. E., and Daniels, J. C. (eds.): Serum Protein Abnormalities—Diagnostic and Clinical Aspects. Boston, Little, Brown and Co., 1975.

Rose, N. R., and Friedman, H. (eds.): Manual of Clinical Immunology. Washington, D.C., American Society of Microbiology, 1976.

Rose, N. R., and Bigazzi, P. E. (eds.): Methods in Immunodiagnosis. New York, John Wiley & Sons, 1973, pp. 1-30.

Ruddy, S., and Austen, K. F.: Complement and its components. *In* Cohen, A. S. (ed.): Laboratory Diagnostic Procedures in the Rheumatic Diseases, 2nd ed. Boston, Little, Brown and Co., 1975, pp. 131-157.

Singer, J. M.: Standardization of the latex test for rheumatoid arthritis serology. Bull. Rheum. Dis., *24*:762, 1973-74.

Sternberger, L. A.: *In* Osler, A., and Weiss, L.: Immunocytochemistry. Englewood Cliffs, N.J., Prentice-Hall, Inc. 1974.

Tucker, E. S., III: The role of complement and other biochemical mediators in immunologic disease. *In* Nakamura, R. M. (ed.): Immunopathology: Clinical Laboratory Concepts and Methods. Boston, Little, Brown and Co., 1974, pp. 104-137.

Weir, D. M.: Immunochemistry. *In* Handbook of Experimental Immunology, 2nd ed., vol. 7. London, Blackwell Scientific Publications, 1973.

Williams, C. A., and Chase, M. W. (eds.): Methods in Immunology and Immunochemistry, vol. III. New York, Academic Press, Inc., 1970.

4

36

THE IMMUNOGLOBULINS: BIOLOGY AND STRUCTURE

Manuel J. Ricardo, Jr., Ph.D.

The cornerstone of any immunologic response is the distinction between *self* and *non-self*. An immunocompetent individual is generally able to recognize foreign substances called *antigens*. These substances are usually complex molecules which are capable of triggering an immune response. Such responses are characterized by *specificity* and *memory*, which are fundamental features of all immune reactivities. Specificity is the adaptability of the immune system to alter its response to match the antigenic stimulus. Memory is the ability to react to a second exposure to the same antigen more rapidly and more intensely. The secondary response is often sustained longer than that stimulated by the first antigen exposure. Rarely do we suffer twice from such diseases as measles, mumps, chicken-pox, and whooping cough.

The immune system can be conveniently divided, for the sake of simplicity, into two major types of effectors: (1) soluble substances, *antibodies*, that are released into the bloodstream and secretions to complex with antigen (humoral immunity) and (2) certain classes of cells that may or may not require antibodies to act more effectively against antigens (cellular immunity).

Antibodies are globular proteins which bind antigen. The association of antibody activity with the gamma (γ) globulin fraction of serum was first shown years ago by Tiselius (1939). He hyperimmunized rabbits with pneumococcal polysaccharides to produce high titers of circulating antibody (Fig. 36–1; the dashed curve indicates the increased γ-globulin in hyperimmune serum) and subsequently examined the effect of absorbing the serum with antigen on the electrophoretic profile. Only the γ-globulin fraction was significantly reduced after removal of specific antibody (Fig. 36–1; the solid line in the γ-region depicts the normal level of globulin, which consists mostly of immunoglobulin G (IgG)).

We now recognize that heterogeneity exists in the types of molecules that can function as antibodies and that their exquisite specificity appears to rest solely in the amino acid sequence of their N-terminus. These gamma globulins are now called immunoglobulins. In each species, the immunoglobulin molecules can be divided into different classes or *isotypes* based on their differences in amino acid sequence of the carbon part of the molecule (C-terminus). For example, in humans five major *isotypes* can be distinguished: immunoglobulin M (IgM), IgG, IgA, IgE, and IgD.

CHARACTERIZATION OF ELECTROPHORETIC MOBILITY

One of the characteristic features of purified immunoglobulins is their inherent electrophoretic heterogeneity. Therefore, the classification of immunoglobulins based strictly on electrophoretic mobility is inadequate because certain classes of antibodies exhibit electrophoretic mobility from α^1 to γ^2 (Fig. 36–1). Human IgG purified from serum displays a broad range of mobilities when subjected to electrophoresis (Table 36–1). This heterogeneity is related to a further subclassification of IgG and to distinct biologic activities. The population of IgG antibodies in serum consists of four subclasses (isotypes) of immunoglobulin molecules (Table 36–2), each possessing a unique antigenic determinant (epitope) which permits their identification by serologic analysis. Subgroups have also been described for IgM and IgA. These subclassifications are based again upon minor chemical differences located in the C-terminal half of the molecule.

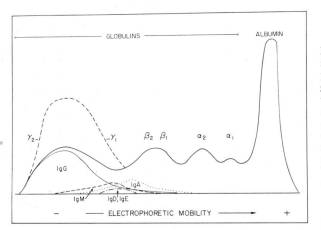

Figure 36–1. Electrophoretogram of normal and hyperimmune serum. The cathodal end shows the distribution pattern of the five major classes of human immunoglobulins. Association of antibody activity with the γ-globulin serum fraction is depicted by the broken curve (hyperimmune serum). Absorption of the hyperimmune serum with the appropriate antigen will reduce only the elevated γ-globulin (dotted line) fraction to normal concentrations (solid line) of which IgG is the major component with a γ_2 to γ_1 mobility as indicated. The other four immunoglobulin classes preferentially show an γ_1 mobility.

Table 36-1. PHYSICAL PROPERTIES OF HUMAN IMMUNOGLOBULINS

WHO DESIGNATION	IgM	IgG	IgA	IgD	IgE
Heavy chains	μ	γ	α	δ	ε
Heavy chain subclasses	μ_1, μ_2	$\gamma_1, \gamma_2, \gamma_3, \gamma_4$	α_1, α_2	–	–
Light chains	κ or λ	κ or λ	κ or λ	κ or λ	κ or λ
Molecular formula	IgM(κ) $(2\mu2\kappa)_5$ IgM(λ) $(2\mu2\lambda)_5$	IgG(κ) $2\gamma2\kappa$ IgG(λ) $2\gamma2\lambda$	IgA(κ) $(2\alpha2\kappa)_{1-3}$ IgA(λ) $(2\alpha2\lambda)_{1-3}$ IgA(κ) $(2\alpha2\kappa)_2 S^b$ IgA(λ) $(2\alpha2\lambda)_2 S$	IgD(κ) $2\delta2\kappa$ IgD(λ) $2\delta2\lambda(?)$	IgE(κ) $2\varepsilon2\kappa$ IgE(λ) $2\varepsilon2\lambda$
Number of 4-chain units per molecule	5	1	1–3	1	1
Heavy chain molecular weight, daltons	65,000	50,000–55,000	62,000	70,000	73,000–75,000
Light chain molecular weight, daltons	23,000	23,000	23,000	23,000	23,000
Sedimentation coefficient, S_{20w}	18.0–19.0	6.7–7.0	6.6–14.0	6.9–7.0	7.9–8.0
Molecular weight, daltons	900,000	143,000–160,000	159,000–447,000	177,000–185,000	187,000–200,000
Electrophoretic mobility	γ^1–β^1	γ^2–α^1	γ^2–β^2	γ^1	γ^1
Carbohydrate content, per cent	7–14	2.2–3.5	7.5–9.0	12–13	11–12
Heavy chain allotypes	–	Gm	Am	–	–
Light chain allotypes	Km(κ)	Km(κ)	Km(κ)[a]	Km(κ)	Km(κ)
Valency for antigen binding	5(10)	2	2	?	2
			(? polymeric forms)		

[a] Formerly designated Inv marker.
[b] Dimer in external secretions carries secretory component -S.

Table 36-2. PROPERTIES ASSOCIATED WITH SUBCLASSES OF HUMAN IMMUNOGLOBULIN G

COMBINED PROPERTIES OF IgG SUBCLASSES	IgG_1	IgG_2	IgG_3	IgG_4
Per cent distribution of total normal serum IgG	66 ± 8	23 ± 8	7.3 ± 3.8	4.2 ± 2.6
Synthetic rate, mg/kg/d, in serum	25	?	3.4	?
Fractional catabolic rate, per cent/d (day),	8	6.9	16.8	6.9
(half-life, d)	(23)	(23)	(7)	(23)
Ratio of κ:λ	1.4–2.4	1.0–1.1	1.1–1.3	5.0–7.0
Allotypic markers (Gm types)	1, 2, 3, 4, 17	23	5, 6, 10, 11, 13, 14, 21	?
Complement-fixing capacity	+2	+	+3	–
Heterologous skin-binding capacity	+	–	+	+
Placental transfer to fetus	+	±	+	+
Macrophage receptor	+	–	+	–
Reaction with protein A	+	+	–	+
Dominant antibody activities:				
Antitetanus toxoid	+2	+	+	±
Antidiphtheria toxoid	+2	+	+	±
Antithyroglobulin	+2	+	+	±
Anti-DNA	+2	+2	±	±
Anti-Rh	+2	–	+	±
Anti-Factor VIII	–	–	–	+
Antidextran	–	+	–	–
Antilevan	–	+	–	–
Antiteichoic acid	–	+	–	–
Number of interheavy chain disulfide bonds in hinge region	2	4	5	2
Position of light-heavy chain disulfide bond on the heavy chain	N214	N131	N131	N131

4

PARAPROTEINS AND ANTIBODIES

The important breakthrough with respect to understanding immunoglobulin structure was the understanding of paraproteins. These proteins are present in high concentration in the serum of individuals with neoplastic and proliferative diseases of lymphoid cells (B-lymphocytes) and plasma cells. They are products of monoclonal proliferation, unlike normal antibodies in serum, which are derived from a polyclonal expansion. The electrophoretic mobilities of the paraproteins, therefore, are homogeneous. Plasma cells in myeloma patients produce homogeneous serum paraproteins generally of either IgG or IgA isotype. In Waldenström's macroglobulinemia, the lymphoid tumors produce monoclonal IgM serum proteins (see Chap. 30, p. 1084).

Paraproteins are not considered true antibodies, since monoclonal expansion is not from known specific antigen stimulation. However, some paraproteins have been reported to bind certain chemically defined substances (ligands). The existence of paraproteins of every immunoglobulin isotype has thus allowed the isolation of large quantities of unique populations of immunoglobulins and their subsequent physiochemical and biologic characterization. With refinement of technology, the structural features and biologic activities of

Table 36-3. PHYSIOLOGIC PROPERTIES OF HUMAN IMMUNOGLOBULINS

WHO DESIGNATION	IgM	IgG	IgA	IgD	IgE
Physiologic properties					
Normal adult serum concentration mg/ml	1.2–4.0	8.0–16.0	0.4–2.2	0.03	17–450 ng/ml
International units/ml	69–322	92–207	54–268	–	< 100
Per cent total immunoglobulin	13	80	6	1	0.002
Intravascular distribution, per cent	41	48	76	75	51
Synthetic rate, mg/kg/d	27	26	5.7	0.4	0.003
Catabolic rate in serum, per cent/d (day)	25	6	15	37	65–90
(or half-life, d)	(5–6)	(18–23)	(5–6.5)	(2.8)	(2.3)

Table 36–4. BIOLOGIC PROPERTIES OF
HUMAN IMMUNOGLOBULINS

WHO DESIGNATION	IgM	IgG	IgA	IgD	IgE
Biologic properties					
Agglutinating capacity	+4	±	+2	–	–
Complement-fixing capacity	+4	+	–	–	–
Homologous anaphylactic hypersensitivity	–	–	–	–	+4
Heterologous guinea pig anaphylaxis	–	+	–	–	–
Fixation to homologous mast cells and basophils	–	±	–	–	+4
Cytophilic binding to macrophages	–	+	–	–	–
Placental transport to fetus	–	+	–	–	–
Rheumatoid factor-binding activity	–	+	–	–	–
Tumor-blocking activity	?	+	?	?	?
Present in external secretions	±	+	+4	–	+2

Other characteristic properties:

  IgM—Produced early in immune response, first effective defense against
    bacteremia.

  IgG—Combats microorganisms and their toxins in extravascular fluids.

  IgA—Defends external body surfaces.

  IgD—Present on lymphocyte surface of immunocompetent cells, important for
    B cell activation (?), and/or immunoregulation (?).

  IgE—Raised in parasitic infections, responsible for symptoms of atopic
    allergy.

immunoglobulin molecules first elucidated with paraproteins have been confirmed using antigen-specific antibody proteins. A summary of the differences in the physiologic and biologic properties of the various immunoglobulin isotypes is illustrated in Tables 36–3 and 36–4. Evaluation of patients with monoclonal immunoglobulins is discussed in Chapter 42, p. 1382.

SUMMARY OF
ANTIBODY STRUCTURE

Antibody molecules in man and other animals are composed of a basic four-chain unit of two identical light and heavy chains (Figs. 36–2 and 36–3). The isotypes of immunoglobulin are defined by the heavy chain constant regions (γ_1, γ_2, γ_3, γ_4, μ_1, μ_2, α_1, α_2, ε, or δ). All immunoglobulins share either kappa (κ) or lambda (λ) light chains. IgM exists as a polymer of five identical subunits (IgM's) linked to each other or to a J chain by intersubunit disulfide bonds. Polymeric forms of IgA (dimers and trimers) also contain a J chain and may contain an additional polypeptide chain (secretory component), synthesized by lumen epithelial cells, if found in extracellular secretions. The domain structure of immunoglobulins is intimately related to its function. The

variable domain at the N-terminal end of the molecule is responsible for antigen binding. The specialized constant region domains are implicated in a number of biologic functions, such as complement binding and control of turnover rate. A more detailed discussion of antibody structure is presented on p. 1230.

BIOLOGIC ACTIVITIES
OF IMMUNOGLOBULINS

Immunoglobulin M. Structural studies of IgM have been done with proteins obtained from patients suffering from Waldenström's macroglobulinemia. They have served as a model for structural analysis of IgM antibodies, just as myeloma proteins and Bence Jones proteins are models for IgG antibodies and light chains respectively. Human IgM's are referred to frequently as macroglobulin because they have a molecular weight of about 900,000 daltons (see Table 36–1). Each molecule can be dissociated into five similar subunits (IgM$_s$), each having a molecular weight of 180,000 daltons and bearing an extra C_H domain (Fig. 36–3). As with IgA, polymerization of the IgM$_s$ subunits appears to be a process involving the addition of J chain and carbohydrate groups immediately prior to or coinciding with its release from the cell. The mono-

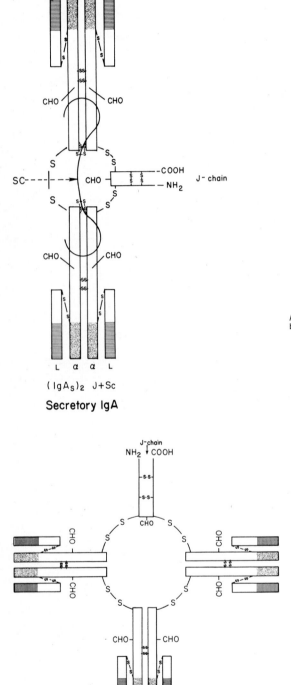

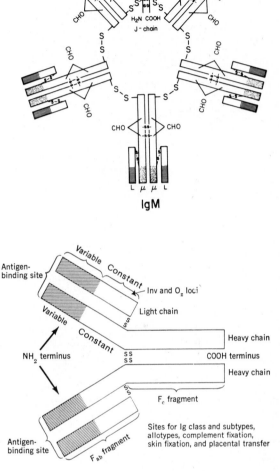

Figure 36–2. Representative structures of the polymeric immunoglobulins (IgA and IgM). The basic immunoglobulin unit consists of two light and two heavy chains. These units may be present in pairs, triads, or pentamers. The accessory J-chain is associated with each of the polymers and is believed to be linked by disulfide bonds to two of the subunits. The secretory component (SC) is found only in secretory dimeric IgA and may or may not be disulfide linked. The linkage shown in the diagram is hypothetical. The positions of the oligosaccharide groups are indicated by CHO. The variable regions of both heavy and light chains are delineated by dots and horizontal lines, respectively. In humans, IgM is always found as a pentamer and IgA as a monomer, dimer, or trimer in serum. *Lower right,* Schematic diagram of an immunoglobulin molecule (From Harness, D. R.: Postgrad. Med., *48:*66, 1970).

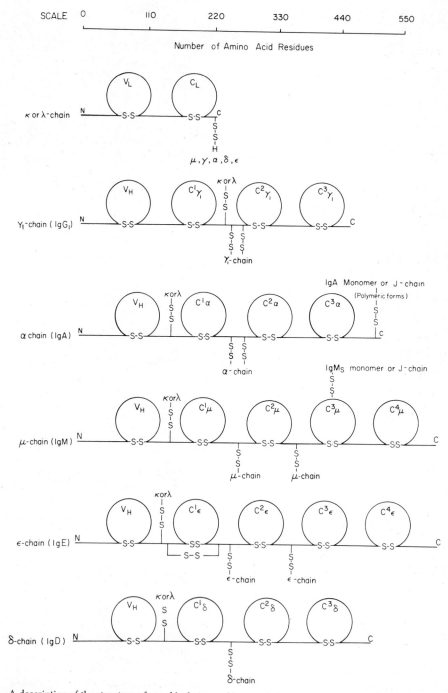

Figure 36–3. A description of the structure of κ and λ chains and heavy chain isotypes. The differences in heavy chain lengths, number of domains, and positions of cysteine residues involved in interlight linkage is illustrated. The number and positions of the interheavy and intraheavy chain disulfide bonds are also illustrated. Each of the domains is identified according to its generic term.

mers are joined through an intersubunit disulfide bond on each μ chain or the J chain to form a pentamer. This circular pentameric arrangement illustrated in Figure 36-2 has been confirmed by electron microscopy studies. The theoretical combining valency of IgM is 10, but this is observed only on interaction with small haptens; with larger antigens the effective valence falls to 5 and may be attributable to some form of steric restriction. Because of their high valence, IgM antibodies are extremely efficient agglutinating and cytolytic antibodies. A summary of the physical and biologic properties associated with IgM is given in Tables 36-1, 36-3, and 36-4 (Metzger, 1970).

There is evidence that IgM antibodies were the first to evolve, and they are usually the first to appear in ontogeny. In the lower vertebrates, however, IgM antibodies do exist as monomeric subunits and not as a pentamer as in mammals. In humans, IgM constitutes approximately 10 per cent of normal serum immunoglobulins. They appear early in response to infection, and it is likely that they play a role of particular importance in cases of bacteremia. IgM proteins predominate in certain humoral immune responses such as antibodies to blood group antigens (isohemagglutinins), the Wasserman antibodies in syphilis, antibodies to the typhoid O antigen, and many antibodies to microbial antigens.

Approximately six days after birth, the serum concentration of IgM rises sharply. This rise normally continues for about a month, diminishes somewhat, then continues to rise until adult levels are achieved by about one year of age. Macroglobulins are distributed predominantly in the intravascular pool in both humans and rabbits. Unlike IgG antibodies, no extensive maternal-fetal transport of IgM takes place.

Membrane-bound IgM, which exists as a monomer subunit, is the first immunoglobulin to be detected on B-lymphoid cells. The elegant studies done in the chicken bursa (a cloacal structure in aves containing lymphoid elements presumed to govern the production of humoral antibodies) have shown that several days after the detection of IgM a few lymphoid cells carry IgG on their surface. As the lymphoid cells mature, they leave the bursa and relocate in peripheral tissues. When these peripheral lymphoid cells are tested for membrane immunoglobulins, the order in which they appear in these distal sites is found to be similar to that in which they developed within the bursa (IgM $\rightarrow$ IgG $\rightarrow$ IgA). In humans, monomer IgM (with IgD) is the major immunoglobulin expressed on the surface of B-lymphocytes (Wigzel, 1974). This is also discussed on p. 1304, Chap. 39.

IgM and IgG antibodies are responsible for most of the specific activities classically associated with antibodies in general, including precipitation, agglutination, transfusion reactions, hemolysis, and complement fixation. On the surface of cells a single molecule of IgM suffices to fix C1q, whereas two antibody molecules are required for fixation by IgG. Differences in C1q activation by IgM and IgG also become apparent when the temperature is varied. The C1q is efficiently activated by IgG at both 4° and 37°C., whereas IgM is very efficient at the lower temperature. (Complement activation is discussed on p. 1246, Chap. 37.)

The plasma cells of patients with macroglobulinemia generally contain intracellular IgM in the 19S polymer form. In most systems studied, the IgM appears in the vascular fluids in its final 19S form, while intracellularly it is in the IgM_S (7S) form. However, in human autoimmune disorders, such as systemic lupus erythematosus, the 7S form can be detected in significant amounts in serum. Selective IgM deficiency is a rare disorder associated with the absence of IgM and normal levels of other immunoglobulin classes (Chap. 42). The cause of this immunologic disorder is unknown. The absence of IgM and presence of IgG and IgA contradict the theory of sequential immunoglobulin development.

Immunoglobulin G. IgG is the major immunoglobulin class (80 per cent) found in human and animal serum (Table 36-3). There are four subclasses which were first distinguished by antigenic differences (p. 1228) in their Fc portion (C-terminus) (Fig. 36-4). These subclasses also show distinct peptide and biologic differences, which are summarized in Table 36-2. The biologic individuality of different immunoglobulin classes, including the IgG subclasses, is dependent on the heavy chain regions, particularly Fc. Nevertheless, the relationship between biologic activity and difference in primary structure is unclear. IgG_1 and IgG_4 molecules differ in their constant region by 14 residues, 11 of which are located in the C_H2 domain. The types of amino acid replacements observed in the Fc fragment of IgG_4 can explain its highly anionic

4

electrophoretic mobility compared with that of the other IgG subclasses, but it is not possible yet to ascribe a particular biologic function to a unique primary sequence.

Complement activation through binding of C1q is most efficient with IgG_1 and IgG_3 antibodies, although the IgG_2 is also active. The IgG_4 antibodies generally are not active in binding complement through the classic pathway. However, IgG_4 can bind complement by the alternative pathway in which the C-terminal end of the C_H1 domain seems to be involved. Another biologic activity with selective subclass distribution is the fixation of IgG to heterologous skin. This reaction can easily be obtained with all subclasses of IgG except IgG_2.

Immunoglobulin G is the only class of antibody that clearly passes through the placenta. The degree of placental transfer of the four IgG subclasses is, however, still a matter of uncertainty. Some reports have shown that IgG_1, IgG_3, and IgG_4 are present in the cord blood in quantities corresponding to those of the mother, while IgG_2 levels generally are lower. The ability of IgG to cross the placenta provides a major line of defense against infection for the first weeks of a child's life, a defense which may be further reinforced by the transfer of colostral IgG across the gut mucosa in the neonate. Normally, the human fetus begins to receive significant quantities of maternal IgG transplacentally at around 12 weeks gestation, although small amounts have been detected in the fetus as early as 8 weeks. The quantity increases steadily until, at birth, cord serum contains a concentration of IgG comparable to or greater than that of maternal serum. Barring any immunologic disorders, adult levels of IgG are reached in the child six or seven years after birth and remain relatively constant throughout life with IgG_1 the dominant isotype.

Immunoglobulin G_3 makes up only about 7 per cent of the total IgG pool in serum but has a number of special properties that appear significant in disease. IgG_3 shows a striking concentration-dependent aggregation which probably is involved in its affinity for C1q. In addition, hyperviscosity of serum may result from relatively low levels of this subclass because of this aggregation. This property of IgG_3 has been implicated in a significant number of clinically important hyperviscosity states. Also, the IgG_3 antibodies apparently are selectively retained in the sera of a number of patients with generalized hypogammaglobulinemia.

IgG antibodies have a high diffusion coefficient, which enables it to diffuse more readily than other immunoglobulin classes into the extravascular body spaces. IgG, being the predominant immunoglobulin in these spaces, carries the major burden of neutralizing bacterial toxins and of binding to microorganisms to enhance their phagocytosis. The complexes of bacteria with IgG antibody can adhere to phagocytic cells because these cells (macrophages and neutrophils) have specialized surface receptors for sites on the Fc portion of the IgG molecule. Furthermore, only IgG antibodies coating target cells (i.e., bacteria) will sensitize them for extracellular killing by specialized K-cells (killer cells). A summary of the physical and biologic properties of IgG is given in Tables 36-2 to 36-4 (p. 1217).

Immunoglobulin A. Interest in IgA has increased in recent years because it is the principal antibody in most external secretions. It is the main immunoglobulin made by plasma cells in glands and mucous membranes. In the lamina propria of human gastrointestinal tract, there are approximately 20 IgA cells per IgG cell in close contact with the overlying glandular epithelium. By contrast, in peripheral lymph nodes and spleen the ratio is about 1:3 (IgA:IgG). In humans serum IgA is mostly monomeric (7S) and of the IgA1 subclass (90 per cent), while in other animal species serum IgA tends to be dimeric but lacks secretory component. In the mucosa, secretory IgA, mostly of the α_2 heavy chain isotype (60 per cent), apparently plays an important role as the first line of defense to protect the body against both microbial infections and the entrance of other foreign macromolecules. It has been postulated that IgA inhibits the adherence of microorganisms to the surface of mucosal cells, thereby preventing their entry into the body tissues. This diminution in absorption may protect the individual against harmful antigens by forming non-absorbable complexes which could be degraded by proteolytic enzymes on the surface of the intestine. Usually, IgA can be found in saliva, tears, and other secretions earlier than in serum. Secretory IgA also reaches adult levels sooner than serum IgA. The IgA system in the intestinal tract of humans, for example, may be fully developed by 2 years of age, while serum IgA levels do not normally reach adult concentrations until 12 years of age. The factor(s) responsible for the slower maturation of the serum IgA system are not understood. Because of this difference in the maturation rate and the unique role of secretory IgA antibodies, it seems reasonable to consider the secretory immune system as a separate entity and not merely as an offshoot of the humoral immune system, where IgG predominates.

The biologic properties of human IgA are summarized in Table 36-4. Whether IgA antibodies can mediate any secondary effector functions following the union of their combining sites with antigen remains unclear. More studies are needed to determine if differences do exist between IgA_1 and IgA_2 antibodies and between serum-type and secretory IgA antibodies. IgA immunoglobulins apparently cannot fix complement by the classic pathway. However, a number of reports indicate that both serum IgA_1 and IgA_2 and secretory IgA are effective activators of the complement alternative pathway if experimentally aggregated. Secretory IgA antibodies have been reported to interact with complement and lysozyme together to bring about bacteriolysis. Antiviral activity by IgA antibodies has been demonstrated in individuals given either of the polio vaccines. The oral Sabin vaccine resulted in a significant coproantibody response. In rats, secretory IgA is believed to play an important role in preventing dental caries. In the alimentary tract, IgA antibodies are undoubtedly being formed against a myriad of environmental antigens. For example, IgA immunodeficiencies, discussed in Chapter 42, can lead to increased levels and incidence of humoral antibodies directed against antigens derived from food and intestinal organisms. It is believed that these antibodies are formed because the antigens are not being absorbed in the epithelial wall of the intestine by IgA and penetrate the intestinal lining and enter the circulation. Secretory IgA thus appears particularly suitable for performing this absorption function for two reasons: (a) its dimeric nature allows for greater antigen binding and (b) the presence of secretory component appears to increase the molecule resistance to proteolysis, which allows it to function in an enzyme-rich milieu.

Although the gut-associated lymphoid tissue is probably the major source of polymeric IgA in serum, there are probably other sites of origin. A small number of IgA precursor cells, which can differentiate into cells that synthesize polymeric IgA, have been localized in peripheral lymph nodes, spleen, and bone marrow cells. In addition, some cells committed to IgA production may migrate to extraintestinal lymphoid tissue from the gut. The serum monomeric IgA may originate from either the spleen, lymph node, bone marrow, or gut (Lamm, 1976).

The structure of IgA is similar to that of the other immunoglobulins. However, the IgA_2 immunoglobulin is unique in that it lacks light-heavy disulfide bonds. The light chains are linked to each other by a disulfide bridge. The association of the light and heavy chain dimers is by strong non-covalent interactions. Other important physical properties of the IgA molecule are given in Tables 36-1 and 36-3 (pp. 1216 and 1217).

Immunoglobulin D. Compared to other immunoglobulins, IgD is a relatively minor component in serum (Table 36-3). The normal human population can be divided into three groups. The major group, which represents 70 per cent of the population, has a concentration of IgD of 20 to 50 μg/ml in serum. The other two groups, each of which represents 15 per cent of the population, contain very low levels of IgD (3 μg/ml) or very high levels of IgD (100 to 400 μg/ml). The reason for the large differences in IgD serum concentration, both in children and in adults, is not known. IgD usually is detected in serum at about six months of age. However, analysis of some human cord sera showed that it contained IgD, and comparison of the concentrations of maternal vs. cord serum IgA, IgM, and IgD suggested that the fetus is capable of synthesizing IgD.

In disease states, the IgD concentration can vary greatly. In chronic infections, IgD levels increase, as do those of the other immunoglobulins. To date, no specific increase of IgD has been associated with a particular disease. Patients with allergies and autoimmune diseases do not show an abnormal IgD concentration. IgD is usually absent in hypogammaglobulinemic individuals. IgD has not been found in secretory or body fluids other than serum. Only about 2 per cent of patients suffering from multiple myeloma produce IgD paraproteins, generally with concentration levels lower than those of IgG, IgA, and IgM myeloma proteins. IgD myelomas are usually of lambda (λ) chain type (80 to 90 per cent), and almost all patients have considerable Bence Jones protein in their urine.

The lability of IgD to heat and acid resem-

4

bles IgE and thus differs from IgG, IgA, and IgM. Both IgD and IgE are present in the serum in very low concentrations and are rapidly catabolized. Neither of these isotypes can bind complement. It now appears that cell-bound IgD is probably biologically far more important than serum IgD.

Antibody activity in IgD has been difficult to demonstrate in spite of its structural similarities to other immunoglobulins. However, IgD activity against insulin, penicillin G, milk protein, diphtheria toxoid, nuclear antigens, bovine gamma globulin, and thyroid antigens has been reported. But absorption of activity with antiserum to IgD has not been demonstrated. The biologic function of serum IgD is still unknown (Spiegelberg, 1972).

Recent observations have demonstrated that significant proportions of human, mouse, and monkey immunoglobulin bearing peripheral blood B-lymphocytes carry both IgM and IgD on their surfaces. These findings have been extended to B-lymphocytes in spleen and newborn (cord) blood lymphocytes. In all these cases the number of IgD$^+$ cells was much greater than would be expected from only a consideration of the concentration of IgD in normal serum. The possibility that IgD on the cells was acquired by passive adsorption was excluded by the demonstration that after proteolytic stripping of membrane-bound IgD, it was regenerated. The finding that both IgD and IgM are simultaneously present on a high proportion of lymphocytes was unexpected. Surface IgD and IgM were both shown to have the same light chain, idiotype, and antibody specificity and, hence, presumably variable region sequences. These membrane-bound immunoglobulins are thus likely to act as distinct receptors for the same antigen. Following antigen or mitogen stimulation, there is a rapid decrease of surface IgD in stimulated cells. Eight days after stimulation, no IgD$^+$ B-lymphocytes can be detected. These findings have caused considerable speculation about the role of surface IgD in the induction of humoral response and tolerance. It has been postulated that immunocompetent B-lymphocytes bearing only IgM are susceptible to tolerance upon antigen exposure, while IgM- and IgD-bearing cells upon exposure to antigen lead to B cell differentiation and maturation. The role IgD plays would be viewed as turning on, turning off, or modulating (controlling) B cell division and/or differentiation. The regulatory influence of IgD could be linked to a suppression of surface IgD or to a release or cleavage of the surface IgD during the triggering process. The latter possibility seems attractive, since IgD has a remarkable susceptibility to degradation, which may account for its very short half-life in the body (see Table 36-3).

Among the human immunoglobulins, IgD has two unique structural features. In both the intact molecule and the Fc fragment, the globular domains appear to be less compact than in other immunoglobulins. This difference in conformation may account in part for increased susceptibility to proteolysis. The other feature is the presence of only one interheavy chain disulfide bond (Fig. 36-3).

Immunoglobulin E. This class of antibody represents a minor but distinct isotype of proteins in serum of man and higher primates. IgE was first discovered in the sera of patients with hay fever. It is now firmly established that reaginic hypersensitivity reactions in atopic diseases are mediated by IgE antibody. Homocytotropic antibodies, which are similar to human IgE antibodies, have now been detected in experimental animals (rabbits, dogs, mice, guinea pigs, monkeys, pigs, horses, and cattle). The physiochemical properties of the reaginic antibodies in these animals are similar to those of human IgE and different from the other human isotypes (Bennich, 1971).

Immunoglobulin E levels can be elevated up to 30 times normal in various diseases, among which atopic disorders and parasitic infestations appear to be the most prominent. Elevated amounts of monoclonal IgE have also been found in the serum of patients with IgE myeloma. IgE levels have also been investigated in sera from patients with malaria and syphilis. The present results indicate that IgE does not play a major role in the immunity of these diseases. The main physiologic role of IgE is still uncertain. Persistence of the immunoglobulin class through evolution suggests that it might be important in the survival of the individual, but obviously atopic diseases do not seem to promote the survival of the species. Perhaps its importance is to be found in the widespread occurrence of IgE-mediated immune reactivity in parasitic (helminthic) infection. It is thought that histamine release resulting from contact of parasite antigens with mast-cell bound IgE antibody in the gut wall facilitates rejection of the intruders.

Only a very small proportion of plasma cells in the body are synthesizing IgE at any given time. The IgE-forming cells were first detected in primate lymphoid tissues by using a fluorescent antibody technique. In non-atopic individuals, recurrently infected tonsils and adenoids removed by surgery possess a large number of plasma cells which stain with anti-IgE. Bronchial and peritoneal lymph nodes, as well as the gastrointestinal mucosa, contain some IgE-forming plasma cells. By contrast, IgE-forming cells are scarce in human spleen, subcutaneous lymph nodes, and respiratory mucosa.

The role of IgE antibodies in immediate hypersensitivity reactions is due to their attachment to membrane receptors on mast cells and basophilic granulocytes. This cytotropic property has been shown to be located in the Fc fragment. Upon combining with certain specific antigens, called allergens, on the surface of these cells, IgE antibodies trigger the degranulation of mast cells, with the release of pharmacologic mediators (vasoactive amines) responsible for the characteristic wheal and flare skin reactions evoked by the exposure of the skin of allergic individuals to allergens (Type I hypersensitivity). IgE antibodies provide a striking example of the bifunctional nature of antibody molecules. The Fc portion of the molecule binds to the target cells, while the Fab portion binds the allergen. Type I hypersensitivity is discussed on p. 1385 in Chapter 42.

A comparison of the molecular weight of ε-chain to the other isotypes of heavy chain indicates that it is larger by an amount corresponding to one domain. Both IgE and IgM appear to possess an extra domain (Fig. 36–3) based on their molecular size and cysteine content. Like IgG and IgD, IgE normally exists only in monomeric form. The physiochemical and biologic properties of IgE are given in Tables 36–1, 36–3, and 36–4.

DISTRIBUTION AND CONCENTRATION OF IMMUNOGLOBULINS IN BODY FLUIDS

The concentration of a given antibody class in serum is dependent on a number of factors. First, there is a direct relationship between the concentration of a particular immunoglobulin class or subclass in body fluids and the number of plasma cells secreting that particular isotype. For some unknown reason, the number of plasma cells forming immunoglob-

ulins of each class is different. Second, the rate of synthesis of a given antibody per plasma cell can differ, but generally the rates are similar for all classes. Therefore, this factor plays a minor role in influencing the concentration of a particular immunoglobulin. On the other hand, the rate of catabolism of a given antibody class plays a major role in determining the concentration of serum immunoglobulins. The constant region of an immunoglobulin heavy chain is involved in this catabolism and, therefore, in regulating the distribution and levels of immunoglobulins in body fluids. Finally, the rate at which immunoglobulin exchange occurs between intra- and extravascular spaces will also affect the concentrations of antibody. The rate of exchange between plasma and lymph space depends primarily upon the diffusion coefficient of the immunoglobulin. For example, IgG has a high diffusion coefficient and can predominate in extravascular spaces, whereas IgM has a low diffusion coefficient and is found predominantly in serum. Relatively large amounts of IgD have been reported in the intravascular space, suggesting that it has a low diffusion coefficient. This may well result from asymmetry of the molecule caused by the three oligosaccharide moieties. IgA is relatively more concentrated in lymph than in serum, probably due to the local synthesis of IgA in the intestines and drainage into the thoracic duct. The average concentrations of human immunoglobulin classes and subclasses of IgG are shown in Tables 36–2 and 36–3. The concentrations can vary considerably from individual to individual for any of the antibody isotypes. In some animals, such as guinea pigs and rats, immunoglobulin concentrations are lower than for man, whereas rabbits, goats, and horses have similar levels.

The external fluids of saliva, tears, bronchial secretions, colostrum, and intestinal secretions all have much lower concentrations of immunoglobulin than does serum. The major class of immunoglobulin in these secretions is IgA. The average concentration ratios of IgA to IgG in secretions is 20:1, compared with 1:5 in serum. IgM is the only other known immunoglobulin that is capable of interacting with secretory component. In some instances, agammaglobulinemic individuals, who lack both IgG and IgA, have a compensatory increase in IgM. IgE immunocytes are more frequently found in lymphoid tissue around secretory glands than in lymph nodes and

4

spleen. Because of this, IgE may also be more concentrated in secretions.

In man, the concentration of immunoglobulin in the cerebrospinal fluids is very small. The IgG concentration in these fluids is about $1/100$ of that in serum and makes up approximately 12 per cent of the total proteins in cerebrospinal fluid. The levels of both IgA and IgM are equally small, and IgD and IgE apparently are undetectable in these fluids. Immunoglobulin entry into the cerebrospinal fluid may occur by passive diffusion across the blood-brain barrier and/or by direct entry after synthesis by plasma cells in the central nervous tissue.

Man and most animals are unable to form appreciable quantities of antibody until sometime after birth, when they become immunologically mature. Therefore, immune protection is provided to the offspring by the transfer of IgG from the mother to the young. In man and other primates, prenatal transfer of immunoglobulin to the fetus appears to be the major route, and only IgG is transferred. Although human colostrum is rich in IgA, this immunoglobulin is probably not transferred to serum but rather plays an important role in immune function within the gastrointestinal tract. In some animals, such as mice, rabbits, and rats, only IgG is transferred via the yolk sac during pregnancy and additional IgG present in their colostrum is transferred to the young by intestinal absorption in the first 24 postnatal hours (Spiegelberg, 1974).

METABOLISM OF IMMUNOGLOBULIN

Immunoglobulins are constantly being synthesized and catabolized in the body. The synthetic rates and average half-life in days of human immunoglobulin are summarized in Tables 36-2 and 36-3. IgG_1 has one of the highest synthetic rates and the longest half-life of the IgG subclasses. IgG_3, however, has a much shorter plasma half-life and a much faster turnover rate. Several studies of IgG_3 myeloma protein have established that the rapid turnover of IgG_3 is a property of this IgG subclass and seems intimately related to the structural difference in the Fc portion of the γ_3 chain and the number of interheavy disulfide bridges. IgG turnover studies in a number of diseases support the concept of the concentration-catabolism effect, which states that the catabolic rate of IgG is related directly to its serum concentration. A low fractional turnover rate is seen with reduced serum IgG levels and high fractional turnover rate with high serum IgG levels. In some cases, abnormalities in metabolism can be associated with a normal serum immunoglobulin level. This is seen in patients with various connective tissue diseases, such as systemic lupus erythematosus, rheumatoid arthritis, polymyositis, and various forms of vasculitis. These individuals have increased IgG fractional turnover rates and shortened half-lives, indicating hypercatabolism. However, a simultaneous increase in synthesis may counteract this hypercatabolism and result in elevated serum IgG levels (Waldman, 1969).

The fractional turnover rate of IgM is independent of the serum concentration and, thus, differs from IgG metabolism. IgM proteins derived from either monoclonal or polyclonal proliferation have similar catabolism rates. However, the fractions of the IgM pool which have cold agglutinin properties generally are catabolized more rapidly. Patients with chronic idiopathic cold agglutinin syndrome synthesize IgM at about 10 times the normal rate. Individuals subjected to repeated malarial infection, characterized by splenic enlargement (tropical splenomegaly syndrome) also display markedly increased IgM synthesis.

IgA_2 molecules are catabolized more rapidly with a shorter plasma half-life than IgA_1. The reported synthetic and catabolic rates for IgA in Table 36-3 are for IgA_1 subclass, since IgA_1 comprises the majority of the IgA pool in serum.

A distinguishing feature of IgD metabolism is its high fractional turnover rate and short plasma half-life (see Table 36-3). Currently, it remains unclear whether IgD catabolism follows the concentration-catabolism effect.

Immunoglobulin E has the lowest serum concentration of the five classes of antibodies and its metabolic pool size is approximately 10^5 times smaller than that of IgG. The low level of IgE in plasma is the result of the highest turnover rate, the shortest half-life, and the lowest synthetic rate (1/1000 that of IgG) of the immunoglobulins (see Table 36-3). It is possible that the fixation of IgE to cell surface receptors of various tissues may also be involved in the catabolism of IgE. Therefore, saturation of IgE cell surface receptors may lead to prolonged survival of unbound IgE molecules in the serum.

Markedly decreased rates of IgE synthesis are found in patients with hypogammaglobulinemia. Deficiencies of IgE are frequently associated with IgA deficiencies.

The rate at which immunoglobulins are catabolized is dependent in part on the structure of the constant region of their respective heavy chain. The Fc fragments of IgG are catabolized relatively slowly and are only moderately increased from that of intact IgG. Heavy chain disease proteins generally have half-lives similar to those of native IgG, but their turnover rates, like those of Fc fragments, are generally higher than those of intact IgG. Fc fragments survive approximately 40 times longer in plasma than purified L chain monomers or dimers and Fab or $F(ab')_2$ fragments (Fig. 36-4). The fractional turnover rate of monomer L chain is about 100 times that of native IgG molecule. However, the L chain dimers are catabolized more slowly than the L chain monomers. Fab or $F(ab')_2$ fragments are rapidly metabolized, with half-life in plasma of about four hours. The mechanism(s) of immunoglobulin catabolism is not understood at present.

Corticosteroids and azathioprine are two common *immunosuppressive* drugs frequently used to alter the manifestations of abnormal immune function in patients with various diseases. A summary of immunoglobulin metabolism in a number of disease states is given in Table 36-5. The great majority of subjects receiving standard therapeutic dosages of immunosuppressive drugs show the features of hypercatabolism: an increased fractional turnover rate and a shortened plasma half-life. This leads to a reduction in immunoglobulin concentration. A number of disorders are associated with a reduction of antibody levels (hypogammaglobulinemic state) rather than an increase in immunoglobulin levels (Table 36-5). These are discussed further in Chapter 42.

FACTORS WHICH MAY CAUSE VARIATIONS IN IMMUNOGLOBULIN LEVELS

Valid interpretation of serum immunoglobulin levels requires recognition of biologic variations which exist throughout the life

Table 36-5. ABNORMALITIES IN IMMUNOGLOBULIN METABOLISM ASSOCIATED WITH CERTAIN DISORDERS

CLASSIFICATION	METABOLIC STATE	DISEASE STATE
Hypogammaglobulinemia	Decreased immunoglobulin synthesis	Ataxia—telangiectasia (IgA) Chronic lymphocytic leukemia (CLL) Congenital and acquired hypogammaglobulinemia Selective immunoglobulin deficiency Wiskott-Aldrich syndrome (IgM)
	Excessive loss of immunoglobulin	Gastrointestinal loss (a) lymphatic abnormalities (b) ulcerating conditions (c) unknown Nephrotic syndrome
	Hypercatabolism	Cryoglobulinemia Familial idiopathic hypercatabolic hypoproteinemia Multiple myeloma Myotonic dystrophy Wiskott-Aldrich syndrome (IgG)
Hypergammaglobulinemia	Polyclonal gammopathy	Connective tissue diseases Cirrhosis Infection
	Monoclonal gammopathy	Benign monoclonal gammopathy Multiple myeloma Waldenström's macroglobulinemia
	Decreased catabolism	Renal tubular disease (a) cystinosis (b) adult Fanconi's syndrome

span of the individuals. The most important of these variables are age, sex, and race.

The first indication that normal immune function may decline with *age* came from histologic studies which showed that in man and lower animals, the thymic lymphatic mass decreased with age. This normal atrophy of the thymus begins at the time of sexual maturity. Additional age-related histologic changes in lymphatic tissues are the diminishing numbers of germinal centers and increases in the amount of reticulum and the number of plasma cells and phagocytes. Several reports have also indicated that the number of circulating lymphocytes in humans decreases progressively during or after middle age. This decrease is apparently due to a decline in the absolute number of circulating thymic-derived (T) lymphocytes, while the number of B-lymphocytes remains essentially the same. This suggests a possible reduction in cellular immunity (T-lymphocyte mediated) rather than humoral immunity antibody production (B-lymphocyte mediated). Some investigators have reported a decrease in delayed hypersensitivity to common skin test antigens in previously sensitized individuals. In general, when assessed with an antigen to which the individual has not been sensitized previously, it appears that T-lymphocyte functions decline with age. Supportive evidence for this association comes from both *in vivo* and *in*

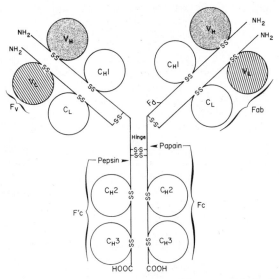

Figure 36–4. Schematic representation of immunoglobulin G molecule. The relative positions of the *interchain* disulfide bonds and the *intrachain* disulfide bonds which form the loop regions are shown. Each of the loops delineates the domain of the light and heavy chain labeled accordingly. The probable sites of enzymatic cleavage in the "hinge" region by papain or pepsin are indicated. The papain fragments are designated Fab and Fc. The pepsin fragments are Fc' and Fab'2 (two Fab fragments disulfide linked). Digestion of Fab with pepsin under the proper conditions will yield the fragment Fv (V_H and V_L non-convalently associated). The part of the heavy chain which contributes to the Fab fragment is designated Fd. See text, p. 1230, for further details.

Table 36–6. SERUM IMMUNOGLOBULIN CONCENTRATIONS

AGE (YEARS)	MEAN IgG (mg/ml)		MEAN IgA (mg/ml)	
	White Male	White Female	White Male	White Female
5–9	10.28	11.05	1.09	1.10
10–14	10.41	11.13	1.16	1.15
15–19	10.55	11.20	1.23	1.21
20–24	10.69	11.28	1.32	1.28
25–29	10.83	11.35	1.40	1.35
30–34	10.98	11.43	1.50	1.42
35–39	11.12	11.50	1.59	1.49
40–44	11.27	11.58	1.70	1.57
45–49	11.42	11.66	1.81	1.65
50–54	11.57	11.74	1.93	1.74
55–59	11.72	11.81	2.06	1.83
60–64	11.88	11.89	2.20	1.93
65–69	12.04	11.97	2.34	2.03
70–74	12.20	12.05	2.49	2.14
75+	12.36	12.13	2.66	2.26

The data were derived from 3213 serum samples collected from an unselected group of subjects from a single health community (Tecumseh, Michigan) (Cassidy, 1974).

vitro studies of lymphocytes from old mice and elderly humans, showing a decreased ability to mount a graft-vs-host reaction and to proliferate when stimulated by mitogens (Kay, 1976).

Results in aging rodents have shown that antigen-induced primary antibody responses decrease with age, but the secondary antibody responses need not necessarily be impaired. The onset of decline in primary antibody responses can occur as early as the period of thymus involution. This again suggests that in primary antibody responses, aging may be affecting the regulatory T-lymphocytes and not B-lymphocytes directly.

In mice the number of B-lymphocytes in the spleen and lymph nodes does not seem to change significantly with age. These findings parallel the results obtained in human peripheral lymphoid cells. The serum IgG and IgA in man tend to increase with age (Table 36-6), whereas serum IgM may remain relatively constant. Antibody production with certain antigens has been reported to decrease markedly. This could arise from a decrease either in the number of antigen-sensitive immunocompetent cells within the B-lymphocyte pool or in the immunologic burst-size of antigen-stimulated B-lymphocyte clones.

Studies on a large unselected group of healthy white subjects (3213) from a single community (Tecumseh, Michigan) have shown that the mean concentrations of IgG and IgA increase with age, with slight but significant differences between the sexes. Females were reported to have higher serum levels of IgG and lower levels of IgA (Table 36-6). Although these *sex differences* for IgG and IgA are statistically significant, their biologic meaning is not apparent. The IgM levels in these subjects remained relatively constant with age. However, females had higher mean levels of IgM (1.06 mg/ml) compared with males (0.77 mg/ml). Other results document the occurrence of a relative hypoglobulinemia in healthy older individuals.

Several studies have reported that immunoglobulin levels and more recently the specific immunoglobulin levels are higher in persons with *pigmented skins*. Table 36-7 presents the results obtained in a healthy biracial population in Evans County, Georgia. Negroes had higher levels of the three major immunoglobulins (IgM, IgG, and IgA) than did Caucasians. The most prominent difference was in IgG. No urban-rural difference in immunoglobulin levels was noted in this study. White and blue-collar workers in Rochester, New York, had serum levels of IgM and IgG similar to those of white subjects in rural Georgia. All Negroes and white women in the Evans County community had a higher prevalence of anti-IgG globulin (rheumatoid factors) than did white men. Similar results have been obtained in other rural and urban communities. A triracial study in Durban, Natal, has shown that Bantu male adults have significantly higher levels of IgM (32 per cent more), IgG (40 per cent more), and IgA (32 per cent more) in their sera than comparable whites in this community, born in the same year and having the same ABO blood group. Healthy Asiatic male adults had about 20 per cent more IgG, 23 per cent more IgA, and 7 per cent more IgM than comparable whites. Control groups used in these studies were matched for age, sex, and race, as well as for several environmental factors.

In addition to the above-stated biologic factors which may influence immunoglobulin levels in serum, very recent data indicate that the concentration of all four human subclasses of IgG appear to be under *genetic control*, affected to some extent by the Gm phenotype of the individual. The data

Table 36-7. SERUM IgG CONCENTRATION IN A BIRACIAL POPULATION

SEX	AGE (YEARS)	NO. SAMPLES TESTED	WHITES MEAN (±SE) (mg/ml)		NO. SAMPLES TESTED	NEGROES MEAN (±SE) (mg/ml)	
Men	15–34	17	11.2	(7.3)	21	13.4	(6.5)
	35–54	17	10.8	(5.9)	19	13.5	(9.0)
	55–74	20	10.9	(7.4)	20	13.3	(5.8)
Women	15–34	19	10.6	(6.3)	18	15.6	(8.0)
	35–54	19	12.3	(3.4)	15	15.4	(6.4)
	55–74	20	10.9	(6.1)	16	14.2	(9.6)

The data are representative of subjects living in Evans County, Georgia (Lichtman, 1967).

indicate that, in Caucasians, individuals homozygous for the allelic factors Gm4, Gm23, and Gm5 found on IgG_1, IgG_2, and IgG_3 molecules, respectively (see Table 36–2), have higher levels of these immunoglobulin isotypes than do individuals homozygous for the allelic factors Gm1 (IgG_1), Gm17 (IgG_1), and Gm21 (IgG_3). Furthermore, certain Gm factors apparently affect the concentration of other immunoglobulin classes. For example, Caucasians homozygous for Gm4 and Gm5 have lower serum IgD levels than those homozygous for Gm1 and Gm21. Extension of these studies into non-Caucasian subjects may eventually be correlated with the differences seen in immunoglobulin levels among the races. Since the Gm factors are located on the heavy chain constant regions responsible for the many biologic activities of the antibody molecule, it seems likely that the selective force(s) for constant-region genes would be associated with the biologic activity of the immunoglobulin molecules.

BASIC STRUCTURAL FEATURES OF IMMUNOGLOBULINS

Serum Antibodies. The immunoglobulin fraction of normal serum consists mainly of IgG antibodies with molecular weight of approximately 150,000 daltons and a sedimentation coefficient of 7S (see Table 36–1). The other major antibody population in serum is IgM, a polymer immunoglobulin, with a molecular weight of about 900,000 daltons and a 19S sedimentation value. The physical properties of the other antibodies (immunoglobulins) found in serum are given in Table 36–1.

Reductive Cleavage of Antibodies. Edelman (1961) showed by zone electrophoresis under denaturing and reducing conditions that rabbit IgG antibodies consisted of two types of polypeptide chains. Likewise, Porter described two sizes of polypeptide chains by gel filtration (molecular sieving) (Fig. 36–5) under conditions similar to those used by Edelman (Fleishman, 1962). The 50,000 dalton polypeptide was called heavy (H) chain and

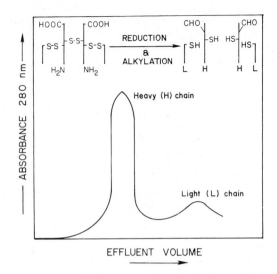

Figure 36–5. Gel filtration of reduced and alkylated immunoglobulin G on Sephadex G75 in 1N acetic acid. The heavy and light chain fractions are labeled. A simple scheme of the reductive cleavage is shown (Modified from Fleishman, 1962).

contained covalently attached carbohydrate. The lower molecular weight polypeptide (23,000 daltons) was designated light (L) chain and lacked carbohydrate. From these studies, the basic structure of an IgG molecule was formulated as 2 H-chains and 2 L-chains based on the amount of both polypeptides recovered from the molar amount of native IgG reduced (Fig. 36–5). Subsequent studies with other human immunoglobulin isotypes as well as with animal species have shown that all possess the same fundamental disulfide-linked, four-chain structure. Cleavage of these molecules with mercaptans (dithiothreitol, 2-mercaptoethanol) followed by alkylation, yields identical molar ratios of the two constituent polypeptide chains, i.e., one light chain for each heavy chain recovered. However, differences do occur between antibody molecules in the number of four-chain units per immunoglobulin protein and the additional appearance of accessory polypeptides (J chain, secretory component). The structure of polymeric immunoglobulins is illustrated in Figure 36–2.

Figure 36–6. Structural analysis of the immunoglobulin hinge region. Partial sequences of the hinge region are shown for human IgG_1 paraprotein Eu, rabbit IgG, guinea pig IgG_2, and mouse IgG_2. The sequences are aligned for maximum homology. The dots indicate possible deletion positions. The solid lines indicate the extent of sequence homology of the various proteins

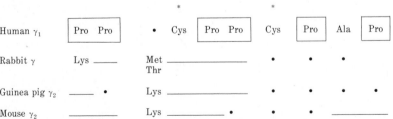

with the human sequence. The positions of non-homology are identified by the specific amino acid substitutions. The cysteine residues involved in the interheavy disulfide linkage are marked by an asterisk. The two proline-rich peptides are delineated by solid boxes separated by the small glycine-rich peptide (dashed box).

Enzymatic Cleavage of Antibodies. Immunoglobulins can be split by the proteolytic enzyme papain into two major 3.5S components. The fragment capable of combining with antigen to form a soluble complex, which will not precipitate because it is univalent, was designated Fab (fragment antigen binding) by Porter (1959). The other fragment, which lacks binding affinity for antigen, is termed Fc (fragment crystallizable), even though these Fc fragments (N225-N446) do not crystallize readily (Fig. 36-4, p. 1228).

Another proteolytic enzyme, pepsin, cleaves the intact IgG molecules above the interheavy chain disulfide bond toward the C-terminus, generating a 5S component consisting of two Fab fragments and designated Fab'2, which is bivalent and can still precipitate with antigen (Nisonoff, 1960). Extensive reduction of Fab'2 or Fab with mercaptans yields an Fd' or Fd fragment (N-terminal half of the heavy chain), respectively, and free light chain. The abridged Fc fragment is called pFc' (N334-N446). Frequently, though, the Fc part of the molecule is completely digested. The enzyme-sensitive portion of antibody molecules is designated the "hinge" region. Using appropriate digestion conditions, pepsin cleavage can also be restricted to the interdomain segment between C_H2 and C_H3, yielding the fragment Facb (fragment antigen and complement binding) which spans residues N1-N330. Furthermore, pepsin cleavage of Fab'2 or Fab fragment can yield an Fv (fragment variable) fragment under carefully controlled conditions (Fig. 36-4, p. 1228).

Disulfide Bonds. With few exceptions, immunoglobulins possess both interchain H-L and H-H disulfide bonds (Fig. 36-5). The light chain cysteine residue that contributes to the H-L linkage is at the C-terminus of the chain (human κ) or adjacent to it (human λ). This contrasts to the position of the H-L linking cysteine residues in the heavy chain at position 131 or about 214, depending on isotype and animal species (Fig. 36-6). While these disulfide bonds stabilize the structure, they apparently are not essential in every case, since some IgA monomers and IgD molecules lack the H-L bonds. On the other hand, the H-H disulfides are critical, along with their high proline content, in giving the "hinge" region of the molecule a degree of inflexibility (Fig. 36-6). This structural feature is important in allowing the Fab arms of the molecule to rotate 180 degrees (segmental flexibility) in solution or on the surface of cells for antigen interaction.

All immunoglobulin proteins have intrachain disulfide bonds which are essential in establishing the domain structure in both polypeptide chains (Figs. 36-3 and 36-4). Reduction of these intrachain bonds followed by sequence analysis has revealed that each domain segment contains a single disulfide loop which spans 60 to 80 amino acid residues. The average length of each domain segment is approximately 110 residues, which includes the amino acid residues of the disulfide loop. The light chains of human IgG have two loop sections per polypeptide chain, while the heavy chains have four loop sections. Heavy chains derived from human IgM (μ) and IgE (ϵ) paraproteins contain an additional loop section (see Fig. 36-3, p. 1220) which is responsible for the higher molecular weight of these chains.

The polymeric immunoglobulins are characterized by possessing *intersubunit* disulfide bonds, which are essential in maintaining the structure of their polymeric form. In addition, they contain the accessory polypeptide J chain, which is also disulfide linked between two monomer units (see Fig. 36-2) (Mestecky, 1974). The secretory component or transport (T) piece found exclusively in dimeric secretory IgA may be disulfide linked to the monomers (Underdown, 1977) (see p. 1220).

VARIABILITY IN STRUCTURE RELATED TO ANTIBODY SPECIFICITY

Sequence Analysis. Amino acid analysis of a number of purified paraproteins and induced antibodies has revealed that, within a given major immunoglobulin isotype, the N-terminal amino acid (N1-N110) portions of both heavy and light chains show considerable variation, whereas the remaining part of the chains is relatively constant in structure. A comparison of light chain sequences has revealed that residues around positions 30, 50, and 90 are hypervariable (Fig. 36-7). These

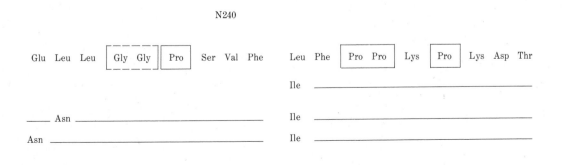

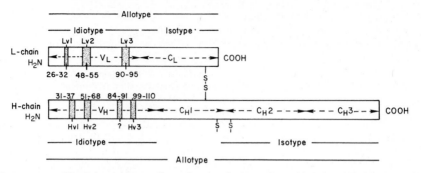

Figure 36–7. The structure of the light and heavy chains showing the positions and lengths of the hypervariable regions in the V_L domain (designated Lv1, Lv_2, Lv_3) and V_H domain (designated Hv1, Hv2, Hv3). The amino acid residues are numbered starting from the N-terminal. In some heavy chains an additional (?) hypervariable region (N89-N91) has been observed. The diagram also illustrates the region(s) where the major immunoglobulin variants may be found. The idiotypic determinants are found exclusively in the V_L and V_H domains and the isotypic marker in the constant regions of both chains. The allotypic markers can occur throughout the entire length of both chains.

"hot spots" on the light chains are designated L_v1, L_v2, and L_v3, respectively. A similar conclusion was reached for the heavy chain after extensive sequence analysis of V_H regions. The relative positions of the three heavy chain hypervariable segments (H_v1, H_v2, and H_v3) in the variable region of the molecule are illustrated in Figures 36-7 and 36-8. An additional segment of hypervariability (positions 86 to 91) has been described for some heavy chains.

The Antigen-binding Site. Several studies have shown that the proteolytic fragments Fab or Fab'2 obtained from induced antibodies contain the antigen-specific binding sites, thus implicating the variable domains (V_L/V_H) or the constant domains (C_L/C_H1) in antigen recognition. Further digestion of the Fab fragments from a mouse myeloma protein (having DNP-lysine specificity) with pepsin yielded the Fv fragment, which contains only the V_L/V_H domain held together by non-covalent interactions (Fig. 36-4) (Wells, 1973). Thus, the V_L/V_H domain was capable of binding DNP-lysine and contained the idiotypic specificity (see idiotypy).

Indirect evidence that the variable region is part of the antigen-binding site has resulted from the work of Wu (1970) and others. In these studies the amino acid sequences of variable regions of both light and heavy chains derived from paraproteins or induced antibodies were analyzed for the extent of residue variation. The degree of variability in each of the V_H positions is illustrated in Figure 36-8. Similar results have been obtained for the V_L region. More direct evidence that the variable region on both heavy and light chains contributes to antibody specificity is suggested by experiments in which isolated chains were examined for their antigen-combining potential. Isolated heavy chains demonstrate varying degrees of residual activity, but light chains show relatively little. However, on recombination there was always a significant increase in antigen-binding capacity.

Significant insight into the nature and location of antibody-combining sites has come from affinity-labeling experiments first pioneered by Singer (Singer, 1966; Thorpe, 1969). In this method, radioactive chemical labels similar to the antigen used to elicit the antibody response are allowed to attach to amino acid residues in or very near the active sites of the antibody molecule. The reactive residue(s) can then be identified by isolating the labeled peptides from the antibody molecule or by limited sequence analysis of each hypervariable region in both heavy and light chains. In general, each of the six hypervariable regions in the V_L/V_H domain has been implicated in binding radiolabeled ligands. Lysyl, arginyl, tyrosyl, and tryptophanyl residues frequently are tagged with site-directed affinity labels in antibodies with different specificities.

Poljak has reported the three-dimensional structure of the Fab' fragment of a human paraprotein (1973). This work provides the most precise view into the combining site which involves the variable regions of both light and heavy chains (Fig. 36-9). This study and others revealed a molecule with four globular subunits that correspond to the homology regions of the light chain V_L and C_L and the heavy chain V_H and C_H1. The four homology subunits of Fab' closely resemble each other, sharing a basic pattern of polypeptide chain folding (Fig. 36-9). The existence of this underlying structural pattern further supports the postulate that a gene duplication mechanism gave rise to the subunit structure of immunoglobulins (Fig. 36-10). The regions of the hypervariable sequences in the light and heavy chains occur in close spatial proximity to each other and form a shallow groove (15 × 6 Å, with a depth

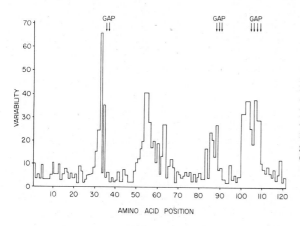

Figure 36-8. An analysis of human heavy chain variable region sequences. Variability in a given residue position is defined as the number of different amino acids found in that position divided by the frequency of the most common amino acid at that position. GAP indicates positions at which insertions have been found. The frequency of insertions ($\downarrow$) is greatest in the Hv3 region (N100-N110) (Modified from Capra, 1975).

of 6 Å) at an exposed end of the molecule, in a region where the coiled polypeptide chains are least subject to structural constraints (Fig. 36-9). The number and nature of the amino acid residues present in this region will determine the geometry of this area, the antigen binding, and the idiotypic specificities of immunoglobulins and antibodies. The position of residues frequently modified in affinity-labeling experiments falls within the binding groove (Givol, 1973).

4

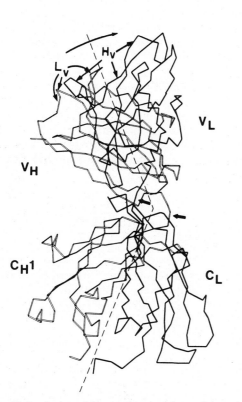

Figure 36-9. A view of the α carbon backbone of the polypeptide chain of Fab' domain of human IgG, (λ) protein based on x-ray crystallography. The open line indicates the light chain (V_L and C_L) and the solid line indicates the V_H and C_H1 domains of the heavy chain. The two short arrows indicate the V-C switch region of both chains. The longer arrow indicates a possible motion of the V and C_1 domains. The approximate positions of the light and heavy chain hypervariable regions are indicated. Note the difference in the angle between the V_L and C_L subunits and that between the V_H and C_H1 subunits. The twofold axes of symmetry are depicted by the dashed line (Reproduced with permission Poljak, 1974).

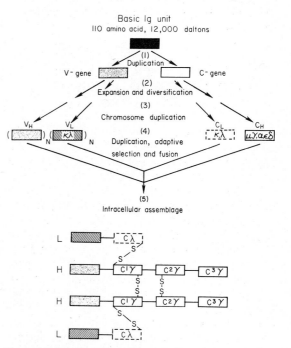

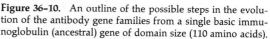

Figure 36-10. An outline of the possible steps in the evolution of the antibody gene families from a single basic immunoglobulin (ancestral) gene of domain size (110 amino acids).

Idiotypy. Amino acid substitutions in the variable domains of antibody molecules give rise to structurally different antigen-combining sites. Such variable region structures, when injected into heterologous species, have elicited antibodies against individual antigenic determinants referred to as idiotypes. Attempts to correlate a specific variable region amino acid sequence to a given idiotypic determinant are inconclusive. This has strengthened the supposition that a given idiotype may consist of a set of reactivities and that tertiary structure requiring both chains is needed for full idiotypic expression (Natvig, 1973).

An examination of streptococcal antibodies in a large number of immunized rabbits revealed that related rabbits produce streptococcal antibodies with the same idiotype, while unrelated rabbits did not. These studies were extended to mice, and proof was obtained that idiotypes are inherited, indicating the inheritance of variable genes (V-genes) responsible for the chemical structure associated with the binding site of antibodies. The inheritance of identical or similar idiotypes is not always demonstrable because an idiotype is a complex phenotype. What has, in fact, become evident in recent years is the interrelationships between hypervariable regions, idiotypy, and the antibody-combining site. The location of idiotypic determinants in immunoglobulin G molecules and that of the other two major immunoglobulin variants is illustrated in Figures 36-7 and 36-8.

STRUCTURAL CORRELATES UNRELATED TO ANTIBODY SPECIFICITY

The constant domains of immunoglobulin molecules (C_L, C_H1, C_H2, C_H3, and C_H4 for μ and ε chains only) are not directly involved in antigen binding. However, they do show considerable heterogeneity in primary structure but to a far lesser extent than the hypervariable segments of the V_L/V_H domain. Variability in the constant regions has been observed in both polypeptide chains and in all immunoglobulin isotypes regardless of their origin. The detection of these structural differences in the constant domains of immunoglobulin molecules was made possible first by use of specific antisera and subsequently by sequence analysis. These specific antisera detect characteristic chemical groups associated with either isotypic or allotypic determinants.

Light Chains. The light chains (about 214 amino acids) are common to all immunoglobulin isotypes. Structural examination of light chains was made possible by the discovery that some individuals with myeloma disease have in their urine a monoclonal dimeric form of light chains called Bence Jones protein. The dimer polypeptide chain is derived from the light chain pool in the synthesis of the myeloma immunoglobulin protein. Serologic analysis with antisera raised in rabbits against Bence Jones proteins from several patients led to the discovery of two isotypic forms of light chains (κ and λ). The isotypic determinant of κ or λ resides in the C_L domain. As one would expect, the parent myeloma protein and its complementary Bence Jones protein would react only with either κ or λ antisera, never both. The reaction of normal globulin (normal serum antibodies) with these reagents showed that molecules with κ or λ chains are present. The two isotypic specificities were never found on the same molecule. The ratio of $\kappa:\lambda$ in normal serum is 2:1, although this ratio can vary in different species, as well as between different populations of antibodies (see Table 36-2). Interestingly, the number of reported cases of myeloma protein carrying κ or λ chains is also approximately 2:1 (65 per cent:35 per cent) suggesting that the cells producing κ or λ chains are at equal risk for neoplastic conversion.

The first 22 amino acids of the N-terminal end of light chains are relatively invariant. Based on numerous sequence analyses, κ chains can be classified into at least 3 subgroups (κI, κII, and κIII) (Table 36-8). Positions N9 and N13 contain characteristic amino acids for each of the κ subgroups (Figure 36-11). Similar results were obtained for λ chains, classifying them into 5 subgroups (λI-V). Thus, sequencing light chains up to residue N110 is generally sufficient for typing them, since V_κ is always found with C_κ (N111-N120) and V_λ with C_λ.

In human κ chain, specific amino acid substitutions determine the isotypic variants associated with subtyping the κ chain into three subtypes, Km 1-3 (see Tables 36-1 and 36-8). Leucine is always present for specificity Km 1 and 2 and valine for specificity Km 3. The λ chain has been also subtyped into Oz^+ and Oz^- (Table 36-8) by amino acid substitutions in the $C\lambda$ domain. In λ Oz^+ chains, positions 154 and 191 are occupied by serine and lysine respectively. More extensive sequence analyses have further classified Oz^- chain into three sub-subtypes.

As indicated earlier, κ chains terminate in cysteine at position 214 and λ chains terminate in serine at position 215 with a penultimate cysteine residue. These cysteine residues are involved in H-L

Table 36–8. SUMMARY OF IMMUNOGLOBULIN VARIANTS

TYPE OF VARIATION	DISTRIBUTION	VARIANT	LOCATION	EXAMPLES
Isotypic	All variants present in serum of a normal individual	Classes Subclasses Types Subtypes Subgroups	C_H C_H C_L C_L V_L, V_H	IgM, IgE IgA$_1$, IgA$_2$ κ, λ $\lambda 0z^+, \lambda 0z^-, \kappa$Km (1)-(3) $V_{\kappa I}$-$V_{\kappa I}$, $V_{\lambda I}$-$V_{\lambda VI}$
Allotypic	Allelic forms not present in all individuals	Allotypes	Mainly C_H/C_L Occasionally V_H/V_L	Gm group (human) b$_4$, b$_5$, b$_6$, b$_9$ rabbit light chain
Idiotypic	Antigenic individuality specific to each Ig molecule	Idiotypes	V_H/V_L	Determinant identified by antibody specific to an individual myeloma protein or antibody molecule

Modified from Roitt, 1977.

chain linkage. The cysteine residues involved in intrachain disulfide loop formation in both chains are conserved in the same positions.

Allotypy. Allotypic variations have been localized in the C_L and H chain domains in rabbit IgG (Table 36–8). The so-called group b allotypic variants occur on κ chains and group c variants with λ chains; therefore, these are mutually exclusive on a single molecule. Heavy chain allotypes are considered below in the discussion of heavy chains. If allotypes represent primary genetic differences, then there must be differences in primary protein structure associated with allotypic variation. The most acceptable explanation for the existence of allotypes is that they represent the accumulation of non-deleterious mutations in replicate copies of an ancestral immunoglobulin gene.

Heavy Chains. Similar studies using specific antisera prepared against normal and myeloma proteins have established the existence of five major classes of heavy chains (μ, γ, α, δ, and ε) in the human, each of which gives

rise to a distinct immunoglobulin isotype of either κ or λ origin. Although all five isotypes of human immunoglobulins have the same basic four-chain structure in the monomeric form, they differ characteristically in the amino acid sequence of their class-specific heavy chain. This difference is restricted to the constant region sequences, which are homologous but unique to each class of heavy chain. Furthermore, the constant region sequences of heavy chains determine such characteristic differences in immunoglobulin class structure as (a) the length of the chain and the number of domains, (b) the number and location of the interchain, intrachain, and intersubunit disulfide bridges, (c) the position, number, and kind of oligosaccharides attached to the heavy chain, and (d) the degree of polymerization of the immunoglobulin molecules (Fig. 36–3).

Antibodies generally exhibit two sets of interlinked functions in which the heavy chain is the major participant: (a) specific binding of antigen at the Fv region of the molecule and (b) biologic or effector activities.

				N$_5$				*	N10				*	N15				N20			
$V_{\kappa I}$	Asp Asx	Ile	*Gln* *Glx*	Met Leu	Thr	Gln Glx	Ser	Pro	*Ser*	Ser Thr	Leu	Ser	*Ala* *Thr*	Ser Val	*Val*	Gly	*Asp*	Arg	*Val* Ile	Thr	Ile	*Thr*
$V_{\kappa II}$	*Glu* Glx Lys	Ile Met	Val	Leu Met	Thr	Gln Glx	Ser	Pro	*Gly* *Ala*	Thr	Leu	Ser	*Leu*	Ser	Pro	Gly	Glu Glx	Arg	Ala	Thr Ala	*Leu*	Ser
$V_{\kappa III}$	Asp	Ile	Val	Met Leu	Thr	Gln	Ser Thr	Pro	*Leu*	Ser	Leu	*Pro*	*Val*	*Thr*	Pro	Gly	Glu	*Pro*	Ala	*Ser*	Ila	Ser

Figure 36–11. The subtyping of human κ chains based upon amino acid sequence analyses. The residues underlined indicate subtype-specific amino acid substitutions. The asterisk marks positions N9 and N13 where subtype-specific substitutions occur in all three types of κ chains. Glx or Asx signifies the presence of either the amide or acidic form of glutamyl or aspartyl (From Hood, 1971).

The latter functions are localized at the Fc part of the molecule and under physiologic conditions come into effect only after antigen binding. The current consensus is that the binding of antigen by the Fab transmits a signal through the "hinge" region, causing an allosteric change in the conformation of the Fc structure. This change in conformation is believed to be responsible for amplifying the specific effector activity associated with a given Fc structure. Hydrodynamic studies further suggest that the Fab fragments of human, rabbit, guinea pig, and mouse are linked to the Fc domains through a flexible "hinge" region. Chemical studies have confirmed that the "hinge" region contains two relatively inflexible proline-rich peptide sequences connected by a highly flexible glycine-rich region (see Fig. 36-6). This distinctive structural arrangement may permit the more facile movement of Fab fragment *vis-à-vis* the Fc and seems responsible for the susceptibility of immunoglobulin molecules to proteolytic cleavage at the "hinge" region (see Fig. 36-4).

Structural examination of all human γ_1 myeloma heavy chains has shown that they share an identical amino acid sequence from N111 to the C-terminal end except for a few changes which account for the heavy chain constant region allotypic markers, Gm (see Tables 36-1 and 36-2). Similar to the κ chain Km allotypes, these structural differences can be distinguished serologically. The γ_1 constant domains (C_H1, C_H2, and C_H3) show very little amino acid sequence homology with any other heavy chain (including those of γ_2, γ_3, and γ_4). These polypeptide chains, in turn, have their own characteristic constant region sequences and isotypic and allotypic markers (see Table 36-2). All γ_1 Gm allotype markers can, in some cases, be defined by specific sequences. The Am allotype marker is found in the Fc region of α_2 chains (see Table 36-1). In rabbits, group a allotypic markers have been assigned to the heavy chain V_H domain (see Fig. 36-7).

Analogous to the light chain, the N-terminal 22 amino acid sequences of heavy chains fall into four subtypes (V_HI to V_HIV). However, the heavy chain subtypes appear to be shared by all heavy chain classes, which is in contrast to the light chain, where subtype association with a given light chain class occurs.

In summary, immunoglobulins can, therefore, be classified according to three different parameters related to different antigenic and biochemical structures (see Table 36-1): (a) Heavy chain constant regions constitute the basis for the different classes and subclasses.

(b) Light chain C regions specify the types or subtypes. (c) Variable regions of both heavy and light chains can be divided into different groups and subgroups.

Immunoglobulin Domain. The domain hypothesis proposed by Edelman (1962) has provided an important conceptual framework upon which to build our understanding of the structural and functional properties of immunoglobulins and antibodies. Primary sequence data provided the first impetus toward the formulation of a domain concept. Complete amino acid sequences have been determined for κ, λ, γ, μ, α, and ε chains of human immunoglobulins. Taken together, these sequences have indicated that both heavy and light chains could be divided into contiguous homology regions. The extent of sequence homology between the regions is variable. The light chain homologous subunits were designated V_L and C_L. The heavy chains have one V_H domain and three or four constant region domains, C_H1 to C_H4 (see Fig. 36-3).

Another evidence in favor of the domain hypothesis is the linear, periodic arrangement of the intrachain disulfide bonds. X-ray crystallography of several Fab fragments has shown that these bonds are important in allowing each homology region to assume a compact globular structure. The four homology subunits of Fab' closely resemble each other, sharing a basic pattern of polypeptide chain folding (see Fig. 36-9). The angle between the major axes of the C_L and V_L homology subunits is greater than 90 degrees, whereas the angle between the axes of the C_H1 and V_H subunits is smaller than 90 degrees (see Fig. 36-9). As a result, the Fd' chain (N-terminal half of the heavy chain) is more folded over itself, displaying a closer association between the V_H and C_H1 subunits than is the case for the V_L and C_L subunits of the light chain. The linkage between the V-domain (V_L/V_H) and the C_1 domain (C_L/C_H1) occurs by more loosely folded stretches (see Fig. 36-9). Analogous to the "hinge" region, this structural arrangement may allow a possible relative motion of the V and C_1 domain, as well as susceptibility to enzymatic cleavage yielding the Fv fragment (Poljak, 1975).

In formulating the domain concept, Edelman proposed that each domain has evolved to perform a specific function(s). Recent experimental data have lent support to this viewpoint. A summary of the current state of knowledge regarding the functional differentiation of immunoglobulin domains is given in Table 36-9. Although a number of biologic properties of immunoglobulins have not been

Table 36-9. BIOLOGIC PROPERTIES
OF IMMUNOGLOBULIN DOMAINS
(Dorrington, 1974)

DOMAIN	KNOWN OR PROBABLE FUNCTION

C_H3	1. Cytotrophic reactions involving:
	   (a) Macrophages and monocytes
	   (b) Heterologous mast cells
	   (c) Cytotoxic killer (K) cells
	   (d) B cells

C_H2	1. Binding of complement (Clq) 2. Control of catabolic rate
C_H1/C_L	1. Non-covalent bonding of heavy and light chains 2. Site of heavy-light chain disulfide bond 3. Spacers between interdomain interactions involving antigen binding and effector functions 4. Influences the segmental flexibility of the molecule (?)
V_H/V_L	1. Antigen binding 2. Non-covalent bonding of heavy and light chains

From Dorrington, K. J., and Painter, R. H.: Functional
domains of immunoglobulin G. *In* Brent, L., and Holborow, J. (eds.): Progress in Immunology II. Amsterdam,
North Holland Publishing Co., 1974.

ascribed to a particular domain yet, it has
become evident that the concept of struc-
tural-functional domains now stands as one
of the basic principles of immunoglobulin
biology.

Accessory Polypeptide Chains. Recent
studies on polymeric immunoglobulins have
shown the presence of a polypeptide chain, the
J chain, in addition to the H and L chains that
compose the monomer unit. The presence of
the J chain in polymeric immunoglobulins and
its absence from monomeric immunoglobulins
suggest that it may be important in facilitating the polymerization of the IgA and IgM
subunits into their appropriate polymeric
form (Inman, 1974). In the case of secretory
IgA, the presence of J chain is clearly mandatory for the association of the secretory component (SC). The binding site for SC is probably in the Fc structure, the conformation of
which is dependent on the presence of J chain
(see Fig. 36-2).

The J chain is a small glycopeptide with a
distinctive acidic property and a fast electrophoretic mobility in alkaline gels. The J polypeptide contains significantly large amounts
of arginine (9 residues), aspartic acid (20 residues), and glutamic acid (13 residues) per molecule, has a molecular weight of 15,000 daltons,

and represents less than 5 per cent of the total
polymer protein.

The J chain is a very hydrophilic protein, with
charged amino acids and amides of carboxylic acids
constituting about 40 per cent of the total residues,
whereas the other immunoglobulin polypeptide
chains and secretory component have a greater
number of hydrophobic amino acids. Such data
strongly suggest that the J chain has evolved independently of all other immunoglobulin chains and
secretory component. However, studies of polymer
biosynthesis by mouse plasma cell tumors have
shown that J chain is manufactured in the same
cells as the H and L chains of either μ or α cell
lineage. The J chains isolated from human polymeric IgA and IgM have been shown to be identical
in amino acid composition, peptide maps, and antigenicity. The carbohydrate content and composition are similar to those found in μ chains themselves, but they lack galactosamine. Quantitative
measurements indicate that there is a single
J chain in each IgM pentamer or polymeric IgA
molecule. The J polypeptide is covalently bonded to
the penultimate cysteine residue of α and probably
μ chains linking only two of the subunits of these
polymeric immunoglobulins (see Fig. 36-2). Physiochemical studies have indicated that the J chain is
a very elongated molecule. This is based on its low
diffusion coefficient (approximately 8) and a large
minimum axial ratio of about 18, while with other
known globular proteins of similar molecular
weight the converse occurs.

The *secretory component* is preferentially
associated with dimeric IgA in external secretions but is not bound to any protein in serum,
including serum type IgA. The secretory component may exist in free form or bound to
secretory IgA by strong non-covalent interactions. The binding does not usually involve
covalent bonding, although disulfide bonds
have been implicated in a small fraction of
human secretory IgA molecules (see Fig. 36-
2). Bound and free secretory components have
been isolated and compared in human and
rabbit, and within each species they were reported to be similar in molecular weight
(71,000 daltons for human and 70,000 daltons
for rabbit), peptide maps, amino acid sequences of the first 14 residues, and antigenic
determinants. The secretory component is a
single glycopeptide with a high carbohydrate
content and an electrophoretic mobility in the
fast β range. At present, it is not possible to
speculate on the evolutionary origin of secretory component, since it does not have homology to any known protein.

Much of the IgA secreted by the plasma cells
in exocrine glands and mucous membranes is

4

dimeric. The secreted IgA passes from the interstitial tissues across the epithelial basement membrane into epithelial layer. At some point prior to its secretion into the lumen it combines with secretory component, which is made in epithelial cells. Thus, the fully assembled secretory IgA molecule is the synthetic product of two distinct types of cell (α plasma cells and epithelial cells), both of which reside locally in the mucous membrane or gland. The exact site where dimeric IgA couples with secretory component is not known but may well be inside the epithelial cell or at its surface.

Carbohydrate Moieties of Immunoglobulins. One of the striking differences in the structure of immunoglobulin is the number, sequence, kind, and location of carbohydrate groups. Carbohydrate is found usually in the constant regions of heavy chains, most frequently in the C_H2 domain. Rarely do the V_H domain and light chain have carbohydrate.

Most human α chains contain two or three oligosaccharide groups, but all of them contain at least one group attached at asparagine 297. Secretory IgA has a higher carbohydrate content than serum IgA because the secretory component contains more carbohydrate than the α chain.

Studies on monoclonal immunoglobulins have indicated that IgG has only one oligosaccharide group and that both IgM and IgE generally have an average of five groups. This agrees with the overall carbohydrate of immunoglobulins, since IgM, IgD, and IgE have the largest amounts of oligosaccharide, followed by IgA and then by IgG (see Table 36-1, p. 1216).

Each of the constant domains of human μ chain contain at least one carbohydrate moiety. The $C_\mu2$ domain has two oligosaccharide groups whose structures are heterogeneous. One group consists of a linear unbranched polymer (simple form), while the other displays an extensively branched polymeric form (complex). Like the α chain carbohydrate, all the μ chain oligosaccharides are attached to an asparagine residue in the obligatory sequence Asn-X-Ser/Thr through an N-glycosidic bond involving N-acetylglucosamine. Carbohydrates can attach to this sequence wherever it occurs in the immunoglobulin molecule. Should the sequence occur by chance in the V_H region or light chain, then carbohydrate would also attach there. A small number of immunoglobulin polypeptide chains having carbohydrate in the V_H region have been reported. Another, less common type of linkage is the O-glycosidic bond between an amino sugar of

an oligosaccharide side chain and a serine residue of the polypeptide chain.

Only IgA and IgD have both N-acetylgalactosamine and N-acetylglucosamine. Other carbohydrate residues common to immunoglobulin oligosaccharides are fucose, mannose, galactose, and sialic acid.

The hydrophilic nature of carbohydrates suggests that they are on the surface of immunoglobulin affecting perhaps the conformation of the Fc and the solubility of the molecule. Although the precise function of the carbohydrate moiety is poorly understood, it seems almost certain to play an important role in the secretion of antibodies by plasma cells and in biologic functions associated with the Fc fragment.

TWO GENES,
ONE POLYPEPTIDE CHAIN

The recognition of variable and constant regions led to the hypothesis that separate variable (V) and constant (C) genes code for the two regions of light and heavy chains (Dreyer, 1965). This hypothesis has not been disproved, and the idea that two structural genes code for each immunoglobulin polypeptide chain has become widely accepted as a basis for theories of anibody diversity. In heavy chains, the C_H gene is believed to have duplicated and fused before linking with the V_H gene (see Fig. 36-10). Both sequence data and high resolution x-ray analysis of Fab fragments have indicated that the domain is the obvious unit of immunoglobulin gene evolution.

Experimental support for the two-gene hypothesis has come from various laboratories and from many studies. Based on physiochemical properties, amino acid sequence, and individual specific antigenic determinants, two paraproteins (IgM$_\kappa$ and IgG$_\kappa$) isolated from the same serum were shown to share three of the four genes (V_L, C_L, and V_H) controlling the biosynthesis of these two myeloma proteins. As mentioned earlier, paraproteins are homogeneous products of a single clone of malignant plasma cells. A plausible interpretation of these results would be that a genetic switching event must have occurred in one or more cells involving only the C_H gene. Extensive genetic studies have now clearly established that the C regions of μ and γ chains are synthesized by different structural genes. The sharing of identical V regions by the μ chain and the λ chain is consistent with a number of biologic observations. It is well-known that maturation of an immune response is accompanied by a change in the dominant antibody isotype produced (IgM → IgG). During this "switch" period a number of immunocytes are frequently found which synthesize both IgM and IgG molecules. In an attempt to explain these observations at the molecular level, immunogeneticists have proposed a "genetic switch" hypothesis. It states that following a primary immunization, a given V_H gene is translocated to a C_μ gene to initiate the synthesis of IgM antibody. With the maturation of the response in one or more of the immunocytes, this same V_H gene becomes linked to a C_γ gene to initiate the synthesis of IgG antibody. In these immunocytes, then, the C_γ gene is derepressed, the C_μ gene is repressed, and the genes controlling the variable portions of the light and heavy chain and constant part of the heavy chain remain unchanged. Furthermore, it is believed that the two genes which code for the variable (V) and constant (C) portions are not adjacent.

The a1, a2, and a3 allotypic markers of rabbit heavy chains are of great interest because they occur in the V_H regions of different classes of heavy chains (γ, α, μ, etc.) and thus are frequently interpreted as indirect evidence in support of the existence of separate V_H genes, which, together with fewer C_H genes, specify a complete polypeptide chain. Complementary pedigree analysis of rabbits with both V region and C region allotype markers showed that V region allotypes are linked to the C region allotypes with predictable genetic recombinations. In light of these and the above results, it seems unlikely that a single gene codes for both the V region and C region of rabbit heavy chain.

The most recent and most powerful evidence in support of the two-gene hypothesis has come from molecular hybridization studies of mouse light chain (κ) genes. The pattern of mRNA-DNA hybridization was completely different in the genomes of mouse embryo cells and adult mouse plasmacytoma cells (Hozumi, 1976). The pattern of embryo DNA showed two components, one of which hybridized with C gene sequences and the other with V gene sequences. The pattern of the adult tumor DNA showed a single component that hybridized with both V gene and C gene sequences. These results can be interpreted to mean that in the embryo genome the V_κ and C_κ genes are some distance away from each other, while in the adult genome they have undergone rearrangement, narrowing the distance between themselves during differentiation of lymphocytes. How this somatic-rearrangement event occurs during lymphocyte differentiation remains an enigma. Recent development in *in vitro* recombinant DNA technique has allowed the cloning of this same mouse V_κ gene from embryo tissue, and its nucleotide sequence is being determined.

A hypothetical scheme for the evolution of immunoglobulin V and C genes is given in Figure 36-10. An early gene duplication gave rise to the primordial V and C genes. The V gene library was expanded through discrete duplications into three V region families (V_λ, V_κ, and V_H). The primordial C gene, in turn, gave rise to the C_λ and C_κ genes, whereas contiguous duplications gave rise to C_H genes (μ, γ, α, ε, and ∂) which consist of three or four homology units the size of the original primordial gene. The lack of sequence homology between the products of V and C genes stresses their early divergence from a common ancestral gene.

ASSEMBLAGE OF IMMUNOGLOBULINS

The synthesis and assembly of immunoglobulins follow the general rules established for proteins that are to be exported from the cell of origin. The assembly may follow any of three possible pathways:

(a) $H + L \longrightarrow HL + HL \longrightarrow H_2L_2$

(b) $H + H \longrightarrow H_2 + L \longrightarrow$
$$H_2L + L \longrightarrow H_2L_2$$

(c) $H + L \longrightarrow HL + H_2L + L \longrightarrow H_2L_2$

There is no single assembly pathway that operates for all cells or all immunoglobulins of any one class. Fully assembled IgG may be secreted 30 to 40 minutes after the initiation of synthesis. Several factors affect the rate of immunoglobulin assembly: (a) the concentration of heavy and light chains at individual sites in the cisternae, (b) the extent of complementarity between the newly synthesized heavy and light chains, particularly their variable regions, (c) the rate of disulfide bond formation, and (d) the rate of glycosylation just prior to secretion. Assembly is more quickly accomplished if equimolar amounts of complementary heavy and light chains are present in balanced concentration in the cisternae (Bevan, 1972).

METHODS FOR DETECTION OF ANTIGENS AND ANTIBODIES

The techniques used for detecting antigens differ depending on whether the antigen of interest is soluble or cell bound. Several of these methods are described in more detail in Chapter 35.

The methods most commonly used to quantitate immunoglobulins in the clinical laboratory are radial immunodiffusion (RID), both Fahey and Mancini variations; electroimmunodiffusion (EID); laser nephelometry; and radioimmunoassay (RIA) for IgE and IgD. Concentrations of immunoglobulin may be estimated by immunoelectrophoresis (IEP), but this is a poor choice to the other methods. On the other hand, of these techniques, only IEP provides a qualitative appraisal of the immunoglobulin, i.e., whether it is monoclonal or polyclonal. Thus, IEP has its greatest use in identifying monoclonal immunoglobulins, while the other methods provide more reliable determinations of the total serum concentration of the immunoglobulin isotope being measured.

IgG, IgA, and IgM are present in the serum in high enough concentrations that RIA is not needed. The choice among the other systems depends on the number of samples and nature of the laboratory facility. Radial immunodiffusion is relatively easy to perform. Systems are commercially available. Variation of technical personnel in reading the plates may be high, however. This seems to be more of a problem with the time-related Fahey method. The plates must be read after a specified elapsed time in this system, a factor that may present a problem to some laboratories. With the Mancini technique, the plates go to completion and thus time of reading is not as critical as long as the reaction is finished. There may be less variation in reader perception of these plates, but the plates may take more than 72 hours—especially for IgM—to be completed.

Electroimmunodiffusion is an excellent technique in the research laboratory, where the number of specimens is not large and the variation in protein concentration not broad. However, the clinical laboratory may need to assay many specimens, and the serum concentrations of immunoglobulins cover a wide range. Thus, EID requires investment in equipment and an appreciation of the levels of immunoglobulins acceptable for the antibody concentration in the plates being used. EID may have a smaller coefficient of variation than RID systems, and results may be obtained within hours after the assay has been initiated.

Laser nephelometry is a relatively new technique for quantitating immunoglobulins. It has the major disadvantage of requiring a moderate investment in equipment. However, it has the potential of being automated, and, being meshed with electronic data processing, it has a lower coefficient of variation than RID, gives results within minutes, and costs about the same per assay as RID, excluding the capital investment in equipment.

Ring Test. This assay is a useful qualitative method for the rapid detection of either soluble antigen or precipitating antibody. It involves carefully overlaying a solution of antibody (antiserum) with a solution of antigen in such a way that a sharp liquid interface is formed. A ring of precipitation occurs near the interface, usually in the antibody layer. An immunologic reaction is called precipitation when the combination of antibody and antigen in solution results in a visible aggregation. The ring test is not a quantitative method. Either antigen or antibody can be detected quickly in amounts as small as $1\,\mu g$ of protein if care is taken in carrying out the test. The reaction is less dependent upon critical initial ratios of antibody and antigen than when these materials are mixed for other immunoprecipitation tests (discussed below and on p. 1186).

Quantitative Precipitation. Immunoprecipitation is the simplest and most direct means of demonstrating antigen-antibody reactions in the laboratory. This occurs when a multivalent antigen reacts with divalent or multivalent antibody. Precipitation depends upon the formation of large insoluble three-dimensional lattices formed by multiple connections of antigen and antibody molecules (see p. 1188).

Gel Immunodiffusion Tests. The gel diffusion test involves a precipitation reaction in a semisolid medium (agar) rather than in a liquid medium (as in the ring test). The object of the immunodiffusion test is to bring together, through diffusion, optimal concentrations of antigen and antibody to form visible precipitation arcs. This test is a valuable guide to purification of either antigen or antibody, since it provides resolution and identification of components in mixtures. The number of precipitin lines indicates the minimal number of antigen-antibody systems present in a given sample, provided that artifacts due to temperature and concentration are excluded and that non-specific reactions are controlled with preimmunization serum. The major advantage of gel diffusion lies in the detection of more than one antigen-antibody system. The test has a high degree of sensitivity, the lower level of detection being a few micrograms of antigen and antibody. Limitations of the gel diffusion technique are of two kinds: (1) its failure to resolve components in some complex mixtures and (2) its failure to detect non-precipitating antibody.

Three gel diffusion assays widely used in clinical immunology laboratories are the Oudin, Preer, and Ouchterlony tests. The tube method developed by

Oudin involves one-dimensional diffusion of one reagent. In small tubes containing a layer of agar in which antiserum (0.5 to 1.0 mg/ml) is uniformly dispersed, the antigen solution is placed on top. As the antigen diffuses into the agar, bands of precipitate develop from reaction of antigen with specific antibody. Since only one reagent diffuses (the antigen), this is called a single-diffusion method. The Preer method is also one-dimensional, but both antigen and antibody diffuse. In this test, undiluted antiserum is placed in the bottom of a small tube previously coated with agar, a layer of agar is placed directly above the serum, and antigen solution is placed on top of the agar layer. Bands of precipitate develop in the agar layer between the two solutions, to which both antigen and antibody migrate. This method involves double diffusion, since the reaction occurs in that part of the tube where neither reactant was originally present. The plate method of Ouchterlony is a powerful but simple technique which allows qualitative detection of antigens in solution and also allows one to determine antigenic relationships between different antigens.

Radial Immunodiffusion. This is a quantitative gel immunoprecipitation technique in which the agar containing the antiserum is poured onto a plate, as in the Ouchterlony method, and wells are cut into it. The radial immunodiffusion test is used routinely, particularly for immunoglobulin (IgM, IgG, and IgA) determinations and also for components such as C3 (third component of complement), C-reactive protein, and many other proteins. Radial immunodiffusion plates are commercially available for the quantitation of the various human serum protein levels. Generally, standards containing known amounts of the protein in question are placed in the same plate as the unknown sample and a standard curve is constructed for them (p. 1190.)

In many cases, when quantitating immunoglobulin levels in pathologic sera, the radial immunodiffusion may be highly inaccurate. For example, polymeric forms of immunoglobulin, such as occurs in multiple myeloma or Waldenström's macroglobulinemia, diffuse more slowly than native monomers, resulting in underestimation of immunoglobulin concentrations in these diseases. Furthermore, high-molecular immune complexes which may circulate in cryoglobulinemia or rheumatoid arthritis will result in falsely low values of immunoglobulins by a similar mechanism. In sera of patients with macroglobulinemia, systemic lupus erythematosus, rheumatoid arthritis, and ataxia telangiectasia, low molecular weight forms of IgM (7S IgM) may be present and thus cause an overestimation of their IgM concentrations. This results from the fact that 7S IgM diffuses more rapidly than 19S IgM parent molecules, which are used as the standard. In some cases of IgA deficiency, patients may have in their serum antibodies to ruminant proteins (including anti-immunoglobulin antibodies). Testing such sera in the radial

immunodiffusion assay will lead to falsely high values of immunoglobulin concentrations because diffusion and precipitation occur in two directions simultaneously.

Conventional Immunoelectrophoresis. Identification and approximate quantitation can be accomplished by these methods for about 30 individual proteins present in serum, urine, or other biologic fluids. Immunoelectrophoresis is a diagnostic tool frequently used, especially in the detection of monoclonal gammopathies (p. 235).

Rocket Immunoelectrophoresis. This technique is a quantitative method which involves electrophoresis of antigen into a gel-containing antibody (see Chap. 35, p. 1193). This test is rapid but restricted to detection of antigens that move to the positive pole on electrophoresis. Thus, it is suitable for proteins such as albumin, transferrin, and ceruloplasmin.

Two-dimensional Immunoelectrophoresis (Crossed Immunoelectrophoresis). This assay can be regarded as a combination of the electrophoretic separation method used in conventional electrophoresis and electroimmunodiffusion (electrophoretic induction of antigen migration to enhance the establishment of a precipitin zone). The antigen mixture is first separated electrophoretically in agarose, as described for immunoelectrophoresis. The strip of agarose containing the separated antigens is then placed on a second slide and an antibody-containing agarose solution is allowed to solidify adjacent to it. Electrophoresis, as described for the rocket system, is then performed at right angles to the original electrophoretic separation, giving rise to peaks. Quantitation is possible with this technique by comparing the surface areas of the precipitated peaks with those given by known amounts of standard antigens.

Radioimmunoelectrophoresis. This assay combines immunoelectrophoresis and radioautography for the detection of radiolabeled antigens. It has been applied most often to the study of proteins or immunoglobulins which are intrinsically labeled with radioactive ^{14}C or ^{3}H amino acids during cellular biosynthesis in tissue culture. Plasma cells or lymphoblastoid cells from continuous cell lines are grown in tissue culture with radioactive amino acids. The supernatant of these cultures contains radioactive protein synthesized and exported by these cultured cells. Concentrated culture supernates are then subjected to electrophoresis according to the conventional immunoelectrophoresis method. The troughs are filled with either antiserum to human serum or with specific antisera for immunoglobulin light or heavy chain. After the precipitation lines have developed, the plate is dried and overlaid with x-ray film. After a period of exposure, the film is developed and the resultant pattern compared with the normal serum proteins present on the stained immunoelectrophoresis plate.

This technique can also be useful in the detection of soluble antigen-antibody complexes.

4

Radioimmunoassay. The most sensitive techniques in use in immunology are the various kinds of radioimmunoassays for the detection and quantitation of antigens. Radioimmunoassays have been developed for the determination of many different substances, such as hormones, immunoglobulin allotypes, carcinoembryonic antigen, hepatitis B (Australia) antigen, steroids, and morphine-related drugs. Radioimmunoassay is discussed in Chapter 13 (p. 385).

Farr Radiobinding Assay. This method assesses antibody level by determining the capacity of an antiserum to complex with radioactive antigen. The point should be stressed that it is not possible to define the absolute concentration of antibody in a given serum because each serum contains immunoglobulins with a range of binding affinities, and the estimation of the amount of antigen bound to antibody depends upon the concentration and affinities of the antibodies as well as the sensitivity of the test. In the Farr technique, the radiolabeled antigen-antibody complexes are separated from the unbound radio-antigen by salt precipitation with 50 per cent ammonium sulfate. This test, however, is applicable only to those antigens soluble at this salt concentration.

Antiglobulin Coprecipitation Assay. In this technique the radio-antigen bound to antibody is precipitated together with the rest of the immunoglobulin by an antiglobulin serum, leaving free antigen in the supernatant. An advantage of this method is that it allows investigators to determine the distribution of antibody among the classes. This is made possible by use of antiserum made against the various immunoglobulin classes and subclasses instead of an antiglobulin reagent. For example, addition of a radio-antigen to human serum followed by a precipitating rabbit antihuman IgA, would indicate how much antigen had been bound to the serum IgA.

Quantitative Immunoadsorption. This method assesses antibody level by measuring the amount of immunoglobulin binding to an insoluble antigen preparation. Generally, reagents such as bisdiazobenzidine or glutaraldehyde are used to insolubilize the antigen(s) by cross-linking them. After the antibody has adsorbed to the insoluble antigen, it is washed thoroughly to remove contaminants, and the antibody is subsequently dissociated from the complex by centrifugation. All the protein present in the supernatant is now specific antibody. With the aid of the single radial immunodiffusion test, the quantitative distribution of antibody classes can be determined in the immunoglobulin pool present in the supernatant. The quantitative immunoadsorption method has proved useful for routine determination of antiglobulin factors in cases of rheumatoid arthritis.

Complement Fixation. Fixation of complement occurs during the interaction of antigen and antibodies and is described in Chapter 37.

The complement fixation tests have received widespread application in both research and clinical laboratory practice. In diagnostic laboratories, it is often used for detection of the Wasserman reaction for syphilis and the *Coccidioides immitis* antigen. Many of the autoantibodies to insoluble subcellular components (for example, antiplatelet antibodies and anti-DNA antibodies) may be detected by the complement fixation test.

Immunofluorescence. Immunofluorescence, a very sensitive histochemical or cytochemical technique for detection and localization of cellular antigens, whether they are cytoplasmic, nuclear, or on the plasma membrane, is discussed on p. 1199 in Chapter 35.

The availability of fluorescein and rhodamine dyes greatly increases the flexibility of immunofluorescence, particularly for studying membrane antigens using the technique of capping. Capping is an energy-requiring process whereby certain membrane molecules accumulate over one pole of a cell (in particular lymphoid cells) when specific antibody molecules bind to them. If an antiserum (IgG fraction) conjugated with fluorescein is used to induce capping, the cap will appear green under the ultraviolet microscope. The capped cells are then subsequently exposed to a second antiserum whose IgG fraction is rhodamine under conditions not allowing further capping. If the two antisera react with the same membrane antigenic complex, the cap will appear green and red under ultraviolet light. On the other hand, if the cap is only green and the rest of the cell surface appears red, this means that the two antisera reacted with different membrane markers. This double labeling technique has been employed to prove that membrane-bound immunoglobulin on mouse B-lymphocytes is not associated with H-2 (major histocompatibility complex) antigens and that the various H-2 antigens coded by different genes are not associated with each other on the membrane.

Enzyme-linked Antibody Technique. In place of fluorescent dyes, investigators have developed methods in which enzymes such as peroxidase or phosphatase are coupled to antibodies, and these can be visualized by conventional histochemical methods at both the light microscope (an advantage) and electron microscope levels. The conjugates used in this test are both immunologically and enzymatically active (p. 1205).

Ferritin-coupled Antibody Technique. Ferritin-conjugated antibody has also been used for ultrastructural localization of antigens; its distribution can be readily seen from its electron density and the characteristic tetrameric appearance of the iron core. This conjugate can be used for either direct or indirect tissue staining. Other electron-dense particles such as gold or uranium have also been introduced chemically into specific anti-tissue antibodies. These reagents have also been applied in immunoelectronmicroscopy.

Autoradiography. Iodinated (^{125}I) immunoglobulins provide highly sensitive probes for the localization of tissue antigens. The antigens are detected visually after tissue staining by overlaying or coating slides with photographic emulsion. Generally, after one to two weeks of exposure, silver grains (as black dots) appear on the photographic plate. This record has been used for subcellular localization of antigen at the light and electron microscope levels. Autoradiography has also been utilized to detect proteins or immunoglobulins synthesized by cells in culture.

Agglutination. Whereas the cross-linking of soluble multivalent protein antigens by antibody leads to precipitation, cross-linking of cells or large insoluble particles by antibody directed against surface antigens leads to agglutination (p. 1196).

Hemolytic Plaque Assay. This test serves to detect and enumerate antibody-producing cells rather than to detect antibodies or antigens. Cells producing hemolytic antibodies (complement binding antibodies) are the most readily detected. For example, in this test antibody-secreting lymphoid cells from mouse spleen, which have been immunized with sheep erythrocytes, are mixed with target sheep erythrocytes in a warm (46°C.) isotonic 0.6 per cent w/v agarose solution. The cell agarose suspension is then overlayered on preformed 1.2 per cent w/v agarose in a Petri dish. The plates are then incubated at 37°C. in a humid atmosphere for two hours, during which time IgM and IgG secreted by the antibody-producing cells diffuse and bind to the target erythrocytes. On addition of complement and further incubation, the erythrocytes which have bound IgM antibody will lyse, causing visible clear plaques in the red agarose lawn, with a plasma cell at the center of each plaque. IgG antibodies do not cause lysis because of their lower lytic and complement-fixing activity. However, including an anti-immunoglobulin serum in the top agarose layer enhances complement binding and hemolysis by specific anti-sheep erythrocyte IgG. Cells which secrete IgM give direct plaques. While IgG-secreting cells require development with the appropriate anti-immunoglobulin, supplemented serum gives indirect plaques. The flexibility of the plaque assay can be increased to include a variety of other non-erythrocyte antigens by modification of target red blood cells, as in the passive hemagglutination assay.

Nephelometry. Nephelometry (see p. 1240) is an old technique recently refined especially with the use of a laser beam to measure immunoglobulins. This technique is described in Chapters 4 (p. 93) and 9 (p. 236).

4

REFERENCES

Bennich, H., and Johansson, S. G. O.: Structure and function of human immunoglobulin E. Adv. Immunol., *13*:1, 1971.

Bevan, M. J., Parkhouse, R. M. R., Williamson, A. R., and Askonas, B. A.: Biosynthesis of immunoglobulins. Prog. Biophys. Mol. Biol., *25*:131, 1972.

Capra, J. D., and Kehoe, J. M.: Hypervariable regions, idiotypy and antibody-combining site. Adv. Immunol., *20*:1, 1975.

Cassidy, J. T., Nordby, G. L., and Dodge, H. J.: Biologic variation of human serum immunoglobulin concentrations: Sex-age specific effects. J. Chron. Dis., *27*:507, 1974.

Dorrington, K. J., and Painter, R. H.: Functional domains of immunoglobulin G. *In* Brent, L., and Holborow, J. (eds.): Progress in Immunology II. Amsterdam, North Holland Publishing Co., 1974.

Dreyer, W. J., and Bennett, J. C.: The molecular basis of antibody formation: A paradox. Proc. Natl. Acad. Sci., *54*:864, 1965.

Edelman, G. M., and Gally, J. A.: *In* Schmitt, F. O. (ed.): The Neurosciences Second Study Program. New York, Rockefeller University Press, 1962.

Edelman, G. M., and Poulik, M. D.: Studies on structural units of the γ globulins. J. Exp. Med., *113*:861, 1961.

Fleishman, J., Pain, R. H., and Porter, R. R.: Reduction of γ-globulins. Arch. Biochem. Biophys., (Suppl. 1):174, 1962.

Givol, D.: Structural analysis of the antibody combining site. *In* Reisfeld, R. A., and Mandy, W. J. (eds.): Contemporary Topics in Molecular Immunology, vol. 2. New York, Plenum Press, 1973.

Hood, L., and Prahl, J.: The immune system—a model for differentiation in higher organisms. Adv. Immunol., *14*:291, 1971.

Hozumi, N., and Tonegawa, S.: Evidence for somatic rearrangement of immunoglobulin genes coding for variable and constant regions. Proc. Natl. Acad. Sci., *73*:3628, 1976.

Inman, F. P., and Mestecky, J.: The J chain of polymeric immunoglobulins. *In* Ada, G. L. (ed.): Contemporary Topics in Molecular Immunology, vol. 3. New York, Plenum Press, 1974.

Kay, M. M. B., and Makinodan, T.: Immunobiology of aging: Evaluation of current status. Clin. Immunol. Immunopathol., *5*:5, 1976.

Lamm, M. E.: Cellular aspects of immunoglobulin A. Adv. Immunol., *22*:223, 1976.

Lichtman, M. A., Vaughan, J. H., and Hames, C. G.: The distribution of serum immunoglobulins, anti-γ-G globulins and antinuclear antibodies in white and Negro subjects in Evans County, Georgia. Arthritis Rheum., *10*:204, 1967.

Mestecky, J., Schrohenloher, R. E., Kulhavy, R., Wright, G. P., and Tomana, M.: Site of J chain attachment to human polymeric IgA. Proc. Natl. Acad. Sci., *71*:554, 1974.

Metzger, H.: Structure and function of γ M macroglobulins. Adv. Immunol., *12*:57, 1970.

Natvig, J. B., and Kunkel, H. G.: Human immunoglobulins—classes, subclasses, genetic variants and idiotypes. Adv. Immunol., *16*:1, 1973.

Nisonoff, A., Wissler, F. C., Lipman, L. N., and Woernley, D. L.: Separation of univalent fragments from the bivalent rabbit antibody molecule by reduction of disulfide bonds. Arch. Biochem. Biophys., *89*:230, 1960.

Poljak, R. J.: X-ray diffraction of immunoglobulins. Adv. Immunol., *21*:1, 1975.

Poljak, R. J., Amzel, L. M., Chen, B. L., Phizackerley, R. P., and Saul, F.: The three-dimensional structure of Fab′ fragment of a human myeloma immunoglobulin at 2.0-Å resolution. Proc. Natl. Acad. Sci., *71*:3440, 1974.

Poljak, R. J., Amzel, L. M., Avey, H. P., Chen, B. L., Phizackerley, R. P., and Saul, F.: Three-dimensional structure of the Fab—fragment of a human immunoglobulin at 2.8-Å resolution. Proc. Natl. Acad. Sci., *70*:3305, 1973.

Porter, R. R.: The hydrolysis of rabbit γ-globulin and antibodies with crystalline papain. Biochem. J., *73*:119, 1959.

Roitt, I.: *In* Essential Immunology, 3rd ed. Oxford, Blackwell Scientific Publications, 1977, p. 21.

Singer, S. J., and Doolittle, R. F.: Antibody active sites and immunoglobulin molecules. Science, *153*:13, 1966.

Spiegelberg, H. L.: Biological aspects of immunoglobulins of different classes and subclasses. Adv. Immunol., *19*:259, 1974.

Spiegelberg, H. L.: γ D immunoglobulin. *In* Inman, F. P. (ed.): Contemporary Topics in Immunochemistry, vol. 1. New York, Plenum Press, 1972, p. 165.

Thorpe, N. O., and Singer, S. J.: The affinity-labeled residues in antibody active sites. II. Nearest-neighbor analyses. Biochemistry, *8*:4523, 1969.

Tiselius, A., and Kabat, E. A.: An electrophoretic study of immune sera and purified antibody preparations. J. Exp. Med., *69*:119, 1939.

Underdown, B. J., DeRose, J., and Plaut, A.: Disulfide bonding of secretory component to a single monomer subunit in human secretory IgA. J. Immunol., *118*:1816, 1977.

Waldman, T. A., and Strober, W.: Metabolism of immunoglobulins. Prog. Allergy, *13*:1, 1969.

Wells, J. V., Fudenberg, H. H., and Givol, D.: Localization of idiotypic antigenic determinants in the Fv region of murine myeloma protein MOPC-315. Proc. Natl. Acad. Sci., *70*:1585, 1973.

Wigzell, H.: On the relationship between cellular and humoral antibodies. *In* Cooper, M. D., and Warner, N. L. (eds.): Contemporary Topics in Immunobiology, vol. 3. New York, Plenum Press, 1974, p. 77.

Wu, T. T., and Kabat, E. A.: An analysis of the sequences of the variable regions of Bence Jones proteins and myeloma light chains and their implications for antibody complementarity. J. Exp. Med., *132*:211, 1970.

37

COMPLEMENT

Thelma A. Gaither, B. S.,
and Michael M. Frank, M. D.

4

The complement system is composed of a series of circulating blood proteins which serve as mediators of the inflammatory response. In addition, the complement proteins are important in the opsonization of foreign particulate matter, including bacteria, and in cytotoxic reactions toward cells and bacteria. Thus, the complement system has evolved as a complex interacting series of proteins designed to mediate host defense reactions and to protect against infections. In general, there are very few individuals deficient in one of these proteins. Furthermore, the absence of a component generally is not overtly responsible for manifestation of a disease state. This is in sharp contrast to inherited defects in the coagulation cascade. The usual role of the complement system in disease is to produce tissue damage. In these situations, the complement system is functioning normally, but it is being activated under abnormal circumstances. For example, circulating immune complexes may be deposited in the kidneys of patients with systemic lupus erythematosus, and these circulating complexes may activate complement in a perfectly normal fashion. This normal activation process may lead to renal inflammation and glomerular damage. In this case,

the complement system is functioning normally but, nevertheless, is intimately associated with the development of disease.

STRUCTURE AND FUNCTIONAL RELATIONSHIPS

The proteins in the complement system are given either numerical or letter designations. These proteins circulate as inactive precursors in serum and are activated in a very precise order of biochemical reactions. In many cases, activation of the proteins is associated with cleavage of the protein component. The larger fragment produced by the protein cleavage is responsible for continuation of the complement sequence. The smaller fragment often has the function of promoting the inflammatory response. There are a number of ways in which complement proteins can be activated. For example, proteolytic enzymes, such as those released from certain bacteria, may cleave a complement protein, leading to the uncovering of the active site and the propagation of the complement sequence. More often, antigen-antibody complexes on microbial or viral surfaces are the inciting agents. The processes which transpire when these agents interact with complement have been examined in detail.

SEQUENCE OF REACTIONS OF THE CLASSIC PATHWAY

This pathway is responsible for the lysis of most antibody-sensitized cells. In many of the assays where the classic pathway is studied, the presence of a functionally active component is indicated by the lysis of sheep erythrocytes sensitized with rabbit antibody. Sheep erythrocytes are particularly advantageous for use because, for reasons that are not completely understood, they are much more easily lysed by antibody and complement than are erythrocytes from other species. Sheep erythrocytes have on their surface a potent lipopolysaccharide antigen, the Forssman antigen. This antigen is widely distributed in nature. The critical antigenic grouping in this lipopolysaccharide is a specific sugar linkage which is seen as very foreign in animals that do not have the enzymes to form this linkage. Rabbits are a Forssman-negative species and respond to the injection of sheep erythrocytes by producing enormous amounts of anti-Forssman antibody. Thus, high titer antiserum to the sheep erythrocyte is easily obtainable and sheep erythrocytes themselves, being easily lysed by fresh serum, are sensitive indicator particles for the presence of lytic complement activity.

Activation of the classic complement pathway is initiated by the interaction of antigen with C1-fixing antibody. Not all classes of immunoglobulin activate the classic pathway. IgM and IgG subclasses IgG_1, IgG_2, and IgG_3 are the immunoglobulins that bind and activate C1. This reaction has been studied in detail in several model systems. The precise molecular nature of the antigen-antibody-C1 interaction is not clear, but it is known that C1 binds to the Fc fragment of antibody in the antigen-antibody complex by a non-covalent, easily reversed linkage. C1 itself is a complex protein composed of three subunits, C1q, C1r, and C1s, which are held together in the presence of calcium.

The portion of the C1 molecule which interacts with immunoglobulin is the C1q subcomponent. The ability of C1q to interact with aggregated immunoglobulin has provided the basis for a number of new tests designed to detect the presence of soluble immune complexes in the blood of patients with a variety of diseases. Radiolabeled C1q is added to the serum or plasma sample, and one of a number of techniques is used to differentiate free C1q from that bound to protein components of serum. The presence of bound C1q suggests the presence of immunoglobulin complexes in the serum or plasma sample. These techniques are discussed further on p. 1274 (Zubler, 1976).

The binding of C1 to antibody in turn leads to activation of C1. It appears that a single molecule of most IgM antibodies can "fix" and activate one molecule of C1. The activated component in each case is indicated by (‾); thus, activated C1 is designated as C$\bar{1}$. Although C1 binding by a single IgG molecule has been described, C1 binding usually requires an IgG doublet, two molecules side by side, in most of the experimental models studied.

The fact that the binding of C1 by IgG requires cooperative interaction of several IgG molecules has consequences of clinical importance. Since IgG molecules bind to a cell surface in a random fashion, it may require the attachment of hundreds or thousands of IgG molecules to obtain a C1-fixing site. This is thought to be the explanation for the fact that anti-Rh antibodies of the complement-fixing subclasses do not effectively provide a site for complement fixation when they bind to human erythrocytes. The appropriate Rh antigens are sparsely scattered on the erythrocyte surface, and this precludes the formation of antibody doublets, with subsequent complement fixation. Thus, complement activation is not noted in most anti-Rh mediated hemolytic states, whereas it is noted in hemolytic states mediated by cold agglutinins and anti-A, B, and O blood group substance antibodies.

The activation of C1 leads to the generation of an enzymatic site which in model systems has been shown to have esterase activity. This activation is associated with cleavage of one of the protein chains in C1r and C1s. The activated antigen-antibody C1 complex now is capable of interacting with the next component in the complement sequence, C4. C4 is cleaved by C1 acting as an enzyme, and two cleavage fragments are formed. The larger fragment is highly reactive for a few moments after its formation and appears to bind to any suitable receptor in the microenvironment. Some of the activated C4 molecules bind to the erythrocyte cell membrane as a cluster around the antigen-antibody-C1 site. Therefore, one antibody site can lead to the deposition of many C4 molecules. The antibody C1-C4 complex can, in turn, bind to and activate the next component in the sequence, C2. Again, this important reaction involves cleavage of the component. In this case, C1 esterase in association with C4 and in the presence of Mg^{++} can cleave C2, leading to the formation of a $C\overline{142}$ complex. This complex is unstable. However, in the presence of C3, the hemolytic sequence is continued and C3 is cleaved into two fragments, C3a and C3b. C3a is released and C3b is bound to the erythrocyte membrane. Again, amplification is an important part of the C3 reaction in that hundreds of C3b molecules may be deposited at each complement-fixing site. If C3 is not present, the $C\overline{142}$ complex decays to $C\overline{14}$, releasing an inactivated fragment of C2. Many of the remaining reactions in the complement sequence follow this general formulation. The $C\overline{1423b}$ complex can bind and then cleave C5 into two fragments, C5a and C5b. Again, C5b attaches to the cell membrane and continues the hemolytic sequence, and the C5a fragment is released. This general pattern is continued for C6, C7, C8, and C9; however, the reactions differ in detail. Activation of several of these components does not appear to be accompanied by cleavage. When all of the complement components have reacted with a site on the cell surface, the cell membrane may be damaged in such a way that the cell lyses.

BIOLOGIC FUNCTIONS ASSOCIATED WITH ACTIVATION

As discussed above, the complement system subserves many functions which do not involve cell lysis. Many of the features of the inflammatory response are promoted by complement fragments, and complement plays a key role in opsonization. Table 37-1 lists the most widely accepted biologic functions of complement components and complement fragments. Most of these biologic properties are self-explanatory. It should be mentioned that anaphylatoxic factors cause mast cells to degranulate and release their various mediators in the absence of cytotoxicity. The opsonic properties of the complement proteins appear to depend on the presence of specific receptors on the surface of phagocytic cells. Foreign materials with opsonically active

Table 37–1. BIOLOGIC ACTIVITIES OF THE COMPONENTS OF THE COMPLEMENT SYSTEM OF MAN

C1	Increases affinity of some antibodies
C1q	Aggregation of antigen-antibody complexes
C1,4	Viral neutralization
C4	Immune adherence receptors on lymphocytes and PMN's
C2	Cleavage product may have kinin-like properties
C3a	Chemotactic and anaphylatoxic
C3b	Opsonic immune adherence receptors on B-lymphocytes, PMN's and macrophages
C3d	Receptor on lymphocytes and macrophages
C5a	Chemotactic, anaphylatoxic
C567	Chemotactic
C8,9	Lysis

fragments on their surface interact with these receptors, leading first to membrane adherence and, as a second step, to phagocytosis.

Many of the biologic properties of these complement fragments are controlled by the presence in serum of specific protein inhibitors. Thus, the enzymatic activity of activated C1 is destroyed by the C1 esterase inhibitor, the integrity of the opsonically active protein C3b is destroyed by the C3b inactivator, and an inactivator of cell-bound C6 exists. There is also an inactivator of the vasoactive material, anaphylatoxin, which destroys the activity of C3a and, to a lesser extent, C5a. Other regulatory proteins exist which are beyond the scope of this review.

ALTERNATIVE COMPLEMENT PATHWAY

In recent years, it has become clear that there is another mechanism for the activation of complement which does not utilize the classic complement components, C1, C4, and C2 and which does not have an absolute requirement for antibody. When many microorganisms are exposed to fresh serum, they activate and bind to their surface the opsonically important complement component, C3, as well as the later components in the complement series which mediate bacterial lysis. Further analysis of this mechanism has demonstrated that there exists a pathway of complement activation which is phylogenetically older than the classic pathway and which bypasses the early components of the classic pathway. This

4

Table 37–2. A MORE COMPLETE VERSION OF THE CLASSIC AND ALTERNATIVE PATHWAYS

Classic Pathway

1. $EA + C1qrs \underset{}{\overset{Ca^{++}}{\rightleftharpoons}} EAC1 \rightarrow EA\overline{C1}$

   $\| Ca^{++}$

   C1q, C1r, C1s

2. $EA\overline{C1} + C4 \rightarrow EA\overline{C14}b + C4a$

3. $EA\overline{14} + C2 \xrightarrow{Mg^{++}} EA\overline{C142}a + C2b$

   $\downarrow$

   $EA\overline{C14} + C2a^d$

4. $EAC\overline{142} + C3 \rightarrow EAC\overline{1423}b + C3a$

   $\diagup C2a^d$

   $EAC143b$ (see below for C3b decay)

5. $EAC\overline{1423} + C5 \rightarrow EAC\overline{14235}b + C5a$

   $\diagup C2a^d + C5b^d$

   $EAC143$

6. $EAC\overline{14235} + C6 \rightarrow EAC\overline{142356}$

   $\diagup C2a^d$

   $EAC14356 \rightleftharpoons EAC143 + C56$

7. $EAC\overline{142356} + C7 \rightarrow EAC\overline{1423567}$

8. $EAC\overline{1423567} + C8 \rightarrow EAC\overline{12345678} \rightarrow$ slow lysis

9. $EAC14235678 + C9 \rightarrow EAC1\text{-}9$

10. $EAC1\text{-}9 \xrightarrow{37^\circ C} E^* \xrightarrow[\text{Inhibited}]{0.09 \text{ M EDTA}}$ Lysis

Subunit and fragment letter designations are used only when they first appear. C2 is required to maintain active enzymatic activity through the C5 step. Superscript "d" indicates a decay product. EAC1-7 is stable with regard to the action of C8 and C9. The build-up of C5-9 on and in the lipid bilayer leads to the development of a transmembrane pore. The bar is over the active enzyme. E* refers to a cell which has reacted with all of the components of complement and which will go on the lysis.

   EA = erythrocyte plus antibody
   EAC = erythrocyte plus antibody plus complement

pathway is composed of a series of proteins which resemble the classic complement components in their mechanism of action. The details of the protein interactions which make up this pathway are still not completely clear. As shown in Figure 37–1 (p. 1250), there are a number of components in the *alternative or properdin pathway* which are analogous to the components of the *classic complement path-* *way* and which function to form a C3 cleaving enzyme. Properdin factor D is analogous to C1 of the classic complement pathway. It forms a DFP (diisofluorophosphate)-inhibitable active enzyme which is heat labile, as is C1. Properdin factor B is analogous to C2. This component of the alternative pathway also is heat labile and forms a non-stable enzyme complex which is important in the cleavage of C3. It

Table 37-2. (*Continued*). A MORE COMPLETE VERSION OF THE CLASSIC AND ALTERNATIVE PATHWAYS

Alternative Pathway

Bacteria, fungi, antigen-antibody complexes, zymosan (Z), inulin, PNH erythrocyte surface initiate, but the mechanism of initiation is still not certain.

One possibility is shown in line 1. Once C3b is generated, the sequence continues as in line 2.

1. $Z + C3 + D + B + P \xrightarrow{Mg^{++}}$ Small quantity $Z\overline{C3bBb} + \overline{D}$

2. $Z + B + \overline{D} + C3b \xrightarrow{Mg^{++}} Z\overline{C3bBb}$

3. $Z\overline{C3bB} \searrow Z\overline{C3bBb} \longrightarrow ZC3b + Bb^d$
   $\quad Ba \quad)$

4. $Z\overline{C3bBb} \xrightarrow{Properdin} Z\overline{C3bBb}$ (stabilized)

   $\xrightarrow{C3NeF}$

5. $Z\overline{C3B} + C3 \rightarrow Z\overline{C3BC3b} + C3a$

6. $ZC3BC3 + C5 \rightarrow Z\overline{C3B35b} + C5a$

7. $ZC3B35 + C6 \ldots\ldots$ as in 6 above

C3NeF appears to represent IgG anti C3bBb

$\sim$ represents the activated component before cleavage occurs

C3b Inactivation Sequence

4

1. $EAC1\text{-}3b + \beta1H \rightarrow EAC1\text{-}3b\beta1H$

2. $EAC1\text{-}3b\beta1H + C31NA \rightarrow EAC1\text{-}3b^i\beta1H$

3. $EAC1\text{-}3b^i\beta1H + $ Serum trypsin-like enzyme $\rightarrow EAC1\text{-}3d + \beta1H + C3c$

Superscript "i" represents partial cleavage with inactivation of site.

β_1H appears to occupy the same site as B on C3b and can displace B.

$$D = \text{Factor D}$$
$$B = \text{Factor B}$$
$$P = \text{Properdin}$$

appears that a C3 cleavage product, C3b, serves the same role in the alternative pathway that C4 serves in the classic pathway. C3b, in combination with properdin factors B and D, forms an enzyme which is capable of cleaving C3. Thus, if a small amount of cleaved C3 can be generated, a major amplification of C3 cleaving capacity can be achieved via C3b interacting with components of the alternative pathway.

There are at least two regulatory proteins which are important in preventing the C3 cleaving enzyme formed by alternative pathway activation from decaying, thereby increasing the effectiveness of the cleaving enzyme. These two proteins are properdin and so-called C3 nephritic factor. The latter factor derives its name from the fact that it was first discovered in the sera of patients with membranoproliferative glomerulonephritis and low serum C3. When this factor is added to normal fresh serum with intact alternative pathway mechanisms, marked C3 cleavage results, with a dramatic fall in C3 titer. When the C3 nephritic factor was first discovered, it was hoped that this agent would provide an explanation for the low C3 and concomitant nephritis seen in membranoproliferative glomerulonephritis, but it is now clear that this protein simply serves a regulatory role in alternative pathway activation.

The mechanisms for activation of the alternative pathway are under active investigation. Although bacterial and fungal surfaces

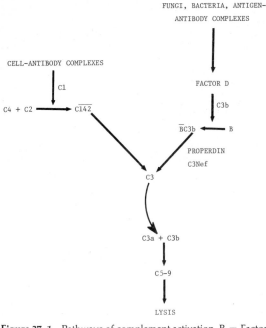

Figure 37-1. Pathways of complement activation. B = Factor B. C3Nef = C3 nephritic factor. The activated complement complex is indicated by the bar above the letter and numbers. The classic pathway of activation utilizes C1, C4, and C2, and the alternative pathway utilizes factors D, B, and C3b.

with repeating polysaccharide subunits are important in activating the alternative complement pathway, aggregated immunoglobulins and, presumably, antigen-antibody complexes of a number of types perform a similar function. Thus, complexes containing IgM, IgG, IgA, and IgE can activate the alternative pathway, although in the absence of classic pathway activation rather large amounts of complexes are required. The biochemical interactions which comprise alternative pathway activation and the biologic consequences of this activation are still being defined. However, they appear to be very similar to those which result from classic pathway activation. As will be made clear subsequently, there are a number of diseases which appear to be associated with classic pathway activation and a number of diseases which are more commonly associated with activation of the alternative pathway. It is in identification and definition of these diseases that the clinical pathologist will often be asked to aid the clinician. A more detailed version of complement activation is presented in Table 37-2.

COMPLEMENT IN DISEASE STATES

As mentioned previously (p. 1245), in most disease states complement functions normally in producing inflammation and tissue damage. When complement plays a role in the development of a disease, it is often being activated by an abnormal antibody, immune complex, or foreign material. It is frequently of importance to assess the level of one or another component of complement as a means of following the activity of a disease process. Thus, patients with active lupus erythematosus may have depressed levels of C3 and C4, and these component levels may be followed as a rough index of disease activity.

When one determines the levels of a component in serum, it is important to recognize that this represents a static measurement of serum proteins which are turning over rapidly. Even in the normal individual, the fractional catabolic rate of most of the components which have been measured is on the order of 2 per cent per hour. Many of these proteins behave as acute phase reactants, and their levels in serum may rise dramatically in inflammatory states. Their rates of catabolism may increase greatly in various autoimmune diseases. The finding of a decreased level of a component may raise suspicion that the complement system is participating in tissue damage but does not prove it. The finding of a normal serum level of a component does not preclude the participation of complement in tissue injury. For example, patients with primary biliary cirrhosis have an increased catabolic rate of C3, and it has been suggested that C3 may play some role in the development of this disease. Nevertheless, the level of C3 in the serum of patients with primary biliary cirrhosis is almost always elevated. In this case, increased synthesis obscures the increased catabolism. It should also be recognized that complement function in various body compartments may differ. Complement activity in the blood of patients with seropositive rheumatoid arthritis may be normal or elevated; however, the complement activity of joint fluid may be severely depressed.

The final general concept to be discussed is that of the "complement profile." Earlier sections have introduced the classic and alternative complement pathways and their mechanisms of action. In recent years, an attempt has been made to determine which pathway of complement activation predominates in mediating tissue damage or depressed component levels in one or another illness. The simplest approach to this problem examines the levels of various components and assumes that decreased levels of a component of one or the other pathway are more likely to occur when that pathway is activated. Therefore, if a patient has depressed levels of C3 and C4 and normal levels of properdin factor B and properdin, the classic pathway is likely to be involved. If a patient has decreased levels of C3 and factor B and/or properdin and normal levels of C4, alternative pathway activation is most likely. In this way, determining the levels of a limited number of components can provide a great deal of information. Except in the case of the genetically controlled complement abnormalities, one never needs to know the levels of all complement components, except for investigational purposes.

There is now considerable interest in the detection of decay products in various body fluids. Thus, C3 decay products have been found in sera of patients with primary biliary cirrhosis, rheumatoid arthritis, and lupus erythematosus at the time of this review, and this list will probably grow rapidly.

A detailed discussion of the levels of complement components in various disease states (Frank, 1975) is beyond the scope of this review. Nevertheless, a brief statement as to the role of complement in various groups of illnesses will be provided. It is fair to state that the role of complement in each of these disease groups is under active investigation.

DIAGNOSIS OR ASSESSMENT OF CLINICAL ACTIVITY IN DISEASE

Rheumatologic Diseases. The most straightforward example of a rheumatologic disease mediating many of its effects via complement activation is that of *systemic lupus erythematosus*. Circulating immune complexes activate complement and are deposited in a variety of tissue sites, leading to tissue damage. It has been suggested that determination of levels of C3 and C4 is helpful in following the activity of this disease. Depressed levels of complement in joint fluid have been shown to exist in a number of other rheumatologic conditions, including rheumatoid arthritis.

Normal or elevated serum complement levels are found in juvenile rheumatoid arthritis, most patients with adult onset rheumatoid arthritis, palendromic arthritis, pseudogout, gout, Reiter's syndrome, and gonococcal arthritis.

Depressed CH_{50} and cleavage products of C3 and properdin factor B are thought to represent intra-articular activation in the synovial fluid of almost all patients with seropositive rheumatoid arthritis and many patients with seronegative rheumatoid arthritis, SLE, pseudogout, gout, Reiter's syndrome and gonococcal arthritis. This is not true of fluids obtained from patients with degenerative arthritis (Hunder, 1977).

Infectious Diseases. As previously discussed, one major function of the complement system is to protect against infection. Patients with gram-negative septicemia are often depleted of C3 and components of the alternative pathway, as are patients with certain fungal diseases, such as cryptococcal septicemia. A major area for future investigation concerns the role of complement in the tissue damage associated with chronic infection. This is an area which is only beginning to be explored. It is known that patients with HB_S Ag-positive infectious hepatitis have an early fall in serum C3, which later returns to normal. This may be associated with signs of immune complex disease, i.e., arthralgia, etc. In a similar fashion, complement appears to play an important role in a number of parasitic infections, including malaria. In patients with vivax malaria C1, C4, and C2 may be depressed. In patients with falciparum malaria, C3 may be depressed as well.

Renal Diseases. Complement is thought to be of key importance in glomerular damage in a variety of the glomerulonephritides (Michael, 1974). This is usually demonstrated by the deposition of C3 and/or other components in the vicinity of the glomerular basement membrane (Table 37-3). Many of these patients will show activation of the alternative pathway on serum analysis. The role of complement in interstitial and tubular disease is less clear. However, there are those who believe that complement may have some function in these disorders as well.

Dermatologic Diseases. As in the other groups of diseases listed, complement is thought to play a part in the ongoing tissue damage in a variety of dermatologic illnesses. These include pemphigus vulgaris, bullous

Table 37-3. COMPLEMENT LEVELS IN SELECTED RENAL DISEASES

	C1	C4	C2	C3	P	B
Acute glomerulonephritis	N	D	D	D	D	N or D
Systemic lupus erythematosus	D	D	D	D	N or D	D
Membranoproliferative glomerulonephritis	N	N	N	D	N or D	N or D
Post-streptococcal glomerulonephritis	Normal in initial sera ($<$10 days) in some studies					
″ Later	D	D slight	D slight	D	D	N or D
Idiopathic nephrotic syndrome	N	N	N	N		D
Anaphylactoid purpura with nephritis	N or D low levels transient	N or D	N	—	N or D	N

Note: The syndrome of partial lipodystrophy may be associated with C3 depression, C3NeF in serum, and membranoproliferative glomerulonephritis.

B = Factor B; D = depressed; N = normal; and P = properdin.

pemphigoid, and herpes gestationis. It should be noted that serum complement levels are usually normal or elevated in these chronic inflammatory states, and the importance of complement is suggested by immunofluorescent analysis of tissue biopsies and by studies of blister fluid.

Hematologic Diseases. In many types of autoimmune hemolytic anemia, complement plays an important role in opsonization of erythrocytes, leading to their clearance by cells of the reticuloendothelial system. However, even in those cases in which complement is clearly involved, serum complement levels are often normal. Complement is particularly important in the clearance of cells coated by IgM cold agglutinins antibody with anti-I specificity. Another complement-related hematologic problem is paroxysmal nocturnal hemoglobinuria (PNH). In this illness, the patient's erythrocytes and other blood cell elements develop a membrane defect which renders them exceedingly susceptible to complement-mediated lysis. This acquired cellular defect is associated with cytotoxicity and clearance due to activation of the alternative pathway by the cell membrane.

GENETIC DISORDERS

As discussed previously, the number of patients with genetically controlled complement disorders is few, and these patients are of greatest interest because they allow us to determine the role of complement components in various biologic phenomena and in various disease states. In general, the absence of the components follows simple mendelian genetics and is inherited as an autosomal recessive trait. Thus, heterozygous patients tend to have half normal levels or less and homozygous-deficient patients have little or no de-

Table 37-4. INBORN ERRORS OF THE COMPLEMENT SYSTEM OF MAN

C1q: Deficiency not complete: thymic alymphoplasia, hypogammaglobulinemia

C1r: Systemic lupus erythematosus, glomerulonephritis

C1s: Systemic lupus erythematosus

C4: Systemic lupus erythematosus

C2: Most common deficiency—discoid lupus erythematosus, systemic lupus erythematosus, glomerulonephritis, anaphylactoid purpura, dermatomyositis, vasculitis

C3: Frequent infections—all pyogens—resemble congenital hypogammaglobulinemia

C5: Systemic lupus erythematosus

C6: Repeated *Neisseria* infections

C7: Scleroderma, *Neisseria* infections

C8: *Neisseria* infections, systemic lupus erythematosus

C9: Not identified

C1 inhibitor: Hereditary angioedema. *Note:* C1 normal or depressed, C3 always normal. Occasional patients with lymphoid malignancies or autoimmune disease may consume or destroy their C1 esterase inhibitor and develop the clinical picture of hereditary angioedema.

C3 inactivator: Recurrent infections

Deficiencies of C1-9 are associated with CH_{50} of 0. Deficiencies of C1, C4, C2 associated with systemic lupus erythematosus often have negative LE preps. Deficiencies of C3-9 are associated with the absence of bacteriocidal activity of serum. Deficiency of C3 or C5 is associated with absent or diminished chemotactic activity of serum and may be associated with absent leukocyte response to infection. The genes for C2, C4, and properdin factor B are clearly linked to HLA. All inheritance patterns studied to date are autosomal recessive with the exception of C1 inhibitor deficiencies.

tectable component activity. As shown in Table 37-4, deficiencies are known for almost every component of the classic pathway. Most of these patients present with one or another manifestation of autoimmune disease, and the role of complement deficiency in the development of these diseases is under active investigation. One interesting hypothesis is that autoimmunity may be a manifestation of chronic viral illness. If complement aids in viral neutralization, an interruption of those pathways of activation may promote chronic viral infection. It is striking that deficiencies other than C3 deficiency are not generally associated with the presence of acute infectious diseases. This is attributed to the fact that the alternative pathway is available for opsonization of microorganisms in most of the deficiency states. C3 is a key component of both pathways and plays a key role in opsonization. Thus, absence of this component is associated with infection with a wide variety of pathogens, especially in childhood before the development of high titer antibodies. Interestingly, deficiency of a number of the late-acting components is associated with a high incidence of disseminated infection with *Neisseria* organisms (Agnello, 1978).

A number of other deficiency states exist. Patients with hypogammaglobulinemia and/or severe combined immunodeficiency often have depressed levels of C1q. In part, these depressed levels of C1q relate to the low levels of IgG in the circulation. It appears that C1q interacts with IgG in the circulation and that this interaction leads, in turn, to decreased C1q catabolism.

A group of patients with Leiner's syndrome has been evaluated, and it is suggested that these patients have abnormal C5 function. The data on which this conclusion rests are based on highly complex assays, and it appears at present that this conclusion is not warranted. The defect in Leiner's disease could reside at another step in the alternative complement pathway.

ASSAY OF COMPONENTS

GENERAL PRINCIPLES AND TYPES OF ASSAYS

Today, accurate methods are available for measuring each of the nine classic pathway components, most of the alternative pathway components, and several enzymes and inhibitors which regulate the complement system. However, many of these methods are still considered research techniques and are not available on a routine basis. We will confine our attention to techniques which do not require a laboratory skilled in complement research for their performance. In general, two types of techniques are in use: those that measure the complement proteins as antigens in serum and those that measure the functional activity of the components. Both techniques have advantages and disadvantages as research and diagnostic tools, and these will be reviewed.

Methods for antigenic (immunochemical) analysis are generally simpler to perform. These antigenic assays are highly specific and require fewer specialized reagents and considerably less personnel time. Reagents for measuring several proteins of the complement system are commercially available, including C1q, C4, C3, C5, properdin factor B, and C1 inhibitor. In these assays, either serum or plasma can be used, and the commonly available methods of freezer storage ($-20°$C.) are sufficient. For these reasons, antigenic assays are easily adaptable to a routine laboratory. On the other hand, antigenic assays do not provide information on the activity of a component, since they may detect degradation products as well as functionally active components. The presence in serum of small fragments of a protein with antigenic activity may confuse the results. A protein fragment may diffuse more rapidly than the parent molecule, and the usual radial diffusion techniques will indicate falsely high levels. As an example, the most commonly employed antigenic assay for C3 measures its major degradation product, C3c (β1A) by radial immunodiffusion. For accurate measurements of C3c, the specimen should be thawed and incubated at $37°$C. for a number of days to allow for complete conversion of C3 to C3c. In fact, this is not usually done and can present a source of error. There are no commercially available standards for intact C3. In general, antigenic assays are not as sensitive as functional assays and may not detect the presence of a component in certain body fluids, whose presence can be shown by its functional activity. The sensitivity of assays depends to some degree on the strength of the antisera employed, and with the usual assays, as little as 1 to 10 μg/ml of a protein antigen can be measured. Antisera to most components, other than those listed above, are still not generally available except as research reagents.

Functional complement assays may be described as both sensitive and precise tools for providing important information on the activity of a component. Some of these methods may be used to quantitate activity at the molecular level, while others express complement function in arbitrary titration units. Commercial reagents are available for titrating all components of the classic pathway system. However, for the most part, these assays are performed in a limited number of research facilities at this time. Most functional assays involve complex, time-consuming procedures, which require special, relatively highly purified reagents. These reagents are very expensive when compared with those required for antigenic tests.

PROCEDURES FOR EVALUATING FUNCTIONAL ACTIVITY

Handling of Samples

The proper handling of samples is critical for correct functional analysis. For most functional complement assays, serum rather than plasma is chosen for analysis because both chelators (EDTA) and heparin are anti-complementary. EDTA plasma may be used, however, in some functional tests where the sample is diluted enough ($> 1:100$) to overcome the chelating effect of EDTA. To obtain serum for functional assays, a fresh blood sample is allowed to clot at room temperature for $\frac{1}{2}$ hour and then in the cold for about one hour. If C1q binding studies are needed, the sample is allowed to clot two hours at room temperature. In this case, complete clot polymerization appears to facilitate accurate assay. If cryoprecipitating antibodies are suspected, clot formation and centrifugation of the specimen should proceed at $37°C.$, since complement fixation may occur if the specimen aliquot is chilled. To separate serum, the clot is rimmed and usually is centrifuged in the cold. Serum should be stored in multiple aliquots to avoid thawing and refreezing. The serum aliquots should be stored immediately at $-40°C.$ to $-70°C.$ Serum aliquots can be stored for long periods at $-70°C.$ without loss of activity. When sera are to be transported, they should be well sealed before being packed in a container with large quantities of dry ice.

Reagents and equipment

Almost all functional analyses can be performed with equipment limited to a spectro-

Table 37–5. SOLUTIONS COMMONLY USED IN COMPLEMENT ASSAYS

Stock solutions

1. *Veronal-buffered saline (Stock VBS)*
   To prepare 2 liters, dissolve 83.0 g NaCl and 10.19 g Na-5,5' diethyl barbiturate in 1.5 liters of distilled water. Mix vigorously while titrating to pH $7.35 \pm .05$ with 1 N HCl. Bring to 2.0 liters volumetrically with distilled water. This solution is five times the concentration of an isotonic solution and may be stored at $4°C.$ for at least one month. It is diluted immediately before use.

2. *0.10 M disodium ethylenediamintetraacetate (Stock EDTA)*
   Dissolve 37.2 g in about 800 ml of distilled water. Adjust the pH to $7.65 \pm .05$ with 2 N NaOH and bring to 1.0 liter with distilled water. Store at $4°C.$ Stock EDTA may be used for at least three weeks.

3. *Dextrose with Ca++, Mg++, and gelatin (D)*
   A 5 per cent solution of dextrose in distilled water (D5W) is obtained from commercial sources. Approximately 1 liter is measured volumetrically, 1.0 ml of Stock Solution 6 is added, and the solution brought to 1.0 liter. 100 to 200 ml of the mixed solution is added to 1 g of gelatin in an Erlenmeyer flask and heated until all of the gelatin granules have dissolved. After the remaining solution is added, the D is well mixed and stored at $4°C.$ D may be used for one week.

4. *2.00 M MgCl₂ solution*
   Prepare about 200 ml of solution containing $MgCl_2$ at approximately 3 M. Measure the specific gravity of the solution and determine the $MgCl_2$ concentration from the *Handbook of Chemistry and Physics* (conversion tables for concentrated values of aqueous solutions). Adjust the concentration to 2.00 M by adding distilled $H_2O.$

5. *0.300 M CaCl₂ solution*
   About 200 ml of an approximately 0.5 M solution of $CaCl_2$ is prepared. Measure the specific gravity of this solution and determine $CaCl_2$ concentration as described above. Adjust to 0.300 M by adding distilled $H_2O.$

6. *Stock metals*
   A solution containing 1.0 M $MgCl_2$ and 0.15 M $CaCl_2$ is prepared by combining equal volumes of Solutions 4 and 5.

Working solutions

1. *Isotonic VBS with gelatin and metals (VBS)*
   To prepare 1 liter add 200 ml of Stock Solution 1 to a 1 liter volumetric flask. Add 1.0 ml Stock Solution 6 and bring to 1.0 liter with distilled $H_2O.$ Add 0.1 per cent gelatin as in Stock Solution 3. VBS should be prepared fresh every 3 to 5 days and stored at $4°C.$

2. *Isotonic VBS-dextrose of lowered ionic strengths (DVBS)*
   Buffers of varying ionic strengths are prepared by mixing Stock solution 3 with Working Solution 1 in varying proportions. 0.065μ DVBS is prepared by mixing three parts of the former solution with two parts of the latter. DVBS should be prepared fresh.

3. *Isotonic VBS-EDTA buffer (EDTA)*
   Mix nine parts of Working Solution 1 without metals with one part of Stock Solution 2. This solution is stable for at least one week at $4°C.$

4. *C-EDTA*
   Dilute fresh guinea pig serum (titer of at least 170) 1:25 in Working Solution 3. This reagent is stable for one week at $4°C.$

photometer, pH meter, conductivity meter, precision balance, refrigerated centrifuge, and water baths which can be regulated with precision at 37°C. and 30°C. The usual array of calibrated pipettes, graduated beakers, etc., is needed, and it should be mentioned that it is advisable to avoid using mouth pipetting with blood samples from diverse sources. Methods for preparing solutions commonly used in functional complement assays are outlined in Table 37-5. Two basic reagents are required for titrating lytic activity. They are washed and standardized sheep erythrocytes (E) and rabbit antiserum to sheep erythrocyte stroma (A).

Preparation of Sheep Erythrocytes (E).

Sheep blood is drawn aseptically into an equal volume of sterile Alsevers solution. This preparation of sheep cells is commercially available. The anticoagulated whole blood is stored for at least one week at 4°C. before use and may be used for up to six weeks if sterility is maintained. Studies have shown that the age of sheep cells can greatly influence the titers of most complement components (Gaither, 1973), and titers may be falsely low with fresh cells. An appropriate volume of cells is removed for washing under sterile conditions. After centrifugation, the supernatant and buffy coat are removed. Cells are suspended in 0.01 M EDTA buffer and incubated at 37°C. for 10 minutes. The cells are washed in EDTA, followed by three washes in VBS. The washed, packed cells are then diluted about 15-fold in VBS. To determine cell concentration, a small sample of the cells is diluted 1:25 in distilled water. The optical density (O.D.) of the lysate is determined at 541 nm. In general, an O.D. of 0.420 corresponds to a sheep cell concentration of 1×10^9 cells/ml. Cells at this concentration, which are stored in VBS, are designated as "E." E may be stored at 4°C. and utilized for approximately one week. Additional washes immediately before use may be required to remove any lysed cells from the preparation. For some studies, 1.5×10^8 red cells/ml are required. A 1:25 dilution of such cells in distilled water corresponds to an O.D. of 0.560 at 412 nm.

Preparation of Anti–Sheep Erythrocyte Antibody (A).

Two types of anti-sheep erythrocyte antibody are in common use: antibody to whole sheep erythrocytes and antibody to the Forssman antigen on the erythrocytes. Both types are commercially available. Either appears to be satisfactory for studies of "whole" complement activity (CH_{50}). Most workers who report functional titrations of individual components utilize rabbit anti-Forssman antibody, and there are no studies that we know of which systematically compare the usefulness of the various types of antibody. It is known, however, that many of the anti-whole erythrocyte antibody preparations contain low avidity antibody which can transfer from site to site on the erythrocyte surface, thereby influencing the kinetics and end points of various titrations. Antibody with a high degree of specificity for the Forssman antigen of sheep erythrocytes can be prepared by immunizing rabbits with boiled sheep erythrocyte stroma. The method of immunization influences the class of antibody produced. Intravenous injection is optimal for the preparation of antibody in which the predominant hemolysin is IgM. Antigen in Freund's adjuvant is best for IgG hemolysin. The procedures for preparation of stroma and rabbit immunization are explained fully in Kabat's textbook (1961). For the purpose of the complement studies presented here, the immunization schedule and procedure should be designed to produce antisera in which most of the hemolytic activity is in the IgM fraction. Before use, the complement activity of the antiserum is destroyed by heat inactivation for 30 minutes at 56°C. Antisera with acceptable activity may be diluted, usually to 1:100, in normal saline and stored at −20°C. for many months or at 4°C. for short periods of time.

A 15-minute kinetic assay is used to titrate anti–Forssman antibody (Table 37-6). The unit of hemolytic antibody, AB_{50}, is defined as that amount of antiserum which, under the described conditions, lyses half of the red cells in exactly 15 minutes. A series of accurately prepared dilutions of the antiserum is prepared in VBS. A dilution of pooled guinea pig complement, usually diluted 1:7.5 in VBS, is the complement source. The guinea pig serum complement must be preadsorbed with E to remove natural hemolysin. In the assay, 0.5 ml E (5×10^8/ml) is mixed with 0.5 ml of the appropriate dilutions of antiserum. After 15 minutes at 37°C., 0.25 ml of the diluted guinea pig complement is added, and the mixture is incubated further at 37°C. In this and all other titrations discussed, the cells are mixed frequently to maintain a uniform cell suspension. After exactly 15.0 minutes, the

Table 37-6. PROTOCOL FOR TITRATION OF ANTIBODY AND SAMPLE DETERMINATIONS

	TEST TUBE					
	1	2	3	CB	CBC	100%
E (5×10^8 ml)	0.5	0.5	0.5	0.5	0.5	0.5
Hemolysin, 0.5 ml	1:20,000	1:40,000	1:80,000	–	–	–
			Incubate 10.0 minutes 37°C.			
Guinea pig complement, 1:7.5	0.25	0.25	0.25	–	0.25	–
			Incubate 15.0 minutes 37°C.			
EDTA buffer, ml	2.5	2.5	2.5	2.75	2.5	–
H_2O (ml)	–	–	–	–	–	2.75
Absorbance (O.D.) 541 nm	0.454	0.137	0.040	0.003	0.014	0.698
Absorbance (O.D.) Corr.	0.440	0.123	0.026	–	–	0.695
$y/1 - y$	1.73	0.215	0.039	–	–	–
Titer, AB_{50}	24,000	–	–	–	–	–

E = sheep erythrocytes
CB = sheep erythrocytes with buffer alone
CBC = sheep erythrocytes plus complement
y = absorbance (corrected) of test sample/absorbance (corrected) of 100% lysed sample
AB_{50} = amount of antiserum which under described conditions lyses half of the erythrocytes in exactly 15 minutes.

reaction is stopped with the addition of 2.5 ml of ice cold EDTA, mixed, and centrifuged. The supernatants are analyzed photometrically at 541 nm and the titers determined using the Von Krogh equation (see below). Controls include E plus complement (CBC), E with buffer alone (CB), and E lysed 100 per cent in distilled H_2O.

Titration of complement requires sheep E sensitized with an optimal amount of antibody (A). An optimally sensitized preparation contains sufficient antibody so that the complement titer is independent of antibody concentration. To determine the optimal amount of antibody, 0.5 ml of a series of two-fold falling dilutions of antibody is added to an equal volume of E with careful mixing. After incubating the sensitized cells for 10 minutes at 37°C., 5.5 ml VBS and 1.0 ml of a dilution of fresh frozen guinea pig serum complement (1 CH_{50} Unit) are added. After incubating the mixture at 37°C. for one hour, the cells are sedimented, the absorbance (O.D.) of the supernatant is determined at 541 nm, and the percentage of lysed cells determined. The per cent lysis is plotted versus the log of the dilution of the antiserum. A strong antiserum will cause optimal lysis at a dilution of $>1:500$. Sheep erythrocytes sensitized with optimal amounts of antibody are designated EA. Sensitization is accomplished using a very standardized procedure. A volume of E is placed in a container which allows for easy mixing. The diluted antiserum is slowly pipetted in a dropwise fashion into an equal volume of cells, with constant swirling of the contents to ensure an even distribution of antibody on the cells. Antibody is always added to E. EA are generally incubated for 15 minutes at 30°C. or 37°C. before use. They remain stable when stored at 4°C. but may require additional washes in VBS if spontaneous cell lysis occurs.

Cellular intermediates in the complement system with membrane-bound components are also used for functional assays. EAC4 have cell-bound C4 and may be used as a reagent for measuring the remaining eight components. There are a number of methods available for forming this intermediate. Each begins with the preparation of EA. Some investigators recommend that twice the optimal concentration of antibody be used. The procedure used in our laboratory is as follows: A 10 ml volume of EA containing 5×10^8 cells/ml is chilled to 0°C., and partially purified guinea pig C1 (500 to 1,000 C1 effective molecules or sites per ml of suspension) is added (e.g., if the commercially supplied C1 has a titer of 10,000 units, it would be diluted 1:10 to yield 1,000 sites/cell). Guinea pig C1 is compatible with the early human components and is generally chosen for preparing both guinea pig and human intermediates. The EAC1 solution is mixed well and held at 0°C. for 15 minutes to form the complement cell intermediate EAC1. A solution containing 2 ml of fresh or fresh frozen human serum complement and 18 ml of EDTA buffer is prepared, heated at 37°C. for 15 minutes to ensure chelation of all calcium and magnesium, and then cooled to 0°C. This ice cold solution is added to 0°C. EAC1 with vigorous mixing. After 15 minutes incubation at 0°C., the cells are washed two times in EDTA in the cold and three times in VBS. During the 15 minute incubation, two competing reactions occur. C4 functions in the absence of metals. On the other hand, EAC1 is EDTA sensitive and C1 dissociates from the intermediate in the absence of calcium. Thus, two reactions proceed:

$$\text{EAC1} + \text{Serum} \underset{\nearrow}{\overset{\text{EDTA}}{\searrow}} \begin{array}{l} \text{EAC14} \xrightarrow{\text{EDTA}} \text{EAC4} \\ \qquad\qquad\qquad + \text{C1q r \& s} \\ \text{EA} + \text{C1q r \& s} \end{array}$$

Under the condition of the procedures, adequate amounts of C4 combine with EAC1 before the C1 is stripped from the cellular intermediate. The EAC4 cells are suspended in VBS to $1.5 \times 10^8/\text{ml}$ and stored at 4°C. They retain C4 on their surface indefinitely and can be used as long as the preparation can be washed free of the hemoglobin, which represents non-specific lysis of some of the stored cells. Before use, EAC4 should be tested to determine if the cells have a sufficient number of C4 sites. A simple test in which the remaining eight components are added in excess is sufficient. To a 0.2 ml volume of EAC4, add C1 at 500 sites/cell. After ten minutes at 30°C., 100 units of C2 (a 1:10 dilution of C2 with a titer of 1:1000) are added and the reaction is continued at 30°C. for ten minutes. A 1:25 dilution of serum treated with EDTA provides the late components. Two ml of this solution is added and the mixture is stirred well and immediately transferred to 37°C. EAC4 should lyse completely within five minutes. More precise information on the number of EAC14 sites available for interaction with C2 can be obtained from t_{max} determinations (Kabat, 1961; Rapp, 1970). The t_{max} measurement refers to a complex kinetic reaction in which the time for maximum lysis of a specific cell mixture is related to the number of C4 sites/cell. A short t_{max} indicates a large number of sites. EAC4 reagents which have acceptable t_{max} values are commercially available (Cordis Laboratories, Miami, Florida). The EAC14 intermediate is prepared by adding partially purified guinea pig C1 to EAC4 suspended in DVBS at an ionic strength of $0.065\,\mu$. EAC4 are prepared as described. To saturate EAC4 with C1, at least 200 to 400 molecules of C1 per cell are added. C1 is allowed to react with EAC4 for 10 minutes at 30°C. To remove free C1 and other contaminating components, the EAC14 cells are then washed with $0.065\,\mu$ DVBS. The washed cells are stored in the same buffer, generally at $1.5 \times 10^8/\text{ml}$. EAC14 remains stable when stored at 4°C. under these conditions for days to weeks. It should be noted that it is possible to prepare EAC1, EAC14, and EAC4 and store these cells for prolonged periods of time in liquid nitrogen (Rowe, 1965; Hunsicker, 1975). Such cells are perfectly acceptable for use in functional comple-

ment titrations. The EAC4 intermediate may also be prepared by adding partially purified components directly to EA. EA, described above, are suspended in $0.065\,\mu$ DVBS to $1.5 \times 10^8/\text{ml}$. Guinea pig C1 is added in excess (500 to 1000 sites/cell), and the mixture is incubated at 30°C. for 15 minutes. After one wash in $0.065\,\mu$ DVBS, EAC1 are resuspended in the same buffer. Partially purified human C4 is added at a concentration which yields 100 sites per cell, and the mixture is brought to 37°C. for 30 minutes. EAC14 may be washed in DVBS and used for complement assays where that intermediate is required, or they may be converted to EAC4 cells by removing the C1 with several EDTA washes.

The simplest functional assay of the classic pathway measures total hemolytic complement. The absence of any one of the nine components results in a total hemolytic complement titer (CH_{50}) of zero. However, a normal value does not exclude reduced levels of individual components. When a patient's history and symptoms suggest a possible deficiency, hemolytic titrations of individual components may be required.

The procedure for total complement evaluation is outlined in the sample titration (Table 37–7). The titer is expressed in CH_{50} units (the reciprocal of the dilution of complement which lyses 50 per cent of the EA). In this case, the 50 per cent end point is determined from the Von Krogh transformation. This empirically derived formula converts the S-shaped dose-response curve into a linear curve. Values of $y/1 - y$ are calculated, in which y equals the percentage of red cells lysed in a test dilution. A graph is constructed in which the log of the relative volume of complement is plotted against the log of $y/1 - y$ values. Usually, a straight line is obtained, and the titer is calculated by determining the relative volume of complement at which $y/1 - y$ equals 1.0 (the point where 50 per cent lysis is obtained). That value is divided into the original serum dilution (1:60 for human serum) to calculate the concentration of serum complement which lyses 50 per cent of the cells. The reciprocal of this value is the complement titer. It expresses the number of 50 per cent hemolytic units which are present in 1.0 ml of undiluted serum.

To measure most complement components individually, partially purified components are required. However, C4 and C6 are exceptions because of the availability of C4-deficient guinea pig serum (C4D) and C6-deficient rabbit serum (C6D). These assays are based on

4

Table 37-7. PROTOCOL FOR TITRATION OF WHOLE COMPLEMENT AND SAMPLE DETERMINATIONS

| | TEST TUBE | | | | | | | |
	1	2	3	4	5	CB	CC	100%
VBS (ml)	5.5	5.3	5.0	4.5	4.0	6.5	5.5	–
5×10^8/ml EA	1.0	1.0	1.0	1.0	1.0	1.0	–	1.0
Serum (1:60)	1.0	1.2	1.5	2.0	2.5	–	2.0	–
H_2O (ml)	–	–	–	–	–	–	–	6.5
				Incubate 1 Hour 37°C.				
Absorbance (O.D.) 412 nm	0.102	0.185	0.322	0.490	0.596	0.008	0.003	0.664
Absorbance (O.D.) Corr.	0.094	0.177	0.314	0.482	0.588	–	–	0.656
$y/1 - y$	0.167	0.370	0.918	2.77	8.65	–	–	–
Titer, CH_{50}	39.5	–	–	–	–	–	–	–

VBS = veronal-buffered saline (see Table 37-5)
 CB = sheep erythrocytes with buffer alone
CBC = sheep erythrocytes plus complement
   y = absorbance (corrected) of test sample/absorbance (corrected) of 100% lysis sample

the principle that the deficient sera are good sources of the remaining components, which they possess at normal or near normal concentrations. The assays for C4 and C6 are, thereby, greatly simplified and can be performed easily if the deficient sera are available. The deficient sera must be fresh or frozen fresh to prevent loss of complement activity.

The C4 assay is performed in 0.084 μ DVBS. C4D is diluted 1:75 and kept ice cold until used. A broad range of serum dilutions is prepared—1:1,000, 1:10,000, and several two-fold falling dilutions, starting at 1:50,000. EA are prepared as described and suspended to 1.5×10^8/ml. Generally, a 0.2 ml volume of the serum dilution is added to 0.2 ml of EA and 0.2 ml C4D. The mixture is incubated at 37°C. for one hour; 2.0 ml of EDTA is added, the tubes are centrifuged, and the supernatant is analyzed spectrophotometrically at 412 nm. Controls include EA plus C4D, EA plus buffer, and a 100 per cent lysis control. A standard serum should be in-

Table 37-8. PROTOCOL FOR TITRATION OF C4 BY C4D METHOD AND SAMPLE DETERMINATION

| | TEST TUBE | | | | | |
	1	2	3	CB	C4D	100%
EA (1.5×10^8/ml)	0.2	0.2	0.2	0.2	0.2	0.2
Serum, 0.2 ml starting with 1:100,000	1:1	1:2	1:4	–	–	–
C4D serum 1:75	0.2	0.2	0.2	–	0.2	–
0.084 μ DVBS	–	–	–	0.4	0.2	–
			Incubate 1 Hour 37°C.			
EDTA	2.0	2.0	2.0	2.0	2.0	–
H_2O (ml)	–	–	–	–	–	2.4
Absorbance (O.D.) 412 nm	0.847	0.559	0.330	0.011	0.024	1.087
Absorbance (O.D.) Corr.	0.823	0.535	0.306	–	–	1.076
Z	1.45	0.688	0.335	–	–	–
Titer	141,380	–	–	–	–	–

EA = sheep erythrocytes with antibody
  E = sheep erythrocytes
 CB = sheep erythrocytes and buffer alone
C4D = C4-deficient serum
  Z = average number of sites damaged by complement per sheep erythrocyte

cluded each time this assay is performed because several variables may affect the titer on a given day. This method and the procedure for calculating C4 titer are outlined in Table 37-8.

C6 assays are performed by similar methods. C6 deficient rabbit serum is diluted 1:20 in the 0.065 μ DVBS diluent. A reagent consisting of EA and an equal volume of C6D is prepared and incubated at 37°C. for $\frac{1}{2}$ hour to allow the early components in the rabbit serum to interact with the sensitized cells. Diluted serum samples ranging from 1:100 to 1:1000 are prepared. 0.2 ml of a serum dilution is added to 0.4 ml of the EA-C6D reagent. The reaction is completed in 90 minutes at 37°C., at which time 2.0 ml of EDTA is added.

The assay for serum C4 is extremely efficient, yielding titers which are greater than titers obtained by the more complex standard procedure. However, the C6 assay using deficient rabbit serum is not efficient. When this

method is applied, titers are reduced approximately by a factor of 10. However, this method is perfectly acceptable for determining normal C6 levels when a control standard serum is assayed simultaneously.

Standard procedures for measuring the hemolytic activity of each of the components of the classic pathway are outlined in Table 37-9. The following general methods apply to these assays:

1. Low ionic strength buffer (0.065 μ DVBS) is utilized.
2. The cellular intermediate is suspended to 1.5×10^8 cells/ml.
3. All serum and complement dilutions are prepared fresh and held at 0°C. to 4°C.
4. Reaction mixtures are frequently mixed to ensure adequate cell suspensions.
5. When individual components are required

Table 37-9. STANDARD HEMOLYTIC ASSAYS OF CLASSIC PATHWAY COMPONENTS

COMPONENT		VOLUME (ml)	COMPONENT		VOLUME (ml)
C1	Test dilution	0.2	C4	Test dilution	0.2
	EAC4	0.2		EAC1	0.2
	1 hour 30°C.			20 min. 37°C.	
	C2	0.2		C2	0.2
	10 min. 30°C.			10 min. 30°C.	
	CEDTA 1:25	2.0		CEDTA 1:25	2.0
	1 hour 37°C.			2 hours 37°C.	
C2	Test dilution	0.2	C3	Test dilution	0.2
	EAC14	0.2		EAC14	0.2
	30°C. t_{max}			C5,6,7 reagent*	0.2
	CEDTA 1:25	2.0		C2	0.2
	1 hour 37°C.			30 min. 30°C.	
C5	Test dilution	0.2		C8,9 reagent	0.2
	EAC14	0.2		1 hour 37°C.	
	C367 reagent	0.2		EDTA	2.0
	C2	0.2	C6	Test dilution	0.2
	30 min. 30°C.			EAC14	0.2
	C89 reagent	0.2		C357	0.2
	1 hour 37°C.			C2	0.2
	EDTA	2.0		30 min. 30°C.	
C7	Test dilution	0.2		C89	0.2
	EAC14	0.2		1 hour 37°C.	
	C356	0.2		EDTA	2.0
	C2	0.2	C8	EAC14	0.2
	30 min. 30°C.			C2	0.2
	C89	0.2		C3567	0.2
	EDTA	2.0		30 min. 30°C.	
C9	EAC14	0.2		Test dilution	0.2
	C2	0.2		C9	0.2
	C3567	0.2		1 hour 37°C.	
	30 min. 30°C.			EDTA	2.0
	Test dilution	0.2			
	C8	0.2			
	1 hour 37°C.				
	EDTA	2.0			

*If each of the components in the mixed reagent has a titer of 1000, 1.0 ml C5, 1.0 ml C6, and 1.0 ml C7 may be mixed and brought to a total volume of 10.0 ml. This reagent contains the recommended 100 sites/cell for each component.

in excess, C1 is added at a concentration which yields from 500 to 1000 C1 sites/cell, and the remaining eight components are added at concentrations which yield 100 sites/cell. Often, the titers of commercial complement components are expressed as CH_{50} units/ml. The CH_{50} titer is the reciprocal of the dilution yielding 50 per cent lysis, at which point the Z value is approximately 0.70 site per cell (see below).

Immune hemolysis is the result of a complex series of reactions which occur on the cell surface. Photometric measurements show the proportion of cells lysed by this series of reactions. The principle of Poisson distribution is applied to relate the degree of hemolysis to the molecular events which occur on the cell surface. This approach is based on the assumption that the interaction of cell-bound antigen, antibody, and complement occurs in random fashion and that the amount of lysis is the sum of a large number of interactions in which limited quantities of the component being titrated interact with other components which are all in excess. It is well established that one lesion on the erythrocyte surface which has interacted with hemolytic antibody and all of the complement components can cause cell lysis. The Poisson distribution is used to relate the number of lysed cells (cells with one or more lesions) to the concentration of the antibody or complement reactant being titrated. The average number of damaged sites per red cell is expressed as Z. The equation relating this value to lysis is: $Z = -\ln(1 - y)$, where y is the percentage of lysed cells. To calculate the titer of the component being measured, Z values are plotted on the ordinate against serum concentration plotted on the abscissa on an arithmetic or a log-log graph. The titer is the reciprocal of the dilution of serum which corresponds to a Z value of 1.0 or one hit per cell.

COMPLEMENT LEVELS BY ANTIGENIC ASSAY

For use in antigenic assays, the specimen should be refrigerated or frozen. Bacterial contamination may cause protein denaturation or fragmentation, while freezing and thawing do not usually have an adverse effect on antigenic levels. For certain complement assays, the specimen is diluted in saline to achieve the correct concentration range for accurate quantitation. When C3 is assayed and precise titrations are desired, using C3c standards, sterile sera should be incubated at 37°C. for several days prior to analysis.

Antigenic analysis of complement proteins makes use of one of several immune precipitin techniques. Single radial immunodiffusion (RID) is the most commonly employed method for specific quantitation of protein. Basically, one of two approaches is used: that of Mancini (1965), or that of Fahey (1965). In both methods, antigen is loaded into wells in a gel containing antibody and rings of precipitation are formed. In the Fahey method, the time at which results are read is critical because the antibodies in the gel matrix are not in excess and, therefore, diffusion end points are not reached. This can lead to inaccurate evaluations of antigenic complement. The technique of Mancini, considered to be both sensitive and accurate, employs the more simplified end point methodology with antibody excess in the gel. The Mancini method is used by most commercial firms in the preparation of immunodiffusion plates. These methods are discussed further in Chapter 35, p. 1186.

Radial immune diffusion kits are commercially available for several complement components, including C3, C4, and factor B. These kits consist of plates which contain a thin layer of 2 per cent agarose containing monospecific antibody. Protein standard serum, a stabilized pool of normal human serum, is supplied, usually in prediluted solutions. Each standard solution contains a specific amount of the particular protein being measured for use in construction of the reference curve. A delivery device (a microliter syringe or calibrated pipetter), which can accurately measure and deliver lambda quantities of serum, is useful; and a calibrated magnifier, which is accurate to 0.1 mm, is needed.

Another method of assessing complement activation is discussed on page 1208.

COMPLEMENT FIXATION TESTS

A detailed consideration of this procedure will not be presented here, since a complete discussion of this topic is available (Kabat, 1961). Nevertheless, complement fixation reactions are of great importance in clinical diagnosis and will be mentioned briefly. The test procedure depends on the ability of fresh serum complement to interact with antigen-antibody complexes. In the first step of the reaction, the complement is incubated with the materials which may contain antigen and antibody. If antigen-antibody complexes are formed, they will interact with complement in much the same way as a complex of antibody and a cell surface antigen interact with complement. The complement is activated, components are fragmented, and the complement is "used up" or "fixed." In the second stage, sensitized sheep cells (EA) are added, and the mixture is incubated at 37°C. for one hour. If the serum contains antibody to the antigen used, complement is fixed and is, therefore, no longer available to lyse the EA. Thus, the absence of lysis indicates a positive reaction, while complete lysis indicates a negative result.

There are two general approaches to complement fixation tests. In the first one, concentrated, fresh serum is the complement source; and the amount of complement fixed is determined by titration of the serum before and after fixation. In the second one, a dilution of serum is used that will provide either just enough complement for lysis of the EA or slightly more than enough (3 to 5 CH_{50} Units). In this case, the sensitized cells are added without further dilution. Incubation of the test materials with complement can take place at 37°C. for one hour or overnight in the cold. In general, cold incubation leads to higher titers.

Complement can be inactivated by a number of agents other than antigen-antibody complexes, such as bacteria, endotoxins, yeast, and aggregated gamma globulins. Therefore, controls are necessary to demonstrate that neither the serum nor the antigen alone will fix complement. The complement fixation test is particularly valuable in that it does not require that antigens or antibodies be present in highly purified form, both soluble and particulate antigens may be utilized, and antigens as well as antibodies may be measured.

4

REFERENCES

Agnello, V.: Complement deficiency states. Medicine, *57*:1, 1978.

Fahey, J. L., and McKelvey, E. M.: Quantitative determination of serum immunoglobulins in antibody agar plates. Immunology, *94*:84, 1965.

Frank, M. M.: Complement. *In* Current Concepts. Scope Publication, 1975, pp. 1–48.

Gaither, T. A., and Frank, M. M.: Studies of complement-mediated membrane damage: The influence of erythrocyte storage on susceptibility to cytolysis. J. Immunol., *110*:482–489, 1973.

Hunder, G. G., McDuffie, F. C., and Mullen, B. J.: Activation of C3 and factor B in synovial fluids. J. Lab. Clin. Med., *89*:160, 1977.

Hunsicker, L. G., and Mayes, E. R.: Preservation of antibody and complement bearing sheep erythrocytes (EA and EACH) by glycerol freezing. Fed. Proc., *34*:955, 1975.

Kabat, E. A., and Mayer, M. M.: Experimental Immuno-chemistry, 2nd ed. Springfield, Ill., Charles C Thomas, Publisher, 1961.

Mancini, G., Carbonara, A. O., and Hermans, J. T.: Immunochemical quantitation of antigens by single radial immunodiffusion. Int. J. Immunochem., *2*:235, 1965.

Michael, A., and McLean, R.: Evidence for activation of the alternate pathway in glomerulonephritis. Adv. Nephrol., *4*:49, 1974.

Rapp, H. J., and Borsos, T.: Molecular Basis of Complement Action. New York, Meredith Corporation, 1970.

Rowe, A. W., and Allen, F. H., Jr.: Freezing of blood droplets in liquid nitrogen for use in blood group studies. Transfusion, *5*:379, 1965.

Zubler, R. H., and Lambert, P. H.: The ^{125}I-Cq binding test for the detection of soluble immune complexes. *In* Bloom, B. R., and David, J. R., (eds.): In Vitro Methods in Cell-Mediated and Tumor Immunity. New York, Academic Press, 1976, pp. 565–572.

38

AUTOIMMUNITY AND AUTOIMMUNE DISEASE

Burton Zweiman, M.D.,
and Robert P. Lisak, M.D.

CURRENT CONCEPTS

An understanding of current concepts of autoimmunity and its pathogenic mechanisms requires a brief discussion of the regulation of immune responses. The latter depends on a highly complex set of interactions among antigen, antibody, immune complexes, complement, macrophages, and one or more subpopulations of lymphocytes (Thaler, 1977). These interactions are described in Chapter 34; however, for the purposes of this discussion it should be mentioned that components include (1) genetic control through immune response genes linked directly or indirectly to the histocompatibility complex; (2) cellular cooperation between macrophages and lymphocytes and between T- and B-lymphocytes themselves (Nossal, 1975; Gershon, 1974; Shortman, 1975); (3) a primary regulatory role of T-lymphocytes in both the initiation (helper T cell function) and prevention/termination (suppressor T cell function) of a particular immune function. This important regulatory function determines the degree of antibody formation

by B cells or conversion of such cells to plasma cells, the normal switch from IgM to IgG antibody production against a particular antigen, and the degree of direct T cell-mediated reactivity, among other functions. The end result of an effective functional immune response would be the harmonious appearance of normal immune reactivity expressed appropriately with self/non-self discrimination (Talal, 1977).

Autoimmunity represents a breakdown of such self/non-self discrimination which may or may not result in adverse effects in the host. Some consider it a termination of the natural unresponsive (tolerant) state (p. 1181). Currently, many investigators believe that such tolerance is induced by at least two mechanisms involving contact between antigen and immunocompetent cells: (1) elimination of the small clone of immunocompetent cells "programmed" to react with the antigen (Burnet's clonal selection theory), and (2) induction of unresponsiveness in the immunocompetent cells through excessive antigen binding to them (Nossal, 1975) and/or through triggering of a suppressor mechanism (Gershon, 1974; Tada, 1975; Thaler, 1977).

There is increasing evidence that much of tolerance to tissue antigens is an active process involving T cells (p. 1175). B cells with surface receptors for DNA and other tissue components are present in small numbers in the normal circulation. The reason why immune responses to such substances develop weakly or belatedly in normals may relate to the experimental observation that tolerance in the T cell population is achieved much more readily than in B cells with the low concentrations of antigen that would be released from tissues in normal catabolism (Howard, 1975; Allison, 1974). In this "T cell tolerance," (a) the "helper" T cell function to concentrate antigens more effectively for presentation to the B cell may be depressed; (b) suppressor T cells may reduce the helper T cell function that does persist; (c) there is lack of conversion of IgM to IgG antibody synthesis by those B cells which may be activated directly by certain antigens.

It is also apparent that tolerance is terminated more readily, as well as induced with more difficulty, in B lymphocytes. Therefore, in many cases, B cells are ready to produce autoantibodies at any time, and frequently do this weakly in normals, especially with increasing age. However, such autoimmune reactivity increases markedly and prematurely when helper T cells are made responsive (or lose tolerance) to autoantigens. Conditions which may lead to such T cell responsiveness include (1) exogenous alterations of normal host components by agents such as the type C viruses which incorporate membrane components as they bud from the infected cell (Talal, 1977); (2) haptens which may complex to tissue proteins acting as a carrier (Weigle, 1973); (3) tolerance to tissue components which may also be lost when immune responses are induced to a foreign antigen, which cross-reacts with normal tissue components (Weigle, 1973); (4) non-specific stimulation of helper T cells by adjuvants or depression of the regulating suppressor T cell activity (Allison, 1971).

The lack of normal regulation of immune responses may play a role in the increased production of autoantibodies by mutant lymphoid clones in lymphoproliferative and immune deficiency states. In this regard, clinical autoimmune disease may commonly reflect a form of immunologic deficiency. Because of absent or defective lymphocytes, invading microorganisms may not be handled normally, persisting in and altering tissue cells with resultant uncovering of previously sequestered antigenic sites or formation of "neo-antigens." It is of note that in selective IgA deficiency, a particularly high prevalence of autoimmune disorders is seen (Wells, 1975). This may relate to a defective barrier to entry of foreign substances at mucosal surfaces associated with the IgA deficiency.

Although most agree that the T and B cell populations are generally exposed to only low levels of tissue components during development, the previous concept that elements of organs like the thyroid, adrenal, and testis are sequestered from contact with the immune apparatus has been questioned by evidence of the normal circulation of such components even in the adult stage. It is becoming increasingly evident that the capacity for autoimmune reactivity is likely constantly present in normal individuals (Allison, 1974). Expression (or lack of it) appears to be modulated by a complex set of interacting factors such as (1) *sex*—autoimmune responses are more common in the female (Talal, 1977); (2) *genetics*—there is an increased evidence of autoimmune antibodies in the sera of near relatives of those with certain autoimmune diseases (DeHoratius, 1975); (3) *age*—many autoantibodies (e.g., rheumatoid factor, antinuclear antibodies, antithyroglobulin antibodies) are found more commonly in asymptomatic aged than in young individuals; (4) *thymic control*—evidence that thymus plays a role in autoimmunity includes the observations that (a) the onset in life of naturally occurring autoimmune disease and immunodeficiency in NZB/W mice is accelerated by neonatal thymectomy (Steinberg, 1974), and (b) thymic hyperplasia is seen in at least some clinical autoimmune states (Burnet, 1972); (5) *exogenous factors* (sunlight, drugs, certain virus infections) may "trigger" a prominent autoimmune response by T cell activation or some other mechanisms (Phillips, 1975).

Autoimmune responses do not necessarily result in disease. Several investigators have adapted Koch's postulates in an attempt to relate autoimmunity to disease. These might include:

1. Demonstration of an immune response (humoral and/or cellular) to a well-defined tissue antigen alone or complexed to a foreign agent.

2. Induction of an immune response to that

Table 38-1. PRESUMPTIVE CLINICAL EVIDENCE SUGGESTING AN AUTOIMMUNE MECHANISM IN A HUMAN DISEASE

1. Pathologic picture similar to that in experimental autoimmune states
2. Presence of humoral or cell-mediated immune response to tissue antigens
3. Decrease in serum complement component(s)
4. Presence of other possible autoimmune disease
5. Familial prevalence of the same or other putative autoimmune disease
6. Clinical improvement following steroid or cytotoxic ("immunosuppressive") therapy

antigen in experimental animals, resulting in lesions similar to those seen in disease.

3. Transfer of the disease to normal recipients with products of the experimental autoimmune response.

It has been difficult to meet all these criteria in suspect human diseases. Therefore, some have postulated that an autoimmune mechanism is likely when several clinical manifestations are present. Some of these are listed in Table 38-1 with the understanding that no one criterion specifically identifies autoimmunity.

The immunogenic stimulus in autoimmunity may be (1) foreign substance which induces an immune response that cross-reacts against tissue components; (2) a complex of the foreign substance with the tissue, sometimes in a hapten-carrier relationship; (3) an endogenous material, sometimes restricted to one organ; (4) no obvious antigen defined. To a major degree, the nature and locale of this immunogenic stimulus will determine whether the disease manifestations are localized or systemic. Those localized predominantly to one organ system include endocrine (Hashimoto's thyroiditis, Addison's disease), gastrointestinal tract (pernicious anemia, autoimmune liver disease), and neuromuscular system (certain demyelinating diseases, myasthenia gravis). However, although the autoantibodies are organ- (and sometimes species-) specific, it is not unusual to find other antitissue antibodies in the serum of patients with disease manifestions in only one organ system (Irvine and Barnes, 1975). For example, antithyroglobulin antibodies are more commonly found in the sera of those with pernicious anemia; however, only a minority of such patients develop concomitant thyroiditis. In addition, there is an increased familial prevalence not only of the particular organ-associated autoimmune disease, but also of the antibodies against components of other organs.

What mechanism underlies this association of anti-organ antibodies in these patients or their near relatives? The answer is not clear. However, based on our foregoing discussion of T- and B-lymphocyte activities, it is conceivable that genetically controlled B cell hyperactivity against certain organ components characterizes this patient population, with resultant modest increase in T cell responses against one particular organ. This may result in marked increases in humoral (and possibly cell-mediated) immune responses that are associated with disease induction. The role of cell-mediated immunity in human autoimmune disease states is not well-defined (Stiller, 1975).

In a second group of diseases, the autoimmune response is not directed against organ- or species-specific antigens (DNA and other nuclear antigens, mitochondria). Rather, they seem to reflect a generalized abnormal humoral hyper-reactivity, possibly because of defective suppressor T cell function. The lesions are likely due at least in part to deposition of immune complexes containing tissue components, often with complement, with involvement of multiple organs. Therefore, it is not surprising that there is significant overlap in the clinical manifestation of this collagen-vascular disease group (e.g., SLE, rheumatoid arthritis).

However, these distinctions are by no means clear-cut. There are instances in which autoimmunity appears primarily organ-directed, but is also expressed as multiple antibodies against organ non-specific antigens. Examples of this are biliary cirrhosis and Sjögren's syndrome. In addition, tissue components may be released from an organ damaged by an organ-specific autoimmune reaction; these components may also combine with preformed antibodies to form a pathogenic immune complex damaging formed elements (e.g., hemolytic anemias) or the glomerulus.

AUTOIMMUNITY AND COLLAGEN-VASCULAR DISORDERS

The term collagen-vascular disorders has been commonly applied to a group of disorders with multisystemic manifestations even though prominent blood vessel involvement is only sometimes seen, and primary involvement of collagen rarely. Most observers would include systemic lupus erythematosus, rheumatoid arthritis, periarteritis nodosa, and probably scleroderma. Common features are inflammatory reactions, a potential for involvement of any organ system, and an understandable merging of one clinical presentation into another. These considerations should be kept in mind when evaluating the diagnostic and prognostic significance of one or more of the immunologic findings present in these disorders. The observer will then be more understanding of the overlap in prevalence of immunologic as well as clinical findings. In this regard, it should be emphasized that the result of any one laboratory determination is still only partial evidence to confirm a clinical impression and not diagnostic by itself. Because of the chronic inflammatory reactivity, likely owing at least in part to antigenic stimulation, it is not surprising to find elevated sedimentation rates and polyclonal increases in serum gamma globulins detected by one or more methods. It is to some of the antibody activities in these gamma globulins that we will first direct our attention.

ANTINUCLEAR ANTIBODIES (ANA)

Antibodies directed against a large number of tissue components have been found in systemic lupus erythematosus (SLE). Of them, the antinuclear antibodies have been the center of most interest because of their diagnostic usefulness and pathogenic implications. Since the discovery of the L.E. cell, an ever-increasing number of nuclear components have been isolated which react to varying degrees with lupus sera, utilizing techniques that presumably measure antigen-antibody activity. A list of the currently described major nuclear "antigens" is shown in Table 38-2. Because of their widespread clinical use, immunofluorescence techniques of detection of ANA will be discussed first and in greater detail.

Table 38–2. NUCLEAR ANTIGENS DETECTED BY IMMUNOFLUORESCENCE ANTI-NUCLEAR ANTIBODY TESTING

Particular or soluble nucleoprotein
DNA
Sm antigen
Nuclear ribonucleoprotein
Low molecular weight RNA (4-6S)
Histones
Others?

IMMUNOFLUORESCENT METHOD

Binding of gamma globulins to a variety of cell nuclear substrates has been demonstrated with considerable utility in many laboratories using immunofluorescent techniques. Immunofluorescence is a histochemical method for detecting antigens in tissue (direct technique) or antibodies which bind *in vitro* to tissue antigens (indirect technique). The mechanisms underlying this technique are discussed in Chapter 35. However, a common approach for detecting ANA includes:

Mammalian cells—fixed gently
↓ washed with buffered saline
Incubation with test or control serum
↓ washed with buffered saline
Incubation with fluorescein-conjugated antihuman immunoglobulins (previously absorbed with tissue powder)
↓ washed with buffered saline
Counterstain with diluted Evans blue or rhodamine (optional)
↓ washed with buffered saline
Mount cover slip with buffered glycerol and read in microscope adapted for fluorescence.

This technique is relatively simple; with the development of interference filters, availability of an ultraviolet light source is no longer required. There are many minor variations and adaptations of this technique, with no one uniformly superior to the rest (Rothfield, 1976). However, several *technical factors* and *potential pitfalls* must be kept in mind. Nuclear substrates from a variety of cell cultures, blood smears, tissue imprints, and tissue sections have been used with varying degrees of sensitivity (Barnett, 1970). Some substrates appear to be preferable in exhibiting certain fluorescence patterns. Leukocyte-specific preferential ANA has been reported in Felty's syndrome. Mild fixation (e.g., acetone for 10 minutes) retards "leaking out" of aqueous-extractable nuclear antigens during the washing procedures. Some commercially prepared antisera tend to be heavily conjugated with high fluorescein:protein ratios and will therefore bind more non-specifically to the tissue substrate. This may make interpretation of nuclear staining more difficult. Use of gamma globulin fraction of the antiserum which has been extensively dialyzed and column fractionated will reduce the non-specific effects. Each lot of fluoresceinated antiserum should be standardized using a chess board technique (Hale, 1971).

Advantages of the immunofluorescent detection of ANA (Rothfield, 1976) are several. It is a very sensitive screening test. Tests are positive in significant titer in greater than 95 per cent of patients with active untreated SLE. A persistently negative ANA by this method effectively rules out this diagnosis, although exceptions do occur. It detects anti-

4

Table 38-3. PREVALENCE OF POSITIVE*
ANA TESTS BY IMMUNOFLUORESCENCE
IN SOME CLINICAL STATES

Systemic lupus erythematosus	>95%
Rheumatoid arthritis	25–30%
Juvenile rheumatoid arthritis	20%
Sjögren's syndrome	50–60%
Progressive systemic sclerosis	60–70%
Dermatomyositis/polymyositis	<10%†
Periarteritis nodosa (typical)	<10%
Myasthenia gravis and/or thymoma	30–50%
Drug-induced states‡	
Hydralazine	35–50%
Procainamide	50–70%
Anticonvulsants	8–15%
Normals	<5%
Normals, elderly (>70 yrs.)	10%

.* Positive in at least 1:10 serum dilution.

† High incidence of an apparently unique ANA in one report (see text).

‡ Results vary considerably in reports which may reflect, in part, population treated and duration of treatment.

bodies present against all nuclear components and it can be semiquantitated using serum dilution titers. Relatively large numbers of sera can be tested at one time and where needed, immunofluorescence tests for other anti-tissue antibodies (discussed later) can be performed with the appropriate substrates at the same time, at considerable saving in technician time.

However, there are *disadvantages* of the immunofluorescent ANA technique. It is not very specific for SLE. After one has determined a minimal dilution (generally 1:8 to 1:16) in which an acceptably low percentage of normals, the serum is reactive, positive responses are seen in a sizable number of disease states other than SLE and in up to 10 per cent of elderly "normal" individuals (Table 38–3). Sera from many patients treated with hydralazine and procainamide, and to a lesser extent with several other drugs, will also be positive. Detection of all ANA by immunofluorescence, while advantageous in screening, does not allow a consistent distinction of antibodies against individual nuclear components. Finally, the very sensitivity of the immunofluorescent technique contributes to its inconsistency as a parameter to follow activity of the disease and effects of therapy (Rothfield, 1976; Weitzman, 1977).

Attempts have been made to improve the diagnostic specificity of immunofluorescent ANA determinations by the use of serial dilution titers. It is true that higher ANA

titers (often >1:160) are found in active SLE compared with other conditions (Ritchie, 1967), but there is considerable overlap, particularly in "highly expressed" rheumatoid arthritis and Sjögren's syndrome. Certain patterns of fluorescent staining of the nucleus have been found to correspond fairly well, but not uniformly, to certain nuclear components (Table 38–4 and Fig. 38–1). The "peripheral rim" or "shaggy" pattern has been more commonly but not uniformly associated with anti-DNA antibodies found in active SLE (Tan, 1967; Weitzman, 1977). However, the frequent concomitant presence of antinucleoprotein antibodies may also give rim patterns at times; it also may result in an intense diffuse fluorescence, making the rim pattern difficult to see. The nucleolar staining pattern seen with binding of certain sera from scleroderma and SLE patients (Ritchie, 1967) may also be masked by intense diffuse nuclear staining.

The L. E. cell phenomenon bears special mention because of its original role in expanding immunologic knowledge about SLE and the continued widespread use of the L.E. phenomenon (Zweiman, 1976). This is essentially an *in vitro* phenomenon; L. E. cells are rarely found *in vivo* except in bone marrow or in inflammatory exudates. In a commonly used technique, heparinized blood is agitated with glass beads or by other mechanical means so that nuclei are released from disrupted leukocytes. When these nuclei interact with antinucleoprotein antibodies in the serum, they are altered, with loss of chromatin pattern and a resultant homogenous appearance (hematoxylin bodies). The hematoxylin bodies are

Table 38-4. NUCLEAR ANTIGENS AND IMMUNOFLUORESCENCE PATTERNS IN SOME CLINICAL STATES

IMMUNOFLUORESCENCE PATTERN	ANTIGEN	CLINICAL STATES*
Diffuse	Nucleoprotein Others?	SLE, RA, SS, Sj, drug-induced
Rim (shaggy)	DNA Nucleoprotein	SLE, occasionally others
Speckled	Nuclear RNA-protein Sm Histone Others	SLE, MCTD, SS, Sj, RA, drug-induced

*SLE = systemic lupus erythematosus; RA = rheumatoid arthritis; SS = progressive systemic sclerosis; Sj = Sjögren's syndrome; MCTD = mixed connective tissue disease.

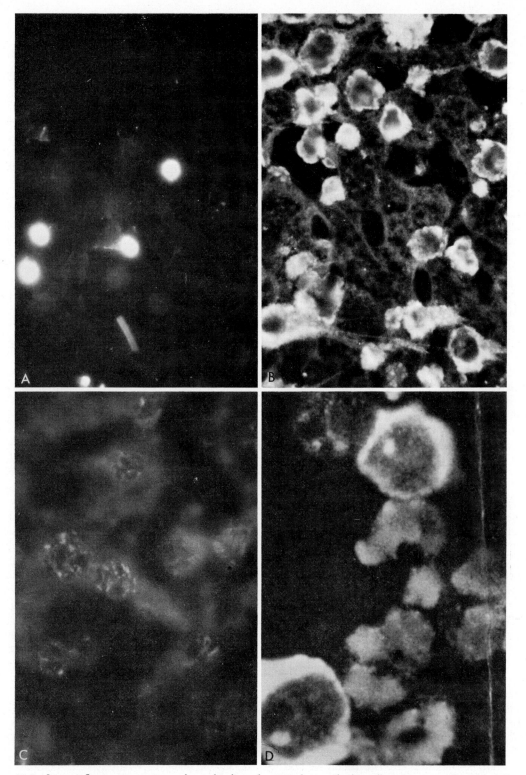

Figure 38–1. Immunofluorescence patterns due to binding of anti-nuclear antibodies, all at 600× magnification. *A*, Inverse diffuse fluorescence. *B*, Peripheral rim pattern. *C*, Speckled pattern. *D*, Nucleolar and cytoplasmic fluorescence.

phagocytized by remaining viable leukocytes in a complement-dependent reaction resulting in blood granulocytes with cytoplasm stretched and nucleus displaced by a homogenous inclusion which is stained light blue by Wright's stain.

Cells containing nuclei with well-preserved chromatin ("tart cells") or partially preserved chromatin do not convey the same diagnostic significance as true L. E. cells. A positive L. E. cell test (generally considered when at least four typical L. E. cells are found in a 20 minute search) is found in about 50 to 80 per cent of SLE patients and is therefore a much less sensitive screening test. L. E. cell tests also become negative more readily than immunofluorescent ANA tests in steroid-treated individuals. Other disadvantages include the relatively time-consuming nature of the tests performed in large numbers of patients, including the tedious reading period (for at least 20 minutes) and sometimes subjective elements in visual interpretation. Positive L. E. cells tests are more specific for SLE but are also found in about 5 per cent of rheumatoid arthritics, in some scleroderma patients (particularly those with vasculitis), and in some with drug-induced reactions. Its diagnostic usefulness has generally been surpassed by other tests.

SEROLOGIC TESTS FOR NUCLEAR ANTIGENS

Major recent advances in diagnostic specificity have come from attempts to quantitate antibodies against individual nuclear components.

Antibodies against native double-stranded DNA (anti-nDNA) are thought by most investigators to be present in significant amounts, predominantly in those with active SLE (Talal, 1976). Although it is currently debated whether such reactivity is directed partially against small amounts of contaminating single-stranded DNA (ss DNA), the observation of presumptive anti-DNA antibodies has been used pragmatically to help diagnose and follow the activity of SLE. There is some debate as to how often anti-nDNA antibodies in significant quantity are found in the sera of those with diseases other than active SLE. Different results may reflect technical variables described below.

Early methods of detection, such as precipitin or complement fixation reactions, were limited by the considerations mentioned

above for these techniques such as insensitivity or anti-complementary activity of serum. More recent techniques include hemagglutination and DNA binding assays.

Hemagglutination tests using DNA-coated tanned sheep erythrocytes have been employed with success by some groups (Inami, 1973). Major *advantages* of this approach are that no specialized equipment is needed, and at least semiquantitative measurements by serial dilutions of serum are feasible. *Disadvantages and possible pitfalls* of the techniques include variables in hemagglutination technique which may lead to lack of reproducibility. It should be stressed that any heterophil antibodies against sheep antigens must be removed by thorough absorption of all sera with sheep erythrocytes or use of other adaptations. In addition, close attention to pH and other factors is required to keep the DNA securely attached to the erythrocyte. DNA coating of erythrocytes must be done at the time of the assay.

In *DNA binding assays*, attempts have been made to demonstrate by immunofluorescence binding of human gamma globulins to either purified DNA solutions ("DNA spot test") or DNA-rich microorganisms. However, for a variety of reasons, binding of putative antibodies in sera to radiolabeled (^{3}H or ^{14}C) DNA has been used most extensively in both research and clinical studies in recent years. In most assays, radiolabeled DNA is incubated at 37°C. and then at 4°C. with test and control sera. Any resultant DNA-gamma globulin complex is separated from the free DNA by either precipitating DNA-gamma globulin complex with 50 per cent saturated ammonium sulfate (Farr technique: Pincus, 1969) or by trapping the DNA-gamma globulin complex on cellulose filters during gentle vacuum filtration (Talal, 1976).

In either method, the radiolabeled bound DNA (in the precipitate or on the filter) is counted in a scintillation counter and generally expressed as a percentage of the labeled DNA added to the serum.

Although each method has intrinsic advantages and disadvantages, the major overall *advantages* of the binding assay are several. It measures presumptive antigen-antibody interaction directly without requirement for a secondary reaction (hemagglutination, complement fixation, etc.) that may add technical and biologic variables. Radiolabeled or DNA preparations (now commercially available) are stable at $-20°$C. and can be used almost immediately in the test. Semiquantitation is feasible and inhibition studies with "cold" DNA (or with a test serum presumably containing DNA) can be performed.

However, several *disadvantages and pitfalls* of the binding techniques should be kept in mind. First, the selectivity of the test for SLE requires that the antigen preparation contain little contaminating single-strand DNA (ss-DNA); there is considerable binding to ss-DNA of sera in a number of disease and drug-induced states, and in some normals as well. There is some debate as to the degree of contamination of "native" DNA preparations with ss-DNA, and whether the activity we call "anti-DNA" is really directed against such contaminants. However, in experienced hands, this technique is pragmatically useful, provided that each new lot of labeled DNA is calibrated. Second, DNA binds to serum components other than gamma globulins (Aarden, 1976). Prior $56°$C. incubation of sera should be done to inactivate the first component of complement, a major nonimmunologic binder of DNA. Low degrees of binding occur when the technique is carried out effectively; normal sera should bind <10 per cent of the added labeled DNA. Binding of >20 per cent is generally positive in most laboratories. In Table 38–5, the prevalence of such binding in different disease states is listed, with the understanding that variable results have been reported by different groups, possibly because of technique variables. Third, although DNA binding can be quantitated, the pattern is non-linear. However, a comparison of test serum binding with a standard curve obtained with a positive control at each determination is helpful. For following individual patients with SLE, it may be preferable to establish ranges of binding percentages which are then indicated as strongly, moderately, and weakly (but definitely) positive, equivocal, and negative.

Occasionally, anti-DNA tests will be negative in sera obtained at the peak of an acute exacerbation of SLE. Robitallie (1973) has shown free circulating DNA (antigen excess) in some such situations. He has modified immunodiffusion and hemagglutination techniques utilizing patient sera with high anti-DNA titers as a reagent to detect DNA present in at least moderate amounts. Others recommend assaying the increased capacity of serum treated with DNAse to bind radiolabeled DNA as a measure of complexes containing DNA (Bardana, 1975).

As mentioned earlier, speckled patterns in the immunofluorescent ANA test have been found in a variety of disease and drug-induced states, and likely reflected binding to one or more nuclear components which were at least partially extracted by aqueous solvents, so called extractable nuclear antigens (ENA). More recently, the nature and diagnostic significance of at least two of these components have been defined (Tan and Peebles, 1976; Maddison, 1977). The *Sm antigen* is a nonhistone, nuclear protein, devoid of nucleic acids against which antibodies are found predominantly, if not entirely, in active SLE, particularly when there is renal involvement present. Antibodies against nuclear *ribonucleoprotein (RNP)* are found in sera of some SLE patients, generally with milder disease. (Sharp, 1971). However, these antibodies are also found in other collagen-vascular diseases, including a high percentage of those with an overlapping clinical picture consisting of some manifestations of scleroderma, polymyositis, and SLE without a typical clinical pattern for any of these more defined syndromes. In this disorder, called the "mixed connective disease syndrome" by some (Sharp, 1972), major renal involvement is unusual and the clinical response to relatively low doses of corticosteroids is good.

Detection of antibodies against both the Sm and RNP is generally carried out using a hemagglutination assay involving tanned sheep erythrocytes (RBC) coated with the reactant. For screening purposes, Tan and Peebles

Table 38–5. PREVALENCE OF ELEVATED ANTI-DNA ANTIBODY IN SOME CLINICAL STATES

	PERCENTAGE OF SERA WITH ELEVATED BINDING OF nDNA
Active SLE	65–80%
Questionable SLE	30%
Discoid LE	15–20%
Rheumatoid arthritis	10%
Other collagen vascular diseases	5–15%
Drug-induced positive ANA	10%
Normals	0–2%

Modified from Pincus, T., Schur, P. H., Rose, J. A., Decker, J. K., and Talal, N.: Measurement of DNA-binding activity in SLE. N. Engl. J. Med., *281:*701, 1969, and Talal, N.: Immunologic and viral factors in autoimmune disease. Med. Clin. North Am., *61:*205, 1977.

(1976) extract a relatively impure saline-soluble extract of rabbit thymus; portions of this extract are pretreated with RNAse (to inactivate the RNP). Although other components are likely present, Tan believes that almost all of the antibody reactivity against the extract is directed to Sm and/or RNP.

In this assay (assuming negative control tests with extract coated sheep erythrocytes in buffer and with uncoated sheep erythrocytes in test serum), agglutination by a serum of extract-coated sheep erythrocytes indicates antibodies against the Sm and/or RNP components.

Agglutination by the same serum titer of sheep red blood cells coated with RNAse treated extract indicates that the antibody is directed against the Sm antigen. A titer lower than that against the untreated antigen indicates the presence of antibody activity against both Sm and RNP. No agglutination by the same serum of sheep erythrocytes coated with RNAse treated extract indicates antibodies against only RNP.

The major *advantages* of this assay are the use of relatively defined nuclear components rather than an immunofluorescence pattern, relative ease of performance without specialized equipment, and semiquantitation by serum serial dilution. *Disadvantages and possible pitfalls* include variables in any hemagglutination technique already noted in the discussion of anti-DNA antibody techniques and the need to adjust pH very carefully for consistent binding of the extract to the erythrocytes and for RNAse inactivation. In addition, the lack of standardized, commercially prepared "antigen" components has generally limited the use of this technique to date to a few research-oriented laboratories. For this reason, Sharp (1972) has recommended carrying out immunofluorescent ANA tests comparing responses in regular and RNAse treated cellular substrates. Speckled nuclear fluorescence seen in the former and not in the latter suggests that anti-RNP reactivity is present in the serum. Counterimmunoelectrophoresis has also been suggested as a technique to detect these antibodies. However, techniques of this type hold great promise in the continuing search for assays which will increase the specificity of diagnosis of collagen-vascular disorders and/or provide laboratory guidelines for prognosis and treatment. Examples of the latter appear to be the improved prognosis in SLE generally associated with the presence of anti-RNP antibodies and the absence of anti-Sm activity. Also, Sharp reported that lupus nephritis associated with anti-RNP as well as anti-DNA antibodies is more likely to respond to treatment than when anti-DNA antibodies are persistent and anti-RNP are absent.

Antibody reactivity against another nuclear component detected by immunodiffusion has been reported in sera of about 60 per cent of those with polymyositis and even more commonly in those with the mixed connective disease syndrome (Wolfe, 1977). Akizuki (1977) has found antibodies against an acid nuclear protein antigen in 70 to 85 per cent of patients with the sicca syndrome with or without SLE but infrequently in SLE alone.

Use of ANA Determination in the Differential Diagnosis of SLE

Screening for the diagnosis of SLE—perform immunofluorescent ANA test first:

a. Consistently *negative* test (<1:8 or 1:10 titer)—strong evidence against the diagnosis of active, untreated SLE.

b. *Borderline* positive (1:8 to 1:16) suggests:

(1) SLE—inactive and/or under treatment with steroid and/or cytotoxic therapy.

(2) Certain other diseases or drug-induced states. If this test becomes negative after drug withdrawn (may take months), suspect drug-induced reaction, especially if anti-nDNA tests are negative. Otherwise, suspect underlying SLE.

c. *Strong positive*—SLE or (less likely) other conditions

(1) Check titer—the higher the titer, the more likely the patient has SLE (but consider highly expressed rheumatoid arthritis, Sjögren's syndrome)

(2) Perform anti-DNA antibody—if >20 per cent by binding assay, strongly suggests diagnosis of SLE. If binding is <20 per cent this suggests: (a) SLE inactive or (sometimes) activity limited to skin or musculoskeletal system; (b) SLE being treated with large doses of steroids; (c) SLE in some major acute flare-ups—anti-DNA antibodies complexed *in vivo* with DNA; search for circulating DNA; (d) Other disease states—assay for rheumatoid factor and anti-Sm, anti-RNP, if available.

There is a further discussion of nuclear antigens on page 1211 of Chapter 35.

RHEUMATOID FACTORS AND RHEUMATOID ARTHRITIS

Gamma globulins with demonstrable anti-gamma globulin activity have long been called rheumatoid factors (RF) because of their occurrence in sera of over 80 per cent of those with rheumatoid arthritis. However, our current knowledge of these anti-gamma globulins leads us to believe that rheumatoid factor was an unfortunate choice of name. Not only are they not found uniformly in typical rheumatoid arthritis, as noted above; they are commonly found in significant amounts in a number of other diseases frequently characterized by hypergammaglobulinemia, as well as in a sizable percentage of asymptomatic elderly individuals (Vaughn, 1969) (Table 38-6). It should be emphasized that the diagnosis of rheumatoid arthritis, like SLE, is based on a constellation of clinical manifestations with laboratory studies confirming clinical impressions.

First, we must define exactly what we mean by rheumatoid factors. Highly purified immunoglobulins are only weakly immunogenic, particularly in the same species. The observations that the serum of many rheumatoid arthritis patients agglutinated sheep erythrocytes coated with rabbit anti-sheep red blood cell antibody (Rose-Waaler test) led to the finding that similar binding by rheumatoid arthritis serum to heat-aggregated human gamma globulin coated on inert particles like latex beads or bentonite resulted in the agglutination or flocculation (respectively) of the latter. The responsible serum factor was found to be an IgM gamma globulin, which could be quantitated by serial dilution of the test serum. Earlier, observers thought that rheumatoid factors reacted with unique antigenic determinants uncovered or formed when normal gamma globulins were altered by exogenous factors, possibly an infection. A form of autoimmunity would then result. More recent findings have suggested that the situation is much more complex.

Although RF production may be induced by exogenously altered autologous gamma globulin, the usual rheumatoid factors react with determinants found in both aggregated and native IgG. Reactivity with the aggregated form is more likely because of the multivalent antigenic sites achieved during the process of aggregation (Winchester, 1976). Indeed, the presence of normal (unaggregated) IgG in the test serum may competitively inhibit to some degree the *in vitro* binding of the aggregated IgG reagent to IgM rheumatoid factors in the same specimen (Winchester, 1976).

RF can be of any immunoglobulin class; most of the clinically applied methods reflect the amount of IgM RF because of the greater efficacy of pentavalent IgM molecules in agglutination reactions (Winchester, 1976). RF of the IgG and IgA class may be very important in both diagnosis and understanding of immunopathology (Pope, 1974). However, their bivalency makes for weak binding and their detection requires much more sensitive, complex, and time-consuming techniques still generally limited to research laboratories (Hay, 1975).

RF found in rheumatoid arthritis and chronic infectious/inflammatory states is generally polyclonal. However, monoclonal (paraprotein) rheumatoid factors may be found in paraproteins formed in multiple myeloma, Waldenström's macroglobulinemia, purpura hyperglobulinemia, and in certain other lymphoproliferative states (Capra, 1971). A cold-reactive RF forms mixed cryoprecipitates with native IgG. It is seen in some patients with SLE, Sjögren's syndrome, and infectious mononucleosis, and in the "mixed cryoglobulinemia" syndrome (see later section) presenting with vasculitis, arthritis, and frequently progressive glomerulonephritis.

RF are produced actively in the synovium of involved joints (Johnson, 1975). It is present, along with IgG, in the neutrophils, and sometimes in cryoprecipitable complexes, in the inflammatory joint fluid. RF here are generally IgM but may be IgG or IgA as well. Antinuclear antibodies (even anti-DNA antibodies) have been found in joint fluid at a time when the serum does not contain them. Likewise, fluid complement levels are generally quite depressed, with evidence of complement

Table 38-6. RHEUMATOID FACTOR—POSITIVE LATEX FIXATION TESTS IN VARIOUS CLINICAL STATES

CLINICAL STATES	PERCENTAGE POSITIVE ($\geq$ 1:160 dilution)
Rheumatoid arthritis	80%
Juvenile rheumatoid arthritis	20%
Ankylosing spondylitis	<15%
Infections	
SBE	48%
Viral disease, non-specific	15%
Infectious hepatitis	24%
Tuberculosis	11%
Leprosy	24%
Lung Diseases	
Bronchitis	62%
Asthma	17%
Silicosis	15%
Idiopathic pulmonary fibrosis	32%
Miscellaneous Disease	
Sarcoid	17%
Cirrhosis of liver	36%
Sjögren's syndrome	>90%
Myocardial infarction	12%

deposition (along with IgG and IgM) in involved synovial tissue while serum complement levels are generally normal in rheumatoid arthritis of mild to moderate severity without prominent extra-articular manifestations.

Therefore, it is not too surprising that the complexes of RF and "substrate" IgG found in the serum appear to differ in several respects from those in the joint fluid (possibly involving antigen-IgG immune complexes or self-associating IgG rheumatoid factors as well) and generally do not bind C1q well. The latter probably at least partially explains why depressed serum complement levels and glomerulonephritis are so much less common in rheumatoid arthritis than in SLE.

The pathogenic significance of RF is still debated. Some have speculated that RF may exert a protective role in promoting phagocytic clearance of circulating immune complexes (Tesor, 1970). Serum rheumatoid factors are absent in some patients with classic rheumatoid arthritis, even when detailed searches are also made for non-IgM and "hidden" rheumatoid factors (Winchester, 1976). About 30 per cent of these with hypogammaglobulinemia and with little IgM or IgG and no rheumatoid factors develop a rheumatoid arthritis-like picture. This has suggested that RF may be an abortive protective mechanism and that the high (sometimes extremely high) RF levels found in highly expressed rheumatoid arthritis (RA) with a worse prognosis reflects a very potent pathogenic process to which RF production is a response. However, it is conceivable that in such patients the large IgG-IgM complexes are pathogenic (since depressed serum complement levels are more common then). Indeed, therapeutic attempts have been made to reduce the levels of RF, and presumably the toxic complexes, with penicillamine.

Clinical Application of Rheumatoid Factor Determinations

The major reason for looking for RF is when RA is suspect. In this regard RF determination should be considered only in light of the clinical picture, evidence of inflammatory reaction (sedimentation rate, possibly serum protein electrophoresis), appropriate joint x-rays, and examination of the joint fluid for appearance, cell count, crystals, mucin clot and protein levels, complement levels, and culture where appropriate. Several technical approaches to measure RF are used, some of which will be discussed here.

In most clinical laboratories, the latex fixation test of Singer (1975) is still preferred for RF determinations. *Advantages* are the relative simplicity and speed of performance. *Disadvantages and possible pitfalls* are: (1) it gen-

erally detects mainly IgM RF; (2) low levels are present in normals, particularly with increasing age. These may be a heterogeneous group of antigammaglobulins (Singer, 1975). Therefore, normal ranges have to be established for each laboratory; (3) a titer of $\geq 1:80$ is a reasonable starting point; observers feel that the extensively marketed and commonly used "slide latex" tests are less sensitive and reproducible than the tube latex test. The slide tests should be used only for screening purposes, if at all; (4) false positive RF tests may be seen in sera which are hyperlipidemic, contain bulky cryoglobulins, or in which the first component of complement has not been inactivated.

True "positive" RF tests are found, generally in lower titer, in a number of inflammatory conditions other than RF, such as subacute bacterial endocarditis, sarcoidosis, infectious mononucleosis, and SLE (Table 38-6). However, most of these conditions are characterized by prominent hypergammaglobulinemia, in helpful distinction to the normal or slightly elevated levels seen in typical RA. The highly expressed RA patients with nodules in subcutaneous areas, vasculitis, and sometimes involvement of the heart, lungs, and eyes, are generally not difficult to distinguish clinically; serum RF levels are often very high here. The distinction between RA and SLE on clinical grounds is sometimes difficult, especially in the early stages. A helpful point is that almost all the 20 to 25 per cent of RA patients whose serum is ANA positive also have prominently elevated serum RF levels as well; by contrast, RF appears in only about 20 per cent of SLE patients (generally in modest titer), while positive ANA tests are seen in >95 per cent of cases, and hypergammaglobulinemia is also common.

A number of clinical pictures considered in the diagnosis of RA may present with negative RF determination. Included among them may be:

(a) *Early RA*—significantly elevated RF titers may not be seen in the serum for the first several months; RF may be found in the inflammatory joint fluid before it is seen in the serum.

(b) *Juvenile RA*—positive latex RF tests are found in about 30 per cent of typical cases. In additional patients, RF or IgG, and IgA classes are found by specialized techniques. RF are seen more commonly with (1) onset past age 10, (2) fever, subcutaneous nodules, and antinuclear factors. The latter are found more commonly when iridocyclitis is present. Evidence of currently or recently antecedent streptococcal infection should be looked for where appropriate.

(c) *Arthritis associated with certain systemic diseases* (Thaler, 1977)—such as Marie-Strumpell ankylosing spondylitis, Reiter's syndrome, colitic arthropathy, and psoriatic arthritis. The initiating events likely differ in these individuals, but spondylitis, sacroileitis, ocular involvement, and increased incidence of histocompatibility type B 27 are seen in all. RF levels and complement levels in both serum and joint fluids are usually normal.

(d) In some "definite" and a few "classic" RA cases (using the clinical criteria of the American Rheumatism Association) (Ropes, 1956), RF levels are consistently negative.

CRYOGLOBULINS

Cryoglobulins are immunoglobulins (Ig) of a single class, or complexes consisting of more than one Ig class, which are altered by some process which makes them insoluble to varying degrees at temperatures below 37°C. (Brouet, 1974; Barnett, 1970a). This alteration may involve binding with presumptive antigens and/or complement components either prior to or during the process of cryoprecipitation. Although such precipitation generally is most striking at 4°C., some degree of it occurs at temperatures of 30 to 31°C. reached in some distal small vessels—of obvious biologic significance. A great deal of study in recent years reveals that cryoglobulins are very heterogeneous in type and formation and may play important roles in vasculitis and nephritis associated with systemic disease. Cryoglobulins may be classified as follows:

Single monoclonal immunoglobulin (cryoglobulin 1)—these are paraproteins most commonly IgG (in multiple myeloma) and IgM (in macroglobulinemia, some lymphomas), but IgA and "Bence-Jones" types have been described (Brouet, 1974). Such cryoglobulins are also sometimes seen in "benign" monoclonal gammopathy, which may or may not be followed by overt lymphoproliferative malignancy years later. Single monoclonal cryoglobulins are generally present in high (>5 mg/ml) concentration in the serum.

Mixed polyclonal-monoclonal (cryoglobulin 2)—these are complexes of a polyclonal "antigen" (generally IgG) and monoclonal IgM with anti-IgG (rheumatoid factor activity). The monoclonal anti-IgG may occasionally be in the IgG or IgA class (Brouet, 1974). This polyclonal-monoclonal complex is often associated with IgM lymphoproliferative states, with certain IgM antibody activities (cold agglutinins, heterophil antibody) also present in the complex. This type of cryoglobulin is present in moderate to high (>1 mg/ml) levels in the serum.

Mixed polyclonal-polyclonal (cryoglobulin 3)—in this complex, both components are polyclonal (most commonly IgG-IgM, occasionally IgG-IgM-IgA). Complement components are frequently present (particularly C1q), and various antigenic and antibody activities in the cryoprecipitate have been described. These cryoglobulins are present in low (<1 mg/ml) levels in the serum and constitute over half the cases of cryoglobulinemia. Very low levels (<80 μg/ml) are found in up to 50 per cent of normal sera. The exact constituents of cryoprecipitate vary not only between conditions but also among individual patients with the same condition. It has now been appreciated that the Ig components with rheumatoid factor activity may be binding to the Fc portion of another Ig molecule which is also bound in an immune complex.

Mixed cryoglobulins may be found in certain infections such as HBs antigen-positive hepatitis, cytomegalic virus, infectious mononucleosis, and lepromatous leprosy. Antigenic determinants of the infectious organism may be found in some cases when dissociation of the complex is feasible. The immunoglobulin (Ig) here is frequently IgM, especially in certain viral infections.

Cryoprecipitates commonly encountered in sera of SLE patients have been found to contain different component patterns in different studies (Barnett, 1970a). IgG-C1q complexes without other complement components and antilymphocyte as well as anti-IgG in IgM components of mixed cryoglobulins have been found (Winfield, 1977). The IgM with rheumatoid factor activity appears to be deposited in tissue lesions as part of the complex. Opinions vary as to the frequency with which DNA-anti-DNA complexes are present (Barnett, 1970a; Winfield, 1977).

4

MECHANISMS AND CLINICAL MANIFESTATIONS ASSOCIATED WITH CRYOGLOBULINEMIA

Cryoglobulins, types 1 and 2, occur mainly in immunoproliferative disorders (about 5 per cent of those with multiple myeloma, and an even higher per cent of patients with macroglobulinemia, lymphomas, and lymphocytic leukemias). Types 2 and 3 cryoglobulins are generally associated with conditions in which prominently elevated rheumatoid factor levels are seen, including certain acute and chronic infections and autoimmune disorders. However, in at least one third of cases, cryoglobulins appear in the absence of overt associated disease and are called "essential." Symptoms which occur depending on the nature of the cryoglobulin generally are due to the *precipitability* in cooler parts of the body. These include Raynaud's phenomenon and acrocyanosis; in more severe cases with high levels of cryoglobulins (or exposure to very cold temperatures) digital necrosis with gangrene can occur. Cryoglobulins may be found in up to 20 per cent of patients with cold-induced urticaria. Purpura in the lower extremities is common because of cooler skin temperatures and effects of stasis. *Hyperviscosity* may lead to sludging in certain vessels (most readily observed in the retinal and conjunctival areas) and may contribute to the ischemic changes, including those in the nervous system. *Immune complexes* may also contribute to symptoms. Twenty per cent of patients with cryoglobulins (not including those with SLE) may have renal disease, most commonly a diffuse glomerulonephritis. In these cases immunoglobulin and complement are found in a granular pattern in the glomerulus. This is most commonly seen in type 2 cryoglobulins, without any correlation between the type of cryoglobulin and precise pattern of renal histopathology. Immune complex patterns of manifestation may include joint symptoms with mixed cryoglobulins, especially type 3, and intra-abdominal vascular involvement.

Thus one can find manifestations that appear to be due to the cryoglobulins per se without associated defined collagen-vascular or "autoimmune disease." This is best exemplified in the "mixed cryoglobulin" syndrome originally described by Meltzer (1966), with joint and skin involvement and sometimes progressive glomerulonephritis. On the other hand, there is increasing evidence for the role of cryoglobulins, not only in collagen-vascular lymphoproliferative disorders but also in other putative "immune-complex" mediated diseases, such as acute post-streptococcal glomerulonephritis (McIntosh, 1975). In the latter, the cryoprecipitates may contain Ig with anti-streptococcal antibody, and their presence seems to correlate with active or persistent disease.

The *techniques* for detection of cryoglobulins are relatively straightforward and easy to carry out in all clinical laboratories, provided certain simple precautions are observed: (1) The blood should be allowed both to clot and to be transported at as close to body temperature as feasible to avoid losing small amounts of cryoglobulin, which occurs when clotting takes place at cool temperatures; (2) for the same reason, serum separation should be carried out in a warm environment; (3) serum then stored at 4°C. should be observed for at least four days before a negative report is submitted; (4) to be definitely identified as a typical cryoprecipitate, the cold-precipitable material must be in a clear serum specimen obtained by complete clotting and should redissolve completely on warming of the chilled specimen. The amount of cryoglobulin can be roughly quantitated by determination of protein content in the cryoprecipitate. A more gross screening method has been the "cryocrit" determination in which the serum is cold-incubated in a hematocrit tube, which is then centrifuged in the cold after maximal cryoprecipitation has occurred. The relative volume occupied by the cryoprecipitate is then expressed on a percentage basis.

IMMUNE COMPLEXES AND THEIR MEASUREMENT IN DISEASE STATES

With increasing interest in the possible role of immune complexes in a variety of disease states, including postulated "autoimmune" disorders, great efforts have been made to develop methods that will measure circulating immune complexes. To date, such efforts have been limited by several considerations (Agnello, 1976). Most, if not all, techniques applicable to clinical use measure putative immune complexes by indirect methods and not by direct measurement. The techniques often involve biologic assays with the problem of intrinsic variability that may result. Because immune complexes likely vary considerably in both components and certain biologic properties, one technique may not accurately meas-

Table 38-7. SOME APPROACHES TO THE
MEASUREMENT OF CIRCULATING
IMMUNE COMPLEXES

Anticomplementary activity of serum
Techniques involving first component of complement (C1)
    C1 precipitin
    C1 binding radioimmunoassay
Techniques utilizing rheumatoid factors (RF)
    Inhibition of binding of RF to aggregated IgG
    Inhibition of the aggregation by RF of IgG-coated latex
    particles
Techniques involving cellular substrates
    Inhibition of binding of aggregated IgG to Raji cells
    Binding to peritoneal macrophages
    Platelet aggregation

ure all types of immune complexes. Conversely, aggregation of immunoglobulins by physical means not involving immune mechanisms may well mimic the reactivity of true immune complexes with any of the methods described, since at least some of the activities of immune complexes in these assays is secondary to aggregations of immunoglobulins that seem to occur during formation of the complex.

Many assays have been described or are under development. The discussion here will be limited to those under intensive use or study in this country (Table 38-7).

COMPLEMENT-RELATED ASSAYS

Anticomplementary Activity of the Serum. For years, it had been noted that complement-fixation serologic tests for syphilis and other infectious diseases were frequently not feasible because of "anticomplementary activity" of the serum itself (in the absence of antigenic material in the medium) (Johnson, 1975). It is now recognized that, in many of those cases, the serum involved bound added complement, probably to an immune complex contained therein. In some of the cases, hemolytic complement activity of the serum itself was reduced, suggesting *in vivo* binding of complement. This demonstration has generally not turned out to be suitable for clinical diagnostic use. However, an extension of that, the C1q binding test, has been used extensively.

The C1q Precipitin Assay. The C1q molecule, a subunit of the first component of complement, binds with monomeric IgG (in the IgG_1, IgG_2, IgG_3 sub-classes) and IgM. The binding of C1q is markedly increased if the IgG is aggregated, even when (in certain situations) the aggregated Ig is soluble. When large amounts of C1q binding aggregated Ig are present, a precipitin reaction in gel diffusion set-up can be observed. However, the relative insensitivity of this technique has limited its diagnostic applicability to conditions like SLE in which relatively large amounts of circulating complexes are present.

Complement-Binding Assays. This modification employs the binding of radiolabeled C1q to a test serum in comparison with binding of this labeled reagent to a standardized soluble preparation of aggregated IgG (Nydegger, 1974; Hay, 1976). Because such interaction generally does not result in an insoluble reaction product, separation of the bound C1q has been accomplished by means such as the addition of appropriate concentrations of polyethylene glycol (PEG). This addition results in precipitation of complexes (including bound C1q) over 200,000 dalton m.w., whereas the unbound C1q ($<$200,000 m.w.) remains in the supernatant. Normal sera generally bind up to 11 per cent of added C1q. This technique (Woodrofe, 1977) is more sensitive than the precipitin assay, but several *disadvantages* and *potential* pitfalls must be considered: (1) C1q may be bound by Ig molecules which are physically aggregated (such as occurs sometimes during storage). Freshly obtained sera or sera stored at $-70°$C. should be used whenever possible (Woodrofe, 1977). (2) Substances other than Ig complexes may bind C1q. For example, double-stranded and single-stranded DNA (which may be found in serum and pathologic fluids) bind C1q, as do certain other polyribonucleotides, heparin, and endotoxins. Prior heat inactivation of the serum will eliminate some of this non-immunologic binding of C1q. However, it also reduces the binding of the aggregated IgG, decreasing the sensitivity of the test. Some (Zubler, 1976) have used EDTA-treatment of serum rather than heating, with reportedly increased sensitivity; (3) There are relatively low molecular weight complexes in high antigen-excess which may or may not contain Ig molecules found in the sera of some SLE patients that do not react to alkylation/reduction methods as one would expect in the case of immune complexes (Woodrofe, 1977) (4) Relatively pure preparations of C1q are required; the lack of ready availability of C1q has generally limited this technique to suitably equipped research laboratories. (5) C1q tends to aggregate during radiolabeling; separation techniques may increase the subsequent nonspecific precipitation of C1q in polyethylene glycol.

METHODS INVOLVING
RHEUMATOID FACTORS

The principle underlying these techniques is that rheumatoid factors (particularly monoclonal ones occurring in macroglobulinemia or as components of certain cryoglobulins described above) will bind to immune complexes. In a situation analogous to that seen with C1q, a precipitin-in-agar reaction can be observed if the high levels of immune complexes are present (Winchester, 1971). However, more recently, a binding inhibition approach has been tried, using one of two modifications.

A solid-phase radioimmunoassay (Luthra, 1975) utilizes monoclonal rheumatoid factor bound to an insoluble support such as polystyrene tube or microcrystalline cellulose. The ability of the test serum when first applied to block the subsequent binding of a standardized ^{125}I-labeled aggregated gamma globulin is measured in comparison with the blocking ability of unlabeled aggregated gamma globulin. The latter is used in several concentrations so that a standard curve can be derived. By plotting the degree of binding-inhibition which results from use of the test serum against the standard curve, one can estimate the activity equivalent to a certain amount of soluble aggregated Ig complexes.

In a second modification, single latex particles of a particular size are coated with soluble aggregated IgG (Levinsky, 1977). Such particles would ordinarily be aggregated by addition of a rheumatoid factor. If the test serum is incubated with the rheumatoid factor (RF) in advance, the binding of the RF to any immune complexes in the serum will reduce the aggregation of the coated latex particles subsequently added to the mixture. The number of non-agglutinated particles is counted.

These rheumatoid factor binding techniques are very sensitive but have major *limitations* and *potential pitfalls:* (1) They do not measure immune complexes directly; as with C1q, physically aggregated and monomeric IgG elements in the serum may prevent subsequent binding of the RF to either the labeled aggregated IgG or IgG-coated latex particles. (2) The use of aggregated IgG (either labeled or on latex particles) to simulate an immune complex may not always be valid, depending on the nature of the immune complex. (3) Different RF do vary in the degree of affinity for complexed IgG and aggregated IgG. The greater the affinity; the more sensitive the assay. In most cases, it appears that monoclonal RF without cryoglobulin properties seem to work most effectively with good sensitivity. This variance may present a major problem because of the limited amount of monoclonal RF from a single patient donor available for long-term use. Use of the more readily available polyclonal RF will result in a sensitive assay; however, polyclonal RF which may be present in test sera will affect the determination. (4) Methods utilizing RF reagents may preferentially detect smaller circulating immune complexes not picked up by other techniques. This may result in the more common reporting of positive results in rheumatoid arthritis sera which seem to contain disproportionately more of these smaller complexes.

PLATELET AGGREGATION TESTS (Myllyla, 1973)

Since immune complexes tend to aggregate platelets, aliquots of pooled washed platelets from normal donors may be incubated with serial dilutions of test and positive control (immune complex-containing) sera overnight, generally at 37°C. Although sensitive, this assay is sometimes quite variable from day to day, possibly relating to platelet sources used, among other factors.

THE RAJI CELL ASSAY

Principle of the Raji Cell Assay (Theofilopoulos, 1976). Different B lymphoblastoid cells maintained in culture retain varying densities of the surface membrane Ig (SIg) receptors for the Fc portion of IgG and for C3. The Raji line cells have no SIg, low avidity Fc receptors, and high density of receptors for C3. These characteristics have been used to determine the amount of gamma globulin from a test or control serum which binds to a prescribed number of Raji cells, detected by the subsequent attachment of radiolabeled anti-human IgG. The principle underlying this assay is that the relatively weak binding of circulating Ig to the Fc receptor serves as a fair estimate of the "background" binding of monomeric Ig when there is little or no immune complex alteration of the Ig. More IgG which is part of a circulating immune complex with antigen and complement binds to the Raji cells than does monomeric IgG, because the complex binds not only to the weaker Fc receptor but also to the strong C3 receptor. In this way, the binding of test sera can be compared with a standard curve derived from the binding of measured amounts of aggregated IgG (with bound complement).

The major *advantages* of the Raji cell assay are (Woodrofe, 1977): (a) It is very sensitive. As little as 5 μg of bound aggregated IgG can be detected. In comparison, the usual sensitivity of C1q binding assays and monoclonal RF assays are to levels of 50 and 25 μg, respectively. (b) Determinations are not altered in sera which is heated to 56°C., stored in the frozen state, or to which is added heparin, DNA, or endotoxin. (c) No unique reagents like highly purified C1q or monoclonal RF are required. ^{125}I anti-IgG is needed, but the capacity for preparation of this reagent is more readily available with likelihood that it can be supplied to clinical laboratories.

Disadvantages and potential pitfalls (Woodrofe, 1977) of this technique include the following: (a) There is a need to maintain a lymphoblastoid cell line in continuous culture. This is technically not too difficult. However, the varying results obtained in different laboratories using this technique may be due in part to different cell receptor characteristics which developed when aliquots of what was originally one cell line have been maintained by different groups. (b) The great sensitivity of the technique is accomplished by higher binding of normal IgG than is seen with other techniques. (c) More day-to-day variation in the binding equivalents requires establishing a standard curve with each test run (Woodrofe, 1977). (d) Cytotoxic anti-lymphocyte antibodies may cause some lysis of the cultured cells.

A VIEW OF THE CURRENT SIGNIFICANCE OF ASSAYS FOR IMMUNE COMPLEXES

This field is one characterized by rapid change, with findings of uncertain significance. There appears to be little question that serum of many patients with active SLE contains putative immune complexes by almost any technique employed; estimation of such levels may help in determining prognosis and response to therapy. Consistent findings seem to be present in some stages of hepatitis, "essential mixed cryoglobulinemia," and certain other vasculitis patterns. However, there have been increasing, and sometimes bewildering and contradictory, reports of presumptive circulating immune complexes detected by one technique or another. These include a variety of infections, malignancy, and childhood nephrotic syndrome to name a few. It is certainly conceivable that circulating immune complexes do occur quite commonly in disease and may be of varying degrees of pathogenic importance. It is also likely that optimal immune complex detection may require concomitant use of several techniques, each with its own intrinsic advantages and disadvantages. For example, the Raji cell assay is very sensitive for detecting the presence of relatively large complexes with bound C3. By comparison, monoclonal RF techniques are better for detecting smaller complexes, and the C1q binding assays are sensitive for complexes which effectively bind that complement component. However, it is also possible that the indirect assays available may be binding to something besides an immune complex, even if that "something" contains IgG. Analytical studies of materials considered as immune complexes will help clarify the picture.

ORGAN-DIRECTED AUTOIMMUNE STATES

ENDOCRINE DISORDERS

THYROID

The thyroid appears to be one of the best examples of how a postulated autoimmune pathogenesis might cause organ-directed disease (Volpe, 1977). Although there is much still to be learned about the exact mechanisms involved, current theories suggest that normal thyroglobulin (presumably released from the thyroid) circulates systemically in very low amounts. This may be sufficient to induce a "low-zone" (low dose) T-lymphocyte tolerance in normals, with weak production of antithyroglobulin by those B cells with receptors for thyroglobulin, increasing gradually (particularly in females) with age. Likely because of some alteration of the thyroid by infections or chemical or other factors, there is induced in the (genetically?) predisposed individual immune responses to one or more thyroid components. These immune responses may or may not cause tissue destruction, but are frequently valuable as diagnostic markers.

Some consideration of the major thyroid disorders in which immunologic study is of assistance will be helpful before considering the individual tests. Hashimoto's thyroiditis is an inflammatory condition occurring mainly in middle-aged women and characterized by gland enlargement due to marked lymphocytic inflammatory changes. The latter may consist of lymphoid follicles with active germinal centers, in which much of the antithyroglobulin antibody appears to be synthesized. Normal thyroid glandular structures are adversely altered, and in prominent cases, progressive disease may lead to thyroid atrophy and myxedema. In *thyrotoxicosis*, the thyroid may contain small areas of lymphoid infiltration as well as evidence of the typical glandular hyperactivity. Graves' disease is a multisystemic disorder, particularly in young to middle-aged females, consisting (to varying degrees) of (1) hyperthyroidism with diffuse hyperplasia of the thyroid (the most common pattern seen with diffuse toxic goiter); (2) a myopathy; (3) an infiltrative ophthalmopathy, frequently leading to exophthalmos; (4) presence of long-acting thyroid stimulator (LATS).

As with all the organ-oriented diseases associated with autoantibody production, it is very important to determine when the antibodies under discussion are pathogenic or are epiphenomena, reacting to antigens liberated as a result of tissue damage owing to nonimmune causes. A third possibility is that the immune reactivity is not the primary pathogenic event but, once present, causes further tissue damage. Evidence against a primary pathogenic role for thyroid autoantibodies in Hashimoto's and Graves' diseases is (1) the lack of correlation between the level of autoantibody and the severity of disease in individual cases, and (2) the lack of development of thyroid disease in infants born with high levels of antithyroid antibodies because of placental transfer. The failure to transfer disease when antibodies are present in the serum may mean that the pathogenic antibodies had been bound by thyroid tissue in the serum donor (Nakamura, 1969).

In terms of laboratory evaluation, the best *screening* test for all antithyroid antibodies appears to be immunofluorescence using frozen section of primate thyroid tissue, preferably obtained from thyrotoxic glands of blood group O humans (Tung, 1974). This technique can detect with reasonable sensitivity antibodies to thyroglobulin, with a floccular pattern seen in the colloid, the "second colloid antigen" (CA-2) resulting in a diffuse staining, and microsomal antigens of thyroid epithelial cells leading to cytoplasmic (but not nuclear) staining of these cells but not of epithelial cells of other organs like the kidneys.

The technique employed is similar to that used in other indirect immunofluorescent techniques with the understanding that use of methanol-fixed (for colloid antigens) and unfixed (for epithelial antigens) sections of primate thyroid tissue is essential, and specificity for thyroid cells must be demonstrated.

Positive binding is seen in low dilutions of normal sera, possibly related to asymptomatic focal lymphocytic thyroiditis. Positive tests are found in up to 90 per cent of those with active Hashimoto's thyroiditis, and a persistently negative test mitigates strongly against this diagnosis, in comparison with the weakly positive or negative reactions seen commonly in other types of non-toxic goiter and thyroid tumors. Positive staining is seen with a majority of sera from those with idiopathic myxedema (although more sensitive techniques may sometimes be required). On the other hand, the immunofluorescence technique is the only current method available for detection of antibodies to the CA-2 antigen of colloid. The latter antibodies are still of uncertain significance; however, some report their presence in 5 to 8 per cent of thyroiditis patients in the absence of other demonstrable anti-thyroid antibodies (Bigazzi, 1976). However, positive CA-2 reactions are also seen with sera of 30 to 50 per cent of those with De Quervain's thyroiditis, Graves' disease, and thyroid cancer.

However, strongly positive binding of serum antibodies specific for colloid or epithelial cells does not make a diagnosis of lymphocytic thyroiditis and/or idiopathic myxedema. One or more antithyroid antibodies (particu-

larly those directed against thyroid epithelial cells) are found in a minority of those with other thyroid disorders, other "antitissue" autoimmune states like pernicious anemia, myasthenia gravis, SLE, and highly expressed rheumatoid arthritis (Bigazzi, 1976).

Measurement of *anti-thyroglobulin antibodies* by the tanned cell *hemagglutination* test is used extensively. Its major *advantages* are (a) the specificity of the reaction for a particular antigenic group; (b) its great sensitivity (likely greater than immunofluorescence). A very high antibody titer ($>1:1000$) suggests a diagnosis of Hashimoto's thyroiditis or "primary" myxedema, rather than other thyroid or non-thyroid conditions. *Disadvantages* of this technique are (a) the requirement for relatively pure thyroglobulin. However, this need appears to be currently met from commercial sources, including some kits which have been used with good results; (b) the need to consider heterophil antibodies against the carrier cells. However, this is generally not a major problem, since diagnostic titers of anti-thyroid antibodies are generally present at much greater serum dilution than is the case for the heterophil antibodies; (c) like screening immunofluorescence, it is not too specific. Some reactivity is seen with sera of normals, especially in older females, possibly reflecting "silent" thyroiditis. Once upper limits of normal have been established in each laboratory, positive responses are seen in 75 per cent of those with Hashimoto's disease and idiopathic myxedema and in 40 per cent of those with Graves' disease and thyroid tumors (Table 38-8). However, titer differences noted above may help in the differential diagnosis.

Anti-thyroglobulin antibodies have also been measured by the precipitin and latex agglutination technique. Both of these are insufficiently sensitive for diagnostic screening purposes; however, positive responses in significant titer are more specific for Hashimoto's thyroiditis and idiopathic myxedema.

The screening immunofluorescence test is currently the most sensitive method for detecting antigens from lipoprotein membranes of microsomes in the cytoplasm of thyroid epithelial cells (from an unfixed thyrotoxic gland) in the measurement of *antithyroid microsomal antibody*. The apical staining in the epithelial cells can generally be distinguished readily from the colloid staining noted above and from the cytoplasmic staining due to antimitochondrial antibodies. It is positive in 70

Table 38–8. PREVALENCE OF ANTI-THYROID
ANTIBODIES IN SOME DISEASES

CLINICAL STATE	ANTIBODIES		
	Thyroglobulin	CA-2*	Thyroid epithelial
Hashimoto's	75–95%	40–70%	70–90%
Idiopathic myxedema	75%	40%	65%
Graves	40%	5–10%	50%
Non-toxic goiter	20–30%	–	20%
Thyroid cancer	40%	10%	15%
Pernicious anemia	25%	–	10%
Normals	10%	–	10%
Normals > 70 years old	20%+	–	20%+

Modified from Bigazzi, P. L., and Rose, N. R.: Tests for antibodies to tissue-specific antigens. *In* Rose, N. R., and Friedman, H. (eds.): Manual of Clinical Immunology Washington, American Society of Microbiology, 1976; Tung, K. S. K., Ramos, C. V., and Deodhar, S. D.: Anti-thyroid antibodies in juvenile lymphocytic thyroiditis. Am. J. Clin. Pathol., *61*:549, 1974; and Doniach, D.: *In* Bastenie, V. A., and Gepts, W. (eds.): Immunology and Autoimmunity in Diabetes Mellitus. Amsterdam, Excerpta Medica, 1974.
*CA-2 = colloid antigen, or "second antigen of the colloid."

to 90 per cent of those with active thyroiditis, 65 per cent of those with idiopathic hypothyroidism, 50 per cent of those with thyrotoxicosis, and about 17 per cent of those with thyroid tumors (Table 38–8). The complement fixation assay is less sensitive, but more specific, generally being positive only in those with active thyroiditis.

Long-acting thyroid stimulator (LATS) is a polyclonal gamma globulin which appears to bind to a receptor on thyroid cells with a pattern similar to any antigen-antibody reaction (Smith, 1970). It stimulates thyroid activity and is assayed by measuring the release of radioactive iodine from mouse thyroid at 8 to 24 hours (compared to the two-hour release period for TSH). It is present in the sera of about 50 per cent of those with Graves' disease where it is thought to be involved in its pathogenesis without feedback inhibition of its synthesis by thyroid hormone. LATS is absent or present only in small amounts in patients with nodular toxic goiter or other thyroid disorders.

**Summary—use of thyroid immunology
tests in diagnosis (Table 38–8)**

Immunofluorescence Screening Test. Negative staining of colloid and epithelial cytoplasm is strong evidence against diagnosis of active Hashimoto's thyroiditis or primary myxedema, in comparison with other types of thyroiditis, nodules, or tumors. Positive response, not diagnostic for thyroiditis, is seen in other thyroid disorders and other autoimmune states.

Thyroglobulin Hemagglutinin Test. This is not specific, but high (>1:1000) titers are unusual except in Hashimoto's thyroiditis.

Complement Fixation Tests for Microsomal Antigen. When positive, these tests strongly suggest active Hashimoto's thyroiditis.

ADRENAL

More than two thirds of cases of Addison's disease are idiopathic; evidence suggests that many of these are autoimmune in etiology, analogous to Hashimoto's thyroiditis (Volpe, 1977). In about 40 to 70 per cent of those with Addison's disease, the serum contains antibodies (generally in <1:100 titer) against cortical elements, probably microsomal, as detected by immunofluorescence (Bigazzi, 1968) and other techniques (Irvine, 1967). These antibodies, generally present in low titer, are not a simple reflection of adrenal cell damage, since they are present in only 7 to 18 per cent of those with adrenals markedly involved by tuberculosis, and in only 1 per cent of normals (Bigazzi, 1976). These antibodies generally bind to components in the whole adrenal cortex, but may occasionally involve only individual zones.

There is a striking incidence (over 40 per cent) of autoimmune involvement of other endocrine glands in patients with Addison's disease (Blizzard, 1967): (1) thyroid (Hashimoto's and Graves' diseases, asymptomatic anti-thyroid antibodies); (2) ovary with antibodies reacting with steroid-producing cells in the theca interna. These cells may contain antigens that cross-react with antigens in the adrenal cortex; (3) pernicious anemia; (4) diabetes; (5) hypoparathyroidism. It is of interest that the converse situation is not the case; anti-adrenal antibodies are unusual in other autoimmune disorders unless there is associated adrenal gland involvement.

OVARY AND TESTIS

Antibodies against cytoplasmic components of different cells of the ovary have been described in Addison's disease and in premature ovarian failure (Irvine, 1969). These techniques are generally still limited to research laboratories and are not standardized for clinical use.

Antisperm antibodies have been investigated in the sera of infertile couples by a variety of techniques (Shulman, 1976). Several agglutination techniques utilize semen of either the patient or a homologous male (if enough sperm of adequate motility are not available from the former). In studies from several laboratories, appropriately diluted (generally >1:8) sera of about 18 per cent and 9 per cent of infertile males and females, respectively, agglutinate test sperm, provided that several approaches are used and borderline response tests are repeated. By contrast, such reactivity is found in only 3 per cent of normal sera (Shulman, 1976). Elevated serum antisperm antibody levels are found after vasectomy, but only occasionally in males with primary testicular agenesis. Sperm immobilization tests (Isojima, 1972) have been used less extensively, with need for more comparative studies in large patient groups. It appears that extensive experience with either technique is required to make valid interpretations of the sometimes subjective findings.

DIABETES MELLITUS

Because of the relatively high incidence of autoimmune disorders in those with diabetes, an immunologic basis for this common condition has been sought (Doniach, 1974). Although the results have generally been negative, antibodies reacting with all cells of the islets have been found in those patients with diabetes accompanying "autoimmune endocrine" disorders. There appears to be a higher incidence of these anti-islet cell antibodies in groups of patients with insulin-dependent diabetes. Indeed, some feel the presence of these antibodies is a marker of insulin dependency (Irvine, 1977). In addition to the common appearance of anti-insulin antibodies in insulin-treated subjects, the same antibodies have also been found in sera of some untreated diabetics. Such antibodies have also been found in sera of a small group of patients with normal fasting blood sugar and postprandial hypoglycemia. An immunoglobulin in the sera of insulin-resistant diabetics appears to bind to a tissue receptor for insulin, preventing some of the insulin biologic effects (Flier, 1976).

GASTROINTESTINAL DISORDERS

PERNICIOUS ANEMIA AND ATROPHIC GASTRITIS

The histopathologic picture in atrophic gastritis that almost always accompanies pernicious anemia is characterized by lymphocytic infiltrate and absence of parietal and chief cells (Irvine, 1975). Associated with the lesion is decreased synthesis of gastric acid and intrinsic factor. The latter normally binds ingested vitamin B_{12} at one site and binds to receptors in the distal ileum at another of its sites. In this manner, vitamin B_{12} transport across the ileum is affected.

Besides the histologic picture, several other immunologic findings suggest an autoimmune pathogenesis of pernicious anemia. Antibodies against cytoplasmic component of gastric parietal cells are detected by immunofluorescence in up to 90 per cent of those with pernicious anemia, in a lower percentage (about 60 per cent) of those with atrophic gastritis without hematologic abnormalities, and in those with other autoimmune diseases like thyroiditis. These antibodies, like certain other anti-tissue antibodies, are unusual in young normals but are found with increasing frequency in the asymtomatic older age group (15 per cent in those >60 years old).

Autoantibodies to intrinsic factor are found less commonly (40 to 60 per cent) in pernicious anemia, but appear more specific for this disorder (Strickland, 1971). A radioimmunoassay technique is required. The antibody may well be pathogenic and not just a result of gastric mucosal damage, since transplacental transfer of anti-intrinsic factor antibody can result in defective vitamin B_{12} absorption in the infant without any atrophic gastritis (Bar-shany, 1967).

LIVER DISEASE

Autoimmune responses as a possible cause of chronic liver disease remain a fascinating enigma (Paronetto, 1976). Several commonly occurring manifestations suggest an organ-localized autoimmune pathogenesis, based on the criteria listed earlier in this chapter, e.g., hypergammaglobulinemia, prominent lymphocyte and plasma cell inflammatory responses occurring mainly in the liver, familial occurrence, one or more circulating anti-tissue antibodies, and response (sometimes) to therapies effective against experimental autoimmune disorders. Yet most of the autoantibodies are neither liver- nor species-specific; indeed, they react less with liver tissue than with some other tissue sources. Therefore, the pathogenetic significance of these antibodies is uncertain; however, they are of certain pragmatic value in the diagnosis and prognosis of certain conditions noted here.

Chronic active hepatitis is an inflammatory condition that may occur at any age, but most commonly in young women (deGroote, 1968). It is characterized by prominent lymphocyte and plasma cell inflammatory changes which start in the portal tracts. In the more benign ("persistent hepatitis") form, it is limited to those areas. In the more aggressive form, both acute and chronic inflammatory changes (with histiocytes and ductal proliferation) disrupt the limiting plate with resultant "piecemeal necrosis" of adjacent liver parenchyma. Associated with this are clinical and laboratory signs of continued liver inflammation and dysfunction. There are also a number of immunologic abnormalities present to varying degrees, in addition to the commonly occurring hypergammaglobulinemia and increased sedimentation rate. In some patients, joint, skin, and serosal manifestations may appear, along with serologic findings such as positive ANA and L.E. cell tests, suggestive of SLE. This pattern, occurring predominantly in young women, has been called "lupoid hepatitis" (Mackay, 1956). In some patients (generally not the "lupoid hepatitis" group), chronic active hepatitis appears to reflect chronic infection with the hepatitis B virus (Paronetto, 1976; Blumberg, 1977). Overall, the prognosis in aggressive chronic active hepatitis is not good, with significant mortality reported at five years.

Idiopathic biliary cirrhosis (Husby, 1977) is a progressive condition starting with apparently non-infectious inflammation in the bile ducts of young to middle-aged women and manifested initially as painless jaundice with itching. There is progressive ductal occlusion and resultant cirrhosis which may progress to end-stage liver failure. Familial incidence, immunologic abnormalities, and associated "autoimmune disorders" are all increased in frequency in this syndrome. A major differential diagnosis is biliary cirrhosis secondary to extrahepatic obstruction.

Idiopathic cirrhosis (Husby, 1977) is an ill-defined entity that may actually represent a collection of disorders characterized by the gradual onset of hepatic dysfunction with varying degrees of jaundice. There is no past history of definite antecedent hepatitis, alcoholic abuse, or other toxic or nutritional factors.

More recently, an autoimmune basis has been postulated for certain *drug-induced hepatotoxicity* (Paronetto, 1970) reactions such as those associated with repeated halothane use. However, the evidence is still quite indirect and circumstantial. Four types of antibody determinations, all non-specific for liver disease, have been found to be of some prognostic value (Table 38-9).

Anti-smooth muscle antibodies (Whittingham, 1966) are of IgM or IgG class, are non-organ- and non-species-specific, and are assayed most commonly by immunofluorescence using unfixed frozen section of either rat stomach or human esophogeal or uterine tissue. A uniform diffuse fluorescence of the muscle fibers is seen with sera diluted at least 1:10 in <5 per cent of normals but up to 90 per cent of those with chronic active hepatitis and 25 to 40 per cent of those with biliary cirrhosis and idiopathic cirrhosis. Serum anti-smooth muscle antibodies are also found transiently in many (as high as 80 per cent) cases of viral hepatitis without any temporal or immunologic relationship to known viral antigens. Anti-smooth muscle antibodies are also common in infectious mononucleosis (up to 80 per cent of those with high titer heterophil antibodies), certain malignant tumors, and perhaps intrinsic asthma (Holborow,

Table 38-9. PREVALENCE OF AUTOANTIBODIES IN LIVER DISEASE

DISEASE	ANTI-SMOOTH MUSCLE	ANTIMITOCHONDRIAL	ANA
Chronic active hepatitis	70–90%	30–60%	60%
Chronic persistent hepatitis	45%	15–20%	15–30%
Acute viral hepatitis	10–30%	5–20%	20%
Acute alcoholic hepatitis	0	0	0
Biliary cirrhosis	30%	60–70%	5%
Cryptogenic cirrhosis	15%	30%	0
Alcoholic (Laennec's) cirrhosis	0	0	5%
Extrahepatic biliary obstruction	5–10%	5–10%	5%

Modified from Whittingham, M. B., Irwin, J., Mackay, I. R., and Smalley, M.: Smooth muscle autoantibody in "autoimmune" hepatitis. Gastroenterology, *51*:499, 1966, and Husby, G., Skrede, J., and Blomhoff, J. P.: Serum Ig and organ non-specific antibodies in diseases of the liver. Scand. J. Gastroenterol., *12*:297, 1977.

1972). However, titers of at least 1:100 suggest progressive chronic active hepatitis (Husby, 1977). By contrast, sera of SLE patients with strong antinuclear antibody reactivity are rarely positive for anti-smooth muscle antibody. *Possible pitfalls* of this technique include false negative results when insufficiently fresh or fixed tissue substrates are used.

Antimitochondrial antibodies may be IgG, IgM, or IgA and are also not specific for organ or species source. Fresh unfixed sections of rat kidney are used most commonly as substrates in a standard immunofluorescence technique with intense diffuse staining of the cytoplasm of ductal tubules at serum dilutions of at least 1:10 considered positive. Such positive reactions are seen in <1 per cent of normals but in up to 90 per cent of those with biliary cirrhosis, and 25 per cent of those with chronic active hepatic or idiopathic cirrhosis. Titers of >1:160 are generally limited to biliary cirrhosis. A very helpful distinguishing point in the differential diagnosis of obstructive jaundice is that antimitochondrial antibodies are absent in early infectious hepatitis, alcoholic cirrhosis, or extrahepatic biliary obstruction.

Antinuclear antibodies (ANA) are commonly found in the three liver conditions described but are unusual in viral hepatitis or alcoholic cirrhosis. A helpful distinguishing point is that ANA in liver diseases is generally accompanied by positive anti-smooth muscle and negative anti-DNA tests, whereas the ANA in SLE is commonly accompanied by anti-DNA antibodies, while anti-smooth muscle antibodies are infrequent.

One of the perplexing aspects of putative autoimmune liver disease is that it has been very difficult to demonstrate antibodies specific for liver cells in the sera of such patients, which frequently contain one or more non-tissue-specific autoantibodies (Paronetto, 1976). Recently, Diedrichsen (1977) has reported by immunofluorescence techniques a deposition pattern of immunoglobulin (Ig) at the peripheral hepatocytes in certain liver diseases. In perhaps a more definitive study, Hopf (1976) has reported that two different immunologic patterns may be seen in chronic hepatitis. In the first, HB_s antigen is present in the serum, and a granular Ig deposition pattern is seen in the hepatocytes that are undergoing progressive damage. In the second pattern, HB_s antigen is absent. Ig is deposited along the peripheral membrane of the hepatocytes, and antibodies to the cell membrane itself are present in the serum. If these findings are confirmed, an important step in our understanding of autoimmune processes in the liver will have been made.

Summary

1. Anti-smooth muscle antibody determinations help distinguish lupoid hepatitis from SLE; when present in high titer, the antibodies may indicate progressive liver disease. There is no evidence that this antibody is pathogenic, but may reflect "uncovering" of antigenic sites in the small amount of muscle elements in liver cells damaged by inflammation.

2. Antimitochondrial antibodies help distinguish biliary cirrhosis from extrahepatic obstruction, viral hepatitis, and alcoholic cirrhosis.

3. ANA are positive in several liver diseases as well as in SLE. Anti-DNA are generally negative, whereas anti-smooth muscle and/or antimitochondrial antibodies are positive in liver disease.

INFLAMMATORY BOWEL DISEASE

In a review of this field, Solomon (1976) pointed out that antibodies reacting with colon components are commonly found in the sera of patients with chronic ulcerative colitis, Crohn's disease of the colon, and in some cases of regional ileitis. The antigenic determinant in at least some of the cases is a mucopolysaccharide localized in the cytoplasm of the epithelial cells of the mucosa. These determinants may cross-react with lipopolysaccharides in *Escherichia coli*, which is commonly found in the bacterial flora of the gut.

However, such anticolon antibodies are not cytotoxic for human fetal colon tissue; nor do their titers correlate well with the severity, duration, course, or extent of disease. There is more evidence that lymphocytes from some patients with inflammatory bowel disease are cytotoxic for human fetal colon tissue. A finding of uncertain significance is the depressed capacity to express delayed hypersensitivity (anergy) which occurs commonly, but not uniformly, in inflammatory bowel disease.

SKIN DISORDERS

The skin may be involved in positive autoimmune reactions in at least three ways: first, inflammatory involvement of cutaneous vessels with secondary effects such as some lesions in SLE, hypersensitivity angiitis, and the syndrome of urticaria and "palpable purpura" with or without mixed cryoglobulinemia (Sofer, 1976) already referred to; second, deposition of putative circulating immune complexes in the skin as may occur in SLE; and third, localized autoreactivity against skin components, as may be seen in certain primary skin disorders. Patterns of response are summarized in Table 38-10.

In the majority of both systemic (SLE) and discoid (DLE) forms of lupus erythematosus, deposition of immunoglobulin (mainly IgG) and complement can be demonstrated by immunofluorescence in a granular pattern just beneath the dermal-epidermal junction of involved skin corresponding to the area of histologic involvement (Wertheimer, 1976). (Fig. 38-2). A fascinating finding of diagnostic and likely great pathogenetic importance is that similar deposition patterns can be found in uninvolved skin in 50 to 60 per cent of SLE patients but not in patients with DLE or other skin disorders. The latter deposition pattern is seen more commonly in those with active systemic disease; it is currently debated whether it correlates well with prominent renal involvement (Gilliam, 1974). A major portion of the immunoglobulin deposited appears to have antinuclear (and possibly anti-DNA) activity, suggesting the presence of immune complexes deposited from the circulation or formed locally. Immunoglobulin in the serum from such patients does *not* bind *in vitro* to the dermal-epidermal junction of normal skin (Tan, 1976).

Bullous pemphigoid is a chronic, relatively benign disorder (Lever, 1969). It is characterized by numerous subepidermal bullae forming at the dermal-epidermal junction. Immunofluorescence study shows deposition of IgG and complement in a *linear* pattern along the basement membrane, unlike the granular, or "lumpy," pattern seen in SLE (Landry, 1973). Also in contrast to the situation in SLE, serum IgG and complement from most bullous pemphigoid patients will bind *in vitro* to the dermal-epidermal junction of skin from a variety of species (Landry, 1973); they will also bind *in*

Table 38-10. AUTOIMMUNITY AND THE SKIN

DISORDER	PATTERN ON DIRECT IMMUNOFLUORESCENT STAINING	SERUM ANTIBODY ACTIVITY
Systemic lupus erythematosus	Ig* and complement at dermal-epidermal junction in affected, sometimes normal skin	Immune complexes, some nuclear antigens
Discoid lupus	As in SLE, but only in affected skin	? Probably same as SLE
Bullous pemphigoid	Linear deposition Ig and complement in basement membrane of lesions	Anti-basement membrane
Pemphigus group	Ig and complement deposited in intercellular spaces of epidermis (varying patterns)	Against 1 or more epidermal components (keratinocytes, bridges)
Dermatitis herpetiformis	Granular deposition IgA and alternative complement path. components	? Related to jejunal antigens?

*Ig = Immunoglobulin

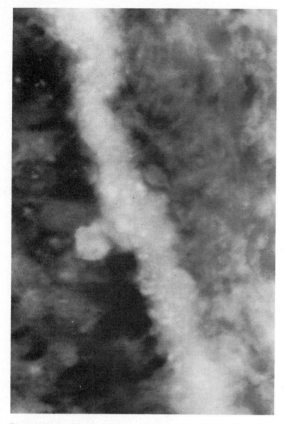

Figure 38-2. Immunofluorescence study of SLE skin lesion. Deposition of IgG in an irregular fashion along dermal-epidermal junction (×600).

vivo when the serum is transferred to normal subhuman primates, but no lesions have been observed at these sites. This observation and the inconsistent correlation between titer of anti-basement membrane antibody and extent of disease have suggested to some that these humoral responses are secondary events, possibly to virus-induced tissue damage. The increased incidence of malignant tumors in those with bullous pemphigoid has been noted, but searches for cross-reacting antigens in skin components and tumors have not turned up impressive findings to date.

Pemphigus represents a group of disorders of varying grades of severity (Lever, 1969), including pemphigus vulgaris, pemphigus vegetans, pemphigus foliaceous (brazilian and erythematous forms) characterized by intra-epidermal bullae likely due to loss of integrity of the prickle cell layer (acantholysis) of the epidermis. Immunofluorescence study shows deposition in 90 per cent of patients of Ig (mainly IgG) and possibly complement (debated) in the intercellular spaces of the epi-

dermis and in the blister fluid (Jordan, 1976). The sera of a large majority of such patients contain immunoglobulin which reacts with intercellular substances of the prickle cell layer, possibly the glycocalyx of the keratinocytes. A diverse pattern of specificity for antigen localization and species of the substrate skin may be seen with the use of sera from patients with different pemphigus subtypes. These antibodies may be pathogenetic, since the titer correlates with activity of the disease, immunoglobulin deposition is frequently seen in the epidermis of skin with little or no inflammatory involvement, the depth within the epidermis of the *in vitro* binding of the serum immunoglobulin appears to correlate with the primary locus of the lesion in the serum donor, and high-titered sera can transfer to rabbits or monkeys a predisposition to the formation of pemphigus-like lesions.

Dermatitis herpetiformis is a chronic disease characterized by intense pruritic and subepidermal bullae similar to those seen in bullous pemphigoid. Immunofluorescence also shows deposition of immunoglobulins and complement at the dermal-epidermal junction, most prominently at the tips of the dermal papillae. However, several differences from the findings in bullous pemphigoid have been observed: (1) The deposition pattern is granular, suggesting an immune complex rather than anti-basement membrane activity. A circulating 10 S putative immune complex has been described. (2) The predominant immunoglobulin detected has been IgA, with evidence of activation of the alternative complement pathways. This unusual pattern has strengthened the association of this apparently localized skin condition to gluten-sensitive enteropathy (Gebhard, 1974). Elevated serum IgA and antigluten levels are common, and similar jejunal lesions are seen in both conditions, although clinical intestinal manifestations are unusual in the skin disorder. (3) The serum of dermatitis herpetiformis patients does not bind to the basement membrane; in a minority of cases an antireticulin antibody has been described.

Finally, we will consider *other skin or mucosal disorders.* In recurrent aphthous stomatitis and the possibly related Behçet's syndrome, ulcerative lesions of the mucosa and skin are characterized by non-specific inflammation and severe patterns of immune reactivity directed against cells of skin and mucosa from a variety of sources. No diagnostic or pathogenic significance of such responses has been definitely shown. The same conclusion may be drawn about a cytotoxic antibody against the superficial epidermis of homologous skin, which is found in the serum of many patients with generalized eczema and exfoliative dermatitis.

Clinical immunologic approach to skin disease

A. Skin biopsy for histopathologic changes with immunofluorescence

(1) Deposition of immunoglobulin along dermal-epidermal junction

(a) In lesions—seen in several diseases

(b) Granular deposition of IgG and other immunoglobulins, complement in lesions, and sometimes in uninvolved skin—suspect SLE

(c) Granular deposition of IgA close to epidermal-dermal junction in and near involved skin at tips of papillae—suspect dermatitis herpetiformis

(d) Linear deposition of Ig and complement—suspect bullous pemphigoid

(2) IgG deposition in intercellular areas (intracellular bridges, other loci) within epidermis—suspect pemphigus

B. Serum studies

(1) Ig binding to dermal-epidermal junction area—positive in bullous pemphigoid, negative in SLE and dermatitis herpetiformis

(2) Ig binding to intercellular areas—suspect pemphigus

(3) Search for ANA—positive in SLE, less commonly in herpetiformis and bullous pemphoid—anti-DNA points to SLE

(4) Rheumatoid factor—frequently positive in pemphigus, bullous pemphigoid

(5) Complement profile—prominent decreases suggest immune complex deposition pattern associated with vasculitis, palpable purpura, SLE

C. Technical factors and possible pitfalls

(1) Choice of fresh skin lesions without extensive destructive changes, including normal skin, will lead to more likely detection by immunofluorescence

(2) Non-specific binding of fluorescein to damaged skin requires careful control

(3) Indirect (serum) assays may detect high titer anti-blood group antibodies or ANA localized on skin cells that may make interpretation difficult unless adequate controls are carried out

RENAL DISEASE

The kidney has long been suspected as a locus of human immune disease (Wilson, 1977). These impressions have been based mainly on the extrapolation from impressive experimental animal findings, and more limited findings in a few human diseases. However, much of the evidence is circumstantial, based on the findings by immunohistochemical techniques of the deposition of immunoglobulins and complement components in the glomerulus. Therefore, it must first be determined that such localization does not simply reflect just the deposition of any serum protein in a highly vascular tissue damaged by non-immune mechanisms. A test of whether immunoglobulins found in the kidney glomerulus (or any inflamed tissue area, for that matter) could consist of these sequential steps:

1. Determination that immunoglobulins and/or complement components are present in higher concentration than a serum protein like albumin thought to be uninvolved in immune reactions. Evidence of fibrinogen deposition is less helpful in this regard, since it probably can be seen in both immune and non-immune responses.

2. Determination that immunoglobulins eluted from involved tissues have antibody activity *in vitro*. If the antibody activity per milligram of gamma globulin in the tissue eluates is greater than seen in the serum obtained concomitantly from the patient, preferential tissue localization of the antibody is suggested.

3. Identification of the antigen in the lesion.

4. If the antibody isolated is detected against a component of kidney tissue, such activity should be demonstrated *in vitro* (by immunohistochemical or serologic study), or by passive transfer to animals.

Unfortunately, logistic and ethical considerations in human disease frequently limit demonstration to only the first steps, resulting in the circumstantial nature of the evidence. Comparisons with the experimental autoimmune kidney disease models have led to exciting hypotheses.

It is generally accepted (Wilson, 1977) that most immunologically mediated renal diseases fall into several categories (Table 38-11). In the *first*, antibodies are induced *in vivo* against the basement membrane (BM) of the glomerulus (and possibly the renal tubule or

Table 38-11. CATEGORIES OF "IMMUNOLOGIC" RENAL DISEASE

Associated Anti-Glomerular Basement Membrane Antibody
  Most cases of Goodpasture's syndrome
  Some rapidly progressive glomerulonephritis
  Altered membrane by virus? drugs?

Associated with Circulating Immune Complex
  SLE
  Certain other vasculitis
  Certain infections—bacterial, treponemal viral, parasitic
  Tumors?
  Ig/anti-Ig

Membranoproliferative Glomerulonephritis
  Alternative complement activation
  ? Genetic factors

Tubulo/Interstitial Nephritis
  Drugs, infection?
  Associated with immune complex-mediated disease
  Involvement of transplanted kidneys

lung basement membrane). The factors making such membranes autoantigenic in humans are not well-defined. However, it appears likely that binding of drugs like methicillin, certain infectious agents, and even the renal damage caused by other immune mechanisms may lead to such responses. The end result may be direct damage to the BM with or without complement activation. The production of anti-BM antibodies appears to be self-limited, lasting weeks to months after removal of the inciting agent with nephrectomy. This characteristic may be of practical importance, to be discussed later.

In the *second* category, immune complexes composed of non-renal antigens and corresponding antibodies are deposited in one or more of several loci in the glomerulus, possibly dependent on the size and other characteristics of the complex. For example, immune complex deposits localized in the mesangium should be relatively large and cleared readily with mild disease. Complexes localized in the subepithelial area would be larger but still not as damaging as those trapped on the subendothelial side of the GBM where inflammatory responses are most prominent.

Immune complex activation of complement in glomerular basement membrane (GBM) may be augmented by the presence of cells with receptors for C3 located in that area. The result of this activation likely involves release of biologically active products, including those which attract granulocytes to the site. The end result of this chain of events is an inflammatory response type of tissue injury.

There is increasing evidence that non-immunologically activated complement may cause another category of glomerular disease. In these cases, activation of the alternative complement pathway (p. 1247) appears to be the mechanism involved, analogous to the *in vitro* activation of C3 by certain bacterial products and polysaccharides.

However, it should be stressed that current knowledge indicates that the term "glomerulonephritis" is non-specific insofar as pathogenesis, with inclusion of a variety of glomerular disorders. We will now look at a few such disorders.

DISORDERS WITH ANTI-GLOMERULAR BASEMENT MEMBRANE (GBM) ANTIBODY

These likely represent less than 5 per cent of glomerular disorders (Wilson, 1977). They are characterized by a *linear* deposition of immunoglobulin and sometimes complement along the GBM (Wilson, 1976) (Fig. 38-3). Histologically, prominent epithelial cell proliferation around the capillary loop frequently leads to a rapidly progressive proliferative glomerulonephritis with marked crescent formation.

Goodpasture's syndrome is an uncommon disease which shows involvement of alveolar and glomerular basement membranes such as anti-GBM antibody leading to alveolar hemorrhage and almost invariably fatal glomerulonephritis. More recently, milder forms of the disease have been recognized (McPhaul, 1976). However, it must be noted that Ig linear deposition patterns by immunofluorescence may not always be diagnostic in anti-GBM disease. (1) Finely granular deposits may look linear unless high magnification is employed. (2) Linear patterns may occasionally be due to deposition of Ig which have no anti-GBM activity, such as in early SLE. (3) In later stages of Goodpasture's syndrome, glomerular damage may mask the typical linear pattern with a more lumpy appearance on immunofluorescence. In occasional patients, Goodpasture's syndrome appears to be associated with immune complex deposition (Wilson, 1977).

More recently, passive hemagglutination and radioimmunoassays have been used to determine anti-GBM antibody. The sensitivity of such techniques and the correlation of antibody titers obtained with the severity of

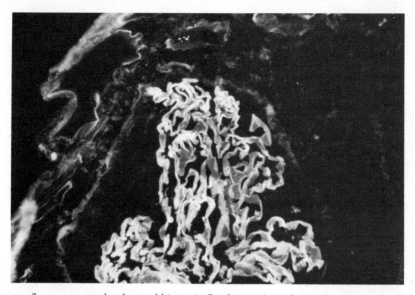

Figure 38-3. Immunofluorescence study of a renal biopsy in Goodpasture's syndrome. Deposition of IgG in a smooth linear pattern along the glomerular basement membrane ($\times 600$).

disease has varied among investigators. Wilson (1977) has reported what appears to be a highly sensitive and specific radioimmunoassay for antibodies to the non-collagenous protein of the GBM. Positive results were seen in sera from 76 of 78 patients with Goodpasture's syndrome and 43 of 52 patients with other forms of anti-GBM nephritis. In contrast, only a low incidence was seen in those with either immune-complex type (2 of 393) or negative (1 of 222) immunoglobulin deposition patterns in the GBM.

Measurement of the anti-GBM antibodies may turn out to be of considerable assistance not only in diagnosis but also in monitoring a new therapeutic approach (plasmapheresis to remove anti-GBM antibodies), which has been shown experimentally to cause the glomerular damage (Lang, 1977). However, such techniques are not yet available for use in the clinical laboratory.

IMMUNE COMPLEX-MEDIATED GLOMERULONEPHRITIS

The characteristic finding in this category is the immunofluorescent demonstration of Ig and C3 deposited in and near the GBM in an irregular pattern varying from granular to large globular accumulations. It has been estimated (Wilson, 1976) that such patterns are seen in 70 to 80 per cent of those with human glomerulonephritis. In about one third of those with "immune complex type" immunofluorescent immunoglobulin (Ig) deposition patterns, a putative circulating immune complex was detected by one or another of the techniques described earlier in this chapter.

The strongest evidence for immune complex pathogenesis comes in *SLE*, in which irregular deposits of Ig and complement components are found in almost all cases with glomerular involvement (Fig. 38-4). Eluted Ig has been shown in some cases to exhibit strong antibody activity against ribosomes and a variety of nuclear antigens, including DNA (Winfield, 1975). There is also at least indirect evidence that DNA is present in involved areas of the capillary as well. Although a linear deposition may be seen in the GBM of early lupus nephritis, anti-GBM activity in either the tissue eluates or serum of such patients is unusual (Wilson, 1977).

Several histologic patterns have been described with the understanding that progression from less prominent to more severe involvement may occur in individual patients (Baldwin, 1977). In *focal* glomerulonephritis, mesangeal and endothelial cell proliferation occurs in isolated capillary loops of some glomeruli. Immunoglobulin (Ig) and C3 deposition is generally limited to the mesangium. The clinical presentation is relatively benign, with urinary sediment abnormalities and proteinuria but without frank nephrotic syndrome or renal insufficiency. In the uncommon

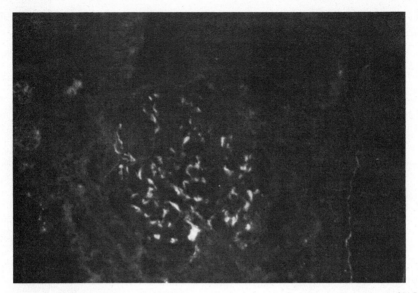

Figure 38-4. Immunofluorescence study of a renal biopsy in systemic lupus erythematosus. Deposition of IgG in an irregular, granular pattern along the glomerular basement membrane ($\times$600).

membranous glomerulonephritis presentation, there is a diffuse hypertrophy of the basement membrane with little cellular proliferation other than in the mesangium. A diffuse, finely granular deposition of IgG and complement is seen throughout the glomeruli with electron-dense deposits on the epithelial aspects of the membrane. The nephrotic syndrome with a slowly progressive course is the usual presentation.

The *diffuse proliferative glomerulonephritis* picture is the most abnormal with the worst prognosis. Almost all glomeruli are involved with irregular proliferation of both mesangeal and endothelial cells. Irregular thickenings in the basement membrane may result in the "wire loop" appearance of the clinically described lesion. There is heavy irregular deposition of Ig and of components of both the classic and alternative pathways. Large electron-dense deposits starting in the subendothelial area may also be found in the basement membrane itself. The clinical picture is that of severe renal disease, often progressing to end-stage renal failure within a period of months to several years.

OTHER EXAMPLES OF IMMUNE COMPLEX-MEDIATED DISEASE

Putative immunohistochemical evidence of immune complex deposition in the kidney has been reported in at least some patients with systemic disorders with or without evidence of joint, skin, or vessel inflammation (Wilson, 1977). Examples include: (1) HB$_s$ antigen-positive hepatitis, sometimes also with urticaria, joint symptoms, or evidence of vasculitis elsewhere. These extrahepatic manifestations may be most prominent during the time period before obvious clinical signs of hepatic inflammation become obvious. (2) Infections with beta-streptococci, spirochetes, *Plasmodium malariae, Salmonella typhosa, Mycobacterium leprae, Schistosoma mansoni, Toxoplasma* (Gamble, 1975; Ward, 1969; Tesor, 1970), and certain viruses such as lymphocytic choriomeningitis and Epstein-Barr. (3) Chronic infections of heart valves or shunts with *Staphylococcus, Corynebacterium bovis* or *Enterococcus* (Strife, 1976). (4) Thyroglobulin and possibly other tissue antigens to which prominent antibody responses occur in autoimmune diseases. Tumor-antitumor antibody has also led to deposition of complexes (Lewis, 1971). This list will undoubtedly increase as intensive studies are carried out in a wide variety of disease states. It may even be that the transient "febrile proteinuria," long noted in association with certain infectious diseases, may reflect in part a self-limited glomerular inflammatory reaction due to circulating complexes.

A similar deposition pattern is seen in kidneys from some patients with *idiopathic glomerulonephritis*. It is not clear whether immunologic mechanisms play a role in the latter situation. In *acute post-streptococcal glomerulonephritis*, deposition of C3 and properdin, and only sometimes IgG, is seen. In the severe and often rapidly fatal *rapidly progressive glomerulonephritis*, fibrinogen deposition is especially heavy, along with IgG, C3 and prominent epithelial crescents.

Membranoproliferative glomerulonephritis

In about 10 per cent of kidneys examined by immunofluorescence, deposits of complement components in the absence of Ig are found in the glomeruli. Some of these cases appear to be examples of advanced stages of immune-complex-induced nephritis with possible activation of the alternative complement pathway by previously damaged GBM (Wilson, 1977). There appears to be a subgroup of patients described originally by West and his colleagues (1966) with a membranoproliferative glomerulitis, "tram track" changes of the GBM seen in ultramicroscopy, and markedly decreased levels of the latter complement components. In at least some of these patients, a circulating non-immunoglobulin (?) gammaglobulin ("C3 nephritic factor") appears to activate C3 by the alternative pathway. This mechanism is described elsewhere in this text. However, the ultimate result of this activation is progressive glomerular damage with subsequent renal insufficiency.

Immune tubulointerstitial disease

An experimental autoimmune inflammatory disease in the renal tubules can be induced by appropriate sensitization to renal tubule BM (TBM), analogous to that seen with GBM. In some instances, there is cross-reactivity between GBM and TBM in these experimental models. Likewise, anti-TBM antibodies are found in about 70 per cent of those with Goodpasture's syndrome and more commonly than anti-GBM in renal transplant recipients (Wilson, 1977). Linear deposits of Ig are found in the renal tubules. Such deposits are also found in some patients with methicillin-induced tubular disease. Anti-TBM antibodies without anti-GBM antibodies are found in a minority of patients with immune complex-induced glomerulonephritis and may play a role in the peritubular and interstitial inflammatory cell responses seen in some cases of SLE and certain other disorders.

CLINICAL LABORATORY APPROACH TO THE STUDY OF SUSPECTED AUTOIMMUNE RENAL DISEASE

Direct immunofluorescence studies of renal tissue from patients comprise the main approach available. Proper processing of specimens for frozen section preparation is critical here. Only a limited number of glomeruli are available in many needle biopsy specimens and all are needed for study when the disease involvement is focal. Mild fixation (95 per cent alcohol or acetone for short periods) is generally helpful, but excessive fixation must be avoided. One should look for deposition of "non-immunologic" serum proteins like albumin, using similar immunofluorescent techniques. As in any immunofluorescent method, the quality of the fluorescein-conjugated antiserum (preferably the Ig fraction of the latter) is an important determinant of both sensitivity and selectivity. One must determine periodically that the reagents used do not bind non-specifically to kidney tissue which is normal or damaged by non-immune mechanisms. Fluorescein-antibody techniques are discussed on p. 1198.

Measurement of anti-GBM antibodies is also performed. The only technique readily available is that of indirect immunofluorescence. Acetone-fixed frozen sections of normal kidney are incubated with test and control sera; after appropriate washes, the section is incubated with fluorescein-conjugated antiserum to one or more human Ig components. Although serial dilution studies have been reported, it is not clear how quantitative this technique is for anti-GBM antibodies. Some (Evans, 1975) have pointed out that a non-specific faint linear fluorescein pattern may result from the binding of normal serum components to the GBM of normal human kidneys. They have suggested the use of normal monkey kidney tissue to obviate this problem.

Passive hemagglutination tests and radioimmunoassays for anti-GBM antibody depend upon the nature and quality of the GBM component used as the antigen. Findings with use of one preparation by Wilson (1977) have already been described. Others (Evans, 1975) have noted that such serologic assays may be more sensitive than indirect immunofluorescent approaches, but there may be real technical problems with breakdown of GBM components used in the assays.*

---

*Complement components in renal diseases are discussed in Chapter 37, p. 1251.

CARDIAC DISORDERS

An immunologic basis for *rheumatic heart disease* (RHD) has been suspected for a long time. The sera of many patients with RHD contain antibodies which bind *in vitro* to foci in the myocardium and heart valves (Kaplan, 1969). Antimyocardial antibodies may be responsible for the deposition of immunoglobulin and complement components found in the same area of RHD tissues at autopsy. These antibodies appear to be strongly cross-reactive with streptococcal antigens and are not toxic to heart tissue unless the latter is damaged previously by some other cause. Because anti-heart antibodies are commonly found in those with recent streptococcal infection without cardiac sequellae, detection of such antibodies has not been a particularly useful diagnostic test.

About 3 per cent of those with a recent myocardial infarction will manifest a clinical syndrome including fever and chest pain, often with signs of pleuritis and pericarditis and musculoskeletal symptoms (Kaplan, 1969). Antiheart antibodies, not cross-reacting with streptococci, are found in the sera of about 30 per cent of such individuals. A similar picture may be seen in some individuals who had undergone recent surgical procedures on the heart. The pathologic or diagnostic significance of such antibodies has not been demonstrated.

NEUROMUSCULAR SYSTEM

There are several important neurologic diseases in which the immune system may play an important role in the pathogenesis and/or etiology. There have been a number of investigations of serologic and cellular immune abnormalities in these entities. In some instances these findings are helpful in confirming the clinical diagnosis; in others, the immunologic phenomena are primarily investigative at this time. In one disorder, myasthenia gravis, there is an assay for an autoantibody which will soon become part of the diagnostic armamentarium.

MULTIPLE SCLEROSIS

Multiple sclerosis is a common demyelinating disease of the central nervous system.

Table 38–12. EVIDENCE FOR AUTOIMMUNITY IN MULTIPLE SCLEROSIS

1. Antibodies to myelin and myelin contituents.
2. Antibodies to oligodendroglia
3. *In vitro* myelinotoxicity and glial toxicity of serum and CSF (cerebrospinal fluid)
4. Oligoclonal increase in CSF Ig
5. *In vitro* cell-mediated immunity by blood and CSF cells to myelin components
6. Similarity of MS and experimental allergic encephalomyelitis
7. Increase in certain HL-A and Ia antigens (HL-A A3, B7, DW2, and DRW2)

Important pathologic changes consist of (a) perivenous cuffs of mononuclear inflammatory cells; (b) perivascular and periventricular confluent areas of myelin loss called plaques, with relative preservation of neurons and axons; (c) astrocytic proliferation (Adams, 1977). Current research into the etiology and pathogenesis of multiple sclerosis relates to viral and autoimmune factors (Paterson, 1973).

There is much evidence, largely indirect, that viruses may be etiologic agents in multiple sclerosis. However, there is considerable controversy in the literature related to this evidence as regards reproducibility and interpretation of the findings. An equally large and indirect body of experimental evidence suggests an autoimmune pathogenesis (Table 38–12). However, the lack of reproducible findings has made for varying interpretations concerning the cause of multiple sclerosis. The lack of specificity of many of these viral and immune-related abnormalities limits the diagnostic and prognostic usefulness of most of these assays.

Various theories have been advanced to tie the seemingly conflicting data related to viruses, autoimmunity, and immunogenetics together. These include (1) shared antigenicity between viruses and myelin constituents; (2) release of a hidden antigen by a subclinical infection; (3) attempts by the immune system to destroy a virus within a nervous system cell; (4) molecular mimicry between virus and an HL-A or Ia antigen; (5) virus combining with or directing the synthetic apparatus of host cells to form or produce a neoantigen; (6) virus acting as a hapten and triggering a response against the self tissue, the carrier molecule.

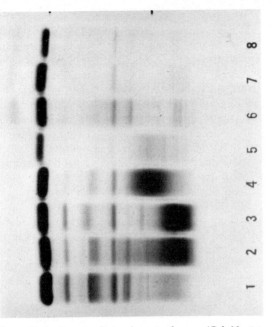

Figure 38–5. Agarose electrophoresis of serum (Gels No. 1 to 4 and cerebrospinal fluid (Gels 5 to 8). Left is anode. The dense band seen on the right of Nos. 1 to 4 is gammaglobulin. No. 8 shows no bands in that region, but Nos. 5, 6, and 7 demonstrate oligoclonal bands characteristic of multiple sclerosis. (Courtesy of Doctor Dean Arvan.)

Laboratory measurements in the diagnosis of multiple sclerosis (MS)

Protein Studies in the Cerebrospinal Fluid (CSF). The laboratory measurement of current greatest diagnostic use is analysis of CSF for the percentage of immunoglobulin (Ig), as well as the Ig pattern. It has been found that spinal fluid Ig is increased (>15 per cent of total protein) in the CSF of 65 to 75 per cent of MS patients at some time during the course of the disease (Tourtellotte, 1971). Various methods have been used to characterize the immunoglobulin in CSF. Of these, electrophoresis in agarose currently seems to be the most useful technique (Link, 1971; Johnson, 1977). A picture of a typical CSF pattern in MS is shown in Figure 38–5. *Advantages* of this technique include (a) use of commercially available prepoured agarose plates and simple, relatively inexpensive electrophoretic apparatus; (b) the ability to determine the total protein, percentage, and amount of Ig using a gel scanner and the presence of an oligoclonal pattern in a single assay; (c) the high sensitivity of the technique, being positive in 80 to 94 per cent of patients with multiple sclerosis

and in about 50 to 60 per cent with the first attack; (d) treatment of the agarose slide with anti-human immunoglobulin prior to staining for protein may further enhance demonstration of the bands (Cawley, 1976); (e) electrophoresis in agarose is more sensitive than that in agar or on cellulose acetate in demonstrating oligoclonal bands when the total Ig percentage is normal; (f) other techniques do not have the utility of agarose electrophoresis; for example, radial immunodiffusion, tube precipitin reactions, and electroimmunodiffusion cannot demonstrate the protein patterns; (g) isoelectric focusing and acrylamide gel electrophoresis and isotachyphoresis are more technically difficult, require more expensive equipment, and may not have the diagnostic specificity of agarose techniques. A radioimmunoassay has recently been described which allows the demonstration of IgM and IgA as well as IgG elevations (Mingioli, 1978), but these techniques are not yet adapted to clinical use.

The major *disadvantage* of agarose electrophoresis is the need to concentrate CSF prior to use. In addition, all assays for oligoclonal CSF proteins should be interpreted with the understanding that such CSF paraproteins are not found exclusively in MS (Table 38–13). However, the combination of clinical manifestations and evidence of infection with either syphilis or other infectious agents may be of aid in distinguishing these other diseases from MS. Oligoclonal bands have been shown to be present in the spinal fluid of patients with optic neuritis (Sandberg-Wollheim, 1975). Some of these patients have gone on to develop multiple sclerosis, but only after 5 to 20 years will we know if all optic neuritis patients with oligoclonal bands are destined to develop clinical multiple sclerosis.

It is necessary with all of the above techniques to perform simultaneous assays on sera

Table 38–13. CONDITIONS ASSOCIATED WITH OLIGOCLONAL CEREBROSPINAL FLUID (CSF) GAMMAGLOBULINS

1. Multiple sclerosis
2. Neurosyphilis
3. Subacute sclerosing panencephalitis
4. Chronic mycobacterial and fungal meningitis
5. Chronic viral meningitis and meningoencephalitis (uncommon)
6. Acute viral meningitis (uncommon)
7. Optic neuritis
8. Acute disseminated encephalomyelitis (?)

to insure that the abnormal pattern or increased spinal fluid immunoglobulin levels do not simply mirror an abnormality of serum globulins.

The nature of the antigen(s) to which the majority of these immunoglobulin bands of presumed antibody are directed is not known. This is in contradistinction to subacute sclerosing panencephalitis where incubation of spinal fluid with cell lines bearing measles virus antigens results in absorption of most of the bands (Mehta, 1976).

Serum Autoantibodies in MS. Several *serum autoantibodies* have been reported to occur frequently in MS. The diagnostic usefulness of these findings is limited by the occurrence of such antibodies in other diseases. Antibodies to myelin, demonstrated by immunofluorescence, occur in elevated titer in multiple sclerosis, with relatively good correlation with disease activity. However, myelin-binding activity occurs in low titer in normal sera, in high titer in amyotrophic lateral sclerosis, where myelin loss is secondary, and in Guillain-Barré syndrome, where demyelina-

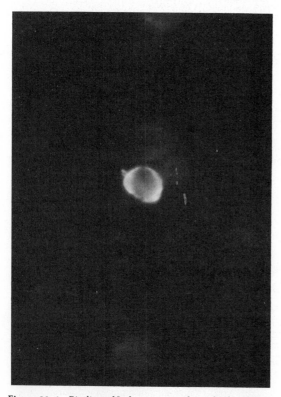

Figure 38–6. Binding of Ig from serum of a multiple sclerosis patient to surface of bovine oligodendroglial cell; immunofluorescent study (×600).

tion is limited to the peripheral nervous system (Edgington, 1970; Lisak, 1975b). Antibodies to oligodendroglia (Fig. 38-6) occur in the serum of patients with MS and not in normals; however, they are found in other disorders in which myelin or oligodendroglia are affected, such as subacute sclerosing panencephalitis and acute disseminated encephalomyelitis (Abramsky, 1977). In addition, this antibody is most easily demonstrated using suspension cultures of bovine oligodendroglia, a technique which is not yet feasible for most clinical laboratories.

Measles-lymphocyte Studies. It has been observed by some that the peripheral blood lymphocytes of patients with multiple sclerosis form a greater number of rosettes with a cell line containing measles virus, when compared with normals or patients with other neurologic diseases. Since there was no overlap between the results in multiple sclerosis and other diseases, it was suggested that this examination could be used for the diagnosis of multiple sclerosis (Levy, 1976). However, other groups have found such overlap between multiple sclerosis patients and normals (Offner, 1976). In addition, this examination does not lend itself to widespread laboratory use at this time.

Neurophysiologic Tests. *Neurophysiologic tests*, including visual, auditory, and somatosensory evoked potentials, are useful in demonstrating silent lesions and thus documenting dissemination of neurologic lesions, but abnormalities of any single test are not sufficient to make the diagnosis of multiple sclerosis.

GUILLAIN-BARRÉ SYNDROME

Guillain-Barré syndrome is an acquired disease of peripheral nerve and roots often associated with recent viral illness or immunizations or, rarely, with surgery, systemic lupus erythematosus, lymphoma, or pregnancy (Asbury, 1969; Arnason, 1971). The pathologic features include an inflammatory perivascular infiltrate consisting of lymphocytes, monocyte macrophages, and segmental demyelination. The lesions are virtually identical with those seen in experimental allergic neuritis, a disease induced in animals by sensitization with peripheral nerve in Freund's complete adjuvant. Considerable controversy exists over the nature of the peripheral nerve myelin constituent responsible for induction of the experimental disease and the relative roles of cell-mediated and humoral immune responses. A similar situation pertains in Guillain-Barré syndrome; various investigators have reported antibodies and cell-mediated immunity to myelin or components of myelin. Currently, there is no specific immunologic diagnostic test for Guillain-Barré syndrome. The diagnosis is still based on the clinical picture and supported by an increase in cerebrospinal fluid total protein.

MYASTHENIA GRAVIS

Myasthenia gravis (MG) is a disorder of the neuromuscular junction characterized by neurophysiologic and immunologic abnormalities (Penn, 1971; Lisak, 1975a; Linstrom, 1977). Current findings suggest an anatomic abnormality at the neuromuscular junction muscle endplate with an accompanying decrease in the receptor for acetylcholine (Frambrough, 1973), leading to an apparent postsynaptic defect. Clinical manifestations include motor weakness, especially on repetitive stimulation, and frequent thymic enlargement seen radiographically.

Several lines of evidence suggest that autoimmune mechanisms may play a role in the pathogenesis of MG (Table 38-14). Histologic abnormalities of the thymus are found in most patients with myasthenia. This is generally a lymphoid cell hyperplasia with germinal centers; however, in a minority of cases, a lymphoid thymoma is present. Increased B-lymphocytes and other immune abnormalities of the thymus (Abdou, 1974) are discussed subsequently. There is an increased prevalence of co-existent disorders of presumed autoimmune etiology (e.g., thyroiditis, pernicious anemia, SLE) and an even higher prevalence of circulating autoantibodies in MG (Table 38-15). Several of these autoantibodies are directed

Table 38-15. SOME AUTOANTIBODIES ASSOCIATED WITH MYASTHENIA GRAVIS

1. Anti-acetylcholine receptor	60-85%
2. Antimuscle	30% (90% with thymoma)
3. Antithyroblobulin	30%
4. Antinuclear antibodies	20-40%
5. Cold reactive antilymphocyte	40%
6. Coomb's positive anti-red cell	10%
7. Anti-gastric parietal cell	10%
8. Rheumatoid factor	7%

against components of the neuromuscular system and bear more detailed discussion because of possible pathogenic and diagnostic significance.

Early immunofluorescence studies (Lisak, 1975a) showed antibodies to one or more structural components of normal muscle in >1:60 titer in about 30 per cent of myasthenics, 90 per cent of those with MG plus thymoma, and 30 per cent of those with thymoma alone (Fig. 38-7). The latter finding is likely related to the observation that the anti-

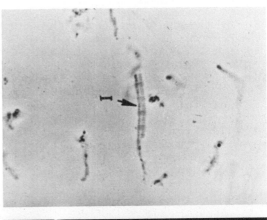

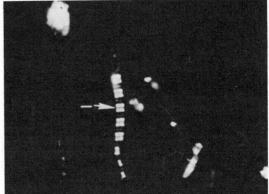

Figure 38-7. Binding of IgG from serum of myasthenia gravis patient to muscle structural bands (arrow); immunofluorescence (bottom) and phase (top) study (×400). (Courtesy of Doctor Donald Schotland.)

Table 38-14. IMMUNOPATHOGENESIS OF MYASTHENIA GRAVIS

1. Thymic hyperplasia with germinal follicles (70%)
2. Thymoma (10-15%)
3. Antibodies to acetylcholine receptor and muscle
4. Transfer of neuromuscular block to mice with myasthenic Ig
5. Other (non-neuromuscular) antibodies
6. Association with other "autoimmune" diseases
7. Cell-mediated immunity to muscle and acetylcholine receptor
8. Increase in thymic B cells
9. Autologous mixed leukocyte reaction between thymus and blood cells
10. Increase in HLA-A1, A3, B8, and DW3

muscle antibodies bind to the thymic myoid elements. Some have postulated that the thymus is primary immune stimulus for production of such antibodies. These antibodies do not appear to be pathogenic for the endplate but may be responsible for the inflammatory cell changes seen in muscle fiber areas of some myasthenics.

More recently, it has been reported that immune reactivity to the acetylcholine receptor (AChR) is seen in most myasthenics and may be of major pathogenic importance (Linstrom, 1977). First, it was shown that myasthenic muscle had less AChR, as assayed by the binding of alpha-bungarotoxin (Frambrough, 1973). The muscle endplate shows pathologic changes, with deposition of Ig and C3 (Engel, 1977). The serum of 60 to 85 per cent of myasthenics contains anti-AChR antibodies as detected by one or more assays (Linstrom, 1977). Such sera passively transfer a myasthenic neuromuscular block to mice (Toyka, 1977). It is not yet clear how such anti-AChR antibodies might be pathogenic. They apparently do not bind to the AChR molecule at the combining site for acetylcholine. It has been suggested that steric hindrance and effects on AChR turnover or damage of the motor endplate may all be elements in the antibody effect. Evidence of increased reactivity to AChR in the blood lymphocytes of myasthenics (Abramsky, 1975; Richman, 1976) suggests that cell-mediated immune responses may play a role in pathogenesis.

Of great potential importance is the discovery of an experimentally induced model of autoimmune reactivity to AChR in several animal species (Linstrom, 1977), with clinical, immunologic, and pathologic similarities to MG. These include elements of both humoral and cell-mediated immune responses to AChR.

Laboratory Diagnosis of Myasthenia Gravis

The diagnosis of myasthenia gravis is based on the clinical picture and confirmed by pharmacologic (improvement with edrophonium and/or neostigmine; worsening with low dose curare) and clinical electrophysiologic (decremental response to low frequency repetitive electrostimulation) tests. The antibodies against structural muscle components, found in 30 per cent of all patients with myasthenia, have not proved to be sensitive enough to aid in diagnosis nor to be of definite prognostic value. A recently developed radioimmunoassay for anti-AChR antibody (Linstrom, 1977) promises to be a sensitive and highly specific test in the diagnosis of MG, being positive in a large majority of sera from patients with this disorder, and only rarely positive in the sera of

normals and those with other muscle disorders.

DERMATOMYOSITIS AND POLYMYOSITIS

Polymyositis and dermatomyositis are acquired inflammatory myopathies of unknown etiology (Bohan, 1975). Although often considered together, each almost certainly represents several distinct albeit related syndromes. Dermatomyositis includes (a) childhood dermatomyositis, a disease in which pathologic evidence for vasculitis is quite prominent and (b) adult dermatomyositis with or without associated neoplasm. It is not clear that the presence or absence of associated solid tumor implies a different pathogenesis. Polymyositis is a syndrome which can be either idiopathic, not associated with any other disease, or associated with clinical and/or serologic evidence of other "collagen-vascular" or "autoimmune" diseases, including scleroderma, rheumatoid arthritis, systemic lupus erythematosus, and Sjögren's syndrome. There is little evidence for any association of polymyositis with neoplasm. Polymyopathy is a term best applied to acquired myopathies, including polymyositis, as well as other acquired myopathies such as sarcoid, metabolic, endocrine, and non-inflammatory carcinomatous myopathies.

The prominent vasculitis noted in childhood dermatomyositis in muscle and other organ systems strongly suggests that immune complexes may be involved in the pathogenesis of this disease. The demonstration of immunoglobulin and complement in the vessels of such patients (Whitaker, 1972) lends support to this hypothesis. Vasculitis is not generally a prominent feature of adult dermatomyositis. Although vasculitis is seen in some muscle biopsies of patients with idiopathic polymyositis and polymyositis associated with other collagen-vascular diseases, it is not common or usually prominent. There is *in vitro* evidence for cell-mediated immunity to muscle in polymyositis (Currie, 1971) and for the presence of virus-like particles as well. Serum antibodies to muscle are not found in dermatomyositis and polymyositis.

Patients with dermatomyositis and polymyositis with or without associated neoplasm or other collagen-vascular diseases often have serologic abnormalities, including increased erythrocyte sedimentation rate, increased serum immunoglobulins, and increased antinuclear antibodies. Depression of serum complement is not usually seen unless associated with the accompanying collagen-vascular disease, even in childhood dermatomyositis. It has been reported that sera of about 50 per cent of patients with dermatomyositis and polymyositis react with nuclear material extracted from calf thymus which is not RNA or DNA (Reichlin, 1976; Wolfe, 1977).

To date, other diseases associated with antinuclear antibodies do not seem to react with this antigen unless myositis is part of the clinical picture in the patient. If the presence of this antibody can be confirmed by other groups, it will be of aid in helping to distinguish polymyositis from the larger spectrum of acquired myopathies. Currently, the diagnosis of dermatomyositis and polymyositis is based on the clinical picture and confirmed by (a) elevation of serum enzymes, especially creatinine phosphokinase; (b) myopathic and "irritative" patterns on electromyography; and (c) inflammatory myopathic muscle biopsy with or without vasculitis.

LYMPHOCYTES

ANTILYMPHOCYTE ANTIBODIES

Circulating antibodies of the IgG type which react with lymphocytes have long been detected in the sera of some polytransfused subjects and multiparous females. The antibodies appear to be directed against HLA (histocompatibility locus antigen) components in the donor cells, and react best at room temperature or at 37°C. In addition, a different type of antilymphocyte antibody of the IgM type exerts cytotoxic effects on human lymphocytes most strongly at 15°C. (Kunkel, 1975). The latter antibodies react predominantly with T-lymphocytes, but anti–B-lymphocyte activity may be seen in some sera. Lymphocytes of different normal donors show varying susceptibility to the cytotoxic effects of these cold-reactive antibodies, not based on the usual HLA specificities. Cold-reactive antibodies have been found in SLE patients and close household contacts of such individuals (De Horatius, 1975a), in rheumatoid arthritis, scleroderma, MG, MS, Hodgkin's disease, and solid tumors, and in normal subjects with recent viral infection or immunizations. In some cases (e.g., SLE) IgG warm-reactive antilymphocyte antibodies are found as well.

The biologic significance of such antibodies is not well-defined. Some evidence suggests correlation of levels of such antibody with degree of "autoimmune" disease activity and/or depressed CMI, but further study is required to clarify the matter.

There is a further discussion of organ-specific autoantibodies on p. 1277.

MIXED LYMPHOCYTE REACTIONS (MLR)

When lymphocytes from two histoincompatible humans are cultured together, the cells of one or both individuals will proliferate as a manifestation of immune reactivity of the T-lymphocytes to histocompatibility antigens on cells of the other subject (Bach, 1976). This reactivity is discussed elsewhere (p. 1394). Pertinent to our discussion are observations that these antigens (at the "D" locus) are contained on B- and likely on T-lymphocytes. Such MLR are valuable indicators of tissue "self" and "non-self" insofar as organ transplantation is concerned. Therefore, it is noteworthy that positive MLR responses have occasionally been seen when human blood lymphocytes obtained during acute exacerbations of leukemia or viral infections (and then freeze-stored in the viable state) react with cells of the same individual obtained during remission.

It is not clear whether such autoreactivity is directed against "neoantigen" that may be formed in virus-altered blood lymphocytes, or whether "hidden" (e.g., fetal) antigens are expressed in the abnormal cells. Positive MLR responses have been reported in at least two of the putative autoimmune disorders discussed here. MLR responses between autologous synovial fluid and blood lymphocytes of some rheumatoid arthritis patients have been reported (Griffiths, 1974). Also, the hyperplastic thymic cells of some myasthenic patients will stimulate blood lymphocytes of the same individuals in a positive MLR (Abdou, 1974). Again, the mechanisms involved are not well-defined. However, the MLR may not reflect only allogeneic histoincompatibility in normals. Recent reports (Opelz, 1975) suggest that modest reactivity is induced in T-lymphocytes of normals by B cell–enriched fractions of the same blood. It appears that the autologous MLR stimulated by thymus cells in myasthenia noted previously cannot be explained as simply a matter of increased B cells in the myasthenic thymus.

In summary, techniques for measuring antilymphocyte antibodies and MLR are fre-

4

quently available in clinical laboratories, at least on a regional basis, related to organ transplantation programs. However, the diagnostic usefulness of the findings in autoimmune disease is not defined sufficiently to recommend application at present.

SOME OTHER CONSIDERATIONS IN THE APPROACH TO AUTO-IMMUNE DISEASES

The emphasis in this chapter has been predominantly on assays for humoral autoimmune reactivity detected in the test tube or in tissue. However, findings in experimental autoimmunity models suggest that cell-mediated immune responses may play a major pathogenetic role in some of the conditions already discussed here. At least part of the reason for the emphasis on humoral immunity assays is that the techniques involved have been available for a longer period of time and can be performed relatively easily and reproducibly in the sizable numbers of cases seen in clinical situations. Yet it is conceivable that at least some of these humoral responses to tissue antigens are epiphenomena or occur secondary to tissue damage due to non-immune causes.

Detection of human cell-mediated immune (CMI) responses to the same tissue antigen has been explored in any depth only in recent years. First, one must know whether the individual can manifest CMI responses to exogenous antigens. The most straightforward approach has been the determination of whether subjects with a particular disease manifest less recall-delayed hypersensitivity skin test responses to a panel of ubiquitous antigens as compared with an age-matched control population. Depressed responses (Kantor, 1975), called anergy, are seen in some putative autoimmune disease states, but not commonly enough to be of real diagnostic value. Testing for primary sensitization to contact-sensitizing agents like dinitrochlorobenzene (Chretien, 1973) are still research procedures. Determinations of the relative and absolute numbers of lymphocyte subpopulations and assays of the *in vitro* functional capabilities of such cells are discussed in another chapter in this section and will not be dealt with here. Suffice it to say that any abnormalities detected in human autoimmune disease have not yet been of sufficient diagnostic value to warrant inclusion of these more time-consuming techniques in a clinical laboratory approach. It should be mentioned that evidence by one or another techniques of *in vitro* blood leukocyte reactivity to components of glomeruli, liver, and colon (in certain types of glomerulonephritis, hepatic disease, and ulcerative colitis, respectively) have been impressive at times. These *in vitro* reactions may reflect pathogenetically important *in vivo* events. However, these assays do not seem to be at the level where they can be applied reproducibly in clinical diagnosis.

Alterations in the complement system have also not been discussed in detail, since this is the subject of Chapter 37. However, it should be stressed that complement activation appears to be involved in a number of the autoimmune reactions described here.

REFERENCES

Aarden, L. A., Lakmaker, F., and Fetkamp, T. E. W.: Immunology of DNA. I. The influence of reaction conditions in the Farr assay as used for the detection of anti-ds DNA. J. Immunol. Methods, *10*:27, 1976.

Abdou, N. I., Lisak, R. P., Zweiman, B., Abrahamsohn, I., and Penn, A. S.: The thymus in myasthenia gravis. Evidence for altered cell populations. N. Engl. J. Med., *291*:1271, 1974.

Abramsky, O., Aharonov, A., and Webb, C.: Cellular immune response to acetylcholine receptor-rich fraction in patients with myasthenia gravis. Clin. Exp. Immunol., *19*:11, 1975.

Abramsky, O., Lisak, R. P., Silberberg, D. H., and Pleasure, D. E.: Antibodies to oligodendroglia in patients with multiple sclerosis. N. Engl. J. Med., *297*:1207, 1977.

Adams, C. W. M.: Pathology of multiple sclerosis: Progression of the lesion. Brit. Med. Bull., *33*:15, 1977.

Adler, M. K., Baumgarten, A., Hecht, B., and Siegel, N. J.: Prognostic significance of DNA binding capacity in patients with lupus nephritis. Ann. Rheum. Dis., *34*:344, 1975.

Agnello, V.: Detection of immune complexes. *In* Rose, N. B., and Friedman, H.: Manual of Clinical Immunology. Washington, American Society of Microbiology, 1976.

Agnello, V., Winchester, J. R., and Kunkel, H. G.: Precipitin reactions of the C1q component of complement with aggregated Ig globulin and immune complexes in gel diffusion. Immunology, *19*:909, 1970.

Akizuki, M., Boehm-Truitt, M. J., Karsan, S. S., et al.: Purification of an acid nuclear protein antigen and demonstration of its antibodies in subsets of patients with the sicca syndrome. J. Immunol., *119*:932, 1977.

Allison, A. C., Denman, A. M., and Barnes, R. D.: Cooper-ating and controlling functions of thymus-derived lymphocytes in relation to auto-immunity. Lancet, *2*:135, 1971.

Allison, A. C.: *In* Katz, D. H., and Benacceraf, B. (eds.): Immunologic Tolerance. New York, Academic Press, 1974.

Almon, R. R., Andrew, C. G., and Appel, S.: Serum globulin in myasthenia gravis: Inhibition of bungarotoxin binding to acetylcholine receptors. Science, *186*:55, 1974.

Arnason, B. G. W.: Idiopathic polyneuritis (Landry-Guillain-Barré Strohl syndrome) and experimental allergic neuritis: A comparison. *In* Rowland, L. P. (ed.): Immunological Disorders of the Nervous System. Baltimore. The Williams and Wilkins Company, 1971.

Asbury, A. K., Arnason, B. G. W., and Adams, R. W.: The inflammatory lesion in idiopathic polyneuritis: Its role in pathogenesis. Medicine, *48*:173, 1969.

Bach, F. H.: Mixed leukocyte cultures: A cellular approach to histocompatability testing. *In* Bach, F. H., and Good, R. A. (eds.): Clinical Immunology, vol. 3. New York, Academic Press, 1976, p. 273.

Baldwin, D. S., Gluck, M. C., Lowenstein, J., et al.: Lupus nephritis—Clinical course as related to morphologic forms and their transitions. Am. J. Med., *62*:12, 1977.

Baldwin, D. S., Rothfield, N., McCluskey, R. M., et al.: The clinical course of the proliferative and membranous forms of lupus nephritis. Ann. Intern. Med., *73*:929, 1970.

Bardana, E., Harbeck, R. J., Hoffman, A. A., Pirofsky, B., and Carr, R. I.: The prognostic and therapeutic implications of DNA: Anti-DNA immune complexes in SLE. Am. J. Med., *59*:515, 1975.

Barnett, E. V., Bluestone, R., Cracchiolo, A., Goldberg, L. S., Kantor, G. L., and McIntosh, R. M.: Cryoglobulinemia and disease. Ann. Intern. Med., *73*:95, 1970a.

Barnett, E. V.: Substrates for antinuclear factors. *In* Holborow, E. J. (ed.): Standardization in Immunofluorescence. Oxford, Blackwell Scientific Publications, 1970b.

Bar-shany, S., and Herbert, V.: Transplacentally acquired antibodies to intrinsic factor with a vitamin B_{12} deficiency. Blood, *30*:777, 1967.

Benacerraf, B., and Katz, D. H.: The nature and function of histocompatability-linked immune response genes. *In* Benacerraf, B. (ed.): Immunogenetics and immunodeficiency. Baltimore, University Park Press, 1975, p. 117.

Bigazzi, P. L., Andrada, J. A., Andrada, E., et al.: Immunofluorescence studies on Addison's disease. Int. Arch. Allergy Applied Immunol., *34*:455, 1968.

Bigazzi, P. L., and Rose, N. R.: Tests for antibodies to tissue-specific antigens. *In* Rose, N. R., and Friedman, H. (eds.): Manual of Clinical Immunology. Washington, American Society of Microbiology, 1976.

Blizzard, R. M., Chee, D., and Davis, W.: The incidence of adrenal and other antibodies in the sera of patients with idiopathic adrenal insufficiency. Clin. Exp. Immunol., *2*:19, 1967.

Blumberg, B. S.: Non-A, Non-B hepatitis. Ann. Intern. Med., *87*:111, 1977.

Bohan, A., and Peters, J. B.: Polymyositis and dermatomyositis. N. Engl. J. Med., *292*:344; 403, 1975.

Brouet, J. C.: Biological and clinical significance of cryoglobulins. Am. J. Med., *57*:775, 1974.

Burnet, M.: The clonal selection theory of acquired immunity. Cambridge, Cambridge University Press, 1959.

Burnet, M.: Autoimmunity and autoimmune disease. Philadelphia, F. A. Davis Company, 1972.

Capra, J. D., Winchester, R. J., and Kunkel, H. G.: Hypergamma globulinemic purpura. Studies on the unusual anti-gamma globulin characteristics of the sera of these patients. Medicine, *50*:125, 1971.

Castleman, B.: The pathology of the thymus gland in myasthenia gravis. Ann. N. Y. Acad. Sci., *135*:496, 1966.

Cawley, L. P., Minard, B. J., Tourtellotte, W. W., Ma, B. I., and Chelle, C.: Immunofixation electrophoretic techniques applied to identification of proteins in serum and cerebrospinal fluid. Clin. Chem., *22*:1262, 1976.

Chorzelski, T. P.: Immunofluorescence studies in the diagnosis of dermatitis herpetiformis and its differentiation from bullous pemphigoid. J. Invest. Derm., *56*:373, 1971.

Chretien, P. B., Twomey, P. L., Trahan, E. E., and Catalana, W. J.: Quantitative dinitrochlorbenzene contact sensitivity in pre-operative and cured cancer patients. Natl. Cancer Inst. Monogr., *39*:263, 1973.

Currie, S., Saunders, M., Knowles, M., and Brown, A. E.: Immunologic aspects of polymyositis. Q. J. Med., *40*:63, 1971.

de Groote, J., Desmet, V. J., Gedgik, P., et al.: A classification of chronic hepatitis. Lancet, *2*:626, 1968.

De Horatius, R. J., and Messner, R. P.: Lymphocytotoxic antibodies in family members of patients with systemic lupus erythematosus. J. Clin. Invest., *55*:1254, 1975a.

De Horatius, R. J., Pillarisetty, R., Messner, R. P., et al.: Anti-nuclei acid antibodies in SLE patients and their families. J. CLin. Invest., *56*:1149, 1975b.

Diedrichsen, H.: Peripheral immunofluorescence of hepatocytes. Acta Pathol. Microbiol. Scand., *85*:399, 1977.

Doniach, D.: *In* Bastenie, V. A., and Gepts, W. (eds.): Immunology and Autoimmunity in Diabetes Mellitus. Amsterdam, Excerpta Medica, 1974.

Edgington, T. S., and D'Alessio, D. J.: The assessment by immunofluorescence methods of humoral antimyelin antibodies in man. J. Immunol., *105*:248, 1970.

Engel, A. G., Lambert, E. H., and Howard, F. M.: Immune complexes (IgG and C3) at the motor end-plate in myasthenia gravis. Ultrastructural and light microscopic localization and electrophysiologic correlations. Mayo Clin. Proc., *52*:267, 1977.

Evans, D. J., and Mangenella, P.: Demonstration of circulating antibodies to glomerular basement membrane. Ann. N. Y. Acad. Sci., *254*:600, 1975.

Flier, J. S., Kahn, C. R., Jarrell, D. B., et al.: The immunology of the insulin receptor. Immunol. Commun., *5*:361, 1976.

Frambrough, D. M., Drachman, D. B., and Satyamurti, S.: Neuromuscular function in myasthenia gravis: Decreased acetylcholine receptors. Science, *182*:293, 1973.

Francis, T. C.: Recurrent aptithous stomatitis and Behcet's disease. Oral Surg., *30*:465, 1970.

Gamble, C. N., and Reardan, J. B.: Immunopathogenesis of syphilitic glomerulonephritis. N. Engl. J. Med., *292*:449, 1975.

Gebhard, R. L.: Dermatitis herpetiformis. J. Clin. Invest., *54*:98, 1974.

Gershon, R. K.: T cell control of antibody production. *In* Cooper, M. D., and Warner, N. L. (eds.): Contemporary Topics in Immunology, 3rd ed. New York, Plenum Publishing Co., 1974.

Gilliam, J. N., Cheatum, D. E., Hurd, E. R., et al.: Immunoglobulin in clinically uninvolved skin in SLE. Association with renal disease. J. Clin. Invest., *53*:1434, 1974.

Griffiths, M. M., and Williams, R. C.: In vitro peripheral blood and synovial fluid lymphocyte interactions. Arthritis Rheum., *17*:111, 1974.

Hale, W. L., and Bergquist, D. N.: Chessboard analyses with antinuclear antibodies. Ann. N. Y. Acad. Sci., *177*:354, 1971.

Hay, F. C., Nineham, L. J., and Roitt, I. M.: Routine assay

4

for detection of IgG and IgM antiglobulins in seronegative and seropositive rheumatoid arthritis. Br. Med. J., *3*:203, 1975.

Hay, F. C., Nineham, L. J., and Roitt, I. M.: Routine assay for the detection of immune complexes of known Ig class using solid phase C1q. Clin. Exp. Immunol., *24*:396, 1976.

Holborow, E. J.: Standardization. *In* Immunofluorescence. Oxford, Blackwell Scientific Publications, 1970.

Holborow, E. J.: Smooth-muscle antibodies, viral infections, and malignant disease. Proc. R. Soc. Med., *65*:481, 1972.

Holman, H., and Deicher, H. R.: The reaction of the lupus erythematosus (L. E.) cell factor with deoxyribonucleoprotein of the cell nucleus. J. Clin. Invest., *38*:2059, 1959.

Hopf, V., Meyer zum Buschenfelde, K. H., and Arnold, W.: Detection of a liver-membrane auto-antibody in HBs antigen-negative chronic active hepatitis. N. Engl. J. Med., *294*:578, 1976.

Howard, J. G., and Mitchison, N. A.: Immunological tolerance. Prog. Allergy, *18*:43, 1975.

Husby, G., Skrede, J., and Blomhoff, J. P.: Serum Ig and organ non-specific antibodies in diseases of the liver. Scand. J. Gastroenterol., *12*:297, 1977.

Inami, Y. H., Nakamura, R. M., and Tan., E. M.: Micro hemagglutination test for detection of native and single-strand DNA antibodies and circulating DNA antigen. J. Immunol. Methods, *3*:287, 1973.

Irvine, W. J.: The association of atrophic gastritis with autoimmune thyroid disease. Clin. Endocrinol. Metab., *4*:351, 1975.

Irvine, W. J., Steward, A. G., and Scarth, L.: A clinical and immunological study of adrenocortical insufficiency (Addison's disease). Clin. Exp. Immunol., *2*:31, 1967.

Irvine, W. J., Chan, M. M., and Scarth, L.: Further characterization of auto-antibodies reactive with extra-adrenal steroid producing cells in patients with adrenal disorders. Clin. Exp. Immunol., *4*:489, 1969.

Irvine, W. J., and Barnes, E. W.: Addison's disease, ovarian failure and hypoparathyroidism. Clin. Endocrinol. Metab., *4*:379, 1975.

Irvine, W. J., McCallum, C. J., Gray, R. S., Campbell, C. J., Duncan, L. J. P., Forquhar, J. W., Vaughan, H., and Morris, P. J.: Pancreatic islet cell antibodies in diabetes mellitus correlated with duration and type of diabetes, coexistent autoimmune diseases and HLA type. Diabetes, *26*:138, 1977.

Isojima, S. K., Tsuchiya, K., Koyama, C., et al.: Further studies on sperm-immobilizing antibody found in sera of unexplained cases of sterility in women. Am. J. Obstet. Gynecol., *112*:199, 1972.

Jokinen, E. J., and Jukinen, J.: DNA hemagglutination test in the diagnosis of SLE. Ann. Rheum. Dis., *24*:477, 1965.

Johnson, A. H., Mowbray, J. F., and Porter, K. A.: Detection of circulating immune complexes in pathological human sera. Lancet, *1*:762, 1975.

Johnson, K. P., Arrigo, S. C., Nelson, B. J., and Ginsberg, A.: Agarose electrophoresis of cerebrospinal fluid in multiple sclerosis. A simplified method for demonstrating cerebrospinal fluid oligoclonal immunoglobulin bands. Neurology, *27*:273, 1977.

Jordan, R. E.: Complement activation in pemphigus and bullous pemphigoid. J. Invest. Dermatol., *67*:366, 1976.

Kantor, F. S.: Infection, anergy and cell-mediated immunity. N. Engl. J. Med., *292*:629, 1975.

Kaplan, M. H., and Frengley, J. D.: Autoimmunity to the heart in cardiac disease. Am. J. Cardiol., *24*:459, 1969.

Klein, F., Valkenborg, H. A., and Cats, A.: On standardi-

zation of the latex fixation test. Bull. Rheum. Dis., *26*:866, 1975.

Kuntz, M. M., Innes, J. B., and Weksler, M. E.: Impaired immune surveillance in chronic lymphatic leukemia (CLL) and systemic lupus erythematosus (SLE). Clin. Res., *24*:448A, 1976.

Kunkel, H. G., Winfield, J. B., Winchester, R. J., and Wernet, P.: Antibodies to lymphocytes in human sera. *In* Williams, R. W. (ed.): Lymphocytes and Their Interactions. New York, Raven Press, 1975, p. 183.

Landry, M., Sams, W. M., and Jordon, R. E.: Bullous pemphigoid: Elution of *in vivo*-fixed antibody. J. Invest. Derm., *61*:348, 1973.

Lang, C. H., Brown, D. C., Staley, N., et al.: Goodpasture syndrome treated with immunosuppression and plasma exchange. Arch. Intern. Med., *137*:1076, 1977.

Lever, W. F., and Hashimoto, K.: The etiology and treatment of pemphigus and pemphigoid. J. Invest. Derm., *53*:373, 1969.

Levinsky, R. J., Cameron, J. S., and Soothill, J. F.: Serum immune complexes and disease activity in lupus nephritis. Lancet, *1*:564, 1977.

Levy, N. L., Auebach, P. S., and Hayes, E. C.: A blood test for multiple sclerosis based on the adherence of lymphocytes to measles infected cells. N. Engl. J. Med., *294*:1423, 1976.

Lewis, M. D., Loughridge, L. W., and Phillips, T. M.: Immunological shades in nephrotic syndrome associated with extrarenal malignant disease. Lancet, *2*:134, 1971.

Link, H., and Muller, R.: Immunoglobulins in multiple sclerosis and infections of the nervous system. Arch. Neurol., *25*:324, 1971.

Linstrom, J. M.: An assay for antibodies to human acetylcholine receptor in serum from patients with myasthenia gravis. J. Immunol. Immunopathol., *7*:36, 1977.

Lisak, R. P.: Immunologic aspects of myasthenia gravis. Ann. Clin. Lab. Sci., *5*:288, 1975a.

Lisak, R. P., Zweiman, B., and Norman, M. E.: Antimyelin antibodies in neurologic diseases. Immunofluorescent demonstration. Arch. Neurol., *32*:163, 1975b.

Luthra, H. S., McDuffied, F. C., Hunder, G. G., et al.: Immune complexes in sera and synovial fluids of patients with rheumatoid arthritis: Radioimmunoassay with monoclonal rheumatoid factor. J. Clin. Invest., *56*:458, 1975.

Mackay, I. R., Taft, C. I., and Cowling, D. C.: Lupoid hepatitis. Lancet, *2*:1323, 1956.

Maddison, P. J., and Reichlin, M.: Quantitation of precipitating antibodies to certain soluble nuclear antigens in SLE. Arthritis Rheum., *20*:819, 1977.

McIntosh, R. M.: Cryoglobulins III. Q. J. Med., *44*:285, 1975.

McPhaul, J. J., and Mullins, J. D.: Glomerulonephritis mediated by antibody to glomerular basement membrane. J. Clin. Invest., *57*:351, 1976.

Mehta, P. D., Kane, A., and Thomas, H.: Relationship between homogeneous IgG fractions and measles virus antibody activities in subacute sclerosing panencephalitis brain. J. Immunol., *117*:2053, 1976.

Meltzer, M., and Franklin, E. C.: Cryoglobulins, rheumatoid factors and connective tissue disorders. Arthritis Rheum., *10*:489, 1967.

Mingioli, E. S., Strober, W., Tourtellotte, W. W., Whitaker, J. N., and McFarlin, D. E.: Quantitation of IgG, IgA, and IgM in the CSF by radioimmunoassay. Neurology, in press.

Myllyla, G.: Aggregation of human blood platelets by immune complexes in the sedimentation pattern test. Scand. J. Haematol., *19* (Suppl.): 1, 1973.

Nakamura, R. M., and Weigle, W. O.: Transfer of experimental autoimmune thyroiditis by serum from thyroidectomized donors. J. Exp. Med., *130*:263, 1969.

Nossal, G. J. V., and Schrader, J. W.: B lymphocyte antigen interactions in the initiation of tolerance or immunity. Transplant Rev., *23*:138, 1975.

Nydegger, V. E., Lambert, P. H., Gerber, H., and Miescher, P. A.: Circulating immune complexes in the serum in systemic lupus erythematosus and carriers of hepatitis B antigen. Quantitation by binding to radiolabelled C1q. J. Clin. Invest., *54*:297, 1974.

Offner, H., Konat, G., and Clausen, J.: A blood test for multiple sclerosis. N. Engl. J. Med., *296*:451, 1976.

Ooi, Y. M., Vallota, E. H., and West, C. D.: Serum immune complexes membranoproliferative and other glomerulonephritides. Kidney Int., *11*:275, 1977.

Opelz, G., Kuichi, M., Takosugi, M., and Terasaki, P. Y.: Autologous stimulation of human lymphocyte sub-populations. J. Exp. Med., *142*:1327, 1975.

Paronetto, F., and Popper, H.: Lymphocyte stimulation induced by halothane in patients with hepatitis following exposure to halothane. N. Engl. J. Med., *283*:277, 1970.

Paronetto, F., and Popper, H.: Two immunologic reactions in the pathogenesis of hepatitis. N. Engl. J. Med., *294*:606, 1976.

Paterson, P. Y.: Multiple sclerosis: An immunologic reassessment. J. Chron. Dis., *26*:119, 1973.

Patrick, J., and Linstrom, J.: Autoimmune response to acetylcholine receptor. Science, *180*:1973.

Penn, A. S., Schotland, D. H., and Rowland, L. P.: Immunology of muscle disease. *In* Rowland, L. P. (ed.): Immunologic Disorders of the Nervous System. Baltimore, The Williams and Wilkins Company, 1971.

Phillips, P. E.: The virus hypothesis in systemic lupus erythematosus. Ann. Intern. Med., *83*:709, 1975.

Pincus, T., Schur, P. H., Rose, J. A., Decker, J. K., and Talal, N.: Measurement of DNA-binding activity in SLE. N. Engl. J. Med., *281*:701, 1969.

Pope, R. M., Teller, D. C., and Mannik, M.: The molecular basis of self-association of antibody to IgG (rheumatoid factor) in rheumatoid arthritis. Proc. Natl. Acad. Sci. U.S.A., *71*:517, 1974.

Reichlin, M., and Mattioli, M.: Description of a serological reaction characteristic of polymyositis. Clin. Immunol. Immunopathol., *5*:12, 1976.

Richman, D. P., Patrick, J., and Arnason, B. G. W.: Cellular immunity in myasthenia gravis. N. Engl. J. Med., *294*:694, 1976.

Ritchie, R. F.: The clinical significance of titered antinuclear antibodies. Arthritis Rheum., *10*:544, 1967.

Robitallie, P., and Tan, E. M.: Relationship between deoxyribonucleoprotein and deoxyribonucleic acid antibodies in systemic lupus erythematosus. J. Clin. Invest., *52*:316, 1973.

Ropes, M. W., et al.: Proposed diagnostic criteria for rheumatoid arthritis. Bull. Rheum. Dis., *7*:121, 1956.

Rothfield, N. F.: Detection of antibodies to nuclear antigens by immunofluorescence. *In* Rose, N. R., and Friedman, H.: Manual of Clinical Immunology. Washington, American Society for Microbiology, 1976.

Sandberg-Wollheim, M.: Optic neuritis: Studies on the cerebrospinal fluid in relation to clinical course in 61 patients. Acta Neurol. Scand., *52*:167, 1975.

Sharp, G. C., Irwin, W. S., Laroque, C., et al.: Association of autoantibodies to different nuclear antigens with clinical patterns of rheumatic disease and responsiveness to therapy. J. Clin. Invest., *50*:350, 1971.

Sharp, G. C., Irvin, W. S., Tan, E. M., et al.: Mixed connective tissue disease—an apparently distinct rheumatic disease syndrome associated with a specific antibody to an extractable nuclear antigen (ENA). Am. J. Med., *52*:48, 1972.

Shortman, K., von Boehmer, H., Lipp, J., and Hopper, K.: Subpopulations of T-lymphocytes. Transplant Rev., *25*:163, 1975.

Shulman, S.: Antigenicity and autoimmunity in sexual reproduction: A review. Clin. Exp. Immunol., *9*:267, 1971.

Shulman, S.: Human anti-sperm antibodies and their detection. *In* Rose, N. R., and Friedman, H.: Manual of Clinical Immunology. Washington, American Society of Microbiology, 1976.

Singer, J.: On standardization of the latex fixation. Bull. Rheum. Dis., *26*:868, 1975.

Smith, B. R.: The interaction of the LATS in thyroid tissue *in vitro*. J. Endocrinol., *46*:45, 1970.

Sofer, N. A.: Clinical presentations and mechanisms of necrotizing angiitis of the skin. J. Invest. Derm., *67*:354, 1976.

Solomon, G. E.: Auto-immune factors in inflammatory bowel disease. Mt. Sinai J. Med., *43*:602, 1976.

Steinberg, A.D.: Pathogenesis of autoimmunity in New Zealand mice. V. Loss of thymic suppressor function. Arthritis Rheum., *17*:11, 1974.

Stiller, C. R., Russell, A. S., and Dosseter, J. B.: Autoimmunity, present concepts. Ann. Intern. Med., *82*:405, 1975.

Strickland, R. G., Baur, S., Ashworth, L. A., E., et al.: A correlative study of immunological phenomena in pernicious anemia. Clin. Exp. Immunol., *8*:25, 1971.

Strife, C. F., McDonald, B. M., Reiley, E. J., et al.: Shunt nephritis. J. Pediatr., *88*:403, 1976.

Tada, T., Taniguchi, M., and Takemori, T.: Properties of primed suppressor T cells and their products. Transplant. Rev., *26*:106, 1975.

Talal, N., and Pillarisetty, R.: Radioimmunoassay for antibodies to deoxyribonucleic acid. *In* Rose, N. R., and Friedman, H. (eds.): Manual of Clinical Immunology. Washington, American Society of Microbiology, 1976.

Talal, N.: Immunologic and viral factors in autoimmune disease. Med. Clin. North Am., *61*:205, 1977.

Tan, E. M.: An immunologic precipitin system between soluble nucleoproteins and serum antibody in systemic lupus erythematosus. J. Clin. Invest., *46*:735, 1967.

Tan, E. M.: Relationship of nuclear staining patterns with precipitating antibodies in SLE. J. Lab. Clin. Med., *70*:800, 1967.

Tan, E. M., and Peebles, C.: Quantitation of antibodies to Sm antigen and nuclear ribonucleoprotein by hemagglutination. *In* Rose, N. R., and Friedman, H. (eds.): Manual of Clinical Immunology. Washington, American Society of Microbiology, 1976.

Tan, E. M.: Immunopathology and pathogenesis of cutaneous involvement in SLE. J. Invest. Derm., *67*:360, 1976.

Tesor, J. T., and Schmid, F.: Conversion of soluble immune complexes into complement fixing aggregates by IgM-rheumatoid factor. J. Immunol., *105*:1206, 1970.

Thaler, M. S., Klausner, R. P., and Cohen, H. J.: Medical Immunology. Philadelphia, J. B. Lippincott, Co., 1977.

Theofilopoulos, A. N., Wilson, C. B., and Dixon, F. J.: The Raji cell radioimmunoassay for detecting immune complexes in human sera. J. Clin. Invest., *57*:169, 1976.

Tourtellotte, W. W.: Cerebrospinal fluid immunoglobulins and the central nervous system as an immunological organ particularly in multiple sclerosis and subacute sclerosing panencephalitis. Rowland, L. P. (ed.). Baltimore, The Williams and Wilkins Company, 1971.

4

Toyka, K. V., Drachman, D., Griffin, D. E., Pestronk, A., Winkelstein, J. A., Fischbeck, K. H., and Kao, I.: Myasthenia gravis. Study of humoral immune mechanisms by passive transfer to mice. N. Engl. J. Med., *296*:125, 1977.

Tung, K. S. K., Ramos, C. V., and Deodhar, S. D.: Antithyroid antibodies in juvenile lymphocytic thyroiditis. Am. J. Clin. Pathol., *61*:549, 1974.

Vaughn, J. H.: Summary: Rheumatoid factors and their biological significance. Ann. N. Y. Acad. Sci., *168*:204, 1969.

Vincent, A., Pinching, A. J., and Newsom Davis, J.: Circulating anti-acetylcholine receptor antibody in myasthenia gravis treated by plasma exchange. Neurology, *27*:364, 1977.

Volpe, R.: The role of autoimmunity in hypoendocrine and hyperendocrine function. Ann. Intern. Med., *87*:86, 1977.

Ward, P. A., and Kibukamusoke, J. W.: Evidence for soluble immune complexes in the pathogenesis of the glomerulonephritis of quartan malaria. Lancet *1*:283, 1969.

Weigle, W. O.: Immunological unresponsiveness. Adv. Immunol., *16*:61, 1973.

Weitzman, R. J., and Walker, S. E.: Relation of titered peripheral pattern ANA to anti-DNA and disease activity in SLE. Ann. Rheum. Dis., *36*:44, 1977.

Wells, J. V., Michaeli, D., and Fudenberg, H. H.: Autoimmunity in selective IgA deficiency. Birth Defects, *11*:144, 1975.

Wertheimer, D., and Barland, P.: Clinical significance of immune deposits in the skin in SLE. Arthritis Rheum., *19*:1249, 1976.

West, C. D., Davis, N. C., Forestal, J., Herbst, J., and Spitzer, R.: Antigenic determinants of human B1c and B1q globulins. J. Immunol., *96*:650, 1966.

Whitaker, J. N., and Engel, W. K.: Vascular deposits of immunoglobulin and complement in idiopathic inflammatory myopathy. N. Engl. J. Med., *286*:333, 1972.

Whittingham, M. B., Irwin, J., Mackay, I. R., and Smalley, M.: Smooth muscle autoantibody in "autoimmune" hepatitis. Gastroenterology, *51*:499, 1966.

Whittingham, S., Irwin, J., Mackay, I. R., Marsh, S., and Cowling, D. C.: Autoantibodies in healthy subjects. Aust. Ann. Med., *18*:130, 1969.

Wilson, C. B., and Dixon, F. J.: Anti-glomerular basement membrane antibody-induced glomerulonephritis. Kidney Int., *3*:74, 1973.

Wilson, C. B., and Dixon, F. J.: The renal response to immunologic injury. *In* Brenner, B. M., and Rector, F. C., Jr. (eds.): The Kidney. Philadelphia, W. B. Saunders Company, 1976.

Wilson, C. B.: Recent advances in the immunological aspects of renal disease. Fed. Proc., *36*:2171, 1977.

Winchester, R. J., Kunkel, H. G., and Agnello, V.: Occurrence of gamma-globulin complexes in serum and joint fluid of rheumatoid arthritis patients. J. Exp. Med., *134*:2865, 1971.

Winchester, R.: Tests for detection of rheumatoid factors. *In* Rose, N. R., and Friedman, H. (eds.): Manual of Clinical Immunology. Washington, American Society of Microbiology, 1976.

Winfield, J. B., Winchester, R. J., Wernet, P., and Kunkel, H. G.: Specific concentration of anti-lymphocyte antibody in serum cryopathies of SLE. Clin. Exp. Immunol., *19*:44, 1977a.

Winfield, J. B., Faiferman, I., and Koffler, D.: Avidity of anti-DNA antibodies in serum and IgG glomerular eluates from patients with SLE. J. Clin. Invest., *59*:90, 1977b.

Winfield, J. B., Koffler, D., and Kunkel, H. G.: Specific concentration of polynucleotide immune complexes in the cryoprecipitates of patients with systemic lupus erythematosus. J. Clin. Invest., *56*:563, 1975.

Wolfe, J. F., Adelstein, E., and Sharp, G. C.: Antinuclear antibody with distinct specificity for polymyositis. J. Clin. Invest., *59*:176, 1977.

Woodrofe, A. J., Borden, W. A., Theofilopoulos, A. N., et al.: Detection of circulating immune complexes in patients with glomerulonephritis. Kidney Int., *12*:268, 1977.

Zubler, R. H., Lange, G., Lambert, P. H., et al.: Detection of immune complexes in unheated sera by a modified ^{125}I-C1q binding test: Effect of heating on the binding of C1q by immune complexes and the application of the test to SLE. J. Immunol., *116*:232, 1976.

Zweiman, B., and Hebert, J.: The L. E. cell phenomenon: Mechanisms and significance. Int. J. Dermatol., *15*:121, 1976.

39

LYMPHOCYTES

David T. Rowlands, Jr., M.D.,
Theresa L. Whiteside, Ph.D.,
and Ronald P. Daniele, M.D.

STRUCTURE OF LYMPHOCYTES

HETEROGENEITY OF LYMPHOCYTES

RELATIONSHIP OF LYMPHOCYTES TO IMMUNE RESPONSES

DIFFERENTIATION OF THE LYMPHOID SYSTEM

PROPERTIES USEFUL FOR STUDIES OF LYMPHOCYTES

TECHNIQUES USEFUL IN THE CLINICAL LABORATORY

MEASUREMENT OF FUNCTIONAL CAPACITIES OF LYMPHOCYTES

APPLICATION OF IMMUNOLOGIC METHODS TO HUMAN DISEASES

4

Lymphocytes localized to tissues or circulating in blood or lymph make up the cellular system principally responsible for the array of immune reactions now recognized in vertebrates. The principal tissue sites where lymphocytes are found may be divided into *primary lymphoid organs* (the thymus and bone marrow), in which antigen-independent processes of division and differentiation create new lymphoid cells, and *secondary lymphoid organs* (lymph nodes, spleen, and portions of the gastrointestinal tract), in which antigen-driven antibody production and generation of effector cells takes place. Maximal expression of immune responses by lymphocytes often requires interactions with macrophages or their products.

Our intention is to discuss the cellular and tissue architecture of the immune system, the interrelationships of the cells making up this system, the development and properties of lymphocytes, and their roles in mediating or influencing human disease. The latter objective can be faced only with some degree of timidity because of the almost daily enlargement of basic knowledge of immunology, leading to the rapid alterations in applications and interpretations of the clinical situations in which immune processes take part.

STRUCTURE OF LYMPHOCYTES

General Characteristics. Lymphocytes, stained with conventional histologic stains and seen through the light microscope, have deceptively homogenous appearances. They are approximately the same size as other leukocytes (8 to 12 μm), and their distinctly defined cellular membranes are responsible for rounded and regular contours. Their nuclei are equally uniform, having dense nuclear chromatin which on detailed examination appears clumped. The cytoplasm of lymphocytes has a bland appearance due to the paucity of cellular organelles. The lack of staining of the cytoplasm led early students of lymphocytes to believe that these cells had little functional activity. The existence of small, medium, and large lymphocytes was not attributed to function but simply marked a maturation stage. Today, large lymphocytes are thought to be activated cells. Lymphoblasts, seen in tissue sections or in smears of peripheral blood, are larger by at least twofold than their mature counterparts. In addition to a large nucleolus, they have a large cytoplasmic volume with numerous polyribosomes and well-developed Golgi zones. The two main lymphocyte subpopulations (T and B cells) are indistinguishable by light microscopy.

Examination of lymphocytes using the increased magnification capabilities of the electron microscope highlights the clumped appearance of the nuclear chromatin. As might be expected from light microscopy, the cytoplasm is found to contain a few lysozomes, sparse mitochondria, a small Golgi zone, and poorly formed aggregates of RNA. The plasma membrane of a lymphocyte is a typical unit membrane. Early studies suggested that certain classes of lymphocytes (B cells) could be distinguished from other lymphocytes by the presence of long cytoplasmic processes or villous projections. However, more recent information suggests that this finding was factitious, that the method of preparation may influence the morphology of lymphocytes, and that the surface characteristics of these cells may change depending on the external environment.

Plasma cells are derived from lymphocytes and, unlike their progenitors, clearly represent cells designed for the synthesis of immunoglobulins. Plasma cells are of about the same size as lymphocytes and have equally sharply defined cell walls. Their nuclei are eccentrically placed within the cell and, except for a small indentation, are round in appearance. The nuclear chromatin is as intensely stained as that of lymphocytes, but the chromatin is distributed more regularly along the nucleus in a pattern resembling the spokes of a wheel ("cartwheel nucleus"). The cytoplasm, except for one small area, stains intensely with pyronin, reflecting the large quantities of RNA available in the cellular cytoplasm. The unstained zone in the cytoplasm corresponds to the indented portion of the nucleus and is the site of the well-developed Golgi apparatus. As might be anticipated by its pronounced pyroninophilia, abundant and highly organized ribosomes are found in the cytoplasm of plasma cells. Well-developed plasma cells may contain small granules or bodies which stain with eosin or other acidic dyes and are called Russell bodies. The plasma cells containing Russell bodies have an especially notable cytoplasm with the endoplasmic reticulum appearing as large cisternae by electron microscopy. Unu-sually large amounts of immunoglobulins lie within these cisternae. Plasma cells not only produce antibodies, but also actively release or secrete them.

Cell Surfaces. The structural features of lymphoid cells discussed above are significant with regard to the performance of these cells as synthesizers of highly specialized products such as immunoglobulins and lymphokines. Clearly, receipt of appropriate signals and the transmission of their message to the internal portions of these cells are of great importance. In recent years, it has become clear that recognition of specific as well as non-specific stimuli occur at the cell surface of the lymphocyte. The surface properties of lymphocytes are then of paramount importance in cell biology of lymphocytes, inasmuch as cellular responses to environmental stimuli are dependent on the expression of specific receptors on lymphocyte surfaces. The presence of these receptors on lymphocytes permits identification and enumeration of subsets of lymphocyte subpopulations and allows for some understanding of the roles these cells play in normal as well as disease processes.

The cell surface of lymphocytes is regarded as a fluid mosaic permitting extensive rearrangement of surface molecules (Singer, 1974). Recent evidence suggests, however, that molecules that are intercalated into the lipid bilayer are also under variable degrees of restriction and modulation by a submembranous apparatus consisting of microfilaments and microtubules. This submembranous or cytoskeletal apparatus is now believed to be involved in the modulation of surface antigens and molecules. Such a modulation of surface antigens affords a means for controlled interactions between cells and their milieu. The dynamic nature of the lymphocyte membrane is best illustrated in a phenomenon of "capping" (Schreiber, 1976). In several animal species and man, immunoglobulin (Ig) molecules are evenly distributed over the surfaces of certain lymphocytes (B cells), as determined by using fluorescein-labeled anti-Ig. Upon reaction with the specific antibody, microclusters of Ig-anti-Ig begin to flow rapidly to one pole of the cell in an energy-requiring process which results in the formation of a polar cap. The cytoplasm underneath the cap contracts, leading to the formation of a uropod at the opposite pole and a flow of cytoplasm away from the cap. The result is a transient motion of the entire lymphocyte along its substratum, accompanied by endocytosis or internalization of the surface Ig-anti-Ig complexes. Capping in lymphocytes is thought to be dependent on the membrane-cytoplasm interaction because myosin—a component of microfilaments which form a cytoskeleton—shifts in close apposition to the Ig-anti-Ig microclusters. In addition, nucleotides and calcium appear to be involved in this modulation. The precise mechanism and physiologic role of capping are not understood as yet, but recognition of the phenomenon has provided a useful tool for analysis of the interrelationships between surface receptors on lymphocytes.

The opportunity for modulation of molecules within the plane of the membrane implies that surface receptors expressed by a lymphocyte may differ depending on the state of cellular activation, differentiation, and even distinct phases of the cell cycle. This appears to be so, as exemplified by the studies of one subpopulation of murine lymphocytes (T cells). Immunologically immature murine thymocytes express several surface receptors (G_{1X}, TL, Thy_1, Ly_1, $Ly_{2,3}$, Lys, H_2) (Cantor, 1975). Maturation and differentiation of these cells into antigen-reactive cells are associated with the loss of several surface receptors. Further specialization into functionally committed effector cells leads to an additional change in surface properties so that only one or two of the early receptors are retained. There are indications that the expression of surface Ig may be a function of cellular activity, because antigen- or mitogen-activated T-lymphocytes bear surface Ig's, in contrast to a majority of T cells, which are devoid of easily detectable Ig receptors. The presence of surface Ig on activated T cells appears to be derived from the exogenous binding of IgG to acquired Fc receptors on these cells (Yoshida, 1972). Plasma cells, which actively produce and secrete Ig, are nevertheless devoid of surface Ig receptors. The latter are ubiquitous on membranes of B lymphocytes. T lymphocytes activated by allogeneic stimulation express *de novo* an insulin receptor, while, as noted above, Fc receptors are detectable on T-lymphocytes when stimulated into G and S phases of the cell cycle by different agents. It is now clear that surface receptors are not constant or invariable features of lymphoid cells. Rather, qualitative and/or quantitative changes in these receptors may occur at any stage of cellular development and are closely related to the membrane interaction with the environment, cell metabolism reflecting cellular events, or functional capabilities of lymphocytes.

Antibody- or ligand-mediated redistributions of surface molecules may lead to a reversible removal of these molecules from the membrane. The removal may be accomplished by either or both of the following mechanisms. It appears that as a result of surface membrane turnover, some surface constituents are continually shed to the outside of the cell, a process known as exocytosis (Schreiber, 1976). In contrast, pinocytosis involves the internalization and perhaps reutilization of the molecules being removed from the surface. Little is known about the mechanisms and significance of these processes in lymphoid cells. They are energy-dependent, for metabolically inhibited cells do not undergo pinocytosis. It may be speculated that continual removal of the "used up" receptors, enzymes, and other membrane constituents keeps the cell surface in a virgin state, freed from all the complexes formed between surface sites and environmental factors, free to accept new stimuli or messages.

The biochemical characteristics of surface receptors on lymphocytes have been incompletely explored. Those receiving most attention have been the surface immunoglobulins. It has already been mentioned that when these are altered, as by aggregation using immunoglobulin-specific antisera, they are very rapidly taken into the lymphocyte by pinocytosis and/or shed from the cell surface. Such specific and reversible antibody-mediated removal or alteration of surface antigens on lymphocytes is called antigenic modulation. It may involve a variety of surface antigens other than immunoglobulins, and it may represent an important control mechanism in the generation and regulation of immune responses. Surface immunoglobulin, due to its established specificity, is the most likely candidate for that surface receptor which is responsible for the reaction of a lymphocyte with an antigen.

Lymphocytes are the key cells of the immune system. By virtue of their surface receptors, they are responsible for the recognition of antigens and for the appropriate response to these antigens. They are qualified not only to *initiate* specific antibody-mediated immune responses, but also to gear their cellular machinery to elaborate and release a variety of other factors that are capable of acting as effector molecules. These effector molecules, in turn, may in a specific or non-specific way affect other lymphocytes, other leukocytes (e.g., monocytes), and other tissue cells. Lymphocytes are capable of and required to establish an effective cooperation with other cells of the reticuloendothelial system for the immune response to take place. In order for the immune system to function efficiently, a high degree of regulation must be built into it, and there is a large body of evidence to suggest that certain subpopulations of lymphocytes (e.g., suppressor cells) are involved in and/or responsible for this regulation. Finally, lymphocytes must be responsible for maintaining immunologic memory. It is clear now that an extraordinary degree of functional heterogeneity exists among lymphocytes and that the three morphologically identifiable types of lymphocytes (small, medium, and large) cannot account for the host of functions required of them.

HETEROGENEITY OF LYMPHOCYTES

The immune response comprises a complex and not yet fully understood series of events which are antigen-driven and which result in the synthesis and secretion of humoral antibodies ("humoral immunity") and/or the delayed-type hypersensitivity reactions broadly referred to as ("cell-mediated immunity"). Lymphocytes mediate all phases of the immune response; however, not *all* lymphocytes participate in *all* stages of this response at *all* times. The remarkable "division of labor" takes place among lymphocytes in the course of the immune response. It is only in recent years that this form of functional diversity has been successfully correlated with recognizable and distinct components of the lymphoid system.

The broadest separation of lymphocyte compartments can be made by designating one portion as T cells (thymus-dependent) and the other portion as B cells (bursal or bone-marrow derived). The former term (T cell) has its origin in experimental studies carried out in the early 1960's, when it was shown that surgically removed thymuses in very young animals of several species resulted in the failure of development of portions of the immune response and lymphoid tissues located in lymph nodes and spleen. The latter term (B cell) followed the classic experimental work of

Glick (reviewed in Cooper, 1974), who showed that removal of the bursa of Fabricius in chickens resulted in a loss of certain other lymphocyte-dependent functions. Similarly, Claman (1966), at a later date, showed that B cell functions in mammals could be supplied by cells of the bone marrow. These studies also led to a concept that will be enlarged upon later—namely, that cellular interactions between T and B cells were required for complete expression of the immune response.

T and B lymphocytes are heterogeneous not only in their functional activities (Table 39-1), but also in their origin, lifespan, migration patterns, anatomical distribution, and surface characteristics.

B-lymphocytes.   These cells ultimately synthesize and release immunoglobulins. It is generally accepted that B lymphocytes have easily detectable immunoglobulin (Ig) on cell membranes. There is diversity within the B cell category such that various subpopulations are relatively restricted in the types of antibodies which they can synthesize and release. In man, there are four subclasses of IgG and two of IgA. If a given mature B-lymphocyte or plasma cell is capable of producing only one class of immunoglobulin, there must be at least nine different types of B-lymphocytes: for example, there are IgG_2 B-lymphocytes and IgM B-lymphocytes. The situation is further complicated by the fact that each type of B-lymphocyte probably produces Ig receptors with a single and unique antigen specificity. Thus, there are many types of B-lymphocytes with different antigen specificities. Approximately 10 to 15 per cent of circulating blood lymphocytes are immunoglobulin-bearing cells, and the immunoglobulins most frequently seen on these cells are IgM and IgD (Rowe, 1973). IgG- and IgM-positive lymphocytes are found primarily in organized lymphoid tissues, while the sites of external immunoglobulin secretion contain many IgA- and IgE-bearing cells. The foregoing emphasizes the enormous complexity of the Ig-bearing B-lymphocyte population.

B cells also have receptors on their surfaces which recognize the Fc portion of immunoglobulins (the Fc receptors), as well as receptors which are able to recognize and react with components of the complement system (C3 receptors) (Ross, 1973). Neither the chemical nature of these receptors nor their physiologic roles are clear at this time, except that they may be significant in cellular interactions. In

Table 39–1. BIOLOGIC REACTIONS MEDIATED BY
LYMPHOCYTES

REACTION	B-LYMPHOCYTE ANTIBODIES	T-LYMPHOCYTE SENSITIZED CELLS
Protection against infection	Encapsulated bacteria (streptococci, pneumococci, meningococci, *H. influenzae*)	Intracellular pathogens (viruses, bacteria, fungi, protozoa)
Transplant rejection	Major cause of hyperacute rejections Also important in acute and chronic rejections—may be protective of the graft	Major mechanism for chronic rejection
Graft versus host reaction	Not involved	Involved
Tumor immunity	May enhance tumor growth	Main mechanism for eliminating tumor cells
Autoimmunity	Mediate "immune-complex" diseases and autoimmune diseases of formed elements of blood	Involved in pathogenesis of solid organ disease (thyroiditis, adrenalitis)
Tolerance	May participate through feedback and/or immune complex inhibition	Generation of suppressor lymphocytes

4

any case, they provide the basic tools for identifying and enumerating B cells in man.

There is evidence that C3 receptors and Ig receptors and perhaps Fc receptors are found on the same or most B-lymphocytes (Ehlenberger, 1976). That is not to say, however, that all B-lymphocytes carry all three receptors. Some SIg-positive B-lymphocytes may not express C3 receptors or Fc receptors or both. Thus, B cells are no more homogenous than lymphocytes as a whole. It appears that the B cell compartment is actually made up of various populations of cells having one or more of the surface markers described above.

Exposure of B cells to antigens *in vitro* may lead to proliferation of a limited extent. In most species, this proliferation accounts for activation of as much as 2 to 3 per cent of the B cells in response to a particular antigen. Considering the vast array of antigens to which an animal can respond *in vivo*, such responsiveness to individual antigens implies that recognition is relatively rather than rigidly specific for the antigens in question. Surface receptors other than immunoglobulins are also related to immunity. Thus, B cells may be stimulated into metabolic activity and proliferation by a variety of agents termed mito-

gens (Greaves, 1972a). These agents are nonspecific stimulators in the sense that prior sensitization is not a requirement for recognition and activation and the responsive cells are not as limited in number as were antigens. However, in some cases the recognition of mitogens appears to be species-related. For example, lipopolysaccharide (LPS) may serve in mice as a non-specific B cell mitogen, but the B cells of man seem to be unresponsive to polyclonal mitogens, such as LPS. Similarly, anti-immunoglobulins serve as a proliferative stimulus in several animal species excepting man. In fact, one is hard put to identify a general B cell mitogen in man. Certain plant lectins, such as PHA, which, as we shall see, is a potent mitogen for T cells, readily stimulate B cells when they are made insoluble (Greaves, 1972b). Another lectin, pokeweed mitogen (PWM), thought to be a selective stimulator for B-lymphocytes, has been shown to act on both B and T cells in man (Greaves, 1972a).

As indicated earlier, plasma cells represent the extreme maturation form of B-lymphocytes. They are fully equipped for massive protein synthesis and appear to be significantly restricted with regard to the class and specificity of the immunoglobulins which they synthesize and secrete. It appears that each plasma cell makes and secretes an immunoglobulin of one class and with one unique antigenic specificity. Plasma cells differ significantly from their progenitor lymphocytes in having little in the way of immunoglobulin, Fc, or complement surface receptors. Further, a plasma cell antigen (PC1) is found only on antibody-secreting cells and not on B-cell precursors.

T-Lymphocytes. These cells are responsible for reactions of cellular immunity. Because cell-mediated immunity is antigen-directed, T cells must have surface receptors which recognize antigens exercising a degree of specificity similar to that of B cells. The nature of these receptors is less clear than is that of B cells, with the principal controversy concerning the presence of immunoglobulins on T cells. Immunoglobulins on surfaces of T cells are not easily detected by conventional procedures, perhaps because they are buried in the membrane, are sparse, or are present as monomers or polypeptide chains. The argument is not resolved at this time, and it may only be stated that little or no exposed immunoglobulin can be detected on T cells, although in activated T cells the amount of surface immunoglobulin may increase to easily detectable levels, probably by the binding of IgG via Fc receptors.

An important surface property of human T-lymphocytes from the standpoint of clinical medicine is the receptor for sheep erythrocytes (E). This surface receptor is selective for human T-lymphocytes, but its detection is to some extent temperature-dependent. Fc receptors are generally absent from surfaces of circulating T cells, but activated T-lymphocytes may express them. T-lymphocytes also express their receptors for PHA and concanavalin A, as evidenced by their marked proliferative response to appropriate concentrations of these mitogens. Interestingly, B cells and other lymphoid cells also express receptors for these mitogens, but their proliferative response may be negligible or nil. In addition, T cells respond by proliferation to alloantigens related to the major histocompatibility complex and expressed on allogeneic cells, including B cells. Finally, some T-lymphocytes may express specific differentiation antigens, such as theta antigen in the mouse, and antigens identifiable with anti-thymocyte or anti-brain sera in man (Cantor, 1976).

Other Lymphocytes. Cells which cannot be labeled as T or B cells on the basis of their surface properties constitute a "third lymphocyte population." The existence of this third population has been deduced from the lymphocyte enumeration studies, where the sums of identifiable T and B lymphocytes seldom exceed the figure of 90 per cent. Indeed, more careful search resulted in the discovery of lymphocytic cells which could not be "tagged" by any of the available reagents. These are referred to as *"null" cells*. The name should not be taken to mean that these cells are functionless. Rather, it means that at a given time null cells do not bear any receptors recognizable by the methods at hand. Whether null cells represent undifferentiated stem cells, immature T or B cells, or those lymphocytes that have lost their recognizable surface receptors remains to be discovered. There is some evidence, for example, that about half of human lymphocytes that lack identifiable markers for T or B cells will eventually synthesize demonstrable surface Ig when cultured *in vitro* for seven days (Chess, 1975).

A second type of lymphocyte, which fits with neither T, B, nor null cells, has been identified in human peripheral blood. These are *"L cells,"* so named because of the labile surface IgG they bear (Lobo, 1975; 1976). They have high-affinity Fc receptors, which differ from those on B cells by being resistant to digestion with trypsin. L cells do not have surface receptors for C3 and they fail to adhere to nylon wool columns. They are non-phagocytic, non-adherent to glass, and negative for non-specific esterases, making it unlikely that they are monocytes. The functional properties of L-lymphocytes are unlike those of T cells, B cells, or monocytes. They do not proliferate in response to mitogens or soluble antigens, but are capable of enhancing *in vitro* responses of T-lymphocytes supplemented with monocytes. L-lymphocytes have a cytotoxic potential but cannot develop into antibody-producing cells. The site of origin and role of L-lymphocytes in the immune response is unknown. The importance of these cells rests in the fact that for some time, unless certain technical precautions were taken (*vide infra*), they were classified as B cells because of the binding of labile exogenous Ig via their Fc receptors.

A third type of non-T, non-B-lymphocyte, possibly related to L-lymphocytes, consists of *killer (K) lymphocytes* which mediate antibody-dependent cytotoxicity (ADCC). The presence of C3 receptors distinguishes these cells from L-lymphocytes, according to some investigators (Perlmann, 1975). Several others contend that both B cells and "null" cells have K cell activity. In addition, naturally occurring cytotoxic cells have been recently described in the mouse. These have a wide array of target specificities, are independent of previous active immunizations, are implicated in defensive mechanisms against tumors, and are somewhat akin to the K cells. There is also evidence that a cell similar in surface properties to the K cell may exercise suppressive activity on cytotoxic lymphocytes in man. The real nature of cells responsible for antibody-mediated cytotoxicity remains to be elucidated. It must be emphasized that cells of T lineage are also capable of target-cell killing, but they react directly with the target cells and that reaction is presumably independent of antibody.

It can be clearly seen, then, that the division of lymphocytes into two separate compartments—T cells and B cells—does not entirely or realistically account for all the different subpopulations of lymphocytes. While emphasizing the differences between the two lymphocyte populations, this compartmentalization fails to stress the enormous heterogeneity seen within each, as well as the fact that T and B cells have a common origin, intimately interact with each other, and inhabit the same lymphoid organs.

RELATIONSHIP OF LYMPHOCYTES TO IMMUNE RESPONSES

The essence of the immune response is that "antigens" are recognized by appropriate cells in the lymphoreticular system. Recognition is followed by an intricate, but as yet only partially understood, series of cell-to-cell and intracellular events culminating in the synthesis and release of effector molecules.

Substances which serve best as antigens are relatively large ($\geq 10,000$ M.W.), have relatively complex and rigid structures (e.g., proteins and polysaccharides), and are foreign to the host. Immune responses to certain small molecules (haptens) can be mounted only when the haptens are attached to larger (carrier) molecules. Haptens may be extremely small but can be recognized with exquisite sensitivity. In this way, haptens may be equated with

the various antigenic determinants (epitopes) on more complex antigens.

Studies in recent years have demonstrated that both T- and B-lymphocytes are ordinarily needed for antibody synthesis (Miller, 1968). The key experiment in this regard was that which Claman and his colleagues (1966) carried out in mice. They showed that reconstitution of lethally irradiated mice sufficient to permit an immune response required both bone marrow cells and thymic cells. Repopulating of these animals with thymic or bone marrow cells alone did not restore immune competence. The conclusion drawn from this and similar experiments is that cellular cooperation between T and B cells is necessary for the immune response to at least some antigens.

Using the murine model, it was demonstrated that, although both cell types were required for full expression of the antibody response to sheep red blood cells, only the bone-marrow derived cells produced antibodies. The mice used in these experiments had a unique chromosome marker so that bone marrow cells could be identified as antibody producers. In this and other reconstitution experiments in neonatally thymectomized animals, it was demonstrated that the reconstituting thymus cells act as "helper" cells in the development of immune responses. Thus, there exists a clear division of labor within the immune system, with B cells producing antibody and T cells exercising amplifying and, under certain circumstances, suppressive effects.

T-Cell Help. The precise mechanism of *T-cell help* is not fully understood (Feldmann, 1974; Gershon, 1974). It has been demonstrated that T-cell help is not required for immune responses to certain antigens. Studies of immune responses to hapten-carrier conjugates indicated that most antigens and molecules contain two types of determinants: carrier determinants, which are recognized by helper T cells, and haptenic determinants, with which antibody-producing cells (B cells) react directly (Fig. 39-1). If an animal is competent to produce B cells capable of recognizing the haptenic determinants on the antigen molecule but for some reason is unable to produce T cells for recognition of the carrier determinant, only a limited antibody response will ensue. The antibody produced in this situation is hapten-specific IgM. On the other hand, if the responding animal's T cells are competent to recognize and react with the

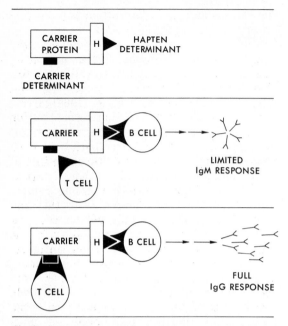

Figure 39-1. The proposed relationship between carrier proteins, haptens (H), T cells, and B cells is illustrated. In most cases, a full immune response occurs only when there is appropriate recognition of the carrier by T cells and the hapten by B cells. A more limited IgM response may be seen when B cells recognize the hapten without T cell help.

carrier determinant, a full-strength anti-hapten IgG response takes place. Thus, it appears that a main consequence of a T cell–B cell interaction is to provide a mechanism for regulating the magnitude and quality of the immune response. We do not know why certain antigens are "T-dependent" and others "T-independent," but the repetitive subunit structure of all T-independent antigens (such as pneumococcal polysaccharides) suggests that spatial orientation and/or molecular conformation of the antigen may be important for B-cell recognition.

A large body of evidence supports the contention that both T and B cells possess specific receptors for antigens and cooperate in the synthesis of antibody in response to thymus-dependent antigens. There are two theories to explain the nature of cooperation between helper T cells and antibody-producing B cells. In one, a T cell, having reacted with a carrier determinant, elaborates a soluble factor which can stimulate B cells into producing anti-hapten antibody. In the other, direct contact and interaction of T and B cells, during which the T cell presents antigen to B cells of appropriate specificity, is postulated. There is evi-

dence that both antigen-specific and non-specific factors are involved in the production of antibodies to thymus-dependent antigens. The three factors that are likely candidates include (reviewed in Basten and Mitchell, 1976):

a. Allogeneic effect factor (AEF), which is not antigen-specific and is elaborated by those T cells that are specific for and react with the carrier portion of the antigen. The subsequent reaction of the B cell with the hapten and AEF is a signal for the B cell to proliferate and differentiate into an antibody-producing cell. AEF is probably a product of the immune response genes linked to the H-2 complex in the mouse.

b. IgT, which is an immunoglobulin with specificity for the carrier determinant on the surface of T cells. The antigen-IgT complex is then shed from the T-cell surface and its hapten portion is presented to the B cell via a macrophage.

c. Ia factor, which is an antigen-specific soluble product of the I region released by the T cell after it reacts with the carrier portion of the antigen. The Ia factor then reacts with B cells.

No firm conclusions can be drawn at present regarding the manner in which T and B cells cooperate in the immune response. Helper cells may influence effector cells by one or several soluble factors and/or cell-to-cell interactions. The participation of a "third-party" cell in the process of cooperation is also likely.

Probably more than one type of host cell recognizes antigens.

Macrophages. Macrophages as well as lymphocytes can recognize antigens. Macrophages are large reticuloendothelial cells whose main biologic role is that of a scavenger: they phagocytose foreign materials. Macrophages adhere to glass or plastic surfaces and are found fixed in tissues or free in peritoneal exudates and circulation of all known multicellular species of animals. It is well known that efficient phagocytosis of bacteria by macrophages depends upon the presence of antibody molecules (opsonins), which can react with these bacteria. The bacterial antigen-antibody complexes are recognized by the Fc receptors for IgG on the cell surfaces of macrophages, with the complex being taken up and processed by them. The C3 receptors, present on macrophages, and Fc receptors have an evident physiologic role of enhancing phagocytosis by macrophages. A major portion of antigen recognized by macrophages is taken up by the phagocyte and digested. However, approximately 1 per cent of antigen presented to the macrophage may remain on the surface of the cell, serving as an available site for stimulating lymphocytes, which are capable of recognizing (i.e., equipped with appropriate surface receptors) this antigen (Unanue, 1972). While the specificity in the immune response is brought about by lymphocytes, the macrophage is essential in antigen processing, cell interactions, and optimal functioning of lymphocytes; however, macrophages appear not to be antigen-specific.

It has been clearly demonstrated in animal experiments and in *in vitro* antibody-generating or mitogen-responding systems that the presence of macrophages is essential for antibody production and cell-mediated and mitogen responses (Basten, 1972). Figure 39–2 schematically represents T- and B-cell cooperation involving macrophages and an antigen-specific factor (T-cell immunoglobulin, IgT), which concentrates the antigen on the surface of macrophages for presentation to B cells with antigen-specific surface receptors. It may be noted that T cells and macrophages not only are involved in the help-type responses, but also exercise suppressive effects as indicated. Antibody responses are not indefinite: suppression is, thus, a part of normal immune responses. Neither the mechanism of suppression nor the nature of the suppressor cell is clearly understood. We know from studies of murine models that T cells with certain surface characteristics (Ly 2, 3 surface antigens) (Cantor, 1975) mediate this suppression and that macrophages may be involved through elaboration of specific or non-specific suppressive factors (Basten, 1976). Also, suppression of the immune response may be initiated by external antigens if these are given at certain crucial concentrations (low- vs. high-zone tolerance) or have a tolerogenic conformation. Suppression may also be internal as, for example, when antigen-antibody complexes generated *in situ* block the antigen-specific receptors on T cells involved in regulation of the immune response. In addition, the interactions between T cells, B cells, and macrophages appear to be under genetic control, with immunoregulating genes linked to the major histocompatibility complex exercising this control (Benacerraf, 1975). The immune reactions to thymus-dependent antigens are

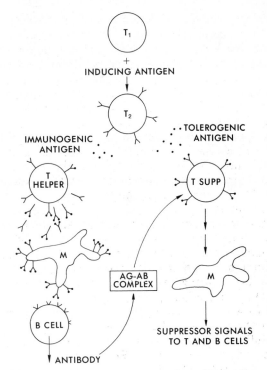

Figure 39–2. T_1 represents virgin T cells, and T_2 represents antigen-specific T cells.

complex, dynamic responses including many factors, many cells, and mechanisms of stimulation, suppression, and feedback regulation.

Effector and helper cells that are responsible for the synthesis of products active in the immune response and that provide controls for such synthesis must interact with antigens through antigen-specific receptors on their surfaces. It is generally accepted that immunoglobulin is the receptor for antigen on B cells. The chemical nature of the T-cell receptor is not established.

Since B cells have easily identifiable surface immunoglobulins, it has been assumed that these molecules are antigen receptors and transmit a signal for proliferation to the cell. As we pointed out, IgM and IgD are the predominant classes of surface Ig on B cells. It has been suggested that a possible role for IgD may be that of a receptor for antigens. Detailed studies of the synthesis of immunoglobulins have been done, and they indicate that a B cell synthesizes and secretes antibodies of the same class as that on its surface. In contrast to secreted immunoglobulins which are 19S in the case of IgM, membrane-bound IgM is 7S. Although the basic structure of all monomeric immunoglobulins is similar, with characteristic four-chain structures comprising V (variable) and C (constant) domains, their antigenic heterogeneity (differences in amino acids of polypeptide chains) allows us to categorize them on the basis of class as IgG, A, M, D, and E. Further heterogeneity, which is genetically controlled within the species, is responsible for *allotypic* differences within each class. Most important, heterogeneity within a variable, antigen-combining site results in *idiotypic* determinants that provide a basis for unique antigenic specificity of every immunoglobulin molecule. Thus, idiotype is a unique antigen-binding site on an antibody molecule (see Chap. 36, p. 1232). It has been emphasized recently that the regulation of immune responses may occur through a network of antibodies to idiotypes (Jerne, 1973). Also, the association of surface immunoglobulins with products of the major histocompatibility complex (HLA in man, H-2 in mice) indicates participation of genetic factors in the immune responses (Benacerraf, 1975).

The antigen that recognizes a receptor specific for it on the surface of a lymphocyte is capable of the activation of a small number of precursor cells. These cells then proliferate, generating a clone of lymphocytes committed to respond to the specific antigen. The nature of signals or chemical mediators that are needed to accomplish the antigen-driven proliferation is not certain. A number of *in vitro* experiments involving a variety of soluble antigens and mitogens have amply demon-

strated that the interaction of antigen with the surface receptor generates the signal for proliferation. However, it is not clear how the signal is transmitted from lymphocyte membrane to cellular machinery, what cellular products are made, and how these products affect other cells in the course of helper-effector processes. There is a possibility that one signal, i.e., the antigen-receptor union, is not sufficient for initiation of these events and that a second signal must be supplied by a helper cell for the immune response to occur. In fact, it has been suggested that tolerance (state of immunologic unresponsiveness) occurs if the first signal is not followed appropriately by the second one from the helper cell.

Suppressor T Cells. The role of these lymphocytes in the regulation of immune responses has been recently emphasized (Gershon, 1974). It is thought that this cell is involved in the control of both cellular immunity and antibody synthesis through soluble factors it elaborates. There is evidence that, in the mouse, suppressor T cells are a distinct subpopulation of T lymphocytes with unique surface determinants (Ly 2, 3 antigens) (Cantor, 1975). In Figure 39-3 a representative T cell is shown to be capable of providing a number of factors and performing a variety of functions. It is more likely that T cells specialize in different functions. For example, helper T cells can be distinguished from suppressors by the presence of Ly 1 antigens. Interactions between cells participating in the immune response may result in cooperation, regula-

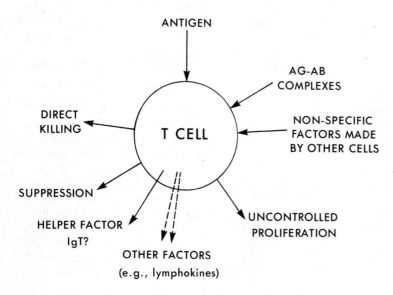

Figure 39-3. The varieties of input to T cells are indicated, as are the possible functions of these stimulated cells.

Table 39-2. INTERACTIONS BETWEEN CELLS INVOLVED
IN THE IMMUNE REACTIONS

INTERACTION	RESULT	DEFECT	CONSEQUENCE
Cooperation	Antibody response	Excess	Autoimmunity
		Not enough	Infections
Regulation	Balance of immune responses	Control	Tolerance or immune deficiency
		Control	Autoimmunity or escape from control
Suppression	Immunologic unresponsiveness	Excess	Infections or tumor growth
		Not enough	Autoimmunity

tion, or suppression of immune responses (Table 39-2). A defect in any of these may lead to excessive or inadequate immune responses.

DIFFERENTIATION OF THE LYMPHOID SYSTEM

Experimental studies with thymectomized animals and bursectomized birds, as well as observations on patients with various immunodeficiency disorders, indicate that, from a developmental viewpoint, the lymphoid system can be divided into three compartments. The first, the pool of undifferentiated stem cells, is a source of ancestral lymphoid cells capable of extensive proliferation and maturation into functionally competent cells. The second, the central or "primary" lymphoid tissues (thymus and bursa or bursa-equivalent in mammals), controls the development of lymphoid cells and is the site of intense, antigen-independent lymphopoiesis. The third compartment encompasses peripheral or "secondary" lymphoid organs (spleen, lymph nodes, gut-associated lymphoid tissue) and is made up of mixed populations of functionally differentiated T and B cells. In the peripheral lymphoid organs, T and B cells are located in distinct anatomic locations. In lymph nodes, for example, B cells populate the follicular areas, while T cells are found in the paracortical region. It must be emphasized that at any given time a great majority of lymphocytes (80 per cent or more) exist outside of the lymphoid tissues, i.e., in the blood and tissues.
Embryonic Origin of Lymphocytes. Lymphoid cells make their first appearance in yolk sac or fetal liver, along with other hema-

topoietic stem cells (Cooper, 1974). All lymphocytes are derived from a primitive pluripotential stem cell to be found in the blood islets of the yolk sac. In fetal life, the liver is a source of stem cells and later, in postnatal life, bone marrow becomes a pool of pluripotential stem cells. In the mouse, the spleen may also act as a source of these cells. It appears that two distinct pluripotential stem cells exist. One, capable of forming colonies *in vivo* (CFU-S) and at a later stage of development *in vitro* (CFU-C), is a progenitor of myeloid and erythroid elements. The other, unable to grow *in vitro* under any known conditions, is an ancestral cell for lymphocytes. Both of these stem cells are derived from a more primitive cell whose existence is suspected but not proved. Lymphoid cells capable of producing immunoglobulins can be detected around the eighth week of human embryonic life. In the mouse fetal liver, the first sign of B cells is glimpsed through the appearance of cells with IgM in their cytoplasm and, a bit later, on their surfaces. Similar cells are detectable in human bone marrow. This indicates that the commitment process may take place before the developing lymphoid cells reach their microenvironments or that differentiated lymphocytes may return to and perhaps influence the site of hematopoiesis. It is not known how or what directs developing lymphoid cells to either the thymus or the lymphoid tissue that is an equivalent of the bursa in chickens. It is possible that the gut-associated lymphoid tissue ("GALT") in man may be this equivalent. The migration from fetal liver or adult bone marrow to primary lymphoid tissues must occur via the blood stream. Once there, the progenitor cells come under the inductive influences thought to be mediated by epithelial elements of the lymphoid tissue and become committed to the lymphoid pathway of differentiation. Little is known about the properties of these inductive factors, but it is possible that humoral factors, such as erythropoietin in the marrow and thymosin in the thymus, play important roles.

The first organs to become inhabited by lymphocytes during development are the thymus, fetal liver, and bursa-like tissue. In the thymus, and bursa in the chicken, a very high mitotic index can be observed even before the fetus is born. A similar phenomenon is seen in germ-free animals. These observations have been taken as evidence that lymphopoiesis is dependent on a supply of stem cells. When the thymus is depleted of lymphocytes by irradiation or cortisone treatment, only the influx of stem cells results in repopulation with lymphocytes and further development of immune responsiveness. Mature lymphocytes or even thymocytes cannot effectively repopulate the thymus. Removal of primary lymphoid organs early in development results in absent or defective immune responses, as pointed out earlier. On the other hand, removal of these organs in an adult does not influence the immune competence unless the pool of immunocompetent lymphocytes is depleted by irradiation or other measures. In such cases, the repair of the immune system is dependent on both the supply of stem cells and the presence of primary lymphoid organs. Thus, central lymphoid tissues are needed for the development of immunologic competence but not for maintaining such competence.

The presence of epithelial cells in the primordial thymus and persistence into adult life of these cells suggests that they serve as a hormonal source acting locally to induce maturation of lymphocytes from appropriate mesenchyme. Experiments to distinguish between hormonal mechanisms and simple maturation from primitive stem cells in the thymus have been devised. When thymic epithelial cells are placed opposite appropriate mesenchymal cells on either side of a cell-impermeable millipore filter, maturation of lymphocytes from mesenchymal cells is readily demonstrated. Similarly, the observation that transplants of thymuses into animals after thymectomy function when only thymic epithelial cells are present adds support to the concept of participation of humoral factors in lymphocyte maturation. More recently, extracts of thymuses

containing a hormone-like substance, "thymosin," have been shown to restore thymus-like activity in otherwise thymus-free animals (Bach, 1971). These preparations have even been used successfully in the treatment of some children with congenital thymic deficiencies. The epithelial elements constitute the microenvironment of the thymus needed for development of functionally competent lymphocytes.

Experimental studies in bursectomized chickens as well as studies of immunologically defective humans made it clear that sites other than the thymus were important in the maturation of the B cell series of lymphocytes. Following this demonstration, an extensive search for the bursal equivalent in mammals was made. As might be supposed, lymphoid masses with associated epithelial cells became prime candidates, since similar cellular relationships were recognized in both the thymus and the bursa of Fabricius. Various tissues along the gastrointestinal tract (e.g., tonsils and Peyer's patches) suited this theory. None of these tissues, however, has been shown conclusively to be bursal equivalents in mammals. It would now seem that the bone marrow is the most likely source of B-cell precursors, with the liver producing such cells quite early in development.

Development of Lymphocytes.   Production of new immunocompetent T- and B-lymphocytes continues throughout life, although the rate slows down (Cooper, 1974). As Figure 39-4 illustrates, pro-T and pro-B cells migrate to the thymus and the bursa-like lymphoid tissue, respectively, where cytodifferentiation commences. This differentiation undoubtedly involves many steps, alterations in surface markers, and changes in functional properties of maturing lymphocytes. Through the use of antisera specific for differentiation antigens on maturing cells, it is possible to identify and actually isolate the functional subpopulations of T cells in the mouse. Figure 39-5 depicts in a schematic way the maturation of murine T cells.

The phenotype of maturing murine T cells undergoes continual changes as it develops from a primitive, null prothymocyte into a functionally specialized circulating T cell. The first antigen to be identified as characteristic of thymic lymphocytes was the θ or Thy 1 antigen in the mouse. This antigen is carried by thymic lymphocytes into peripheral lymphocyte pools such as the spleen and lymph

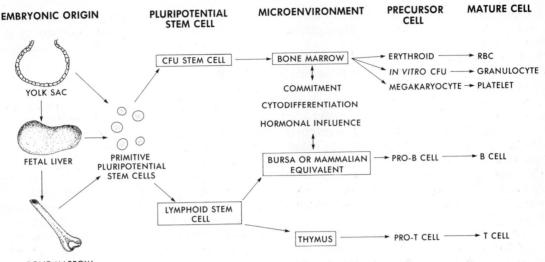

Figure 39-4. Illustration of the relationships between sources of stem cells and the sites of maturation of hematopoietic cells and lymphocytes.

nodes. Its presence on the surface of a cell is used to distinguish thymus-derived from other lymphocytes. When the thymocyte leaves the thymus for the peripheral lymphoid tissue, it still has Thy 1 antigen, but in much decreased quantities. A series of antigens designated as Ly antigens are also demonstrable on T cells, and their presence can be correlated with different functional subpopulations of T cells. The Ly 1 cells control delayed hypersensitivity, are involved in responses to the MHC antigens (MLC-reactive cells), and serve as helper cells in immune responses to T-dependent antigens. Ly 2, 3 cells appear to effect cell-mediated lympholysis and include a population of suppressor cells (Cantor, 1975). The suppressor T cells are Ia$^+$ (a surface antigen

coded for by immune response genes), while the cytotoxic T cells are Ia$^-$. The functions of T cells carrying all three antigens (Ly 1,2,3) have yet to be defined. They are viewed by some as antigen-reactive cells which are not committed functionally. The thymus leukemia (TL) antigen is a classic differentiation antigen, as it is expressed exclusively on thymocytes and not on circulating T cells. Thus, the development of T cells can be traced in the mouse (but not in humans due to lack of defined alloantisera) to include a thymus-sponsored conversion of null prothymocytes into thymocytes bearing a full complement of T-cell markers and eventually into at least three sets of T cells, each programmed for a different function and each bearing unique surface

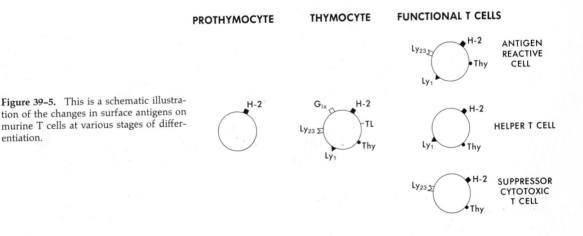

Figure 39-5. This is a schematic illustration of the changes in surface antigens on murine T cells at various stages of differentiation.

alloantigens. In humans, T-lymphocytes can now be divided into two functional subpopulations. The first comprises cells with receptors for the Fc portion of IgM (T_μ) and with helper activity for the proliferation and differentiation of PWM-stimulated B cells to plasma cells (Moretta, 1977). T-lymphocytes with the receptors for IgG (T_γ), which are capable of suppressing the polyclonal B-cell differentiation induced by PWM, represent the second functional subpopulation. The two human T-cell subpopulations can also be distinguished by their differential sensitivity to corticosteroids, irradiation, and thymopoietin (Gupta, 1977).

Present concepts of the maturation of B cells also include a pro-B cell which arises from the stem cell in the marrow or fetal liver. It is thought that the pro-B cell, like pro-thymocyte, has no detectable surface markers (is "null") (Vogler, 1976). The first marker to appear on maturing B cells is immunoglobulin M (Raff, 1976). Immunoglobulin D appears on these IgM-positive cells at a somewhat later time in both the mouse and man. These precursors of antibody-producing cells have been most extensively studied in the mouse. In adoptive transfer experiments, primitive lymphoid cell populations (e.g., fetal liver or bone marrow cells) were injected into irradiated syngeneic animals. Subsequent analysis of their capacities to form colonies and/or produce antibodies indicated that the earliest cells to be recognized as B cells by these methods appear in the liver early in development of the embryo and then go through further developmental stages in the spleen or other lymphoid organs. It seems clear that the ability of these cells to recognize antigens pre-

cedes their abilities to synthesize antibodies. It has been hypothesized that IgD may be the "early" cell surface receptor for antigens (Rowe, 1973).

The sequence for development of B-lymphocyte surface receptors appears to be surface immunoglobulin → receptors for the Fc portion of immunoglobulin → receptors for C3 (Fig. 39-6). The B cell emerges from the maturation process bearing receptors for an antigen, which in fact are antibody molecules inserted into the surface membrane. During cell maturation, "switchover" of membrane immunoglobulin may occur, so that B cells which initially express only IgM or IgD on their surfaces switch to an IgG or IgA phenotype. During the switchover, there may be brief periods when two immunoglobulins or no membrane immunoglobulins are present on the cell. Although it has been suggested that the immunoglobulin type on a lymphocyte reflects the extent of differentiation of B cells, experimental evidence for the switchover theory is fragmentary and open to criticism.

Other surface receptors that characterize the B-cell line include plasma cell antigen (PC1) found on antibody-secreting cells but not on B-cell precursors and p 23,30 antigen, which is a glycoprotein molecule found on human B cells, myeloid progenitor cells, and a variety of human leukemic lymphocytes (Schlossman, 1976).

Maturation and differentiation of lymphocytes are not completely understood as yet. They involve a complex series of progressive and regressive changes in surface receptors under the control of hematopoiesis-inducing microenvironment. The many unanswered questions about differentiation include those

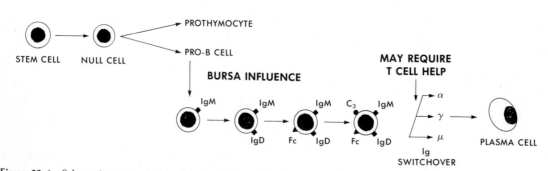

Figure 39-6. Schematic representation of differentiation of B cells in terms of changes in surface properties and synthesis of immunoglobulins.

having to do with the nature and properties of prolymphocytes, the commitment process, the influences exerted on developing cells by their microenvironments, the role of antigens in the differentiation process, and synchronization of surface properties with functional maturation of developing lymphocytes.

Recirculation of Lymphocytes (Sprent, 1977). Lymphocytes are not permanent residents of any one lymphoid tissue. Rather, they briskly move throughout all tissues of the body. As many as 80 per cent of small lymphocytes in the blood of adult animals are long-lived cells capable of extensive and long-term recirculation. Both small T- and B-lymphocytes recirculate. The pathway of recirculating lymphocytes takes them from the blood stream to the extravascular connective tissue spaces and peripheral lymphatic vessels and back to the blood via the lymphatic system (Fig. 39-7).

"Blood-to-lymph recirculatory" includes those blood-borne cells which extravasate from blood to lymph within the lymph nodes. In the lymph nodes, the small lymphocytes are continually added to the lymph: about 10 per cent of lymphocytes which enter a node in the arterial blood do not exit via the venous route, but instead extravasate to the lymph. This passage from blood to lymph is initiated at the special segments of postcapillary venules with a high cuboidal epithelium (HEPCV = high epithelium postcapillary venules) shortly after

blood-borne cells enter the node (i.e., near the cortico-paracortical junction). The migration through the node occurs via one of the three routes: (1) A paracortical sinus route where the cells enter a subfollicular sinus, pass through sinuses in paracortex and medulla, and leave the node via the efferent lymphatic. (2) A paracortical cord route which takes longer than the sinus route and is principally taken by T cells. Most of these cells leave the cords at the paracortex-medulla junction to enter the medullary sinuses and reach the efferent lymphatic. (3) The perifollicular route followed mainly by B cells which pass through a series of perifollicular capillaries and eventually end up in the subfollicular sinuses (Kelly, 1975). The minimum transit time of a population of labeled small lymphocytes from blood to lymph is about two to four hours in the rat.

In the spleen, the migrating small lymphocytes pass through the pores of the marginal sinus to enter periarteriolar lymphocyte sheaths. From there they exit, probably via the marginal zone channels. During the two-to-four-hour passage through the spleen, there are ample opportunities for lymphocytes to extravasate into the splenic tissue in much the same way as in the lymph nodes. In the gut lymphoid tissue, the cells migrate from the blood via postcapillary venules into interfollicular lymphoid tissue and out via the lacteals. It is of interest that either in the lymph nodes, spleen, or gut-associated lymphoid tissue re-

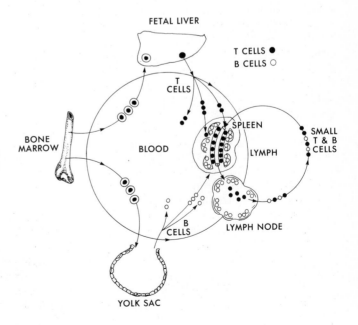

Figure 39-7. Recirculation of lymphocytes showing the interrelationships of T and B cells with various lymphoid tissues.

circulating lymphocytes do not migrate through the follicles or germinal centers.

From the fragmentary information at hand, it appears that the single most important factor determining which lymphocytes recirculate lies in the cell surface characteristics. Experiments in which treatments with trypsin or neuraminidase were shown to radically alter the migration patterns of lymphocytes support this view. Exposure to viruses, bacteria, other microorganisms, and antigens also alter cell surface characteristics of lymphocytes and, thus, play an important role in modifying their migration patterns through lymphoid tissues.

The physiologic significance of the rapid exchange of lymphocyte populations between blood and lymphoid tissues is that immunologically competent cells may be concentrated within short periods of time at the sites of antigen stimulation. In fact, within the confines of the complex and intricate architecture of the lymphoid system, the cellular interactions are not understood, but it is suspected that they are important in generating new memory B cells.

Responses to Antigenic Stimulation. The initial introduction of antigen into an intact animal produces profound changes in peripheral but little change in central lymphoid tissues. The sites of maximal alterations of the peripheral lymphoid tissues after injection of antigens are determined in large measure by the route of injection of antigen. If the injection is subcutaneous, regional lymph nodes are most extensively modified, while an intravenous injection of antigen causes profound alterations of the splenic lymphoid follicles. Other factors, such as the nature of the antigen, its speed of degradation within macrophages, and whether there is a pre-existing antibody all determine where and for how long antigens are retained in the lymphoid tissues.

Antigens injected subcutaneously enter the regional lymph node through the afferent lymphatics. Much of the antigen uptake in the node is by the sinus-lining macrophages. They degrade much of the antigen, although some of it remains in a surface-associated, native form. Antigen which passes through the first node is in a biologically screened state and as such remains in the circulation until specific antibody appears.

Within two to three days after subcutaneous administration of an antigen, the draining lymph node is characterized by enlarged paracortical cords and the presence of many blast cells. This is followed by the formation of active germinal centers and the appearance of plasma cells in the medulla. The sequence of events may be reconstructed as follows. First, the draining lymph node swells visibly owing to a reduction in the number of cells exiting via the efferent lymph. "Sinus plugging," which refers to filling up of the sinuses in paracortex with aggregates of lymphocytes, also contributes to the node swelling. The traffic through the sinuses becomes very sluggish because of the stickiness and enlargement of macrophages lining the sinuses in the paracorticomedullary junction. Next, the paracortical cords begin to fill uniformly with lymphocytes and swell until the entire paracortex becomes spherical. The lymphocytes stacked up in the paracortical cords undergo extensive mitotic activity. Both T- and B-lymphocytes divide, although the peak of mitotic activity of B cells lags behind that of T cells. Shortly after the onset of mitoses, plasmablasts may be seen at or near the paracorticomedullary junction. Some of these blast cells leave the node through medullary sinuses emptying into the efferent lymphatics, but the majority differentiate into sessile plasma cells within the medulla.

The magnitude and length of "lymphocyte trapping" by the activated node depend on the amount and physical characteristics of antigen and are self-limiting. On about day four or five, the trapping ends with outpouring of cells from the congested paracortical sinuses into the medullary sinuses and out of the node so that its lymphocyte output rises to 5 to 10 times that of a normal level. Paracortical cords decrease in size, and a week or 10 days after antigenic stimulation, the number of cells in the efferent lymph returns to normal. Although both proliferation and differentiation of the lymphocytes may be observed in the node within 24 to 48 hours of injection of an immunizing dose of antigen, antibody formation is not detected until the second to fourth day in the deep paracortex or medulla. Germinal centers do not appear until after five to seven days in primary and four to six days in secondary responses. This means that germinal centers are not involved in the initiation of antibody synthesis. Once synthesis starts, immune complexes composed of specific antibody and eliciting antigen localize on surfaces of dendritic cells within follicles. This is followed by the accumulation of large pyroninophilic dividing cells at the site. They are surrounded by a cuff of medium and small lymphocytes. It is uncertain what happens to the progeny of the dividing cells in germinal centers. They probably pass slowly into the follicular paracortex. They may be memory B-lymphocytes, since elimination of germinal centers results in normal antibody production but a failure to develop immunologic memory in experimental models.

Much of what we know about responses of lymphocytes to antigens in lymphoid tissues is fragmentary and incomplete. The exact time sequence of events following antigenic stimulation and coordination of the local events with systemic appearance of antibody molecules, as well as details of cellular cooperation, interaction of antigens with various lymphoreticular cells, effects of lymphocyte products, and the microenvironments of lymphoid tissue compartments on these events, remain to be worked out.

PROPERTIES USEFUL FOR STUDIES OF LYMPHOCYTES

Analysis of subpopulations of lymphocytes is a two-step process. The first requires separation of lymphoid cells from others. This step ordinarily depends upon physical characteristics of the cells (e.g., size or density) or cell surface properties which determine their differential adherence to substrates such as glass or to specific ligands such as immunoglobulins. The conditions chosen for such separations are of critical importance and should be selected with an eye to the purpose of the study. Some methods of separation may provide a good cell recovery, while others may be more effective in preserving the metabolic qualities of the purified cells.

The second process in analysis of subpopulations of lymphocytes is the quantitation of these cells. Quantitation depends on the presence of receptors located on the cell surfaces. It must be remembered that mononuclear cells other than lymphocytes may express the same receptors as lymphocytes. This is particularly important with respect to monocytes and macrophages. Therefore, it is important to remove such cells prior to the study of lymphocytes, or to identify the non-lymphocytes as contaminants of a given lymphocyte population. The receptors which permit enumeration of lymphocytes include receptors for Fc

portions of immunoglobulins, receptors for complement components, surface immunoglobulins (SIg), and receptors for sheep red blood cells (E) (Jondai, 1973; Aiuti, 1974). None of these is specific for lymphocytes. Surface immunoglobulins, although synthesized exclusively by lymphocytes, may be absorbed to surfaces of other cells (e.g., monocytes). The receptor for E, thought to be specific for human T cells, has recently been detected on a variety of human tissue cells, although not on other mononuclear cells (Woda, 1977).

Functional properties of lymphoid cells have been used only sparingly in enumerating the enriched cell populations of lymphocytes. Stimulation of lymphocytes with mitogens, such as PHA, Con A, or pokeweed, have been used to identify responsive T or B cells, and only in the case of PHA have these methods been modified to permit actual enumeration of T cells based on their responsiveness to PHA (Nowell, 1975). Similarly, mixed lymphocyte cultures have been used in a semiquantitative manner to determine the capacities of lymphocytes to stimulate the proliferation of other lymphocytes or to respond to other lymphocytes. Measurement of synthetic properties of lymphocytes (i.e., production of immunoglobulins or lymphokines) have been used sparingly to this point. Other functional properties, such as antibody-dependent or antibody-independent cytotoxicity, have also served as a guide for characterizing the T or B cell components of lymphocytes.

The analytical methods mentioned thus far deal with lymphocytes in suspensions. The desirability of identifying subpopulations of lymphocytes in solid tissues is obvious, especially where it relates to diagnosis of lymphomas and to pathogenesis of other tumors. Methods for such studies are now available and include immunomicroscopy with labeled antisera specific for T and B cells and rosetting techniques. The latter may be carried out using only frozen sections and until very recently were, for technical reasons, limited to the detection of B cells. Rosetting studies and immunofluorescence can now be used to detect T cells in tissues.

Identification and enumeration of lymphocytes, whether in suspensions or in tissues, are of limited clinical importance unless the functional status of identified cells can be simultaneously discerned. Even then, the value of *in vitro* analysis of lymphocyte populations remains dubious because clinically meaningful correlations between *in vitro* procedures and *in vivo* behavior of lymphoid cells in patients are still lacking.

TECHNIQUES USEFUL IN THE CLINICAL LABORATORY

Isolation of Lymphocytes.   Lymphocytes can be separated from other formed elements of the blood by velocity sedimentation or by density-gradient centrifugation. Velocity sedimentation uses gradients of protein such as albumin, dextran, or fetal calf serum, and the separation is a function of the radius of the cellular elements. Whether the separation is carried out by gravity or under the influence of centrifugation, the end result is an enrichment of the upper layers with mononuclear cells—especially T and B cells. The second method, density gradient centrifugation, depends upon the specific gravity of a gradient (either linear or discontinuous), made up by solutions such as albumin or Ficoll. The lighter cells (those with the greatest nucleus/cytoplasm ratio) band nearest the top of the gradient, with each cell population seeking that specific gravity that corresponds to its own in the gradient.

Among the various methods available for separation of lymphocytes, the Ficoll-Hypaque technique of Boyum (Boyum, 1968; 1974) has been used with greatest apparent success. For the Ficoll-Hypaque (F/H) technique (Fig. 39-8), bloods should be collected in heparin free of preservative, diluted (1:3) with a balanced salt solution, layered onto a Ficoll-sodium metrizoate gradient with density of 1.077 g/ml, and centrifuged at 400 g for 30 minutes at 22 to 25°C. It is important to ensure that centrifugation of blood preparation occurs at the same temperature at which the specific gravity of the Ficoll-Hypaque gradient has been established.

Separated lymphoid cells are collected from the interface by means of a Pasteur pipette and washed three times using calcium-free saline to minimize clumping. Under certain circumstances, it may be necessary to incubate the cells collected at the interface at 37°C. for periods between 2 and 24 hours. This allows exogenous immunoglobulin to be eluted from the surface of lymphocytes and monocytes which may occur by two mechanisms: (1) the absorption of either immunoglobulin or antigen/antibody complexes via the Fc receptor, or (2) the directing of antibodies toward determinants of the mononuclear cells (Lobo, 1975; Daniele, 1976).

The shape or dimensions of the tube used to form the gradient do not affect the results of cell separation. Provided that the conditions of separation are adhered to rigorously, recovery of nearly 90 per cent of the cells applied to the gradient can be anticipated. Losses of as many as 30 per cent of the cells may occur, usually owing to poor initial recovery at the interface or to improper washing procedures. Yields of less than 60 per cent are unacceptable and may lead to distortions in the T and B cell ratios of the final preparation.

It should be pointed out that these procedures for separation have been developed largely using peripheral blood from normal subjects. Separations of lymphocytes from patients with lymphoproliferative or other disorders may require modifications. In those circumstances, the physical characteristics of lymphocytes may be altered, and careful adjustment of the purification procedure may be necessary.

Monocyte contamination of lymphocyte preparations may represent another serious problem, since monocytes may account for as much as 40 per cent of the mononuclear cells isolated from the peripheral blood using Ficoll-Hypaque technique (Zucker-Franklin, 1974). These cells are especially significant, since they carry certain surface receptors also seen on B cells. Thus, a quantitative assay (e.g., for C3 receptors) could result in an overestimation of the B-cell population if significant contamination with monocytes is present. Monocytes can be easily distinguished from lymphocytes on morphologic or histochemical grounds by their ability to phagocytize and the high concentrations of hydrolytic enzymes in monocytes. However, identification of these cells may be more difficult in the disease state.

Techniques for Separation of Monocytes from Lymphocytes.   The first of these methods depends on phagocytic properties of monocytes. The cell preparation containing lymphocytes and contami-

ISOLATION OF MONONUCLEAR CELLS
ON FICOLL-HYPAQUE GRADIENTS

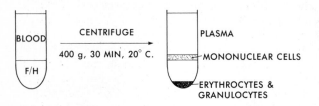

Figure 39–8. Blood collected in preservative-free heparin is layered on Ficoll-Hypaque. After centrifugation, the mononuclear cells appear as a discrete layer.

nating monocytes is incubated at 37°C. with iron particles coated with poly-L-lysine or with uniformly sized (0.8 μm in diameter) latex particles coated with IgG for a period of time sufficient for phagocytosis (30 to 60 min). The monocytes are then separated from the lymphocytes either by centrifugation or by the passage of cells over a strong magnet.

The second method depends on the adherence of monocytes to glass surfaces. It is best done before gradient centrifugation using leukocyte-rich plasma or whole peripheral blood. A suitable adherent surface may be provided by Petri dishes, glass slides, or a flask with a flat surface. The cell preparation containing lymphocytes and contaminating monocytes is incubated in a Petri dish or glass flask (flat-bottom) for 45 to 60 minutes at 37°C. The addition of human or fetal calf serum aids in monocyte adherence. Non-adherent cells (lymphocytes) are gently washed away from the glass surfaces. To isolate monocytes, cells adhering to glass or plastic surfaces are teased off with a rubber policeman. The removal of adherent cells may be facilitated by prior incubation in the cold with 5 mM EDTA. These methods yield lymphocyte preparations of high purity (90+ per cent) but have a disadvantage of large lymphocyte losses (up to 50 to 60 per cent) with reference to the starting material. Losses of lymphocytes are greatest in the methods relying on phagocytosis and are due to non-specific adherence of the foreign particles to the surfaces of lymphocytes. The purification method based on adherence of monocytes to glass surfaces causes less non-specific loss of lymphocytes but is cumbersome when large volumes of cells are to be processed.

The one general method of correcting for contamination of suspensions or tissues with monocytes depends on enumeration of monocytes using histochemical procedures (i.e., peroxidase stain) (Zucker-Franklin, 1974). The other corrective method depends on conventional light microscopy but can be done with greater certainty when various monocyte markers are provided to aid the morphologist. In general, this can be done by permitting monocytes to phagocytize particles, such as latex, carbonyl iron, or antibody IgG-coated red blood cells, before doing differential counts. Errors

may occur due to non-specific attachment rather than to adsorption of latex particles or iron to the surfaces of lymphocytes. Antibody-coated red blood cells are better than latex for this purpose, since extracellular red blood cells may be eliminated by osmotic lysis before the differential counts are done.

Enumeration of Lymphocytes. The presence of cell surface markers has provided the basis for enumerating subpopulations of lymphocytes. In applying the techniques based on these characteristics to the quantitations of lymphocytes and in interpreting the results so achieved, it is necessary to understand that the expression of surface markers is subject to continual changes, as it depends on metabolic activities of the cells. Therefore, these techniques are not fool-proof and, in fact, much variability may be seen among different laboratories engaged in lymphocyte quantitations using the same protocols. These methods are new and have, perhaps, made a premature transition from the research to the clinical laboratory.

The markers used to detect B cells are surface immunoglobulins, receptors for Fc portions of IgG, and receptors for activated third component of complement. The methodology for each of these assays is currently subject to considerable refinement, so that it is difficult to select one general method applicable to all laboratories and all clinical situations. With this in mind, the methods outlined below will include brief descriptions of those assays that are most reliable and most widely used. However, we wish to stress that even these may be subject to some uncertainty.

DETECTION OF SURFACE IMMUNOGLOBULINS. The principle of this method is based on quantitative detection of immunoglobulins, represented on the cell surface of B cells other than mature plasma cells, using antisera specific for the heavy chain or the light chain classes of human immunoglobulins. Quantitation is possible by labeling the antisera with compounds such as fluorescein or rhodamine

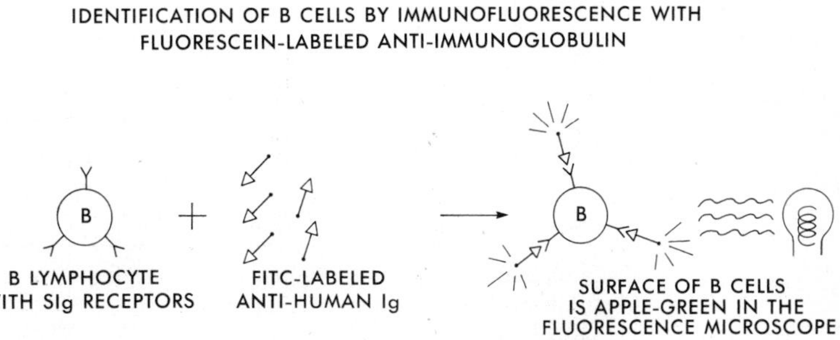

IDENTIFICATION OF B CELLS BY IMMUNOFLUORESCENCE WITH
FLUORESCEIN-LABELED ANTI-IMMUNOGLOBULIN

Figure 39-9. Appropriately labeled antibodies to human immunoglobulins can react with surfaces of B lymphocytes and are then detected by fluorescence.

B LYMPHOCYTE
WITH SIg RECEPTORS

FITC-LABELED
ANTI-HUMAN Ig

SURFACE OF B CELLS
IS APPLE-GREEN IN THE
FLUORESCENCE MICROSCOPE

and counting positively stained lymphocytes (Fig. 39-9). Clearly, it is necessary that the antisera be highly specific and that they be adequately fluoresceinated. When commerical reagents are used, it is essential that the specificity of antisera be checked against reliable standards, as described on page 1200 in Chapter 35. Such standards include myeloma cells or beads to which are coupled established myeloma proteins. Specificity then can be ascertained by agglutination of erythrocytes coated with the immunoglobulin, staining of coated beads, or inhibition of staining of lymphocyte surfaces (Aiuti, 1974). Precautions must be taken to wash the cells adequately so as to remove serum components adsorbed to their cell surfaces by virtue of the Fc receptors. Several methods have been proposed to determine cells which truly synthesize surface Ig and, therefore, by definition are B cells. Cells may be incubated overnight after controlled trypsinization of the cell to remove all surface immunoglobulins without injury to the cell. The cells are allowed to incubate in serum-free medium for periods of 6 to 24 hours to permit resynthesis of surface immunoglobulins (Rowlands, 1974; Lobo, 1975).

Immunofluorescent assay involves incubation of washed and/or trypsinized lymphocytes with fluoresceinated monospecific antisera at 4°C. for 30 minutes (sodium azide may aid in preventing capping). A fluorescence microscope (preferably with epi-illumination) is necessary for enumeration of the stained lymphocytes. It is recommended that monospecific antibodies to the various heavy and light chains rather than a polyvalent serum be used for quantitations. This allows for enumerations of B cells bearing different immunoglobulin classes and of lambda- and kappa-positive cells. Since the proportions of cells expressing different immunoglobulins may deviate from normal in disease

(Table 39-3), such enumerations may be clinically important. It has been suggested that the fluoresceinated F(ab')$_2$ fragments of monospecific antisera be used to avoid binding of these reagents to B cells through the Fc portions of their heavy chains (Winchester, 1975). This precaution seems to be particularly necessary when cells obtained from neoplasms are evaluated. All antisera used for enumerations of B cells must be checked for monospecificity by the established immunologic procedures and must be centrifuged (100,000 g) immediately prior to staining to remove aggregates that may have high binding affinity for the Fc receptors. Table 39-3 shows the distribution of normal immunoglobulin-bearing (SIg$^+$) cells in human blood and selected lymphoid tissues.

It should be noted that there is considerable variation in the literature with regard to the relative proportion of SIg$^+$ cells detected in the human peripheral blood (range 10 to 20 per cent or more). The decreasing proportion of SIg$^+$ cells reported in recent years undoubtedly reflects the increasing specificity of commercially available antisera and measures aimed at eliminating exogenous Ig. It is essential that individual laboratories establish their own lymphocyte panels to serve as normal controls. When peripheral blood lymphocytes are studied with regard to SIg, each of the major immunoglobulin classes can be identified on these cells. However, the dominant classes of immunoglobulins are likely to be IgM and IgD, and the normal ratio of $\kappa +/\lambda +$ cells is 2/1. In disease states, these proportions may change (Table 39-3).

DETECTION OF Fc RECEPTORS. The receptors for Fc portions of immunoglobulins can be detected using immunomicroscopy or rosetting techniques. The former is an exact duplicate of the method outlined above, except that labeled aggregated human IgG is used in place of anti-immunoglobu-

Table 39-3. DISTRIBUTION OF SURFACE MARKERS ON LYMPHOCYTES ISOLATED FROM NORMAL CONTROLS AND PATIENTS WITH LYMPHOPROLIFERATIVE DISEASES*

SURFACE MARKER	NORMAL BLOOD	NORMAL LYMPH NODE	CHRONIC LYMPHOCYTIC LEUKEMIA (CLL)	MALIGNANT NODE (PDLL-N)
IgG	3	12	2	54
A	2	8	1	4
M	12	16	80	60
D	10	14	75	10
K	8	20	83	63
L	5	11	1	2
E	68	70	10	34
EAC	25	30	30	50
EA	14	16	12	4

*Data from representative cases. Monocytes were not removed from the peripheral blood. Figures are expressed as per cent of positive cells.
PDLL-N = Poorly differentiated lymphocytic lymphoma—nodular type.

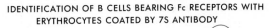

IDENTIFICATION OF B CELLS BEARING Fc RECEPTORS WITH
ERYTHROCYTES COATED BY 7S ANTIBODY

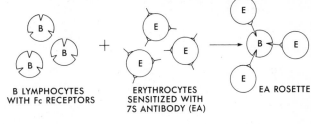

B LYMPHOCYTES
WITH Fc RECEPTORS

ERYTHROCYTES
SENSITIZED WITH
7S ANTIBODY (EA)

EA ROSETTE

Figure 39–10. B cells when mixed with anti-body-coated erythrocytes form rosettes.

lin. There are several rosetting techniques available for detection of Fc receptors, all based on the principle that antibodies of the IgG class, when placed on the surface of an erythrocyte, present their altered Fc portions to those cells that carry appropriate receptors. These cells bind to the antibody-coated erythrocytes (Fig. 39-10), forming easily recognizable rosettes. The number of EA rosettes formed by lymphoid cells depends on many factors, such as purity of the antibody used to coat the erythrocytes. The spatial orientation and concentration of Fc receptors for IgG vary among lymphoid cells. For example, a subpopulation of lymphocytes (L cells) with Fc receptors that are resistant to digestion with trypsin and that have a high affinity for altered Ig has been identified in the human peripheral blood (Fig. 39-11). These cells (L) apparently do not synthesize immunoglobulin, do not have a receptor for an E rosette, and do not bear the characteristics of phagocytic cells (e.g., adherence, phagocytosis). The precise functional role of these cells remains to be determined (Lobo, 1976). It is, however, important to consider that such cells may interfere with or give spuriously high values for SIg-positive cells unless certain precautions are taken to allow exogenous Ig to be

removed from the membrane (e.g., either by an incubation in the absence of autologous serum or trypsinization as described above).

DETECTION OF COMPLEMENT RECEPTORS. Complement receptors are detectable on many different cell types, including lymphocytes and monocytes. Those on B cells may be of at least two types. One recognizes the C3d and the other the C3b fragment of C3. A rosetting method employing sheep erythrocytes sensitized with anti-SRBC subagglutinating antibody sensitized with components of complement (EAC) is used for detection of cells bearing receptors for C3 (Fig. 39-12).

Two systems have been used to determine the complement receptor on B lymphocytes (Ross, 1973). In the first method, mouse complement is used. This has the advantage of detecting both C3d and C3b on neoplastic cells. An alternative technique is similar to that described for EAC mouse, except human complement is used and multiple incubation steps are required for the preparation of indicator cells. This is accomplished by incubating sheep red blood cells first with subagglutinating concentrations of anti-SRBC serum followed by incubation with purified human C1, C4, C2, and C3 in that order.

A FLOW DIAGRAM OF A SEPARATION PROCEDURE BASED ON CELL
SURFACE PROPERTIES FOR HUMAN PERIPHERAL BLOOD LYMPHOCYTES

Figure 39–11. The diagram represents the ways in which cell surface properties may be used to separate and categorize subsets of human B and T lymphocytes.

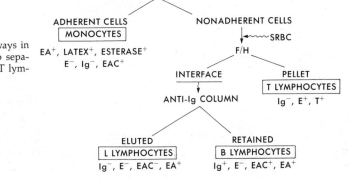

F/H PURIFIED LYMPHOCYTES

ADHERENT CELLS
MONOCYTES
EA$^+$, LATEX$^+$, ESTERASE$^+$
E$^-$, Ig$^-$, EAC$^+$

NONADHERENT CELLS
SRBC
F/H

INTERFACE
ANTI-Ig COLUMN

PELLET
T LYMPHOCYTES
Ig$^-$, E$^+$, T$^+$

ELUTED
L LYMPHOCYTES
Ig$^-$, E$^-$, EAC$^-$, EA$^+$

RETAINED
B LYMPHOCYTES
Ig$^+$, E$^-$, EAC$^+$, EA$^+$

IDENTIFICATION OF B CELLS BEARING RECEPTORS FOR C3 WITH
EAC INDICATOR CELLS

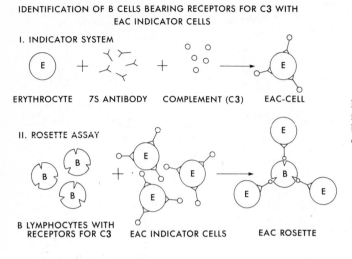

Figure 39–12. B cells can be detected by rosette formation using sheep erythrocytes which have been treated with appropriate antibody and complement.

The mean value for EAC-positive lymphocytes in the circulation of healthy adults is 15 per cent (range of 10 to 19 per cent), but this figure varies among laboratories, and it is essential for each to establish its own normal mean and range.

Certain general requirements apply to this and other rosetting techniques. Thus, a lymphocyte reacting with three or more indicator cells forms a rosette; at least 200 lymphocytes must be counted to determine a proportion of rosetting cells; since cells other than lymphocytes have C3 or Fc receptors, lymphocytes must be purified prior to rosetting; trypsinization of SRBC prior to sensitization is recommended to avoid errors due to spontaneous rosette formation; a subagglutinating dose must be determined for each batch of antierythrocyte serum; controls with E and EA coated with 7S and 19S antibody are required. The foregoing serves to emphasize that rosetting techniques, although simple in principle, are technically demanding and time-consuming.

ENUMERATION OF T CELLS. Human T-lymphocytes are capable of forming spontaneous rosettes with unmodified sheep erythrocytes (E). The T rosette assay is simple and thus accessible to all clinical laboratories. It calls for washed lymphocytes and washed SRBC (E) in a 1 per cent suspension to be mixed and centrifuged briefly (Fig. 39–13). The critical factor in the optimal determination of T-lymphocytes using unsensitized sheep erythrocytes is the ratio of sheep cells to lymphocytes. It has been recommended that a ratio of 50 to 100 to one yields optimal results (Aiuti, 1974). The tube is then placed in a refrigerator (4°C.) for at least 16 hours. Resuspended cells are then counted in a hemocytometer, and the proportion of rosetting cells is determined by microscopy.

This rosetting technique may be affected by many factors and is reproducible only if performed under carefully controlled conditions. The percentages of E rosettes in normal human peripheral blood generally range from 60 to 80 per cent, depending on the laboratory. Normal controls must always be included. A variety of modifications that have been described undoubtedly measure different subpopulations of T-lymphocytes. The best known modification consists of mixing SRBC with the lymphocytes only for a brief period during centrifugation and measures "active E rosettes." The latter are formed by a subpopulation of T cells, which have "high affinity" receptors for SRBC and which may be altered in number or in their capability to rosette with SRBC in disease states. Thus, both the determination of total T rosettes (long-term incubation at 4°C.) and active T rosettes (brief incubation) may be clinically significant. Approximately 25 per cent of human blood lymphocytes form active rosettes. It has been suggested that the active T rosettes are more sensitive in detecting defects in T cell function than total T cells (e.g., overnight incubation at 4°C.).

Little is known about the nature of the T-rosette phenomenon. Recent experiments indicate that the binding of SRBC to human T cells represents a

IDENTIFICATION OF T CELLS WITH
UNTREATED SHEEP ERYTHROCYTES

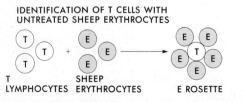

Figure 39–13. Human T cells can be detected by rosette formation using untreated sheep erythrocytes.

receptor-ligand interaction rather than a non-specific electrical charge event. The receptor for SRBC appears to be a protein which can be isolated by controlled enzymatic proteolysis from the surfaces of T- but not B-lymphocytes.

A second method for enumeration of T cells depends on the availability of specific anti-human T-cell sera. T-cell antisera have been made by injecting experimental animals with human thymocytes, human brain (in rodents, T-lymphocytes bear the theta antigen which is also present in the brain), and/or peripheral T-lymphocytes purified by various techniques from blood or lymphoid tissues (Whiteside, 1976). These antisera generally have many specificities directed to cells other than T-lymphocytes and must be rigorously and extensively absorbed with human erythrocytes, human serum components, human tissues, and finally human B cells. The specificity of absorbed anti-human T cell sera for T-lymphocytes must then be demonstrated by immunologic procedures. With certain of the antisera, complement-dependent lysis of lymphocytes might be used to determine the relative proportion of T cells in a given preparation of cells. To date, reliable anti-human T cell serum is not available for routine diagnostic use. In addition, the relationships between the T-lymphocyte populations identified by the E rosetting method versus immunofluorescence with the anti-T cell sera are not established. It seems likely that each method identifies populations of T cells that probably overlap but are not identical. Human T cells may also be identified by histochemical techniques (see Chap. 30).

DETERMINATION OF Ia ANTIGENS.   Detailed analysis of the major histocompatibility locus in mice shows a distinct and now well-defined association with Ia (immune-associated) antigens. That a similar association will be defined in man seems certain. The alloantisera that are used for detection and definition of the human Ia antigens are being defined in several laboratories. Ia antigens are expressed on B cells and on certain other non-lymphoid cells, namely, monocytes and endothelial cells. As an analogue of the mouse system, it is

likely that human Ia antigens are associated with Fc receptors for aggregated IgG which appear on B-lymphocytes.

Determination of Lymphocytes in Tissue Sections by Rosetting Techniques.   Indicator cells (E, EA, and EAC) prepared for the enumeration of lymphocytes in suspensions may be used for their identification in cryostat sections. Figure 39-14 illustrates the rosetting technique in sections. It should be performed only on freshly embedded tissues or tissues stored in liquid nitrogen. For T rosettes in sections, erythrocytes treated with a sulfhydryl reagent, 2 amino-ethylisothiuronium bromide (AET), should be used in order to stabilize lymphocyte-E binding. Further, caution is advised while performing E rosettes, because the E receptor seems to be labile and the rosetting conditions must be carefully controlled. Rosetting in sections allows for studies of the distribution of T cells, B cells, and macrophages in normal and pathologic tissues and the identification of effector cells in cellular infiltrates, and offers possibilities for the combination of cytochemical and immunologic procedures.

The methods for enumerations of T- and B-lymphocytes that we chose to present here can, at this time, be applied in a clinical laboratory with a fair degree of success. It is essential to bear in mind, however, that there is much we do not understand about surface properties of lymphocytes, that there may be overlaps in surface markers between T- and B-lymphocytes or lymphocytes and other mononuclear cells, and that a judicious interpretation of results requires proper controls, must be performed in the light of clinical facts, and calls for a highly trained and experienced interpreter.

Methods for Separation of Lymphocyte Populations.   Nearly all of the techniques described so far can be applied to separations and isolations of individual subpopulations of lymphocytes. For example, using rosetting and Ficoll-Hypaque gradients, E-positive lymphocytes can be centrifuged and recovered in a pellet, leaving the non-E rosetting population at the gradient interface. This latter population can, in turn, be rosetted with EA

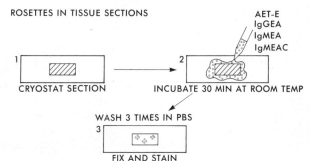

Figure 39-14. Cryostat tissue sections when incubated with various erythrocyte preparations show rosette formation.

Table 39-4. METHODS FOR SEPARATION OF HUMAN
LYMPHOCYTE SUBPOPULATIONS ON THE BASIS OF CELL
SURFACE PROPERTIES

METHOD OF SEPARATION	WAY OF RECOVERY	LYMPHOCYTE SUBPOPULATION
I. Rosetting followed by gradient centrifugation*	In the pellet	E
		EA
		EAC
	In the interface	Unrosetted cells
II. Immunoadsorbent column charged with		
(a) anti-Ig	Retained	SIg$^+$
	Eluted	SIg$^-$
(b) anti-T cell	Retained	T cells
	Eluted	B, L, null cells
III. Adherence to glass, nylon, wool, etc.	Adherent	B cells
	Non-adherent	T and L cells
IV. Cytotoxicity with anti-lymphocyte sera:		
(a) anti-B cell	Not killed	T, null, L cells
(b) anti-T cell	Not killed	B, null, L cells
(c) anti-null cell	Not killed	T, B, L cells

*The unrosetted cells from the interface of Ficoll-Hypaque gradients can be rosetted again and separated further on another gradient.

or EAC indicator cells, so that EA- or EAC-positive lymphoid cells, respectively, are recovered following the second gradient centrifugation. Other techniques frequently utilize differential adherence of lymphocytes to various solid surfaces or to appropriately charged columns as well as cytotoxic potentials of selective antilymphocyte sera in the presence of complement. Table 39-4 lists those separation techniques that have been most widely used in recent years. It is essential to monitor cells undergoing separation procedures for their surface characteristics in order to quantitate the recovered subpopulations and estimate their purity. Figure 39-11 further illustrates how surface properties of lymphocytes may be used for the separation of different lymphocyte subpopulations.

MEASUREMENT OF FUNCTIONAL CAPACITIES OF LYMPHOCYTES

Functional properties of lymphocytes, such as *in vitro* responsiveness to mitogens, soluble antigens, allogeneic cells, and abilities to produce immunoglobulins or lymphokines and to effect cell-mediated or antibody-dependent cytotoxicity may be used for identification and, to a certain extent, for quantitative purposes. Some of these *in vitro* assays require sophisticated equipment and, thus, are not accessible to a majority of clinical laboratories.

Still, these assays are necessary for an accurate appraisal of the immune status in man, because it is the functional competence of lymphocytes, not their number, that ultimately determines immune responsiveness. We wish to emphasize, however, that the functional *in vitro* assays may not always reflect the *in vivo* situation at hand. For example, a normal *in vitro* response to an antigen (e.g., mumps) does not mean that the responsive lymphocytes are immunologically competent *in vivo*. Many factors in the body (serum components, cellular products, enzymes, inhibitors, hormones) may influence functional capabilities of lymphocytes. Until better correlations are established between various *in vitro* assays and *in vivo* responsiveness, their clinical significance must remain limited. None of the *in vitro* assays mentioned earlier can, at this time, be recommended as the best functional assay: we do not know whether lymphocytes secreting lymphokines or effecting cell-mediated cytotoxicity *in vitro* can do the same *in vivo* and how important these functions may be in any one biologic reaction mediated by lymphocytes *in vivo*. Functional properties of lymphocyte subpopulations isolated from normal peripheral blood by procedures similar to those in Figure 39-11 are listed in Table 39-5.

Table 39-5. FUNCTIONAL PROPERTIES OF THE LYMPHOCYTE SUBPOPULATIONS ISOLATED FROM HUMAN PERIPHERAL BLOOD

	POPULATION OF CELLS TESTED				
	T cells	B cells	L cells*	T + B	T + L
In Vitro Proliferation					
Mitogen					
PHA	+++	+	−	++++	++++
CON A	++	+	−	++++	++++
PWM	+	++	−	++++	+
MLC					
Stimulator	+	++++	+		
Responder	++++	+	−		
ANTIGENS	++	+	−	++++	++++
PWM-induced					
Ig synthesis	−	+	−	++++	−
Antibody-dependent					
cytotoxicity	−	+	++++		

*Some investigators designate these as K cells.

PHA = Phytohemagglutinin.
Con A = Concanavalin A.
PWM = Pokeweed mitogen.
MLC = Mixed lymphocyte culture.
+ = Degree of reaction.
− = No reaction.

4

Lymphocyte Proliferation. Responses to soluble plant lectins—in particular phytohemagglutinin (PHA) and Concanavalin A (Con A)—are thought to measure a functional potential of human T cells and have been widely used. These mitogens can be particularly useful probes of T cell function, since T cells which respond to antigens may represent less than 1 per cent of the T cells employed in the *in vitro* culture, whereas as many as 50 to 60 per cent of the T cells will respond to PHA and Con A. Furthermore, a number of *in vitro* studies have established that mitogen responsiveness is fundamentally similar to antigen responses and may be used as a model of antigen stimulation (Greaves, 1972).

The principle of mitogenic stimulations is illustrated in Figure 39-15. The stimulation index gives a semi-quantitative measure of the response. Normal controls must be run simultaneously with a patient's lymphocytes. It is necessary to stimulate

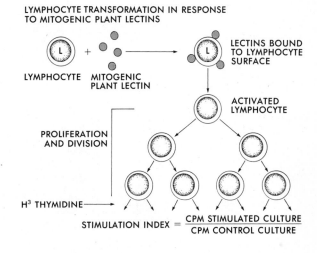

Figure 39-15. Lymphocytes may be stimulated into proliferation by antigens, allogeneic lymphocytes, or non-specific lectins. The response to allogeneic lymphocytes is called the mixed lymphocyte culture (MLC).

LYMPHOCYTE TRANSFORMATION IN RESPONSE TO MITOGENIC PLANT LECTINS

LYMPHOCYTE   MITOGENIC PLANT LECTIN

LECTINS BOUND TO LYMPHOCYTE SURFACE

ACTIVATED LYMPHOCYTE

PROLIFERATION AND DIVISION

H³ THYMIDINE

$$\text{STIMULATION INDEX} = \frac{\text{CPM STIMULATED CULTURE}}{\text{CPM CONTROL CULTURE}}$$

lymphocytes at several different PHA concentrations, because the optimal response is often concentration-dependent. Three- and seven-day incubations are necessary because normal cells respond optimally on day 3, while the peak response of a patient's cells may be delayed. Extreme care must be taken in evaluating these responses to avoid misinterpretation of dilutional effects. For example, when cells from patients with CLL were stimulated with PHA, delayed responses were observed and thought to be caused by defective T cells in these patients. However, when the technique was modified to measure the numbers of cells going into mitosis as a function of time by adding colchicine at the start of the culture and H³ thymidine two hours before its termination, it appeared that the T cells from CLL patients were functionally normal. Thus, the poor proliferative response to T cell mitogens in patients with CLL appears to be due to a reduction in the number of responsive T cells and concomitant increase in neoplastic B cells (Rowlands, 1974).

The example of PHA stimulation illustrates the difficulties inherent in all assays of functional properties of lymphocytes, interpretation being the key. To complicate matters, it now appears that certain B cells, in addition to subpopulations of T cells, are responsive to PHA and Con A. It is noteworthy, however, that when lymphocyte responses are measured at their peak, for example, at three or four days, the responding lymphocytes are almost entirely T cells (Greaves, 1972). Significant B cell

proliferation appears to occur later in the proliferative response, sometime between five and seven days. Con A probably stimulates a different subpopulation of T-lymphocytes than does PHA, and pokeweed mitogen (PWM), formerly considered primarily a B-cell mitogen, activates both T and B cells. Human lymphocytes do not proliferate in response to endotoxin or antihuman Fab. It is now held that T-lymphocytes are primarily responsible for specific antigen-mediated proliferations. Fractionations of lymphocytes and removal of different lymphocytic and monocytic subpopulations seem to affect *in vitro* responses to mitogens and/or antigens, and contributions of the different fractions to full-scale *in vitro* responses are now being evaluated. For example, optimal responses to both mitogens and antigens may require the presence of monocytes or factors produced by monocytes.

Allogeneic stimulation, also known as mixed lymphocyte culture (MLC), has been widely employed in clinical laboratories in histocompatibility testing preceding transplantations (Chap. 41). If lymphocytes from two individuals differ at the genetically determined D locus, they will stimulate each other into proliferation under optimal culture conditions. By preventing one set of lymphocytes from division (irradiation or mitomycin C), it may be determined whether they act as stimulators or responders in this system. When the kidney recipient's lymphocytes respond by proliferation to the donor's lymphocytes, chronic rejection of the kidney graft may be anticipated. In contrast, in bone

CELL-MEDIATED CYTOLYSIS IN WHICH SPECIFICALLY IMMUNIZED CYTOTOXIC T LYMPHOCYTES (CTL) INTERACT DIRECTLY WITH TARGET CELLS. THE QUANTITATIVE ASSAY MEASURES ⁵¹Cr RELEASE FROM ⁵¹Cr-LABELED TARGET CELLS FOLLOWING THE INCUBATION OF TARGET CELLS WITH THE APPROPRIATE NUMBER OF CTL'S. ONE CTL MAY KILL MORE THAN ONE TARGET CELL.

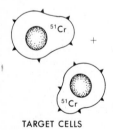
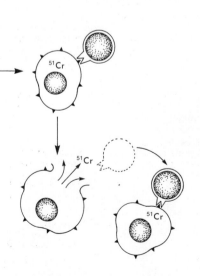

Figure 39-16. Cell-mediated cytolysis is produced when cytotoxic T cells interact with appropriate target cells. Cytotoxicity is evidenced by release of ⁵¹Cr from labeled target cells.

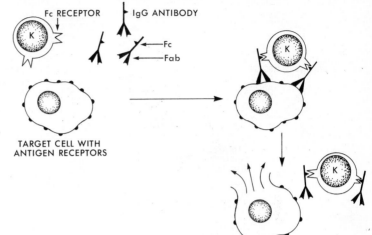

ANTIBODY-DEPENDENT CYTOLYSIS. INTERACTION BETWEEN THE K CELL AND
TARGET CELL IS MEDIATED BY THE IgG ANTIBODY WITH SPECIFICITY DIRECTED
TO AN ANTIGEN ON THE TARGET CELL SURFACE. K CELL HAS HIGH-AFFINITY
RECEPTORS FOR THE Fc PORTIONS OF IgG BOUND TO THE TARGET CELL.

Figure 39-17. Antibody-dependent cytolysis results when a K cell having high affinity receptors for Fc portions of Ig bind to target cells through associated IgG antibodies.

marrow transplantations, where graft versus host rejections are the danger, proliferation of the donor's lymphocytes in response to the recipient's indicates a poor prognosis. The lack of response in MLC indicates compatibility at the D locus.

Cytotoxicity. Cytotoxicity assays measure the capabilities of lymphocytes to kill target cells in the reactions not involving complement. Three types of lymphocytotoxicity are recognized: (a) cell-mediated lympholysis (CML), in which cytotoxic, specifically sensitized T-lymphocytes may be shown to release radioactive chromium from the labeled target tissue (Cerottini, 1974). CML is an energy-dependent process which requires direct contact between a target cell and cytotoxic T-lymphocytes (Fig. 39-16); (b) antibody-dependent lympholysis which is mediated by SIg$^-$ cells with high-avidity Fc receptors called K (killer) cells (Cerottini, 1974; Perlmann, 1975). The K cell recognizes and reacts with antibody coating the target cell, so that the specificity of this cytotoxic reaction is determined by the anti-target antibody (Fig. 39-17); (c) cytotoxicity mediated not by cells but by cellular products of these cells. A variety of such products are known to be released by activated lymphocytes, and they are collectively labeled as lymphocytotoxins because of their injurious effects on cells. The biologic importance of these three cytotoxic reactions is not clear, although there is some evidence that CML may play a particularly significant role in allogeneic transplant systems and in viral infections. The presence of naturally occurring cytotoxic cells has been recently correlated with defense against syngeneic tumors in the mouse. The existence of such cells in humans is not established.

Lymphocyte Products. Lymphocytes activated by mitogens or antigens release a variety of substances (Table 39-6), some of which are antigen-specific. Although antibody synthesis in response to antigens can be easily measured in experimental animal systems using plaque assays, these are not suitable for human use. Quantitative *in vitro* assay for synthesis of immunoglobulins by isolated human lymphocytes has recently been developed (Choi, 1977). Human B and T cells are cultured in a medium containing labeled amino acids and the stimulatory concentration of PWM. The B cells which differentiate into immunoglobulin-synthesizing plasma cells can be estimated morphologically and/or labeled immunoglobulins in the culture

Table 39-6. A PARTIAL LISTING OF SOLUBLE FACTORS RELEASED BY ACTIVATED LYMPHOCYTES

MIF	Macrophage Inhibition Factor
MAF	Macrophage Activating Factor
MCF	Macrophage Chemotactic Factor
BF	Blastogenic Factor
TF	Transfer Factor
PF	Permeability Factor
ECF	Eosinophil Chemotactic Factor
LTF	Lymphocytotoxic Factor
NCF	Neutrophil Chemotactic Factor
LIF	Leukocyte Inhibition Factor
CIF	Cloning Inhibition Factor
I	Interferon
SRF	Skin Reactive Factor

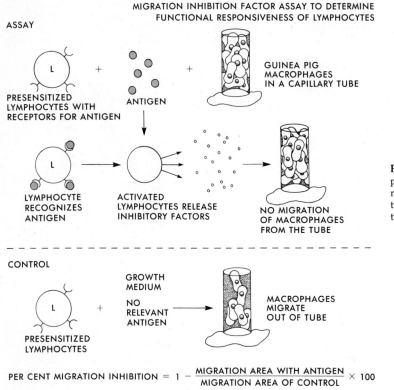

MIGRATION INHIBITION FACTOR ASSAY TO DETERMINE
FUNCTIONAL RESPONSIVENESS OF LYMPHOCYTES

ASSAY

PRESENSITIZED
LYMPHOCYTES WITH
RECEPTORS FOR ANTIGEN

ANTIGEN

GUINEA PIG
MACROPHAGES
IN A CAPILLARY TUBE

LYMPHOCYTE
RECOGNIZES
ANTIGEN

ACTIVATED
LYMPHOCYTES RELEASE
INHIBITORY FACTORS

NO MIGRATION
OF MACROPHAGES
FROM THE TUBE

CONTROL

PRESENSITIZED
LYMPHOCYTES

GROWTH
MEDIUM

NO
RELEVANT
ANTIGEN

MACROPHAGES
MIGRATE
OUT OF TUBE

$$\text{PER CENT MIGRATION INHIBITION} = 1 - \frac{\text{MIGRATION AREA WITH ANTIGEN}}{\text{MIGRATION AREA OF CONTROL}} \times 100$$

Figure 39-18. Interaction of appropriate antigen and lymphocytes causes release of MIF, which alters the migration of macrophages from a capillary tube.

supernatant can be quantitated. The T cells play a regulatory role in this system by either helping the B cells in carrying on Ig synthesis or, under certain conditions, suppressing this synthesis. It has been demonstrated that the defective T cells from patients with hypogammaglobulinemia suppress Ig synthesis by normal B cells in this *in vitro* system (Waldmann, 1974). The suppressor role of human T cells is currently being evaluated in relation to those human diseases that may have autoimmune or hyperimmune etiologies.

The production of lymphokines affords another way of estimating responsiveness of lymphocytes to external stimuli. As illustrated in Figure 39-18, only lymphocytes presensitized to an antigen are capable of elaborating the soluble factors when exposed to this antigen *in vitro*. Lymphokines are recognized by their effect on other cells, e.g., macrophages, whose migration they inhibit. The quantitative *in vitro* assay (migration inhibition factor (MIF) assay, Fig. 39-18) was developed to measure the release of certain lymphokines by lymphocytes isolated from the peripheral blood. The assay is laborious, technically demanding, and time consuming. As such, it does not lend itself to clinical situations, and various simplified versions, such as the leukocyte migration inhibition microdroplet technique, are used instead. Studies indicate that neither the MIF assay nor its modifications corre-

late with other *in vitro* assays of cell-mediated immunity, with *in vivo* skin tests, or with clinical observations. It has been established that B cells, as well as T cells, are capable of producing MIF after stimulation with antigens and mitogens (Rocklin, 1974).

Skin Tests. These assay the ability of the patient's lymphocytes to recognize and respond *in vivo* to an antigen. Unlike the *in vitro* procedures discussed earlier, intradermal skin tests offer an opportunity to determine a delayed hypersensitivity response in the presence of all inhibitory or stimulatory factors that are present in the body but not in a test tube. Delayed hypersensitivity skin tests are valuable in the overall assessment of immunocompetence. Inability of the skin to react to a battery of common antigens to which the subject could have expected to be exposed is termed *anergy*. Antigens included in such a battery may vary and should include at least five antigens, for example: PPD, candida, mumps, streptokinase-streptodornase, Trichophyton. A skin response to antigens to which lymphocytes in a healthy adult are likely to be sensitized must be distinguished from a response to new antigens such as DNCB (dinitrochlorobenzene). The former estimates immunologic memory; the latter is a measure of ability to mount an immune response following sensitization with a new antigen. Skin tests with DNCB appear to give a better estimate of immunocompetence than those with recall antigens. The DNCB skin test requires a local sensitization with the chemical which is followed 10 to 14 days later by a challenge dose applied to the skin surface.

Delayed hypersensitivity skin tests are read 24 to 48 hours following intradermal injection of the antigens. The diameter of an area of induration is an index of cutaneous hypersensitivity, and it must equal or exceed 5 mm for the test to be positive. Negative response to a preliminary (low) dose of an antigen should be always confirmed by testing with higher concentrations of the same antigen. Also, negative responses indicate anergy only if the patient's inflammatory response (which is a component of a delayed hypersensitivity reaction) is unimpaired. Rebuck's skin-window technique or local irritants, such as croton oil, may be used to assess a patient's inflammatory responses. Skin tests with recall antigens are of no value in establishing the diagnosis of defective cell-mediated immunity during the first year of life. Infants may fail to react because of lack of previous contact with a given antigen. Occasional patients may develop marked local reactions to skin tests. Topical corticosteroids may be used to relieve these local symptoms. Skin test results may or may not correspond to results of other *in vitro* functional assays. Skin tests are also discussed in Chapter 42, p. 1402.

There are many assays available today for enumeration and functional assessment of lymphocytes. Only some of these assays were discussed here. We wish to emphasize that there are many components to cell-mediated and humoral immunity. Because of poor correlations observed between various *in vitro* assays, *in vivo* skin tests, and clinical data, it may be that each test measures only one component or a limited number of components. Our ability to assess immunocompetence is thus limited. Our understanding of how the various components influence each other or are affected by other factors *in vivo* is also limited. Therefore, while enumerating lymphocytes or determining their functional responses in patients, it is necessary to remember these limitations and to use judgment in applying the obtained data to diagnostic or prognostic considerations. These assays and their uses are also discussed in Chapters 34 and 42.

APPLICATION OF IMMUNOLOGIC METHODS TO HUMAN DISEASES

It is apparent, even at this early stage, that immunologic techniques, such as those described, have contributed to an increased understanding of the role of the immune processes in human diseases. In some instances, these techniques have also provided a rationale for therapy. The effectiveness of immunologic methods in studying diseases can best be illustrated in three groups of diseases: immunodeficiency states, lymphoproliferative malignancies, and autoimmune phenomena.

Immunodeficiency Diseases. Although the first description of immunodeficiency was made only 25 years ago, present-day clinicians are able to recognize and diagnose a wide spectrum of syndromes having distinct clinical features, unique immunologic defects, and characteristic biochemical abnormalities. Further, corrective measures have become available for many of these diseases. It is through the study of immunodeficiencies in humans and in animals that the first glimpse of functional divisions within the lymphoid system was obtained. Today, immunodeficiencies are known to be a result of derangements in differentiation and functional diversification of T- and/or B-lymphocytes. These derangements or "blocks" in lymphoid cell differentiation may be genetically determined, induced by external factors, or secondary to a physiologic imbalance of the normally differentiated lymphoid system. Evaluation of patients with immunodeficiency is discussed in Chapter 42, p. 1396.

Lymphoproliferative Diseases. This group of diseases has been extensively studied by immunologic methods in recent years (Aiuti, 1974; Ross, 1973). In some instances these methods are an important diagnostic tool; in the majority of lymphoproliferative malignancies, they are helpful in characterization of malignant subpopulations and in shedding some light on their nature and derivation. For the purpose of this discussion, we have arbitrarily selected a few diseases which illustrate the usefulness of the procedures available to a clinician.

It is reasonable to think of lymphoproliferative diseases as representing monoclonal proliferations of lymphoid cells at one particular stage of normal differentiation. In this context, a tremendous heterogeneity in properties of lymphoid cells in different cases of the same disease can be conveniently explained in terms of errors at different stages of differentiation. Contributions of the neoplastic process itself and of the milieu in which the neoplastic differentiation occurs to this heterogeneity must not be overlooked. In the case of T-cell malignancies, the lack of knowledge regarding differentiation markers on T-lymphocytes makes a similar analysis difficult at present.

Multiple myeloma (MM), Waldenstrom's macroglobulinemia (WM), and heavy chain diseases are the three instances in which the contribution of immunologic techniques to diagnosis cannot be overemphasized. All three represent proliferations of cells in the B-cell lineage, with the plasmacytoid lymphocytes in WM being less differentiated than neoplastic plasma cells in MM. While the clinical features and histopathology of all three diseases are characteristic, serum protein electrophoresis, immunoelectrophoresis, and immunofluorescence studies of bone marrow biopsies are virtually diagnostic. Even a small number of plasma cells in the bone marrow biopsy indicates MM, if all contain the same homogenous protein demonstrated in the patient's serum.

In applying immunologic techniques to studies of leukemias and lymphomas, it is necessary to be aware of certain difficulties: (1) The performance of E rosette test requires special attention, since a minor technical modification may cause major variations in the results. The temperature, quantity of SRBC, incubation time, and addition of decomplemented and SRBC-adsorbed human serum may all alter the results. For example, there are leukemic ALL blasts that express the receptor for SRBC and form E rosettes at 37°C., while a majority of normal human T cells do not. (2) The detection of SIg on a lymphocyte does not mean that it synthesizes that SIg. A possibility of surface adherence by free Ig, aggregated Ig, or antigen-antibody complexes through the Fc receptors must be borne in mind. The adhering products may originate in the patient's serum (surfaces of leukemic blasts are generally "sticky") or may be introduced with the antisera used for immunofluorescence. Thus, a proof of synthesis (i.e., presence of intracellular Ig, ability to resynthesize the SIg after trypsin treatment) is necessary for interpretation of the immunofluorescence tests. (3) Applications of techniques used for normal circulating cells to neoplastic tissues must be done cautiously. There is always a possibility of a selective loss during purification procedures, as cellular characteristics of malignant mononuclear cells may be different from those of normal cells. Also, the presence of both normal and tumor cells requires careful morphologic controls when cell markers are studied to ascertain which cells express the marker. (4) Results of cell marker studies should be correlated to other diagnostic methods such as histology, clinical picture, and conventional and scanning electron microscopy. These points emphasize the necessity for a battery of immunologic tests, rather than any single one, when evaluating the neoplastic lymphoid cells.

When chronic lymphocytic leukemia (CLL) is studied by immunologic techniques, a majority of cases fall into a B-cell category because the membrane phenotype of these neoplastic cells is $SIg^+FcR^+C3R^+E^-$. The majority of the SIg^+ cells have monoclonal IgM on their surface, and this IgM is often associated with an IgD having the same light chain. The quantities of SIg^+ on CLL cells are low compared with normal cells. All SIg^+ CLL cells do not necessarily have the Fc receptors and C3 receptor. In fact, subgroups of CLL have been described with $SIg^+FcR^+C3R^-E^-$ and $SIg^+FcR^-C3R^+E^-$ cells. Also, a small proportion of CLL's have cells with the SIg FcR^+C3R^+E phenotype. To make things even more complicated, rare CLL cases appear to be T-cell neoplasms, because their neoplastic lymphocytes express E rosette marker rather than SIg. On the basis of the foregoing, it appears that chronic lymphocytic leukemia, although classified as a B-cell neoplasm, represents a mixed immunologic entity. The studies of *in vitro* behavior of these neoplastic cells support this conclusion.

Acute lymphocytic leukemias (ALL) appear to be as heterogeneous as chronic leukemias. The majority of ALLs (80 per cent) fall into the category of the "null"-cell diseases, with the membrane phenotype: $SIg^-FcR^-C3R^-E^-$. This does not imply that these neoplastic cells are devoid of all immunologic markers. In fact, various leukemia-associated antigens as well as Ia-like antigens may be detected on these cells with appropriate immunologic reagents. The second group of patients with ALL (20 per cent) have what appears to be a T-cell malignancy, and the cellular phenotype is $SIg^-FcR^-C3R^-E^+$. Also, a small proportion of ALL cases have been described with neoplastic cells of the B-cell type (SIg^+). These studies of surface markers on ALL cells show that ALL is a heterogeneous disease with at least three subtypes. Correlations between immunologically defined subgroups and prognosis have been conflicting. Markers characteristic for both T- and B-lymphocytes are occasionally seen on the cells of patients with lymphocytic leukemias. The immunologic analysis of leukemias indicates that our present attempts at classification of these and other lymphoid neoplasms must await further antigenic, biochemical, and immunogenetic studies. The most important task now is to correlate the available immunologic findings to cytology, morphologic data, and clinical as well as prognostic observations in hope of focusing on effective therapeutic means for these diseases.

Among the non-Hodgkin's lymphomas, Sezary's syndrome has received considerable attention recently. It is a T-cell cutaneous lymphoma characterized by progressive infiltrations of skin, lymphoid tissues, and visceral organs by malignant lymphocytes exhibiting surface characteristics of T cells: the absence of SIg, complement, and Fc receptors and the ability to form E rosettes. *In vitro* studies of isolated Sezary's cells show them to be defective in proliferative responses to plant mitogens or in mixed lymphocyte culture as well as in killing of target cells in the cytotoxicity assays. These cells spontaneously release a lymphokine resembling MIF, so that some patients may have detectable circulating levels of this factor. Recently, using the *in vitro* system for studies of Ig synthesis in the presence of PWM, it was possible to show that the T-lymphocytes from these patients fail to regulate *in vitro* synthesis of Ig in a normal manner. Isolated Sezary's cells continued exercising helper activity even at such high lymphocyte concentrations as are suppressive in normal controls. This led to a theory that Sezary's syndrome represents a malignant proliferation of helper cells. Presumably, these abnormal helper cells are also responsible for excessive lymphokine production.

Cutaneous T-cell lymphomas may at times be difficult to differentiate from non-malignant exfoliative erythrodermas and other skin diseases. The application of the rosetting and immunofluorescence techniques to cryostat sections may be helpful in the positive identification of malignant T cells in cutaneous lymphoid infiltrates.

There is little doubt that application of immunologic techniques to studies of lymphoproliferative diseases, as in immunodeficiencies, has been most successful in identifying and partially characterizing abnormal lymphoid populations. We have tried to show the reader how such identification can be achieved and interpreted. It is also obvious that there are many uncertainties as to the clinical significance of such analyses. On the positive side is the fact that immunologic characteristics of neoplastic lymphocytes may be indicative of prognosis. In ALL, the 80 per cent or so of patients with "null" cell disease have a much better prognosis and response to chemotherapy than the 20 per cent of patients with the T-cell leukemia who require more intensive therapy. Lymphoproliferative diseases are also discussed in Chapter 30.

Autoimmune Diseases. Immunologic evaluation of patients for autoimmune diseases begins with the search for the humoral or cellular immune component that is directed against the patients' own tissues. Traditionally, the demonstration of high titers of autoantibodies to the affected organ has been a hallmark and the diagnostic feature of autoimmune disease. High levels of antithyroid antibodies in Hashimoto's thyroiditis or of antierythrocyte antibodies in autoimmune hemolytic anemia (AIHA) illustrate the point. Both serologic and immunofluorescence techniques are available for the detection of autoantibodies. However, it has become apparent recently that autoantibodies to multiple organs are often detectable in patients with autoimmune diseases and that these autoantibodies may not be pathogenic. Thus, the presence of autoantibody does not necessarily mean that a relevant lesion exists. For example, in patients who recovered from an infection with *Mycoplasma pneumoniae*, cold agglutinins reactive with autologous red cells are detectable, but hemolytic anemia is only an infrequent complication. Healthy elderly individuals often have autoantibodies (rheumatoid factors, antinuclear antibodies) in the sera. Patients with chronic liver diseases often have antibodies to smooth muscle, mitochondria, and nuclear antigens. Antinuclear antibodies have been detected in patients treated with certain drugs who do not have any signs of SLE. Finally, healthy relatives of patients with SLE frequently produce antinuclear antibodies. This means that the presence of autoantibodies may be a result of infections, drugs, aging, or genetic susceptibility and is not a sufficient reason to diagnose autoimmune disease.

Many autoimmune disorders are now believed to be mediated by cellular immune mechanisms rather than humoral immunity. Several well-studied animal models, such as allergic encephalitis or the NZB/NZW mouse model, support this concept.

The *in vitro* techniques we discussed can now be applied to the evaluation of cell-mediated immunity in patients with autoimmune diseases. It may be expected that lymphocytes which become sensitized to autoantigens as a result of a traumatic event (e.g., infection or other tissue damage) are capable of inflicting an injury to the relevant tissue or organ. Indeed, such autosensitized lymphocytes have been demonstrated in patients with pernicious anemia, thyroiditis, diabetes mellitus, and others. For example, lymphocytes from patients with pernicious anemia respond *in vitro* to intrinsic factors, to other gastric antigens, or to both, as assessed by the release of MIF or by proliferation in culture. Lymphocyte transformation in response to thyroglobulin has been described in patients with thyroiditis. The leukocyte migration inhibition tests are generally positive when thyroid extracts or thyroid microsomes are used to stimulate cells from patients with Hashimoto's disease, primary myxedema, or thyrotoxicosis. Leukocytes from these patients were also reported to exercise a direct cytotoxic effect on thyroid cells in monolayer cultures. The leukocyte migration inhibition tests and lymphocyte transformation to pancreatic antigens appear to be positive in a majority of patients with diabetes mellitus. The presence of autosensitization of lymphocytes demonstrable *in vitro* in patients with autoimmune disorders implies their involvement in tissue-damaging processes, but it does not implicate them in the pathogenesis of the disease. It is not clear whether the autosensitization is secondary to the pathogenic event.

A characteristic feature of many autoimmune diseases is their well-documented association with malignancies and with immunodeficiencies: AIHA with chronic lymphocytic leukemia, Sjögren's syndrome with its numerous serologic abnormalities and its tendency toward malignant deterioration, and autoimmune polyendocrine deficiencies with immunoglobulin abnormalities provide well-known examples of this thesis. Also, every autoimmune disease is characterized by an association with *multiple autoantibodies*. Clinical observations show that all autoimmune diseases form *clusters* of related syndromes: polyendocrinopathies, sequential AIHA and immune thrombocytopenia, Hashimoto's thyroiditis together with Graves' disease, and others. These features indicate that a fundamental disturbance in the regulation of the immune response may be a basic abnormality in autoimmune diseases.

Through the use of immunologic methods, the nature of the abnormal immunoregulation in autoimmune individuals is beginning to be elucidated. It appears that a selective absence of one subpopulation of T-lymphocytes, the suppressor cells, may account for the spectrum of abnormalities listed above. This has been demonstrated in the New Zealand mouse model as well as in patients with SLE. In the latter, the selective loss of a suppressor T cell may be due to anti-T cell antibodies in the circulation. It is not known what leads to the loss or decrease in the suppressor T-cell population in other autoimmune diseases. In all, the result is deranged immune responsiveness to auto- as well as exogenous antigens. This view of autoimmune phenomena, brought about by recent developments in immunology, may fundamentally alter our treatment of this group of diseases. Immunosuppression, currently a standard therapeutic modality in autoimmune diseases, may have to be replaced by controlled and preferably selective immunostimulation with the hope of activating T-lymphocytes that are not doing their job. Autoimmunity is discussed further in Chapter 38.

REFERENCES

Aiuti, F., Cerottini, J. C., Coombs, R. R. A., Cooper, M., Dickler, H. B., Froland, S. S., Fudenberg, H. H., Graves, M. F., Grey, H. M., Kunkel, H. G., Natvig, J. B., Preud'homme, J. L., Rabellino, E., Ritts, R. E., Rowe, D. S., Seligman, M., Siegal, F. P., Stjernsward, J., Terry, W. D., and Wybran, J.: Identification, enumeration, and isolation of B and T lymphocytes from human peripheral blood. Scand. J. Immunol., *3*:521, 1974.

Bach, J. F., Dardenne, M., Goldstein, A., Guka, A., and White, A.: Appearance of T cell markers in bone marrow rosette forming cells after incubation with thymosin, a thymic hormone. Proc. Nat. Acad. Sci. (Wash.), *68*:2734, 1971.

Basten, A., and Mitchell, J.: The role of macrophages in T-cell-B-cell collaboration in antibody production. In Nelson, D. S. (ed.): Immunobiology of the Alveolar Macrophage. New York, Academic Press, 1976.

Benacerraf, B., and Katz, D.: The histocompatibility-linked immune response genes. Adv. Canc. Res., *21*:121, 1975.

Boyum, A.: Separation of blood leucocytes from blood and bone marrow: Introduction. Scand. J. Clin. Lab. Invest., *21* (Suppl. 97):77, 1968.

Boyum, A.: Separation of blood leucocytes, granulocytes and lymphocytes. Tissue Antigens, *4*:269, 1974.

Cantor, H., and Boyse, E. A.: Functional subclasses of T lymphocytes bearing different Ly antigens. II. Cooperation between subclasses of Ly cells in the generation of killer cell activity. J. Exp. Med., *141*:1390, 1975.

Cantor, H., and Weissman, I.: Development and function of subpopulations of thymocytes and T lymphocytes. Prog. Allergy, *20*:1, 1976.

Cerottini, J. C., Brunner, K. T.: Cell-mediated cytotoxicity, allograft rejection and tumor immunity. Adv. Immunol., *18*:67, 1974.

Chess, L., MacDermott, R. P., and Schlossman, S. F.: Immunologic functions of isolated human lymphocyte subpopulations. VI. Further characterization of the surface Ig negative, E rosette negative (null cell) subset. J. Immunol., *115*:483, 1975.

Choi, Y. S.: Serological precipitation method for studying biosynthesis and secretion of immunoglobulin by human peripheral blood lymphocytes. J. Immunol. Methods, *14*:37, 1977.

Claman, H. N., Chaperon, E. A., and Triplett, R. F.: Immunocompetence of transferred thymus-marrow cell combinations. J. Immunol., *97*:928, 1966.

Cooper, M. D., and Lawton, A. R.: The development of the immune system. Sci. Am., *231*:559, 1974.

Daniele, R. P., and Rowlands, D. T., Jr.: Lymphocyte subpopulations in sarcoidosis: Correlation with disease activity and duration. Ann. Intern. Med., *85*:593, 1976.

Ehlenberger, A. G., McWilliams, M., Phillips-Quagliata, J. M., Lamm, M. E., and Nussenzweig, V.: Immunoglobulin-bearing and complement-receptor lymphocytes constitute the same population in human peripheral blood. J. Clin. Invest., *57*:53, 1976.

Feldmann, M.: Antigen-specific T cell factors and their role in the regulation of T-B interaction. *In* Sercarz, E., Williamson, A. R., and Fox, C. F.: The Immune System: Genes, Receptors, Signals. New York, Academic Press, 1974, p. 497.

Gershon, R. H.: T cell control of antibody production. Contemp. Top. Immunobiol., *3*:1, 1974a.

Gershon, R. K.: T cell control of antibody production. *In* Cooper, M. D., and Warner, N. L.: Contemporary Topics in Immunobiology 3. New York, Plenum Publishing Corporation, 1974b.

Greaves, M., and Janossy, G.: Elicitation of selective T and B lymphocyte responses by cell surface ligands. Transplant. Rev., *11*:87, 1972a.

Greaves, M. F., and Bauninger, J.: Activation of T and B lymphocytes by insoluble phytomitogens. Nature [New Biol.], *235*:67, 1972b.

Gupta, S., and Good, R. A.: Subpopulations of human T lymphocytes. I. Effect of thymopoietin, corticosteroids, and irradiation. Cell. Immunol., *34*:10, 1977.

Jerne, N. K.: The immune system. Sci. Am., *229*:52, 1973.

Jondal, M., Wigzell, H., and Aiuti, F.: Human lymphocyte subpopulations: Classification according to surface markers and/or functional characteristics. Transplant. Rev., *16*:163, 1973.

Kelly, R. G.: Functional anatomy of lymph nodes. I. The paracortical cords. Int. Arch. Allergy Appl. Immunol., *48*:836, 1975.

Lobo, P. I., and Horwitz, D. A.: An appraisal of Fc receptors on human peripheral blood B and L lymphocytes. J. Immunol., *117*:939, 1976.

Lobo, P. I., Westervelt, F. B., and Horwitz, D. A.: Identification of two populations of immunoglobulin-bearing lymphocytes in man. J. Immunol., *114*:116, 1975.

Miller, J. F. A. P., and Mitchell, G. F.: Cell to cell interaction in the immune response. I. Hemolysin-forming cells in neonatally thymectomized mice reconstituted with thymus or thoracic duct lymphocyte. J. Exp. Med., *128*:801, 1968.

Moretta, L., Webb, S., Grossi, C., Lydyard, P. M., and Cooper, M. D.: Functional analysis of two human T-cell subpopulations: Help and suppression of B-cell responses by T cells bearing receptors for IgM or IgG. J. Exp. Med., *146*:184, 1977.

Nowell, P. C., Daniele, R. P., and Winger, L. A.: Kinetics of human lymphocyte proliferation: Proportion of cells responsive to phytohemagglutinin and correlation with E rosette formation. J. Reticuloendothel. Soc., *17*:47, 1975.

Perlmann, P., Perlmann, H., Larsson, A., and Wahlin, B.: Antibody-dependent cytolytic effector lymphocytes (K cells) in human blood. J. Reticuloendothel. Soc., *17*:241, 1975.

Raff, M. C., Megson, M., Owen, J. J. T., and Cooper, M. D.: Early production of intracellular IgM by B-lymphocyte precursors in mouse. Nature, *259*:224, 1978.

Rocklin, R. E., MacDermoth, R. P., Chess, L., Schlossman, S. F., and David, J. R.: Studies on mediator production by highly purified human T and B lymphocytes. J. Exp. Med., *140*:1303, 1974.

Ross, G. D., Rabellino, E. M., Polley, M. J., and Grey, H. M.: Combined studies of complement receptor and surface immunoglobulin-bearing cells and sheep erythrocyte rosette-forming cells in normal and leukemic human lymphocytes. J. Clin. Invest., *52*:377, 1973.

Rowe, D. S., Hug, K., Forni, L., and Pernis, B.: Immunoglobulin D as a lymphocyte receptor. J. Exp. Med., *138*:965, 1973.

Rowlands, D. T., Daniele, R. P., Nowell, P. C., and Wurzel, H. A.: Characterization of lymphocyte subpopulations in chronic lymphocytic leukemia. Cancer, *34*:1962, 1974.

Schlossman, S. F., Chess, L., Humphreys, R. E., and Strominger, J. L.: Distribution of Ia-like molecules on the surface of normal and leukemic human cells. Proc. Natl. Acad. Sci. U.S.A., *73*:1288, 1976.

Schreiber, G. F., and Unanue, E. R.: Membrane and cytoplasmic changes in B lymphocytes induced by ligand-surface immunoglobulin interaction. Adv. Immunol., *24*:37, 1976.

Singer, S. J.: Molecular biology of cellular membranes with applications to immunology. Adv. Immunol., *19*:1, 1974.

Sprent, J.: Recirculating lymphocytes. *In* Marchalonis, J. J. (ed.): The Lymphocyte: Structure and Function. New York, Marcel Dekker, 1977.

Unanue, E. R.: The regulatory role of macrophages in antigenic stimulation. Adv. Immunol., *15*:45, 1972.

Vogler, L. B., Pearl, E. R., Gathings, W. E., Lawton, A. R., and Cooper, M. D.: B lymphocyte precursors in bone marrow in immunodeficiency state. Lancet, *2*:376, 1976.

Waldmann, T. A., Broder, S., Blaese, R. M., Durm, M., Blackman, M., and Strober, W.: Role of suppressor T cells in pathogenesis of common hypogammaglobulinemia. Lancet, *2*:609, 1974.

Whiteside, T. L., and Rabin, B. S.: Surface immunoglobulin on activated human peripheral blood thymus-derived cells. J. Clin. Invest., *57*:762, 1976.

4

Winchester, R. J., Fu, S. M., Hoffman, T., and Kunkel, H. G.: IgG on lymphocyte surfaces; technical problems and the significance of a third cell population. J. Immunol., *114*:1210, 1975.

Woda, B. A., Fenoglio, C. M., Nette, E. G., and King, D. W.: The lack of specificity of the sheep erythrocyte-T lymphocyte rosetting phenomenon. Am. J. Pathol., *88*:69, 1977.

Yoshida, T. O., and Andersson, B.: Evidence for a receptor recognizing antigen complexed immunoglobulin on the surface of activated mouse thymus lymphocytes. Scand. J. Immunol., *1*:401, 1972.

Zucker-Franklin, D.: The percentage of monocytes among "mononuclear" cell fractions obtained from normal human blood. J. Immunol., *112*:234, 1974.

40

PHAGOCYTIC CELLS

Polymorphonuclear Cells and Monocytes

Eufronio G. Maderazo, M.D., and
Peter A. Ward, M.D.

As the name implies, phagocytes are cells that are endowed with the ability to engulf particles. In general these include the polymorphonuclear granulocytes (neutrophils and eosinophils), the monocytes of the blood, and, at the tissue level, the macrophages. Although other cells such as certain endothelial cells and the alveolar lining cells are also known to internalize particles, we will concern ourselves only with the blood-associated phagocyte cells: neutrophils and monocytes.

PHYSIOLOGY OF PHAGOCYTES

Although evidence is fragmentary, it is generally believed that monovalent and divalent cations, metabolic fuels such as ATP and GTP, cyclic nucleotides, and microtubules and microfilaments are responsible for the translation of chemical and electrical energy into mechanical work. The precise role of these various factors and their interplay are poorly understood.

Both *microtubules* and *microfilaments* are filamentous cytoplasmic structures that are currently believed to play important roles in cellular functions. Microtubules are hollow filaments made up of polymers of a well-known protein, tubulin. The interaction of microtubules with membranes controls the movement and distribution of membrane transport proteins and cell surface receptors. These effects suggest their importance as regulators in the movement of substances through the cell membrane and in membrane-membrane or membrane-substrate interactions in cell adherence and locomotion (both random and chemotactic). In addition, microtubules also direct the traffic of cytoplasmic inclusions and thereby influence the release of intracytoplasmic substances, particularly lysosomal granule contents (Goldstein, 1973). The effects of microtubule disturbance on cell function are seen in Chédiak-Higashi cells (Oliver, 1976) and in cells treated with the antitubulin drug, colchicine (Rinehart, 1977).

Microfilaments are smaller in diameter than the microtubules and are made up of actin polymers. These structures are arranged randomly or oriented in subplasmalemmal bundles. It is hypothesized that cell-substrate contact activates actin-binding protein and myosin which gels and contracts the actin fila-

1335

ments (Stossel, 1978). The importance of microfilament in cell adherence, locomotion, phagocytosis, and degranulation has been shown in cells treated with low concentrations of cytochalasin B (Rinehart, 1977), which dissolves actin gels and in cells from a child with dysfunctional leukocytic actin (Boxer, 1974).

To facilitate engulfment, the phagocytes have to be brought in close proximity to their target particles. This requires leukocytic mobilization, a phenomenon that involves two events, adherence to endothelial surfaces and locomotion. Adherence to endothelial cells allows the phagocyte to gain a foothold in the vascular network. This is an important prerequisite to the mobilization of leukocytes into extravascular sites. Adherence to endothelial cells is also important for locomotion itself, since the phagocyte moves in a "head over heels" fashion, which requires that a part of the cell be firmly anchored. The regulatory mechanism of adherence is at present mostly unknown. A list of conditions and drugs that affect granulocyte adherence is given in Table 40-1.

Cell locomotion is either "random" or "chemotactic." Random locomotion is similar to the movements of a blind man left in the middle of an open field. The probability of his moving in one direction would be equal to the probability of his going in any other direction. Chemotaxis is the unidirectional response to a concentration gradient of a chemical attractant. This is similar to the same blind man going in the direction of the sound he hears. Random locomotion is either non-stimulated or stimulated (chemokinetic or a non-oriented response to the presence of chemotactic or other chemical substances). To differentiate these responses of leukocytes from responses of other cells such as bacteria and amebae, the terms leukotaxis and leukokinesis were introduced. The most important source of chemotactic factors is the complement system from which are derived the chemotactic fragments of C3 and C5, and the $C\overline{567}$ complex. Cell-derived chemotactic factors such as those from lymphocytes, granulocytes, and macrophages have also been described (Ward, 1974). The humoral regulation of leukocyte locomotion has been studied more extensively than regulators of other leukocyte functions, such as phagocytosis. These regulators include the chemotactic factor inactivator (CFI) (Ward, 1974) and the cell-directed inhibitor of leukotaxis (CDI) (Maderazo, 1977).

The chemotactic factor inactivator is a regulator that is present in normal human serum. It acts directly on chemotactic factors to bring about their inactivations. Two types of inactivators have been identified recently, both of which are heat-labile and non-dialyzable, one being an α-globulin with specificity against the C5 chemotactic fragment and the other a β-globulin with specificity against the C3 chemotactic fragment. Elevations of serum CFI have been associated with chemotactic defects and have been observed in patients with Hodgkin's disease, cirrhosis, sarcoidosis, and lepromatous leprosy (Table 40-2).

The cell-directed inhibitor of leukotaxis (CDI) is another regulator of cell locomotion which is present in normal serum. It acts directly on both polymorphonuclears and monocytes to inhibit locomotion and phagocytosis. Present evidence suggests that CDI is an IgG. Also, polymeric IgA has been described to have similar activity (Van Epps and Williams, 1976). Elevations of CDI in serum have been associated with abnormal leukocyte locomotion and have been observed in patients with anergy, cirrhosis, cancer, and recalcitrant adult periodontitis (Table 40-2).

A low molecular weight cell-directed specific inhibitor against monocytes has been described in patients with cancer (Snyderman, 1976). This material differs from the heavy molecular weight CDI described above by its molecular weight (8,000 to 12,000 daltons), by being dialyzable, by its lack of activity against polymorphonuclear cells, and by its lack of effect on phagocytic function of leukocytes.

Table 40-1. DISORDERS OF GRANULOCYTE ADHERENCE*

Decreased Adherence

Diseases:	Dysglobulinemia
	Myelogenous leukemia
	Diabetes mellitus (Bagdade, 1976)
	Post streptococcal glomerulonephritis (Ruley, 1976)
Drugs:	Alcohol, prednisone, aspirin, colchicine, and epinephrine
Others:	Glycolytic inhibitors, bradykinin, cyclic AMP inducers, and cyclic GMP blockers

Increased Adherence

Diseases:	Endotoxemia
Drugs:	Levamisole, aminoglycoside antibiotics (Seklecki, 1978), propranolol
Others:	Hemodialysis, cyclic AMP blockers, and cyclic GMP inducers

*References not cited are available in several papers (MacGregor, 1974; 1977).

Table 40-2. DISORDERS OF PHAGOCYTE LOCOMOTION OF HUMANS*

Cellular defects
  Congenital
    Chédiak-Higashi syndrome
    "Lazy leukocyte" syndrome
    Down's syndrome (Kahn, 1975)
    Dysfunctional leukocytic actin
    Other defects—periodontosis (Maderazo, 1976)
  Acquired
    Metabolic—diabetes mellitus
    Infections—bacterial, viral
    Malignant tumors and leukemia
    Other—lymphoid defects, rheumatoid arthritis, hyperimmunoglobulinemia E
  Others
    Neonates (Miller, 1973)

Humoral defects
  Inhibitor of cells
    Drugs (Quie, 1977)
    ↑Cell-directed inhibitor (Maderazo, 1977) found in patients with malignant tumors, cirrhosis, periodontitis, anergy
  Inhibitor of chemotactic factors
    ↑Chemotactic factor inactivator found in patients with Hodgkin's disease, cirrhosis, sarcoidosis, lepromatous leprosy
  Deficiency of substrates for chemotactic factors
    Congenital and acquired complement deficiencies

*References not cited are available in two reviews (Ward, 1974; Clark, 1978).

Phagocytosis is initiated by attachment of a particle to the surface of the phagocyte, followed by invagination of the particle along with a portion of the cell membrane. Two major enhancers of phagocytosis have been described: the opsonins which coat the target particles to render them palatable to the phagocyte (Winkelstein, 1973) and tuftsin, which acts directly on the cell to stimulate its phagocytic activity (Najjar, 1975). The heat-stable specific opsonin is specific antibody acting alone or in combination with complement activated via the classic pathway. The heat-labile opsonin includes the complement system and its C3b and C5b products which are generated via activation of the classic or alternative complement pathways. It is not clear how opsonins enhance phagocytosis, but it appears that immunoglobulin can act as a ligand that attaches to the bacterial surface antigen via its F(ab)$_2$ portion and to specific receptor sites on the phagocyte cell surface via the Fc portion of the Ig molecule. Presumably, C3b can also act as a ligand, since both neutrophils and monocytes have receptors for C3b. Opsonic deficiencies have been described in newborn infants, in sickle cell disease, and in deficiency

states of C3 and C5 components of complement.

The other phagocytosis-enhancing material present in normal serum is called tuftsin. This is a tetrapeptide (L-threonyl-L-lysyl-L-prolyl-L-arginine) and acts directly on the cell to stimulate phagocytosis of opsonized bacteria. Two types of tuftsin disorders have been described: one was congenital owing to the presence of an abnormal (mutant) peptide which competitively inhibits normal tuftsin; and another a deficiency state which has been observed in splenectomized patients owing to the lack of a tuftsin-releasing enzyme derived from the spleen (Najjar, 1975). Conditions that are associated with abnormal phagocytosis are listed in Table 40-3.

Once the microbe is phagocytosed a series of events within the neutrophil leads to the eventual *killing* and *digestion* of the microbe (Spitznagel, 1977). First, the phagosomal membrane will fuse with the lysosomal granule membrane forming the phagolysosomes, resulting in the release of lysosomal granule contents into the phagocytic vacuole. This is followed by a burst of metabolic activity leading to killing and digestion of the microbe. For simplicity, this microbicidal mechanism can be categorized under oxygen-dependent and oxygen-independent systems. The former consists of myeloperoxidase and cofactors (halides, thiocyanate, thyroxine, and triiodothyronine), hydrogen peroxide, superoxide anions, hydroxyl radicals, and singlet oxygen. This system, by a series of powerful oxida-

Table 40-3. DISORDERS OF PHAGOCYTOSIS*

Intrinsic defects
  Congenital
    Dysfunctional leukocytic actin
    Down's syndrome (Rosner, 1973)
  Acquired
    Leukemia (Goldman, 1972)
  Others
    Neonates (Miller, 1973)
Extrinsic defects
  ↑Cell-directed inhibitor (Maderazo, 1977)
  Opsonic deficiencies: (Winkelstein, 1973) sickle cell disease, immunoglobulin abnormalities, and complement abnormalities
  Tuftsin abnormalities (Najjar, 1975)
  Others: drugs (steroids, levorphanol, ethanol) toxins (staphylococcus protein A and alpha toxin)
  Ill-defined defects: severe infections, diabetes mellitus, rheumatoid arthritis

*References not cited are available in several reviews (Stossel, 1977; Cline, 1975; Baehner, 1975).

Table 40–4. DISORDERS OF PHAGOCYTE
MICROBICIDAL FUNCTION*

Intrinsic defects
  Congenital
    Chronic granulomatous disease
    Down's syndrome (Gregory, 1972)
    Chédiak-Higashi syndrome
    G-6-PD deficiency
    Myeloperoxidase deficiency
  Acquired
    Leukemia
    Lymphoproliferative disorders
  Others
    Neonates (Miller, 1973)

Extrinsic defects
  Drugs: levorphanol, phenylbutazone, hydrocortisone
  Ill-defined defects: rheumatoid arthritis, protein-calorie
    malnutrition, severe infections, diabetes mellitus

*References not cited are available in several reviews
(Quie, 1975; Baehner, 1975).

tion-reduction reactions, is assumed to destroy
and digest phagocytosed microbes. The oxygen-independent system includes low pH, lysozyme, lactoferrin, and cationic proteins.
These factors are microbicidal or microbistatic
per se. For example, acid-sensitive organisms
may be killed by the low pH achieved in the
phagocyte vacuole, lysozyme lyses bacterial
cell wall, lactoferrin binds iron and deprives
the organism of an essential nutrient, and
cationic proteins may interfere with microbial
metabolism by binding to acidic groups of the
microbial surface. Various disorders that have
been found to be associated with an abnor-

mality of microbial killing function by phagocytes are listed in Table 40–4.

Since the same factors and resources of the
cells often subserve various cell functions, it is
common to observe multiple dysfunctions resulting from a single subcellular abnormality.
Examples of conditions associated with multiple phagocyte dysfunctions are listed in Table
40–5. As noted previously, the patient with
leukocytic actin dysfunction had problems in
granulocyte locomotion, phagocytosis, and degranulation, since all these functions require
normal microfilament activity. Leukocyte adherence studies were not reported, but that
too would be expected to be affected, since
adherence also requires microfilament activity. Chédiak-Higashi cells have dysfunctions
of chemotaxis and microbial killing owing to
an abnormality of microtubule assembly. The
defective chemotaxis reflects the importance
of microtubule function in membrane and
membrane-substrate activities and in sensing
chemotactic stimuli, whereas the defective
microbial killing function reflects the requirement of microtubules for the control of cytoplasmic granule traffic, lysosomal granule and
phagosome membrane fusion, and lysosomal
enzyme release. Because of the cell surface
activity of microtubules, Chédiak-Higashi cells
would also be expected to have decreased adherence. The explanation of phagocyte dysfunctions observed in the other conditions
listed in Table 40–5 is not known.

Certain disorders not associated with multiple dysfunctions are also included in Table

Table 40–5. EXAMPLES OF CONDITIONS ASSOCIATED WITH
MULTIPLE PHAGOCYTE DYSFUNCTIONS

DEFECT	ADHERENCE	LOCOMOTION	PHAGOCYTOSIS	MICROBIAL KILLING
Congenital				
Leukocytic actin dysfunction	Unknown	Decreased	Decreased	Unknown
Chédiak-Higashi syndrome	Unknown	Decreased	Normal	Decreased
Down's syndrome	Unknown	Decreased	Decreased	Decreased
Chronic granulomatous disease	Unknown	Normal	Normal	Decreased
Myeloperoxidase deficiency	Unknown	Normal	Normal	Decreased
Tuftsin deficiency	Unknown	Normal	Decreased	Normal
Acquired				
Leukemia, acute myelogenous	Decreased	Decreased	Decreased	Decreased
Diabetes mellitus	Decreased	Decreased*	Decreased	Decreased
Rheumatoid arthritis	Unknown	Decreased	Decreased	Decreased
Protein-calorie malnutrition	Unknown	Decreased	Normal*	Decreased
Severe infections	Unknown	Decreased*	Decreased	Decreased
Other				
Neonates	Unknown	Decreased	Decreased	Decreased

*Controversial

40–5 because they are typical examples of specific dysfunctions. For example, chronic granulomatous disease of childhood and myeloperoxidase deficiency typify phagocytic disorders of microbial killing, and tuftsin deficiency exemplifies disorders of phagocytosis.

RELATIONSHIPS BETWEEN THE HOST AND THE MICROBES

Although there is increasing and convincing evidence that the host defenses also protect the host from proliferation of malignant neoplasms, we will concern ourselves with the host defenses against infection only. To better understand some of the manifestations of phagocyte abnormalities, a review of the relationships between the host defenses and the microbe is presented.

The diagram shown in Figure 40–1 shows a balance in which microbial factors are on one side and the host factors are on the other side. The microbial factors include microbial virulence and microbial quantity. Virulence includes all the factors that make the microbe detrimental to the host, such as toxins, enzymes that may increase invasiveness of microbes, substances that may neutralize the host defenses, and others. On the other side of the balance are the host factors consisting of local, humoral, and cellular defenses. Under normal conditions this balance is tilted in favor of the host. The angle of the tilt is the host reserve which favors host defense over microbial factors. Off the horizontal, the microbial factors predominate with resulting infection. Therefore, given a normal host, infection can occur in one of several conditions. The quantity of the microbe can be increased to overwhelm even a normal host. For instance, in one of the "Earth Day" celebrations (Fass, 1971) epidemic histoplasmosis occurred in a large group of young, apparently normal individuals who were exposed to high concentrations of dust contaminated with bird droppings. Because of increased virulence, infections can also occur in the normal host even if the amount of exposure is not overwhelming. For example, most normal individuals exposed to *Neisseria gonorrheae*, *Shigella*, or *Vibrio cholera* will be infected. On the other hand, infections can also occur if the host is defective, even if there is little or no change in the microbial factors. An example of this is patients with extensive burns who have increased susceptibility to skin bacteria such as *Staphylococcus aureus* or *Streptococcus*. This increased susceptibility can be diminished by replacing the lost skin cover with dressings, with synthetic materials, or with pig skin. Infections also occur as a result of abnormalities in humoral factors, such as in patients with immunoglobulin or complement deficiencies. Individuals who develop granulocytopenia as a reaction to certain drugs often have sore throat as their initial complaint. The sore throat in this case may be due to pharyngitis from overgrowth of the patient's normal microflora.

INTERACTION OF HOST FACTORS

The epithelial cover, together with the antimicrobial substances in secretions and the phagocytes and lymphocytes in the subepithelial mucosal regions, provides local defenses against penetration by microbes. The importance of this first line defense is shown by infections that occur when the skin is broken, such as in wounds and burns, abnormalities of

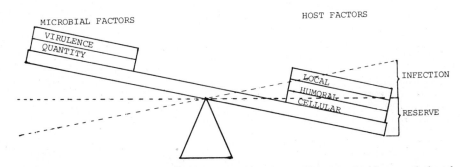

Figure 40–1. Diagram showing the preferable relationship between the host and the microbial factors—the host factors exceed the microbial factors. Changes from this relationship that favor the microbe will tilt the see-saw in the opposite direction, resulting in infection.

drainage due to obstruction, and ciliary immobility in the upper airways.

The major components of the humoral defenses are the immunoglobulins (antibodies) and the complement system. The immunoglobulins function mainly as a trigger for complement activation and as a potentiator of cellular function, particularly phagocytosis, by opsonization of target particles. Antibody can also inactivate microbial toxins by its neutralizing or antitoxin activity. The complement system, like the antibodies, also functions mainly by regulating or potentiating cell function by generation of the complement-derived chemotactic factors and the phagocytosis-enhancing factors. But by itself complement can also directly lyse bacteria, which is probably important for the defense against gram-negative organisms, particularly against the *Neisseria* species.

The cellular factors are made up of the polymorphonuclear cells, monocytes and macrophages, and lymphocytes. The lymphocytes function mainly by their ability to secrete a wide variety of substances (lymphokines and immunoglobulins) with a broad spectrum of activities. Lymphocytes also contain immunologic memory and probably represent the principal cells involved in identifying a foreign material as "non-self." Lymphocytes also have profound influences on the activities of other cells such as monocytes and macrophages and even other lymphocytes. Together with other cells, particularly the macrophages,

lymphocytes are the main cells involved in cell-mediated immunity, which is expressed in cutaneous delayed hypersensitivity reaction, protection against extracellular organisms, protection against neoplasms, and graft rejection.

As can be seen from the above organization of the host defense system, the various host factors do not act independently, but rather act in concert with one another.

CLINICAL MANIFESTATIONS OF PHAGOCYTE ABNORMALITIES

Table 40-6 shows that the infecting organism often signals the host abnormality. In general, recurrent infections owing to extracellular organisms are manifestations of abnormalities of immunoglobulins, complement, or polymorphonuclear cells. Infections owing to intracellular organisms suggest disorders of monocytes, macrophages, and lymphocytes; and also immunoglobulins and complement. Therefore, any recurrent infection should require the evaluation of phagocytes (either polymorphonuclear cells, monocytes, or both), immunoglobulins, and the complement system.

Aside from the signs and symptoms specifically attributable to the myriad conditions associated with phagocyte abnormalities (Tables 40-1 to 40-4), in our experience certain manifestations signal the presence of a phagocyte dysfunction.

Table 40-6. PATHOGENIC AGENTS THAT MAY SIGNAL UNDERLYING HOST DEFENSE DISORDER

OBSERVED PATHOGEN	SUSPECTED DISORDER

Extracellular bacteria
  Staphylococcus
  Streptococcus
  Hemophilus
  Meningococcus
  Enterobacter
  Pseudomonas
  Serratia
  Others
	Serum: antibody, complement
	Cells: granulocytes

Intracellular agents
  Bacteria: *Salmonella, Brucella*
    Listeria, Nocardia,
    Actinomyces, Myco-
    bacteria
  Viruses: *Herpes, CMV, Vaccinia,*
    Influenza, etc.
  Fungi: *Cryptococcus, Aspergillus,*
    Histoplasma, Candida,
    etc.
  Protozoa: *Toxoplasma, Pneumocystis,* etc.
	Serum: antibody, complement
	Cells: macrophage, monocyte, and
	    lymphocyte

Recurrent or frequent infections are the most common manifestation that results in referral for phagocyte function testing. The most common site of the infection is the skin and adjacent soft tissues, and the most frequent pathogens are *Staphylococcus aureus* and hemolytic streptococci. The next most frequent site of involvement is the upper and lower respiratory tract, followed by infections in other locations, including the blood stream.

Any severe or life-threatening infection, especially if no apparent increase in the microbial factors (virulence and quantity) is present and no obvious breaks in the local defenses (epithelial linings, secretory immunoglobulin) are evident. Contrary to some reports, patients who develop *Listeria* meningitis, for example, should be considered abnormal.

Inappropriate response to infections in patients with serious bacterial infections. Absence of fever and other signs of infection in a patient with systemic infection can indicate a host disorder.

Low white blood cell count in acutely infected body fluids. This should be considered an obvious sign of abnormal host cell mobilization. The low white cell count in ascitic fluid of cirrhotics with spontaneous peritonitis is one example.

Infections that do not respond to seemingly appropriate therapy such as bacteremic *Pseudomonas* pneumonia. One series showed a mortality of 100 per cent regardless of antibiotic therapy (Iannini, 1974). Many (30 per cent) of his patients were leukopenic and some had diseases associated with granulocyte dysfunctions. If the white cell count is normal in a non-responsive patient, a qualitative defect of phagocytes should be suspected.

"Cold" abscess owing to organisms that ordinarily cause "hot" abscesses, such as "cold" abscess formation due to staphylococci in patients with chronic granulomatous disease of childhood, and in some patients with the syndrome of eczema, hyperimmunoglobulinemia E, and leukotactic abnormality (Hill, 1975).

Granulomatous reaction to a non-granulomatous infection suggests a host defect. Analyses of factors that lead to granuloma formation indicate that such a reaction occurs if one of two conditions exists: (a) the phagocytosed particle is resistant to intracellular enzymes and is not effectively destroyed, or (b) the phagocytes have an abnormal digestive mechanism. Thus, granuloma formation occurs as a response to mycobacterial infections or peritoneal contamination with glove powder, since these particles are difficult for phagocytes to digest. On the other hand, easily digestible organisms, such as staphylococci and *Escherichia coli,* can cause granuloma formation in the presence of phagocytes with bactericidal disorders, such as those in patients with chronic granulomatous disease of childhood and in malakoplakia.

PHAGOCYTE FUNCTION TESTS

The preceding section tells us when to suspect the presence of a phagocyte abnormality and for whom (most likely patients) to request specific determinations. The next step is to decide what measurements and examinations are needed. To this end, several manifestations are important, since they allow immediate focus on certain dysfunctions: for example, a patient who develops a granulomatous reaction as a result of infection from non-granuloma-forming bacteria will require tests for microbial killing; a patient with "cold" abscesses owing to staphylococci or streptococci should be tested for phagocyte leukotaxis and microbial killing; a patient with acute bacterial meningitis with inappropriately low granulocyte count in the cerebrospinal fluid not due to a parameningeal focus may have a granulocyte mobilization defect and requires testing for leukotaxis; the same is true in acute bacterial peritonitis with low cell counts in ascitic fluid. Most other manifestations do not allow the pinpointing of specific dysfunctions and, therefore, will require screening procedures for all four major phagocyte functions (adherence, locomotion, phagocytosis, and microbial killing). Granulocytes are tested if the organisms responsible for the infectious problem are "extracellular bacteria," whereas monocytes are best tested first if the pathogens are "intracellular agents" (Table 40-6).

A flow schema is shown in Table 40-7. For screening purposes, testing up to Step 1 is all that is necessary. Beyond Step 1 studies require sophisticated and well-supported laboratories in terms of personnel and expertise.

PREPARATIONS OF HUMAN LEUKOCYTES

Polymorphonuclear Cells

Venous blood is collected into a plastic syringe containing 50 units of preservative-free

Table 40-7. LABORATORY DIAGNOSTIC STEPS IN PATIENTS WITH SUSPECTED PHAGOCYTE DYSFUNCTION*

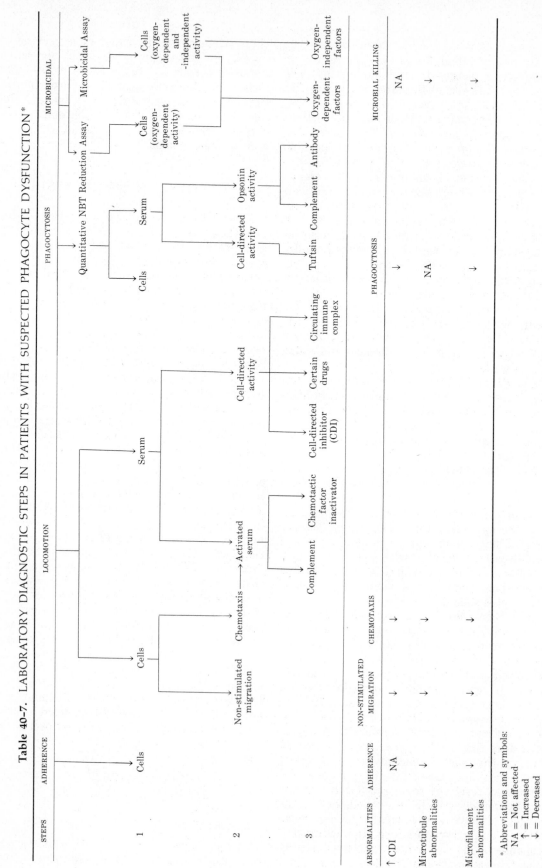

ABNORMALITIES	ADHERENCE	NON-STIMULATED MIGRATION	CHEMOTAXIS	PHAGOCYTOSIS	MICROBIAL KILLING
↑ CDI	NA	↓	↓	↑	NA
Microtubule abnormalities	↓	↓	↓	NA	↑
Microfilament abnormalities	↓	↓	↓	↓	↓

* Abbreviations and symbols:
NA = Not affected
↑ = Increased
↓ = Decreased

heparin (sodium) per milliliter of blood. The syringe is stood on its plunger to allow the red cells to sediment by gravity for 30 to 60 minutes. The leukocyte-rich plasma is then collected into a plastic 40 ml test tube, using a bent needle (or a polyethylene catheter attached to the tip of the syringe needle), and centrifuged at low speed (500 g) for 10 minutes. The cell button is resuspended in Medium 199 (pH 7.4) and the concentration is adjusted to 5×10^6 cells/ml.

In some subjects (frequently males) in whom erythrocytes sediment very slowly or not at all, sedimentation can be hastened by adding an equal volume of 6 per cent dextran in saline to the heparinized blood sample.

Monocytes

Monocytes are prepared by density gradient centrifugation in Ficoll-Hypaque, as described on p. 1318.

LEUKOCYTE ADHERENCE ASSAY

Various methods of determining leukocyte adherence are known; among these are *in vivo* procedures such as determinations of the marginating pool of granulocytes using injected epinephrine (Athens, 1961), and *in vitro* methods using glass beads. The easiest and most reproducible assay, however, is that using scrubbed nylon fibers (MacGregor, 1974). A modification of this technique is used in our laboratory. In this method, when washed leukocyte samples as described above and 40 mg of nylon fibers are used, most normal individuals have a 90 per cent or greater adherence. Values below 80 per cent are abnormal. An increasing number of conditions and drugs have now been found to influence granulocyte adherence (see Table 40-1).

This assay system is highly reproducible if several variables are closely monitored. First, washing of cells will increase adherence by approximately 10 to 20 per cent. Therefore, if one uses heparinized whole blood or leukocyte-rich plasma in which the cells are not washed, the normal values have to be correspondingly lowered or, preferably, determined in each laboratory beforehand. Second, the amount of nylon fibers used should be weighed as accurately as possible. In experiments using various amounts of fibers, it was shown that adherence increases directly with the weight of fibers used, peaks at approximately 50 mg, and plateaus thereafter. The use of 40 mg of fibers is therefore sensitive in detecting decreased adherence values, but insensitive to increases in adherence. To detect adherence greater than normal, lesser amounts of fibers (e.g., 20 mg) should be used. Another critical factor to control is the length of the packed fiber column, since the shorter the column, the greater the adherence, and vice versa.

Materials

1. Leukocyte preparations from the patient and normal individual
2. Plastic tuberculin or insulin syringes (Pharmaseal)
3. Scrubbed nylon fibers (Fenwall)
4. TC Medium 199, pH 7.4 (Difco)
5. Counting chamber
6. Micropipette counting system (Unopette, B-D)

Method

Scrubbed nylon fibers (40 mg) are packed into plastic tuberculin (or insulin) syringes, and the packed column adjusted to 15 mm in length. The leukocyte preparation (0.5 ml) with a known granulocyte count is then applied to the top of the column and allowed to filter through. The filtrate is collected and recounted by gravity. This can be accomplished in a 2 to 3 minute period. The percentage adherence is then calculated as follows:

$$\text{Percentage adherence} = \frac{\substack{\text{Granulocyte count of original sample} - \\ \text{Granulocyte count of filtrate}}}{\text{Granulocyte count of original sample}} \times 100$$

LEUKOTAXIS ASSAY

The easiest and the most available *in vivo* assay for leukocyte mobilization appears to be the delayed cutaneous hypersensitivity reaction. Another *in vivo* method is the Rebuck skin window technique (Rebuck, 1955). The chief problems with these procedures include their non-specificity, the difficulty in standardization and reproducibility, and their inconvenience.

Various *in vitro* procedures are available, the most popular being the Boyden micropore filter technique because of its relative simplicity, convenience, and applicability to performance of many experiments in one day. This method uses a chamber which is divided by a micropore filter into an upper (or cell) and a lower (or chemotactic factor) compartment. The cells are placed in the upper compartment

Table 40-8. METHODS OF MICROPORE FILTER LEUKOTACTIC ASSAY

	METHOD 1	METHOD 2	METHOD 3
Mechanics	*Number* of cells that have reached a predetermined distance	*Distance* migrated by the fastest cells	Average distance migrated per cell
Examples	1. Distal surface cell count (Boyden, 1962) 2. Radioassay-double filter technique (Gallin, 1973) 3. Cell count distal to cell monolayer (Ward, 1968) 4. Distal surface cell count with correction for detached cells (Keller, 1972; Frei, 1972)	"Leading front technique" (Zigmond, 1973)	"Distance per cell technique" (Maderazo, 1978)
Problems due to:			
1. Cell detachment from distal filter surface	Yes (Method 1, Example 1.)	No	No
2. Magnification and minification of defects	Yes	No	No
3. Large variability	Yes	No	No
4. Susceptibility to bias	More	Less	Least
5. Inability to detect defects of mass migration	No	Yes	No
6. Laboriousness	Less	Less	More

and allowed to migrate from the proximal to the distal surface of the filter. Three methods have been used to evaluate polymorphonuclear cell locomotion into the micropore filter (summarized in Table 40-8). The first method involves the enumeration of the number of cells that have reached a predetermined distance. The second method measures the distance reached by the fastest or the deeper-most cells. The third method incorporates both the *number* of cells and the *distance* of migration. An example of the first is the original method described by Boyden in which cells are allowed to migrate completely through the filter. Those cells that have reached the distal surface are then counted. Modifications of the first method include counting of all cells that have moved distal to the cell monolayer, the radioassay double-filter technique using radioactive chromium-labeled granulocytes, and the distal filter surface counts with corrections for detached cells (which is done by using a second filter to catch cells that have detached from the distal surface of the upper filter or by

cell counts in the fluid in the lower compartment). The second method, known as the "leading front" technique, was described by Zigmond (1973). In this method the cells are not allowed to penetrate completely the thickness of the filter. The distance migrated by the fastest cells is recorded and used as the measure of locomotion.

There are problems with these methods. With the first method the most widely known problem is cell detachment from the distal filter surface. This detachment is variable, increases with time of incubation, and is probably indirectly related to leukocyte adherence. The second problem is the magnification or minification of leukotactic defects. Magnification occurs because only those cells that have reached the distal surface are counted and are given a grade of 100 per cent migration, whereas those cells that do not reach the distal surface are not counted and are given a grade of 0 per cent migration regardless of how close to the distal surface they have migrated. In our experience this has led to the clinical laboratory discrepancy in which a relatively well patient has a greater than 90 per cent inhibition of leukotaxis. This has resulted in some individuals questioning the relevance of leukotaxis assays, because many patients with chemotactic inhibition approaching 100 per cent did not die when they had serious infections. In addition to magnification of abnormalities, errors are also magnified. Reduction to the point that a previously obvious defect is not detected has been observed less frequently. This occurs on prolonged incubation of chambers, where the slowly moving (abnormal) cells are allowed enough time to reach the distal surface, at the same time that an increasing number of normal cells on the distal surface are detaching. The third problem of this method is the error created by nonuniformity of the cell distribution on the filter. Unless the total area of the filter is counted, representative areas of low or high counts could be selected for counting depending upon the bias of the reader. Yet if fields are not selected the variation often becomes so great that in many instances the data cannot be evaluated. The radioassay double filter technique will correct this problem because the total number of radiolabeled cells detached from the distal surface of the upper filter is counted.

The second method ("leading front" technique) depends on accepting the concept that the cell population is homogeneous in its migration characteristics through the micropore filter, and that, therefore, the fastest migrating cells represent the total cell population. We have found that this concept is not true, since at least two types of cells with different behaviors of migration in micropore filters exist. In addition, since it is mainly a measure of distance migrated by a few representative cells, it may not detect disorders of mass migration.

The method presented will incorporate measurements of both the cell number and the distance migrated by the cells.

Materials

1. Leukocyte and serums from the patient and normal control
2. Leukotactic chambers (Ahlco Corporation, Southington, CT) (Fig. 40-2)
3. Micropore filters, 13 mm diameter and 5 μm pore size (Sartorius)
4. Sodium heparin, preservative-free
5. TC Medium 199, pH 7.4 (Difco)

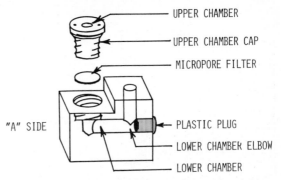
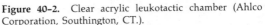

Figure 40-2. Clear acrylic leukotactic chamber (Ahlco Corporation, Southington, CT.).

6. Staining cassettes for micropore filters (Ahlco Corporation, Southington, CT) (Fig. 40-3)
7. Staining chemicals:
   a. Acid alcohol (70%, 90%, and 100%)
   b. Acid hematoxylin (4 ml concentrated acetic acid/100 ml hematoxylin)
   c. Acid alcohol (3 drops HCl/200 ml 70% isopropyl alcohol)
   d. Bluing agent (20 g $MgSO_4$ + 2 g $NaHCO_3$ in 1 l water)
   e. Xylene
8. Preparation of chemotactic factors:
   a. Bacterial chemotactic factor: *Escherichia coli* is incubated in Medium 199 at 37°C. for 24 to 48 hours. After incubation the bacteria are removed by ultracentrifugation at 20,000 rpm for 20 minutes. The filtrate is then saved and tested for chemotactic activity. The least amount producing the most activity is used in subsequent experiments.
   b. Activated serum: Normal serum is activated by incubation with zymosan (1 ml serum and 5 mg zymosan) at 37°C. for 5 minutes. This procedure will generate complement-derived chemotactic factors in the serum. A 3 per cent concentration of this material is used in the lower compartment to test chemotactic function. Besides zymosan, other substances have been used to activate serum, such as endotoxin and immune complexes.

Method

A micropore filter is placed on the floor of the upper chamber compartment and the upper chamber cap is placed and tightened slightly. (Excessive tightening may produce corrugations of the filter which result in irregular deposition of cells). The lower compartment is filled with the properly diluted chemotactic factor such as zymogen-activated serum or *Escherichia coli* supernate up to the elbow; 0.1 ml of the cell suspension containing

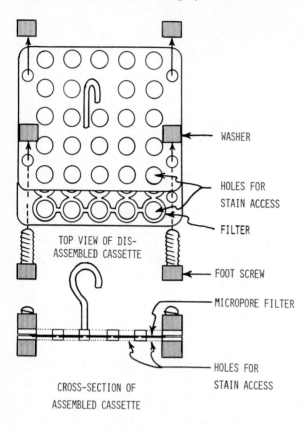

WASHER

HOLES FOR
STAIN ACCESS

FILTER

TOP VIEW OF DIS-
ASSEMBLED CASSETTE

FOOT SCREW

MICROPORE FILTER

HOLES FOR
STAIN ACCESS

CROSS-SECTION OF
ASSEMBLED CASSETTE

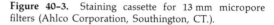

Figure 40-3. Staining cassette for 13 mm micropore filters (Ahlco Corporation, Southington, CT.).

5×10^6 cells/ml is added to the upper compartment, which is then filled completely with Medium 199. Following this, the lower compartment is filled similarly with Medium 199. (Filling the lower compartment completely before the upper compartment is filled will lead to seepage of the chemotactic factor through the filter into the upper compartment.) The prepared chambers are incubated in air at 37°C.

The optimum incubation time is one that will allow the fastest migrating cells to reach at least halfway, but not completely penetrate the thickness of the filter. Periods that do not allow suffi-

cient penetration into the depths of the filter are insensitive in detecting defects, except for the more severe ones. Table 40-9 shows the usual protocol for polymorphonuclear cell migration and incubation times. In our laboratory, cells tested in the absence of serum or plasma in the upper compartment are incubated for 90 minutes, while cells tested with serum or plasma are tested for 60 minutes. Disallowing cells from completely penetrating the filter avoids the variability of cell loss owing to cell detachment from the distal surface.

After incubation, the filters are removed, placed in specially made staining cassettes (Fig. 40-3),

Table 40-9. PROTOCOL FOR PHAGOCYTE LOCOMOTION WORK-UP

UPPER COMPARTMENT (CELLS + SERUM)		LOWER COMPARTMENT (FACTOR)	TO TEST OR SCREEN FOR:
Normal	+ No	No	⎰Nonstimulated
Patient's	+ No	No	⎱Locomotion
Patient's	+ No	Activated* Normal serum	⎰Chemotaxis,
Normal	+ No	Activated* Normal serum	⎱Complement-derived chemotactic
Normal	+ No	Activated* Patient's serum	factor, and chemotactic factor inactivator
Normal	+ Normal	No	⎰Cell-directed inhibitor
Normal	+ Patient's	No	⎱of leukotaxis and leukokinesis
Patient's	+ Normal	No	enhancing factor

*See p. 1345 for serum "activation" by zymosan.

Table 40-10. CALCULATION OF
LEUKOTACTIC INDEX (LI)*

DISTANCE FROM ORIGIN (A) (in μm)	NUMBER OF CELLS (B)	(A × B)
0 (monolayer)	15	0
10	37	370
20	12	240
30	10	300
40	13	520
50	7	350
60	8	480
70	9	630
80	4	320
90	6	540
100	0	0
Total excluding monolayer count:	106	3750†
Total including monolayer count‡:	121	

*LI (− m) excluding monolayer = $3750 \div 106 = 35.38 \, \mu$m
LI (+ m) including monolayer = $3750 \div 121 = 30.99 \, \mu$m
†This number is the total distance migrated by all the
cells in cell-μm.
‡Inclusion of monolayer count in calculation of LI improves sensitivity of the method in assessment of non-
stimulated migration and responses to chemotactic factor.

and, without being allowed to dry, quickly fixed in
100 per cent isopropyl alcohol for 30 seconds. The
filters are then stained in hematoxylin for 2 minutes, rinsed in water, decolorized in acid alcohol for
30 seconds, rinsed in water again, immersed in the
bluing agent for 30 seconds, rinsed in water, dehydrated successively in 75 per cent, 95 per cent, and
absolute isopropyl alcohol for 30 seconds each, and
finally cleared in xylene for 5 to 10 minutes. The
stained filters are mounted on slides with Permount and covered with a thin cover slip.

The cells are counted (using 400× magnification)
at every 10 μm interval from the proximal cell
monolayer to the distal surface. The number of
cells counted per level is multiplied by the distance
of that level to the proximal cell monolayer. Then
the products obtained are added and the sum is
divided by the total number of cells counted. The
number obtained is the leukotactic index (LI, which
is the average distance (in micrometers) migrated
by the cells within the allotted chamber incubation
time). Refer to Table 40-10 for sample calculation.
Three or more fields are counted and the LI for
each duplicate or triplicate filter is calculated.

Evaluation of Results. Because of large
day-to-day variability that occurs if the several variables are not stringently controlled,
normal controls are performed simultaneously
with each experiment. Variability also exists
among normal cells and serums. In our laboratory, cell indices less than 64 per cent and

serum values below 72 per cent of control values are abnormal. It is preferable, however, to
retest the patient using a different normal
control before making a final determination.

PHAGOCYTOSIS ASSAY

The methods chosen for discussion here are
used in our laboratory because of their relative
simplicity, sensitivity, precision, and reproducibility. We do not use methods of quantitation by direct microscopic counting of "phagocytized" particles, despite their greater
simplicity, because of difficulty in differentiating between *surface* and *internalized* particles.

The phagocytosis radioassay is quite complex and involved but is included because of its
sensitivity and precision. For screening purposes, however, the quantitative nitroblue tetrazolium reduction test is sufficient. The NBT
reduction test is simple, rapid, sensitive, and
reproducible; it requires fewer cells for testing; it is better known and more widely applied; and it requires equipment that is
generally available in most, if not all, laboratories. Chemiluminescence (CL) assay is an
equivalent, more recently described examination that uses light emission (probably derived
from singlet oxygen formation in phagocy-
tizing leukocytes) as the indicator of phagocytic and oxygen-dependent microbicidal activities (Allen, 1972). The CL assay requires
more cells to produce optimally detectable
light emission; red cell contamination interferes with its measurement, requiring greater
cell handling; and finally, a scintillation spectrophotometer, not generally available, is required for measurement of luminescence.
Hence, CL will not be discussed further.

PHAGOCYTOSIS RADIOASSAY

In this method iodine-125–labeled bovine
serum albumin antigen-antibody (immune
complex) precipitate is used as the particles
for engulfment (Ward, 1973). This method
cannot be used to test opsonizing activity of
serum. The most important technical aspect to
monitor is the efficiency of removing extracellular immune precipitate from cells containing
ingested immune precipitate. Two controls are
performed simultaneously to quantitate this
efficiency.

Materials

1. Patient's and normal polymorphonuclear leukocytes
2. Bovine albumin in Cohn Fraction V (Mann Research Laboratory)
3. Crystalline bovine serum albumin (BSA) (Pentex)
4. Deep-well crystal scintillation gamma detector and scaler counter
5. Ethylenediaminotetraacetic acid (EDTA)
6. TC Medium 199, pH 7.4 (Difco)
7. Phosphate-buffered saline, pH 7.4 (PBS)
8. Preparation of radiolabeled immune precipitate:
   a. Antibody to BSA is prepared from rabbits immunized by repeated intradermal injections of 10 mg crystalline BSA.
   b. The IgG fraction is obtained by DEAE cellulose fractionation of the hyperimmune serum.
   c. With the use of quantitative precipitin analysis, the equivalence point of antigen-antibody binding is determined.
   d. Next BSA (bovine serum albumin) is labeled with iodine-125 by incubation of 1 mg BSA with 0.5 mC of ^{125}I (New England Nuclear).
   e. An approximate quantity of labeled and unlabeled BSA is added to the antibody to form a dense precipitate, which is incubated at 37°C. for 2 hours and then kept at 4°C. overnight. The precipitate is washed and suspended in phosphate-buffered saline (PBS) to give 600 μg antibody nitrogen/ml.

Method

1. Cells ($1 \times 10^7/0.25$ ml in Medium 199), immune precipitate (0.20 ml containing 20 to 30 μg antibody nitrogen with antigen at equivalence and radioactivity of about 10 to 15×10^3 cpm), and 0.20 ml of PBS are mixed and the initial radioactivity is counted and recorded.
2. The mixture is incubated at 37°C. for 30 minutes in a shaking water bath following which 0.1 ml of 0.2 M EDTA is added to stop the reaction. Then excess BSA (0.1 ml of 400 mg BSA/ml) is added to solubilize extracellular immune precipitate, and the mixture is incubated for another 30 minutes at 37°C. in the water bath. After incubation, the mixture is diluted with 3 ml PBS and centrifuged at 1000 g for 20 minutes. The supernatant fluid is discarded and the residual radioactivity is determined in the deep-well scintillation counter.
3. Both EDTA and BSA controls are used to monitor the efficiency of separating extracellular from intracellular immune complexes. The closer the values to background activity, the greater the efficiency.
   a. EDTA is added to the cells prior to incubation with immune precipitate.

b. Excess BSA is added to immune precipitate prior to incubation with cells.

4. For calculation of phagocytosis, the uptake of radiolabeled immune complexes by normal (reference) control cells is determined in duplicate and the average value obtained. The ratio of the corresponding value derived from patient cells to that value as described above (preceding sentence) multiplied by 100 gives per cent phagocytosis by patient cells as compared with normal cells.

Thus, per cent phagocytosis can be calculated:

$$\% \text{ phagocytosis} = \frac{\text{uptake by patient cells}}{\text{uptake by control cells}} \times 100$$

If this assay is properly performed, the coefficient of variation is less than 1 per cent. Percentage reduction exceeding 10 per cent of normal, especially if consistent on repeat studies with different normal controls, is abnormal. The variability of phagocytosis in a normal population has not been determined.

QUANTITATIVE NITROBLUE TETRAZOLIUM (NBT) TEST

The quantitative NBT assay is an indirect test used to screen for disorders of phagocytosis and bacterial killing (oxygen-dependent bactericidal system). Defects of bacterial killing function owing to abnormalities of the oxygen-independent factors will not be detected by this assay. The method is slightly modified from that by Baehner (1968).

Materials

1. Normal and patient's polymorphonuclear cells
2. Zymosan (Sigma) is opsonized with serum (2 mg zymosan with 0.05 ml serum) by incubation at 37°C. for 5 minutes.
3. Nitroblue tetrazolium Grade III (Sigma)
4. Potassium cyanide, 0.01 M
5. Hydrochloric acid, 0.5 N
6. Pyridine (Fisher Scientific)
7. Spectrophotometer

Method

1. Polymorphonuclear cells (2×10^6 cells in 0.4 ml Medium 199) are mixed with 0.05 ml of opsonized zymosan and 0.1 ml of 0.01 M of potassium cyanide and incubated in a shaking water bath at 37°C. After 10 minutes, 0.1 ml of NBT (2 mg/ml in saline) is added and incubation is con-

tinued. After 15 minutes, the reaction is stopped with 4 ml of 0.5 N hydrochloric acid.

2. The tubes are centrifuged at 1000 g at 4°C. for 10 minutes, the supernatant fluid is discarded, and the reduced NBT (formazan) is extracted from the cell button with 4 ml of pyridine in a boiling water bath for 10 minutes under an exhaust hood.

3. The absorption of the extract is then determined in a spectrophotometer at 550 nm using pyridine as the blank control.

4. As a control a tube of cells without opsonized zymosan is run simultaneously to correct for spontaneous NBT reduction, which is high in certain conditions (Lace, 1975). The corrected NBT reduction is obtained by subtracting the control value from results obtained in the presence of opsonized zymosan. (For determination of serum opsonizing activity, use a control consisting of cells and unopsonized zymosan).

5. The per cent decrease of NBT reduction can then be determined as follows:

Per cent decrease of NBT reduction =
$$\frac{\text{Normal NBT} - \text{Patient's NBT}}{\text{Normal NBT}} \times 100$$

where normal NBT = A_{550} of extracted blue formazan in normal cells and patient's NBT = A_{550} of extracted blue formazan in patient's cells. Variability within a small group of normals has not exceeded 25 per cent.

Phagocytosis assay using radiolabeled immune precipitate can be combined with NBT assay to differentiate between a defect of phagocytosis and an inability to generate reducing activity for NBT dye. This can be done by replacing 0.05 ml of opsonized zymosan with 0.025 ml of immune complex.

BACTERIAL KILLING ASSAY

Most methods of quantitating bacterial killing by phagocytes are laborious, expensive, and require practice to obtain reproducible results. The method we use is a modification of a technique described previously (Tan, 1971), which uses *Staphylococcus aureus* as the test organism and lysostaphin to kill extracellular

Table 40-11. SCHEMATIC ILLUSTRATION OF LEUKOCYTE BACTERICIDAL ASSAY

Staphylococcus aureus
(4×10^8 B/ml)

0.5 ml B		0.5 ml B
+ 0.5 ml Medium 199		+ 0.4 ml PMN
		+ 0.1 ml Serum
1.0 ml B		1.0 ml B/PMN/Serum
(2×10^8 B/ml)		(2×10^8 B and
		2×10^6 PMN/ml)

Incubate, 37°C. × 1 hr

| 0.1 ml B | 0.1 ml B/PMN/Serum | 0.1 ml B/PMN/Serum |
| + 1.9 ml Sterile water | + 0.1 ml lysostaphin | + 1.9 ml sterile water |

Incubate, 37°C. × 20 min
+ 0.1 ml trypsin

Incubate, 37°C. × 10 min
+ 1.7 ml sterile water

Dilutions	2.0 ml (1×10^7 B/ml)	2.0 ml (1×10^7 B/ml)	2.0 ml (1×10^7 B/ml)
10^{-0}			
	Estimated bacteria/ 0.1 ml of each dilution	Plate Dilutions 10^{-0}, 10^{-1}, and 10^{-2}	Plate Dilutions 10^{-3} and 10^{-4}
10^{-4}	100		
10^{-5}	10		
10^{-6}	1		
	(A) = Initial inoculum	(B) = Live intracellular bacteria	(C) = Total live bacteria

organisms. With this technique it is possible to define separately the engulfment and the bactericidal process. To facilitate understanding of this complicated method, it is illustrated in Table 40–11.

Materials

1. Patient's and control polymorphonuclear leukocytes
2. 18-hour trypticase soy broth culture of *Staphylococcus aureus*
3. Mueller-Hinton agar plates. These are used because they are transparent, which allows counting of the colonies through the agar without opening the plates.
4. Sterile plastic tubes with caps
5. Isotonic saline
6. TC Medium 199, pH 7.4 (Difco)
7. Lysostaphin, 10 units/ml (Schwarz-Mann, Becton-Dickinson)
8. Trypsin, 2.5%
9. Distilled water
10. Sonifier (W-140, Branson Sonic)
11. Spectrophotometer

Method

1. An 18-hour broth culture of *Staphylococcus aureus* in trypticase soy broth is washed twice with sterile distilled water. The bacterial button is resuspended in 4 ml of distilled water and then sonicated for 15 seconds at 45 watts to disaggregate the bacteria. The solution is then adjusted to an absorbance of 0.75 at 650 nm using a spectrophotometer. This solution should contain 4×10^8 bacteria/ml.

2. To a 0.5 ml aliquot of bacterial suspension in a capped plastic tube, 0.4 ml of PMN solution (containing 5×10^6 cells/ml) and 0.1 ml of serum are added and incubated in a shaking water bath at 37°C. for 1 hour.

3. After incubation, 1.8 ml of distilled water is added to 0.1 ml of the bacteria-PMN-serum mixture. Serial 10-fold dilutions are then carried out with distilled water and 0.1 ml portions from each of the 10^{-3} and 10^{-4} dilutions are plated by spreading evenly over Mueller-Hinton agar plates using a smooth sterile L-shaped glass rod spreader. This will enumerate the *total live bacteria* (live extracellular and intracellular bacteria).

4. Into another 0.1 ml portion of the incubated bacteria-PMN-serum mixture is added 0.1 ml of lysostaphin (10 units/ml) and incubated in the water bath at 37°C. for 20 minutes. After incubation, 0.1 ml of 2.5 per cent trypsin is added to inactivate the lysostaphin and the mixture reincubated at 37°C. for another 10 minutes. Two serial 10-fold dilutions with distilled water are carried out and 0.1 ml of the undiluted and the two 10-fold dilutions are plated. This will enumerate only *live intracel-*

lular bacteria, since lysostaphin will destroy all bacteria not within cells.

5. To determine the number of live bacteria in the *initial inoculum,* 0.5 ml of the bacterial suspension is mixed with 0.5 ml of Medium 199. Serial 10-fold dilutions are made and 0.1 ml portions of the 10^{-4}, 10^{-5}, and 10^{-6} dilutions are plated.

6. The plates are incubated in air at 37°C. for 18 to 24 hours and the number of colonies on each plate is counted. Counts from countable higher dilutions are used. Calculation of killed intracellular (D) and total phagocytosed bacteria (E) can then be made from A (initial inoculum), B (live intracellular bacteria), and C (total live bacteria), thus:

D (killed intracellular bacteria) = A − C
E (phagocytosed bacteria)   = B + D

Values that exceed the control by one log or greater are abnormal.

To test for phagocytosis and bacterial killing of gram-negative organisms, antibiotics can be used to eliminate extracellular bacteria. For example, to test for *Escherichia coli* phagocytosis and killing, gentamicin can be used. Antibiotic concentration five times higher than the minimum inhibitory concentration (MIC) for the strain of the organism is used in step 4, so that during the lysis procedure the 1:10 dilution of the mixture (0.2 ml to 2 ml) with distilled water will sufficiently lower the antibiotic concentration below the MIC.

MONOCYTE FUNCTION TEST

The preceding paragraphs have discussed testing of polymorphonuclear cell function. With few modifications the same techniques can be applied for monocytes. Monocytes are generally more adherent than polymorphonuclear cells so that testing monocyte adherence requires lowering the amount of nylon fibers, for example, from 40 to 30 mg per column.

For testing monocyte locomotion, these modifications are necessary: (1) use micropore filters of 8 μm porosity, (2) use specific chemotactic factor for monocyte response, since monocytes do not usually respond to most *E. coli*-derived chemotactic factors, and (3) incubate the chamber for three hours. For screening purposes, testing non-stimulated migration and chemotactic responsiveness is all that is necessary.

Increasing the incubation time of the cell-immune precipitate mixture to 60 minutes is the only modification necessary when testing monocyte phagocytosis using the radioassay method, but the values are generally lower than those obtained for polymorphonuclear cells. NBT reduction by monocytes is also lower and slower. The incubation period of the cell-opsonized zymosan mixture is extended to 60 minutes. The amount of formazan extracted is consistently four to six times less than that obtained in the same number of polymorphonuclear cells incubated for the same period of time. Increasing zymosan or NBT dye concentration does not significantly increase NBT reduction.

Comparative studies between the bactericidal powers of monocytes and polymorphonuclear cells have been reported (Steigbigel, 1974). In general, the former is said to be less active than the latter. No modification of the microbicidal assay is necessary when testing monocytes.

REFERENCES

Allen, R. C., Stjerholm, R. L., and Steele, R. H.: Evidence for the generation of an electronic excitation state(s) in human polymorphonuclear leukocytes and its participation in bactericidal activity. Biochem. Biophys. Res. Commun., 47:679, 1972.

Athens, J. W., Raab, S. O., Haab, O. P., Mauer, A. M., Ashenbrucker, H., Cartwright, G. E., and Winthrobe, M. M.: Leukokinetic studies. IV. The total blood, circulating, and marginating granulocyte pools and the granulocyte turnover rate in normal subjects. J. Clin. Invest., 40:989, 1961.

Baehner, R. L.: Microbe ingestion and killing by neutrophils: Normal mechanisms and abnormality. Clin. Haematol., 4:609, 1975.

Baehner, R. L., and Nathan, D. G.: Quantitative nitroblue tetrazolium test in chronic granulomatous disease. N. Engl. J. Med., 278:971, 1968.

Bagdade, J. D., and Stewart, M.: Impaired granulocyte adherence: Another defect in host defense in diabetes mellitus. Clin. Res., 24:340A, 1976.

Boyden, S.: The chemotactic effect of mixtures of antibody and antigen on polymorphonuclear leukocytes. J. Exp. Med., 115:453, 1962.

Boxer, L. A., Hedley-Whyte, E. T., and Stossel, T. P.: Neutrophil actin dysfunction and abnormal neutrophil behaviour. N. Engl. J. Med., 291:1093, 1974.

Clark, R. A.: Disorders of granulocyte chemotaxis. In Gallin, J. I., and Quie, P. G. (eds.): Leukocyte Chemotaxis. New York, Raven Press, 1978.

Cline, M. J.: The White Cell. Cambridge, Mass., Harvard University Press, 1975.

Fass, R. J., and Saslaw, S.: Earth day histoplasmosis. A new type of urban pollution. Arch. Intern. Med., 128:588, 1971.

Frei, P. C., Baisero, M. H., and Ochsner, M.: Chemotaxis of human polymorphonuclears in vitro. II. Technical study. J. Immunol. Methods, 1:165, 1974.

Gallin, J. I., Clark, R. A., and Kimball, H. R.: Granulocyte chemotaxis. An improved in vitro assay employing ⁵¹Cr-labelled granulocytes. J. Immunol., 110:233, 1973.

Goldman, J. M., and Catovsky, D.: The function of phagocytic leukocytes in leukemia. Br. J. Haematol., 23(Suppl.):223, 1972.

Goldstein, I., Hoffstein, S., Gallin, J., and Weissmann, G.: Mechanisms of lysosomal enzyme release from human leukocytes: Microtubule assembly and membrane fusion induced by a component of complement. Proc. Natl. Acad. Sci. U.S.A., 70:2916, 1973.

Gregory, L., Williams, R., and Thompson, E.: Leukocyte function in Down's syndrome and acute leukemia. Lancet, 1:1359, 1972.

Hill, H. R., and Quie, P. G.: Defective neutrophil chemotaxis associated with hyperimmunoglobulinemia E. In Bellati, J. A., and Dayton, D. H., (eds.): The Phagocytic Cell in Host Resistance. New York, Raven Press, 1975.

Iannini, P. B., Claffey, T., and Quintiliani, R.: Bacteremic pseudomonas pneumonia. J.A.M.A., 230:558, 1974.

Kahn, A. J., Evans, H. E., Glass, L., Shin, Y. H., and Almonte, D.: Defective neutrophil chemotaxis in patients with Down's syndrome. J. Pediatr., 87:87, 1975.

Keller, H. U., Borel, J. F., Wilkinson, P. C., Hess, M. W., and Cottier, H.: Reassessment of Boyden's technique for measuring chemotaxis. J. Immunol. Methods, 1:165, 1972.

Lace, J. K., Tan, J. S., and Watanakunakorn, C.: An appraisal of the nitroblue tetrazolium reduction test. Am. J. Med., 58:685, 1975.

MacGregor, R. R.: Granulocyte adherence changes induced by hemodialysis, endotoxin, epinephrine and glucocorticoids. Ann. Intern. Med., 86:35, 1977.

MacGregor, R. R., Spagnuolo, P. J., and Lentnek, A. L.: Inhibition of granulocyte adherence by ethanol, prednisone, and aspirin, measured with an assay system. N. Engl. J. Med., 291:642, 1974.

Maderazo, E. G., Lavine, W., Stolman, J., Ward, P. A., and Cogen, R.: Early onset and recalcitrant periodontitis: Manifestation of subtle leukotactic dysfunction. Abstract 106. Proceedings 16th Interscience Conference on Antimicrobial Agents and Chemotherapy, Chicago, Illinois, Oct. 27-29, 1976.

Maderazo, E. G., Ward, P. A., Woronick, C. L., and Quintiliani, R.: Partial characterization of a cell-directed inhibitor of leukotaxis in human serum. J. Lab. Clin. Med., 89:190, 1977.

Maderazo, E. G., and Woronick, C. L.: A modified micropore filter assay of human granulocyte leukotaxis. In Gallin, J. I., and Quie, P. G. (eds.): Leukocyte Chemotaxis. New York, Raven Press, 1978.

Miller, M. E.: Neonatal immunology and related protective mechanisms. CRC Crit. Rev. Clin. Lab. Sci., 4:1, 1973.

Najjar, V. A.: Defective phagocytosis due to deficiencies involving the tetrapeptide tuftsin. J. Pediatr., 89:1121, 1975.

Oliver, J. M.: Impaired microtubule function correctable by cyclic GMP and cholinergic agonists in the Chediak-Higashi syndrome. Am. J. Pathol., 85:395, 1976.

Quie, P. G.: Disorders of phagocyte function. Biochemical aspects. In Greenwalt, T. J., and Jamieson, G. A. (eds.): Progress in Clinical and Biological Research, Vol. 13. New York, Alan R. Liss, Inc., 1977.

Quie, P. G.: Pathology of bactericidal power of neutrophils. Semin. Hematol., 12:153, 1975.

4

Rebuck, J. W., and Crowley, J. H.: Method of studying leukocyte function in vivo. Ann. N.Y. Acad. Sci., 59:757, 1955.

Rinehart, J. J., and Boulware, T.: Microfilament and microtubule function in human monocytes. J. Lab. Clin. Med., 90:737, 1977.

Rosner, F., Kozinn, P. J., and Jervis, G. A.: Leukocyte function and serum immunoglobulins in Down's syndrome. N.Y. State J. Med., 73:672, 1973.

Ruley, E. J., Huang, S. W., Plaut, J., and Morris, N.: Defective phagocyte adherence in acute poststreptococcal glomerulonephritis. Clinical and laboratory observation. J. Pediatr., 89:748, 1976.

Seklecki, M. M., Quintiliani, R., Maderazo, E. G.: Aminoglycoside antibiotics moderately impair granulocyte function. Antimicrob. Agents Chemother., 13:552, 1978.

Snyderman, R., and Pike, M. C.: An inhibitor of macrophage chemotaxis produced by neoplasms. Science, 192:370, 1976.

Spitznagel, J. K.: Bactericidal mechanisms of the granulocyte. In Greenwalt, T. J., and Jamieson, G. A. (eds.): Progress in Clinical and Biological Research, Vol. 13. New York, Alan R. Liss, Inc., 1977.

Steigbigel, R. T., Lambert, L. H., Jr., and Remington, J. S.: Phagocytic and bactericidal properties of normal human monocytes. J. Clin. Invest., 53:131, 1974.

Stossel, T. P.: Phagocytosis: Clinical disorders of recognition and ingestion. Am. J. Pathol., 88:741, 1977.

Stossel, T. P.: The mechanism of leukocyte locomotion. In Gallin, J. I., and Quie, P. G. (eds.): Leukocyte Chemotaxis. New York, Raven Press, 1978.

Tan, J. S., Watanakunakorn, C., and Phair, J. P.: A modified assay of neutrophil function. Use of lysostaphin to differentiate defective phagocytosis from impaired intracellular killing. J. Lab. Clin. Med., 78:316, 1971.

Van Epps, D. E., and Williams, R. C., Jr.: Suppression of leukocyte chemotaxis by human IgA myeloma components. J. Exp. Med., 144:1227, 1976.

Ward, P. A.: Leukotaxis and leukotactic disorders. A review. Am. J. Pathol., 77:520, 1974.

Ward, P. A., and Zvaifler, N. J.: Quantitative phagocytosis by neutrophils. I. A method with immune complexes. J. Immunol., 111:1771, 1973.

Ward, P. A., Lepow, I. H., and Newman, L. J.: Bacterial factors chemotactic for polymorphonuclear leukocytes. Am. J. Pathol., 52:725, 1968.

Winkelstein, J. A.: Opsonins: Their function, identity and clinical significance. J. Pediatr., 82:747, 1973.

Zigmond, S. H., and Hirsch, J. G.: Leucocyte locomotion and chemotaxis. New methods for evaluation and demonstration of a cell derived chemotactic factor. J. Exp. Med., 137:387, 1973.

41

HLA

The Major Histocompatibility Complex

William C. DeWolf, M.D.,
William G. Cannady, and
Edmond J. Yunis, M.D.

4

The human immune system is a complex array of interconnecting checks and balances with amplifying and suppressing systems, much the same as many of the endocrine organs in the body. This concept had not been appreciated until recently when two facts became apparent:

1. The immune system is made up of many subpopulations of lymphocytes such as responder, helper, suppressor, and effector cells with specific functions.

2. Many (and maybe all) of these cells are under the genetic control of loci within the major histocompatibility complex.

Much of the immune dynamics is understood in the mouse histocompatibility system (H-2); however, much less is known of the human major histocompatibility complex (HLA). Currently, great effort is being made to further unravel the HLA complex in order to gain a better understanding of cell-cell interaction, immune function, and immune response, especially as it applies to transplantation, cancer, development, and disease susceptibility. Appreciation of the basic concepts of immunogenetics, then, is desirable in developing a proper understanding of the etiology, pathogenesis, and possible therapy of many human disease states.

This work was supported by NIH Grant Nos. CA 20531 and CA 19589.

Mouse H-2 Complex – Chromosome 17

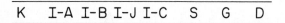

K	I-A	I-B	I-J	I-C	S	G	D

Figure 41–1. Schematic diagram of the mouse MHC region (Benacerraf, 1977). The K and D regions code for antigens stimulating tissue rejection and specific cytolytic T-cells. The S region codes for complement factors and the I region codes for various aspects of immune responsiveness. The G locus codes for an erythrocyte antigen.

BRIEF HISTORY

The origin of immunogenetics as it relates to histocompatibility closely parallels the first scientific realization of the fundamental rule of transplantation, namely, autografts taken from and returned to the same donor succeed, while grafts between two genetically dissimilar individuals fail. This understanding was advanced by the development of inbred strains of laboratory animals; one of the first experiments that established the basic principles of transplantation was performed in inbred strains of mice by Little (1916). He demonstrated that skin grafts *within* inbred strains were successful, while grafts *between* inbred strains (allografts) were not; grafts from either parent strain to first generation (F_1) hybrids grew in all animals; likewise, skin grafts from second generation (F_2) animals or subsequent generations survived on F_1 animals. These and other studies showed that acceptance of allografts depends on common factors (transplantation antigens) between the donor and recipient, which were determined by independent genes. Accordingly, if the combination of factors present in the allograft did not match those of the host, the allograft would not survive.

In 1938 Gorer established that the allograft reaction in the mouse was related to the degree of histocompatibility of alloantigens detected by serologic methods. Snell (1948) named the genes determining the fate of allografts "histocompatibility" or "H" genes, and firmly established the genetic basis of histocompatibility. The second serologic specificity to be studied in any detail, H-2, became the major system in the mouse; thus, today H-2 refers to the major histocompatibility complex (MHC) in the mouse, specifically referring to a small segment on the mouse chromosome 17 carrying genes controlling transplantation antigens, as well as other genes, currently under extensive study, which play an important role in immune regulation (Fig. 41-1).

Genetic analysis in man, as in the mouse, has led to the conclusion that one principal genetic system controls transplantation antigens as well as other important immune functions. This region, known to be the short arm of chromosome 6, is called the HLA complex. It is the major histocompatibility complex (MHC) of man corresponding to H-2 in the mouse (Fig. 41-2).

The discovery of the HLA system was, in fact, done independently of research on the mouse system. Between 1920 and 1950 several publications appeared attempting to demonstrate the existence of antileukocyte activity in the blood of leukopenic patients; from that effort, Dausset (1952) described the existence of antileukocyte antibodies. Shortly thereafter, Dausset (1954) suggested that they may be allospecific, i.e., the antibodies reacted with small number of group O unrelated individuals. A systematic study was then begun to

HLA–Complex – Chromosome 6 (Short arm)

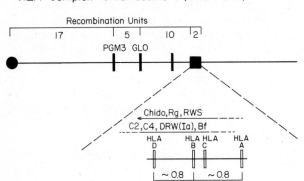

Figure 41–2. Schematic summary of the human MHC region on chromosome 6. HLA-A, B, C, and D loci are shown. GLO (glyoxylase) and PGM_3 (phosphoglucomutase-3) lie to the left of HLA. The Chido locus, the Rodgers (Rg) locus, and the locus controlling susceptibility to ragweed antigen (RWS) are also somewhere to the left of HLA. Bf codes for factor B of the properdin system and C2 and C4 for complement factors. DRw codes for HLA-D related antigens similar to the mouse Ia (immune response associated) antigens.

Table 41–1.   NOMENCLATURE FOR FACTORS OF THE HLA SYSTEM

LOCUS A	LOCUS B		LOCUS C
A1	B5*		CW1
A2	B7†		CW2
A3	B8†		CW3
A9	B12*†		CW4
A10	B13*		CW5
A11			CW6
A25(10)	B14 ⟨ 14.1*	
A26(10)	⟨ 14.2†	
A28	15.1†	
A29	B15 ⟨		**LOCUS D**
AW19	⟨ 15.2*		DW1
AW23(9)	Long*		DW2
AW24(9)	B17 ⟨		DW3
AW30	⟨ Short†		DW4
AW31	B18†		DW5
AW32	B27*		DW6
AW33	B37*		DW7
AW34	B40		DW8
AW36	BW16*†		DW9
AW43	BW21*†		DW10
	22.1†		DW11
	BW22 ⟨	
LOCUS B	⟨ 22.2*	
BW4*(4a)	BW35†		**LOCUS DR**
BW6†(4b)	BW38*(16)		DRW1
	BW39†(16)		DRW2
	BW41†		DRW3
	BW42†		DRW4
	BW44*(12)		DRW5
	BW45†(12)		DRW6
	BW46		DRW7
	BW47†	
	BW48	
	BW49*(21)	
	BW50†(21)	
	BW51*(5)	
	BW52*(5)	
	BW53†	
	BW54(22)	

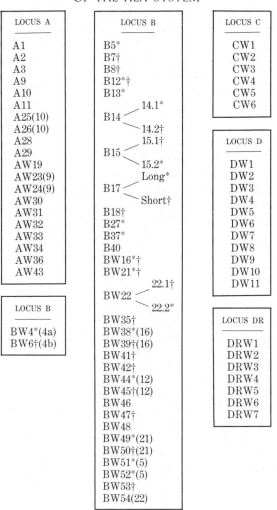

The numbers in parentheses represent previous assignments. Most HLA-B locus antigens can be further typed by their reactivity with HLA-BW4 and HLA-BW6 antisera indicated by * or †.

investigate antibodies that developed after blood transfusion (Payne, 1957), and the first HLA leukocyte specificity—Mac—was then detected using six sera that reacted in a similar but not identical way (Dausset, 1958). The importance of such a finding was immediately recognized because Amos (1953) had proved that H-2 antigens (transplantation antigens) could be detected on mouse leukocytes by leukoagglutination. From then on knowledge concerning the HLA complex accumulated rapidly: van Rood (1958) and Payne (1958) independently discovered antileukocyte antibodies in the sera of multiparous women; shortly thereafter, Payne (1964) described two specificities in a first or LA series, LA1 and LA2 (identical to Mac) which behaved in the population and segregated in families like alleles. Since that time the definition of the HLA complex has grown to what it is today through intense international collaboration involving exchange of sera and cells, so as to combine the increasing amount of information from many laboratories throughout the world into one understandable system (Table 41–1).

PRINCIPLES OF IMMUNOGENETICS APPLIED TO A SINGLE SYSTEM

BASIC GENETICS

In man there are 46 chromosomes made up of 23 pairs; 22 pairs are autosomal chromosomes and one pair is sex chromosomes. The chromosomes of each pair are called homologous chromosomes because the genetic information on each of the two concerns itself with the same phenotypic trait. The region of the chromosome associated with that given trait is called a *locus* and the genetic material at that locus is referred to as a *gene* or *allele*. The term allele is usually used when referring to alternate forms of the gene expressed at that locus, i.e., at the locus determining eye color, there may be a "blue" allele or "brown" allele. An individual who has the same gene or allele at a given locus on both homologous chromosomes is said to be *homozygous* at that locus. On the other hand, when the two alleles are not the same, the individual is *heterozygous;* if both genes in a heterozygous individual are expressed, they are said to be codominant. *Polymorphism* refers to the possible existence of more than one allele at a given locus (for instance, HLA is a highly polymorphic system). Inheritance of alleles involves *segregation,* which refers to the distribution of alleles among offspring. For instance, consider a single genetic locus at which both father and mother are heterozygous (Fig. 41–3). If the father's two alleles are labelled *a* and *b* and the mother's *c* and *d*, then there are four genotypes possible for offspring, i.e.: *ac, ad, bc,* and *bd.* If inheritance is random, then the different genotypes should be present in equal numbers. The chances of one sibling within a family being identical to another is 25 per cent, be-

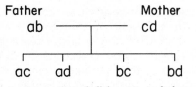

Figure 41–3. Segregation of alleles at a single locus.

cause there are only four possible genotypes. The chance of being identical at one allele only (haploidentical) is 50 per cent, and the chance of being a total mismatch is 25 per cent.

During meiosis, homologous chromosomes pair prior to reduction of the number of chromosomes from 46 (the diploid number) to 23 (the haploid number). It is then possible for recombination to occur, at which time homologous regions of the paired chromosomes exchange genetic material by breakage at corresponding positions and reunion to the non-sister chromosome—commonly known as "crossing over" (Fig. 41-4). The frequency of recombination between two loci is proportional to the distance separating the loci. Loci close together will usually segregate as a unit, and are said to be linked; two loci relatively far apart on a chromosome may show independent assortment.

THE GENETICS OF HLA

The major histocompatibility complex is a small chromosomal region within the genetic makeup of all vertebrates studied thus far; it plays an important role in the expression of transplantation antigens, as well as other associated biologic phenomena such as immune responsiveness, development, and susceptibility to disease. In the mouse, the MHC is located on chromosome 17 (Fig. 41-1) and is called H-2 (Klein, 1975); in the human, the MHC is on the short arm of chromosome 6 (Francke, 1977) (Fig. 41-2) and is called HLA. All nucleated cells have HLA antigens on their cell surface with the possible exception of the trophoblast (Amos, 1975). This is in contrast to the ABO system which also controls strong transplantation antigens and affects graft survival. The ABO system is reviewed in Chapter 43.

Following the 1975 International Histocompatibility Workshop, the World Health Organization (WHO) HLA nomenclature committee provided new terminology for all of the then known 45 HLA-A, -B, and -C antigens and the first 6 HLA-D antigens. An updated summary from the 1977 International Histocompatibility Workshop (Bodmer, 1977a) is shown in Table 41-1. Designations with a "w" mean "workshop" (i.e., Dw3) which identifies a provisional status.

Currently four principal loci have been recognized within the HLA region (Fig. 41-2): HLA-A, HLA-B, HLA-C, and HLA-D. Other associated loci code for complement factors, properdin factor B, and red blood cell groups (Chido and Rogers) and HLA-D related (HLA-DRw) antigens. The HLA region is highly polymorphic, with several antigen specificities known for each of HLA-A (formerly the "first" or "LA" locus), HLA-B (formerly "second" or "fourth" locus), HLA-C ("third," "T," or "A-J" locus), and the HLA-D (MLR-S or LD) locus.

Within a family each child inherits one HLA chromosome or one haplotype from the mother and one from the father; a "haplotype," then,

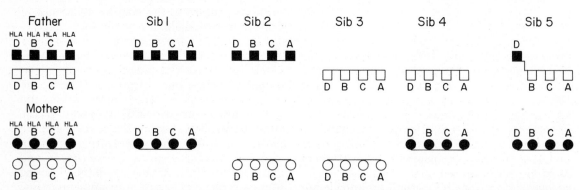

Figure 41-4. HLA haplotype segregation within a family. Sibling 5 is a recombinant between the maternal HLA-B and HLA-D loci. This means that sibling 5 is HLA-A, HLA-B, and HLA-C identical to sibling 4, yet they are reactive to each other in MLC because of non-identity at the HLA-D locus as a result of recombination.

is the genetic composition of one chromosome, and each individual has two haplotypes. Only four different HLA types are possible among children from the same family (assuming no crossovers occur) (Figs. 41–3 and 41–4) and in a family of five children at least two of them will be HLA identical. Statistically, then, 25 per cent of all siblings will be HLA-identical, 50 per cent will have one chromosome (haplotype) in common, and 25 per cent will have two chromosomes (two haplotypes) different. As mentioned, segregation of parental haplotypes usually occurs en bloc with no recombination between the HLA-A and HLA-B loci; however, approximately one gamete in 100 (0.80 per cent) shows recombination between HLA-A and HLA-B; likewise, the frequency of recombination between HLA-B and HLA-D is also 0.80 per cent. Genetic recombination can complicate histocompatibility testing between siblings, as shown in Figure 41–4; i.e., two siblings may be identical for all serologically detectable (SD) antigens (A, B, C loci), but still different at the LD (lymphocyte defined) or HLA-D locus. Thus, they will stimulate each other in mixed lymphocyte culture (MLC) assay, as between siblings 4 and 5. Conversely, there may be another sibling in the same family (such as sibling 1) who has the same HLA-D locus antigens as the sibling with the crossover, and these two siblings will be MLC non-stimulatory in spite of disparity at their HLA-A, B, and C loci.

The value of recombination studies has been enhanced by the discovery of loci closely linked to HLA (Fig. 41–2) (Bodmer, 1976; Bach, 1976a; Snell, 1976a; van Rood, 1976; McKusick, 1977). An example is phosphoglucomutase-3 (PGM-3), which is thought to lie 15 centimorgans (a relative measure of distance based on frequency of recombination between the indicated loci) to the left of HLA; likewise, other associated components of the HLA linkage group includes genes controlling the red blood cell antigens for groups P, Chido, and Rogers, and the erythrocyte isoenzyme glyoxalase I (GLO), as well as structural and regulatory genes such as factor B of the properdin system (Bf) and genes controlling synthesis of the second (C2) and fourth (C4) components of complement. In addition, genes controlling cell surface antigens which cause stimulation in MLC are located near HLA-D. Knowledge of such polymorphic loci closely located within or near the HLA region facilitates study of recombinational events. For example, an unexpected incompatibility between HLA-iden-tical siblings may be associated with a recombinational event outside the MHC, as determined by a detailed typing for some of the HLA linkage alleles. This would help define the presence and position of a yet undetected locus for a transplantation antigen. Such information is needed to explain rejection of kidney transplants between HLA-identical siblings, as well as graft-versus-host (GVH) disease after bone marrow transplantation.

Because the HLA-C and HLA-D specificities are defined in only 50 to 75 per cent of the population, and HLA-D locus typing is as yet imperfect, practical typing for transplantation purposes is basically limited to the HLA-A and HLA-B loci. Because of the limited frequency of recombination, matching for HLA-A and HLA-B *between siblings* is likely to result in matching for the HLA-C and HLA-D locus as well. This, however, does not hold true for unrelated individuals.

The distribution of HLA antigens in the population is not completely random. Genetic theory would predict that, given enough time in evolution, specific alleles of two closely linked loci, such as HLA-A and HLA-B, will be found together on the same chromosome with a frequency about equal to the product of their two independent gene frequencies. However, certain antigens from the different series are associated with each other to a greater degree than would be expected on the basis of their individual frequencies. This unusual association between alleles, more than expected, is called *linkage disequilibrium* or *gametic association*. For example, HLA-A1, B8, and Dw3 occur together on the same chromosome (haplotype) more frequently than chance would predict.

An interesting aspect of population genetics is the difference in frequency of HLA antigens among various racial groups. For example, HLA-A1 and B8 are among the most common antigens in whites, but are almost non-existent in mainland Japanese (Amos, 1975). Such genetic differences may be helpful in tracing population migration and in studying the association of HLA antigens to other traits within populations.

BIOLOGY AND NATURAL HISTORY OF HLA ANTIGENS

The HLA-A, B, and C locus gene products are found on the external cell membrane of almost all tissues except possibly early embryonic cells. The lymphocyte is the main cell of reference because it not only has a high density of surface HLA antigens, but also lends itself well to *in vitro* testing. Studies from both normal and tumor cells in culture indicate that the HLA antigens are indeed ubiquitous and are not differentiation antigens; they do not disappear from cells in continuous culture and are, therefore, a permanent part of cell membranes (Brautbar, 1973; Dausset, 1974b).

The HLA-A and -B locus antigens are glycoproteins. When solubilized with papain from cell surface membranes of lymphoblastoid cell lines, they are composed of two non-covalently bound polypeptide chains, a heavy one with a molecular weight of 33,000 daltons and a light one of 11,000 daltons. The 11,000 dalton polypeptide is identical to beta-2 microglobulin and exhibits structural homology with the $C_H{}^3$ region of the IgG heavy chain (Tanigaki, 1974). Interestingly, despite the intimate relationship of HLA and beta-2 microglobulin on the cell surface, the genetic control for the heavy chain of the HLA molecule exists on the sixth chromosome, while the control for beta-2 microglobulin comes from the fifteenth chromosome (Goodfellow, 1975).

The ubiquitous distribution of the HLA antigens implies that they have an important role in the biology of survival, but the exact nature of this role is not known. The most interesting experimental concept relevant to this problem suggests that the classic HLA-A, B, and C antigens are in some way involved in the interaction of cytotoxic T cells with their targets (Schendel, 1973; Eijsvoogel, 1973). For instance, it is known that when a responding lymphocyte population is stimulated by an allogeneic lymphocyte population, the responder cells will produce killer T cells whose targets are the HLA-A, B, and (to a lesser extent) C antigens of the original stimulator cells; in other words, these antigens are the target determinants with which cytotoxic T cells interact. The biologic role of such a system, however, was not clear until Zinkernagel (1974) provided biologic and evolutionary significance. He showed that cytotoxic spleen cells from H-2^k mice infected with lymphocytic choriomeningitis virus (LCM) will kill H-2^k fibroblasts if they are also infected with LCM virus, but not virus-infected H-2^b (or H-2^d) cells. The superscript refers to a specific genotype within the mouse H-2 system; thus, H-2^k and H-2^d are not genotypically identical, at least at the major histocompatibility complex (MHC). Thus, cytotoxic T cells are lytic only if the target to be lysed carries the specific target antigen and also the same SD antigens (SD = serologically defined antigens, equivalent to HLA-A, -B, and -C gene products in man, and K and D region gene products in the mouse) as the original stimulating cell. This experimental approach has been observed not only with virally infected cells, but also with haptens on chemically modified cells (Shearer, 1976; Shearer, 1977). In other words, the moiety recognized by the cytotoxic T cell is the modifying agent (i.e., a virus or synthetic hapten) in association with determinants (SD antigens) controlled by genes mapping in the MHC. Thus, if an individual becomes infected with an intracellular virus, the SD (serologically or serum defined) antigens on the cell surface play a role in the immune destruction of the virus.

Most of these concepts have been established in the mouse system but not in the human as yet. Further investigation, of course, will be needed to clarify whether or not the SD antigens are actually altered in the process, and their "altered self" antigens are what, in fact, the cytotoxic lymphocytes recognize; on the other hand, the possibility of dual recognition exists in which the cytotoxic lymphocyte recognizes both the SD antigen and the modifying agent (i.e., virus or chemical). This approach presents a logical purpose for the polymorphic and genetic restrictions found in the HLA system; however, much more is needed before a definite understanding is made of the biologic role of HLA.

TECHNIQUES FOR DETECTING HLA ANTIGENS*

Further consideration of the immunogenetics of the HLA system requires knowledge of the two basic methods of assay for HLA disparity: (a) *serologic methods* in which antisera are used to detect cell surface antigens (also called serologically defined or SD antigens), and (b) lymphocyte reactivity in *mixed lymphocyte culture* (MLC) in which cell surface differences are measured by the proliferative response of co-cultured lymphocytes (these structures are sometimes referred to as lymphocyte defined or LD, antigens). In general, the HLA-A, -B, and -C determinants are primarily measured by serologic techniques, and are thus SD antigens, and the HLA-D

---

*Details of methods described by Terasaki (1978).

Figure 41–5.   HLA cross-reactive groups (CREG).

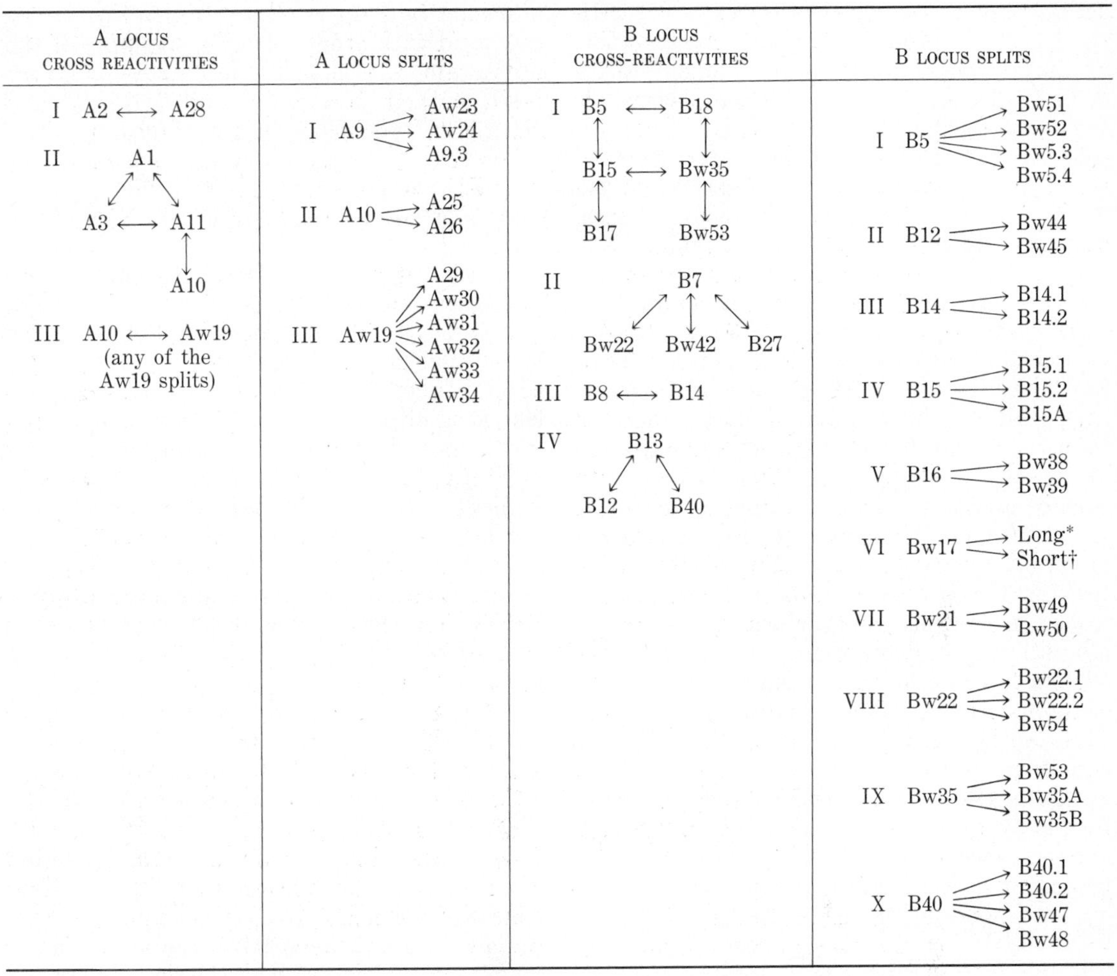

A LOCUS CROSS REACTIVITIES	A LOCUS SPLITS	B LOCUS CROSS-REACTIVITIES	B LOCUS SPLITS
I A2 ⟷ A28 II A1 A3 ⟷ A11 A10 III A10 ⟷ Aw19 (any of the Aw19 splits)	I A9 ⟹ Aw23, Aw24, A9.3 II A10 ⟹ A25, A26 III Aw19 ⟹ A29, Aw30, Aw31, Aw32, Aw33, Aw34	I B5 ⟷ B18 B15 ⟷ Bw35 B17 Bw53 II B7 Bw22 Bw42 B27 III B8 ⟷ B14 IV B13 B12 B40	I B5 ⟹ Bw51, Bw52, Bw5.3, Bw5.4 II B12 ⟹ Bw44, Bw45 III B14 ⟹ B14.1, B14.2 IV B15 ⟹ B15.1, B15.2, B15A V B16 ⟹ Bw38, Bw39 VI Bw17 ⟹ Long*, Short† VII Bw21 ⟹ Bw49, Bw50 VIII Bw22 ⟹ Bw22.1, Bw22.2, Bw54 IX Bw35 ⟹ Bw53, Bw35A, Bw35B X B40 ⟹ B40.1, B40.2, Bw47, Bw48

*Included in Bw4. †Included in Bw6.

locus is measured by methods comparing reactivity in MLC reactions and is considered an LD, or "lymphocyte defined," determinant (Bach, 1976a).

Histocompatibility testing for SD antigens (HLA-A, B, C) is performed by microcytotoxicity methods in which target lymphocytes are incubated with an antiserum and complement. If the lymphocytes carry a cell surface antigen recognized by cytotoxic antibodies in the antiserum, the lymphocytes are lysed. Cellular death is seen by changes in the permeability of the cell membrane as evidenced by the penetration of dyes such as trypan blue or eosin Y, or changes in vital staining by fluorochrome. Current methods include the standard NIH lymphocytotoxicity procedure and the Amos modified procedure (Cannady, 1978b). The NIH standard lymphocytotoxicity assay uses a 30-minute lymphocyte antiserum incubation followed by an additional 60-minute complement incubation period. The entire assay is performed at room temperature. The Amos modified lymphocytotoxicity assay is considered more sensitive and differs from the NIH method in two basic ways. First, the procedure is not performed at room temperature, but rather at 37°C., and second, the antiserum is washed out of the reaction well before complement is added in an attempt to remove any anticomplementary activity that may be present in the antiserum.

Approximately 95 per cent of laboratories performing HLA typing in the United States use the NIH standard technique. Although this assay is less sensitive than the Amos modified method, it is perhaps better suited for routine typing; highly sensitive assays may produce false positive reactions for two reasons: (1) most HLA typing sera contain multiple antibodies at various levels of potency, and on many occasions, using a very sensitive test, may produce false positive reactions from an otherwise monospecific antiserum; (2) there are several crossreactive groups of HLA antigens (i.e., 2-28, 7-W42-W22, 1-3-11, etc.) and an operationally monospecific antiserum, such as anti-B7, in a very sensitive procedure may exhibit a positive reaction with Bw22 cells (Fig. 41-5). While the Amos modified procedure may, in some cases, be too sensitive for routine HLA typing, it is very useful in antibody detection (screening) and crossmatching (compatibility testing).

All lymphocytotoxicity procedures involve complement fixation, which can create a potential source of error in laboratory diagnosis. The most common source of complement is rabbit serum, but there are no standards on age, pool size, or potency. Therefore, quality control procedures by individual laboratories are of primary importance in the preparation of rabbit complement for lymphocytotoxicity testing. Cross-reactivity, as previously mentioned, represents another possible source of laboratory error. This occurs because the HLA system is so highly polymorphic that certain antigens have similar chemical composition. Thus, antibodies directed against specific antigens may crossreact with closely associated antigens (Fig. 41-5). Problems with crossreactivity have become more frequent with the increased sensitivity of HLA-A, B, and C typing procedures. For example, a serum that appears monospecific for the antigen HLA-B5 in the NIH standard HLA procedure may exhibit B5, B18, or Bw35 specificity when used in the Amos modified procedure for HLA typing. This is a major problem in exchanging HLA typing sera when the laboratories are using different typing techniques.

Sometime during HLA typing, an individual may react negatively with a specific antiserum (i.e., anti-B27) and later is shown to be capable of absorbing that antibody from the B27 antiserum. The behavior is referred to as cytotoxicity negative-absorption positive (CYNAP) (van Rood, 1961). The mechanism of this phenomenon is not completely understood, but in some instances it may be attributed to a lack of sensitivity of the typing technique, as might occur with weak typing sera. Occasionally, an HLA typing serum may give a positive reaction only when the test lymphocytes are homozygous for that specific antigen. For these reasons, all HLA typing reagents should be classified as operationally monospecific, as opposed to truly monospecific, because their "monospecific" classification depends on the technique used as well as the dilutions and on whether the antiserum is absorbed with other cells. For example, if the antiserum is a monospecific HLA-A2 in the NIH method, it may exhibit HLA-A2 and HLA-A28 specificity in the Amos modified procedure, or, if an antiserum is a monospecific HLA-A2 in the Amos modified assay, it may be a "short" HLA-A2 by the NIH procedure.

In 1963 van Rood described two determinants, 4a and 4b, which behaved like alleles (Table 41-1). Subsequent testing has proved these specificities to be broad reacting, i.e., several narrower HLA specificities are included in either 4a or 4b. The exact definition of 4a and 4b has been difficult because the antisera that recognize them have not been homogeneous, i.e., their monospecificity has not been established. Recently, however, reagents have improved to the extent that these determinants have been renamed according to WHO nomenclature as HLA-Bw4 (4a) and HLA-Bw6 (4b) (Bodmer, 1977b). Antisera to these determinants are unique because they are "broad reactors" and will react with other specific HLA-B locus determinants to help in their identification (Table 41-1). For example, HLA-B14 may be split into HLA-B14.1 or HLA-B14.2 depending on the reactivity with HLA-Bw4 and HLA-Bw6 antisera. This kind of "cautious" identification of HLA-B locus splits and other HLA-B locus antigens may be important for proper HLA typing in organ transplantation as well as platelet and granulocyte transfusion therapy using unrelated donors.

The procurement of HLA antisera presents an interesting problem because "natural" HLA antibodies do not exist. Sera from nontransfused individuals do not contain this kind of antibody; however, anti-HLA antibodies are frequent in women immunized by pregnancy and occur in about 20 per cent of the cases, depending on factors such as number of births and the degree of genetic disparity between the mother and fetus. The persistence of antibodies in the maternal serum is quite variable but usually lasts only a few months (van Rood, 1961). Immunization by transfusion is also quite frequent and usually depends on the number of transfusions and the HLA types with which the patient is transfused. A third method involving planned immunization has been used primarily outside of the United States (Ferrara, 1975). Healthy volunteers are immunized after taking all possible medical and ethical precautions. The best results have been obtained from immunizations between related individuals differing by only one HLA haplotype or, ideally, by a single HLA antigen, so as to produce the most specific immunization.

In contrast to the preceding review of serologic histocompatibility typing, mixed lymphocyte culture (MLC) matching involves a different principle based on the observations of Bain (1964) and Bach (1964). They noted that when two allogeneic lymphocyte populations are cultured together, the lymphocytes undergo very definite morphologic alterations: the nucleus increases in volume, mitoses occur, and the cells take on the appearance of immature blast cells. The reaction was first established so that the two lymphocyte populations responded to each other (two-way MLC). It was later discovered that treatment with mitomycin C or x-ray could eliminate the ability of a lymphocyte to respond, yet still allow it to stimulate; thus the one-way (unidirectional) MLC was originated in which peripheral blood lymphocytes of one individual (responding cells of a potential recipient) enlarge and divide in response to foreign antigens on the stimulating cells of a second individual (the potential donor) (Bach, 1966). The response to stimulation is measured by the cellular incorporation of radioactive thymidine (^{3}HTdR) added to the system for a matter of hours on the fifth or sixth day of culture. The test, then, measures the capability of the recipient to respond to antigens of the donor.

The primary clinical use of the MLC has been in the selection of compatible donors for transplantation. There has been a good correlation between graft survival and a negative or weak MLC between donor and recipient pairs, especially within families (Thompson, 1977; Bach, 1976b). The standard method uses microplates (O'Leary, 1976). The equipment and supplies used must be sterile because contaminated cultures can lead to false positive or false negative results. Generally the specimen should be used within 24 hours of drawing; otherwise the cells may not stimulate and respond optimally. Lymphocytes are separated on a Ficoll-hypaque density gradient and the stimulating cell population, as previously mentioned, is inactivated with either x-irradiation or mitomycin C so as to block DNA synthesis and, thus, the incorporation of ^{3}H thymidine. The number of stimulator and responder cells per microtiter well varies from laboratory to laboratory, but in general, the most efficient number is 5×10^4 for both responders and stimulators. The plates are incubated for six days in 5 per cent CO_2 in air at 37°C. On the sixth day, the cultures are pulsed for six hours with ^{3}HTdR, and the reaction stopped by cooling to 4°C. The plates are then harvested, the cells recovered, and the amount of ^{3}HTdR incorporated into the cells is measured by scintillation counting.

Each MLC is performed in triplicate and the results can be expressed in a number of ways. The simplest method is the average counts per minute. However, this method fails to take into consideration "background" counts (as determined by autologous stimulation) and day to day variation in counts when two or more studies are being compared. A second general method is to express the response of a particular individual as a "stimulation ratio" (SR) or "stimulation index" (SI), which is the test value (an individual stimulated by another individual) divided by the autologous control (an individual stimulated by himself). This presumably will remove the error produced by "background." The disadvantage of this approach is that the maximal stimulation of each person varies and, therefore, an SR of 10 in one person may be equivalent to an SR of 100 in another. In addition, autologous stimulation in one individual can vary considerably depending on experimental conditions.

The third and perhaps best method of expressing results is to determine some reference value to which a test response can be compared. In concept if the response of cell A to stimulation by cell B is being tested, the first step would be to determine the average maximum responder ability of A. This "reference value," "100 per cent value," or "maximum response value" is best obtained either as the median response to a stimulator panel of unrelated donors or a response to a pool of unrelated donor cells. The second step is to determine the 0 per cent response value (and this should take into account all "background" activity). The best way to establish this value is to stimulate A by its own irradiated cells (autologous stimulation), and whatever value is obtained is arbitrarily called "0 per cent response." The third step is to stimulate cell A with irradiated cell B, measure the cpm, (counts per minute), and then determine its per cent response "relative" to the 100 per cent value (reference value) and the 0 per cent value (autologous value)—hence the term "relative response" or RR. This method is perhaps best because it attempts to quantitate the

4

reaction and is especially evident in intra-family MLC's, which show that all HLA-identical sibling combinations produce less than 5 per cent RR. For one haplotype difference the mean is greater than 50 per cent, and for a two haplotype difference it is approximately 100 per cent (Dupont, 1976).

The genetic control of MLC was found by Bach (1967) to be governed within the same chromosomal region as HLA; later, Yunis (1971), using recombinant families, demonstrated that the principal MLC reactivity was controlled by the HLA-D locus, which was separate and apart from the HLA-A and HLA-B locus and was outside of the HLA-B locus (Chromosome 6).

Our knowledge of the HLA-D series is still rudimentary. Although it is possible to distinguish intrafamily reactivity from non-reactivity and to separate MLC (or HLA-D) identical siblings from non-identical ones, the circumstances become much less defined when dealing with unrelated people. In all probability the HLA-D region is highly polymorphic, with several yet undefined subloci. This hypothesis is compatible with the fact that negative reactions are rare among unrelated individuals (1/10,000) (Snell, 1976b) and that there appears to be a weaker MLC locus near HLA-A (Dupont, 1974). Some intrafamily studies have indicated that there may be several loci controlling MLC reactivity; whether or not this is a result of a few highly polymorphic genes or several less polymorphic genes is not really known (Bach, 1975).

Because of these problems associated with imperfect definition of the gene products of HLA-D (due to the lack of antibodies whose action was strictly associated with MLR), histocompatibility testing for HLA-D has not been as exact as that for SD antigens. One approach to HLA-D typing makes use of the MLC itself, in which the stimulating cells are homozygous for a known D locus specificity (HTC or homozygous typing cells). These cells are found in those families in which the parents possess a common HLA-D haplotype, both of which are passed on to a child, who then becomes homozygous for that D locus antigen. The best cells of genetic purity are from those homozygous individuals who are products of first cousin marriages. These HTC's (homozygous typing cells) can subsequently be used as "reagents" much the same way as a test serum is used. The principle of HLA-D typing with HTC's is that a responding cell, which is the cell to be tested (or the

patient's cell), will not respond to stimulation by an HTC in MLC if the responding cell shares an HLA-D locus specificity with the stimulating HTC. In contrast to typing for SD antigens, which utilizes the principle of a positive antibody-complement lysis response, a positive typing result with the HTC method is defined as the lack of response on the part of a responder cell to stimulation by a homozygous typing cell. Using this technique 11 HLA-D specificities (Table 41-1) have been identified (HLA-Dw1 to HLA-Dw11), all of which continue to retain "workshop" or provisional status because of several basic practical difficulties leading to inconsistencies with this cell-typing technique. The first inconsistency is that stimulation by an HTC is usually not an "all or none" phenomenon, and a responding cell may give a partial or "intermediate" response. A second difficulty relates to the many variables of the procedure that are not completely controlled; examples are: (a) the metabolic status of responding cells, (b) the metabolic status of stimulating cells, and (c) the various day-to-day technical factors concerning the actual performance of the test, all of which are important in regulation of MLC response. These first two difficulties are concerned with the meaning of the term "lack of response" or, in other words, the major difficulty in interpretation of the results concerns the clear definition and separation of *negative* typing response from *positive* responses. The problem has been partially solved by the use of various statistical approaches. If the MLC response of a patient's responding cell to stimulation by a homozygous typing cell is less than 35 per cent of the response to stimulation by a reference pool (i.e., relative response), then that responder is said to give a "typing response" to the HTC, and thus the two cells share the HLA-D determinant specific to the HTC. This method has been derived from other studies of clustering and typing analysis which show that values of RR between 0 and 35 per cent with some HTC are within the 99 per cent confidence level of being a typing response; thus, the 35 per cent cutoff point was established (Yunis, 1975).

The third problem with the HTC method is that the reagents, in this case homozygous typing cells, are not of genetic uniformity. For instance, it is possible for two homozygous typing cells of the same specificity to elicit a strong MLC between each other; this problem is also evidenced when one considers that two typing cells of the same Dw group give different answers when typing a panel of unknown individuals. As yet there is no proven explanation for this phenomenon.

Another approach for detecting and typing for the HLA-D locus specificity is to use the *primed lymphocyte typing* test (PLT). This test is based on the concept that responding cells stimulated in MLC and left in culture for 10 to 14 days (beyond their peak proliferative activity) will give an accelerated proliferative response (secondary response) if restimulated with cells that share the HLA-D allele with the original stimulating donor (Fradelizi, 1975; Sheehy, 1975; Mawas, 1975). Although this test is of significant experimental value in the sense that it has the potential to "trace" a given antigen through different genetic populations, its use as a clinical tool is as yet reserved because of inconsistencies involving false positive and false negative results and, in general, incomplete understanding of all the variables and specificities responsible for a proper PLT response (Bach, 1975; Wank, 1977; Reinsmoen, 1977).

HLA-D RELATED (DRW) B-LYMPHOCYTE ALLOANTIGENS

In addition to the classic serologically defined HLA-A, B, and C locus antigens, another series of cell surface histocompatibility alloantigens has recently been identified. These are expressed predominantly on B-lymphocytes although they are also found on monocytes (Winchester, 1975; Ting, 1976; Stasny, 1977). They are structurally different from the HLA-A, B, and C antigens and made of sialoglycoprotein subunits of molecular weight 29,000 and 34,000 when prepared from detergent-solubilized lymphoblastoid cell lines (p29, 34) (Springer, 1977) or molecular weight 23,000 and 30,000 when prepared from papain-solubilized lymphoblastoid cell lines (p23, 30) (Humphreys, 1976; Schlossman, 1976). This new antigen system is controlled by one and possibly two loci within the HLA region (Mann, 1976). One of these loci is either identical to or in strong linkage disequilibrium with the HLA-D locus; therefore, these alloantigens have been termed DRw (for D related) antigens (Bodmer, 1977b). Thus far seven such antigens have been identified and occur in strong linkage disequilibrium with the corresponding first seven HLA-D specificities (Bodmer, 1977a); i.e., DRw7 is found with HLA-Dw7, etc. Because they still have provi-

sional status, they are termed DRw1-DRw7 (Table 41-1). It is generally agreed that these HLA-D related alloantigens are responsible for most of the stimulating capacity of a cell in MLC (Cresswell, 1975). Therefore, a logical association between HLA-D, as identified by the homozygous typing cell MLC method, and DRw antigens, as identified by dye exclusion cytotoxicity assay, can be made. This association, however, is as yet incompletely understood because DRw antisera are not monospecific and therefore the inhibiting capacity can be broad (Greenberg, 1975). Analogy has been drawn between the DRw antigens and the Ia (immune response associated) antigens in the mouse H-2 system. Control of the many known mouse Ia antigens is from one or more subregions within the I region (Fig. 41-1) of the mouse MHC, and the presence of their gene products on specific subpopulations of lymphocytes has been associated with specific aspects of immune function, such as stimulation in MLC (similar to the DRw1 antigens), suppression, and transfer of information from macrophage to T cell (Schreffler, 1975; Benacerraf, 1972; Murphy, 1976; Thomas, 1977b). The identification of the B cell alloantigen system (DRw antigen) represents the first indentification of antigenic determinants associated with the HLA-D locus as defined by MLC reactivity (Terasaki, 1978).

The antibodies against the DRw antigens are obtained mainly from sera of pregnant women in much the same way that HLA-A, B, and C antisera are obtained, except that the sera must be absorbed with platelets (which are DRw-antigen-negative) to remove any anti-HLA-A, B, or C activity. Anti-DRw activity has always been present in some of the pregnancy antisera but was not identified for a long time because its reaction was weak and poorly reproducible. The reason, of course, was the fact that they reacted only against B-lymphocytes, which ordinarily account for only up to 20 per cent of the peripheral lymphocyte pool. Therefore B cell enriched target population is used when screening sera for the presence of anti-DRw antigen activity as well as for typing lymphocytes for DRw antigen. B cell enrichment can be done by methods utilizing nylon wool (Julius, 1974), rosetting (Weiner, 1973), or anti-F(ab)₂ columns (Chess, 1976), or by using other sources of cells which are predominantly of B cell type, such as lymphocytes from patients with chronic lymphocytic leukemia (CLL) (Chapel, 1977; Gossett, 1977).

Further definition of the HLA-D region will probably reveal the presence of other loci, including immune response loci involved in T- and B-lymphocyte cooperation, and both regulation of help and suppression of the immune response. The observation of reactivity of activated T-lymphocytes with anti-Ia-like antibodies is an important step in that direction (Evans, 1977). Therefore, a more complete definition of the HLA system may then provide a direct pathway to understanding the pathogenesis of many disease states, i.e., as may occur through altered expression of immune response genes or through defective elimination of foreign agents as self-altered antigens.

CLINICAL TRANSPLANTATION

Organ transplantation represents one of the largest frontiers open to medical science, and its essence rests in the field of immunogenetics. Kidney transplantation is a routine procedure in many institutions, with almost 20,000 recorded by the transplant registry (Thirteenth Report, 1977). Bone marrow, heart, liver, and pancreas transplants are also a reality but not yet adaptable to widespread use. The success of these transplants is, in part, a result of immunosuppressive therapy but for the most part depends on the degree of histocompatibility, or tissue matching, between donor and recipient.

RENAL TRANSPLANTATION

Early Genetic Studies. The direct proof that HLA-A, B, and C antigens are important to allotransplantation comes from the observation that allografts are rejected in an accelerated manner when transplantation is performed in the presence of alloantibody specific to antigens of the donor. This, of course, occurs when the donor possesses antigens that are absent on the recipient. The best early demonstration of this phenomenon made use of skin grafts. One such study was by Amos (1969), who showed that HLA disparity within a family as measured by no-haplotype, one-haplotype, or two-haplotype differences has a quantitative effect on survival of skin grafts transplanted within the family. His results demonstrated a mean survival time of 24.9 ± 1.1 days (N = 43) for HLA seroidentical siblings, 14.4 ± 0.3 days (N = 115) for one

haplotype identity, and a mean survival of 11.6 ± 0.5 days (N = 18) for two-haplotype different combinations. Similar skin grafting experiments were also performed across ABO incompatibilities. These demonstrated acceleration of rejection in group O recipients grafted with skin from group A donors as compared with grafts from group O donors (Cepellini, 1969; Rappaport, 1968).

The actual matching of donor and recipient in renal transplantation is commonly expressed by determining the antigens on the recipient and donor cells and "matching" the number of identical antigens. The criteria for an A, B, C, D, or F match as outlined by Terasaki are (Opelz, 1974):

A = no antigen difference

B = no donor antigen mismatched, but not all antigens detected on donor

C = one donor antigen mismatched

D = two donor antigens mismatched

E = three or four antigens mismatched

F = positive crossmatch with donor or ABO incompatibility

This classification refers only to matching between HLA-A and B antigens and is thus becoming somewhat antiquated with the ever-expanding definition of the HLA complex.

The Significance of Antigen Matching. Although the role of HLA in renal transplantation between related individuals is undisputed, the results of matching for HLA-A and HLA-B phenotypes on cadaver (unrelated) transplant survival is not so clear, especially when large groups of transplants are studied. The matching correlations reported in recent surveys range from good in France and England (Dausset, 1974a), to moderate in Scandinavia (Scandia Transplant Report, 1975), to weak in North America (Opelz, 1974), to none at all in San Francisco (Belzer, 1974). However, one of the largest well-controlled cadaver transplant studies from Minnesota shows a definite positive correlation between patient and kidney survival and HLA matching between donor and recipient (Simmons, 1977). The effects of HLA matching on renal transplantation, of course, are much more evident following living related donor (LRD) transplants; in a recent study from over 100 North American transplant centers by the UCLA (University of California at Los Angeles) transplant registry, correlation between haplotype identity and transplant survival was confirmed (Opelz, 1977a). The two-year graft survival between HLA-identical siblings was

80 ± 2 S.E. per cent, while the two-year graft survival between parent and child was 61 ± 1 S.E. per cent; in the same series the two-year cadaver graft survival (0 haplotype identity) was 41 ± 1 S.E. per cent.

Although it is known that the HLA complex has a central role in transplant success, correlation of transplant survival with numbers of incompatible HLA-A or B antigens is not clear cut; hence, investigation next turned to the effect of the HLA-D locus, governing MLC reactivity, on transplant survival. Skin graft prognosis correlates with MLC activity. The lower the MLC activity, the better the prognosis (Hamburger, 1971). Kidney transplant studies with MLC reactivity between recipient and donor also reflect these results both in humans (Cochrum, 1973) and in dogs (Westbroek, 1975). In general, they show that high MLC reactivity correlated with poor graft survival and low MLC reactivity with relatively good graft survival. The inherent difficulty with many of the clinical studies concerning HLA-D, however, is that it is often difficult to control for effects of HLA-A and B similarities and dissimilarities because of linkage disequilibrium between various HLA-D and HLA-B loci; also, prospective matching for the HLA-D locus has not been adequately tried in cadaver transplants for logistic reasons: MLC cultures require six days to perform, which is longer than cadaver kidneys can be preserved. However, MLC typing techniques involving PLT (which require only two to three days) are being investigated and may become clinically available in the near future. Part of the reason for any confusion that may exist regarding the degree of significance of HLA matching in renal transplantation comes from the fact that, despite our relatively advanced knowledge of the HLA linkage group, additional unknown histocompatibility loci probably exist. For example, not all transplants between HLA-identical siblings are successful; approximately 15 per cent of renal transplants between such individuals are rejected within one year (Thirteenth Report, 1977); also, skin grafts between HLA-identical siblings have a prolonged survival, but are eventually rejected (van Rood, 1966; Ceppellini, 1966), and rejection is frequent in bone marrow transplantation between HLA-identical siblings (Storb, 1977a). On the other hand, about one third of completely mismatched cadaver allografts are functioning normally at two years and are not rejected (Opelz, 1977). This information is very suggestive

that loci other than those already identified have an effect on clinical organ transplantation; whether or not they are located near the HLA linkage group on chromosome 6 is not as yet clear.

Other types of antigen matching have been investigated in an effort to improve renal allograft survival. For example, sex-associated transplantation antigens have been well-documented in mice (Galton, 1967; Hildemann, 1970) and have been shown to be of significance in bone marrow transplantation (Storb, 1977b; Bortin, 1977); however, their importance in human kidney transplants has not been demonstrated (Opelz, 1977b).

ABO blood group compatibility antigens have long been known to play an important role in clinical transplantation and should be respected as for transfusion in such a way that transplants must *not* be done with donors of an ABO group incompatible to the isoagglutinin of the recipient (Wilbrandt, 1969). Early studies suggested that O recipients tolerate their graft longer than non-O recipients (Joysey, 1973); however, more recent data from the human renal transplant registry discount this (Thirteenth Report, 1977). Other blood group antigens have also been investigated; for example, Lewis antigens are secreted in the distal convoluted and collecting tubules of the kidney and their presence appears to affect kidney graft survival (Dausset, 1977). The probability of graft survival at two years in le/le homozygous recipients (29 per cent) is much lower than that of Le recipients (58 per cent p < 0.001). Likewise, P antigens are present on leukocytes as well as red cells and, therefore, compatibility of the P system may influence successful organ transplantation. For example, skin graft survival was prolonged from 10.8 days to 12.4 days when donor and recipient were P compatible (Cepellini, 1966); P antigen compatibility may also predict better kidney graft survival (Dausset, 1968).

The HLA Crossmatch. During the early trials of renal transplantation, it became apparent that occasionally some of the grafts underwent rapid and marked rejection, often within a matter of minutes (hyperacute rejection) (Kissmeyer-Nielsen, 1966; Starzl, 1968; Patel, 1969). These were usually associated with disparities in HLA type between donor and recipient. The cause for hyperacute rejection was later associated with the presence of preformed antibody against donor antigens that the recipient had formed, presumably in response to previous polytransfusion or pregnancy. Thus, if a patient is being evaluated as a transplant recipient, his serum should be evaluated and screened for the presence of lymphocytotoxic antibodies by reacting lymphocytes from the donor with serum from the recipient. This is termed the pretransplant crossmatch; it is required of all kidney transplants, and, of course, if positive, is a contraindication to transplantation between that particular donor and recipient. The interpretation of a positive crossmatch must be viewed in light of the possible presence of non-specific autoantibodies against B-lymphocytes; they react maximally at 5°C. and are present in the serum of 20 per cent of normals (Park, 1977). Allogeneic as well as autologous B-lymphocytes may be affected and their presence (autoantibodies) may account for the weakly positive reactions that often occur in the donor-recipient crossmatch (i.e., these weak reactions probably represent the killing of donor B-lymphocytes) (Terasaki, 1978).

Patients without a living related donor (LRD) who are on dialysis awaiting a cadaver allograft to become available are of special concern and interest because they are subject to multiple transfusions, and, therefore, should be more prone to presensitization. An HLA profile is established on such patients and consists of a periodic (usually monthly) screening of the patient's serum to detect the presence of anti-HLA antibodies. The unused portion of the serum specimen should be frozen. The lymphocyte panel ideally consists of enough members, i.e., different lymphocytes, so that most, if not all HLA-A, B, and C antigens will be represented; once the panel is formed, it should remain constant for good quality control. The necessity for monthly screening is that HLA antibody specificity and titers change frequently. When a possible organ is available for transplantation, the HLA crossmatch (patient's serum and donor lymphocytes) should be performed with all of the patient's serum samples (which have previously been frozen) at a minimum of two dilutions. For patients who have been on long-term dialysis, it may be impossible to use every serum sample in the crossmatch and in such situations the most recent and the most reactive serum samples must be used for the crossmatch. Interpretation of the HLA crossmatch is an area of controversy. Originally, most crossmatches were performed using the routine microlymphocytotoxicity assay; however, several newer and more sensitive assays

have been introduced, all of which improved upon the older techniques. The antihuman globulin or AHG (Johnson, 1972) method employs an extra step to add monospecific anti-IgG following antiserum-lymphocyte incubation in order to "boost" the antibody-complement reaction. Other new tests make use of several recommendations for improving sensitivity and include (1) adding subcytotoxic doses of antilymphocyte or antithymocyte globulin (Ting, 1973); (2) using trypsin or other enzyme treatment of cells (Braun, 1972); (3) testing recipient sera in dilution because anticomplementary factor in undiluted sera can cause false negative reactions (Braun, 1976). The proper test to use largely depends on the individual laboratory and other local circumstances.

Preimmunization and Transplant Survival. There are two ways to consider the problems of preimmunization in relation to transplant survival: (1) graft survival in relation to the presence of lymphocytotoxic antibodies as determined by reactivity of recipient serum against a panel of unrelated lymphocytes at the time of transplant, and (2) graft survival in relation to recipient pretransplant transfusion history, specifically, the amount and type of blood transfused (i.e., frozen, packed, etc.).

Initial data regarding the presence of recipient lymphocytotoxic antibodies identified against a panel of cells strongly suggested a parallel between the degree of sensitization and rate of graft rejection (Clark, 1974; van Hooff, 1972); however, more recent data, contrary to expectations, do not indicate a significant difference in graft survival between those individuals sensitized and those not sensitized prior to transplant (Ferguson, 1977; Thomas, 1977b). The reason for this change of findings may be due to more sensitive crossmatch techniques, better antigen-matching techniques between donor and recipient at the time of transplantation, or perhaps to improvements in immunosuppressive treatment, thus overcoming the problems of presensitization.

Clinical trials relating the effects of multiple blood transfusion with graft survival have borne out similar findings. It is, of course, expected that patients who are transfused prior to kidney transplant become preimmunized and thus should reject their graft quicker than untransfused individuals. This is not the case, however. Several well-controlled retrospective analyses (Festenstein, 1976;

Opelz, 1973; van Hooff, 1976) and one prospective study (Opelz, 1976) provide convincing evidence that transfusions have a beneficial effect on kidney graft survival.* The mechanism by which graft survival is prolonged, however, is unknown. The most likely explanation is that it may induce enhancing (or blocking) antibodies. Transfusion of repeated small doses of HLA or related antigens could induce a state of decreased immune responsiveness. Studies of the enhancement phenomenon using skin grafts in mice and kidney grafts in rats point to the possibility that the MHC specificities against which enhancing antibodies are directed may be different from the specificities against which cytotoxic antibodies are directed. In the mouse skin graft system, antisera against all components of the MHC have some enhancing effect. However, antisera directed against the I region of the mouse H-2 complex have a far more obvious effect in prolonging incompatible skin grafts (Staines, 1977). Other studies similar in concept have been done in the rat (Soulillou, 1976).

B Cell Specific Antibodies. B cells constitute up to 20 per cent of the lymphoid population and are now known to have a specific system of alloantigens or HLA-D related (HLA-DRw) antigens. This antigen system may be likened to the mouse Ia (immune response associated) antigen system in that it may be associated with specific types of immune function, such as stimulation in MLC (Bodmer, 1977b; Cresswell, 1975). In the future, more HLA-DRw antigens will presumably be identified on specific subpopulations of lymphocytes, not necessarily just B cells, and will be associated with other aspects of immune function such as suppression and helper activity, as is already known in the mouse Ia antigen system. Curiously, however, transplants done in the face of a positive B-lymphocyte crossmatch (cold antibody) successfully survive without hyperacute rejection (Ettinger, 1976a; Lobo, 1977). However, their subsequent appearance in the post-transplant period can have an entirely different meaning because they coincide with rejection (Ettinger, 1976b). This situation remained a paradox until it became known that sera from as many as 20 per cent of normal males and females have antibodies cytotoxic against autologous as well as allogeneic B-lymphocytes (Park, 1977). These "non-specific" antibodies react

best in the cold and do not seem to influence the outcome of kidney transplants (Ettinger, 1976a). Their function is unknown, although they could well be part of a natural feedback mechanism to inhibit or regulate antibody production by B-cells following an immunization (Terasaki, 1970). The entire picture is unclear and awaits further data before any definite conclusions can be made (Terasaki, 1978).

BONE MARROW TRANSPLANTATION

During the past 25 years, evidence has indicated that animals can be grafted with either suspensions of lymphoid cells or with bone marrow suspensions. Although the procedure is still partially experimental, over 600 have been reported (van Bekkum, 1977). The problems associated with bone marrow transplantation include all of those for renal transplantation and, in addition, those associated with the tendency of the immunocompetent cells in the marrow graft to attack the recipient. The resulting graft-versus-host (GVH) reaction (Elkins, 1971; Simonson, 1962), plus the likelihood of infections makes success difficult. The usual indications for marrow grafting are immune deficiency diseases, aplastic anemia, and, in some cases, leukemia (Thomas, 1977a).

The Choice of a Donor. Except for an identical twin, an HLA genotypically identical sibling is usually the only acceptable candidate. Consequently, there is a major problem in obtaining compatible donors owing to the trend toward small numbers of children among families in societies in which bone marrow transplantation is currently performed. When such a donor does not exist, the search for an HLA-identical, MLR-negative donor can be made through the rest of the family. Among close relatives there is a chance of finding such a donor. If none is found, the last resort is an HLA-identical, MLR-negative unrelated donor. The sex match between donor and recipient can also be important, and although it does not appear to affect graft rejection, it does appear to influence graft-versus-host disease (Storb, 1977b). The identification of HLA-D determinants, as has been mentioned, is based on the degree of response of an individual to homozygous typing cells (HTC) when compared to stimulation by a reference pool. These results of HTC typing are then given in relative responses (RR). HLA-identical sibling

---

*Vincenti, 1978; Opelz, 1978.

combinations produce less than 5 per cent RR. This has become important in donor selection because an RR of more than 1.6 per cent was found to be discriminatory in allograft rejection (Mickelson, 1976). However, when donor and recipient are not genetically identical twins, some degree of histoincompatibility must exist and constitutes a bidirectional immunologic barrier. First, the host may reject the graft; therefore, the host immunologic reactivity must first be suppressed. Total body irradiation (TBI) and various chemotherapeutic agents, such as cyclophosphamide, have been used for this purpose. Bone marrow transplantation is further complicated by the fact that immunologically competent cells of donor origin can react against the "foreign" host to cause a serious or fatal syndrome known as GVH disease.

GVH Disease. The mechanism of GVH disease is unknown. Unfortunately, it is not only the most common complication, occurring in up to 50 per cent of the cases (van Bekkum, 1977) but also the least understood. It is manifested by maculopapular cutaneous eruptions, hepatomegaly, diarrhea with intestinal dysfunction, and occurs 10 to 30 days following transplantation. There is a tendency to correlate GVH with MLC; however, this is not always the case because GVH can occur between HLA-identical, MLC-negative siblings (Dupont, 1977). It seems that differences between genes that are not as yet identified, either within or outside HLA, are also contributing to GVH. These observations are supported by results of experimental bone marrow transplantation in dogs (Storb, 1977c). The median survival time of transplants between littermate DLA-identical (DLA = MHC of dog, corresponding to HLA in human) dogs was 666 days; survival between DLA-identical unrelated animals was only 83 days. Likewise, grafts between pairs of littermates in which one was homozygous and the other heterozygous for antigens of the MHC were also significantly decreased at 29 days. These results support the theory that while many antigens in the MHC play a significant role, other yet-to-be described loci appear to be involved. The presence of non-MHC linked alloantigens between HLA- and MLC-identical bone marrow transplant donors and recipients has been demonstrated (Parkman, 1976). The significance of such antigens is that if the donor and recipient are not identical for that antigen, it acts as a source of sensitization, thus resulting in graft rejection or GVH disease.

Because the identification of these antigens is still experimental, the test procedures used for their identification are not those used in a routine HLA laboratory. Currently, the best method involves cell-mediated lympholysis (CML), which essentially is a two-step process (Lightbody, 1971). The first step involves the generation of killer cells by incubating responder and stimulator cells in an MLC type reaction. The second step involves the killing or lysis of chromium-51–labeled target blast cells. The killer cells which arise from small clones of responding cells are directed against certain antigens on the original stimulating cell and will lyse any cell that contains any or all of these antigens. These "target" antigens are considered to be the gene products, or antigens, controlled by HLA-A and HLA-B (the role of HLA-C antigens has not been clearly defined) (Long, 1975). However, the issue is not completely clear because in the aforementioned studies (Parkman, 1976), cytotoxic cells were generated against the stimulator cells and other related cells, even when the responder and stimulator cells (or individuals) were MHC-identical for all of the antigens for which we commonly type. Thus, again, the conclusion is that other transplantation antigens must exist. Currently, these methods are used to select donors to a greater histoidentity when more than one MHC-identical donor exists, and, in addition, may help to decide on the amount of immunosuppression that may be necessary after transplantation (i.e., if donor and recipient are MHC-identical but the recipient marrow contains cytotoxic cells to the donor cells, immunosuppression to the recipient needs to be increased ahead of time).

HLA AND DISEASE

The biology of HLA in clinical medicine not only includes its role in transplantation, but also its association with many disease states (Table 41-2). This fact first became evident when it was demonstrated that the MHC of the mouse played a deciding role in resistance to oncogenic viruses (Lilly, 1964; Lilly, 1971). The conceptual relationship between the MHC and disease is logical because (1) the MHC of animals is one of nature's best biologic markers and, thus, if any genetic locus, in close linkage with HLA, were the cause of a particular disease, it would lend itself to identification, and (2) the MHC (specifically H-2 in the mouse) has been demonstrated to exert con-

Table 41-2. DISEASES SHOWING POSITIVE HLA ANTIGEN CORRELATION(S)

Ankylosing spondylitis	HLA-B27
Reiter's syndrome	HLA-B27
Acute anterior uveitis	HLA-B27
Reactive arthritis, post- *Yersinia* or *Salmonella* infections	HLA-B27
Psoriatic arthritis	HLA-B27
Multiple sclerosis	HLA-B7 and -Dw2
Complement deficiencies:	
C2	HLA-A10, -B18, and -Dw2
C4	HLA-A2, -B40, -Cw3
Psoriasis vulgaris	HLA-B13 and -Bw17 HLA-Cw6
Idiopathic hemochromatosis	HLA-A3
Celiac disease	HLA-B8 and -Dw3
Dermatitis herpetiformis	HLA-B8 and -Dw3
Myasthenia gravis	HLA-B8
Chronic active hepatitis (childhood onset)	HLA-B8
Chronic active hepatitis (adult onset)	HLA-DRw4

trol on many aspects of immune function and thus may very well have significant influence on the well-being of the host by specific control of the immune system. Thus, over the past few years, numerous reports have appeared attempting to clear up the relationship between HLA and disease. The following text will not attempt to review all of the disease associations, because several excellent reviews are already available (Svejgaard, 1975; Dausset, 1977; McDevitt, 1974; Sasazuki, 1977; Williams, 1978); rather, the basic principles will be emphasized in order to better interpret data pertaining to this subject.

EXPERIMENTAL BASIS FOR THE ASSOCIATION OF HLA AND DISEASE

As mentioned previously, the popular concept that an animal MHC was associated with disease susceptibility began with the work of Lilly (1964), who reported that C3H ($H-2^k$) mice were susceptible to the Gross leukemia virus, while C57BL ($H-2^b$) strains were resistant. This constitutional difference was traced to a gene called Rgv-1 (resistance to Gross virus). Subsequent studies showed that Rgv-1 was located at the Ir-1 locus at the K end of the H-2 complex (Lilly, 1971). These and other

similar studies (Tennant, 1965; Duran-Reynals, 1971; Nandi, 1967) have definitely shown an association between susceptibility to oncogenic virus and the mouse MHC; however, the exact role of the mouse H-2 genes has not been elucidated.

One explanation for the association between H-2 and susceptibility implicated an effect from immune response control genes (Ir genes), which have been shown to be linked to the MHC in several animal species, including mice, rats, guinea pigs, and rhesus monkeys. They have been shown to control IgG antibody production after challenge with synthetic peptides, stimulation in MLC, and other immune functions (Benacerraf, 1977). Reports of Ir genes in man are still controversial; however, HLA has been associated with certain immune responses. For example, there has been reported an association between an increased blastogenic response to streptococcal antigens and the presence of HLA-B5 (Greenberg, 1975). Another more remarkable example of Ir gene control over host integrity in the mouse involves the I-J locus (of the mouse I region), the gene products of which are found on suppressor T cells. When these T suppressor lymphocyte cells are inactivated by I-J antiserum in mice with artificially implanted tumors, the tumors grow less rapidly than otherwise expected (Greene, 1977), presumably because I-J antiserum inhibits tumor growth by abolishing tumor-specific suppressor activity. Although experimental theory suggests the relationship of HLA and disease to be some type of effect involving linkage between genes determining HLA antigens and those controlling inherited deficiencies as a result of decreased or altered "immune responsiveness" of the host (or increased susceptibility of a host), other theories have been suggested and should be mentioned: (1) Sharing of determinants between antigens of the HLA group and those on microbial membranes ("microbial mimicry") leads to "cross tolerance" (Hirata, 1973; Lyampert, 1975; Mittal, 1976). (2) HLA antigens also act as receptors specific for given microbial surface antigens (Crittenden, 1974). (3) Involvement of several genes includes those of the HLA region interacting together and with environmental factors for expression of disease (Mittal, 1976; Drachman, 1976; Alter, 1976). The following sections will divide the relationship of HLA and disease into three basic categories: (1) HLA and malignancy; (2) HLA and infectious disease; and (3) HLA and autoimmunity.

4

HLA AND MALIGNANCY

The oldest association between MHC and malignancy stems from the previously mentioned work by Lilly (1964), who demonstrated a correlation between H-2 and susceptibility to Gross leukemia virus. Similar investigations were then made in man by Kourilsky (1967). The authors were unable to detect any association between HLA and acute leukemia; however, only 10 antigens were tested in that early stage of HLA testing. Since that time several other conflicting reports have appeared regarding the association between HLA and several different types of hematologic tumors, and thus no definite conclusion can yet be made. However, there has been shown an excess of HLA-A2 and HLA-B12 patients among long-term survivors of acute lymphocytic leukemia (ALL), as well as an excess of HLA-Aw19 and HLA-B5 among short-term survivors in Hodgkin's disease (Falk, 1977). It must be remembered that analysis of such data can be difficult because the populations studied must be well controlled for histologic type of tumor as well as for racial difference. In addition, negative associations must be sought because they may suggest that a gene for resistance to cancer may be needed and without it cancer susceptibility will become evident.

The study of other tumors has yielded only a few disease associations. Breast cancer has been thoroughly studied because it was suggested that genetic factors may play a role in its etiology. There is no HLA disease association with the incidence of cancer of the breast (Martz, 1973); however, the frequency of HLA-B8 is twice as high in survivors as in those who have died (Williams, 1978).

HLA AND INFECTIOUS DISEASE

One of the proposed mechanisms whereby HLA influences disease susceptibility is the presumed action of Ir genes or Ir-linked genes. Because host response to infectious disease in general involves the immune system and, in particular, activates immune response functions, an association between HLA and infectious disease has been sought. For example, (1) a positive association has been demonstrated between HLA and infection with *Mycobacterium leprae* (de Vries, 1976);

(2) a low *in vitro* response to primary immunization against vaccinia is associated with HLA-Cw3 (Rene, 1977); (3) a low *in vitro* antibody response to influenza A immunization is associated with HLA-Bw16 (Spencer, 1976); and (4) increased *in vitro* response to streptococcal antigens is associated with HLA-B5 (Greenberg, 1975). Similarly, IgE antibody production specific for ragweed antigen E is in close correlation with particular HLA haplotypes in successive generations in family studies (Levine, 1972), demonstrating that predisposition to hay fever probably is not associated with a particular HLA antigen, but is linked to the HLA complex (Blumenthal, 1974). Indeed, many comparisons between HLA and immune response have also shown no association. An outstanding example cited 10 families and 20 unrelated volunteers (n = 75) who were immunized against diphtheria. The conclusion suggested that the response to immunization is partially controlled by a dominant gene that is not closely linked to HLA (McMichael, 1977).

AUTOIMMUNE AND ENDOCRINE DISEASES

One of the best experimental systems to illustrate the influence of the MHC on autoimmune disease susceptibility and severity is experimental allergic encephalitis (EAE) in the inbred rat (Williams, 1978). EAE is an autoimmune disease which can be elicited by the injection of a defined polypeptide which is known to be present in the central nervous system myelin. Susceptibility in the rat depends on the presence of a single MHC linked gene, e.g., Lewis rats are completely susceptible while BN rats are uniformly resistant. The $(Lew \times BN)F_1$ is susceptible, but develops a disease of diminished severity. The susceptibility gene has been termed Ir-EAE and has been shown to be linked to the MHC of the rat (Williams, 1973). The BN rats may be resistant because of suppressor gene activity or because they simply lack "responder" genes.

An analogous situation in the human, associating disease susceptibility and disease severity with HLA, occurs with multiple sclerosis. HLA-B12 is selectively absent from MS patients. Thus, it is conceivable that an HLA-B12 associated immunoregulatory gene may exist. The function of this hypothetical gene would be to prevent the manifestation of multiple sclerosis (MS) symptoms even in the presence of an otherwise genetically susceptible and environmentally exposed individual. It should be emphasized that the MHC influence may be related to the pathogenesis of the disease and have nothing to do with its etiology. For example, multiple sclerosis might well be caused by a virus, but the lesion may result from an inappropriately regulated immune response to the virus, resulting in autoimmune damage to myelin.

Further evidence to support the association of MS with HLA is the strong association between the disease and the haplotype HLA-A3, B7, Dw2 (Degos, 1974). In addition, the geographic distribution of MS corresponds to that of the HLA-A3, B7 linkage disequilibrium distribution, namely, Northern Europe, especially Scandinavian countries (Snell, 1976c).

Although the phenomenon of genetic linkage disequilibrium is incompletely understood, it is important in the study of disease associations. For instance, it has been mentioned that the haplotype HLA-A3, B7, Dw2 is associated with MS (multiple sclerosis), yet if individual specificities are studied, there is a higher association between MS and HLA-Dw2 than with either HLA-B7 or HLA-A3. This emphasis and importance of the HLA-D locus specificity also holds true for other disease associations: The haplotype HLA-A1, B8, Dw3 is associated with juvenile onset diabetes mellitus, myasthenia gravis, dermatitis herpetiformis, Grave's disease, Addison's disease, and gluten enteropathy; yet when each locus is studied individually, the disease association to HLA-Dw3 is greater than to either HLA-A1 or HLA-B8. These facts suggest two important points: (1) the HLA-D locus is more closely associated with the genetic factors controlling disease susceptibility than is the HLA-A or HLA-B locus, and (2) because the H-2 region of the mouse (corresponding to HLA-D) contains many immunoregulatory genes, it is appropriate to assume that the HLA-D region also contains immunoregulatory genes, including those for disease susceptibility.

A logical extension of the regulatory gene-disease association hypothesis would be to show a relationship to the HLA-DRw antigen system, which, as mentioned previously, is thought to be part of the human equivalent to the Ia (immune response associated) antigen system in the mouse. These antigens are controlled by the HLA-D region that might correspond to the I region of the mouse; the antigens discovered thus far have the immune regulatory function of controlling most of the stimulatory capacity of a cell in MLC. Undoubtedly, if the human system is similar to the mouse, more DRw antigens will be described and associated with other immune functions, such as suppression and cell-cell cooperation. Reports have indicated a strong correlation with MS and DRw2 (Platz, 1977), juvenile onset diabetes mellitus with DRw3 (Mayr, 1977), and chronic active hepatitis with DRw4 (Williams, 1978). On the other hand, a group of diseases is associated with the B locus specificity, HLA-B27. In ankylosing spondylitis, for example, up to 95 per cent of the patients possess HLA-B27, in contrast to only 3 to 7 per cent of the controls; the antigen occurs 15 to 20 times more frequently in patients than in controls (Calin, 1975; Brewerton, 1973; Schlosstein, 1973). Anterior uveitis and Reiter's syndrome are also associated with HLA-B27, which suggests a possible relationship between HLA-B27 and a common etiology to these diseases. Mechanistically, this may involve mimicry of an agent and a receptor on the target organs. These diseases, however, are not found in all HLA-B27 individuals and not all patients have the HLA antigen, which points to the fact that the HLA system, or genes linked to it, is only one of the several genetic factors predisposing to a disease. The knowledge of HLA is incomplete, and therefore it is not possible to determine whether the exceptions in one disease reflect polygenic factors or our inability to type for a disease susceptibility allele. However, even if we were able to detect them, it could not be expected that all individuals bearing the disease susceptibility gene will manifest disease, because other genetic and environmental factors are required to produce clinically detectable disease.

The association between HLA and disease is one of sound experimental foundation and has been found to affect almost every aspect of human disease and development. Effort now is also directed toward identification of the actual loci involved. HLA appears to be a unique region for such analysis because (1) it is highly polymorphic, which means that a gene and its linkage group may be traced not only through a family, but also through a population and geographic region, and (2) the MHC in other animals contain Ir genes; therefore, HLA itself probably is a focus for a large number of regulatory genes such as has been demonstrated for complement components and for stimulating capacity in MLC. Probably functions both related and unrelated to immunology may be regulated from this area. Thus, further understanding should help our eventual concept of disease.

HLA IN CLINICAL BLOOD COMPONENT SUPPORT SYSTEMS

HLA-A, HLA-B, and HLA-C antigens have recently become increasingly important in blood transfusion. These serologically defined antigens lead to immunization in approximately 50 per cent of polytransfused patients and are responsible for 50 to 80 per cent of all non-hemolytic febrile transfusion reactions (Thulstrup, 1971; Cannady, 1978b). The importance of HLA in clinical blood component support specifically concerns (1) platelet transfusion, (2) leukocyte transfusion, and (3) relationship between HLA and blood group antigens (see Chapter 43).

PLATELET TRANSFUSION

The efficacy of platelet transfusion therapy in leukemia, aplastic anemia, and solid tumor patient maintenance has been well documented (Yankee, 1969; Yankee, 1973; Brand, 1978). Platelets carry the HLA antigens on their cell surface and after repeated transfusions of unmatched products there is a high probability of patient sensitization resulting in poor increments after platelet transfusion (Yankee, 1973; Yankee, 1976). Patients may become immunized even in the absence of a demonstrable febrile transfusion reaction. Thus, the goal of effective platelet transfusion is to provide platelets without inducing sensitization (immunity); ideally, the donor should be HLA-identical to the recipient. However, such a donor is usually not available and the donor that is the most HLA compatible, with a negative crossmatch, is used. The same donor should be used as long as possible until immunization occurs. In some cases HLA matching is more important than ABO matching because platelets may be effective for hemostasis even if ABO incompatibility exists (Lohrman, 1974). In practice it is often impossible to provide matched platelets to prevent immunization. Therefore, the use of matched platelets is

indicated in patients who have become refractory to platelet transfusions. In such cases the procedure is based on the transfusion of platelets in the presence of a negative crossmatch. The platelets are usually obtained from matched siblings or HLA-matched unrelated donors.

Measurement of platelet response after transfusion is accomplished by performing a pre-infusion and 20-minute post-platelet infusion count. Normally one would expect a 12- to 16,000 platelets/cu mm increment for each unit of platelets transfused, so that a patient receiving an eight-unit platelet concentrate should have an increment of 96- to 128,000 platelets/cu mm. The response in many patients undergoing prolonged platelet transfusion therapy is initially very satisfactory, but after a period of time begins to diminish.

Platelet collection is very important and should be discussed in detail before proceeding with the relationship of HLA to platelet transfusion therapy. The four primary methods of collection are as follows:

1. *Random pooled* are platelet concentrates removed from whole blood units; a normal concentrate consists of a pool of six to ten units.

2. *Selected pooled* are platelets collected from two or three donors.

3. *Single donor* are platelets collected from one donor, usually on a Haemonetics Model 30 or an IBM machine. Single donor platelets may also be collected using bag pheresis method, but this takes an extremely long time and is very exhausting for the donor.

4. *Single donor HLA matched* are platelets collected from a single individual (related or unrelated) who has been determined to be HLA compatible with the patient.

The choice of collection method is in part determined by the designated use of the platelets: for example, method number one is best suited for a short-term platelet requirement as in a temporary bleeding abnormality secondary to trauma. Methods two and three are used, for instance, in patients with hematologic abnormalities with resultant thrombocytopenia from drug therapy who have not been sensitized to HLA antigens or do not anticipate a long-term need for platelet transfusion. Method four is used on the same group of patients as method three, but who show evidence of HLA sensitization or who will require long-term transfusions.

Failure to increase platelet counts in a patient after repeated platelet transfusions is most likely due to HLA sensitization; however, other possibilities such as fever, infection, splenomegaly, and/or disseminated intravascular coagulation should be considered as a cause before HLA sensitization can be proven responsible.

ABO groups and platelet-specific antigens such as PI and KO apparently have very little effect on the survival of transfused platelets, provided the concentrate is free of red blood cell contamination (Yankee, 1976). A major problem in evaluating the effect of platelet-specific antigens and antibodies in platelet transfusion therapy has been the relative insensitivity of most assays, such as platelet complement fixation, in demonstrating sensitization in patients. Additionally, platelet aggregation using the aggregometer has not solved the problem even though, initially, it was thought to be a more sensitive procedure. In fact, only the HLA system has been documented as adversely affecting repeated long-term platelet transfusions (Yankee, 1969; Brand, 1978). Numerous investigators have demonstrated the correction of diminished platelet survival in refractory patients with HLA-matched platelets. Occasionally a patient becomes refractory to platelet transfusion without demonstrable antibodies present; this may represent an artifact of test procedures which are not sensitive enough to detect low level sensitization. In 1972, Johnson defined the modified antiglobulin lymphocytotoxicity test (AHG), which is more sensitive than the NIH standard lymphocytotoxicity test (STD). Cannady (1974 and 1978b) further demonstrated the increased sensitivity of the AHG procedure with routine HLA typing sera and sera from multitransfused individuals. Current data suggest that the antihuman globulin (AHG) antibody screen and cross-match predicts a poor platelet response in patients approximately 4 to 6 weeks prior to the NIH STD method. In highly sensitized individuals without siblings, the HLA crossmatch may be the only feasible measurement of compatibility.

Current platelet transfusion therapy recommends that the donor platelets possess no foreign HLA antigens with respect to the recipient; a possible exception to this rule is that donor antigens closely related to those of the recipient (i.e., those that are cross-reactive) are tolerated and usually can be used. However Duquesnoy (1977a; 1977b) showed that this was not always true, especially if the recipient was HLA-A2 positive. Such individuals would then require HLA-identical platelets, since platelets matched with CREG* do not produce platelet count increments. This finding is very important because approximately 50 per cent of the American Caucasian population is HLA-A2 positive and theoretically would need exact HLA matches to correct platelet refractory problems; considering that there are now 59 well-defined HLA-ABC antigens with a high number of combinations, a sensitized individual without an HLA identical sibling could require a donor pool of extraordinary size for optimal effectiveness.

LEUKOCYTE TRANSFUSION

The use of neutrophils is a beneficial adjunct in the treatment of infected neutropenic patients (Herzig, 1977; Alavi, 1977). In the 1950's and early 1960's hemorrhage was the major cause of death in patients with aplastic anemia or hematologic malignancies. As platelet transfusion therapy became widely accepted and used as a routine procedure, infection became the major cause of death in this group of patients. In the 1970's leukocyte (specifically granulocyte) transfusion was investigated as an effective method of correcting septic episodes in this high-risk group. Three considerations are important when considering granulocyte transfusion therapy:

1. Condition of the patient
2. Donor selection
3. Method of collection

Condition of Patient. Most centers using therapeutic and/or prophylactic granulocyte transfusions set specific criteria for patient selection. Generally, when the granulocyte count falls below 1000/cu mm the risk for infection is increased. As the count of circulating granulocytes falls below 200/cu mm, the decision must be made whether or not to proceed with a leukocyte transfusion. This decision should take into account the patient's drug therapy. For instance, if the recovery period from a drug-induced aplasia is 14 to 16 days and the granulocyte count falls below 200 (which is the cutoff point) on day 13, it may be feasible to wait one or two days before initiating transfusion therapy in anticipation of marrow recovery. A bone marrow biopsy may also be done at this time to help determine regenerative capacity.

---

* Cross-reactive groups.

Donor Selection. Donor selection is similar to that for platelet transfusion; that is, the use of an HLA-identical sibling is desirable. However, since repeated sessions of leukocyte removal are necessary, usually several donors are required; thus, HLA-matched granulocytes are not routinely used. However, two requirements are essential: the HLA crossmatch should always be negative and the donor and recipient should be at least ABO compatible. Granulocytes, like platelets, have their own cell-specific non–HLA-associated cell surface antigens (Drew, 1978; Lalezari, 1970). However, their identification as well as significance in transfusion is incompletely understood. To be effective, the quantity of leukocytes that are transfused must be in excess of the pulmonary capillary storage capacity; thus, at least 5×10^{10} to 5×10^{11} leukocytes should be given at one time. Leukocyte survival in the recipient is usually short, with only approximately 10 per cent of the transfused granulocytes surviving after six hours. Thus the transfusion must be done frequently, which creates the aforementioned supply problem.

Method of Collection. The two methods for collection of granulocytes are filtration leukopheresis (FL) and continuous flow centrifugation (CFC). *FL concentrates* are pure granulocytes with very little lymphocyte contamination, but there is some doubt concerning their effectiveness because when viewed by electron microscopy, there are vacuoles on the cell surface. Also, some functional properties of granulocytes such as bacterial killing are diminished when they are collected by FL (McCullough, 1976). *CFC granulocyte concentrates* are generally contaminated with lymphocytes and platelets. However, the functional properties of these granulocytes are not diminished and they do not appear damaged when viewed by electron microscopy. The maximum shelf life of granulocyte concentrates is approximately 24 hours. The concentrates are usually kept at 2° to 8°C. prior to infusion; these concentrates cannot, however, be cryopreserved. This suggests the advantage of using monocytes in place of granulocytes because monocytes can be cryopreserved, so that concentrates may be collected in advance and stored until needed. CFC concentrates present a major problem in the possible HLA sensitization of patients, since these concentrates are contaminated with large volumes of lymphocytes; however, the role of HLA in granulocyte transfusion therapy remains unclear.

Donor safety is another consideration because filtration collection may present a hazard. Shortly after filtration begins, the donor becomes neutropenic, a condition similar to hemodialysis-induced neutropenia. Under such conditions, there is an increase in pulmonary marginated neutrophils mediated by complement activation owing to contact of plasma with cellophane, with resultant increase in pulmonary arterial pressure and abnormal gas exchange (Craddock, 1975; Fehr, 1975).

Besides the actual technical procedure of collection, other more practical aspects must be considered, such as cost. Granulocyte transfusion can be an extremely expensive matter when one considers the repetition of donor collection as well as machine and equipment use. Also to be considered is the granulocyte monitoring that is necessary to insure that the neutrophils obtained are of good quality; specifically, this involves sterility, damage, and function. These problems involve long-range solutions and are currently being re-evaluated (Boggs, 1977).

HLA AND BLOOD GROUP ERYTHROCYTE ANTIGENS

In addition to ABO, erythrocytes carry HLA-related histocompatibility antigens known as Bg antigens. These antigens were originally called DBG (Donna-Bennet-Goodspeed) HO, O⁺, and Sturgeon; however, today they are known as Bg^a, Bg^b, and Bg^c (Seman, 1967) and are related to HLA antigens because Bg^a is cross-reactive with HLA-B7, Bg^b to HLA-Bw17, and Bg^c to HLA-A28 (Morton, 1969; Morton, 1971). Likewise, anti-HLA-B8 sera will agglutinate the red blood cells of some but not all HLA-B8 individuals (Nordhagen, 1974).

In repetitive testing of many individuals for the Bg antigen, it is often difficult to reproduce positive results. One explanation is that these antigens are of varying antigenic strengths because they are found primarily on the surface of reticulocytes and their expression is decreased as the erythrocyte matures. The antigenic strength then is directly related to the number of circulating reticulocytes. Another reason is that Bg antigens are soluble in serum (similar to HLA antigens) and may be absorbed onto the surface of mature red cells, which may be responsible for false positive reactions that are often not repeatable.

ABO compatibility is of primary importance

in solid organ transplants, while Rh compatibility is not of significance in organ transplantation. Rh compatibility is important in leukocyte transfusion therapy; immunization must be avoided by proper histocompatibility matching or, in specific cases of Rh negative individuals receiving Rh positive leukocyte concentrates containing red cells, administration of anti-D immune globulin may prevent immunization (International Symposium, 1977).

Lewis (Le) is another erythrocyte histocompatibility antigen system which is thought to be at least in part represented on lymphocytes (Dorf, 1972), and it is possible that sera with anti-Le activity may be lymphocytotoxic. Such reactions may contribute to false positive results in routine HLA typing.

CONCLUSION

The work leading to the concepts of HLA began with the foundations of transplantation, first in mice and then in humans; the eventual realization was that the laws of transplantation were largely controlled by a single genetic system—the major histocompatibility complex—which was found to affect and possibly control other important bodily functions, including immune regulation, development, and in certain cases, susceptibility to disease.

HLA is on the short arm of chromosome six and consists of at least four distinct loci, HLA-A, HLA-B, HLA-C, and HLA-D, that control the expression of a series of cell surface antigens which together form a highly polymorphic system, such that complete identity between two unrelated individuals is rare. It is then especially interesting that Nature should provide such a genetic system; despite the fact that HLA has antigenic expression on essentially all cells and seems to play an important role in maintaining proper body integrity, its exact biologic function remains unknown. Further definition of this genetic region will result in identification of other HLA-linked loci controlling the expression of antigenic determinants, such as the newly described DRw antigens, that will help unravel basic problems relating to cell interactions and immune response. From there, transplant rejection, disease susceptibility, and cancer may be better understood and perhaps more effectively controlled.

4

REFERENCES

Alavi, J. B., Root, R. K., Djerassi, I., Evans, A. E., Gluckman, S. J., MacGregor, R. R., Guerry, D., Schreiber, A. D., Shaw, J. M., Koch, P., and Cooper, R. A.: A randomized clinical trial of granulocyte transfusions for infection in acute leukemia. N. Engl. J. Med., *296*:706, 1977.

Alter, M., Harshe, J., Anderson, V. E., Emme, L., and Yunis, E. J.: Genetic association of multiple sclerosis and HLA determinants. Neurology, *26*:31, 1976.

Amos, D. B.: The agglutination of mouse leukocytes by isoimmune sera. Br. J. Exp. Pathol., *34*:464, 1953.

Amos, D. B., Siegler, H. F., Southworth, J. G., and Ward, F. E.: Skin graft rejection between subjects genotyped for HL-A. Transplant. Proc., *1*:342, 1969.

Amos, D. B., and Ward, F. G.: Immunogenetics of the HLA system. Physiol. Rev., *55*:206, 1975.

Bach, F. H., and Amos, D. B.: Hu-1: Major histocompatibility locus in man. Science, *156*:1506, 1967.

Bach, F. H., and Hirschhorn, K.: Lymphocyte interaction: A potential histocompatibility test *in vitro*. Science, *143*:813, 1964.

Bach, F. H., and Voynow, N. K.: One way stimulation in mixed leukocyte cultures. Science, *153*:545, 1966.

Bach, F., and van Rood, J. J.: The major histocompatibility complex—genetics and biology. N. Engl. J. Med., *295*:806, 1976a.

Bach, F. H., and van Rood, J. J.: The major histocompatibility complex—genetics and biology. N. Engl. J. Med., *295*:927, 1976b.

Bach, F., Sondel, P., Sheehy, M., Wank, R., Alter, B., and Bach, M.: The complexity of the HL-A LD system: A PLT analysis. *In* Kissmeyer-Neilsen, F. (ed.): Histocompatibility Testing 1975. Copenhagen, Munksgaard, 1975, p. 576.

Bain, B., Vas, M. R., and Lowenstein, L.: The development of large immature mononuclear cells in mixed leukocyte cultures. Blood, *23*:108, 1964.

Belzer, F. O., Fortmann, J. L., Salvatierra, O., Perkins, H. A., Kountz, S., Cochrum, K. C., and Payne, R.: Is HL-A typing of clinical significance in cadaver renal transplantation. Lancet, *1*:774, 1974.

Benacerraf, B.: Role of major histocompatibility complex in genetic regulation of immunologic responsiveness. Transplant. Proc., *9*:825, 1977.

Benacerraf, B., and McDevitt, H. O.: Histocompatibility linked immune response genes. Science, *175*:273, 1972.

Blumenthal, M. N., Amos, D. B., Noreen, H., and Yunis, E. J.: Genetic mapping of the Ir locus in man: Linkage to the second locus of HL-A. Science, *184*:1301, 1974.

Bodmer, W. F.: Genetic constitution of chromosome 6 from human gene mapping 3. *In* Third International Workshop on Gene Mapping. Basel, S. Karger, 1976, p. 24.

Bodmer, W. F., Bodmer, J. G., Batchelor, J. R., Festenstein, H., and Morris, P. J. (eds.): Joint Report of the VII International Histocompatibility Workshop. *In* Histocompatibility Testing 1977. Copenhagen, Munksgaard, 1977b.

Bodmer, J., Richards, S., and Bodmer, W. F.: The definition of Ia antigens using 7th Workshop sera. Tissue Antigens, *10*:140, 1977a.

Boggs, D.: Neutrophils in the blood bank. Editorial. N. Engl. J. Med., *196*:748, 1977.

Bortin, M. M., and Rimm, A. A.: Severe combined immunodeficiency disease: Characterization of the disease and results of transplantation. Seventh Report from the International Bone Marrow Transplant Registry. J.A.M.A., 1977.

Brand, A., van Leeuwen, A., Eernisse, J. G., and van Rood, J. J.: Platelet transfusion therapy. Optimal donor selection with a combination of lymphocytotoxicity and plate fluorescence tests. Blood, 1978 (in press).

Braun, W. E.: The new serology of histocompatibility testing and its significance in human renal transplantation. Urol. Clin. North Am., *3*:503, 1976.

Braun, W. E., Grecek, D. R., and Murphy, J. J.: Expanded HLA phenotypes of human peripheral lymphocytes after trypsinization. Transplantation, *13*:337, 1972.

Brautbar, C., Stanbridge, E. J., Pellegrino, M. A., Pellegrino, S., Ferrone, S., Reisfeld, R. A., Payne, R., and Hayflick, L.: Expression of HLA antigens on cultured human fibroblasts infected with mycoplasma. J. Immunol., *111*:1783, 1973.

Brewerton, D. A., Caffrey, M., Hart, F. D., Nicholls, A., James, D. C., and Sturrock, R. D.: Ankylosing spondylitis and HL-A27. Lancet, *1*:904, 1973.

Calin, A., and Fries, J. F.: Striking prevalence of ankylosing spondylitis in "healthy" W27 positive males and females. A controlled study. N. Engl. J. Med., *293*:835, 1975.

Cannady, W. G., DeWolf, W. C., Williams, R. M., and Yunis, E. J.: Laboratory methods in transplantation immunity. *In* Stefanini, M.: Progress in Clinical Pathology, vol. VII. New York, Grune & Stratton, Inc., 1978a, p. 239.

Cannady, W. G., Reckel, R. P., Tripodi, D., Shaw, S., Baldassari, D., and Metz, L.: Sensitivity of various HLA typing techniques. Tissue Antigens, *4*:564, 1974.

Cannady, W. G., Specian, T., Reckel, R. P., Baldassari, D., and Shaw, S.: Leukocyte antibodies in the serum of patients exhibiting febrile transfusion reactions. Results of two lymphocytotoxicity assays. Proceedings of the 6th International Tagung der Gesellschaft fur forensische Blutgruppenkunde. Wurzburg, Schmitt and Meyer, 1978b, p. 139.

Ceppellini, R., Bigliari, S., Curtoni, E. S., and Leigheb, G.: Allotransplantation in man II. The role of A1, A2 and B antigens. Transplant. Proc., *1*:390, 1969.

Ceppellini, R., Curtoni, E. S., Mattiuz, P. L., Leigheb, G., Visetti, M., and Colombi, A.: Survival of test skin grafts in man: Effect of genetic relationship of blood groups in compatibility. Ann. N.Y. Acad. Sci., *129*:421, 1966.

Chapel, H. M., and MacKintosh, L. P.: The use of CLL cells for analysis of the B cell histocompatibility system. Tissue Antigens, *10*:142, 1977.

Chess, L., and Schlossman, S. F.: Methods for the separation of unique human lymphocyte subpopulations. *In* Rose, N., and Friedman, H. (eds.): Manual of Clinical Immunology. Washington, D.C., American Society for Microbiology, 1976, pp. 77–80.

Clark, E. A., Terasaki, P. I., Opelz, G., and Mickey, M. R.: Cadaver-kidney transplant failures at one month. N. Engl. J. Med., *291*:1099, 1974.

Cochrum, K., Perkins, H. A., and Payne, R. O.: The correlation of MLC with graft survival. Transplant. Proc., *5*:391, 1973.

Craddock, P., Fehr, J., Brigham, K., and Jacob, H.: Pulmonary capillary leukostasis: A complement mediated complication of hemodialysis. Clin. Res., *23*:402(a), 1975.

Cresswell, P., and Geier, S. S.: Antisera to human B-lymphocyte membrane glucoproteins block stimulation in mixed lymphocyte culture. Nature, *257*:147, 1975.

Crittenden, L. B., Briles, W. E., and Stone, H. A.: Susceptibility to an avian leukosis sarcoma virus: Close association with an erythrocyte isoantigen. Science, *169*:1324, 1974.

Dausset, J.: Iso-leuco-anticorps. Acta. Haematol. (Basel), *20*:156, 1958.

Dausset, J.: Leuco-agglutinins. IV. Leucoagglutinins and blood transfusion. Vox Sang., *4*:190, 1954.

Dausset, J.: Personal communication, 1977.

Dausset, J., and Nenna, A.: Presence d'une leuco-agglutinine dans la serum d'un cas d'agranulocytose chronique. C.R. Soc. Biol. (Paris), *146*:1539, 1952.

Dausset, J., and Rappaport, F.: Blood group determinants of human histocompatibility. *In* Dausset, J., and Rappaport (eds.): Human Transplantation. New York, Grune & Stratton, Inc., 1968, pp. 383–393.

Dausset, J., and Svejgaard, A. (eds.): HLA and Disease. Copenhagen, Munksgaard, 1977.

Dausset, J., Hors, J., Busson, M., Festenstein, H., Oliver, R. T., Paris, A. M. I., and Sachs, J. A.: Serologically defined HLA antigens and long term survival of cadaver kidney transplants. N. Engl. J. Med., *290*:979, 1974a.

Dausset, J., Singh, S., Gourand, J. L., Degos, L., Solal, C., and Klein, G.: HL-A and Burkitt's disease. Tissue Antigens, *5*:48, 1974b.

Degos, L., and Dausset, J.: Histocompatibility determinants in multiple sclerosis. Lancet, *1*:307, 1974.

de Vries, R. R. P., Lai, A., Fat, R. F. M., and Nijenhuis, L. E.: HLA linked genetic control of host response to mycobacterium leprae. Lancet, *2*:1328, 1976.

Dorf, M. E., Eguro, S. Y., Cabera, E., Yunis, E. J., Swanson, J., and Amos, D. B.: Detection of cytotoxic non-HLA antisera. I. Relationship to Le[al]. Vox Sang., *22*:447, 1972.

Drachman, D. A., Davidson, W. C., and Mittal, K. K.: Histocompatibility (HL-A) factors in familial multiple sclerosis. Is MS susceptibility inherited via the HL-A chromosome? Arch. Neurol., *33*:406, 1976.

Drew, S. I., Bergh, O., McClelland, J., Mickey, R., and Terasaki, P. I.: Antigenic specificities detected on papainized human granulocytes by microgranulocytotoxicity. Vox Sang., *33*:1, 1978.

Dupont, B., Good, R. A., Hansen, G. S., Jersild, C., Staub-Nielsen, L., Park, B. H., Svejgaard, A., Thompson, M., and Yunis, E. J.: Two separate genes controlling stimulation in mixed lymphocyte reaction in man. Proc. Natl. Acad. Sci. U.S.A., *71*:52, 1974.

Dupont, B., Hansen, J., and Yunis, E. J.: Human mixed lymphocyte culture reaction: Genetic specificity and biologic implications. *In* Dixon, F., and Kunkel, H. (eds.): Advances in Immunology, vol. 23. New York, Academic Press, 1976, pp. 108–202.

Dupont, B., Hansen, J., Good, R. A., and O'Reilly, R.: Histocompatibility testing for clinical bone marrow transplantation. *In* Ferrara, G. B., and Kissmeyer-Neilsen, F. (eds.): Proceedings of the International Conference on HLA Systems. In press, 1977.

Duquesnoy, R. J., Filip, D. J., and Aster, R. H.: Influence of HLA-A2 on the effectiveness of platelet transfusions in alloimmunized thrombocytopenic patients. Blood, *50*:407, 1977a.

Duquesnoy, R. J., Filip, D. J., Rodey, G. E., Rimm, A. A., and Aster, R. H.: Successful transfusion of platelets mismatched for HLA antigens to alloimmunized thrombocytopenic patients. Am. J. Hematol., 2:219, 1977b.

Duran-Reynals, M. L., and Lilly, F.: The role of genetic factors in the combined neoplastic effects of vaccinia virus and methyl cholanthrene. Transplant. Proc., 3:1243, 1971.

Eijsvoogel, V. P., du Bois, M. J., Meinesz, A., Bierhorst-Eijlander, A., Zeylemaker, W. B., and Schellekens, P. A.: The specificity and the activation mechanism of cell mediated lympholysis (CML) in man. Transplant. Proc., 5:1675, 1973.

Elkins, W. L.: Cellular immunology and the pathogenesis of graft-versus-host reaction. Prog. Allergy, 15:78, 1971.

Ettinger, R. B., Opelz, G., and Terasaki, P. I.: Successful renal allografts across a positive crossmatch for donor B lymphocyte alloantigens. Lancet, 2:56, 1976a.

Ettinger, R. B., Terasaki, P. I., Ting, A., Malekzadeh, M. H., Pennisi, A. J., Henbogaart, C. U., Garrison, R., and Fine, R. N.: Anti-B lymphocytotoxins in renal allograft rejection. N. Engl. J. Med., 295:305, 1976b.

Evans, R. L., Williams, R. M., and Chess, L.: A subclass of human T cells is activated in MLC to effect ADCC. Fed. Proc., 36:1211, 1977.

Falk, J., and Osoba, D.: The HLA system and survival in malignant disease. Hodgkins disease and carcinoma of the breast. In Murphy, G. P. (ed.): HLA and Malignancy. New York, Alan R. Liss, Inc., 1977, pp. 205–216.

Fehr, J., Craddock, P. R., and Jacob, H. S.: Complement (C') mediated granulocyte (PMN) and pulmonary dysfunction during nylon fiber leukophoresis. Blood, 46:1054, 1975.

Ferguson, R. M., Noreen, H., Yunis, E. J., Simmons, R. L., and Najarian, J. S.: Does responder/non-responder status influence renal allograft success? Transplant. Proc., 9:69, 1977.

Ferrara, G. B., Tosi, R. M., Antonelli, P., and Longo, H.: Serological reagents against new lymphocyte surface determinants. Histocompatibility Testing 1975 Copenhagen, Munksgaard, 1975, p. 608.

Festenstein, H., Sach, J. A., Paris, A. M. I., Pedgrum, G. D., and Moorehead, J. F.: Influence of HLA matching and blood transfusion on outcome of 502 London transplant group renal graft recipients. Lancet, 1:157, 1976.

Fradelizi, D., and Dausset, J.: Mixed lymphocyte reactivity of human lymphocytes primed in vitro. I. Secondary response to allogeneic lymphocytes. Eur. J. Immunol., 5:295, 1975.

Francke, U., and Pellegrino, M. A.: Assignment of the major histocompatibility complex to a region of the short arm of chromosome 6. Proc. Natl. Acad. Sci. U.S.A., 74:1147, 1977.

Galton, M.: Factors involved in the rejection of skin transplanted across a weak histocompatibility barrier: Gene dosage, sex of recipient and nature of expression of histocompatibility genes. Transplantation, 5:154, 1967.

Goodfellow, P. N., Jones, E. A., van Heynigan, V., Solomon, E., and Bobrow, M.: The β2 microglobulin gene is on chromosome 15 and not in the HLA region. Nature, 254:267, 1975.

Gorer, P. A.: The antigenic basis of tumor transplantation. J. Pathol. Bacteriol.. 47:231. 1938.

Gossett, T., Naeim, F., Gatti, R. A., Braun, W. E., Thompson, J. S., Shaw, J. F., and Walford, R. L.: Reactivity of chronic lymphocytic leukemia (CLL) cells, normal B

cells and lymphoblastoid cell lines in the Seventh International Workshop. Tissue Antigens, 10:142, 1977.

Greenberg, L. J., Gray, D., and Yunis, E. J.: Association of HLA-5 in vitro and immune responsiveness to streptococcal antigens. J. Exp. Med., 141:935, 1975.

Greenberg, L. J., Teinsmoen, N., Noreen, H., Chess, L., Schlossman, S. F., and Yunis, E. J.: Serologic analysis of MLC determinants. Transplant. Proc., 9:685, 1977.

Greene, M. I., Dorf, M. E., Pierres, M., and Benacerraf, B.: Reduction of syngeneic tumor growth by an anti I-J alloantiserum specific for suppressor T cells. Proc. Natl. Acad. Sci., 74:5118, 1977.

Hamburger, J., Crosnier, J., and Descamps, B.: The value of present methods used for the selection of organ donors. Transplant. Proc., 3:260, 1971.

Herzig, R. H., Herzig, G. P., Graw, R. G., Bull, M. I., and Ray, K. K.: Successful granulocyte transfusion therapy for gram-negative septicemia. N. Engl. J. Med., 196:701, 1977.

Hildemann, W. H., Morgan, M., and Frautnick, L.: Immunogenetic components of weaker histocompatibility systems in mice. Transplant. Proc., 2:24, 1970.

Hirata, A. A., McIntire, F. C., Terasaki, P. I., and Mittal, K. K.: Crossreactions between HL-A antigens and bacterial lipopolysaccharides. Transplantation, 15:441, 1973.

Humphreys, R. E., McCume, J. M., Chess, L., Herrman, H. C., Malenka, D. J., Mann, D. L., Parham, P., Schlossman, S. F., and Strominger, J. C.: Isolation and immunologic characterization of a human B lymphocyte specific cell surface antigen. J. Exp. Med., 144:98, 1976.

International Symposium: The Nature and Significance of Complement Activation (Ortho Diagnostics, Inc., Raritan, N.J.), 1977.

Johnson, A. H., Amos, D. B., and Ward, F. E.: Mapping B cell specificities with recombinant chromosome 6 families. Tissue Antigens, 10:144, 1977.

Johnson, A. H., Rossen, R. D., and Butler, W. T.: Detection of alloantigens using a sensitive antiglobulin microcytotoxicity test: Identification of low levels of preformed antibodies in accelerated allograft rejection. Tissue Antigens, 2:215, 1972.

Joysey, V. C., Roger, J. H., Evans, D. B., and Herbertson, B. M.: Kidney graft survival and matching for HL-A and ABO antigens. Nature, 246:163, 1973.

Julius, M. H., Simpson, E., and Herzenberg, L. A.: A rapid method for the isolation of functional thymus derived murine lymphocytes. Eur. J. Immunol., 3:645, 1974.

Kissmeyer-Nielsen, F., Olsen, S., Petersen, V. P., and Fieldborg, O.: Hyperacute rejection of kidney allograft associated with pre-existing humeral antibodies against donor cells. Lancet, 2:662, 1966.

Klein, J.: In Biology of the mouse histocompatibility 2 complex. New York, Springer Verlag, 1975, p. 236.

Kourilsky, F. M., Dausset, J., Feingold, N., Dupuy, J. M., and Bernard, J.: Leukocyte groups and acute leukemia. J. Natl. Cancer. Inst., 41:87, 1967.

Lalezari, P., Thalenfeld, B., and Weinstein, W. J.: The third neutrophil antigen. In Terasaki, P. I. (ed.): Histocompatibility Testing. Copenhagen, Munksgaard, 1970, p. 319.

Lawler, S. D., Hockley, A. B., Jones, E. H., Mrazek, I., and Dewar, P. J.: Inhibition of mixed lymphocyte cultures by Ia antibodies. Tissue Antigens, 10:140, 1977.

Levine, B. B., Stembes, R. H., and Fotino, M.: Ragweed hay fever: Genetic control and linkage to HL-A haplotypes. Science, 178:1201, 1972.

Lightbody, J., Bernco, D., Miggiano, V. C., and Ceppellini, R.: Cell mediated lympholysis in man after sensitization of effector lymphocytes through mixed lymphocyte culture. G. Batteriol. Virol. Immunol., *64*:243, 1971.

Lilly, F., Boyse, E. A., and Old, L. J.: Genetic basis of susceptibility to viral leukemogenesis. Lancet, *2*:1207, 1964.

Lilly, F.: The influence of H-2 type on Gross virus leukemogenesis in mice. Transplant. Proc., *3*:1239, 1971.

Little, C. C., and Tyzzer, E. E.: Further experimental studies on the inheritance of susceptibility to a transplantable tumor, carcinoma of the Japanese waltzing mouse. J. Med. Res., *28*:393, 1916.

Lobo, P. I., Westervelt, F. B., Jr., and Rudolf, L. E.: Kidney transplant across a positive crossmatch. Lancet, *1*:925, 1977.

Lohrmann, H. P., Bull, M. I., Delter, J. A., Yankee, R. A., and Grow, R. G.: Platelet transfusion from HLA compatible unrelated donors to alloimmunized platelets. Ann. Intern. Med., *80*:9, 1974.

Long, M. A., Handwerger, B., and Yunis, E. J.: The role of HLA (SD) and MLR (LD) determinants in human cell mediated lympholysis. *In* Kissmeyer-Nielsen, F. (ed.): Histocompatibility Testing 1975. Copenhagen, Munksgaard, 1975, pp. 849–854.

Lyampert, I. M., and Danilova, T. A.: Immunological phenomena associated with crossreactive antigens of microorganisms and mammalian tissues. Prog. Allergy, *18*:423, 1975.

Mann, D. L., Abelson, L., Harris, S., and Amos, D. B.: Second genetic locus in the HLA region for human B cell alloantigens. Nature, *259*:145, 1976.

Martz, E., and Benacerraf, B.: Lack of association between carcinoma of the breast and HL-A specificities. Tissue Antigens, *3*:30, 1973.

Mawas, C. E., Charmot, D., and Sasportes, M.: Secondary response of in vitro primed human lymphocytes to allogeneic cells. I. Role of HLA antigens and mixed lymphocyte culture reaction simulating determinants in secondary in vitro proliferative response. Immunogenetics, *2*:449, 1975.

Mayr, W. R., Schernthaner, G., Ludwig, H., Pausch, V., and Dub, E.: Ia type alloantigens in insulin dependent diabetes mellitus. Tissue Antigens, *10*:194, 1977.

McCullough, J., Weiblen, B. J., Amos, R. D., Boen, J., Fortuny, I. E., and Quie, P. G.: In vitro function and post-transfusion survival of granulocytes collected by continuous flow centrifugation and by filtration leukophoresis. Blood, *48*:315, 1976.

McDevitt, H. O., and Bodmer, W. F.: HL-A, immune response genes and disease. Lancet, *1*:1269, 1974.

McKusick, V., and Ruddle, F.: The status of the gene map of the human chromosomes. Science, *196*:340, 1977.

McMichael, A. J., Sasazuki, T., and McDevitt, H. O.: The immune response to diphtheria toxoid in humans. Transplant. Proc., *9*:191, 1977.

Mickelson, E., Fefer, A., Storb, R., and Thomas, E. D.: Correlation of the relative response index with marrow graft rejection in patients with aplastic anemia. Transplantation, *22*:294, 1976.

Mittal, K. K.: The HLA polymorphism and susceptibility to disease. Vox Sang. (Basel), *31*:161, 1976.

Morton, J. A., Pickles, M. M., and Sutton, L.: The correlation of the Bg^a blood group. Vox Sang., *17*:536, 1969.

Morton, J. A., Pickles, M. M., Sutton, L., and Skov, F.: Identification of further antigens in red cells and lymphocytes. Vox Sang., *21*:144, 1971.

Murphy, D. B., Herzenberg, L. A., Okumara, K., Herzenberg, L. A., and McDevitt, H. O.: A new I subregion (I-J) marked by a locus (Ia4) controlling surface determinants on suppressor T lymphocytes. J. Exp. Med., *144*:699, 1976.

Nardi, S.: The H-2 locus and susceptibility to Bittner virus borne by red blood cells in mice. Proc. Natl. Acad. Sci. U.S.A., *58*:485, 1967.

Nordhagen, R., and Orjasaeten, H.: Association between HLA and red cell antigens. Vox Sang., *26*:97, 1974.

O'Leary, J., Reinsmoen, N., and Yunis, E. J.: Mixed lymphocyte reaction. *In* Rose, N., and Friedmann, H. (eds.): Manual of Clinical Immunology. Washington D.C., American Society of Microbiology, 1976, pp. 821–832.

Opelz, G.: Histocompatibility testing in renal transplantation. Urology (Suppl.), *9*:72, 1977a.

Opelz, G., and Terasaki, P. I.: Prolongation effect of blood transfusions on kidney graft survival. Transplantation, *22*:380, 1976.

Opelz, G., and Terasaki, P. I.: Influence of sex on histocompatibility matching in renal transplantation. Lancet, *2*:419, 1977b.

Opelz, G., and Terasaki, P. I.: Improvement of kidneygraft survival with increased numbers of blood transfusions. N. Engl. J. Med., *299*:799, 1978.

Opelz, G., Mickey, M. R., and Terasaki, P. I.: Calculations on long term graft and patient survival in human kidney transplantation. Transplant. Proc., *9*:27, 1977c.

Opelz, G., Mickey, M. R., and Terasaki, P. I.: HL-A and kidney transplants. Re-examination. Transplantation, *17*:371, 1974.

Opelz, G., Sengar, D. P. S., Mickey, M. R., and Terasaki, P. I.: Effect of blood transfusions on subsequent kidney transplants. Transplant. Proc., *5*:253, 1973.

Park, M. S., Bernoco, D., and Terasaki, P. I.: Autoantibody against B lymphocytes. Lancet, *2*:465, 1977.

Parkman, R., Rosen, F., Rappaport, J., Camitta, B., Levey, R. L., and Nathan, D. G.: Detection of genetically determined histocompatibility antigen differences between HL-A identical and MLC non-reactive siblings. Transplantation, *21*:110, 1976.

Patel, R., and Terasaki, P. I.: Significance of the positive crossmatch test in kidney transplantation. N. Engl. J. Med., *280*:735, 1969.

Payne, R.: The association of febrile transfusion reactions with leukoagglutinins. Vox Sang., *2*:233, 1957.

Payne, R., and Rolfs, M. R.: Fetomaternal leukocyte incompatibility. J. Clin. Invest., *37*:1756. 1958.

Payne, R., Tripp, M., Weigle, J., Bodmer, W. F., and Bodmer, J.: A new leukocyte isoantigen system in man. Cold Spring Harbor Symposium. Quant. Biol., *29*:285, 1964.

Platz, P., Jakobsen, B., Dickmeiss, E., Ryder, L. P., Thomsen, M., and Svejgaard, A.: Ia and HLA-D typing of patients with multiple sclerosis (MS) and insulin dependent diabetes (IDD). Tissue Antigens, *10*:192, 1977.

Rappaport, F. T., Dausset, J., Legrand, L., Barge, A., Lawrence, H. S., and Converse, J. M.: Erythrocytes in human transplantation. Effects of pretreatment with ABO group-specific antigens. J. Clin. Invest., *47*:2206, 1968.

Reinsmoen, N., Hansen, J., Dupont, B., Gatti, R., and Yunis, E.: Antigenic complexity of the HLA-D region as defined by homozygous typing cells (HTC) and primed lymphocyte tests (PLT). Transplant. Proc., 1977, in press.

Rene, R. P., DeVries, R. R. P., Kroettenberg, H. G., Loggen, H. G., and van Rood, J. J.: *In vitro* immune responsiveness to vaccinia virus and HLA. N. Engl. J. Med., *297*:692, 1977.

Sasazuki, T., Grumet, F. C., and McDevitt, H. O.: The

association between genes in the major histocompatibility complex and disease susceptibility. Ann. Rev. Med., *28*:425, 1977.

Scandia Transplant Report: HL-A Matching and kidney graft survival. Lancet, *1*:240, 1975.

Schendel, D. J., Alter, B. J., and Bach, F. H.: The involvement of LD- and SD-region differences in MLC and CML: A "three cell" experiment. Transplant. Proc., *5*:1651, 1973.

Schlossman, S. F., Chess, L., Humphreys, R. E., and Strominger, J. L.: Distribution of Ia like molecules on the surface of normal and leukemic cells. Proc. Natl. Acad. Sci. U.S.A., *73*:1288, 1976.

Schlosstein, L., Terasaki, P. I., Bluestone, R., and Pearson, C. M.: High association of an HL-A antigen W27 with ankylosing spondylitis. N. Engl. J. Med., *288*:704, 1973.

Schreffler, D. C., and David, C. S.: The H-2 major histocompatibility complex and the I immune response region: Genetic variation, function and organization. Adv. Immunol., *20*:125, 1975.

Seman, M. J., Benson, R., Jones, M. N., Morton, J. A., and Pickles, M. N.: The reactions of the Bennet Goodspeed group of antibodies tested with the autoanalyzer. Br. J. Haematol., *13*:464, 1967.

Shearer, G. M., and Schmitt-Verhulst, A. M.: Major histocompatibility complex restricted cell mediated immunity. Adv. Immunol., *25*:1977, in press.

Shearer, G. M., Rehn, T. G., and Schmitt-Verhulst, A. M.: Role of the murine major histocompatibility complex in the specificity of in vitro T cell mediated lympholysis against chemically modified autologous lymphocytes. Transplant. Rev., *29*:222, 1976.

Sheehy, M. J., Sondel, P. M., Bach, M. L., Wank, R., and Bach, F. H.: HLA-LD (lymphocyte defined) typing: A rapid assay with primed lymphocytes. Science, *188*:1308, 1975.

Simmons, R. L., Yunis, E. J., Noreen, H., Thompson, E. J., Fryd, D. S., and Najarian, J. S.: Effect of HLA matching on cadaver kidney function: Experience at a single large center. Transplant. Proc., *9*:491, 1977.

Simonsen, M.: Graft versus host reactions. Their natural history and applicability as tools of research. Prog. Allergy, *6*:349, 1962.

Snell, G. D.: Methods for the study of histocompatibility genes. J. Genetics, *49*:87, 1948.

Snell, G. D., Dausset, J., and Nathanson, S.: *In* Histocompatibility. New York, Academic Press, 1976a, p. 212.

Snell, G. D., Dausset, J., and Nathanson, S.: *In* Histocompatibility. New York, Academic Press, 1976b, p. 230.

Snell, G. D., Dausset, J., and Nathanson, S.: *In* Histocompatibility. New York, Academic Press, 1976c, p. 341.

Soulillou, J., Carpenter, C. B., d'Apice, J. F., and Strom, T. B.: The role of nonclassical, Fc receptor associated Agb antigens (Ia) in rat allograft enhancement. J. Exp. Med., *143*:405, 1976.

Spencer, M. J., Cherry, J. B., and Terasaki, P. I.: HL-A antigens and antibody response after influenza A vaccination: Decreased response associated with HLA type W16. N. Engl. J. Med., *13*, 1976.

Springer, T. A., Kaufman, J. F., Terhorst, C., and Strominger, J. L.: Purification and structural characterization of human HLA-linked B cell antigens. Nature, *268*:213, 1977.

Staines, N. A., Guy, K., and Fish, R.: Passive enhancement and antigens of different regions of the mouse H-2 complex. Transplant. Proc., *9*:941, 1977.

Starzl, T. E., Lerner, R. A., Dixon, F. J., Groth, C. G., Brettschneider, L., and Terasaki, P. I.: Schwartzmann

reaction after human renal homotransplantation. N. Engl. J. Med., *278*:642, 1968.

Stasny, P.: Antigens in human monocytes: Ia like antigens detected in monocytes using Seventh Workshop sera. Tissue Antigens, *10*:147, 1977.

Storb, R., Prentice, R. L., and Thomas, E. D.: Marrow transplantation for treatment of aplastic anemia. N. Engl. J. Med., *296*:61, 1977a.

Storb, R., Weiden, P. L., Prentice, R., Buckner, C. D., Clift, R. A., Einstein, A. B., Fefer, A., Johnson, F. L., Lerner, K. G., Neiman, P. E., Sander, J. E., and Thomas, E. D.: Aplastic anemia (AA) treated by allogeneic marrow transplantation: The Seattle experience. Transplant. Proc., *9*:181, 1977b.

Storb, R., Weiden, P. L., Graham, T. C., Lerner, K. G., and Thomas, E. D.: Marrow grafts between unrelated dogs, homozygous and identical for DLA antigens. Transplant. Proc., *9*:281, 1977c.

Svejgaard, A., Platz, P., and Ryder, L. P.: HL-A and disease associations a survey. Transplant. Rev., *22*:3, 1975.

Tanigaki, N., and Pressman, D.: The basic structure and the antigenic characteristics of HL-A antigens. Transplantation, *21*:15, 1974.

Tennant, J. R., and Snell, G. D.: Some experimental evidence for the influence of genetic factors on viral leukemogenesis. Natl. Cancer Inst. Monogr., *22*:61, 1966.

Terasaki, P. I., Bernoco, D., Park, M. S., Ozturk, G., and Iwaki, Y.: Microdroplet testing for HLA-A, -B, -C, and -D antigens. Am. J. Clin. Pathol., *69*:103, 1978.

Terasaki, P. I., Mottironi, V. D., and Barnett, E. V.: Cytotoxins in disease. N. Engl. J. Med., *283*:724, 1970.

Thirteenth Report of the Human Renal Transplant Registry—Advisory Committee to the Renal Transplant Registry. Transplant. Proc., *9*:9, 1977.

Thomas, E. D.: Bone marrow transplantation for aplastic anemia or acute leukemia. Scand. J. Urol. Nephrol. [Suppl.] *42*:6, 1977a.

Thomas, D. W., Yamashita, Y., and Shevach, E. M.: The role of Ia antigens in T cell activation. Immunol. Rev., *35*:97, 1977b.

Thomas, F., Mendez-Acon, G., Thomas, J., and Lee, H. M.: Quantitation of pre-transplantation immune responsiveness by in vitro T cell testing. Transplant. Proc., *9*:49, 1977c.

Thompson, M., and Dickmeiss, E.: Correlation between mixed lymphocyte culture incompatibility and cadaver kidney graft rejection. Scand. J. Urol. Nephrol., *42*:40, 1977.

Thulstrup, H.: Influence of leukocyte and thrombocyte incompatibility on non-hemolytic transfusion reactions. I. A retrospective study. Vox Sang., *21*:233, 1971.

Ting, A., Hasegawa, T., Ferrone, S., and Reisfeld, R. A.: Presensitization detected by sensitive crossmatch tests. Transplant. Proc., *5*:813, 1973.

Ting, A., Mickey, M. R., and Terasaki, P. I.: B lymphocyte alloantigens in Caucasians. J. Exp. Med., *143*:981, 1976.

van Bekkum, D. W.: Bone marrow transplantation. Transplant. Proc., *9*:147, 1977.

van Hooff, J. P., Kalff, M. W., van Poelgeest, A. E., Persijn, G. G., and van Rood, J. J.: Blood transfusions and kidney transplantation. Transplantation, *22*:306, 1976.

van Hooff, J., Schippers, H., van der Steen, M. A., and van Rood, J. J.: Efficacy of HLA matching in Eurotransplant. Lancet, *2*:1385, 1972.

van Rood, J. J., and van Leeuwen, A.: Leukocyte grouping. A method and its applications. J. Clin. Invest., *42*:1382, 1963.

4

van Rood, J. J., Eernisse, J. G., and van Leeuwen, A.: Leukocyte antibodies in sera from pregnant women. Nature (London), *181*:1735, 1958.

van Rood, J. J., van Leeuwen, A., and Eernisse, J. G.: Leukocyte antibodies in the serum of pregnant women. Vox Sang., *6*:240, 1961.

van Rood, J. J., van Leeuwen, A., Schippers, A., Ceppellini, R., Mattiuz, P. C., and Curtoni, S.: Leukocyte groups and their relations to homotransplantation. Ann. N.Y. Acad. Sci., *129*:467, 1966.

van Rood, J. J., van Leeuwen, A., Termititelen, A., and Keuning, J. J.: The genetics of the major histocompatibility complex in man HLA. *In* Katz, D. H., and Benacerraf, B. (eds.): The Role of the Histocompatibility Gene Complex in Immune Responses. New York, Academic Press, 1976, pp. 31-53.

Vicenti, F., Duca, R. M., Amend, W., Perkins, H. A., Cochrum, K. C., Feduska, N. J., and Salvatierra, O.: Immunologic factors determining survival of cadaver-kidney transplants. The effect of HLA serotyping, cytotoxic antibodies and blood transfusions on graft survival. N. Engl. J. Med., *299*:793, 1978.

Wank, R., Schendel, D., Dupont, B., and Hansen, J.: Typing for HLA-D determinants by 1° homozygous cell typing and 2° restimulation of primed lymphocytes. 1° and 2° HTC responses within Dw4. 1st International Conf. on Primed LD Typing. Bethesda, Md., Naval Med. Res. Inst., 1977.

Weiner, M. S., Bianco, C., and Nussenweig, V.: Enhanced binding of neuraminidase treated sheep erythrocytes to human T lymphocytes. Blood, *42*:939, 1973.

Westbroek, D. L., Vriesendorp, H. M., van den Tweel, J. G., de Gruyl, J., and van Urk, H.: Influence of SD and LD matching on kidney allograft survival in unrelated mongrel dogs. Transplant. Proc., *7*:427, 1975.

Wilbrandt, R., Tung, K. S. K., Deodar, S. D., Nakamoto, S., and Kolff, W. J.: ABO blood group incompatibility in human renal homotransplantation. Am. J. Clin. Pathol., *51*:15, 1969.

Williams, R. M., and Moore, M. J.: Linkage of susceptibility to experimental allergic encephalitis to the major histocompatibility locus in the rat. J. Exp. Med., *138*:775, 1973.

Williams, R. M., and Yunis, E. J.: Genetics of human immunity and its relation to disease. *In* Friedmann, H., and Linna, J. (eds.): Genetics, Infection & Immunity. Baltimore, University Park Press, 1978, in press.

Williams, R. M., Martin, S., Barbosa, J., Falchuk, K. R., Trey, C., Dubey, D. P., Cannady, W. G., Fitzpatrick, D., Noreen, H., Dupont, B., and Yunis, E. J.: Ia like antigens in chronic active hepatitis and diabetes mellitus. Presented at the "Interface Between Immune Mechanisms and Disease" symposium, Brook Lodge, Michigan, 1977.

Winchester, R. J., Fu, S. M., Wernet, P., Kunkel, H. G., Dupont, B., and Jersild, C.: Recognition by pregnancy serums of non-HLA alloantigens selectively expressed on B lymphocytes. J. Exp. Med., *141*:924, 1975.

Yankee, R. A., and Sherwood, A.: The role of histocompatibility in platelet and granulocyte transfusion therapy in HLA typing. A technical workshop, American Association of Blood Banks, San Francisco, Ca., 1976, pp. 27-55.

Yankee, R. A., Graff, R. S., Dawling, R., and Henderson, E. S.: Selection of unrelated compatible platelet donors by lymphocyte HLA matching. N. Engl. J. Med., *288*:760, 1973.

Yankee, R. A., Grumet, G. N., and Rogentine, G. N.: Platelet transfusion therapy—selection of compatible donors by HLA. N. Engl. J. Med., *281*:1208, 1969.

Yunis, E. J., and Amos, D. B.: Three closely linked genetic systems relevant to transplantation. Proc. Natl. Acad. Sci. U.S.A., *68*:3031, 1971.

Yunis, E. J., Page, A., Greenberg, L., Emme, L., Hansen, J., and Dupont, B.: HL-A homozygosity and mixed leukocyte response to 8a homozygous test cells. *In* Histocompatibility Testing 1975, Copenhagen, Munksgaard, 1975, pp. 544-546.

Zinkernagel, R. M., and Doherty, P. C.: Restriction of in vitro T cell mediated cytotoxicity in lymphocytic choriomeningitis within a syngeneic or semiallogeneic system. Nature, *248*:701-702, 1974.

42

GAMMOPATHIES, HYPERSENSITIVITY, IMMUNOLOGIC DEFICIENCY

Russell H. Tomar, M. D.

4

The rapid accumulation of information about normal and abnormal immune responses has just begun to have an impact on clinical medicine. Thus, many laboratory measurements and examinations are evolving or are in trial stage. The intent of this chapter is to provide approaches to selected problems in the diagnosis and management of immunologically related diseases. Determinations already available will be emphasized, with recognition to those measurements or examinations which appear promising.

HYPERIMMUNOGLOBULINEMIA

The biology and structure of immunoglobulins have been described in Chapter 36. Increases in gamma globulin are usually first noted after a serum protein electrophoresis, a measurement of total protein, and/or measurements of albumin and gamma globulin fractions (see Chap. 9). Reference values for the different immunoglobulins vary with age, sex, and race (Tables 36-6 and 36-7). Increases in immunoglobulins are referred to as monoclonal or polyclonal. *Monoclonal immunoglobulins* from any one individual are structurally identical and presumably arise from the expansion of a single immunoglobulin-producing lymphoid cell (clone). *Polyclonal immunoglobulins* in the same individual are structurally different from each other in one or more important ways—by class, as polyclonal IgG, IgA, or IgM; by light chain, κ or λ; or by antigen specificity. Polyclonal immunoglobulins arise from the expansion of several to many different immunoglobulin-producing lymphoid cells.

Polyclonal increases in immunoglobulins have been associated with many disease states (Table 42-1) (Buckley, 1977; Cushman, 1973; Bjorkstein, 1976; Stiehm, 1973; Stites, 1976). Serum protein electrophoresis is often sufficient to establish this condition. Immunoelec-

trophoresis and/or determination of individual immunoglobulins may be of help at times in order to confirm a polyclonal distribution and/or an increased concentration in one or more immunoglobulin classes. Increases in serum immunoglobulins may result from decreased catabolism and/or increased synthesis (Table 36-5). The control mechanisms for these events are not understood. It is likely that in some cases, as with the elevated immunoglobulins in systemic lupus erythematosus, a defect in T-cell regulation exists. The implications of elevated immunoglobulins are also unknown. Most immunoglobulins appear *not* to be directed toward a specific or set of specific antigenic determinants. It also should be noted that most autoantibodies are not monoclonal, but polyclonal. In general, poly-

Table 42-1. POLYCLONAL HYPERIMMUNOGLOBULINEMIAS: SOME ASSOCIATED DISEASE STATES

CONDITION	IMMUNOGLOBULIN CLASSES
Immunodeficiency diseases	
Hyperimmunoglobulin E and recurrent infections	IgE
Wiskott-Aldrich syndrome	IgA, IgE
"Dysgammaglobulinemia Type I"	IgM
Hyperimmunoglobulin A and recurrent infections	IgA
Infections	
Congenital infections (syphilis, toxoplasmosis, rubella, cytomegalovirus)	IgM
Infectious mononucleosis	IgM or all
Trypanosomiasis	IgM or all
Intestinal parasitism	All classes
Several helminthic infections	IgE
Visceral larva migrans	All classes
Chronic granulomatous disease of childhood	All classes
Leprosy	All classes
Chronic infection in general	All classes, with a preference for IgG
Liver diseases	
Chronic active hepatitis	IgG predominates
Acute hepatitis	IgG predominates
Biliary cirrhosis	IgM predominates
Lupoid hepatitis	All classes
Pulmonary disorders	
Pulmonary hypersensitivity syndromes	All classes
Sarcoidosis	All classes
Berylliosis	All classes
"Autoimmune" disorders	
Systemic lupus erythematosus	All classes
Rheumatoid arthritis	IgA or all
Many "autoimmune" states such as thyroiditis	All classes
Scleroderma	All classes
Cold agglutinin disease	IgM
Anaphylactoid purpura	IgA
Miscellaneous	
Down's syndrome	All classes
Amyloidosis	All classes
Narcotic addiction	IgM

Table 42–2. SELECTED CONDITIONS
WHICH HAVE BEEN ASSOCIATED WITH
MONOCLONAL IMMUNOGLOBULINS

Multiple myeloma
Macroglobulinemia of Waldenström
Chronic lymphocytic leukemia
Other leukemias
Lymphomas
"Benign" monoclonal gammopathy
Systemic capillary leak syndrome
Amyloidosis
Chronic liver disease such as chronic active hepatitis,
   primary biliary cirrhosis
Autoimmune disorders, including rheumatoid arthritis,
   systemic lupus erythematosus, thyroiditis, pernicious
   anemia, polyarteritis nodosa, Sjögren's syndrome
Gaucher's disease
Malignancies of various types
Hereditary spherocytosis

clonal increases in gamma globulin are thought to be related to antigenic stimulation of a chronic nature.

Monoclonal immunoglobulins or fragments of immunoglobulins have been associated with a number of conditions (Table 42–2) (Atkinson, 1977; Benbassat, 1976; Ko, 1976; Michaux, 1969; Schafer, 1978; Wells, 1974).

The incidence of monoclonal immunoglobulins (M components) in unselected population studies is estimated to be 0.9 per cent (Bachman, 1965; Axelsson, 1968). Of course, a much higher percentage of "positives" will be found in clinical laboratories where the sera to be tested are preselected. Multiple myeloma and macroglobulinemia of Waldenström account for as few as 2 per cent (Axelsson) and as many as 78 per cent of all subjects with M components. One can expect that at least one half to two thirds of all M components detected will be from patients with these two disorders (Isobe, 1971; Ameis, 1976). In the study by Axelsson (1968), the presence of monoclonal immunoglobulins increased progressively with age: 0.16 per cent of those 25 to 49 years of age; 1.61 per cent of those 50 to 79 years; and 9.2 per cent of those 80 to 89 years of age. In that same study the monoclonal protein was IgG in 61 per cent, IgA in 27 per cent, IgM in 8 per cent, and biclonal in 5 per cent. In other series, light chain myelomas have accounted for up to 25 per cent of all myeloma proteins (Isobe, 1971; Wells, 1974). Multiple myeloma and macroglobulinemia of Waldenström are reviewed in Chapter 30 (p. 1085).

Requests to examine sera for the presence of a monoclonal protein are generated by a physician who recognizes that a patient has clinical symptoms and signs of such disorders, or by the laboratory examination of a serum protein electrophoresis which suggests a monoclonal protein. If there indeed is an M component in a serum protein electrophoresis, a quantitative measurement of immunoglobulins by radial immunodiffusion, nephelometry, or another suitable technique can virtually identify the specific immunoglobulin if only one of the major three isotypes is increased. Of course, this will neither determine the light chain of a monoclonal immunoglobulin nor detect light chain myelomas. There may also be confusion in biclonal immunocytopathies. Quantitative immunoglobulins are useful in monitoring the course of the disease and its treatment. Quantitative immunoglobulins may also be helpful in separating a benign from a malignant condition. Monoclonal immunoglobulin G levels of 2 g/100 ml (220 IU/ml) or immunoglobulin A levels of 1 g/100 (480 IU/ml) (Isobe, 1971) or greater suggest a malignant condition. In many malignant immunocytopathies, the concentration of non-monoclonal immunoglobulins is reduced. Thus, deficiency of polyclonal immunoglobulins is evidence for malignancy. Waldmann and his associates have demonstrated that in many cases this decrease in polyclonal immunoglobulins is due to a macrophage-like suppressor cell (Waldmann, 1978). Paradoxically, then, the patient with a malignant immunocytopathy is immunodeficient while possessing large amounts of a "nonsense" immunoglobulin produced by a poorly controlled clone of lymphoid cells.

Immunoelectrophoresis (IEP) (described on p. 1193 in Chapter 35) is useful in detecting the specific monoclonal protein or proteins. Thus, in patients with suspicious signs, symptoms, or especially hematopathologic findings in the peripheral blood, bone marrow, or lymph node, an IEP may be diagnostic. Whether or not serum protein electrophoresis should precede an IEP depends on the relative availability of these techniques and the sophistication of each in a laboratory. For example, agarose serum protein electrophoresis is probably as sensitive as IEP at detecting most M components. However, electrophoresis on paper or cellulose acetate is not as sensitive. Another way of selecting sera for IEP is by reviewing serum protein electrophoresis determinations. Table 42–3 and Figure 42–1 describe ap-

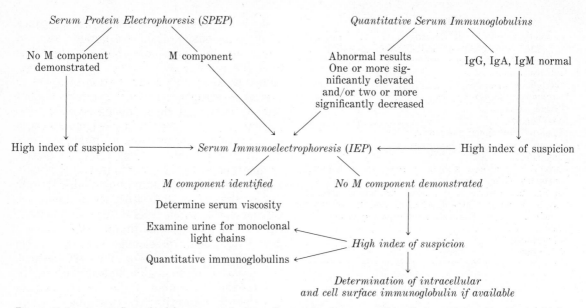

Figure 42-1. Approach to the laboratory evaluation of monoclonal gammopathies. Immunoelectrophoresis should be performed if the serum protein electrophoresis and/or serum immunoglobulin concentrations are abnormal as noted or if there is a high index of suspicion due to the patient's clinical presentation. Quantitative immunoglobulins and serum viscosity are useful measurements for monitoring the patient. Monoclonal light chains in the urine ($>$ 200 mg/24 hours) suggest a malignant condition. This approach supplements hematopathologic and clinical information.

proaches to the diagnosis and management, respectively, of patients with M components.

Immunoelectrophoresis (IEP) is a sensitive, relatively uncomplicated procedure to detect M components and their heavy and light chain components. IEP allows one to semiquantitate the concentration of the immunoglobulins. Technical details of this procedure can be

found in Chapter 35 and elsewhere (Kochwa, 1976; Palmer, 1972). Patients' sera should be compared with normal sera or a normal pool. For example, we pool 100 to 200 ml of blood from normal individuals, quick freeze 1 ml aliquots with dry ice and acetone, and store at $-70°$C. We do not refreeze the unused control sera but discard after retaining for three days

Table 42-3. INTERPRETATION OF SERUM IEP

1. No monoclonal immunoglobulin demonstrated—normal pattern.
2. No monoclonal immunoglobulin demonstrated—polyclonal increase in immunoglobulins of one or more classes.
3. Monoclonal
   a. IgG-κ
      IgG-λ
   b. IgA-κ
      IgA-λ
   c. IgM-κ
      IgM-λ
   with mobility of light chain mirroring that of heavy chain and with normal or decreased quantities of polyclonal immunoglobulins. Examine urine for light chains.
4. Monoclonal light chain only (κ or λ)
   a. IEP with anti-IgE and IgD.
   b. Quantitate IgE, IgD if possible.
   c. No evidence of γ, μ, α, ε, σ heavy chains, then light chain M component.
   d. Examine urine for monoclonal light chains.
5. Monoclonal heavy chain only (α, γ, μ)
   a. Check anti-light chain antisera for potency.
   b. Examine urine for presence of same M component (heavy chain).
   c. IgG heavy chain: gel filtration on G-200 or ultracentrifugation, if available (4S protein compared to 7S whole IgG molecule).

at 4°C. The control sera must be HBsAg-negative.

The following antisera should be used: anti-whole human sera; anti-IgG (γ chains), anti-IgM (μ); anti-IgA (α), anti-κ, and anti-λ (Fig. 42-1). It is important to realize that not all antisera are alike in strength and specificity and that it is possible to be unable to detect an M component with one antiserum, yet find it glaringly present with a second. Thus, each lot of antisera should be compared for titer, such as by gel diffusion against control sera, and specificity against whole human serum in an IEP. Interpretation of an IEP may take considerable experience, but generally one is searching for a disruption of a normally smooth line, i.e., by bowing, thickening, or changed mobility. Examples of IEP's are shown in Figure 42-2. Immunoelectrophoresis is a very useful technique but has limitations. IEP may identify the presence of a heavy and a light chain but does not insure that one indeed has an entire immunoglobulin molecule with the formula of two heavy chains and two light chains.

It is also possible, but unusual, to have monoclonal immunoglobulins present in amounts below the level of detection of the system used. The lower level of detection can be estimated by diluting a known monoclonal immunoglobulin and testing it by IEP. Since monoclonal proteins of IgM, IgA, IgD, and IgE may be present in relatively small quantities compared to IgG, the light chain portion of the whole immunoglobulin may not be detected by IEP. (The inability to detect light chains of immunoglobulins in lesser concentration in the presence of IgG of greater concentration is referred to as an "umbrella effect.") Therefore, other procedures may be required to rule out heavy chain, or "Franklin's" disease. Heavy chain disease is discussed in Chapter 30 (p. 1086). It is possible that the serum being tested and the antibody being used are not in the proper concentrations and that the M component may be missed. Finally, it is possible that the antisera being used will not detect the available determinants on a particular M component. If one has a high index of suspicion, it may be useful to use a second antiserum from another source.

Monoclonal light chains in the urine, Bence Jones protein, may be detected in more than one half of patients with multiple myeloma (Isobe, 1971; Wells, 1974). Polyclonal light chains may be detected in other disorders,

usually as a part of complete immunoglobulin molecules. The detection of Bence Jones protein by heat is reviewed in Chapter 17 (p. 605). Immunoelectrophoresis of urine is more specific and more sensitive than the heat test. IEP on urine with sufficient protein or concentrated by lyophilization or through selective membranes (Minicon, Amicon) can identify monoclonal light chains. This is illustrated in Figure 42-3. Measurement of serum viscosity is discussed in Chapter 30 (p. 1093).

TYPE I HYPERSENSITIVITY REACTIONS—IMMEDIATE HYPERSENSITIVITY

Antibody of class IgE may be formed in response to antigenic stimulation. IgE is cytophilic and binds to basophils and mast cells via its Fc portion (see Fig. 36-3, p. 1221). When antigen (allergen) contacts two or more cell-bound IgE molecules, a sequence of events occurs which results in the release of a number of biologically active substances (Table 42-4) (Johansson, 1972). Cyclic AMP and perhaps cyclic GMP play roles in modulating this process (Fig. 42-4) (Lichtenstein, 1972; Townley, 1975). Vasoactive amines such as SRS-A (slow reacting substance of anaphylaxis) and histamine cause the flow of fluids into the extravascular compartment and contract the smooth muscles. ECF-A (eosinophilic chemotactic factor of anaphylaxis) attracts eosinophils. The effect on the host depends on the site and the extent of damage. These events in the bronchial tree may lead to asthma; in the nasal passages and sinuses, to rhinorrhea or congestion (Frick, 1976). There are three basic methods of detecting anti-allergen IgE: skin testing, either directly or by the passive cutaneous anaphylaxis method (Prausnitz-Kustner); release of histamine from leukocytes; and radioimmunoassay, called the radioallergosorbent test (RAST). These methods are compared in Table 42-5. RAST is safer, less sensitive, but perhaps more specific than skin testing. In several studies it has proved to have a high correlation with bronchial provocative testing using the same antigen (Berg, 1974). A large number of allergens are now commercially available (Pharmacia). Principles of RAST are described in Figure 42-5. The major advantages of RAST are that it is safer by not requiring potentially dangerous skin testing and that it is easier to do on an

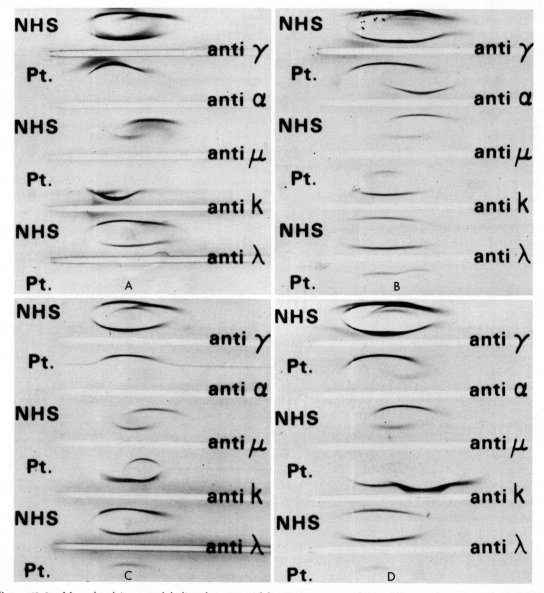

Figure 42–2. Monoclonal immunoglobulins demonstrated by serum immunoelectrophoresis. Aliquots of patient serum and a pool of normal human serum were subjected to electrophoresis on polyacrylamide at pH 8.6 (Poly-E-Film, Pfizer). The separated proteins were reacted overnight with antisera to (1) whole human serum, (2) a combination of IgG, IgA, and IgM, (3) γ, (4) α, (5) μ, (6) κ, and (7) λ chains respectively. The membranes were washed and stained with Amido Black B. *A*, IgG-κ M component. *B*, IgA-λ M component. *C*, IgM-κ M component. *D*, κ light chain M component.

(*Illustration continued on opposite page*)

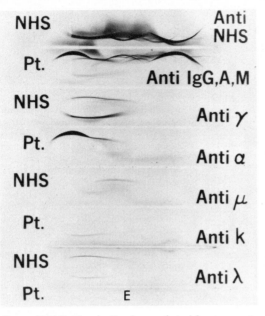

Figure 42–2 *Continued.* E, γ heavy chain M component.

agnosis some 30-fold (1 IU ≅ 2 ng) (Yuninger, 1975). Immunotherapy or desensitization initially leads to an increase in serum IgE, but later IgE declines and blocking antibody of isotype IgG may be found (Lichtenstein, 1973). Not all diseases called "allergic" are mediated through IgE. For example, urticaria and systemic anaphylaxis to penicillin caused by anti-penicilloyl antibodies may be mediated by anti-penicilloyl IgE, but hemolytic anemia is mediated by IgG (cytotoxic antibody—Type II). Serum IgE concentration in a number of disease states is shown in Table 42–6. Allergy, at least to ragweed antigen, appears to be inherited, and familial haplotypes with a predisposition to the development of atopy have been described (Levine, 1972).

uncooperative patient, such as the very young (Evans, 1975).

Serum IgE may be measured as a screen for atopy. About two thirds of non-atopic adults have IgE levels of less than 20 IU/ml; only 1 in 50 has a level greater than 100 IU/ml. This contrasts sharply to atopic adults, virtually none of whom have values of less than 20 IU/ml. Two thirds of adults with allergies have IgE levels of greater than 100 IU/ml. Thus, a serum IgE level of less than 20 IU/ml practically rules out atopy, while one above 100 IU/ml increases the likelihood of this di-

TYPE II HYPERSENSITIVITY REACTIONS—CYTOTOXIC ANTIBODIES

Cytotoxic antibodies are usually of isotypes IgG and/or IgM. Complement is often involved in the mediation of hypersensitivity by this mechanism, either by direct lysis or by attachment to a complement receptor on a phagocytic cell. Cytotoxic antibodies mediate diseases such as autoimmune hemolytic anemia, autoimmune thrombocytopenic purpura, and autoimmune neutropenia, discussed in Chapters 29, 32, and 31 respectively. Antibody-dependent cellular cytotoxicity (ADCC), discussed in Chapter 34, might also be considered a Type II mechanism. It is believed that this mechanism may be operational in some

Figure 42–3. Monoclonal light chains detected by urine immunoelectrophoresis. A spot urine sample is concentrated by drying from the frozen state or through a membrane (Minicon, Amicon). The sample is subjected to electrophoresis and allowed to react with antisera to polyvalent IgG, IgA, and IgM, as well as κ and λ chains. Normal human serum (NHS) is used as a reference. This patient has a monoclonal κ light chain in the urine (Bence-Jones protein).

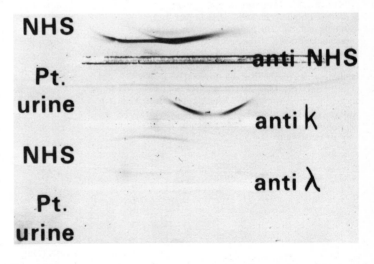

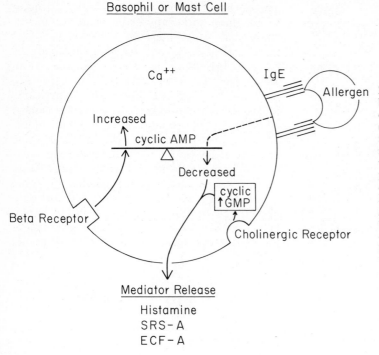

Figure 42–4. Mediator release from cells by allergen-IgE reaction. Two or more cytophilic IgE molecules bind one antigen (allergen) molecule to produce a decrease in intracellular cyclic AMP. This, in turn, incites the release of vasoactive mediators which cause edema, spasm, and eosinophilia in the target tissues. Cholinergic agents, possibly by increasing cyclic GMP levels, may also result in mediator release. β adrenergic agents decrease cyclic AMP, thereby reducing mediator release. SRS-A = Slow Reacting Substance of Anaphylaxis; ECF-A = Eosinophil Chemotactic Factor of Anaphylaxis.

Figure 42–5. The radioallergosorbent test (RAST). The allergen (antigen) is bound to an insoluble material. The patient's serum is reacted with this conjugate. If the serum contains antibody to the allergen, it will be complexed to the conjugate. Radiolabeled anti-IgE is then reacted in the system. If the anti-allergen antibody is of class IgE, the radiolabeled anti-IgE will be added to the conjugate. After appropriate washes, and with proper standards, the amount of anti-allergen IgE in the patient's serum may be determined.

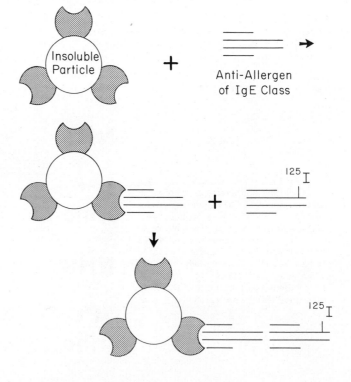

Table 42–4. VASOACTIVE MEDIATORS DERIVED FROM
HUMAN BASOPHILS

MEDIATOR	STRUCTURE	ACTION
Histamine	β-imidazolethylamine Mol. wt. 111	Contracts smooth muscle and increases vascular permeability through histamine type 1 receptors
Slow-reacting substance of anaphylaxis (SRS-A)	Sulfated lipid molecule Mol. wt. 400	Contracts smooth muscle and increases vascular permeability
Eosinophil chemotactic factor of anaphylaxis (ECF-A)	Two tetrapeptides Mol. wt. 1000	Causes selective leucotaxis of eosinophils

Modified from Lichtenstein, L.: Allergy. *In* Bach, F. H., and Good, R. A. (eds.): Clinical Immunology 1. New York, Academic Press, 1972; and Orange, R. P., and Austen, K. F.: Immunologic and pharmacologic receptor control of the release of chemical mediators from human lung. *In* Ishizaka, K., and Dayton, D. H., Jr. (eds.): Biological Role of the Immunoglobulin E System. Washington, D.C., U.S. Government Printing Office, 1972.

organ-specific autoimmune disorders, such as thyroiditis (Allison, 1976). Lymphocytotoxic antibodies have been demonstrated in a number of disorders such as systemic lupus erythematosus, rheumatoid arthritis, and malignancies. Their role in the pathogenesis of disease is unclear and is discussed in Chapter 38 (p. 1295). Techniques for determining most cytotoxic antibodies are not readily available (see Chap. 41, pp. 1358 and 1365).

TYPE III HYPERSENSITIVITY REACTIONS–IMMUNE COMPLEX DISEASES

Complexes of antigen with antibody of isotypes IgG 1, 2, 3 or IgM can fix the first component of complement and activate the complement cascade. As noted in Chapter 37

Table 42–5. COMPARISON OF METHODS USED TO MEASURE ANTIALLERGEN IgE

ASSAY	WITHIN-RUN VARIATION	DAY-TO-DAY VARIATION	SENSITIVITY	CORRELATION WITH BRONCHIAL PROVOCATION
Direct intradermal skin test	$\pm$ twofold	$\pm$ threefold	Excellent	63%
Peripheral leukocyte histamine release	$\pm$ 10%	$\pm$ twofold	Excellent	Good
Radioallergosorbent test	$\pm$ 15%	$\pm$ 25%	Good to excellent	90%

Modified from Berg, T. L. O., and Johansson, S. G. O.: Allergy diagnosis and the radioallergosorbent test. J. Allergy Clin. Immunol., *54*:209, 1974; Yunginger, J. W., and Gleich, G. J.: The impact of the discovery of IgE on the practice of allergy. Pediatr. Clin. North Am., *22*:3, 1975; and Evans, R., III: The radioallergosorbent test (RAST) as a research tool. *In* Evans, R., III (ed.): Advances in Diagnosis of Allergy: RAST. Miami, Symposia Specialist, 1975.

Table 42–6. SERUM IgE LEVELS IN
SELECTED CONDITIONS

Elevated
Atopic dermatitis
IgE myeloma
Hyper-IgE and recurrent infections
Wiskott-Aldrich syndrome
Hodgkin's disease (especially late stages)
Bronchopulmonary aspergillosis
Pemphigoid
Parasites (such as ascariasis)
Leprosy

Elevated to normal
Allergic rhinitis
Allergic asthma
Extrinsic allergic alveolitis
Cystic fibrosis
Aspergilloma
Drug allergies
Severe liver disease
Allergic urticaria
Kawasaki disease
Periarteritis nodosa

Normal
Intestinal lymphangiectasia
Bronchiolitis
Pemphigus
Thyroiditis
Chronic renal failure

Normal to decreased
Leukemias
Multiple myeloma
Isolated IgA deficiency

Decreased
Ataxia-telangiectasia
Sex-linked hypogammaglobulinemia
Congenital hypogammaglobulinemia
Acquired hypogammaglobulinemia
IgE deficiency

Modified from Waldmann, T. A., Strober, W., Polmer, S. H., and Terry, W. D.: IgE levels and metabolism in immune deficiency diseases. *In* Ishizaka, K., and Dayton, D. H., Jr. (eds.): The Biological Role of the Immunoglobulin E System. Washington, D.C., U.S. Government Printing Office, 1972; and Arbesman, C. A.: Clinical implications and metabolism. *In* Ishizaka, K., and Dayton, D. H., Jr. (eds.): The Biological Role of the Immunoglobulin E System. Washington, D.C., U.S. Government Printing Office, 1972.

(p. 1246), activation of this cascade can lead to tissue injury both directly and through the enzymes of the emigrating leukocytes. The Arthus phenomenon, with appearance of erythema and induration at a skin test site two to eight hours after intradermal injection of antigen, results from the injected antigen's binding locally in tissue to antibody and fixing complement. Not only can localized immune complexes bind complement, but also soluble circulating immune complexes may activate complement. Thus, wherever immune complexes locate, determined by their size, shape, and chemical nature, complement is activated and tissue damage may occur (Cochrane, 1973). Immune complexes are soluble only when antigen and antibody are present in certain ratios, as described in Chapter 35 (p. 1186)—generally in modest antigen excess. Von Pirquet and Schick, in their classic study of serum sickness, described the human syndrome of serum sickness produced by injection of horse serum. They noted that precipitating antibody to horse serum is often detectable at the conclusion of these clinical syndromes (Von Pirquet, 1951). Dixon and colleagues clearly demonstrated that precipitating antibody cannot be detected because the available antibody is attached to antigen in a soluble complex (Fig. 42–6) (Dixon, 1971). Theoretically, all antibody-producing immunogens introduced to a host can result in at least a transient appearance of immune complexes. Rarely does this result in overt disease, probably because of the quantity and quality of these complexes. However, there are a number of disorders, such as rheumatologic diseases, drug reactions, postinfectious syndromes, etc., associated with immune complexes (Table 42–7).

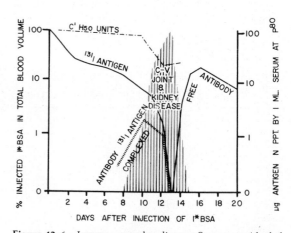

Figure 42–6. Immune complex disease. Symptoms (shaded area) occur 8 to 14 days after the injection of antigen, but precipitating antibody is not detected until about day 14. Prior to that day, antibody is circulating complexed with antigen and activating the complement cascade, resulting in decreased levels of serum complement. (From Dixon, F. J.: Experimental serum sickness. *In* Samter, M. (ed.): Immunological Diseases, 2nd ed., Boston, Little Brown and Company, 1971.)

Table 42–7. SOME DISEASES ASSOCIATED WITH IMMUNE COMPLEXES

A. *Involving endogenous antigens*
    1. Ig: rheumatoid arthritis, mixed cryoglobulins, hypergammaglobulinemic purpura
    2. Nuclear: lupus erythematosus
    3. Specific cellular: tumors, autoimmune diseases
B. *Involving exogenous antigens*
    1. Iatrogenic: serum sickness, drug allergies
    2. Environmental
        Inhaled: extrinsic allergic alveolitis
        Ingested: dermatitis herpetiformis
    3. From infecting microorganisms
        Viral: hepatitis (HBsAg), dengue hemorrhagic fever
        Bacterial: post-streptococcal glomerulonephritis, leprosy, rheumatic fever, endocarditis-related glomerulone-
          phritis, shunt-related glomerulonephritis
        Protozoan: malaria, trypanosomiasis
        Helminthic: schistosomiasis, onchoceriasis
C. *Involving unknown antigens*
    Chronic immune-complex glomerulonephritis
    Vasculitis with or without eosinophilia
    Diffuse interstitial pneumonitis
    Urticaria

Modified from Allison, A. C., Bhamarapravati, N., Cochrane, C. G., Fitch, F. W., Lachman, P., Ngu, J. L., and Winchester, R. J.: The Role of Immune Complexes in Disease, Report of a W.H.O. Scientific Group, Technical Report Series, 606, Geneva, 1972.

In general, findings of cryoglobulinemia and/or decreased complement levels, especially those in the classic pathway such as C4, suggest the presence of immune complexes. As discussed in Chapter 38 (p. 1274), circulating immune complexes may be demonstrated by several techniques. Cryoglobulinemia and complement are also discussed in Chapters 38 (p. 1273) and 37 (p. 1251), respectively. Thus, in the appropriate clinical setting, decreased complement levels alone support the probability of antigen-antibody activation of the complement sequence.

Patterns of the levels of several complement components in renal disease are shown in Table 37-3 (p. 1252). A rise in titer against streptococcal antigens such as streptolysin O or DNAse B (described in Chap. 54, p. 1892) implies prior streptococcal infection and is supportive of the diagnosis of post-streptococcal glomerulonephritis. The absence of such titers using at least two antigen-antibody systems makes that diagnosis much less likely in the otherwise normal individual. Patients with Goodpasture's syndrome or other renal diseases in which antibody is directed against the glomerular basement membrane (GBM) usually have anti-GBM antibody in their sera (Wilson, 1973; 1974). This antibody may be demonstrated by immunofluorescence or by radioimmunoassay—usually by a reference

laboratory. Cryoglobulinemia has been implicated alone and as part of lupus nephritis in the pathogenesis of glomerular dysfunction. Lastly, patients with lupus nephritis should also have antinuclear antibodies in their sera. Renal biopsy findings using light and electron microscopy as well as immunofluorescence may also be of great help in categorizing renal disorders (Heptinstall, 1974).

Of course, the presence of antinuclear antibody (ANA) in high titers, especially of the peripheral rim pattern and circulating anti-native DNA antibodies, strongly support the diagnosis of systemic lupus erythematosus (SLE)—the best studied of the non-iatrogenic immune complex diseases (see Chap. 38, p. 1265). In SLE, native DNA-anti-native DNA may comprise one of the circulating complexes. The combination of anti-native DNA titers and complement levels—especially C4—are believed by some to be particularly useful in monitoring the course of SLE and predicting relapses of lupus nephritis (Appel, 1978; Schur, 1968).

Titering and differentiating the ANA into patterns may be helpful. Identifying antibody to Extractable Nuclear Antigens (ENA) as Sm or RNP help differentiate SLE and mixed connective tissue disease (MCTD), as discussed in Chapter 38 (p. 1266) and shown in Figure 42-7.

Periarteritis nodosa (PAN) is a disorder

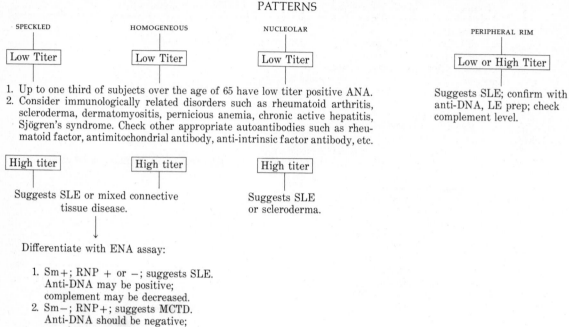

Figure 42–7. Implications of a positive antinuclear antibody (ANA) differentiation with further laboratory studies. Peripheral rim patterns suggest systemic lupus erythematosus (SLE). Other nuclear patterns in low titer are seen in a number of different conditions. The ANA may be divided into antibody to extractable nuclear antigens (ENA) such Sm (Smith) or RNP (ribonucleoprotein), which facilitate the differentiation of mixed connective tissue disease (MCTD) from SLE.

characterized histopathologically by fibrinoid necrosis of small vessels. PAN has many variants: cutaneous PAN, which is a relatively benign disorder; Kawasaki disease, also called mucocutaneous lymph node syndrome; and PAN with circulating hepatitis surface antigen (HBsAg)-anti-HBsAg immune complexes. The relationship of PAN to other vasculitides such as hypersensitivity angiitis and Wegener's granulomatosis is uncertain. It is not clear that immune complexes play a role in the pathogenesis of all variants of PAN. However, in a significant number of patients with clinical visceral PAN (perhaps 50 per cent), HBsAg and/or anti-HBsAg can be detected and HBsAg has been demonstrated at the site of injury (Gocke, 1970; Duffy, 1976). In PAN, however, complement is usually significantly elevated rather than decreased, probably owing to an intense acute inflammatory response. Moreover, serum IgE is often elevated, particularly in the Kawasaki variant (Landing, 1977; Krous, 1974). HBsAg may be deter-

mined in a number of ways, as described on page 1868 in Chapter 52. The fact that gammaglobulin, including anti-HBsAg, is precipitated by 40 per cent saturated ammonium sulfate but HBsAg is not may be used to determine if HBsAg is complexed with its antibodies by assaying the supernatant and precipitate for HBsAg after the "salting out" procedure (Gocke, 1970).

The diagnosis of a number of conditions may be supported by typing at the major histocompatability complex (HLA). Examples are shown in Table 41-2 (p. 1369). Use of these markers in diagnosis is in its infancy but surely will add further understanding of the involved conditions. For example, the association of HLA-B27 with variants of rheumatoid arthritis such as ankylosing spondylitis adds another way of grouping at least some of these disorders, i.e., HLA-B27 positive or B27 negative. The discovery that Reiter's syndrome followed a shipboard outbreak of shigellosis only in those individuals with HLA-

B27 strongly indicates an important role for immunogenetics in the production of such diseases.

Tumor antigens may also elicit antibodies and form antigen-antibody complexes. There have been a number of cases of glomerulonephritis caused by such complexes. In general, these appear to be no different than any other immune complex-caused glomerulonephritis except for the presence of tumor (Couser, 1974; Wells, 1976).

TYPE IV HYPERSENSITIVITY REACTIONS—DELAYED TYPE HYPERSENSITIVITY

Delayed type hypersensitivity (DTH) is most convincingly involved in tissue damage following certain infections, and especially those caused by mycobacteria. The caseous necrosis and cavity seen in tuberculosis is not due to the microorganism proper but to the delayed hypersensitivity response of the host to the mycobacteria. DTH has been implicated in organ-specific autoimmune diseases, in contact dermatitis and of course in tumor immunity. A description and methods for evaluation of cell-mediated immunity are found in Chapter 39 (p. 1325).

INHIBITORS TO THERAPEUTIC AGENTS

Because selected therapeutic agents, such as insulin and coagulation factor VIII, are also immunogenic and may appear as "foreign," it is not surprising that they elicit specific antibodies. At times these antibodies may interfere with biologic activity. Maneuvers such as changing the origin of insulin (as from porcine to bovine or fish), using more purified material, and/or using immunosuppressive agents, may be required (Mattson, 1975). These are discussed further in Chapters 7 (p. 165) and 33 (p. 1150).

ANTIBODIES TO CELL RECEPTORS

Another concept of the pathogenesis of autoimmune disorders involves the presence of antibodies to exposed antigens on cell surfaces. These may be inhibitory, as with anti-insulin receptor or anti-acetylcholine receptor antibodies (myasthenia gravis), or stimulatory, as may be the case with LATS (Graves' Disease) (Cuatrecasas, 1977). These may be a variant of type II reactions (Chapter 38).

HYPERSENSITIVITY REACTIONS OF MIXED TYPE

EXTRINSIC ALLERGIC ALVEOLITIS

Fibrosing alveolitis may be divided into two categories: cryptogenic fibrosing alveolitis and extrinsic allergic alveolitis. Cryptogenic fibrosing alveolitis may be characterized by the absence of both granulomata and giant cells on biopsy of the lung; and the presence of non-organ-specific autoantibodies such as ANA or rheumatoid factor (about 60 per cent) and at times circulating immune complexes. This set of disorders is characterized by alveolar wall infiltration and desquamative pneumonia. It is often a diagnosis of exclusion and a similar disease has been associated with a number of other systemic diseases of unknown etiology, such as rheumatoid arthritis, Sjögren's syndrome, dermatomyositis, scleroderma, chronic active hepatitis, and renal tubular acidosis.

Extrinsic allergic alveolitis is characterized by the presence of granulomata, giant cells, mononuclear cells, and plasma cells and the absence of desquamative pneumonia. Specific precipitants against an antigen can often be detected. The steps leading to development of this set of disorders may be as follows: exposure to an immunogenic material, such as the spores of micropolyspora faeni in moldy hay (Farmer's lung), followed by the formation of 7S serum antibodies. Upon re-exposure, an arthus-type reaction occurs, leading to extravasation of fluid, emigration of leukocytes, and tissue destruction. This episode is acute and not repeated until re-exposure to the antigen. When the antigen is contained within the body, as in colonization of the respiratory tree with *Aspergillus fumigatus* (bronchopulmonary aspergillosis), the reaction may be continuous and the disease either subacute or chronic. Early and intermediate histopathology show epithelioid granulomata, suggesting that the response may be in part type IV rather than type III. In addition, at least 10 per cent of afflicted patients will show a type I or an immediate wheal and flare response to skin testing with the appropriate antigen. Individuals with an immediate response are more likely to have bronchospastic episodes in addition to the more commonly seen symptoms of shortness of breath and malaise. Chronic disease can lead to restrictive pulmonary function, and up to 30 per cent of individuals after an exposure have some remaining symptoms (Pepys, 1975; Nicholson, 1972; Lancet, 1971). This syndrome can be caused by many antigens, some of which are listed in Table 42-8. Workers in certain industries are particularly prone to these disorders. The economic implications extend beyond this, since cattle and possibly horses may also be affected. Some antigens are available for testing either a skin response or serum precipitins. It appears at this time that the most reliable assay for precipitins commonly available is the

microimmunodiffusion test (Flaherty, 1974). The major difficulty in diagnosis is identification of appropriate antigens and the relatively poor sensitivity of the assay systems. The antigenic determinants appear to vary from group to group of microorganisms. Therefore, it is well to use either the specific material to which an individual has been exposed or a pool of materials which are more likely to contain the involved antigens.

Some antigens and kits are commercially available. Caution must be exercised in interpreting results using these systems, since some of the antigens—especially "moldy hay"—contain lipid which appears as a thick, somewhat hazy, precipitant line on a gel diffusion plate. As the antigen is diluted, so is the line giving the appearance of decreasing titers with increasing antigen dilutions. Some *Aspergillus* antigens contain materials which

Table 42-8. EXTRINSIC ALLERGIC ALVEOLITIS

DISEASE	SOURCE OF ANTIGEN	PRECIPITINS AGAINST
Thermophilic actinomycete spores		
Farmer's lung	Moldy hay and produce	*Micropolyspora faeni
Ventilation pneumonitis	Growth in humidified hot-air ventilation system	*Micropolyspora faeni *T. vulgaris
Fog fever in cattle	Moldy hay	*Micropolyspora faeni
Bagassosis	Moldy sugar cane bagasse	T. sacchari
Mushroom worker's lung	Mushroom compost	? uncertain
Fungic spores		
Maple-bark pneumonitis	Moldy maple bark	Cryptostroma corticale
Malt worker's lung	Moldy barley or malt dust	Aspergillus clavus *Aspergillus fumigatus
Cheese worker's lung	Mold on cheese	Penicillium casei
Suberosis	Moldy cork bark	Penicillium frequentans
Sequoisis	Moldy redwood sawdust	Graphium species Aureobosisium pullilons
Paprika-splitter's lung	Paprika dust	Mucus stolonifer
Wood-pulp worker's disease	Contaminated logs	*Alternaria species
B-P mycosis (BP aspergillosis)	Colonization by fungus in respiratory tract	*Antigen from Aspergillus fumigatus, Penicillium, etc.
Animal proteins		
Bird fancier's lung	Bird (pigeon, parrot, hen, budgerigar) droppings, dust	*Antigens in serum, droppings
Pituitary snufftaker's lung	Porcine and bovine posterior pituitary powder	Serum protein and pituitary antigen
Fish meal worker's lung	Fish meal	Fish meal extracts
Insect antigen		
Wheat weevil	Infested wheat flour	Sitophilus granius
Laundry worker's "detergent" lung	Enzymes in detergent	B. subtilis
Furrier's lung	Uncertain	Uncertain
Coffee worker's lung	Coffee beans?	Antigen in coffee bean?
Byssinosis	Cotton	Antigens in cotton

*Commercially available (Hollister-Stier or Greer Laboratories)

Modified from Pepys, J., and Warwick, M. T.: The lung in allergic disease. In Gell, P. G. H., Coombs, R. R. A., and Lachman, P. J. (eds.): Clinical Aspects of Immunology, 3rd ed. London, Blackwell Scientific Publications, 1975; and Fink, J. W.: Hypersensitivity pneumonitis due to organic dust inhalation. N.Y. State J. Med., 72:1834, 1972.

bind to C-reactive protein (CRP) and form a precipitate resembling an Ag-Ab reaction. Patients with high serum CRP levels may appear to have antibody to *Aspergillus* antigens. This *Aspergillus*-CRP reaction requires divalent cations for precipitation to occur. Therefore, solutions containing citrate can prevent or remove such "false positives" (Fink, 1976). Lastly, IgE anti-*Aspergillus* antibody, seen in bronchopulmonary aspergillosis, can be detected through the use of the RAST procedure (p. 1388).

DETECTION OF TUMOR ANTIGENS

There are currently only two readily available systems for detecting antigens associated with tumors. They are carcinoembryonic antigens (CEA) and alpha-fetoprotein (AFP), described in Chapter 34. Briefly, CEA was originally thought to be specific for colonic carcinoma. However, in the ensuing years since its discovery, several facts have emerged. First, CEA is composed of several molecular variants. Second, a number of tumors may be associated with increases in circulating CEA. Third, some non-malignant conditions, such as hepatic dysfunction and even smoking, may also be associated with CEA. Fourth, CEA has been useful in monitoring patients after surgery. Finally, there have been a number of patients who have developed post-transfusion hepatitis not of type A or B, who demonstrated an increase in serum CEA. However, CEA was not detectable in the transfused blood. Several modifications of procedures to measure CEA have been described. These involve differences in extraction procedures (perchloric acid or not); separation of bound and free CEA; quantity of specimen required; time for completion; and normal ranges. An indirect assay, using a perchloric acid extraction, is commercially available (Roche) and measures CEA reliably up to 20 to 25 ng/ml (Zamcheck, 1975).

Alpha-fetoprotein has been associated with hepatoma and with germinal cell tumors. However, its greatest use may be in helping to detect fetuses with neural tube defects. Mothers who have given birth in the past to infants with neural tube defects such as spina bifida or anencephaly probably should have the option of having analysis of amniotic fluid early in pregnancy for alpha-fetoprotein (see Chap. 20). Ataxia-telangiectasia and tyrosinosis have also been associated with the presence of alpha-fetoprotein.

The most sensitive method for detecting these materials is radioimmunoassay, but alpha-fetoprotein may also be detected by gel diffusion or counterimmunoelectrophoresis. Finally, it should be noted that alpha-fetoprotein has been implicated as an *in vitro* suppressor of immune function (McIntire, 1976). There is an intensive search for other and more specific tumor antigens, including those from leukemias, melanomas, and lung cancers, which might be used in diagnosis and management (Herberman, 1973). At this time, none of these can be considered to be a regular laboratory service.

EVALUATION OF THE PATIENT WITH REPEATED INFECTION

The first question to be answered is whether or not the patient truly suffers from an unusual number of infections. This issue may be quite difficult to resolve with certainty, since the average young child may have six viral infections per year. If a good history is insufficient, then a period of observation should help determine to what extent the patient is to be investigated. The type or types of microorganism involved may help guide the direction of study. Since polymorphonuclear cells, antibody, and complement are important in destroying bacteria, repeated bacterial infections suggest a defect in one of these areas. On the other hand, T-lymphocytes seem to be more important in combating intracellular microorganisms such as many viruses, fungi, and some bacteria.

POLYMORPHONUCLEAR CELL DEFECTS

Patients with PMN defects generally suffer from pyogenic bacterial infections. Individuals with chronic granulomatous disease of childhood, however, tend to have difficulty with a more select group of bacteria, i.e., those which are catalase-positive such as staphylococci, *Escherichia coli*, etc. (Baehner, 1975). Phagocytic cell defects are discussed in Chapter 40.

COMPLEMENT DEFECTS

Complement defects may result in bacterial infections. C3 is critical for optimal chemotaxis or phagocytosis. Absence of C3 or of C3 inactivator, which results in utilization of C3, leads to syndromes characterized by multiple bacterial infections. Patients who lack C6, C7, and C8 seem to suffer from infections with *Neisseria* for unknown reasons. Absence of C2 and C4 are not critical for protection from bacterial infection. Complement, including methods of assay, is discussed in Chapter 37.

STEM CELL DEFECTS

Since all of the cellular elements of the blood stream are thought to derive from a primordial stem cell, it is not surprising that deficiencies in lymphoid cells have been associated with deficiencies of erythrocytes, platelets, and polymorphonuclear cells. Virtual absence of these cells has been reported and named reticular dysgenesis or deVaal's syndrome (Hitzig, 1973). Infants with these conditions have not survived beyond a few weeks of life. These represent the most severe manifestations of the complex association between lymphoid cells and hematopoietic tissue (Cline, 1978).

IMMUNOLOGIC DEFICIENCY SYNDROMES

Immunologic deficiencies are usually separated into humoral (B cell), cell-mediated (T cell), and combined (T and B cell). Unfortunately, this convenient separation is often an oversimplification.

Evaluation of immunocompetence: screening procedures

A leukocyte count with differential will reveal if the patient is lymphopenic. Determination of serum immunoglobulin levels will confirm a diagnosis of hypogammaglobulinemia and the specific isotype deficiency. The ability to mount a delayed skin response to recall antigens such as Dermatophytin "O" (Hollister-Stier or Greer Laboratories) or Streptokinase-Streptodornase (SK-SD, Varidase—Lederle) may screen for a T-cell defect. The direction of further evaluation depends on the results of these determinations. Of course, all results must be compared with age-related reference values. This is feasible for lymphocyte counts and serum immunoglobulins. Unfortunately, adequate age-related data are not available for delayed skin test results. By age 15, however, responses should be equal to those of adults. We have found that more than 90

per cent of normal adults will respond to Dermatophytin "O" or SK-SD. In children, skin tests to recall antigens are useful if positive, but difficult to interpret if negative.

Hypogammaglobulinemia, intact delayed type hypersensitivity

The classic form of hypogammaglobulinemia is called Bruton's or *infantile X-linked agammaglobulinemia*. Males are affected, but the disorder is carried silently by the mother. These boys suffer from repeated bacterial infection and have virtually no immunoglobulin of any isotype. They rarely live beyond two years without therapy. T-lymphocyte functions seem intact, but no B-lymphocytes are present in peripheral blood. Lymph nodes have no germinal centers but do have normal paracortical development. Since antibody is also important in some viral infections, these children should receive no live vaccines, viral or otherwise. The diagnosis is established by the personal history; family history, especially that of the child's brothers and his mother's brothers; and the absence of serum immunoglobulins and circulating B cells. These children have no isohemagglutinins and do not produce antibody. A lymph node biopsy may confirm the diagnosis but is an unnecessary hazard if the diagnosis is clear-cut. These children may develop lymphoreticular malignancies or leukemia (Kersey, 1975; Davis, 1973).

The other immunoglobulin deficiencies may be categorized in several different ways: by age of onset—early or late; by the presence of another "primary" disease—primary versus secondary; by isotype(s) of immunoglobulins absent—IgG or IgA or IgM alone or any combination; and by mechanism—lack of B cells (Bruton's), lack of helper function, too much suppressor function, etc. A committee of the World Health Organization has suggested a classification of the immunologic deficiency syndromes (Fudenberg, 1971) (Table 42-9).

The age of onset may merely reflect the severity of the defect, including the type of deficient immunoglobulins, the response to antigen, the exposure to infection of the individual, and the availability and diagnostic acumen of medical personnel. There is controversy about whether these deficiencies, especially those found early in life, are inherited. There is evidence that at least some of the immunoglobulin deficiencies follow viral infections such as rubella (South, 1975). Lymphocytes from individuals with congenital agammaglobulinemia lack the surface enzyme,

Table 42–9. WORLD HEALTH ORGANIZATION STUDY
GROUP CLASSIFICATION OF PRIMARY
IMMUNODEFICIENCIES *

| | DEFICIENCIES | |
	Antibody	CMI
Infantile X-linked agammaglobulinemia	+	
Selective Ig deficiency (IgA)	+	
Transient hypogammaglobulinemia of infancy	+	+
Thymic hypoplasia (DiGeorge syndrome)	(+)	+
Episodic lymphopenia with lymphocytotoxin	(+)	+
Antibody deficiency syndrome with normal or raised Ig concentration	+	+
I.D. with ataxia-telangiectasia	+	+
I.D. with Wiskott-Aldrich syndrome	+	+
I.D. with thymoma	+	+
I.D. with short-limbed dwarfism	+	
I.D. with generalized hematotopoietic hypoplasia (deVaal)	+	+
SCID (autosomal or X-linked)	+	+
Variable immunodeficiency (common, largely unclassified)	+	+

*CMI = cell mediated immunity; I.D. = immunodeficiency; SCID = severe combined immunodeficiency; ( ) = immunoglobulins may be normal.

Modified from Fudenberg, H. H., Good, R. A., Goodman, H. C., Hitzig, W., Kunkel, H. G., Roitt, I. M., Rosen, F. S., Rowe, D. S., Seligmann, M., and Soothill, J. F.: Primary immunodeficiencies. Report of a World Health Organization Committee. Pediatrics, *47*:927, 1971.

Ecto-5′-nucleotidase. Ecto-5′-nucleotidase catalyzes the hydrolysis of purine 5′-nucleotides (AMP, GMP, and IMP) to their respective nucleosides (adenosine, inosine, and guanosine) (Edwards, 1978).

Secondary hypogammaglobulinemia may be associated with a large number of diseases or medications. The best studied are those associated with multiple myeloma, chronic lymphocytic leukemia, and lymphomas (Table 42–10) (Hayward, 1977). Medication, especially the so-called immunosuppressive agents, may alter several functions related to the expression of an immune response. Thus it is difficult to be certain how and to what extent these agents affect T-cell, B-cell, or macrophage function.

It appears as if deficiency of immunoglobulins may exist in any combination. In infantile x-linked agammaglobulinemia, all isotypes are absent or very much reduced. The most common pattern of immunoglobulin deficiency is low serum IgA. Approximately 1 in 500 to 1000 individuals in North America is *IgA deficient* (Ammann, 1971; Buckley, 1975). Secretory IgA is also usually but not necessarily absent in these individuals. Secretory component (SC) is generally present, which demonstrates the independence of production of SC and IgA. Only rarely has IgA been absent in secretions but present in serum. There appears to be an increased incidence of epithelial and lymphore-ticular malignancies in patients with absent IgA. There is an association of absent IgE with absent IgA. Perhaps 70 per cent of patients with ataxia telangiectasia and low serum IgA also lack IgE. The coincidence is lower in other individuals lacking IgA (Ammann, 1971; Buckley, 1975). The pattern of low to absent IgG and IgA with normal to

Table 42–10. CONDITIONS ASSOCIATED
WITH SECONDARY
HYPOGAMMAGLOBULINEMIA

Protein losing
Nephrotic syndromes
Enteropathies
Malnutrition

Reticuloendothelial malignancies
Multiple myeloma
Macroglobulinemia of Waldenström
Chronic lymphocyte leukemia
Other leukemias
Lymphoma
Heavy chain disease

Autoimmune diseases
Rheumatoid arthritis
Lupus erythematosus
Autoimmune thrombocytopenic purpura
Myasthenia gravis
Pernicious anemia

Miscellany
Amyloidosis
Sarcoidosis
Hyperlipoproteinemias

elevated IgM has been recognized. This pattern is called *dysgammaglobulinemia I*. A combination of normal IgG with low IgA and IgM is called *dysgammaglobulinemia II*. Primary *absence of IgM* alone was found in 0.1 per cent of hospital admissions in one study. Nineteen per cent of these patients were asymptomatic and 60 per cent suffered from infections; 22 per cent were atopic, 74 per cent had neoplasms, and 3 per cent had autoimmune diseases (Hobbs, 1975). Serum IgE and IgD are present in such low concentrations that many "normals" may appear to be low or absent in these isotypes. A few patients with recurrent infections have been described with low normal to normal serum IgG levels, but with a deficiency in one or more of the four IgG subgroups (Schur, 1970). Subgroup defects have not been described in IgA.

Finally, there are deficiencies in antibody production to specific antigens. Thus, total immunoglobulin levels may appear normal, but the individual may be deficient in antibody and susceptible to infection with certain microorganisms. There may be poor production of antibody to polysaccharides in the Wiskott-Aldrich syndrome and in multiple myeloma. For example, these individuals seem unable to form antibody to pneumococcal polysaccharides and thus unable to opsonize *Streptococcus pneumoniae*.

Hypogammaglobulinemia is but a final expression of a very complex series of mechanisms for producing antibody. This is described in Chapter 34 (p. 1174). Several immune defects in pathogenesis have been demonstrated and are described in Table 42-11. Some non-immune routes, relating to synthesis and loss of immunoglobulins, are described in Table 36-5 (p. 1228).

Methods of evaluating patients with hypogammaglobulinemia

Immunoglobulins. The essential determination is quantitation of serum immunoglobulins by radial immunodiffusion or nephelometry and comparison with age-matched references. Immunoelectrophoresis provides only a rough estimate. Serum protein electrophoresis may be valuable if a rapid diagnosis is required and the individual has a very low serum immunoglobulin G level. Secretions can be examined for the presence of immunoglobulin and especially IgA by gel diffusion, using anti-alpha chain antibody against saliva or other body fluids. Saliva may be induced by allowing the subject to chew on paraffin. Secretory component (SC) can be measured in the same way, using anti-SC antibody.

Antibodies. Most laboratories can measure isohemagglutinins as part of their reverse ABO erythrocyte typing procedure. Isohemagglutinins usually are not present until about 9 to 12 months of age. Anti-A and anti-B are chiefly IgM; anti-A,B is chiefly IgG. Isohemagglutinins are described in Chapter 43. Anti-streptococcal antibodies (e.g., ASO) are often convenient to determine. Since most children in this country are immunized against diphtheria, tetanus, polio, and pertussis, measurement of antibody to these agents is often available at reference or state laboratories. If the individual has not been immunized against these agents, diphtheria and/or tetanus toxoid can be used as an immunizing agent. Materials with living microorganisms, such as the oral polio vaccine, should not be used in subjects suspected of having an immunologic deficiency syndrome. Pneumococcal polysaccharide might also be used to measure

Table 42-11. IMMUNE PATHOGENESIS OF HYPOGAMMAGLOBULINEMIA

Absence of stem cells	Reticular dysgenesis (deVaal)
Absence of lymphoid cells	Severe combined immunodeficiency ("Swiss")
Absence of B cells	Infantile X-linked agammaglobulinemia (Bruton's)
Absence of T mitogenic factor (from T helper cells?)	Common variable hypogammaglobulinemia
Presence of excess T suppressor cells	Common variable hypogammaglobulinemia
Presence of excess macrophage suppressor cells	Multiple myeloma (polyclonal immunoglobulins)
Presence of antibody to lymphoid tissue	Common variable hypogammaglobulinemia
Dysfunction of B cells	Common variable hypogammaglobulinemia

antibody-forming capacity. For most laboratories, however, it is more convenient to use typhoid vaccines, since *Salmonella* agglutinins (as part of "febrile agglutinins") are commonly available. Side effects such as fever, leukocytosis, and pain at injection site are sometimes observed with this vaccine, however. At least two doses, approximately two to three weeks apart, may be required to elicit antibody formation. Serum specimens should be collected before and two or three weeks after each injection for simultaneous measurement. If serum is collected and frozen in aliquots, one specimen may be tested on several different occasions by using divided aliquots. One agent which has provided further insight is the antigen bacteriophage X174. This phage is a single-stranded DNA virus with a molecular weight of 3×10^6. It is quite symmetrical, being made of 180 structurally identical subunits. Although this is a "live"

organism, it appears to have no harmful effects. Clearance of the organism can be determined by doing phage titers, and the normal individual will develop first an IgM and then an IgG response after primary immunization and a high IgG type response after secondary immunization (Wedgewood, 1975). Table 42–12 is a summary of the work of Wedgewood and his collaborators.

Cellular Mechanisms. In the past several years it has been possible to differentiate B- and T-lymphocytes by their surface markers and thus conveniently enumerate them. These techniques are described in Chapter 39 (p. 1318). Enumeration of cells with complement (EAC) or Fc (EA) receptors may be technically easier and less time-consuming than counting cells with surface immunoglobulins unless one has equipment available for this purpose. EAC or EA determinations are useful

Table 42–12. CLASSIFICATION OF IMMUNE RESPONSE TO BACTERIOPHAGE ΦX174 AND RESPONSES OF PATIENTS WITH PRIMARY IMMUNODEFICIENCY

TYPE	ANTIGEN CLEARANCE	PRIMARY RESPONSE Antibody Quantity	Ig	SECONDARY RESPONSE Antibody Quantity	Ig	SECONDARY > PRIMARY	OBSERVED IN
Normal	Yes	Normal	IgM	Normal	IgG	Yes	Normal controls IgA deficiency Ataxia-telangiectasia
0	None	None		None		No	Severe combined immunodeficiency Infantile X-linked agammaglobulinemia
I	Yes	None		None		No	Common variable hypogammaglobulinemia
II	Yes	Decreased	IgM	Decreased	IgM	No	Combined immunodeficiency (CID) Common variable hypogammaglobulinemia
III	Yes	Decreased	IgM	Decreased	IgM	Yes	Common variable hypogammaglobulinemia including dysgammaglobulinemia I & II Ataxia-telangiectasia
IV	Yes	Decreased	IgM	Decreased	IgM > IgG	Yes	Common variable hypogammaglobulinemia Ataxia-telangiectasia
V	Yes	Decreased	IgM	Decreased	IgG > IgM	Yes	Common variable hypogammaglobulinemia

Modified from Wedgewood, R. J., Ochs, H. D., and Davis, S. D.: The recognition and classification of immunodeficiency diseases with bacteriophage ΦX174. *In* Bergsma, D. (ed.): Immunodeficiency in Man and Animals. Sunderland Mass., Sinauer, 1975.

but not definitive, since surface immunoglobulins are still considered the most reliable marker for B-lymphocytes. These markers are discussed in Chapter 39. A marked decrease in EAC cells usually will indicate a decrease in cells with surface immunoglobulins. However, it is possible to have a "normal" EAC count in the absence of surface immunoglobulins. No cells with surface immunoglobulins are found in SCID, infantile X-linked agammaglobulinemia, and some other cases of hypogammaglobulinemia (see Table 42–13) (Gajl-Peczalska, 1975; Geha, 1975; Griscelli, 1975; Lawton, 1975; Siegal, 1975). It was surprising to find B cells in most patients with decreased immunoglobulins, but it is now apparent that normal B cells require other cells to function properly. Enumerations of cells which rosette with sheep red blood cells (T cells) or those which have surface immunoglobulins or have complement receptors (B cells) are not difficult procedures but cannot be considered to be routine at this time. Even more sophisticated are those procedures which measure immunoglobulin production *in vitro*. Several techniques have been used after stimulation of lymphocytes by a mitogen such as pokeweed mitogen *in vitro*. These include direct measurement of supernatant immunoglobulin by radioimmunoassay; determination of intracellular immunoglobulin by immunofluorescence;

and measurement of anti-sheep erythrocyte antibody by the hemolytic plaque technique. By separating cell populations of normals and patients and then mixing appropriate cells, suppressor and/or helper function in the production of immunoglobulin can be determined in the production of immunoglobulin.

More recently it has been possible to further differentiate human T lymphocytes on the basis of their Fc receptors (Tables 42–13 and 42–14) (Gupta, 1977; Moretta, 1977). We should expect to find as many variations in the mechanisms of immunoglobulin deficiency as there are steps in the production of these proteins. Therefore, we can anticipate an increasing complexity in the pathogenesis of hypogammaglobulinemia.

Other Determinations. Since anemia, neutropenia, and platelet dysfunctions have been associated with hypogammaglobulinemia, a blood count and microscopic review with differential should be performed. Autoantibodies such as ANA and rheumatoid factor or antireticulin antibodies have been described in patients with Ig deficiency. Patients deficient in IgA often have 7S IgM (10 per cent), anti-IgA antibodies (40 per cent), and/or antibodies against proteins in food, especially bovine milk (50 to 60 per cent) or gamma globulin (40 to 70 per cent) (Buckley, 1975; Ammann, 1971). The latter may be one reason

Table 42–13. CELL SURFACE MARKERS IN IMMUNOLOGIC DEFICIENCY DISORDERS*

CONDITION	T CELLS			B CELLS			
	ERL	T_μ	T_γ	EAC	sIgM	sIgG	sIgA
Infantile X-linked agammaglobulinemia	Nl	Nl	Nl-↑	↓↓-↓	O-↓↓	O-↓↓	O
Common variable hypogammaglobulinemia	Nl-↑	↓-Nl	Nl-↑	↓-Nl-↑	↓-Nl	↓-Nl	↓-Nl
Selective IgA deficiency	Nl	Nl	Nl-↑	Nl	Nl	Nl	Nl
DiGeorge syndrome	O-↓↓	–	–	–	↑	↑	↑
Severe combined immunodeficiency	O-↓↓	↓↓	↓↓	↓	↓↓	↓↓	↓↓
Ataxia-telangiectasia	Nl	–	–	↓-Nl	Nl	Nl	Nl
Wiskott-Adlrich syndrome	↓	–	–	↓	Nl	Nl	Nl

*ERL = Erythrocyte (sheep) rosette forming lymphocytes.
T_μ = T-lymphocytes with Fc receptors for IgM.
T_γ = T lymphocytes with Fc receptors for IgG.
EAC = Lymphocytes with receptors for complement.
sIgM = surface IgM.
sIgG = surface IgG.
sIgA = surface IgA.

Table 42–14. CHARACTERISTICS OF T-LYMPHOCYTES WITH SURFACE FC RECEPTORS

	Fc RECEPTOR FOR	
	IgM	IgG
Per cent of circulating T cells	<75	<20
Response to phytohemagglutinin	Less	More
Response to concanavalin A	+	+
Radiosensitive	−	+
Effect on production of immunoglobulins in vitro	Helper	Suppressor

From Moretta, L., Webb, S., Grossi, G. E., Lydyard, P. M., and Copper, M. D.: Functional analysis of two human T-cell subpopulations: Help and suppression of B-cell responses by T-cells bearing receptors for IgM or IgG. J. Exp. Med., *146*:184, 1977.

for the food intolerance so often associated with IgA deficiency. The ability to form anti-IgA antibodies may lead to a blood transfusion reaction and even anaphylaxis. *Giardia lamblia* has been recovered from jejunal or stool specimens from immunoglobulin-deficient patients with malabsorption syndromes. Some patients with the syndrome of malabsorption and immunoglobulin deficiency will demonstrate nodular lymphoid hyperplasia in the gastrointestinal tract (Ammann, 1971).

Impaired delayed type hypersensitivity, normal immunoglobulin levels

Complete absence of thymic function is unusual. Thus, study of syndromes involving impaired T-cell function provides mixed and sometimes confusing results. While *Nezelof's syndrome* is thought to represent "pure" thymic aplasia, some children with this disorder also later develop immunoglobulin abnormalities (Hitzig, 1973).

DiGeorge's syndrome is attributed to dysmorphogenesis of the third and fourth pharyngeal pouches, resulting in a variety of malfunctioning organs. These include parathyroid hypoplasia, anomalies of the great vessels resulting in syndromes such as tetralogy of Fallot, hypertelorism, notched pinnae, and of course aplasia of the thymus. Tetany due to hypocalcemia resulting from hypoparathyroidism is usually the first suggestion of the DiGeorge syndrome. There appear to be at least two forms of this disease: (1) complete absence of thymic function, usually leading to death by infection before the age of two if

untreated, and (2) preservation of some thymic function, in which case the cardiovascular defects may be the most threatening to the individual's life. In both types, it is believed that antibody formation is impaired but that serum immunoglobulin levels are normal. In both Nezelof and DiGeorge syndromes, the thymus is aplastic, although remnants may be found. Lymph node biopsies usually reveal normal germinal centers but absence of lymphoid cells in the paracortical areas (Lischner, 1975).

There are many less complete variants of these syndromes, perhaps reflecting the stages of differentiation of thymic-derived lymphocytes into helper, suppressor, and cytotoxic cells, as described in Chapter 34 (p. 1175). One of these variants is characterized by a lack of the enzyme inosine phosphorylase (also called nucleoside phosphorylase) (Stoop, 1977) (Fig. 42–8). The reason for this association is unknown. Individuals with T-cell defects demonstrate increased susceptibility to infections with organisms such as viruses, fungi, and certain bacteria. One of the best studied conditions with T-cell defects is *chronic mucocutaneous candidiasis* (CMC). This disorder is characterized by fungal infection on the skin and appendages and mucous membranes, unresponsive or only transiently responsive to

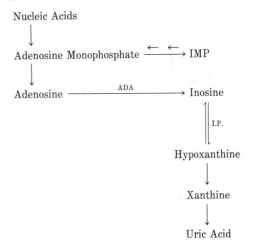

Figure 42–8. Immunodeficiencies associated with absent enzymes in purine catabolic pathways. Absence of adenosine deaminase (ADA) has been demonstrated in some patients with severe combined immunodeficiencies. Absence of inosine phosphorylase, also called nucleoside phosphorylase (IP), has been demonstrated in a few patients who are deficient in thymic derived lymphocyte function. Ecto-5′-nucleotidase (5NT) deficiency has been demonstrated in congenital agammaglobulinemia. This enzyme also catalyzes GMP and AMP to their respective nucleosidases. IMP = inosine monophosphate.

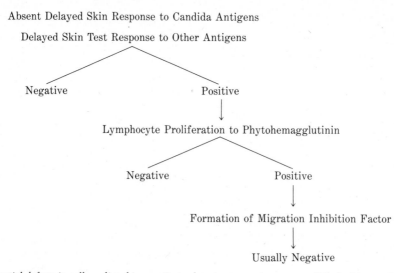

Figure 42-9. Potential defects in cell-mediated immunity in chronic mucocutaneous candidiasis. Most patients identified with this syndrome do not respond to intradermal skin testing with *Candida* antigens, but may respond to other antigens. Other possible malfunctions, particularly those of the endocrine glands, should be studied.

the usual modes of therapy. CMC is often associated with other disorders such as IgA deficiency, hypoparathyroidism, hypoadrenalism, alopecia, and ovarian failure. Patients with CMC generally cannot produce a positive delayed skin response to *Candida* antigens. The cellular defect or defects can be dissected further with *in vitro* and *in vivo* testing (Fig. 42-9) (Valdimarsson, 1973; Kirkpatrick, 1974). Defects in thymic-derived lymphocytes are associated with several other primary disorders, including Hodgkin's disease, sarcoidosis, lepromatous leprosy, disseminated coccidioidomycosis, many, if not all, viral infections.

Methods of evaluation of cell-mediated immunity

In vivo methods

The most convenient way of screening for intact delayed-type hypersensitivity is skin testing with recall antigens. These should be materials to which a large percentage of the population react. Thus, in this country, PPD is of little value. Histoplasmin and/or coccidioidin may be useful in endemic areas. Tricophyton and mumps antigens have been used by several investigators but have not found universal favor. The two most commonly used agents are *Candida* antigen (Dermatophytin "O"—Hollister-Stier or Greer Laboratories) and Streptokinase-Streptodornase (SK-SD, Varidase—Lederle). SK-SD may be used at an initial dilution of 100/25 U/ml with 0.1 ml injected intradermally. If this is negative, some workers have then tested with 400/100 U/ml.

The strength of *Candida* antigens varies greatly from manufacturer to manufacturer and from lot to lot. Dilutions of 1:50 or 1:100 have most commonly been suggested as initial screening concentrations. Children and the elderly are more likely to be non-responsive. Since a skin test requires many steps, such as antigen recognition, inflammatory response, and migration of cells, it is not clear where the defect lies if an individual is unable to respond, i.e., is anergic. We tend to believe that a positive skin test rules out a major defect in cell-mediated immunity; however, there may be defects in other T-lymphocyte functions, such as immunoglobulin production help or suppression.

There are techniques available to test the ability of patients to develop a delayed response to a new antigen. BCG immunization for prevention of tuberculosis leading to a positive PPD (purified protein derivative) is of historical interest but should not be used in immune-deficient patients because BCG contains live acid-fast organisms that may cause a potentially fatal disease called BCGosis. The materials in greatest use for sensitization are dinitrochlorbenzene (DNCB) and dinitrofluorbenzene (DNFB). Most individuals will not react with a contact dermatitis to low concentrations of these substances. However, a subject may be sensitized in about three weeks by one application of a high concentration of material to the skin, usually on the volar aspect of the forearm. The individual can then be retested with a lesser amount of material or a reaction will spontaneously reappear at the site of initial sensitization. Precautions must be taken not to apply too much, since a burn-like reaction often occurs, and not to sensitize oneself. Therefore, gloves, mask, and perhaps gown should be used by the person making up and applying these agents (Hong, 1976). Virtually all normals can be sensitized with DNCB or DNFB.

Another *in vivo* method of evaluating cell-mediated immunity has been through the use of skin grafts. If a graft from an unrelated donor is applied, it should be rejected within one to two weeks. Because of difficulties of standardization, potential problems of graft-vs-host disease (see p. 1179, Chapter 34) and because other techniques are readily available, skin grafting rarely is required.

In vitro methods

Methods of separation and testing of mono-nuclear cell populations have been described in Chapter 39 (p. 1318).

Lymphocyte proliferation

MITOGENS. Mitogenic stimulation of lymphocytes is not truly an immunologic phenomenon. The mitogen, often a plant lectin, binds to a material on the cell surface, often a sugar, and induces the cell to divide. There is no prior sensitization. *Phytohemagglutinin* (PHA) stimulates T-lymphocytes more vigorously than B-lymphocytes. PHA stimulation has become one of the common ways of evaluating T-cell function in humans.

Pokeweed mitogen (PWM) stimulates both T and B cells to respond but T cells less vigorously. B cells will produce immunoglobulins in response to PWM and in the presence of T cells. Thus, pokeweed mitogen has been used to evaluate B-cell or T-cell helper or suppressor functions.

Concanavalin A (Con A) stimulates human T and B cells but T cells more vigorously. There appear to be differences in the ability of subsets of T cells to respond to Con A, but these are not well enough worked out at this time to be clinically useful.

ANTIGENS. In general, T cells respond by proliferation to antigens. Proliferation to antigens, however, is less intensive and takes longer than proliferation to mitogens. The most commonly used soluble antigens are PPD, *Candida,* and SK-SD. The mixed lymphocyte response (MLC) is described in Chapter 41 (p. 1360) and is another way of assaying T-cell function, since it has been well-docu-

mented that the T-lymphocyte is the proliferative cell in this reaction (Oppenheim, 1976).

Lymphokine formation

Lymphokines are biologically active products of lymphocytes. Many have been described (see Table 39-4). There are two general procedures for assaying lymphokines. In the first method, the patient's cells are incubated in the test system directly. In the indirect procedure, the patient's lymphocytes are first stimulated by a mitogen such as PHA or an antigen for 24 to 48 hours. The supernatant containing the lymphokines is then examined in the test system. The leukocyte inhibition factor assay (LIF) is a direct test wherein human buffy coat leukocytes are incubated in capillary tubes in the presence of antigen. Migration at 37°C. is observed after 18 hours (Clausen, 1976). The guinea pig migration inhibition factor assay (MIF) is an example of an indirect procedure whereby the lymphokines produced by human lymphocytes are collected, concentrated—often by lyophilization—and tested for their ability to inhibit the migration of guinea pig peritoneal macrophages from a capillary tube (Rocklin, 1976). It is believed that some of these lymphokines, especially MIF, play an important role in cell-mediated immunity.

Cytotoxic assay

One function of T-lymphocytes is to kill and/or to instruct or "arm" macrophages to kill target cells. This is thought to be important in tumor immunosurveillance. Thus, there exist assays of the cytotoxic ability of T cells as described in Chapter 39 (p. 1327).

Cellular constituents

Human T-lymphocytes are most often enumerated by their ability to rosette with sheep erythrocytes (E rosettes). There are many variations to this simple assay. However, most variations result in a greater or lesser percentage of E rosetting cells. The larger percentage, generally 60 to 80 per cent of mono-nuclear cells, has been called the total T-lymphocyte count. The lesser figure, which varies greatly by technique, has been called the active fraction or the more avid fraction (Wybran, 1973). The total T-lymphocyte figure generally requires fetal calf serum, heating at 37°C. for at least 30 minutes, a high sheep red blood cell/lymphocyte ratio, and overnight incubation at 4°C. The significance of these groups of T cells is not clear but in several disorders, the lesser figure (active T cells) changes with therapy while the total T-lymphocyte count remains relatively constant (Griscelli, 1975; Wybran, 1975). As noted previously, human T cells also have receptors for the Fc portions of IgG and IgM (Tables 42-13 and 42-14). Some laboratories have produced anti-T-cell serum using human thymus, brain, or peripheral T cells. Other laboratories are producing antisera to subgroups of T-lymphocytes, and these should aid in further defining the roles of thymic-derived lymphocytes in a number of disease states (Aiuti, 1975).

Other determinations

A complete blood count and differential should be done to rule out deficiencies of any of the cell types. Immunoglobulins should always be measured to consider coincident immunoglobulin deficiencies. Autoantibodies are common in some of these T-cell syndromes. This is especially true in chronic mucocutaneous candidiasis, in which antibodies to the adrenals, ovaries, and intrinsic factor, among others, have been described. Of course, serum calcium and phosphorus must be examined in patients suspected of having the DiGeorge syndrome because of the associated hypoparathyroidism.

Normal immunoglobulin levels: Intact delayed-typed hypersensitivity

Many patients are in this category initially. Before proceeding, one should re-evaluate the evidence for an immunologic deficiency syndrome, and/or recheck the leukocyte and complement studies. If there appears to be a problem, some considerations might include lack of a humoral or cell-mediated response to a specific antigen not detectable by the usual techniques; a decrease in a subgroup of IgG; dysfunction of a subset of T cells and/or their lymphokines; and the presence of a circulating T-cell inhibitor (Gelfand, 1975).

Hypogammaglobulinemia, absent delayed-type hypersensitivity

Swiss lymphopenic agammaglobulinemia is the classic form of *severe combined immunodeficiency* (SCID) in which the progenitor lymphocytes are absent. In this disease, dif-

ferentiation into T and B cells is possible once a source of uncommitted lymphoid cells is provided, as with a compatible bone marrow transplant. The thymus may be intact. These children have decreased circulating lymphocytes, low serum immunoglobulin levels, and poor to absent delayed-type hypersensitivity. SCID may affect boys or girls but was originally described in boys and inherited in an X-linked pattern. The other mode of transmission appears to be autosomal recessive (Hitzig, 1973). Some patients with autosomal SCID also lack cellular *adenosine deaminase* (ADA). This enzyme is most conveniently measured in erythrocytes but is also normally present in small quantities in lymphocytes. Whether there is a cause and effect relationship between ADA and immunodeficiencies is not clear (Fig. 42-8) (Meuwissen, 1975). However, at least one subject has been described with absent ADA and no immune defects. Deficiencies of T-cell function and an absence of the enzyme inosine phosphorylase have also been described as have deficiencies of B-cell function and absence of Ecto-5'-nucleotidase. Children with SCID often progress to develop lymphoreticular malignancies or leukemia (Kersey, 1975).

Other syndromes in which T- and B-lymphocytes are both involved have also been described. There are two disorders with combined immunodeficiency which should be considered individually. These are the syndromes of ataxia-telangiectasia (AT) and Wiskott-Aldrich (WAS). *Ataxia-telangiectasia* is a complex syndrome involving the central nervous system and skin, in addition to the immune system. Ataxia is usually the first symptom and often becomes apparent between the ages of 12 and 14 months. Telangiectasia of the skin and conjunctiva is first noticed between three and six years of age. Cerebellar and vascular features are present in all patients. Not all suffer from immune defects, however, and three groups may be discerned: one without notable immune defects; a second with a decreased or absent serum IgA; and a third with absent delayed-type hypersensitivity. AT children often have a hypoplastic or absent thymus and hypoplastic lymphoid tissue. Early in life the paracortical lymphoid cells may be present, but they are often lost with time. These children suffer from sinopulmonary infections, often leading to bronchiectasis. They die of infection or lymphoreticular malignancies. Those with IgA also often lack IgE. There is a tendency for AT

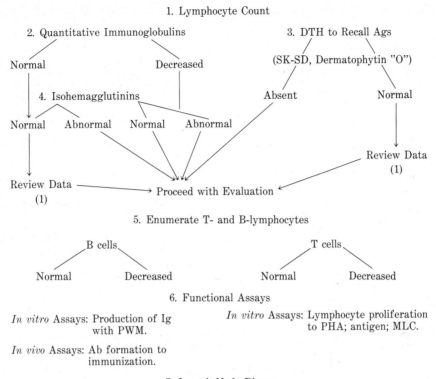

Figure 42-10. Evaluation of immunocompetence. Steps 1, 2, and 3 are screening procedures. Steps 4 through 7 should be considered in light of previous data. (1) Proceeding beyond this part depends on the clinical history and lack of defects in leukocyte or complement function. Consider IgE determination to rule out the syndrome of hyperimmunoglobulinemia E with recurrent infection.

DTH = Delayed type hypersensitivity
Ags = Antigens
Ig = Immunoglobulin
PWM = Pokeweed mitogen
PHA = Phytohemagglutinin
MLC = Mixed lymphocyte culture
Ab = Antibody

to occur in families. Alpha-fetoprotein can often be demonstrated in the serum of these patients (McFarlin, 1972; Boder, 1975).

Wiskott-Aldrich syndrome (WAS) reflects a triad of eczema, thrombocytopenia, and recurrent infections. WAS is inherited by males in an X-linked pattern. These patients cannot make antibody to polysaccharides and some proteins. They have no isohemagglutinins. They often have slightly decreased serum IgM but increased IgG, IgA, and IgE levels. WAS children are often anergic but respond normally to mitogens *in vitro*, but poorly in an MLC or to antigens. There is some controversy about the presence or absence of the Fc receptor on monocytes in WAS patients. Children with this disease die of infection, bleeding, or lymphoreticular malignancies (Cooper, 1968; Blaese, 1975).

Finally, we should note a syndrome called *hyperimmunoglobulin E* with recurrent infections, or Buckley's syndrome. These individuals suffer from recurrent large indolent staphylococcal abscesses. They have a characteristic coarse facies and a very high IgE level. A number of defects in mobility of polymorphonuclears and/or monocytes have been described (Buckley, 1972).

An approach to the evaluation of immunocompetence is described in Figure 42-10.

REFERENCES

Aiuti, F., Cerottini, J. C., Coombs, R. R. A., Cooper, M., Dickler, H. B., Froland, S., Fudenberg, H. H., Greaves, M. F., Grey, I. F. M., Kunkel, H. G., Natvig, J., Preud'homme, J. L., Rabellino, E., Ritts, R. E., Rowe, D. S., Seligmann, M., Siegal, F. P., Stjernsword, J.,

Terry, W. D., and Wybran, J.: International Union of Immunological Societies Report: Identification, enumeration, and isolation of B and T lymphocytes from human peripheral blood. Clin. Immunol. Immunopathol., *3*:584, 1975.

Allison, A. C., Bhamarapravati, N., Cochrane, C. G., Fitch, F. W., Lachman, P., Ngu, J. L., and Winchester, R. J.: The role of immune complexes in disease. Report of a World Health Organization Scientific Group, Technical Report Series 606, W.H.O., Geneva, 1977.

Allison, A. C.: Self tolerance and autoimmunity in the thyroid. N. Engl. J. Med., 295:821, 1976.

Ameis, A., Ko, H. S., and Pruzanski, W.: M components—a review of 1242 cases. Can. Med. Assoc. J., 144:889, 1976.

Ammann, A. J., and Hong, R.: Selective IgA deficiency: Presentation of 30 cases and a review of the literature. Medicine, 50:223, 1971.

Appel, A. E., Sabley, L. B., Golden, R. A., Barland, P., Grayzel, A. I., and Bank, N.: The effect of normalization of serum complement and anti-DNA antibody in the course of lupus nephritis. A two-year prospective study. Am. J. Med., 64:274, 1978.

Arbesman, C. A.: Clinical implications and metabolism. In Ishizaka, K., and Dayton, D. H. (eds.): The Biological Role of the Immunoglobulin E System. Washington, D.C., U.S. Government Printing Office, 1972.

Atkinson, J. P., Waldmann, T. A., Stein, S. F., Gelfand, J. A., MacDonald, W. J., Heck, L. W., Cohen, E. L., Kaplan, A. P., and Frank, M. M.: Systemic capillary leak syndrome and monoclonal IgG gammopathy. Medicine, 56:225, 1977.

Axelsson, N., and Hellen, J.: Frequency of M components in 6995 sera from an adult population. Br. J. Haematol., 15:417, 1968.

Bachman, R.: The diagnostic significance of the serum concentration of pathological proteins. Acta Med. Scand., 178:801, 1965.

Baehner, R. L.: The growth and development of our understanding of chronic granulomatous disease. In Bellanti, J., and Dayton, D. D. (eds.): The Phagocytic Cell in Host Resistance. New York, Raven Press, 1975.

Benbassat, J., Fluman, N., and Zlotnick, A.: Monoclonal immunoglobulin disorders: A report of 154 cases. Am. J. Med. Sci., 271:325, 1976.

Berg, T. L. O., and Johansson, S. G. O.: Allergy diagnoses and the radioallergosorbent test. J. Allergy Clin. Immunol., 54:209, 1974.

Bjorkstein, B., and Lundmark, K. M.: Recurrent bacterial infections in four siblings with neutropenia, eosinophilia, hyperimmunoglobulinemia A, and defective neutrophil chemotaxis. J. Infect. Dis., 133:63, 1976.

Blaese, R. M., Strober, W., and Waldmann, T. A.: Immunodeficiency in the Wiskott-Aldrich Syndrome. In Bergsma, D. (ed.): Immunodeficiency in Man and Animals. Sunderland, Mass., Sinauer Associates, Inc., 1975.

Boder, E.: Ataxia-telangiectasia: Some historic, clinical and pathologic observations. In Bergsma, D. (ed.): Immunodeficiency in Man and Animals. Sunderland, Mass., Sinauer Associates, Inc., 1975.

Buckley, R. H., Wray, B. B., and Belmaker, E. Z.: Extreme hyperimmunoglobulinemia E and undue susceptibility to infection. Pediatrics, 49:59, 1972.

Buckley, R. H.: Clinical and immunological features of selective IgA deficiency. In Bergsma, D. (ed.): Immunodeficiency in Man and Animals. Sunderland, Mass., Sinauer Associates, Inc., 1975.

Buckley, R. H.: In Altman, P. L., and Katz, D. D. (eds.): Human Health and Disease II. Bethesda, Md., FASEB, 1977.

Clausen, J. E.: Leucocyte migration inhibition factor. In Rose, N. R., and Friedman, H. (eds.): Manual of Clinical Immunology. Washington, D.C., American Society of Microbiology, 1976.

Cline, M. J., and Golde, D. W.: Immune suppression of hematopoiesis. Am. J. Med., 64:301, 1978.

Cochrane, C. G., and Koffler, D.: Immune complex disease in experimental animals and man. Adv. Immunol., 16:185, 1973.

Cooper, M. D., Chase, H. P., Lowman, J. T., Krivit, W., and Good, R. A.: Wiskott-Aldrich Syndrome, an immunologic deficiency disease involving the afferent limb of immunity. Am. J. Med., 44:499, 1968.

Couser, W. G., Wagonfeld, J. B., Spargo, B. H., and Lewis, E. J.: Glomerular deposition of tumor antigens in membranous nephropathy associated with colonic carcinoma. Am. J. Med., 57:962, 1974.

Cuatrecasas, P., and Jacobs, S.: Current concepts: Cell receptors in disease. N. Engl. J. Med., 297:1383, 1977.

Cushman, P., and Grieco, M. H.: Hyperimmunoglobulinemia associated with narcotic addiction. Am. J. Med., 54:320, 1973.

Davis, S. D.: Antibody deficiency disorders. In Stiehm, E. R., and Fulginiti, V. A. (eds.): Immunologic Disorders in Infants and Children. Philadelphia, W. B. Saunders Company, 1973.

Dixon, F. J.: Experimental serum sickness. In Samter, M.: Immunological Diseases, 2nd ed. Boston, Little, Brown and Company, 1971.

Duffy, J., Lidsky, M. D., and Sharp, J. J.: Polyarthritis, polyarteritis, and hepatitis B. Medicine, 55:19, 1976.

Edwards, N. L., Magilavy, D. B., Cassidy, J. T., and Fox, I. H.: Lymphocyte Ecto-5′-nucleotidase deficiency in agammaglobulinemia. Science, 201:628, 1978.

Evans, R., III: The radioallergosorbent test (RAST) as a research tool. In Evans, R. III (ed.): Advances in the Diagnosis of Allergy: RAST. Symposia Specialists, 1975.

Fink, J. N.: Hypersensitivity pneumonitis due to organic dust inhalation. N.Y. State J. Med., 72:1834, 1972.

Fink, J. N.: Diseases of the Lung. In Rose, N. R., and Friedman, H. (eds.): Manual of Clinical Immunology. Washington, D. C., American Society of Microbiology, 1976.

Flaherty, D. K., Barboriak, J., Emanuel, D., Fink, J., Marx, J., Moore, V., Reed, C. E., and Roberts, R.: Multilaboratory comparison of three immunodiffusion methods used for the detection of precipitating antibodies in hypersensitivity pneumonitis. J. Lab. Clin. Med., 84:298, 1974.

Frick, O. L.: Immediate hypersensitivity. In Fudenberg, H. H., Stites, D. P., Caldwell, J., and Wells, J. V. (eds.): Basic and Clinical Immunology. Los Altos, Cal., Lange Medical Publishers, 1976.

Fudenberg, H. H., Good, R. A., Goodman, H. C., Hitzig, W., Kunkel, H. G., Roitt, I. M., Rosen, F. S., Rowe, D. S., Seligmann, M., and Soothill, J. F.: Primary immunodeficiencies. Report of a World Health Organization Committee. Pediatrics, 47:927, 1971.

Gajl-Peczalska, K., Lim, S. D., and Good, R. A.: B lymphocytes in primary and secondary deficiencies of humoral immunity. In Bergsma, D. (ed.): Immunodeficiency in Man and Animals. Sunderland, Mass., Sinauer Associates, Inc., 1975.

Geha, R. S., Gatien, J. G., Merler, E., and Rosen, F. S.: Assessment of the B-lymphocyte population in agammaglobulinemia. In Bergsma, D. (ed.): Immunodeficiency in Man and Animals. Sunderland, Mass., Sinauer Associates, Inc., 1975.

Gelfand, E. W., Parkman, R., and Rosen, F. S.: Lymphocytotoxins and immunologic unresponsiveness. In Bergsma, E. (ed.): Immunodeficiency in Man and Animals. Sunderland, Mass., Sinauer Associates, Inc., 1975.

Gocke, D. J., Morgan, C., Lockshin, M., Hsu, K., Bombardieri, S., and Christian, C. L.: Association between polyarteritis and Australian antigen. Lancet, *2*:1149, 1970.

Griscelli, C.: T and B markers in immunodeficiencies. *In* Bergsma, D. (ed.): Immunodeficiency in Man and Animals. Sunderland, Mass., Sinauer Associates, Inc., 1975.

Gupta, S., and Good, R. A.: Subpopulations of human T lymphocytes. I. Studies in immunodeficient patients. Clin. Exp. Immunol., *30*:222, 1977.

Hayward, A. R.: Secondary Immunodeficiency. *In* Immunodeficiency. London, E. Arnold, 1977.

Heptinstall, R. H.: Pathology of the Kidney, 2nd ed. Boston, Little, Brown and Company, 1974.

Herberman, R. B., and Gaylord, C. E. (eds.): Conference and Workshop on Cellular Immune Reactions to Human Tumor-Associated Antigens. NCI Monograph 37. Washington, D.C., 1973.

Hitzig, W. H.: Congenital Thymic and Lymphocyte Deficiency Disorders. *In* Stiehm, E. R., and Fulginiti, V. A. (eds.): Immunologic Disorders in Infants and Children. Philadelphia, W. B. Saunders Company, 1973.

Hobbs, J. R.: IgM Deficiency. *In* Bergsma, D. (ed.): Immunodeficiency in Man and Animals. Sunderland, Mass., Sinauer Associates, Inc., 1975.

Hong, R.: Immunodeficiency. *In* Rose, N., and Friedman, H. (eds.): Manual of Clinical Immunology. Washington, D.C., American Society of Microbiology, 1976.

Isobe, T., and Osserman, E. F.: Pathologic conditions associated with plasma cell dyscrasias: A study of 806 cases. Ann. N.Y. Acad. Sci., *190*:507, 1971.

Johansson, S. G. O., Bennich, H. H., and Berg, T.: The Clinical Significance of IgE. *In* Schwartz, R. S. (ed.): Progress in Clinical Immunology I. New York, Grune and Stratton, Inc., 1972.

Kersey, J. H., Spector, B. D., and Good, R. A.: Primary immunodeficiency and malignancy. *In* Bergsma, D. (ed.): Immunodeficiency in Man and Animals. Sunderland, Mass., Sinauer Associates, Inc., 1975.

Kirkpatrick, C. H., and Smith, T. H.: Chronic mucocutaneous candidiasis: Immunologic and antibiotic therapy. Ann. Intern. Med., *80*:310, 1974.

Ko, H. S., and Pruzanski, W.: M components associated with lymphoma: A review of 62 cases. Am. J. Med. Sci., *272*:175, 1976.

Kochwa, S.: Immunoelectrophoresis (including zone electrophoresis). *In* Rose, N. R., and Friedman, H. (eds.): Manual of Clinical Immunology. Washington, D.C., American Society of Microbiology, 1976.

Krous, H. F., Clausen, C. R., and Ray, C. G.: Elevated immunoglobulin E in infantile polyarteritis nodosa. J. Pediatr., *84*:841, 1974.

Lancet (editorial): Fibrosing alveolitis. *1*:999, 1971.

Landing, B., and Larson, E.: Are infantile periarteritis nodosa with coronary artery involvement and fatal mucocutaneous lymph node syndrome the same? Comparison of 20 patients from North America with patients from Hawaii and Japan. Pediatrics, *59*: 651, 1977.

Lawton, A. C., Wu, L. Y. F., and Cooper, M. D.: A spectrum of B cell differentiation defects. *In* Bergsma, D. (ed.): Immunodeficiency in Man and Animals. Sunderland, Mass., Sinauer Associates, Inc., 1975.

Levine, B. B., Stember, R. H., and Fotino, M.: Ragweed hay fever: Genetic control and linkage to HLA haplotypes. Science, *178*:1201, 1972.

Lichtenstein, L. M., Ishizaka, K., Norman, P. S., Sobotka, A. K., and Hill, B. M.: IgE antibody measurement in ragweed hay fever. Relationship to clinical severity and the results of immunotherapy. J. Clin. Invest., *52*:472, 1973.

Lichtenstein, L.: Allergy. *In* Bach, F. H., and Good, R. A. (eds.): Clinical Immunology, vol. I. New York, Academic Press, Inc., 1972.

Lischner, H. W., and Huff, D. S.: T-cell deficiency in DiGeorge syndrome. *In* Bergsma, D. (ed.): Immunodeficiency in Man and Animals. Sunderland, Mass., Sinauer Associates, Inc., 1975.

Mattson, J., Patterson, R., and Roberts, M.: Insulin therapy in patients with systemic insulin allergy. Arch. Intern. Med., *135*:818, 1975.

McFarlin, D. E., Strober, W., and Waldmann, T. A.: Ataxia telangiectasia. Medicine, *51*:281, 1972.

McIntire, K. R., and Waldmann, T. A.: Alpha-fetoprotein. *In* Rose, N. R., and Friedman, H. (eds.): Manual of Clinical Immunology. Washington, D.C., American Society of Microbiology, 1976.

Meuwissen, H. T., Pickering. R. J., and Pollara, B.: Adenosine deaminase deficiency in combined immunologic deficiency disease. *In* Bergsma, D. (ed.): Immunodeficiency in Man and Animals. Sunderland, Mass., Sinauer Associates, Inc., 1975.

Michaux, J. L., and Heremans, J. F.: Thirty cases of monoclonal immunoglobulin disorders other than myeloma or macroglobulinemia. Am. J. Med., *46*:562, 1969.

Moretta, L., Webb, S., Grossi, G. E., Lydyard, P. M., and Cooper, M. D.: Functional analysis of two human T-cell subpopulations: Help and suppression of B-cell responses by T-cells bearing receptors for IgM or IgG. J. Exp. Med., *146*:184, 1977.

Nicholson, D. P.: Extrinsic allergic pneumonias. Am. J. Med., *53*:131, 1972.

Oppenheim, J. J., and Schecter, B.: Lymphocyte transformation. *In* Rose, N. R., and Friedman, H. (eds.): Manual of Clinical Immunology. Washington, D.C., American Society of Microbiology, 1976.

Orange, R. P., and Austen, K. F.: Immunologic and pharmacologic receptor control of the release of chemical mediators from human lung. *In* Ishizaka, K., and Dayton, D. H. (eds.): The Biological Role of the Immunoglobulin E System. Washington, D.C., U.S. Government Printing Office, 1975.

Palmer, D. F., and Wood, R.: Qualitation and Quantitation of Immunoglobulins. Immunology Series No. 3, Procedural Guide, DHEW (CDC) 74-8102, 1972.

Pepys, J., and Warwick, M. T.: The lung in allergic disease. *In* Gell, P. G. H., Coombs, R. R. A., and Lachman, P. J. (eds.): Clinical Aspects of Immunity, 3rd ed. London, Blackwell Scientific Publications, 1975.

Rocklin, R. W.: Production and assay of human migration inhibition factor. *In* Rose, N. R., and Friedman, H. (eds.): Manual of Clinical Immunology. Washington, D.C., American Society of Microbiology, 1976.

Schafer, A. I., Miller, J. B., Lester, E. P., Bowers, T. K., and Jacobs, H. S.: Monoclonal gammopathy in hereditary spherocytosis: A possible pathogenetic relation. Ann. Intern. Med., *88*:45, 1978.

Schur, P., and Sandson, J.: Immunologic factors and clinical activity in systemic lupus. N. Engl. J. Med., *278*:533, 1968.

Schur, P. H., Borel, H., Gelfand, G. W., Alper, C. A., and Rosen, F. S.: Selective gamma-G globulin deficiencies in patients with recurrent pyogenic infections. N. Engl. J. Med., *283*:631, 1970.

Siegal, F. P., Wernet, P., Dickler, H. B., Fu, S. M., and Kunkel, H. G.: B lymphocytes lacking surface Ig in patients with immune deficiency: Initiation of Ig synthesis in culture of cells of a patient with thymoma. *In* Bergsma, D. (ed.): Immunodeficiency in Man and Animals. Sunderland, Mass., Sinauer Associates, Inc., 1975.

South, M. A., Montgomery, J. R., and Rawls, W. E.: Immune deficiency in congenital rubella and other viral infections. *In* Bergsma, D. (ed.): Immunodeficiency in Man and Animals. Sunderland, Mass., Sinauer Associates, Inc., 1975.

Stiehm, E. R.: Immunoglobulins and antibodies. *In* Stiehm, E. R., and Fulginiti, V. A. (eds.): Immunologic Disorders in Infants and Children. Philadelphia, W. B. Saunders Company, 1973.

Stites, D. P.: Laboratory methods for detection of antigens and antibodies. *In* Fudenberg, H. H., Stites, D. P., Caldwell, J., and Wells, J. V.: Basic and Clinical Immunology. Los Altos, Cal., Lange Medical Publishers, 1976.

Stoop, J. W., Zegers, B. J. M., Hendrickx, G. F. M., Siegenbeek van Heukelom, L. H., Staal, G. E. J., DeBree, P. K., Wadman, S. K., and Ballieux, R. E.: Purine nucleoside phosphorylase deficiency associated with selective cellular immunodeficiency. N. Engl. J. Med., *296*:651, 1977.

Townley, R. G.: Pharmacologic blocks to mediator release: Clinical applications. *In* Adv. Asthma Allergy, *2*:7, 1975.

Valdimarsson, H., Higgs, J. M., Wells, R. S., Yamamura, M., Hobbs, J. R., and Holt, P. J. L.: Immune abnormalities associated with chronic mucocutaneous candidiasis. Cell Immunol. *6*:348, 1973.

von Pirquet, C. F. R. H., and Schick, B.: Serum Sickness. Baltimore, Williams and Wilkins Co., 1951.

Waldmann, T. A., Strober, W., Polmar, S., and Terry, W. D.: IgE levels and metabolism in immune deficiency disease. *In* Ishizaka, K., and Dayton, D. H. (eds.): The Biological Role of the Immunoglobulin E System. Washington, D.C., U.S. Government Printing Office, 1975.

Waldmann, T. A., Blaese, R. M., Broder, S., and Krakaner, R. S.: Disorders of suppressor immunoregulatory cells in the pathogenesis of immunodeficiency and autoimmunity. Ann. Intern. Med., *88*:226, 1978.

Wedgewood, R. J., Ochs, H. D., and Davis, S. D.: The recognition and classification of immunodeficiency diseases with bacteriophage ΦX 174. *In* Bergsma, D. (ed.): Immunodeficiency in Man and Animals. Sunderland, Mass., Sinauer Associates, Inc., 1975.

Wells, J. V.: Immune mechanisms in tissue damage. *In* Fudenberg, H. H., Stites, D. P., Caldwell, J., and Wells, J. V.: Basic and Clinical Immunology. Los Altos, Cal., Lange Medical Publishers, 1976.

Wells, J. V., and Fudenberg, H. H.: Paraproteinemias. DM, February, 1974.

Wilson, C. B., and Dixon, F. J.: Antiglomerular basement membrane antibody-induced glomerular nephritis. Kidney Int., *3*:74, 1973.

Wilson, C. B., and Dixon, F. J.: Immunopathology and glomerular nephritis. Ann. Rev. Med., *25*:83, 1974.

Wybran, J., and Fudenberg, H. H.: Human thymus-derived rosette-forming cells and immunologic disease. *In* Bergsma, D. (ed.): Immunodeficiency in Man and Animals. Sunderland, Mass. Sinauer Associates, Inc., 1975.

Wybran, J., and Fudenberg, H. H.: Thymus-derived rosette-forming cells in various disease states: Cancer, lymphomas, bacterial and viral infections, and other diseases. J. Clin. Invest., *52*:1026, 1973.

Yunginger, J. W., and Gleich, G. H.: The impact of the discovery of IgE on the practice of allergy. Pediatr. Clin. North Am., *22*:3, 1975.

Zamcheck, N., and Kupchik, H. Z.: Summary of clinical use and limitations of the carcinoembryonic antigen assay and some methodological considerations. *In* Rose, N. R., and Friedman, H. (eds.): Manual of Clinical Immunology. Washington, D.C., American Society of Microbiology, 1976.

43

IMMUNOHEMATOLOGY, BLOOD BANKING, AND HEMOTHERAPY

Chang Ling Lee, M.D., and
John Bernard Henry, M.D.

With a section on Therapeutic Pheresis and Plasma Exchange
by Thomas A. Ruma, M.D.

4

INTRODUCTION

The term *immunohematology* refers to immunologic reactions involving blood components. Although it had been used by a few investigators for many years, it was neither well defined nor generally accepted until 1954, when Dr. Israel Davidsohn presented "Immunohematology, A New Branch of Clinical Pathology."

Blood components have been studied intensively. Along with recent advances in immunologic concepts and technology, basic understanding of immunohematology has increased very rapidly. Prior to 1960, major emphasis had been on erythrocytes, whereas since then the immunology of leukocytes, platelets, and plasma components has been the focus of much investigation. The development of new techniques in biochemistry and cytogenetics in the past two decades has also added greatly to the progress of immunohematology.

While the basic sciences were progressing, applications usually developed concurrently. The first and most important application of immunohematology is the safe blood transfusion. The second application is understanding of the pathogenesis, diagnosis, and prevention of Rh immunization (sensitization) associated with pregnancy. In addition, plasma and its derivatives have been used in a number of clinical disorders, and platelet and granulocyte transfusions have saved the lives of many patients. While the precise role of immunohematology in organ transplantation remains unclear, its importance cannot be denied.

In addition to clinical medicine, immunohematology has made important contributions in the areas of human genetics, anthropology, criminology, and, recently, in the resolution of disputed parentage problems. The emphasis of this chapter has been placed on essential basic information as well as important applications pertinent to the practice of laboratory medicine.

The term *blood banking* embraces collection, processing, preservation, preparation, and distribution of blood and blood components and derivatives. Each of these operations has become highly specialized and regulated and requires well-trained personnel and expensive equipment; it is no longer practical to be a small part of every hospital. Currently, more than 80 per cent of blood and blood components are supplied by less than 100 institutions in the United States and by far fewer in many other countries.

The term *hemotherapy* implies selection with preparation and infusion of appropriate blood, blood components, or derivatives for each individual patient. Various types of procedures such as freezing, washing, therapeutic bleeding, and pheresis with special equipment, different types of preservation, more refined techniques for incompatibility testing and antibody identification, increasing number and variety of complex surgical procedures, increasing demand for platelets and granulocytes, plus strict regulation by many professional and governmental agencies, all contribute to the demand for a better *transfusion service* in the hospital.

BASIC IMMUNOHEMATOLOGY

BLOOD GROUP ANTIGENS

The term *blood group* used in this chapter refers not only to groups of erythrocyte antigens but also to other blood components, including leukocytes, platelets, and plasma. The term *antigen* refers to a substance that can initiate an immune response and react with induced antibodies or sensitized lymphocytes. Hence, antigens are also known as immunogens. The term *specificity* refers to the appearance of a substance that can be recognized by immunologic techniques and is commonly used in reference to leukocyte antigens; it may indicate a complex antigen or a fraction of an antigen. The term *factor* has been used to include classic antigens as well as those recognized by immunologic methods not utilizing a specific antibody, e.g., A_2 or A_3. The majority of established antigens or specificities are inherited, follow the rules of inheritance, and serve as useful genetic markers. Those antigens or specificities of blood components that are inherited as a group are referred to as a blood group system. The relationship of genetic markers within a group is reviewed in Chapters 26, 41, and 44.

Biologic properties

Antigen. Complete antigens are substances which can induce, in an animal host, either a humoral or a cellular immune response, or both; they can react with the elicited antibodies or sensitized lymphocytes. An incomplete antigen, which is known as a *hapten,* cannot elicit an immune response by itself but can react with a specific antibody or block a specific antigen-antibody reaction. Haptens, which may be very simple chemicals, have contributed greatly to the study of antigenic determinants.

Antigenicity. The property of an antigen which induces an immune response is known as antigenicity. Antigenicity varies not only with the type of antigen but also with the immunized host. The species and individual condition of an animal host, as well as the route and frequency of immunization, affect the degree of immune response. In general, the host must lack the injected antigen; otherwise, no immune response can be elicited. Blood group antigens are usually far less antigenic than microorganisms; moreover, erythrocyte antigens seem less antigenic than antigens on leukocytes or platelets or in plasma, as evidenced by the occurrence of strongly reactive antibodies in plasma of transfused patients.

Antigens A and B in the ABO system are by far the most antigenic, since individuals who lack either or both antigens almost always have the antibody(ies). The next most potent antigen is perhaps the $Rh_o(D)$ antigen; two thirds of all $Rh_o(D)$ negative persons will develop $Rh_o(D)$ antibodies after sufficient dosage and frequency exposure to the D antigen (Mollison, 1972). Thus, from a clinical standpoint, these three antigens are by far the most important. However, there are many other erythrocyte antigens that are highly antigenic. The relative potency of some clinically important erythrocyte antigens is listed in Table 43-1.

Antigenic Specificity. Besides antigenicity, specificity is also a very important property of an antigen. The basis of dividing human individuals into four basic erythrocyte groups—A, B, AB, and O—is their reactivity with two antisera containing anti-A or anti-B. Erythrocytes of a group A person will be agglutinated by anti-A but not by anti-B, those of group B, by anti-B but not anti-A, those of group AB by both antisera, while those of group O will be agglutinated by neither of them. This type of clear-cut specificity is reflected by most of the established erythrocyte groups and to some extent by the serum protein groups; however, such specificity is less evident in leukocyte antigens. While cross-reactions are common in leukocyte antigens, certain specificities can, nevertheless, be established through cross-absorption. Uncertainties as to the specificity of an antigen-antibody reaction may derive from questionable technical procedures and impure reagents. Therefore, it is of utmost importance to take all precautions before considering the specificity of either an antigen or an antibody.

TABLE 43–1. RELATIVE ANTIGENICITY OF SEVERAL CLINICALLY IMPORTANT BLOOD GROUP FACTORS*

ANTIGEN	RELATIVE POTENCY	ANTIGEN	RELATIVE POTENCY
D	0.70	K	0.10
c	0.041	E	0.0338
k	0.030	e	0.0112
Fy^a	0.0046	C	0.0022
Jk^a	0.0014	S	0.0008
Jk^b	0.0006	s	0.0006

* These figures represent the approximate percentage of persons who are negative for a specific antigen but receive one unit of corresponding antigen-positive blood and develop antibodies to the specific antigen. When relative potency of K antigen is 0.1 as estimated by Korstad (1957), the relative potency of other blood groups can be estimated as shown by Mollison (1972, p. 188).

Physical and chemical properties

Site of Antigen. Biologic differences of various antigens are derived from the differences in their physical and chemical structures; the size, shape, number of available sites, and chemical composition of an antigen are important contributing factors. The smallest *size* of a complete antigen has been shown to have a molecular weight near 4000, while an incomplete antigen can be very small, such as a simple sugar or a benzene ring. Although the shape of blood group antigens remains to be determined, their relationship to the cytoplasmic membrane has been shown to be critical with regard to their activity. For instance, there is an absence of ABO antigen reactivity in the Bombay type of erythrocyte, but the integrity of the red cell membrane seems unaffected. On the other hand, there is evidence indicating the presence of a de-

fective membrane in Rh$_{null}$ individuals who lack all Rh antigens. From these findings, one may assume that the ABO antigens are likely to be extramembranous, whereas the Rh antigens are likely to be intramembranous. These differences may be responsible, at least in part, for the wide differences in the characteristics between the ABO and the Rh antigens.

Number of Antigenic Sites. The number of antigenic sites on erythrocytes for some antigens is known. Using antibodies labeled with radioactive isotopes such as ^{125}I, it is possible to estimate the number of antigenic sites by the number of radioactive antibodies attached to the erythrocytes. Table 43-2 shows some of the estimated antigenic sites on each erythrocyte. The wide variation in the number of sites can explain the diversity of serologic behavior of these antigens. It is also possible to use antibodies labeled with electron-dense particles such as ferritin to count from an electron micrograph the number of antibodies attached to the erythrocyte surface. With immunoelectron microscopy, the findings obtained with radioisotopes have been confirmed (Masouredis, 1973). In addition, the ABO antigens have been shown to cluster, while the Rh antigens remain rather isolated, another contributing factor to their reactivity.

Chemical Composition. The chemical composition of an antigen determines most of its physical and biologic properties. Many of the known complete antigens are proteins, glycoproteins, or lipoproteins. Pure carbohydrate can elicit immune response only in certain animal species, such as man and mouse, whereas pure lipids or free DNA are not antigenic, although they can serve as haptens.

In studies of synthetic peptide chains, the polymers of one type of amino acid may be less antigenic than polymers of different types of amino acids. The presence of specific amino acids, such as glutamic acid, tyrosine, tryptophan, phenylalanine, cystine, and alanine, appears to increase the anti-

Table 43–2. NUMBER OF ANTIGENIC SITES ON EACH ERYTHROCYTE ESTIMATED BY RADIOACTIVE ANTIBODIES

SITE FOR ANTIGEN	PHENOTYPES	NUMBER OF ANTIGENIC SITES	SITE FOR ANTIGEN	PHENOTYPES	NUMBER OF ANTIGENIC SITES
A	A$_1$ adult	810–1170 × 10^3	D	DCce	9.9–14.6 × 10^3
	newborn	250–370 × 10^3		Dce	12–20 × 10^3
	A$_2$ adult	240–290 × 10^3		DcEe	14–16.6 × 10^3
	newborn	140 × 10^3			14.5–19.3 × 10^3
	A$_1$B adult	460–850 × 10^3		DcE	15.8–33.3 × 10^3
	newborn	220 × 10^3		DCcEe	23–31 × 10^3
	A$_2$B adult	120 × 10^3		D--	110–202 × 10^3
B	B adult	750 × 10^3		D^u	0.8–3 × 10^3
	A$_1$B adult	430 × 10^3	c	c+C−	70–85 × 10^3
I	I+	500 × 10^3		c+C+	37–53 × 10^3
Le^a	Le(a+)	4.5–8 × 10^3	e	e+E−	18.2–24.4 × 10^3
K	K+k−	6.1 × 10^3		e+E+	13.4–14.5 × 10^3
	K+k+	3.5 × 10^3	E	e−E+	0.45–25.6 × 10^3

Figures are taken from Mollison (1972).

Table 43–3. SEROLOGIC SPECIFICITY OF ANTIBODIES AGAINST ISOMERS* OF TARTARIC ACID (TA)

HAPTEN	ANTIBODIES AGAINST ISOMERS OF TA		
	l-TA	d-TA	m-TA
l-TA	+++	+/−	+/−
d-TA	−	+++	+/−
m-TA	+/−	−	+++

$$*l\text{-}TA = \begin{array}{c} COOH \\ HOCH \\ HCOH \\ COOH \end{array} \quad d\text{-}TA = \begin{array}{c} COOH \\ HCOH \\ HOCH \\ COOH \end{array} \quad m\text{-}TA = \begin{array}{c} COOH \\ HCOH \\ HCOH \\ COOH \end{array}$$

After Landsteiner (1929).
+ and +++ indicate strength of reaction. − indicates absence of reaction.

genic effect. In general, glycoproteins or lipoproteins are more immunogenic than pure proteins.

While the antigenicity of an antigen depends a great deal on its size as well as other factors, the specificity is determined by the presence of one or a few simple chemicals such as radicals, amino acids, simple sugars, and fatty acids. These simple but critical chemicals are known as antigenic determinants.

Antigenic Determinants. Antigenic determinants were demonstrated by Landsteiner (1929), the father of immunohematology. Using isomers of tartaric acid (T.A.) as the hapten components to produce antibodies in rabbits, Landsteiner clearly demonstrated the specificity and sensitivity of immunologic methods (Table 43-3). Anti-l-TA isomers reacted strongly with l-TA but very weakly with d-TA and m-TA. Anti-d-TA reacted strongly only with d-TA isomers, whereas anti-m-TA reacted strongly with m-TA isomers. The change of position between H and OH radicals attached to the second and third carbons was clearly reflected in the immunologic reactions.

The importance of amino acids as determinants for specificity was beautifully demonstrated by Pauling. The difference between hemoglobin A and hemoglobin S is due to the substitution of one amino acid, glutamic acid for valine in S hemoglobin. Recently, immunoglobulins have been thoroughly studied, not only as antibodies, but also as antigens. The fundamental chemical differences among certain allotypes have been worked out (see Chap. 36). For instance, if the amino acid at No. 153 and No. 191 positions of the kappa light peptide chain are alanine and valine, the specificity of this light chain would be Km(3+); if they are valine and leucine, it would be Km(3−). If the amino acid at No. 214 position of the IgG heavy chain is arginine, the specificity would be Glm(a+); if it is lysine, it would be Glm(a−).

The antigenic determinants of some erythrocyte antigens have also been identified recently. Owing to the difficulty of isolating antigens from the erythrocyte's membrane, most of the work has been done with soluble antigens that share the same specificity as those found on the erythrocytes. These soluble antigens are present in saliva, serum, urine, or other tissue fluids. A summary of these soluble antigens is listed in Table 43-4.

Results of extensive studies by a number of investigators indicate that four sugars, namely, L-fucose, D-galactose, N-acetyl-galactosamine, and N-acetyl-glucosamine are the determinants for H, A, B, Le[a], Le[b], Le[c], and Le[d] antigens (Fig. 43-1). Similar studies reveal that the last three sugars and glucose-ceramide are the antigenic determinants of antigens in the P system; D-galactose and N-acetyl-glucosamine are the determinants for I antigens; D-galactose and N-acetyl-galactosamine and sialic acids are determinants of M and N antigens (Fig. 43-2). These sugars contain a basic unit of six carbons, and each carbon at a specific location has been assigned a number, as indicated in Figure 43-1. A linkage between two sugars can be joined together by two carbons at different locations. For instance, if No. 1 carbon from one sugar is joined to No. 3 carbon of another sugar, it is known as type I (1.3) linkage, whereas No. 1 to No. 4 is known as

Table 43–4. SOME KNOWN SOLUBLE BLOOD GROUP ANTIGENS OTHER THAN SERUM PROTEINS

MAIN SOURCES	A,B,H	I	P	Le[a], Le[b]	Sd[a]	Ch, Rg	HLA-A2,B7	A9
Saliva	4+	1+		3+	1+			
Plasma	1+			2+		3+	2+	2+
Hydatid cyst		1+	3+					
Ovarian cyst	2+	1+						
Amniotic fluid	2+	1+						
Stomach	4+							
Milk		3+		2+				
Urine					4+			2+

1+ to 4+ represent the relative amounts.

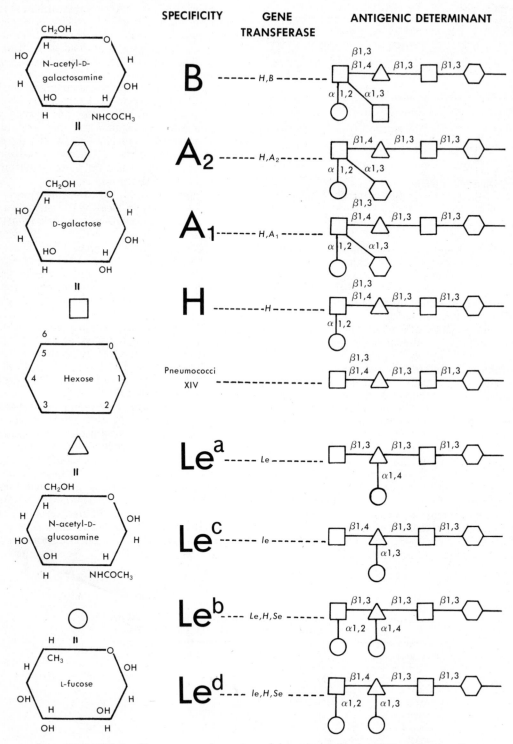

Figure 43–1. Relationships among various proposed determinants for the ABH and Lewis antigens.

type II (1.4) linkage. A change in the type of linkage may be responsible for differences in antigen specificity of A_1 and A_2. Although their determinant sugars are the same, A_1 antigens have type I and II linkages, while A_2 antigens have only type II linkages. The same relationship has been speculated between Le^a and Le^c antigens, as well as Le^b and Le^d antigens.

Figure 43-1 also indicates the precursor substances of ABH or Lewis antigens, which share the same specificity with Pneumococci XIV. Each consists of two D-galactoses, one N-acetyl-glucosamine, and one N-acetyl-galactosamine.

The addition of L-fucose to the terminal sugar through transferase H results in H specificity. If the fucose is added by Le^a or Le^c transferase to the subterminal sugar of the precursor substance, Le^a or Le^c is formed.

It is believed that by the addition of fucose to the subterminal sugar of the H substance, Le^b or Le^d is formed. It is possible, although unlikely, that Le^b or Le^d is formed by the addition of a fucose to the terminal sugar of Le^a or Le^c substance. The formation of Le^b or Le^d substance requires H transferase and Se gene in addition to Le^a or Le^c transferase.

Each transferase is governed by a corresponding gene on the chromosome (see Chaps. 26 and 41).

The addition of N-acetyl-galactosamine to the terminal sugar of H substance by A-transferase results in a substance with A specificity, while the addition of a galactose instead of N-acetyl-galactosamine results in a substance with B specificity. If one compares the structure of galactose with that of N-acetyl-galactosamine, the former has an OH radical at the carbon No. 2 position, while the latter has an $NHCOCH_3$ radical at the same position; this minor chemical difference constitutes the distinct serologic difference between group A and group B erythrocytes.

As shown in Figure 43-2, both galactose and N-acetyl-glucosamine are determinants of I and P_1 antigens. Galactoses are the determinants of P^k antigens. When extracts are made from the erythrocyte membrane, P^k antigens also contain glucose-ceramide, while the P antigen has an additional N-acetyl-galactosamine. When extracts of erythrocytes of type M or N were studied, galactose, N-acetyl-galactosamine, and sialic acid (also known as NANA or N-acetylneuraminic acid) were shown to be the determinants. The basic difference

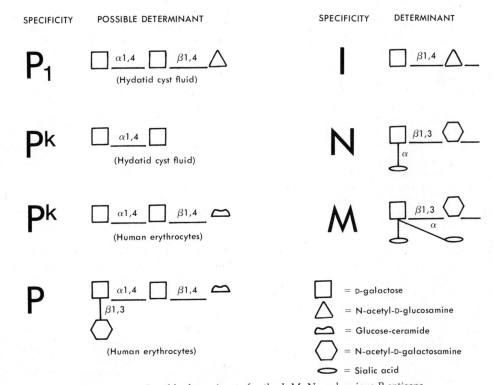

Figure 43-2. Possible determinants for the I, M, N, and various P antigens.

in the specificity of M and N is the number of sialic acid radicals.

Not all antigenic determinants presented in Figures 43-1 and 43-2 are well-established or as clear-cut as the diagram indicates. Our purpose is to present the likely determinants without introducing too many details to confuse the reader. For those who are interested in additional and more exact information, the original reports (Watkins, 1966; Watkins, 1976; Springer, 1977; Feizi, 1971; Dahr, 1977; Cartron, 1978) should be consulted.

Ceramide is not the only lipid that has been shown to be an antigenic determinant related to immunohematology. Caprylate, an octanoic acid derivative, has been shown to be responsible for the so-called "albumin agglutination phenomenon," in which human antibodies agglutinate all human erythrocytes in the presence of bovine albumin. At first albumin was thought to be the responsible antigen; however, an additive used as a preservative for albumin, sodium caprylate, was found to be the determinant (McGinnis, 1972). Anticaprylate antibodies are uncommon but have been observed repeatedly among persons without any known stimulation.

Genetics

The chemical structure of blood group antigens is determined by inheritance. Each antigen is governed by at least a pair of allelic genes, one from the father and the other from the mother. When the pair of genes is identical, it is known as a homozygote; when different, as a heterozygote. If only two alternate allelic genes (P and Q) are responsible for one pair of antigens, three types of zygotes are normally found, P/P, Q/Q, and P/Q; they are known as genotypes. Their corresponding phenotypes would be $P+Q-$, $P-Q+$, and $P+Q+$, which are identifiable serologically. Results of phenotyping a population can be used to predict the phenotypes of children in families. When such predictions are confirmed by actual observation, the allelic relationship of P and Q can be assumed and a blood group system can be assigned.

Population Studies. If a monospecific anti-P serum reacts with erythrocytes of 64 per cent of the population, in the absence of an anti-Q serum, one may assume that the remaining 36 per cent would have the frequency of homozygotes of genotype Q/Q. The frequency of Q (normally represented by q) would be $0.36^{1/2} = 0.6$. Its allelic gene frequency (normally represented by p) would be $1 - 0.6 = 0.4$, since $p + q = 1.0$. These two values may not be the true values, but they can be used as the working parameters to estimate the genotype frequencies:

Frequency of

$P/P = p \times p = 0.4 \times 0.4 = 0.16$ or 16%
$Q/Q = q \times q = 0.6 \times 0.6 = 0.36$ or 36%
$P/Q = 2pq = 2 \times 0.4 \times 0.6 = 0.48$ or 48%

Phenotype frequency of:

$P+ = p \times p + 2pq = 0.16 + 0.48 = 0.64$ or 64%
$Q+ = q \times q + 2pq = 0.36 + 0.48 = 0.84$ or 84%

Since only 50 per cent of the children of a heterozygote (P/Q) are expected to be $P+$ or $Q+$, children of a $P+$ parent are expected to be:

$P+ = 0.16 \times 100\% + 0.48 \times 50\% = 0.625$ or 62.5%
$P- = 1 - 0.625 = 0.375$ or 37.5%

Similarly, children of a $Q+$ parent:

$Q+ = 0.36 \times 100\% + 0.48 \times 50\% = 0.715$ or 71.5%
$Q- = 1 - 0.715 = 0.285$ or 28.5%

Hence, phenotypes of children of different matings can be expected as follows:

MATING	CHILDREN EXPECTED	
	P−	P+
P− × P−	100%	0%
P− × P+	37.5%	62.5%
P+ × P+	$0.375^2 = 14\%$	$1 - 14\% = 86\%$

MATING	CHILDREN EXPECTED	
	Q−	Q+
Q− × Q−	100%	0%
Q− × Q+	28.5%	71.5%
Q+ × Q+	$0.285^2 = 8\%$	$1 - 8\% = 92\%$

Family Studies. All of the above values are estimates based on the assumption that P and Q are allelic genes. This assumption should be verified by studying the members of many families. Owing to sampling problems, the observed values are rarely the same as the expected values, but the validity can be evaluated statistically. If the values obtained from family studies are in agreement with predicted values, the gene frequency of 0.4 for the p and 0.6 for the q can be accepted. Then, one should check other gene frequency values close to 0.4 or 0.6 of known antigens and attempt to establish non-identity. A similar study should be done when and if anti-Q serum is found. Should values from anti-P and anti-Q be in agreement with what was expected, P and Q are likely to be allelic and can be assigned to one blood group system. This is, of course, an oversimplified procedure for the assignment of blood group antigens to one blood group system. Further consideration of basic genetics and blood group genetics appears in Chapters 26 and 44.

Based on the results of genetic studies of various erythrocyte antigens, Race and Sanger have assigned them into 21 major blood group systems and two groups for the so-called "public" and "private" antigens (Table 43-5). These systems, especially those of clini-

Table 43–5.   TIME AND RECOGNITION OF MAJOR
HUMAN ERYTHROCYTE SYSTEMS AND ANTIGENS*

TIME RECOGNIZED	MAJOR SYSTEMS	PUBLIC ANTIGENS	PRIVATE ANTIGENS
1901	ABO		
1902–1925			
1926–1930	MN, P		
1931–1935	Se		
1936–1940	Rh		
1941–1945	Lu		
1946–1950	K, Fy		1
1951–1955	Jk, Le, Di	1	3
1956–1960	Yt	2	2
1961–1965	Au, Xg, Do, Sc, Cs	2	8
1966–1970	Co, Sd, Bg, Ch	6	7
1971–1975		2	7

*Adapted from Race (1975).

cal importance, will be discussed subsequently under erythrocyte blood group systems.

IMMUNE RESPONSE RELATING TO BLOOD BANKING

Immune response is negligible in the unborn and is lacking in germ-free animals; therefore, it is considered developed only after antigenic stimulation. The term *naturally occurring antibodies* does not mean there has been no antigenic stimulation, but rather that it is not identified.

A human host may respond to three types of antigenic stimulation: (1) heterologous antigens, from other species such as microorganisms; (2) isologous antigens, from the same species such as blood components of other individuals; (3) autologous antigens, from the same individual, probably slightly modified by medication or viruses and no longer recognizable as one's own antigen.

Immune responses can be divided into two stages, the primary and the secondary (see Chap. 34). In primary immune response, the host is exposed to the antigen for the first time. It is usually detectable within 7 to 14 days and antibodies are of the IgM class in low titer. In the secondary immune response, the host is re-exposed to the same antigen. It is usually detectable within a week and antibodies are predominately of the IgG class in high titer.

There are two major types of immune responses: the humoral immune response, the production of antibodies, and the cellular immune response, the formation of sensitized lymphocytes. Cells responsible for both types of immune response originate from the stem cells in the bone marrow, but they differentiate under the influence of two different types of lymphoid tissue into two populations of lymphocytes, known as B-lymphocytes or B cells and T-lymphocytes or T cells.

Macrophages are also known to be involved in immune response. Since all three types of cells have been extensively reviewed in Chapters 34, 39, and 40, one table (Table 43-6) and one illustration (Fig. 43-3) are presented here for a brief review.

Immunologic tolerance and enhancement

Although a host may be unresponsive to a normal antigen for many reasons, only three will be mentioned. First, a person may be a non-responder. It has been shown that about one third of Rh_o-negative women are believed to be non-responders and will not develop anti-D despite repeated immunization. Second, when a fetus is injected with a soluble or particulate antigen, the infant will not form antibodies against the specific antigen. Third, a similar type of immunologic tolerance can also be induced in adults. Using the same antigen, tolerance can be induced with a low dose or a high dose, while a very low dose or medium dose would sensitize the host. It is possible that with the high dose level, both the T and B cells are rendered unresponsive. The greater difficulty encountered in making B-lymphocytes tolerant might be related to the high density of surface receptors which require a large number of antigen molecules to become saturated. Cyclophosphamide, a cytotoxic agent for dividing B-lymphocyctes, has been shown to facilitate the induction of tolerance. In general, soluble antigens are more effective in inducing tolerance than are particulate antigens; this may be related to the fact that the latter are readily taken up by macrophages and become more antigenic. Immunologic tolerance can be terminated by the injection of specific antibodies or closely reacting antigens.

Although vaccinations against infectious diseases have been very successful, vaccination against tumor cells often results in early death. This phenomenon is known as immunologic enhancement (see Chap. 34). Many theories have been proposed, but none has been generally accepted.

Table 43–6. MAJOR DIFFERENCES BETWEEN
B- AND T-LYMPHOCYTES

HUMAN LYMPHOCYTES	B	T
Differentiation	Bursa equivalent lymphoid tissue	Thymus
Major immune response	Humoral	Cellular
Helper or suppressor	?	Yes
Distribution		
Blood, lymph, lymph nodes, thymus	25%	75%
Spleen and tonsil	50%	50%
Bone marrow	75%	25%
Surface markers		
SIg*	Abundant	Sparse
Fc receptors*	Yes	No
C3 receptors*	C3b, C3c, C3d	No
Sheep RBC receptors†	No	Yes
Sensitivity to		
Soluble mitogens	?	Yes
Insoluble mitogens	Yes	Yes
X-ray	+ + + +	+
Corticosteroids	+ +	+
Anti-lymphocyte serum†	+	+ + + +

*Useful markers for identifying B-lymphocytes.

†Useful characteristics for identifying T-lymphocytes. A third population of lymphocytes with only Fc markers for IgG are known as null cells or killer (K) cells, which are cytotoxic to antibody-coated cells *in vitro*.

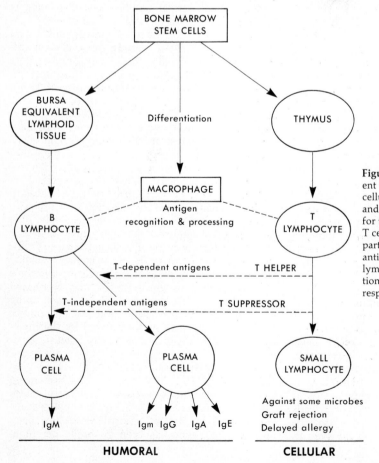

Figure 43–3. Interrelationship among different types of cells involved in humoral and cellular immune response. Bursa equivalent and thymus lymphoid tissues are responsible for the differentiation of stem cells into B and T cells, respectively. Macrophages may play a part in the recognition and processing of antigens, while the plasma cells and small lymphocytes are the effectors in the production of antibodies and in cellular response respectively.

Table 43-7. IMPORTANT PROPERTIES OF FIVE CLASSES OF HUMAN IMMUNOGLOBULIN (Ig)

CLASSES OF Ig	IgG	IgM	IgA	IgD	IgE
Heavy chains	γ	μ	α	δ	ξ
Light chains	κ, λ	κ, λ	κ, λ	κ, λ	κ, λ
Special chains		J	J, Sc		
No. of 4-peptide units	1	5	1-3	1	1
CHO content (%)	3	12	8	13	12
Mol. wt. (monomer)	150,000	900,000	160,000	185,000	200,000
Sedimentation coefficient	7S	19S	7-11S	7S	8S
Inactivated by SH- or heat	+/−	+ + + +	+ +		+ + +
Development in immune response	Late secondary	Early primary			
Half life *in vivo*	22 days	5 days	6 days	3 days	2.5 days
Concentration: mg/ml	8-16	0.5-2	1.4-4	0-0.4	Trace
(%)	(80)	(6)	(13)	(1)	
Distribution other than intravascular	Tissue fluids		Secretions		Secretions
Cross placenta	Yes	No	No	No	No
Induce agglutination	+	+ + + +	+ +		
Fix complement	Both pathways (?)	Classic	Alternate possible		Alternate possible

BLOOD GROUP ANTIBODIES

Immunoglobulins and antigen binding sites

All proteins with antibody activity and proteins having a structure similar to those of antibodies are designated as immunoglobulins (Ig). While Ig's are normal plasma components, antibody activity develops only in response to antigen stimulation. In order to understand antibodies, one must first be familiar with immunoglobulins, which are reviewed in Chapter 36. Information on immunoglobulins that is essential to blood banking is summarized in Tables 43-7, 43-8, and 43-9.

The specificity of an antibody is related to the hypervariable regions of an immunoglobulin. There are four hypervariable regions in heavy chains and three in light chains, as shown in Figure 36-7 (p. 1233). The substitution of amino acids, a modification of the configuration of the peptide chains, or a combination of both determines the specificity of a particular antibody. It is believed that about 20 amino acids are actually in contact with antigens, while only one tetra-peptide may be responsible for the specificity.

An isolated heavy chain from an antibody can bind the corresponding antigen but will do so less strongly than the original molecule. The isolated light chain binds far less well. A recombined light and heavy chain has a much greater affinity to the antigen than either of the isolated chains.

Table 43-8. SOME KNOWN PROPERTIES OF THE FOUR SUBCLASSES OF IMMUNOGLOBULIN G*

SUBCLASSES OF IgG	IgG1	IgG2	IgG3	IgG4
Heavy peptide chain	r1	r2	r3	r4
κ/λ ratio	2.4	1.1	1.4	8.0
Genetic markers	a, x, f, z	n	b0, b1, b3, b4 b5, c3, c5, g, s, t, u, v	4a, 4b
Half life *in vivo* in days	22	22	9	22
Relative serum concentration	64-70%	23-28%	4-7%	3-4%
Cross placenta	+	+/−	+	+
Fix complement	+ +	+	+ + +	+/−
Bind to macrophage	+ + +	+ +	+ + +	+/−
Induce rosette	+		+ + +	
Cryoprecipitation	+	+/−	+ + +	+/−
Spontaneous aggregation	−	−	+ + +	−
Dominant antibodies	Immune anti-A, anti-Rh	Anti-dextrans	Anti-Rh	Anti-AHF

*Modified from Roitt (1974, p. 40).

Table 43–9. VARIANTS OF HUMAN IMMUNOGLOBULINS*

DESIGNATION	MEANING	SUBVARIANTS	DETERMINANT LOCATION	EXAMPLES
Isotypes	Present in all normal human individuals	Classes	C_H	IgG, IgM, IgA, IgD, IgE
		Subclasses	C_H	IgG1, IgG2, IgG3, IgG4 IgA1, IgA2
		Types	C_L	κ, λ
Allotypes	Genetic markers present in some individuals but not in others	IgG1	C_H	G1m(a), (x), (f), (z)
		IgG2	C_H	G2m(n), G2m($-$n)
		IgG3	C_{H3}	G3m(b), (c), (g) . . .
		κ chain	C_L	Km(1), (2), (3)
Idiotypes	Specificity of each immunoglobulin		V_H or V_L	Determinant of individual myeloma protein

*Modified from Roitt (1974, p. 41).

Since one basic 4-peptide unit of Ig contains 2 Fab portions, all untreated antibodies should be bivalent. The valence of polymers would be multiples of 2, such as $5 \times 2 = 10$ for an IgM antibody. Thus, there is no natural univalent antibody.

Alloantibodies

The possible presence of alloantibodies to erythrocytes demands the selection of compatible blood. This is the central issue of blood banking. Alloantibodies to erythrocytes can be (1) naturally occurring; i.e., the antigenic stimuli are unknown; (2) a result of immunization through transfusion; (3) induced by fetal erythrocytes either during pregnancy or at the time of delivery.

Some naturally occurring antibodies appear regularly in persons who lack the corresponding antigen such as anti-A in group B, anti-B in group A, anti-A,B in group O, or anti-P_1PP^k in p persons. It is obvious that these antibodies are of utmost importance for safe blood transfusion therapy. One cannot and must not ignore the presence of these antibodies.

Naturally occurring antibodies may appear only in a certain percentage of the population who lack the respective antigen. For example, 5 to 20 per cent Le(a—b—) persons have anti-Le^a. Other incidences include: 3 per cent with anti-M^g, 2 per cent with anti-Vw, about 1 per cent with anti-Le^b or anti-Wr^a or anti-P_1, about 0.1 per cent with anti-E, about 0.02 per cent with anti-M or anti-N or anti-S (Mollison, 1972). These groups of alloantibodies are usually of low titer with equivocal clinical significance.

Routine compatibility testing (the crossmatch) indicates that there is no detectable incompatibility and usually a match in terms of ABO and Rh$_o$(D) type specificity. Blood transfusion may introduce erythrocytes containing a number of antigens which the recipient lacks. Some of these antigens may be highly antigenic and may induce the production of specific antibodies in the recipient; the clinical significance of these antibodies varies. For a ready reference, Table 43–10 lists the Ig class, optimal reacting conditions, clinical implication, and the chance of finding compatible donors for each antibody. Additional comments can be found in the discussion of each blood group system subsequently.

Alloantibodies to leukocytes or platelets are reviewed elsewhere (p. 1488 and p. 1117, respectively).

Autoantibodies

The term *autoantibody* is used for any antibody that reacts with an antigen of the same subject producing the antibody. It also reacts often with the same antigen of other normal persons. Results from the reaction may induce hemolytic anemia, leukopenia, or thrombocytopenia, but frequently autoantibodies produce no demonstrable signs except laboratory findings. When proper reagents are used, the direct antiglobulin tests are often positive, while the indirect antiglobulin test may or may not be positive. Based upon the optimal reacting temperature, autoantibodies are classified into two general categories: the cold (usually IgM) and the warm (usually IgG).

Table 43–10. SELECTED ERYTHROCYTE ALLOANTIBODIES:
Immunoglobulin class, optimal reaction phase, clinical implications, and chance of finding
a compatible donor

ANTI-	IMMUNOGLOBULIN			OPTIMAL REACTION				HEMOLYSIS IN			COMPATIBLE DONOR*		
	IgM	IgG	IgA	Sal	Alb	AGT	Enz	Vitro	Recipient	Newborn	Type	White (%)	Black (%)
B	3	1	1	4				2	4	2	A,O	85	76
A_1	4			4							A_2,O	48	52
A	3	1	1	4				2	4	2	B,O	56	69
A,B	1	3		4				1	4		O	45	49
H†	4			4				3		0	O_h	very rare	
I	3	1		3			3			0	I−	very rare	
i	3	2	3							0			
P_1	3			3				1	2	0	P_1−	21	6
P		2	2										
P_1PP^k	3	1		3				4	1	1	very rare		
Le^a	3	1		3		2	3	2	1	0	Le(a−)	78	77
Le^b	4			4		3	3	1	1	0	Le(b−)	28	45
Lu^a	3	1		3				0		1	Lu(a−)	92	96
Lu^b	3	1	1	3				0	1		Lu(b−)	<0.1	<0.1
M	3	1		3		1	0	0	1	1	M−	22	30
N	3	1		3			0	0	0‡	0‡	N−	28	26
S	2	2		3		1		0	1	1	S−	45	69
s	1	3				3		0	2	1	s−	11	3
U		3				4		0	2	1	U−	none	1
D	1	3	1	1	3	3	3	0‡	3	4	D−	15	8
C	1	3		1	3	3	3	0	2	1	C−	30	68
DC	1	3		1	3	3	3	0	1	1	DC−	13	7
C^w	2	2		1	3	3	3	0	1	1	C^w−	99	100
c		3			3	3	3	0	2	2	c−	20	1
E	1	3		1	3	3	3	0	2	2	E−	70	98
e		3			3	3	3	0	1	1	e−	2	2
K	1	3		1		3	3	0	2	2	K−	91	97
k		4				3	3	0	1	1	k−	0.2	0.1
Kp^a		4				3	3	0	1	1	Kp(a−)	98	99.9
Kp^b		4				3	3	0	1	1	Kp(b−)	<0.1	0.1
Js^a		4				3	3	0	1	1	Js(a−)	>99.9	81
Js^b		4				3	3	0	1	1	Js(b−)	<0.1	1
Jk^a		4				3	3	0	1	1	Jk(a−)	23	9
Jk^b		4				3	3	0	1	1	Jk(b−)	28	57
Fy^a	1	4		1	3	3	1/0	0	1	1	Fy(a−)	34	90
Fy^b		4			3	3	1/0	0	1		Fy(b−)	17	77
Ch^a	3					3		0			Least incompatible		
Sd^a	3			3		2		0	1	0	Least incompatible		
Yt^a	2	2		3		2		0	1	?	Yt(a−)	<0.1	
Vel	3					3	2	2	0		Vel−	<0.1	
Wr^a	3			3				0	1	1	Wr(a−)	>99.9	

4 = almost all   3 = most   2 = some   1 = few   0 = none
*Approximate values, mostly based on the frequencies in the AABB Technical Manual, 7th ed. (1977).
†In Bombay individuals.
‡Only one case reported.

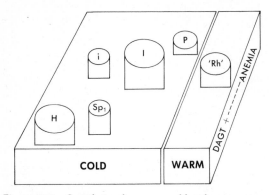

Figure 43–4. Specificity of common cold and warm autoagglutinins which can induce from only a positive direct antiglobulin test (DAGT) to severe anemia in patients. Specificity of autoantibody is indicated in i, I, P, H, Sp$_1$, and Rh (usually e). (Adapted from Mollison, 1972, p. 362.)

Among those autoantibodies producing anemias, about 15 per cent are of the cold variety and the remaining 85 per cent are of the warm variety. Autoantibodies to erythrocytes have been well studied and will be the main subject of discussion (Fig. 43–4). Autoimmune hemolytic anemia is reviewed in Chapter 29.

Cold Autoantibodies. The majority of cold autoantibodies are agglutinins and agglutinate erythrocytes strongly at 4°C., weakly at 24°C., and either very weakly or negatively at 37°C. Cold autoagglutinins can be detected in many normal persons; only a small percentage of them are associated with disease states. However, their clinical significance should not be neglected; cold autoagglutinins often interfere with proper typing and crossmatching. In some cases, it is difficult to establish their specificities; nevertheless, the following specificities can often be identified.

ANTI-H. Low titer anti-H can be demonstrated in many normal persons. These agglutinins clump group O or A$_2$ erythrocytes strongly but react weakly or negatively with A$_1$ or A$_1$B cells, and not at all with O$_h$ cells. They can be neutralized by saliva containing H substance, the exception being the anti-H produced in an O$_h$ individual. There is evidence to indicate that these agglutinins are not immunoglobulins but act very much like properdin, which is an important factor in the alternative pathway of complement activation (Mollison, 1972, p. 363).

ANTI-I. Anti-I is normally an IgM antibody. Those found in normal persons or in cord blood are of low titer and those associated with mycoplasma pneumonia infections are usually of high titer. Anti-I antibodies are separable from antibodies to mycoplasma pneumonia and cannot be absorbed out by mycoplasma pneumonia organisms. Anti-I antibodies react positively with erythrocytes that have I antigens but negatively with those containing only i antigens, including some cord cells. The antibody may sometimes be neutralized with fluids containing I substance, such as milk and saliva. Reactivity of anti-I may be enhanced in the presence of enzyme in the medium or by bovine albumin. The former is a useful criterion for distinguishing anti-I from anti-Sp$_1$, which is usually inactive after enzyme treatment. Anti-Sp$_1$ is a very rare antibody and is probably identical to anti-Pr$_1$ and Pr$_2$.

ANTI-i. Anti-i is normally an IgM antibody but may be IgG or both. Anti-i is often associated with infectious mononucleosis or other types of reticulosis, with or without hemolytic anemia (low incidence). Anti-i antibodies are separable from antibodies specific for infectious mononucleosis.

Serologic differentiation of anti-H, anti-HI, auto anti-I, anti-i, and anti-Sp$_1$ is summarized in Table 43–11.

ANTI-P. Anti-P has been observed primarily in patients with paroxysmal cold hemoglobinuria, a syndrome often associated with syphilis, mumps, or measles, and is known as DL (Donath-Landsteiner) antibody. These antibodies are IgG and are capable of fixing complement on erythrocytes at 4°C. These complement-coated erythrocytes then hemolyze at 37°C.; hence, DL antibody is referred to as an autohemolysin or biphasic hemolysin.

Warm Autoantibodies. Patients with warm autoantibodies usually have a positive direct antiglobulin test (DAGT) and a shortened red blood cell survival, although such patients may not have anemia. Warm autoantibodies can be primary or secondary. Primary means the etiology is unknown, while the secondary is attributed to the presence of other disease conditions. With improvement in the diagnostic procedures, the ratio between primary and secondary has changed from 7:3 to 3:7. Since viruses and medications have been implicated in a number of cases of warm autoantibodies, a similar association may be expected in the remaining so-called "idiopathic" or "primary" warm autoantibodies. It should be remembered that not all hemolytic anemias are due to the presence of autoantibodies; alloantibodies and many other non-immunologic factors can also be the cause (see Chap. 29).

The majority of warm autoantibodies (from

Table 43–11. DIFFERENTIATION OF SPECIFIC
COLD AGGLUTININS

| TEST ERYTHROCYTES | | | | COLD AGGLUTININS | | | | |
Types	H	I	i	Anti-H[1]	Anti-HI[2]	Anti-I[3]	Anti-i[4]	Anti-Sp$_1$[5]
A$_1$i	−	−	+	−	−	−	3+	3+
Oi	+	−	+	3+	−	−	3+	3+
O$_{cord}$	+	−	+	3+	−	+,−	3+	3+
OI	+	+	−	3+	3+	3+	−	3+
A$_2$	+	+	−	1+	2+	3+	−	3+
A$_1$I	−	+	−	−	−	3+	−	3+
O$_h$	−	+	−	−	−	3+	−	3+

[1] Neutralized by H substance.

[2] Neutralized by H substance only in rare types of anti-H-(-i).

[3] Common in mycoplasma pneumoniae infection; some neutralized by I substance.

[4] Common in infectious mononucleosis and other forms of reticulosis.

[5] ?=Anti-Pr$_1$, Pr$_2$: receptors on RBC's are destroyed by proteases.

56 to 100 per cent in various reports) can be demonstrated with the direct antiglobulin test using anti-IgG serum, from 31 to 51 per cent by anti-complement serum as well, and from 11 to 45 per cent by anti-complement serum alone. Although a few examples are detected by anti-IgA alone or concurrently with anti-IgG or anti-complement, a few others are also positive with anti-IgM serum. The eluate from the erythrocytes and antibodies present in the serum of the same patient usually react best at 37°C. by the antiglobulin test. Those antibodies demonstrable with anti-IgG serum are either IgG1 or IgG3. IgG3 antibodies are often associated with overt hemolysis. Anti-complement serum containing anti-C3d has been found most useful.

Usually, the strength of direct antiglobulin reaction shows no correlation with the degree of anemia. In many cases, the specificity of warm autoantibodies cannot be established. In some cases, autoantibodies may react selectively more strongly with cells that have certain Rh or LW antigens, especially hr″(e) antigens. According to their reactivity, autoantibodies have been designated as anti-nl, anti-pdl, and anti-dl. Anti-nl does not react with Rh deletions (Dc−, D−, DC^w−) or Rh$_{null}$ cells; anti-pdl reacts with Rh deletion cells but not Rh$_{null}$ cells, and anti-dl reacts with all cells (Wiener, 1963).

Although many investigators have evaluated this problem with different techniques, the clinical implication of their results remains uncertain. Although one usually tries to avoid transfusing patients with warm autoimmune hemolytic anemia, the use of the least incompatible blood for transfusion of these patients is being generally accepted; however, before such a decision is made, one *must exclude* the possibility of the concurrent presence of alloantibodies.

Autoantibodies against Leukocytes and Platelets. Both cold and warm autoantibodies against leukocytes and platelets are encountered and will be discussed elsewhere (p. 1366 and p. 1367). Cold lymphocytotoxins are quite common if one tests for them, especially with B-lymphocytes (Terasaki, 1977).

Globulins on erythrocytes induced by medication

Many drugs are known to induce a positive direct antiglobulin test (DAGT) and can be classified into the following four categories (Fig. 43–5):

Autoantibodies on Erythrocytes. About 15 per cent of hypertensive patients who receive methyldopa (Aldomet) for 3 to 6 months or longer have been found to have a positive DAGT and about 0.8 per cent of them to have hemolytic anemia. The positive DAGT becomes negative gradually after the termination of methyldopa treatment; it may take from a few months to two years. Serologically, antibodies found on erythrocytes or in serum are indistinguishable from those autoantibodies found in patients with idiopathic autoim-

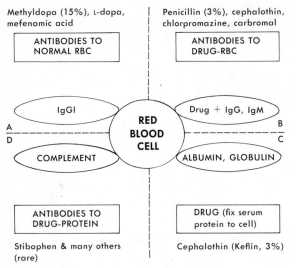

Methyldopa (15%), L-dopa,
mefenamic acid

Penicillin (3%), cephalothin,
chlorpromazine, carbromal

ANTIBODIES TO
NORMAL RBC

ANTIBODIES TO
DRUG-RBC

IgGI

RED
BLOOD
CELL

Drug + IgG, IgM

A
D

B
C

COMPLEMENT

ALBUMIN, GLOBULIN

ANTIBODIES TO
DRUG-PROTEIN

DRUG (fix serum
protein to cell)

Stibophen & many others
(rare)

Cephalothin (Keflin, 3%)

Figure 43–5. Four possible mechanisms for drug-induced positive direct antiglobulin test. Reactive agents on erythrocytes are in ovals; reactive agents in serum are in rectangles. Examples of drugs in each category are given.

mune hemolytic anemia. Antibodies are usually of the IgG subclass with both kappa and lambda light chains and may have Rh or LW specificity. Although several hypotheses have been proposed for the development of these antibodies, none has been generally accepted. About 10 per cent of parkinsonian patients receiving L-dopa, closely related to methyldopa, may develop a positive DAGT, but there has been no report of overt hemolysis in these patients. Although several cases of autoimmune hemolytic anemia have been reported in patients receiving mefenamic acid, an analgesic, a positive DAGT among patients taking this drug is uncommon.

Antibodies on Erythrocytes. About 3 per cent of those patients receiving large doses (for example, 10 million units daily for at least a week) of penicillin intravenously have been found to have a positive DAGT, while only a few of them are found to have hemolytic anemia. The positive DAGT disappears soon after the penicillin is stopped. Cephalothin (Keflin), carbromal, chlorpromazine, and methadone may behave like penicillin. These drugs bind firmly to the red blood cells and react chemically with certain protein groups to form haptenic determinants such as benzylpenicilloyl (BPO). Antibodies are formed against the BPO which are detectable on the erythrocytes and in the serum when penicillin-coated cells are used. Penicillin antibodies may be IgM or IgG. The IgM type may be very common if a very sensitive method is used for detection. This is likely due to exposure to penicillin in many foods. The IgG type may be associated

with the IgM type or by itself. Penicillin antibodies usually do not fix complement; intravascular hemolysis has been seen but is rare. There is no evidence to indicate that IgG penicillin antibodies are associated with the allergic state to penicillin which a patient may have.

Serum Proteins on Erythrocytes. Cephalothin may also fix serum proteins (albumin, globulins including complements) on erythrocytes non-immunologically. About 3 per cent of those patients receiving about 6 gm/day are found to have a positive DAGT. Only two cases of hemolytic anemia have been reported; these were probably due to direct attachment of cephalothin to erythrocytes and subsequent antibody production. Loridine (cephaloridine) as well as other drugs within the cephalothin family may react similarly. Antiglobulin serums of different specificity, including anti-albumin, can give a positive DAGT. Anti-cephalothin (antibodies) in the serum can be detected with cephalothin-coated erythrocytes.

Complement Components on Erythrocytes. Many drugs can form a complex with serum proteins, and antibodies may develop against these drug-protein complexes. As a result of this antibody-drug-protein reaction, complement components, especially C3, are fixed to the erythrocytes through their C3b receptors. Only anti-C3 antiglobulin serum will detect this type of coating on erythrocytes. Antibodies in the serum can be detected only in the presence of the drug-protein complex. The following medications have been reported to give this type of reaction (all are very rare): acetaminophen, aminopyrine (Pyramidon), chloramphenicol, anti-histamines, insecticides, dipyrone, insulin, isoniazid, melphalan, p-aminosalicylic acid, phenacetin, quinine, quinidine, rifampin, stibophene (Fuadin), sulfa drugs, sulfonylurea derivatives, methadone,* streptomycin,* and tetracycline.*

Many drugs have also been incriminated in cases of leukopenia or thrombocytopenia. There is no doubt that mechanisms similar to those for erythrocytes may be involved; however, tests are not yet available at the routine laboratory level.

Lectins

Lectins are specific receptor proteins present in plants (usually their seeds), invertebrate animals (snails, crabs, etc.), and lower vertebrates (fish ova). Although many lectins have been reported (Bird, 1977), only several of them have been found useful in blood banking and are listed in Table 43-12.

The anti-H lectin of *Ulex europaeus* strongly agglutinates group O erythrocytes. It reacts weakly with A_2 cells and very weakly with A_1 or B cells. It is readily inhibited by H substance; some are inhibited by L-fucose and the others by N-acetyl-D-glucosamine. Since the potency of the lectin varies with the source of *Ulex europaeus*, each preparation should be standardized before use. Anti-H lectin is most useful in the study of secretors; saliva of a secretor contains H substances.

The anti-A_1 lectin of *Dolichos biflorus* agglutinates A_1 erythrocytes, an activity which can be inhibited by A substance or N-acetyl-D-galactosamine. Anti-A_1 lectin has been widely used to group A cells and to separate a minor population of A_1 cells from cells of other groups.

The anti-N lectin of *Vicia graminea* agglutinates type N erythrocytes and its activity is inhibited by D-galactose. In addition to typing erythrocytes, anti-N lectin has been useful in elucidating the chemical composition of the M and N antigens.

---

*Mechanism for these drugs is not yet certain.

The anti-T lectin of *Arachis hypogaea* (peanut), anti-Tn of *Salvia sclarea*, and the separable anti-Tn + anti-Cad lectin of *Salvia horminum* are very useful in the study of erythrocyte polyagglutination.

COMPLEMENT AND BLOOD BANKING

Complement concerns blood bankers in two major areas: its involvement in the sensitization of erythrocytes, leukocytes, and platelets *in vivo* and its involvement in the detection of an antigen-antibody and related reactions *in vitro*. Since a detailed description of complement components, their detection and quantitation, and their changes in various diseases is presented in Chapter 37, only a brief outline of complement components that are pertinent to our two subjects will be presented.

Complement consists of at least 19 components that have been fairly well characterized and are listed in Table 37-1 (p. 1247). These components are classified into three groups; two of them are involved in activation and the third is involved in inactivation. A balance of function is achieved between the activators and the inactivators. Activation of complement can be achieved through the classic pathway in which a cell membrane is usually involved, or through the alternate pathway in which the event usually takes place in the fluid phase.

Activation and regulation

The Classic Pathway of Activation of Complement (Fig. 37-1, p. 1250, and Fig. 43-6). Immunoglobulins are usually required for the activation, although other factors such as DNA, RNA, dextran sulfate, trypsin, plasmin, lysosomal enzymes, endotoxins, lymphocyte membranes, and low ionic strength conditions (e.g., 10 per cent sucrose) can also initiate the activation. Among the Ig's, polymeric IgM is most effective; only one molecule is needed to initiate the activation. This is likely due

---

Table 43–12.   LECTINS USEFUL IN BLOOD BANKING*

LECTIN	ACTIVITY INHIBITED BY	SEROLOGIC SPECIFICITY
Ulex europaeus	Fucose N-acetyl-D-glucosamine	Anti-H
Vicia graminea	Galactose	Anti-N
Arachis hypogaea	Galactose	Anti-T, Anti-Tk
Salvia sclarea	N-acetyl-D-galactosamine	Anti-Tn
Salvia horminum	N-acetyl-D-galactosamine	Anti-Tn, Anti-Cad
Dolichos biflorus	N-acetyl-D-galactosamine	Anti-A_1, Anti-Tn, Anti-Cad

*From Bird, 1977.

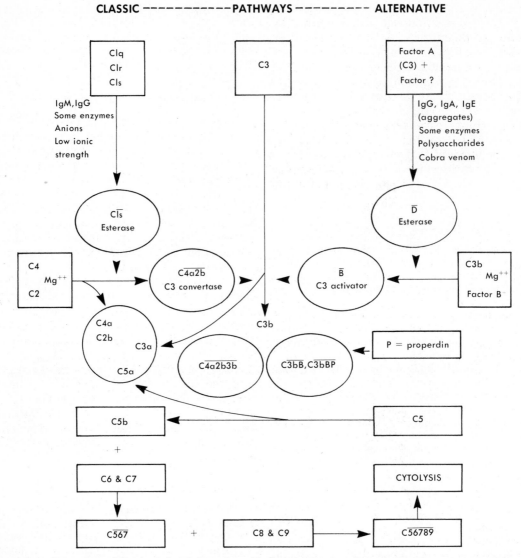

Figure 43-6. Comparison of the classical and alternative pathways of activation of complement. Proenzymes are in squares, activated enzymes are in ovals, activated components in liquid phase are in a circle, and the remaining are in rectangles. C3 and C3b play double roles in the activation process and serve as amplifiers. Properdin (P) serves as a stabilizer for $\overline{C3bB}$ and thus enhances the reaction.

to the fact that one IgM molecule can provide the two Fc portions required for the attachment of a Cl molecule. IgG is much less effective, since two molecules are required to form a doublet for the activation. It has been calculated that on an erythrocyte with 800,000 antigenic sites, approximately 1000 IgG molecules would be needed. The subclass IgG3 is more effective than IgG1; IgG2, IgG4, IgA, and IgE may not activate complement through the classic pathway.

The function of C1 requires the presence of calcium ions too hold C1q, C1r, and C1s together. Any chemicals which bind calcium, such as citrate and EDTA, impair the function of C1 and are commonly used to avoid the involvement of the complement in certain conditions. After C1q attaches to Ig's, C1r and then C1s are activated. Activated C1s which is normally expressed with an upper bar as $\overline{C1s}$ (this sign also applies to other complement components) has the activity of an esterase. In the presence of magnesium ions, $\overline{C1s}$ activates C4 and C2 to form $\overline{C4b2a}$ and releases C4a and C2b into the fluid phase. C4a and C2b may function as kinins, which can dilate the capillaries and contract smooth muscles. $\overline{C4b2a}$, which is known as C3 convertase, can activate many C3's into C3a and C3b. C3a is released into the fluid phase as anaphylatoxin I. C3b may attach to the red cell membrane or form $\overline{C4b2a3b}$. $\overline{C4b2a3b}$, which is also an enzyme, splits C5 into C5b and C5a (anaphylatoxin II in the fluid phase).

C5b appears to bind C6 and C7 by adsorption to form $\overline{C5b67}$, which attaches to the cell membrane and then binds C8 and C9 to form most likely an intramembranous channel resulting in cytolysis. C3a, C5a, and $\overline{C5b67}$ also have the chemotactic activity to attract leukocytes.

The Alternative Pathway of Complement Activation. Aggregated Ig's or Ig-antigen complex can activate complement without attachment to a cell membrane. Ig's include IgG1, IgG2, IgG3, IgG4, IgA1, IgA2, and IgE. Polysaccharides such as inulin, agar, endotoxin, and yeast cell walls, as well as trypsin and cobra venom factor can also activate complement through the alternative pathway.

Factor A, which has been identified as C3, together with other unknown components, may be activated by the above-mentioned factors to form factor $\overline{D}$. Factor $\overline{D}$, similar to $\overline{C1s}$, is also an ester-ase enzyme. Factor B, similar to C2, in the presence of Mg^{++} and C3b (similar to C4b) is activated by factor $\overline{D}$ to form $\overline{B}$. $\overline{B}$, in turn, activates C3 to form additional C3b, which helps to activate more C3's. In this way, the activation process is very much amplified. Furthermore, in the presence of properdin (P), the $\overline{C3bB}$ will form a $\overline{C3bBP}$ complex, which is much more stable than the $\overline{C3bB}$. This amplification system is also believed to involve the classic pathway. After the activation of C3, the subsequent events are identical to those in the classic pathway.

Inactivation of Complement. To achieve a biologic balance, complement activation has to be regulated. At least four inactivators in normal serum have been characterized (Table 43-13). Cl inactivator (C1INA) serves as a check to the $\overline{C1s}$ activity. In patients with C1INA deficiency, excessive activation of complement results in the production of excesses of anaphylatoxin and kinins, a syndrome known as angioedema.

The C3b inactivator (C3bINA) splits C3b into C3c and C3d and serves as a check for the amplification system. While the C3d remains on the cell membrane, the C3c is released into the fluid phase. Since

Table 43-13.   SOME PROPERTIES OF COMPLEMENT COMPONENTS AND INACTIVATORS

NAME	MOLECULAR WEIGHT	SERUM FRACTION	SERUM LEVEL (μg/ml)	SYNONYMS AND COMMENTS
CLASSIC PATHWAY				
C1q	400,000	γ_2	180	18 peptides in 6 subunits attach to Fc of Ig
C1r	170,000	β		+ calcium + C1q + C1s = C3
C1s	90,000	α	110	$\to \overline{C1s}$ = esterase
C2	117,000	β_1	25	$\to$ C2a + C2b(? kinins)
C4	206,000	β_1	600	β1E, one each α, β, γ peptide chain $\to$C4a(? kinins) + C4b($\to$C4d + C4c)
C3	180,000	β_1	1600	β1C, one each α, β peptide chain C3a* + C3b($\to$C3d + C3c)
C5	180,000	β_1	80	β1F, $\to$C5a* + C5b *In fluid with chemotactic and anaphylactoid activity
C6	95,000	β_2	75	C5b + C6 + C7$\to$C$\overline{567}$ attaches to membrane
C7	110,000	β_2	55	C8 & C9 join C567 to form an intramembranous channel resulting in cytolysis
C8	163,000	γ_1	80	
C9	80,000	α	200	
ALTERNATIVE PATHWAY				
Factor A	180,000	β_1		=C3, hydrazine-sensitive factor(HSF)
Factor B	95,000	β_2	200	C3-proactivator(C3PA), Bf Glycine-rich β glycoprotein(GBG)
Factor D	25,000	α		C3PAse, GBGase, B + C3b $\to$ $\overline{D}$ + $\overline{C3bB}$
Factor P	185,000	γ_2	25	Properdin, stabilizing factor for $\overline{C3bB}$ $\overline{C3bB}$ + P $\to$ $\overline{C3bBP}$
INACTIVATORS (INA)				
C1INA	105,000	α_2	180	C$\overline{1}$INA deficiency $\to$angioedema C$\overline{1}$ esterase inhibitor
C3bINA	100,000	β		KAF, splits C3b $\to$ C3d + C3c and $\overline{C3bB}\to$ C3d + C3cB
C3a, C5aINA	300,000	α		Anaphylatoxin inactivator (AI)
C3bBPINA	180,000	β_1	500	β1H, splits $\overline{C3bBP}$ $\to$ C3bP + B

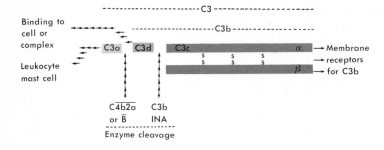

Figure 43-7. Components of C3 consist of one alpha and one beta chain $\overline{C3 + C4b2a}$ or B → C3a + C3b, C3b + $\overline{C3bINA}$ → C3d + C3c; C3a in fluid phase with anaphylactoid and chemotactic activity; C3d binding to cells fixing complement or antigen-antibody complex; C3c binding to receptors for C3b on white and red blood cells.

C3c contains the portion for the receptors on the phagocytes and C3d contains the portion binding erythrocytes, a sensitized erythrocyte may escape phagocytosis by the separation action of C3bINA (Fig. 43-7).

A serum inactivator for C3a and C5a is known as anaphylatoxin inactivator (AI). Anaphylatoxins cause the release of histamine from mast cells and platelets. Histamine increases the permeability of the capillaries, which enables leukocytes to reach target tissue. Many of the symptoms in a hemolytic transfusion reaction such as flushing, pain in the chest, headache, tingling along the vein, etc., may also be related to the release of histamine. AI would serve as a check to these reactions.

Since $\overline{C3bBP}$ is resistant to the action of C3bINA, a serum factor designated as B1H has been demonstrated to split $\overline{C3bBP}$ into C3bP + B. C3bP can then be acted on by C3bINA to form C3cP + C3d (Fearon, 1976).

Complement can be inactivated *in vitro* in a number of ways:

1. Heating at 56°C. for 30 minutes is the classic way, which inactivates basically C1, C2, C5, C8, and C9.
2. Any chelator of calcium, such as EDTA and citrate, would also inactivate the complement activity.
3. Trypsin or human serum containing C3bINA splits C3b into C3c and C3d or C4b into C4c and C4d.

Role of complement in the destruction of erythrocytes in vivo

Antibodies against erythrocyte antigens, either allo- or auto-, are the most common causes for binding complement on erythrocytes *in vivo*. Complement may also be fixed on erythrocytes through an antigen-antibody reaction which may be only partly related to erythrocytes, such as antibodies against penicillin-erythrocyte complex, or completely unrelated, such as antibodies to a chemical-protein complex. Leukocytes and platelets coated with antibodies may also fix complement but have not been well studied.

Intravascular Hemolysis. Intravascular hemolysis is the usual outcome of sensitization of erythrocytes with complement. Lysis of erythrocytes normally occurs through the classic pathway. Erythrocyte stromata which resemble the endotoxins may also initiate an activation through the alternative pathway, which may amplify the reactions of both pathways. This is typical for ABO incompatibility transfusion reactions. Other IgM antibodies, as well as some IgG antibodies (which are able to fix complement), can also induce an intravascular hemolysis.

Extravascular Hemolysis. Extravascular destruction of erythrocytes usually happens through phagocytosis. As shown in Table 43-14, macrophages, monocytes, and granulocytes all have receptors for C3b and C3c/C4. Erythrocytes with bound complement can thus attach to these cells. Those erythrocytes coated with Ig can also attach to these cells through their Fc receptors. Erythrocytes immobilized by macrophages can be completely engulfed or partly engulfed or escape from phagocytosis with the help of serum C3bINA, which splits the C3b and frees the erythrocytes. The incomplete erythrocytes that have escaped from partial phagocytosis may circulate again as spherocytes. Although phagocytosis is not entirely complement-dependent, Mollison (1972, p. 481) has demonstrated that erythrocytes coated with antibodies and complement tend to be destroyed in the liver within a short time, whereas those coated only with antibodies tend to be destroyed more slowly in the spleen. It is generally believed that in the presence of complement, phagocytic activity is enhanced.

The presence of receptors for C3b and C3d on B-lymphocytes and for C3b on other kinds of leu-

Table 43-14. COMPLEMENT RECEPTORS ON HUMAN CELLS

	COMPLEMENT RECEPTORS	
HUMAN CELLS	C3b, C3c/C4	C3d
Macrophages/ monocytes	+	−?
Granulocytes	+	−
Erythrocytes	+	−
Lymphocytes	+	+

kocytes may indicate that complement also plays an important role in the fate of leukocytes.

Role of complement in blood banking test procedures

Hemolysins. To demonstrate the presence of immune anti-A or anti-B or the so-called Donath-Landsteiner antibody (anti-P IgG, fixes complement at 4°C. and lyses the erythrocytes at 37°C.), complement is required. The blood specimen for these tests should not be drawn in tubes containing citrate or EDTA, or be inactivated at 56°C. for 30 minutes. The tests should be done with a fresh specimen. Complement is relatively unstable and deteriorates on storage. More than 50 per cent of its activity is lost in one day at 37°C., in two days at room temperature, or in three weeks at 4°C.; more than 90 per cent activity remains after 4 weeks at $-20°$C. and after 12 weeks at $-55°$C. (Garratty, 1970.)

Detection of Autoantibodies. There is no question about the value of complement in the study of autoantibodies. A certain percentage of autoantibodies can be detected only by anti-C antiglobulin serum; other portions can be detected by anti-C and anti-IgG, and the remaining by IgG only. However, the pattern of direct antiglobulin reaction in general has diagnostic value only in a negative sense; a positive reaction with anti-C is usually not found in patients treated with methyldopa, while a negative reaction is in general against the diagnosis of systemic lupus erythematosus. Various reports have also shown that anti-C3d is the most important component for this purpose. The use of anti-C4d has not been helpful in detecting additional antibodies, but it may pick up some non-specific coating from cold agglutinins after the blood specimen has been drawn from the patient. It is recommended that to detect a true *in vivo* coating of Ig and complement, the blood specimen should be drawn in EDTA tubes to avoid *in vitro* coating. Although so-called broad-spectrum antiglobulin serum, which has an undefined content, is suitable for routine purposes, it should not be used for critical investigative studies.

Detection of Alloantibodies. The role of complement has not been uniformly agreed upon. Few well-documented alloantibodies have been detected with only anti-C serum where other techniques without the use of complement failed to do so. On the other hand, all antibodies detectable in serum could also be detected in citrate and EDTA plasma (Myhre, 1972; Kitagawa, 1978) with equal or higher scores.

In typing erythrocytes, the strength of the antiserum is known and its specificity is defined by recommended techniques. The use of anti-C serum is superfluous and is generally not recommended, since occasionally it may detect some undesirable antigen-antibody reactions. The value of complement in crossmatching has not been generally accepted.

HLA Typing. Complement is required for lymphocytoxicity testing and for complement fixation tests using platelets. Recent demonstration of receptors for C4, and factor B on lymphocyte membranes and of the syntenic location of genes for C2, C4, C8, and factor B with the HLA loci is most interesting.

Hepatitis Testing. Complement fixation has been used in a number of laboratories for studying hepatitis, while the immune adherence test is currently being used in some laboratories for testing HBsAg.

IMMUNOLOGIC REACTIONS INVOLVING ERYTHROCYTES

Hemagglutination, hemagglutination inhibition, and hemolysis, which are the observed phenomena and main concerns of routine blood bank personnel, will be discussed here and the remaining immunologic reactions will be reviewed under each appropriate subject.

Factors affecting hemagglutination

Specific hemagglutination is the single most important reaction in blood banking. There are four groups of factors that can influence the outcome of the reaction: These include (a) the erythrocyte, (b) the serum, (c) the medium, and (d) the physical conditions under which the reaction takes place.

Erythrocytes. The importance of the type, number, and location of antigens on the erythrocytes is illustrated by the ABO and Rh antigens. The number of ABO sites may be close to one million per cell, and they are considered to be extramembranous; thus, erythrocytes are easily agglutinated with the appropriate antibodies. On the other hand, the Rh antigens have only about 10,000 to 30,000 sites per cell and are considered to be intramembranous; thus, they are less easily agglutinated by the appropriate antibodies.

Antibodies. IgG class antibodies often require antiglobulin serum for their demonstration, while IgM antibodies do not. The presence of complement may be required for some reactions. A high concentration of serum globulin or fibrinogen may create rouleaux formation.

Medium. Low pH and low ionic strength medium, such as acidified glucose, accelerate the binding of antibodies onto red blood cells. After 10 years, there has been a resurgence of interest in low ionic strength salt solution (LISS) in antibody screening and crossmatching (Hughes-Jones, 1964; Löw, 1974). Various enzymes, as well as macromolecules, are also used to enhance agglutination.

Physical Conditions. Physical conditions, such as the incubation temperature and time, as well as

4

the duration and speed of centrifugation, markedly affect the agglutination reaction. The above-mentioned factors may influence hemagglutination through their effect on a basic property of erythrocytes, the presence of negative charges on their surface.

Negative Charges. Under normal conditions, erythrocytes remain apart at a distance of approximately 25 nm. This is attributed to the repelling force of negative charges that are present on the surface of the erythrocyte. The presence of these negative charges can be demonstrated by placing the red blood cells in an electrical field and observing their migration toward the positive pole. This migration can be abolished if the cells are treated with certain enzymes capable of degrading sialic acid. Thus, the negative charges on the erythrocyte can be attributed to sialic acid content.

Zeta Potential. The degree of negative charge on an erythrocyte has been expressed by "zeta potential," a term meaning the potential difference between the negative charges on erythrocytes and the cations in the medium. Cations in the medium can be divided into two groups, those which attach firmly to erythrocytes and move together with the erythrocytes and those which move freely in the medium. The boundary between these two layers of cations is known as "Boundary of Shear" or "slip-ping plane." It is at this point that the zeta potential is determined and expressed in $-mV$ (Fig. 43-8). The optimal range for IgM antibodies is -22 to -17 mV, and for IgG, -11 to -4.5 mV. The smaller the numerical values of zeta potential, the shorter the distance between the two erythrocytes (Pollack, 1970).

Inducing hemagglutination

Hemagglutination can be induced in two ways, either by reducing the distance between the erythrocytes or by providing bridges between two short antibodies (Fig. 43-9). In terms of the former, treatment of erythrocytes with enzymes such as neuraminidase, trypsin, papain, bromelin, or ficin irreversibly reduces the sialic acid content and lowers the zeta potential values. Thus, treated cells are readily agglutinated by appropriate antibodies. Since sialic acid is known to be one of the determinants for M and N antigens, enzyme treatment of these cells may destroy these antigens.

The exact mechanism of albumin enhancement in the reaction of certain antibodies is not yet known. One theory is that albumin behaves like electric condensors and has its positive charges neutralizing the negative charges on erythrocytes.

Polybrene and protamine, which are used in AutoAnalyzer systems (Technicon Corporation), pro-

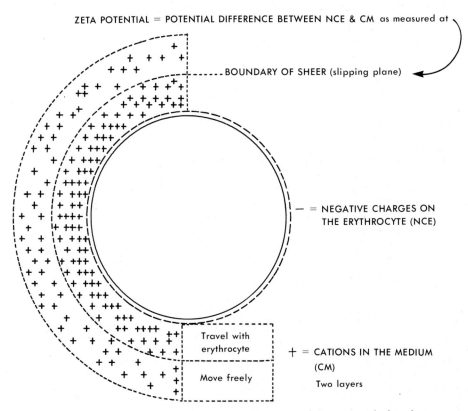

Figure 43-8. Diagramatic presentation on the measurement of Zeta potential of erythrocytes.

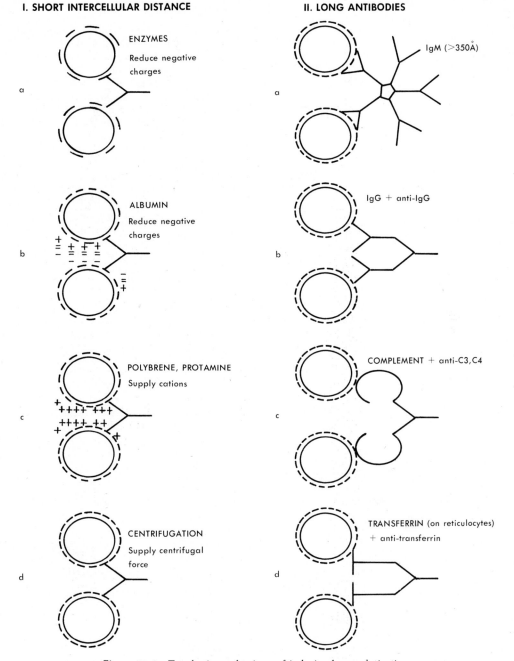

Figure 43–9. Two basic mechanisms of inducing hemagglutination.

vide an excess number of cations which neutralize the negative charges on the erythrocyte and produce non-specific aggregates. Short specific antibodies would then have the chance to touch more than one cell and produce specific agglutination. The addition of certain electrolytes, which counteract the effect of polybrene or protamine, would disperse the non-specific aggregates but not the specific aggregates. In this way, it is possible to detect and identify either the specific antigens or antibodies.

Although further studies are in progress, LISS appears to shorten the incubation time at 37°C. prior to the antiglobulin test and may replace albumin in crossmatching. Experience to date indicates that some antibodies, particularly those with low affinity constants, are detected better or only with LISS (Treacy, 1978).

Centrifugation forces the erythrocytes to come closer together and facilitates hemagglutination.

In terms of inducing hemagglutination by providing bridges between antibodies (Fig. 43-9), IgM antibodies with dimensions greater than 35 nm are able to reach more than one erythrocyte to form aggregates and are known as "complete" antibodies.

IgG antibodies with dimensions usually less than 25 nm can agglutinate only those red blood cells having intracellular distances of less than 25 nm. This may be achieved by any of the previously mentioned factors. Anti-human globulin or anti-complement antibodies may serve as bridges between those antibodies or complement components already attached to individual erythrocytes.

Reticulocytes retain transferrin on their surface in order to transport iron compounds into the erythrocytes to form additional hemoglobin. If the antiglobulin serum also contains anti-transferrin, these antibodies would also serve as bridges to form aggregates of reticulocytes. This reaction may lead to false-positive antiglobulin tests in cases with high reticulocyte counts. However, this is unlikely at the present time owing to improvement in the specificity of anti-human globulin serum.

Non-immune Aggregates. In addition to the non-specific aggregates formed by polybrene and protamine, many other chemicals may induce hemagglutination. A common phenomenon in blood banks is rouleaux formation. Rouleaux are usually induced by a high concentration of dextran, PVP, fibrinogen, or globulin and can be differentiated from true agglutination, either by their microscopic appearance or by their dispersion upon the replacement of serum with saline.

Non-specific aggregates induced by a high concentration of dextrose have been useful in deglycerolyzing frozen red blood cells.

A third type of non-specific agglutination may be found in cord blood contaminated by Wharton's jelly. The presence of hyaluronic acid, together with albumin, has been shown to be responsible and is usually solved by the addition of hyaluronidase.

In conclusion, in any attempt to use hemagglutination reactions to detect antigens or antibodies, appropriate controls must be used to assure the specificity of the reaction.

Hemagglutination inhibition

This reaction is used to detect the presence of soluble antigens such as ABH, Le^a, I, P, Sd^a, and Ch^a in saliva, serum, or other fluids. The use of soluble antigen to neutralize a specific antibody for its identification is in fact a two-stage hemagglutination inhibition. These soluble antigens share the same antigenic specificity as found on the erythrocytes and are capable of neutralizing the corresponding antibodies in the serum. The neutralized serum will then no longer agglutinate the erythrocytes. Consequently, the absence of agglutination in hemagglutination inhibition indicates a positive test and signifies the presence of a specific antigen in the fluid tested. The strength of the antibody used in the test must be adjusted to give not more than a 2+ reaction with the indicator cells. The concentration of the soluble antigen can be determined by titration. An example given in chapter 44 (p. 1526) illustrates the use of saliva in determining the secretor status.

Hemolysis

This is also a very useful reaction in blood banking. It indicates the presence of immune anti-A or anti-B in reverse serum grouping and helps to identify certain antibodies such as anti-P_1, anti-P, anti-PP_1P^k, anti-Jk^a, anti-Le^a, and, sometimes, anti-Le^b and anti-Vel. It may help to exclude Rh antibodies which are generally non-hemolytic. When a 50 per cent end point is used, hemolysis can quantitate soluble A substance with great accuracy. Since complement is required for this reaction, inactivated serum or plasma cannot be used for this purpose. Incubation at 37°C. facilitates this reaction. Precautions must be taken to avoid hemolysis due to non-immunologic factors such as water or chemicals.

ERYTHROCYTE ANTIGENS AND ANTIBODIES

The ABO System

Special characteristics

The ABO system has two unique features which are not found in any other blood group system (Table 43-15): (1) the usual presence of

Table 43-15.   TWO PREDICTABLE SPECIAL FEATURES OF THE ABO SYSTEM

BLOOD GROUP	AGGLUTININS IN SERUM	ANTIGENS ON CERTAIN TISSUE CELLS (SOLUBLE SUBSTANCES IN SECRETORS)
O	Anti-A, anti-B	H(O)
A	Anti-B	H, A
B	Anti-A	H, B
AB	None	H, A, B

strongly reactive agglutinins in the serum of those who lack the corresponding antigen(s), and (2) the regular presence of ABH antigens on many tissue cells and ABH substances in the secretions of secretors. These two unique characteristics make the ABO system by far the most important blood group system in blood transfusion and organ transplantation.

The regular presence of strong anti-A and/ or anti-B (antibodies) in the serum renders the demonstration of A and B antigens on erythrocytes a much easier task. This may be the reason that ABO was the first blood group system to be discovered. It is the only blood group system in which examination of the serum (reverse grouping) can be used reliably to confirm the results of forward grouping of erythrocytes.

Antibodies and agglutinins (Table 43–16)

Human antibodies are readily available, although those from animals and agglutinins from plants are also used in the study of ABO antigens. Human antibodies can roughly be divided into two categories: "natural" and "immune." Both types are the result of immunization. The immunogens of the *"natural"* *type* are probably bacterial in origin, as some bacteria share A or B antigens. This is demonstrated by the fact that anti-A or anti-B antibodies, if any, are of low titer in infants and expected agglutinins are absent in germ-free animals. "Natural" anti-A or anti-B is usually of the IgM class and is readily neutralized by soluble A or B group substances. "Natural anti-A,B" in group O persons is usually of the IgG class and less readily neutralized by A and B substances.

When group O (anti-A,B) serum is absorbed with group A or B cells, the eluate from such cells usually contains anti-A and anti-B. In addition, group O serum often reacts with subgroups of A (A_x) which may be non-reactive with anti-A. Several theories have been proposed to explain these findings, but none has been generally accepted.

Immune anti-A or anti-B is of the IgG class and is usually the result of immunization through fetal-maternal hemorrhage. Likewise, injection of A or B blood group substances for reagent antiserum production usually results in high titers of immune anti-A or anti-B.

Anti-A_1 reacts with A_1 cells but not with A_2 cells. The antibodies can be derived from human anti-A serum absorbed with A_2 cells or from persons of group A_2B, A_2, or A_x who have anti-A_1 in their sera; however, such anti-A_1 (antibodies) are usually weak and unsuitable for reagent purposes. Anti-A_1 (lectin) properly prepared from *Dolichos biflorus* is a very useful reagent for grouping purposes. Transfusion reactions have been reported on occasion in patients whose blood plasma contained anti-A_1 while receiving A_1 erythrocytes (Mollison, 1972, p. 240).

Anti-H strongly agglutinates O cells; however, the reactions are weaker with A_2 or A_3 cells, and weakest or negligible with A_1 or A_1B cells. This antibody can usually be neutralized by H substance. The anti-H found in the serum of persons with the O_h (Bombay) phenotype normally agglutinates and sometimes hemolyzes O cells, while that found in non-O_h persons is usually weak and non-hemolytic.

Anti-H prepared from *Ulex europaeus* provides an excellent reagent for determining

4

Table 43–16.   ABO ANTIBODIES AND AGGLUTININS

SPECIFICITY	SERUM			OTHER SOURCES
	Group	Incidence	Characteristics	
Anti-B	A	All	Usually IgM Titer 1:8-512 Average 64	Colostrum (IgA) Saliva (IgA) Tears Ascitic fluid Anti-A also found in snails and fish roe
Anti-A,B	O, O_h	All	Usually IgG Reacts with A_x, A_3	
Anti-A	B	All	Usually IgM Titer 1:32-2048 Average 256	
Anti-A_1	A_2B A_2 A_x	22-35% 1-8% Most	Few transfusion reactions reported	Anti-A absorbed with A_2 cells *Dolichos biflorus*
Anti-H	O_h Not O_h	All Some	Inhibited by H substance	*Ulex europaeus*, eel, immunized chicken

Table 43-17. DIFFERENTIATION OF COMMON ABO GROUPS

PHENOTYPE	ERYTHROCYTES + ANTI-					SERUM + ERYTHROCYTES				ELUATE ANTI‡	SUBSTANCE IN SALIVA OF SECRETOR
	A	A_1	B	A,B	H	A_1	A_2	B	O		
A_1	4+	4+	−	4+	−	−	−	4+	−	A	H,A
A_{Int}	4+	2+	−	4+	2+	−	−	4+	−	A	H,A
A_2	4+	−	−	4+	2+	†	−	4+	−	A	H,A
A_3	2+*	−	−	2+*	3+	†	−	4+	−	A	H,A
A_m	−/+	−	−	−/+	4+	−	−	4+	−	A	H,A
A_x	−/+	−	−	1−2+	4+	1+ (Usually)	−	4+	−	A	H
B_1	−		4+	4+	4+	4+		−	−	B	H,B
B_3	−		2+*	2+*	4+	4+		−	−	B	H,B
O	−		−	−	4+	4+	4+	4+	−	H	H
O_h	−		−	−	−	4+	4+	4+	4+	−	−

*Minor population of agglutinates.

†May have anti-A_1.

‡Eluate from cells sensitized with anti-A, anti-B, or anti-H should have the specificity of anti-A, anti-B, or anti-H, respectively.

secretor status and detecting H antigens on certain tissue cells. This lectin is usually stronger than human anti-H, and it will react with A or B cells; however, this reagent is usually diluted so that it is non-reactive with A_1 cells.

Common ABO antigens

Although many variants of ABO antigens have been described, only A_1, A_2, and B are of practical importance; A_3, A_m, A_x, B_3, and O_h are seen occasionally, while other subgroups are very rare. Only the first two categories are listed in Table 43-17 and Figure 44-3A (p. 1511) and will be reviewed.

Genetics. The ABO system is controlled by at least three sets of genes: H and h; A_1, A_2, B, and O; and Se and se. Each set is independent of the others and it can be assumed that each has its own locus. Only the ABO locus has been shown to be on chromosome No. 9 (Westerveld, 1976); the two others remain unassigned.

The product of the H gene is fucosyltransferase, which converts the precursor substance to H substance (Figs. 43-1 and 43-10). In the absence of H gene (designated as hh), the precursor substance remains unconverted and O_h or Bombay type results. In this case, despite the presence of ABO genes, A or B antigen will not be formed because H substance, the precursor of the A and B antigens, is absent (see Fig. 44-5A, p. 1532).

There are at least two forms of ABH antigens: soluble glycoproteins found in secretions and plasma and structural lipoproteins which

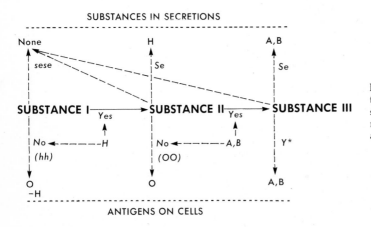

Figure 43-10. Possible genetic pathways in the biosynthesis of ABO antigens and ABH substances. *In the absence of a Y gene, one may have A substance in secretions but no A antigens on erythrocytes.

Table 43-18. ABO SECRETORS AND LEWIS PHENOTYPES

SECRETION STATUS	SECRETOR		NON-SECRETOR	
Frequency	80%		20%	
ABH substance	Present		Absent	
Controlling gene	Se		sese	
Lewis gene	Le	lele	Le	lele
Lewis substance	Le^b + Le^a	None	Le^a	None
Lewis phenotype Le	a−b+	a−b−	a+b−	a−b−

are part of the erythrocyte membrane as well as some epithelial and endothelial cells. Both forms have the same specificity with respect to their reactions with anti-A, anti-B, or anti-H. Soluble ABH antigens can be demonstrated in the secretions of about 80 per cent of the population; these individuals are known as secretors. The secretor status is controlled by a pair of genes *Se* and *se*. In the absence of the *Se* gene (se/se), ABH antigens are not present in the secretions, and these individuals are known as non-secretors (Fig. 43-10).

Since ABH and Lewis antigens share a common precursor (see Fig. 43-1), it is not surprising that the Lewis gene (*Le, le*) is related to the production of ABH antigens. ABH secretors are found to be Le(a−b+) or Le(a−b−), while ABH non-secretors are Le(a+b−) or Le(a−b−) (Table 43-18). In the absence of the H gene, Le^b antigen or substance cannot be formed. This hypothesis is supported by the fact that Le(a−b+) has never been found in a Bombay phenotype (O_h).

Development. Although ABH antigens can be detected on erythrocytes in a six-week-old fetus, they are not fully expressed until a child is 6 to 18 months old. An infant who initially was typed as A_2 may later type as A_1.

Distribution. ABH antigens have been found not only in bacteria but also in some animals. Pig A^p cells have been used to differ-

entiate "immune" and "natural" anti-A; only immune anti-A agglutinins are readily absorbed by A^p cells.

In addition to saliva, ABH substances can also be found in secretions of the upper gastrointestinal tract, ovarian cyst fluid, seminal fluid, and amniotic fluid. With the specific red cell adherence technique, ABH antigens can be found on some epithelial cells as well as on all blood vessel endothelium. The presence of ABH antigens on white blood cells (Gurner, 1958) and platelets (Coombs, 1955) has been reported, but controversy exists in this matter.

ABO grouping

Routine ABO grouping (Table 43-19): Minimum titers of 1:256 are required for anti-A and anti-B reagents used for the forward grouping (cell grouping). Anti-A,B from a group O person is a useful reagent for detecting subgroups of A or B. When a differentiation of A_1 and A_2 is required, anti-A_1 is used (Tables 43-17 and 43-20). Meticulous adherence to manufacturers' directions for use of all reagents is essential for accurate and reproducible results. Further discussion of testing for erythrocyte antigens and antibodies is presented subsequently (p. 1451).

In the reverse grouping (serum grouping) cells of groups A_1, B and O are normally used. O cells serve as a control for unexpected antibodies. A_2 cells should be used when one suspects the presence of anti-A_1.

Table 43-19. ROUTINE ABO GROUPING OF ERYTHROCYTES

CELLS AGAINST SERUM WITH		SERUM AGAINST CELLS OF GROUP			INTERPRETATION	FREQUENCY (%) IN MAJOR U.S. POPULATION*			
Anti-A	Anti-B	A	B	O		Whites	Blacks	American Indians	Orientals
−	−	+	+	−	O	45	49	79	40
+	−	−	+	−	A	40	27	16	28
−	+	+	−	−	B	11	20	4	27
+	+	−	−	−	AB	4	4	<1	5

*Composite figures, calculated from Mourant, 1976.

Table 43-20. DIFFERENTIATION BETWEEN A_1 AND A_2 ERYTHROCYTES

GROUP	A_1	A_2
Quantitative		
Anti-A (weak or diluted)	4+	2+
Antigenic sites: Adult	1,000,000	250,000
Newborn	310,000	14,000
Qualitative		
Reaction with anti-A_1	Positive	Negative
Anti-A_1 in serum	No	Maybe
Antigenic determinant	Type I & II chains	Type II chains only
N-acetyl-galactosaminyl-transferase activity	Max. at pH 6 More active	Max. at pH 7 Less active

Interpretation of ABO grouping results is usually straightforward. Table 43-17 lists the major characteristics. The observation of a minor population of agglutinates (also known as mixed field) to identify A_3 is very helpful. The ability of test cells to adsorb anti-A or anti-B, as well as secretor status studies, may be of great help in the identification of A_m or A_x (Table 43-17). If feasible, the demonstration of acetyl-galactosaminyltransferase, galactosyltransferase, or fucosyltransferase is useful in confirming the presence of *A*, *B*, and *H* genes, respectively.

Some Discrepancies in ABO Grouping

1. Unexpected/additional reactions in cell grouping
   a. Cells modified by bacterial enzymes such as those found in patients with acquired B
   b. Abnormal inheritance such as Cis-AB (In both cases, the cells appear to be group AB with an anti-B component in their serum. See Table 43-21.)
   c. Cells modified by chemicals such as hyaluronic acid found in Wharton's jelly: cord cells agglutinate non-specifically; however, the aggregates will disperse with the addition of hyaluronidase.
   d. Minor population of cells derived from a chimeric twin or a recent non-group specific transfusion

   e. Cells coated with antibodies with subsequent formation of aggregates in the presence of a high-protein medium
   f. Different types of polyagglutinable cells (Table 43-22)
2. Unexpected/additional reactions in serum grouping
   a. The presence of either cold or warm autoagglutinins reacting at room temperature
   b. The presence of alloantibodies such as anti-A_1, anti-H, anti-I, anti-M, anti-Le[a], anti-P_1, and other room temperature-reacting antibodies
   c. The presence of a high concentration of polymers such as gamma globulin, fibrinogen, dextran, or PVP in serum which can induce rouleaux formation (Microscopic examination and/or saline replacement resolves this problem.)
   d. The presence of antibodies directed against (1) lactose or antibiotics such as neomycin or chloramphenicol, which may be present in the reagent red cell preservation solution; (2) caprylate, which is used as a stabilizer for bovine albumin preparations; or (3) acriflavin, which is the dye used in preparations of anti-B reagents
3. Weakened or missing reactions in cell grouping
   a. Subgroups of A or B (see Table 43-17) (Many

Table 43-21. AN AB PERSON WITH ANTI-B

	"CIS-AB"	"Acquired B"
Possible cause Etiology	Inherited	Action of bacteria*
Person (usually)	Healthy	Lower abdominal pathology
Subgroup (usually)	A_2	A_1
Anti-B (usually)	Weak	Strong
Substance in Secretors	A + B	A
Children	A_2B or O	A_1 or O

*Bacterial deacetylase is the most attractive explanation.

Table 43–22. SOME CHARACTERISTICS OF POLYAGGLUTINABLE CELLS

TYPE	T	Tn	Cad
Possible cause	Bacterial neuraminidase?	Unknown (not inherited)	Inherited
Duration	Transient	Persistent	Permanent
Own serum	−	−	−
Cord serum	−	−	−
AB serum	+	+*	+
Polybrene	−	−	+
Arachis hypogea	+	−	−
Salvia sclarea	−	+	−
Salvia horminum	−	+	+

*Minor population of agglutinates is common.

T = Receptors on normal human erythrocytes; when exposed, erythrocytes become polyagglutinable.

Tn = Similar to T receptors, but do not react with anti-T component in the normal serum. The change is permanent.

Cad = Inherited polyagglutinable erythrocytes, probably a strong variant of Sd^a antigen.

other variants have been reported, but they are very rare and of little clinical importance.)

   b. Weakened antigens, A_g or B_g, in certain disease states such as leukemia.

   c. High concentrations of A or B soluble substances in the sera of patients with adenocarcinoma of the stomach. These substances can neutralize the typing serum and give very weak or negative reactions.

4. Weakened or missing expected agglutinins

   a. Hypogammaglobulinemia or agammaglobulinemia

   b. Low titered or absent isoagglutinins, e.g., infants less than six months old or elderly persons

THE RH SYSTEM

The Rh system is perhaps the most complex erythrocyte system in terms of the number of antigens reported, the relationship among these antigens, and the nomenclature proposed by different investigators. Our effort will be to present only essential information. Readers who are interested in more detail should consult Race (1975) and Issitt (1975).

The basic Rh system

The basic information has been derived from five antisera: anti-Rh_o(D), anti-rh′(C), anti-rh″(E), anti-hr′(c), and anti-hr″(e) (Table 43–23). Antigens C and c, as well as E and e, are antithetical; however, the antibody for the antithetical antigen for D has never been found. The term antithetical indicates that the two antigens are controlled by a pair of allelic genes; that is, a person can be C/C or C/c or c/c. A similar condition has been found for the genes E and e. For convenience of expression, the gene allelic to D has been assigned ″d″. Thus, from serologic evidence, the Rh system can be assigned to three loci of genes, and this is basically the proposal of Fisher and Race (Race, 1975, p. 179).

From population and family studies, these three loci are close to each other and inherited as a unit; well-documented crossing-over has not been observed. Therefore, Wiener proposed a one-locus theory: the gene complex (haplotype, or genetic endowment of one of a pair of chromosomes) is really one gene with a product of more than one specificity as determined by different antisera. The serologic factors (antigen expression) were named by Wiener as Rh_o, rh′, rh″, hr′, and hr″ respectively for D, C, E, c, and e. To reflect serologic factors from one gene, he used the term agglutinogen; e.g., Rh_z for the three-antigen complex Rh_o, rh′, and rh″; or rh for the two-antigen

Table 43–23. EXAMPLES OF DIFFERENCES IN CONCEPT AND NOTATION OF THE Rh SYSTEM BY DIFFERENT INVESTIGATORS

PROPOSED FOR	BY	CONCEPT	CHROMOSOME 1a*	CHROMOSOME 1b*
Haplotype	Wiener	1 locus	R^z	r
	Fisher-Race	3 subloci	DCE	dce
Antigens produced by the haplotype	Wiener	1 agglutinogen 2-3 factors	Rh_z Rh_o, rh′, rh″	rh hr′, hr″
	Fisher-Race	2-3 antigens	D, C, E	c, e
	Rosenfield et al.	Numerical	Rh1, Rh2, Rh3	Rh4, Rh5

*A pair of chromosomes.

Table 43-24. EIGHT GENE COMPLEXES (HAPLOTYPES) OF THE Rh SYSTEM*

HAPLOTYPES		ANTIGEN COMPLEX†	FREQUENCIES OF U.S. POPULATION			
Fisher-Race	Wiener	(Agglutinogen, Wiener)	Whites	Blacks	American Indians	Orientals
Dce	R^0	$Rh_0(Rh_0,\ hr'hr'')$	0.04	0.44	0.02	0.03
DCe	R^1	$Rh_1(Rh_0,\ rh'hr'')$	0.42	0.17	0.44	0.70
DcE	R^2	$Rh_2(Rh_0,\ hr'rh'')$	0.14	0.11	0.34	0.21
DCE	R^z	$Rh_z(Rh_0,\ rh'rh'')$			0.06	0.01
dce	r	$rh(hr'hr'')$	0.37	0.26	0.11	0.03
dCe	r'	$rh'(rh'hr'')$	0.02	0.02	0.02	0.02
dcE	r''	$rh''(hr'rh'')$	0.01		0.01	
dCE	r^y	$rh_y(rh'rh'')$				

*Composite figures, calculated from Mourant et al (1976)
†In Fisher-Race nomenclature, antigens as indicated by the letters except 'd'

complex hr′ and hr″. The gene for Rh_z is designated as R^z; that for rh is r. Thus, three closely linked subloci for the Rh gene complex can explain the serologic reactions of blood group factors and genetic endowment of an individual or a population; e.g., gene complex (haplotype) → antigen complex (agglutinogen with multiple specificities). Both types of notations are two different interpretations of the same serologic findings in families and in populations. However, many people find the Fisher-Race notation easier to understand and use. Since the number of Rh antigens is increasing, alphabetical notation is no longer practical; Rosenfield proposed a numerical system—Rh1, Rh2, Rh3, Rh4, and Rh5—to represent the five basic antigens. At the present time, both Wiener (Rh) and Fisher-Race (DCE) notations are commonly used. One should be familiar with both designations.

With the help of the five basic antisera, eight antigen complexes (agglutinogens) are possible (Table 43-24). Each can be assigned to a gene complex or haplotype. The corresponding frequencies of four major American populations are listed. The frequency of dCE is extremely low.

Table 43-25 lists the frequencies of 11 common Rh phenotypes (out of 18 possible phenotypes) as detected by the basic five antisera. Common genotypes within each phenotype and the frequency of each genotype are also

Table 43-25. FREQUENCIES OF COMMON Rh PHENOTYPES*

REACTION WITH ANTI-†					PHENOTYPE		GENOTYPE		FREQUENCIES‡			
D	C	c	E	e	Rh	DCE	Rh	DCE	Whites	Blacks	American Indians	Orientals
+	+	+	+	+	Rh_zrh	DCcEe	R^1R^2	DCe/DcE	0.1176 (89%)	0.0374 (100%)	0.2992 (89%)	0.294 (97%)
							R^1r''	DCe/dcE	0.0084 (6%)		0.0088 (3%)	
							$r'R^2$	dCe/DcE	0.0056 (5%)		0.0135 (4%)	0.0084 (2.8%)
							rR^z	dce/DCE			0.0132 (4%)	0.0006 (0.2%)
+	+	+	−	+	Rh_1rh	DCce	R^1R^0	DCe/Dce	0.0168 (5%)	0.1495 (63%)	0.0176 (15%)	0.042 (50%)
							R^1r	DCe/dce	0.3108 (95%)	0.0884 (37%)	0.0968 (85%)	0.042 (50%)
+	−	+	+	+	Rh_2rh	DcEe	R^2R^0	DcE/Dce	0.0112 (10%)	0.0968 (63%)	0.0136 (15%)	0.0126 (50%)
							R^2r	DcE/dce	0.1035 (90%)	0.0572 (37%)	0.0748 (85%)	0.0126 (50%)
+	+	−	−	+	Rh_1Rh_1	DCe	R^1R^1	DCe/DCe	0.176 (91%)	0.029 (81%)	0.194 (92%)	0.490 (93%)
							R^1r'	DCe/dCe	0.017 (9%)	0.007 (19%)	0.017 (8%)	0.028 (7%)
+	+	−	+	+	Rh_1Rh_z	DCEe	R^1R^z	DCe/DCE			0.053 (100%)	
+	−	+	+	−	Rh_2Rh_2	DcE	R^2R^2	DcE/DcE	0.02 (88%)	0.012 (100%)	0.116 (94%)	0.044 (100%)
							R^2r''	DcE/dcE	0.003 (12%)		0.007 (6%)	
+	+	+	+	−	Rh_2Rh_z	DCcE	R^2R^z	DcE/DCE			0.041 (100%)	
+	−	+	−	+	Rh_0	Dce	R^0R^0	Dce/Dce	0.0016 (5%)	0.1936 (46%)	0.0004 (8%)	0.0009 (33%)
							R^0r	Dce/dce	0.0296 (95%)	0.2286 (54%)	0.0044 (92%)	0.0018 (67%)
−	−	+	−	+	rh	dce	rr	dce/dce	0.1369 (100%)	0.0676 (100%)	0.0121 (100%)	0.0009 (100%)
−	+	+	−	+	rh′rh	dCce	rr'	dce/dCe	0.0055 (100%)	0.0014 (100%)	0.0044 (100%)	0.0012 (100%)
−	−	+	+	+	rh″rh	dcEe	rr''	dce/dcE	0.0028 (100%)		0.0022 (100%)	

*Estimated from haplotype frequencies (p,q from table 43-24) using p^2 for homozygotes and 2pq for heterozygotes.
† + = positive; − = negative.
‡ (%) = per cent of genotypes within a given phenotype.

listed. The zygosity percentage with respect to Rh_o, which is important in the chance of immunization of pregnant mothers by the father, can be determined from these frequencies.

The Rh antibodies

Antibodies in the Rh system differ from those in the ABO system. With few exceptions (anti-C^w and anti-E), they are immune in origin and usually IgG. IgM and IgA Rh antibodies are very rare. With only one known exception, Rh antibodies do not hemolyze erythrocytes (Mollison, 1972, p. 282). Although saline-reacting Rh antibodies are available, most of them react best by albumin, enzyme, or antiglobulin technique. Because of this lack of "naturally occurring" agglutinins, Rh antibodies were not discovered until almost 40 years after the demonstration of ABO antibodies.

Rh_o antibodies develop usually after fetal-maternal hemmorhage and rarely as a result of transfusion with current blood bank technology (routine Rh_o typing of all recipients); however, this may occur when platelet or granulocyte concentrates containing Rh_o-positive erythrocytes are transfused to an Rh_o-negative recipient. Once immunized, antibodies may last for many years and the host responds to secondary exposure very vigorously and promptly.

Zygosity or dosage of D antigen usually cannot be revealed by anti-D titration, whereas certain anti-C, anti-c, or anti-E and anti-e will often show dosage when proper techniques are used. Potent anti-D, anti-E, and anti-c are readily available. Good anti-C and anti-e are less readily available and pure anti-C without anti-C^w is rare.

Quite often, Rh antibodies demonstrate multiple specificities as well as single specificity. Some Rh antibodies react only with antigen complexes such as ce (Rh6, f), CE (Rh22), Ce (Rh7), cE (Rh27), and ce^s (Rh10, V) or CcEe complexes such as Rh17, Rh18, Rh34, and Rh38; or all the Rh antigens such as Rh29 and Rh39 (Table 43-26 and Fig. 43-11). Figure 43-11 also shows all other Rh antigens which have been assigned to the Rh system. Each of them has been discovered by the finding of a specific antibody.

Anti-Rh_o(D) not only serves as a blood typing reagent but may also be used in the prevention of Rh_o immunization. Rh_o immune globulin (Rh_oIg) may be administered to an Rh_o-negative person receiving Rh-positive

Table 43-26. REACTIONS OF FOUR COMPOUND Rh ANTIBODIES WITH ANTIGENS OF EIGHT Rh HAPLOTYPES

HAPLOTYPES	ANTI-			
	CE	Ce	cE	ce(f)
$R^z(DCE)$ $r^y(dCE)$	+	−	−	−
$R^1(DCe)$ $r'(dCe)$	−	+	−	−
$R^2(DcE)$ $r''(dcE)$	−	−	+	−
$R^0(Dce)$ $r(dce)$	−	−	−	+

erythrocytes through either pregnancy or accidental blood transfusion. One vial (about $300\,\mu g$ antibody protein) has been recommended for every 15 ml of Rh_o-positive red blood cells (not whole blood). For instance, if a recipient is estimated to have received 100 ml of red blood cells, 7 vials of Rh_o immune globulin should be given as soon as possible, although satisfactory prevention of immunization has been observed as late as 48 hours after accidental transfusions. When many vials of Rh_o were given to patients receiving large volumes of Rh_o-positive erythrocytes, no harmful side effects were observed (Mollison, 1972) (see also p. 1501).

The Rh antigens

Antigen Rh_o and Its Subunits. Rh_o antigen was established through careful clinical observation and animal experimentation. The first anti-Rh_o serum was produced in rabbits by injecting Rhesus monkey erythrocytes. With this serum, Landsteiner and Wiener found that erythrocytes of 85 per cent of the population react positively and 15 per cent react negatively. The term "Rh" was used to define the antigen discovered.

Besides A and B antigens, Rh_o(D) is the most antigenic. About two thirds of Rh_o(D) negative (−) persons receiving Rh_o(D) positive (+) blood are likely to develop anti-Rh_o(D). It is for this reason that every blood donor and recipient is typed for Rh_o(D) antigen in addition to the A and B antigens.

Results of D typing are not always clear-cut; some D antigens can be detected only by the antiglobulin test and are designated as D^u ($ℜh_o$ Rhw1). There are three types of D^u's: those due to gene interaction, those with an

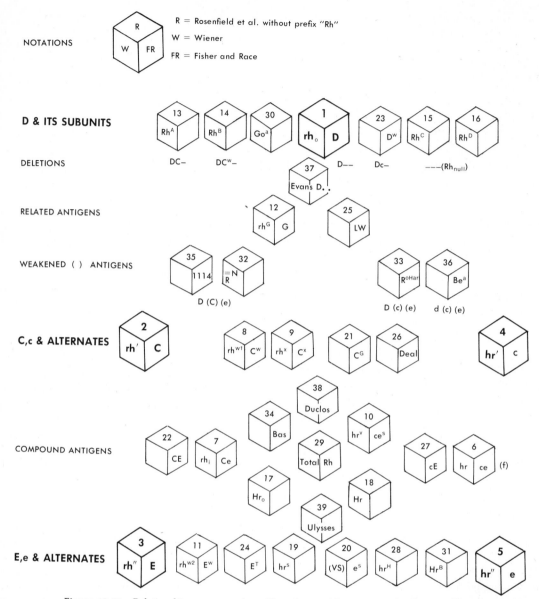

Figure 43–11. Relationships among various Rh antigens with respect to the five specificities.

incomplete D, and those due to another type of inheritance.

One type of D^u is due to the presence of a "C" in the trans position (on the opposite chromosome) such as in the *Dce/dCe* genotype. This person may type as D^u, while her children whose genotype is *Dce/dce* would be typed as a regular D. This type of D^u is fairly common among blacks owing to the high frequency of *Dce* haplotype. People with this type of D^u are unlikely to form anti-D when D+ erythrocytes are transfused.

The second type of D^u has been shown to be an incomplete D antigen. Evidence indicates that $Rh_o(D)$ antigen consists of a mosaic with at least four sub-units: Rh^A, Rh^B, Rh^C, and Rh^D (Fig. 43–11). When one or more of these sub-units is missing, the D antigen reacts as a D^u. In fact, those with a missing unit (such as $Rh^b = Rh^{ACD}$) may develop antibodies against the missing unit (Rh^B). This can explain why a D+ person may develop an alloanti-D.

There are some D^u's that do not belong to either of these two categories and are called "genetic D^u's" (a poor term, since the other two types are also under genetic control).

A slightly stronger D antigen has been observed in the presence of Rh32 antigen, whereas a moderately strong D antigen occurs with Rh30, Rh35, DC−, DC^w, and a greatly enhanced D antigen is seen in D−−.

Antigens C and c and E and e. A person will normally type as C+c+, C−c+, or C+c−; similar reactions are found with E and e. Rare exceptions are produced by the gene complex *DC−*, where E and e antigens are absent. Since DCe and DcE are common phenotypes, anti-CE and anti-Ce are common antibodies formed by the person who has the opposite phenotype. In practice, anti-e and anti-C are often weak and less readily demonstrable. From serologic evidence, one can assume that genes controlling the E and e antigen are close to the genes for C and c antigens rather than to the gene for the D antigen. The logical expression of the gene complex would then be *DCE* instead of *CDE*.

Among the alternate antigens for C and c, C^w can be demonstrated in slightly more than 1 per cent of the white population. Since only a few persons have C^w without C antigen on their erythrocytes and few serums have anti-C without anti-C^w, the exact relationship between C and C^w is not clear.

The antigen G that is often associated with both D and C antigens is not a DC complex. Some persons with D or C antigen may not have the G antigen, while some persons have G antigen without the D or C antigen (r^G). However, many anti-D and anti-C serums also contain anti-G. This explains why mothers immunized only to C antigens produce antibodies reacting with D+ cells as well. Hence, anti-G has been referred to as anti-D and anti-C in some earlier literature.

Among the alternates to E and e antigens (Fig. 43–11), e^s(Rh20, VS) is rare in whites but present in 25 per cent of blacks. Other E or e

variants are very rare. Compound antigens were discussed under Rh antibodies.

Rare weak variants similar to D^u have been reported for C, c, E, and e and are designated as C^u, c^v, E^u, and e^i, respectively. Weakened antigens in a complex (expressed in parenthesis) have been encountered. Examples include Rh35 or $\underline{D}$(C)(e) (whites), Rh 32 or D(c)(e) (blacks, $\overline{\overline{R}}{}^N$), Rh 33 or D(c)(e), (R^{oHar}), and Rh36 or d(c)(e)(Be^a) (Fig. 43–11). Partial deletion of Rh antigens, such as Dc−, DC^w−, D−− and D.. (Rh37, Evans), and LW−, as well as complete deletion Rh$_{null}$, have been reported. For detailed description of Rh variants, Race (1975) and Issitt (1975) give excellent accounts.

Rh Null Syndrome. Erythrocytes lacking all Rh antigens have been found in at least 22 persons in 14 families (Race, 1975). Most Rh$_{null}$ individuals studied presented with a compensated hemolytic anemia and a defect in the erythrocyte (stomatocytes) with shortened red blood cell survival. Rh antibodies with multiple specificities (anti-C, anti-e, anti-Rh29, etc.) may be present in their serum. Anti-Rh29 reacts with erythrocytes of all types except Rh$_{null}$. The M, N, En^a, and i antigens may be enhanced, while S, s, U antigens may be depressed in Rh$_{null}$ people.

Possible genetic pathways in the biosynthesis of Rh and LW antigens are illustrated in Figure 43-12 to explain the two types of Rh$_{null}$ phenotypes. A regulator gene is required to convert substance I to substance II and a *"DCE"* gene complex is required to convert substance II to DCE antigens. In the absence of a regulator gene *X'* (expressed by some as X^oX^o), no substance II is produced and the DCE antigens cannot be formed in spite of the existing *DCE* gene. This is known as the "regulator" type of Rh$_{null}$, who may transmit the *DCE* gene to their children. In the absence of a *DCE* gene (---) from both parents, the children may then be ---/--- and unable to

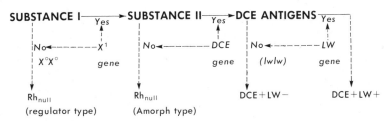

Figure 43–12. Possible genetic pathways in the biosynthesis of Rh and LW antigens. (Modified from Race, 1975.)

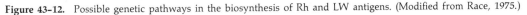

convert substance II to DCE antigens. In this type of Rh_{null}, which is known as "amorph" type, the parents and children have antigens from only one haplotype such as *DCe/---* or *dce/---*.

The LW Antigen. Accumulated data indicate that rabbit anti-Rh_o(D) serum is not identical to the anti-Rh_o(D) found in human serum. With proper techniques, antibodies to erythrocytes of the rhesus monkey will react with both D+ and D− cells (adult cells only, not true with cord cells). Human sera with similar specificity have been found; thus, they react strongly with D+, weakly with D−, and not at all with the patient's own cells. Results of family studies indicate that the antigen detected by these sera is inherited independently from the DCE antigens. This antigen is, in fact, similar to the Rhesus antigen. Since the term Rh has been widely used for D antigen, a term LW was proposed by Levine to honor Landsteiner and Wiener. So far, all Rh_{null} people are LW− also; thus, both antigens must be related. A possible relationship between Rh and LW antigens is illustrated in Figure 43–12.

Anti-LW has been found in LW+ people. In addition, a transient form of LW− has also been observed. There is some evidence to indicate that the LW antigen may be like the D antigen and contain subunits. One must be aware that a person may type as LW-negative by one antiserum and LW-positive by another antiserum. The LW typing serum used in each case, therefore, must be specified.

Rh typing

Routine Rh typing for blood donors and recipients involves only the antigen Rh_o(D). Tests for D^u in D− specimens should be done every time. The term Rh_o-positive or Rh_o-negative refers to D+ or D−. To avoid ambiguity, Rh_o-positive or Rh_o-negative should be used; for simplicity, D+ or D− may serve the same purpose. Erythrocytes with C or E antigen should not be classified as Rh-positive. Meticulous adherence to manufacturers' directions for reagents, including sera, is crucial for accurate and specific Rh erythrocyte typing (p. 1451).

To determine the probable Rh genotype or in the case of antibody problems, tests for C, c, E, and e antigens are usually done. Only human antisera are used for clinical purposes. Saline-reacting antisera are available but are difficult to obtain. Potentiating medium which is usually added to Rh antisera to enhance reactivity may cause non-specific reactions; controls should be included each time. Albumin control, which is still being used in some laboratories, is not identical to diluent control.

Although most Rh antisera react more strongly in the presence of a high-protein medium or enzyme or by antiglobulin test, each serum should be used according to the manufacturer's instructions. A more sensitive method may detect some unwanted weak antibodies.

OTHER ERYTHROCYTE ANTIGENS AND ANTIBODIES

There are about 400 erythrocyte antigens reported in the literature. Race (1975) groups them into 22 blood group systems with separate groups for "public" and "private" antigens (see Table 43–5). Many of these antigens are of academic interest only, at least at the present time. ABO and Rh are by far the most important systems. Other important ones will be described subsequently.

The Lewis system

The ABH and Lewis substances are closely related, as evidenced by:

a. Lewis substances share the same precursor substance as ABH substances (see Fig. 43–1). Since H substance is not detectable in the Le(a+b−) phenotype (non-secretor), competition seems the logical explanation.

b. Le^b substance is probably derived from the H substance rather than from Le^a substance. The fact that no O_h phenotype has ever been observed with an Le(a−b+) phenotype tends to support this view.

c. Some Le^b antibodies react better with group O or A_2 cells (with more H antigen) and are designated as anti-Le^{bH}, whereas others react better with A_1 or A_1B cells and are designated as anti-Le^{bL}.

Since Le(a−b−) cells can be converted to Le(a+b−) or Le(a−b+) cells with the addition of plasma containing the appropriate Lewis substance, Lewis antigens on erythrocytes are thought to be the result of adsorption of soluble antigen in the plasma by the red blood cell.

It should be stressed that there is only one *Le* gene. Its silent allele is *le*, and there is no Le^a or Le^b gene, as the name of the antigen implies. Consequently, Le^a and Le^b are *not* antithetical antigens.

The possible biochemical relationships among Le^a, Le^c, Le^b, and Le^d are shown in Figure 43–1. No clinical significance is yet known for Le^c and Le^d antigens.

Both anti-Le^a and Le^b are usually "natural"

Table 43-27.   PHENOTYPES OF THE LEWIS SYSTEM

| | REACTIONS WITH ANTI- | | FREQUENCY (%) OF U.S. ADULTS | |
PHENOTYPES	Le^a	Le^b	Whites	Blacks
Le(a+b−)	+	−	22	23
Le(a−b+)	−	+	72	55
Le(a−b−)	−	−	6	22
Le(a+b+)*	+	+		

*Encountered occasionally in infants or young children who subsequently become Le(a−b+).

Modified from Miller, 1977, p. 116.

in origin and of the IgM class. These antibodies may react from 4°C. to 37°C., in different types of media, and by various techniques. Quite often anti-Le^a and occasionally anti-Le^b cause hemolysis *in vitro*. Both anti-Le^a and Le^b are unstable at 4°C. or −18°C. Goat anti-Le^a and anti-Le^b have been found satisfactory as typing reagents. Anti-Le^c, anti-Le^d, and anti-Le^x are very rare and of no clinical importance.

The presence of abundant Lewis substance in the serum may neutralize the antibodies *in vitro* during typing or *in vivo* during transfusion. For the former, washed erythrocytes are recommended for typing; for the latter, the Lewis substance may reduce the effect of antibodies on erythrocytes and, thus, benefit the recipient. The infusion of plasma containing Lewis substance has been advocated before the transfusion of Le(a+) or Le(b+) erythrocytes to patients with Lewis antibodies (Mollison, 1972, p. 512).

Hemolytic transfusion reactions due to anti-Le^a have been observed, while those due to anti-Le^b have not been documented. In emergency situations, a number of patients with anti-Le^a have been transfused with Le(a+b−) cells without untoward reactions. Some hospitals do not screen for Le(a−b−) blood for transfusion to patients with anti-Le^b. Perhaps a logical approach would be based on the strength of antibodies. If they are he-

molytic or clearly react by the antiglobulin test, compatible blood would seem to be the first choice.

Since Lewis antigens are poorly developed at birth and Lewis antibodies are IgM (i.e., unable to cross the placenta), hemolytic disease of the newborn has not been implicated with Lewis antibodies.

Common phenotypes of the Lewis system are listed in Table 43-27.

The I and i antigens

Since there are very few I-negative adults in the population, the genetics of these antigens has not been well studied; hence, I and i antigens have not been assigned to a system (Table 43-28). I antigen has also been found in soluble form in saliva, milk, urine, amniotic fluid, ovarian cyst fluid, and hydatid cyst fluid. The antigenic determinant has been shown to contain D-galactose and N-acetyl-D-glucosamine (see Fig. 43-2). Both I and i antigens have been demonstrated on lymphocytes.

Anti-I can be an auto- or alloantibody. Since the frequency of I-negative people is very low, allo anti-I is relatively rare and is found in every ii person as a "natural" antibody. Anti-I is usually of low titer but can be very potent. Auto anti-I is very common and is found in many normal persons as well as in those with acquired hemolytic anemia of the cold anti-

Table 43-28.   I-i ANTIGENS

STRENGTH OF ANTIGEN	FOUND IN ERYTHROCYTES	INCIDENCE
I i		
i$_1$	Whites	Rare
i$_2$	Blacks	Rare
i$_{cord}$	Cord	All
I$_{int}$	Adult (Ii)	Few
I	Adult	Almost all

Table 43–29. SIMILARITY BETWEEN THE
ABO AND THE P SYSTEMS

ABO		P	
Phenotype of erythrocyte	Antibodies in serum	Phenotype of erythrocyte	Antibodies in serum
O_h	Anti-H,-A,-B	p	Anti-$PP_1P^k(Tj^a)$
O	Anti-A($A_1 + A_2$), -B	P^k	Anti-P($P_1 + P_2$)
A_2	Anti-A_1	P_2	Anti-P_1
A_1	None for A antigen	P_1	None

body type. High titered anti-I is usually associated with mycoplasma pneumonia infection.

Anti-i is relatively uncommon but is found in up to 80 per cent of patients with infectious mononucleosis. It may be present in other conditions where the bone marrow is under stress, resulting in premature circulation of erythrocytes. Both anti-I and anti-i are usually IgM but may be IgG. Enzymes usually enhance their reactions with erythrocytes, and both usually react best at 4°C. Strong anti-i may be hemolytic.

Antibodies against a complex of antigens involving I or i antigens have been reported, e.g., IA, IB, IH, IP_1, iH, and iP_1. These antibodies react only when both antigens are present on the cell; they are not a mixture of two antibodies. I antigens are poorly developed at birth, as cord cells usually type as I-negative while adult cells (except those of *ii* people) are I-positive (Table 43–28).

The P system

Biochemically antigens in the P system are related to ABH antigens. The antigenic determinants are composed of three sugars: galactose, N-acetyl-galactosamine, and N-acetyl-glucosamine (see Fig. 43–2). Hydatid cyst fluid can neutralize anti-P_1 and anti-I antibodies. Other similarities between the ABO and P systems are listed in Table 43–29.

Phenotypes p, P^k, P_2, and P_1 in the P system have been likened to O_h, O, A_2, and A_1 in the ABO system, respectively. Both p and O_h are very rare and are considered the precursors of each system; each has "natural" antibodies against other antigens of the same system. P^k people produce anti-P just as group O people produce anti-A; similarly, P_2 people produce anti-P_1, and A_2 people produce anti-A_1.

Anti-P_1 is often found in P_2 persons. It is usually IgM, sometimes hemolytic, and may react at different temperatures and by differ-

ent methods. Anti-P_1 reacts positively with erythrocytes of 79 per cent of whites and 94 per cent of blacks (Miller, 1977, p. 120). Auto anti-P found in patients with paroxysmal cold hemoglobinuria is usually IgG and fixes complement at 4°C. with lysis of cells at 37°C. This is known as biphasic hemolysis. Anti-PP_1P^k (Tj^a) from p people is almost always hemolytic. Anti-P^k is prepared by absorption of anti-PP_1P^k with P_1+, P^k- cells. None of these antibodies has been known to cause hemolytic disease of the newborn; however, a strong anti-P_1 may cause a hemolytic transfusion reaction.

The phenotypes p and P^k are usually very rare; however, p is not uncommon in northern Sweden, whereas cases of P^k have been reported among Finns. The demonstration of P^k antigen on fibroblast cultures of all but p people tends to support strongly the hypothesis that p is the precursor substance of the P antigen.

The MNSs system

Like the P system, M and N antigens were first identified with animal antisera (Table 43–30); these still remain the most useful reagents for M and N typing. Simple sugars, D-galactose, N-acetyl-galactosamine, and sialic acid are the antigenic determinants (see Fig. 43–2). The main difference between M and N antigens is the number of sialic acid residues; M antigen has a greater number of sialic acid residues than the N antigen. This may explain why some anti-M sera also react with N cells and also why enzymes which degrade sialic acid residues destroy the reactivity of M and N antigens.

Anti-M and anti-N are rarely the cause of hemolytic transfusion reactions or hemolytic disease of the newborn. Anti-N-like antibodies have been demonstrated in some patients undergoing renal dialysis (Howell, 1972). Failure

Table 43–30. PHENOTYPES OF THE MNSs SYSTEM

REACTIONS WITH ANTI-					PHENOTYPE	POSSIBLE GENOTYPE	FREQUENCIES(%) IN U.S.A.	
M	N	S	s	U			Whites	Blacks
+	−				M	MM	28	26
+	+				MN	MN	50	44
−	+				N	NN	22	30
		+	−	+	SU	SSU	11	2.7 ⎫ 6.8
						SS^uU	44	4.1 ⎭
		+	+	+	SsU	SsU		23.5
		−	+	+	sU	ssU	45	50.7 ⎫ 68.2
						sS^uU		17.5 ⎭
		−	−	−	S−s−U−	$S^uS^uU−$		1.3 ⎫ 1.5
		−	−	+	S−s−U+	S^uS^uU+		0.2 ⎭

Modified from Miller, 1977, p. 124 and Race, 1975, p. 101.

of some kidney grafts has been attributed to the presence of anti-N agglutinins when a cold kidney is transplanted (Belzer, 1971). The addition of anti-S, anti-s, and anti-U to this system changes that situation somewhat. Both transfusion reactions and hemolytic disease of the newborn have been implicated with all three antibodies.

Genes for S and s appear to be closely linked to M and N genes, although recombination has been observed (Table 43–30). All U− cells are also S−s− (except Rh$_{null}$ cells). However, about 16 per cent of S− and s− cells are U+. Thus, U antigen is not equal to S plus s, as was formerly believed. The phenotype S−s−U− has been found exclusively in blacks; the gene responsible for this phenotype S−s− is assigned as S^u. Three other antigens, M$_1$, Hu, and He, are also predominantly found in blacks (24 per cent, 7 per cent, and 3 per cent, respectively) (Race, 1975, p. 107).

Most human anti-M and anti-N are naturally occurring and IgM, while most anti-S and anti-s are IgG and anti-U is always IgG. Anti-M and anti-N may react better in a acid medium. While anti-s and anti-U behave as typical IgG antibodies, anti-S usually shows decreased reactivity with enzyme-treated S+ cells, just as anti-M and anti-N show decreased reactivity with enzyme-treated M and N cells. There is evidence to suggest that the optimal reacting temperature for IgG anti-s and anti-U is below 37°C. Lectins with anti-M or anti-N specificity are commercially available. By using proper agglutinins, the dosage of M and N and of S and s can often be revealed. For a further discussion of the MN system and rare alleles important in disputed parentage examinations, see Chapter 44 (p. 1514).

The Lutheran system

Genetically, the Lutheran gene has been shown to be linked to the secretor gene providing the first autosomal linkage in blood groups. Lutheran is, so far, the only system in which a dominant gene produces a minus-minus phenotype Lu(a−b−) in addition to an amorphic type of Lu(a−b−).

Clinically, Lutheran antibodies produce very few transfusion reactions or hemolytic diseases of the newborn. Anti-Lu^a may be found after incompatible transfusion, but it is usually transient and weak. Anti-Lu^b is very rare. Both antibodies can be IgG, IgM, or IgA. Some are saline-reactive, while others react after enzyme treatment or in the antiglobulin test. Minor population of agglutinates, which were often described in the literature as a characteristic of anti-Lu^a, has not been observed in our laboratory.

Although at least 10 more Lutheran antigens (Lu^3 to Lu^{12}) have been proposed, they have not been well studied, nor are they of any clinical importance. The common phenotypes are listed in Table 43–31.

Table 43–31. PHENOTYPES OF THE LUTHERAN SYSTEM

PHENOTYPES	REACTIONS WITH ANTI-		FREQUENCIES(%) IN U.S.A.	
	Lu^a	Lu^b	White	Black
Lu(a+b−)	+	−	0.1	0.1
Lu(a+b+)	+	+	6.7	5.2
Lu(a−b+)	−	+	93.2	94.7
Lu(a−b−)	−	−	Very rare	

Modified from Mouront, 1976, p. 514.

Table 43-32. SIMILARITY IN THE POSSIBLE GENETIC
REGULATION OF THE BIOSYNTHESIS OF Rh
AND KELL ANTIGENS

Precursor, unconverted		Rh_{null}	$Kell_{null}$ (K_o, K_x)
Precursor, partially converted		Rh_{mod}	McLeod type*
Original basic haplotype		Dce	kKp^bJs^b (most common)
Number of genes modified within a haplotype	1	dce,DCe,DcE (common)	$KKp^bJs^b,kKp^aJs^b,kKp^bJs^a$ (rare)
	2	dCe,dcE,DCE (rare)	$KKp^aJs^b,KKp^bJs^a,kKp^aJs^a$ (not reported)
	3	dCE (very rare)	KKp^aJs^a (not reported)

*Strong association with X-linked chronic granulomatous disease of boys.

The Kell system

Like the Rh system, the Kell system has become a complex one. Table 43–32 compares the similarity between these two systems. There are six antisera to define three pairs of antithetical antigens—K and k, Kp^a and Kp^b, and Js^a and Js^b. These antigens are assumed to be controlled by a pair of genes and gene complexes as in the Rh system. The lack of Kell antigens (K_{null}, K_o) or poorly developed Kell antigens (McLeod type) similar to Rh_{null} and Rh_{mod} have been described. However, four of the eight possible haplotypes have not been observed. This fact favors the theory that there may be one basic haplotype and other haplotypes are the result of mutations. Thus far, a change in only one of the three genes has occurred in the Kell system, whereas this is not true with the Rh system.

Eighteen Kell antigens have been described; they are either of high incidence or of low incidence (Table 43–33). Only anti-K (9 per cent K+ in whites) and anti-Js^a (20 per cent

$Js(a+)$ in blacks) are relatively common, while the other antibodies are relatively rare.

The antigen K_x, which is also found on neutrophils and monocytes, is probably the precursor substance of other Kell antigens. An X-linked gene (X^1k) is required for its conversion; in its absence, K_x would behave as K_{null} (K_o). If X^1k is replaced by X^2k, the McLeod type (weak k, Kp^b, and Js^b) may be formed. With rare exception, the McLeod phenotype occurs in boys with chronic granulomatous disease (CGD) in whom K_x antigen is no longer demonstrable. Neutrophils of McLeod type without CGD have large amounts of K_x antigen. Thus, the lack of K_x antigen may be related to leukocyte dysfunction (Marsh, 1976).

With few exceptions, Kell antibodies are detectable by antiglobulin test and are not hemolytic or enhanced by enzyme. Numerous hemolytic transfusion reactions (extravascular) and a number of cases of hemolytic disease of the newborn have been attributed to Kell antibodies. Kell antigen is strongly anti-

Table 43-33. PHENOTYPE FREQUENCIES OF KELL ANTIGENS

RELATIONSHIP	HIGH INCIDENCE GROUP			LOW INCIDENCE GROUP		
	Antigen	Whites	Blacks	Antigen	Whites	Blacks
ANTITHETICAL:	k (K2)	99.8%	99.9%	K (K1)	9%	3.5%
	Kp^b (K4)	>99.9%	>99.9%	Kp^a (K3)	2%	<0.1%
	Js^b (K7)	>99.9%	98.9%	Js^a (K6)	<0.1%	19.5%
	Côté(K11)	>99.9%		Wk^a(K17)	0.3%	
UNKNOWN:	Ku (K5)·			Ul^a (K10)	2.6%*	
	KL (K9)·			K^w (K8)	5%	18%
	·	>99.9%				
	K12-K16 ·					
	K18 ·					

*Finnish population.
Modified from Miller, 1977, p. 118.

Table 43-34. PHENOTYPES FREQUENCIES OF DUFFY ANTIGENS

REACTIONS WITH ANTI-				PHENOTYPE	PROBABLE GENOTYPE	FREQUENCY(%) IN U.S.A.	
Fy^a	Fy^b	Fy^{3*}	Fy^4			Whites	Blacks
+	−	+	+/−	Fy(a+b−)	Fy^aFy^a Fy^aFy^4	17	.03 ⎱ 9 8.97 ⎰
+	+	+	−	Fy(a+b+)	Fy^aFy^b	49	1
−	+	+	+/−	Fy(a−b+)	Fy^bFy^b Fy^bFy^4	34	1.36 ⎱ 22 20.64 ⎰
−	−	−	+	Fy(a−b−)	Fy^4Fy^4 (or Fy^4Fy)	Extremely rare	68

*Anti-Fy^5 reacts like anti-Fy^3, but it also reacts with cells of the original anti-Fy donor and does not react with Rh_{null} cells.
Modified from Miller, 1977, p. 121 and Race, 1975, p. 355.

genic and ranks second to D antigen in antigenicity when A and B antigens are excluded.

The Duffy system

The incidence of Duffy antigens shows marked differences between whites and blacks. Among whites, two allelic Fy^a and Fy^b genes can explain the serologic findings. In blacks, at least three allelic genes, Fy^a, Fy^b, and Fy^4, have to be assumed. Phenotypes and possible genotypes for both populations in the United States are listed in Table 43-34.

Anti-Fy^a and anti-Fy^b are usually immune in origin and of the IgG class. Antiglobulin test is normally required for their detection. Enzymes may reduce the reactivity of anti-Fy^a and anti-Fy^b but will enhance the reactivity of anti-Fy^3, Fy^4, and Fy^5. Anti-Fy^3 reacts with all cells with Fy^a or Fy^b but does not react with Fy(a−b−) cells. The one anti-Fy^5 reported gave results similar to those of anti-Fy^3 except that it also reacted with the cells of the original anti-Fy^3 donor but did not react with Rh_{null} cells. Only one or two anti-Fy^3, anti-Fy^4, and anti-Fy^5 sera have been found thus far (Behzad, 1973; Race, 1975, p. 358).

The Duffy genes have been assigned to chromosome No. 1 (Donahue, 1968). They are syntenic but not linked to the Rh genes. Erythrocytes of persons with the phenotype Fy(a−b−) appear to resist *Plasmodium vivax* invasion *in vivo* (Miller, 1975). Thus, Duffy determinants "a" or "b" on the erythrocyte membrane seem essential for the invasion of these malarial parasites.

The Kidd system

Thus far, the Kidd system remains simple. Only two allelic genes, Jk^a and Jk^b, are required to explain the serologic findings. Phenotype Jk(a−b−) has been described in certain populations but is very rare (Race, 1975, p. 366) (Table 43-35).

Anti-Jk^a and anti-Jk^b are usually IgG and detectable usually by the antiglobulin test. Their activities are enhanced by enzymes or by the presence of complement. Although these antibodies may be hemolytic, they are usually weak and accompanied by other antibodies. Hemolytic transfusion reactions and hemolytic disease of the newborn due to Kidd antibodies are not uncommon. These antibodies have also been incriminated in delayed transfusion reactions (Mollison, 1972, p. 562).

Other systems

Other systems with two antithetical antigens and systems with abundant soluble anti-

Table 43-35. PHENOTYPES OF THE KIDD SYSTEM

PHENOTYPE	REACTIONS WITH ANTI-			FREQUENCY (%) IN U.S.A.	
	Jk^a	Jk^b	$Jk^{ab}(3)$	Whites	Blacks
Jk(a+b−)	+	−	+	28	57
Jk(a+b+)	+	+	+	49	34
Jk(a−b+)	−	+	+	23	9
Jk(a−b−)	−	−	−	Very rare	

Modified from Mouront, 1976, p. 601.

Table 43–36. SOME ERYTHROCYTE SYSTEMS WITH TWO KNOWN ANTITHETICAL ANTIGENS

| SYSTEM | PHENOTYPES | | | OPTIMAL REACTION | IMPLICATED IN | |
	Designated	Frequency (%) Whites	Blacks		Hemolytic Transfusion Reaction	Hemolytic Disease of the Newborn
Colton	Co(a+b−)	89.3	100	AGT with		Mild
	Co(a+b+)	10.4		enzyme		
	Co(a−b+)	0.3	<0.1	treated cells		
	Co(a−b−)	<0.1				
Dombrock	Do(a+b−)	17.2	9.4	AGT with		Mild
	Do(a+b+)	49.5	42.5	enzyme		
	Do(a−b+)	33.3	48.1	treated cells		
Diego	Di(a+b−)	<0.1*	<0.1	AGT		Yes
	Di(a+b+)	<0.1	0.5			
	Di(a−b+)	>99.9	99.5			
Scianna	Sc:1,2	< 0.1		Some AGT	Yes	Yes
(Sm-Burrell)	Sc:−1,2	0.3		Some saline		
	Sc:1,−2	99.7	100			
	Sc:−1,−2	<0.1				
Wright	Wr(a+b−)	<0.1	0	Many saline		
	Wr(a+b+)	<0.1	0	All temperatures		
	Wr(a−b+)	>99.9	100	Some AGT		
	Wr(a−b−)	< 0.1				
Cartwright	Yt(a+b−)	91.9	91.6	AGT, 37°C.	Yes	
	Yt(a+b+)	7.8	8.2			
	Yt(a−b+)	0.3	0.2			

*2.5% Chinese, 16% Japanese, 11% Chippewa Indian, 36% Carith Indians.
Modified from Miller, 1977, p. 126.

Table 43–37. SOME ERYTHROCYTE ANTIGENS WITH AN ABUNDANCE OF SOLUBLE FORM*

ANTIGEN	INCIDENCE IN WHITES	REMARKS
Sd^a	98%	Abundant in urine One case of hemolytic transfusion reaction by Sd(a++) cells
Chido (Ch^a)	98%	Abundant in plasma Ch^a syntenic with HLA locus on chromosome No. 6†
Yk^a or Cs^a	88–97%	Present in plasma May be related to leukocyte antigens
Bg^a	29%	Undiluted high titer sera give weak reactions

*From Issitt, 1975, p. 255.
†Antithetical to Rodgers, likely to be identical to C4 (O'Neill, 1977).

Table 43–38. OTHER HIGH (>99.9%) AND LOW (<0.1%) INCIDENCE ERYTHROCYTE ANTIGENS

HIGH INCIDENCE (PUBLIC) ANTIGENS	LOW INCIDENCE (PRIVATE) ANTIGENS*	
Augustine, At^a*	By (Batty)	Ven
En^a**	Good	Zd
Gerbich, Ge:1,2,3**	Heibel	
Gregory, Gy^a**	Hov	
Junior, Jr^a*	Ht^a (Hunt)	
Kn^a**	Rd (Radin)	
Lan**	Rm	
Vel (may lyse cells in vitro)	To^a	

*May cause hemolytic disease of the newborn.
**May cause hemolytic transfusion reactions.

gen, as well as the "public" and "private" antigens, are summarized in Tables 43-36, 43-37, and 43-38, respectively.

TESTING FOR ERYTHROCYTE ANTIGENS AND ANTIBODIES

General considerations

Identification. Proper identification of blood specimens or samples, reagents, and containers is absolutely essential in blood banking. Either the name or the code number of the blood donor must be marked clearly with permanent ink. A printed label must be securely attached to the blood sample. It is forbidden in blood banking to work with unlabeled or improperly marked blood samples. The recipient's blood sample label should include the patient's full name and specimen collection date. During testing, all tubes or other types of containers must also be properly identified.

Reagents. Whenever feasible, licensed reagents or those of equivalent quality should be used. Positive and negative controls should be performed on a daily basis. In selected instances, autocontrols and diluent controls should be performed. Reagents should be stored according to manufacturers' instructions, as frozen storage is not always preferable. In addition, the method of testing recommended by the manufacturer must be carefully followed; the use of an antiglobulin test when it is not recommended may detect other unwanted specificities, resulting in a false-positive test.

Erythrocyte Suspension. With possible exception of ABO and Rh typing (depending on reagents used), 2 to 5 per cent saline suspensions of erythrocytes are usually prepared. Usually one drop of a 4 to 5 per cent or 2 drops of a 2 per cent suspension are used for each test. A minimum sera-to-cell ratio is 1, but a larger ratio is preferable, especially for weak antibodies. Repeated exposure of the same cells to additional serum may enhance the reactivity. For critical typings of ABO, Lewis, Chido, Bg, Yt^a, and Sd^a, washed erythrocytes are preferable, as the presence of the antigen in the plasma may neutralize antibodies in the typing serum.

Procedures. Testing for erythrocyte antigens or antibodies can be done on slides or plastic plates with wells (known as microtiter plates). Similarly, test tubes, capillary tubes, or automated machinery may also be used. Currently, test tubes are the most widely used in blood banks. While microtiter plates are becoming increasingly popular, slide testing has become virtually obsolete (Lapinski, 1978). Unless specified, tests referred to in this chapter are tube tests. Other specific procedures will be mentioned under the specific subjects. Since there are many variations of each type of test, one should use that technique which is most familiar. The AABB Technical Manual (1977) serves as a general reference for various common procedures and alternate techniques.

Incubation. Many tests require a period of incubation to allow the antigen-antibody reaction to occur. Three temperatures are normally used: 4°C., 24°C., and 37°C. When a short incubation period is used, the tubes should be placed in a dry bath or water bath to speed up the equilibrium to the desired temperature (conductivity of air is very poor). Prolonged incubation of enzyme-treated cells should be avoided, as non-specific agglutination may occur.

Enzyme Treatment. Bromelin, papain, trypsin, and ficin are widely used to treat erythrocytes in order to obtain stronger reactions or to provide more effective adsorption of antibodies. Bromelin (0.5 per cent at pH 5.5) or cystein papain (0.1 per cent at pH 6.5) can be used together with serum and cells (one-stage enzyme test). A 0.1 per cent solution of papain, trypsin, or ficin at pH 7.3 may be used to pretreat erythrocytes. Erythrocytes then are washed, resuspended, and tested with the appropriate serum; this is known as the two-stage enzyme test. The two-stage test is much more sensitive than the one-stage test, but it is impractical for crossmatching purposes. In addition, owing to sensitivity of the two-stage test, no centrifugation is required before reading results. A high incidence of false positive reactions, especially when followed by an antiglobulin test, may occur if the test is performed improperly.

Enzymes enhance the reactivity of erythrocytes with certain antibodies, such as those of the Rh, Kidd, Lewis, and P systems. Rare examples of Rh and Kidd antibodies can be detected only with enzyme-treated cells. On the other hand, enzyme treatment may reduce reactivity of M, N, Fy^a, Fy^b, and possibly S antigens; apparently, enzymes affect the antigenic determinants of these antigens.

High-protein Medium. Bovine albumin (22 per cent) has been widely used to potentiate the reactivity of Rh antigens. There is some evidence to indicate that highly polymerized albumin may be more effective. Other polymers such as polyvinylpyrrolidone (PVP) and polybrene have also been used to induce rouleaux or non-specific agglutination in special applications.

LISS. Low ionic strength salt solution (LISS) is being evaluated as a substitute for albumin to enhance antibody uptake and agglutination. LISS appears to function by supplying fewer charged ions in the medium than are present in higher ionic strength solutions, such as 0.85 per cent saline. By enhancement of the association between red blood cells and serum antibodies, LISS appears to have potential in terms of total amount of antibody bound being increased and a reduction in the length of time for the antibody to bind to erythrocytes (Monaghan, 1977; Moore, 1976).

Centrifugation. In the majority of tests, centrifugation is required to reduce the time of incubation and to facilitate reading of results. The time and speed of each centrifuge should be calibrated by using appropriate controls. To avoid breakage of tubes, the number of tubes and the content in each should be balanced within the tolerance of the centrifuge.

Reading of Results. The presence of hemolysis is an indication of a strong reaction and should be recorded. The tube should be tapped gently until the cell button dislodges from the tube before a reading is taken. Proper illumination with a concave mirror is an invaluable aid for macroscopic reading. By placing the tube about 2.5 inches above a 3-inch concave mirror, aggregates can be differentiated easily from the free cells by looking at the mirror (not at the tube). The strength of the reaction can be recorded as follows with score in parenthesis:

H	Hemolysis, presence of free hemoglobin	(10)
4+	One solid aggregate	(10)
3+	One solid aggregate and many small aggregates	(8)
2+	Small aggregates with a clear background	(5)
1+	Small aggregates with a turbid background	(3)

All negative reactions when they are required by the procedure should be read under a microscope and recorded as follows:

+W	Presence of aggregates (1)	
−	Absence of aggregates (0)	
M	Presence of minor population of aggregates (also known as mixed field agglutination mf)	
R	Rouleaux, like a stack of coins, disappears with washing	

Scores are useful when comparison of strengths of two antisera is made.

Records. Information concerning the donor of the blood sample and results of tests should be entered directly onto a laboratory form, preferably in a book. Ink, not pencil, should be used. The date, the time of testing (if known), and the initials of the technologist should also be recorded. Anyone who makes any change in results must put his or her initials next to the change.

Safety. All safety precautions for a clinical laboratory should be observed. Pipetting of blood components by mouth is not acceptable; a mechanical device should be used instead. All blood components are potentially infectious for viral hepatitis and should be treated with respect even though the HB_sAg test may be negative. Whenever feasible, discarded samples of blood components should be autoclaved before final disposal.

Antiglobulin test

Antiglobulin test (AGT) is also known as the Coombs test in honor of one of the investigators who made the test practical (Coombs, 1945). AGT is based on the principle that anti-human globulin antibodies induce agglutination of erythrocytes coated with globulins. AGT has become a powerful tool in the detection of antigens and antibodies undetectable by other techniques. When AGT is used to detect antibodies bound to erythrocytes *in vivo*, it is known as the direct antiglobulin test (DAGT). When AGT is used to detect antibodies in sera by sensitizing erythrocytes *in vitro*, it is known as the indirect antiglobulin test (IAGT).

Antiglobulin Sera (AGS). Antiglobulin sera (AGS) are usually produced in rabbits by immunization. Owing to the different serum components used as immunogens, several types of AGS are available. Broad-spectrum AGS contains antibodies against human immunoglobulins (mainly IgG) and complement components (mainly C3); the activity against each component varies widely among different manufacturers and different lots of the same manufacturer. Monospecific anti-IgG, anti-IgM, and anti-IgA, as well as anti-C3+C4, anti-C3b, anti-C3d, anti-C4b, and anti-C4d are commercially available. Because some rabbits may have antibodies against human erythrocytes or human serum protein, only selected rabbits should be used for immunization. Quite often, rabbit anti-human globulin sera require dilution or absorption or both to achieve required specificity and sensitivity.

Erythrocytes Coated with Globulins. In order to standardize antiglobulin sera and to confirm true negative antiglobulin reactions, two types of coated cells are normally used: those coated with IgG and those coated with C3b or C3d. To sensitize erythrocytes with IgG, Rh antibodies are usually used. To prepare cells coated with C3b, anti-Le^a or anti-I and fresh serum are often employed; additional incubation with fresh serum or trypsin to split C3b will leave cells coated with only C3d. In both cases, an appropriate concentration of antibody must be used to give about a 2+ reaction *only* after the addition of anti-IgG or anti-C3b or C3d, respectively.

Procedure. For the direct AGT, blood samples should be drawn in EDTA to prevent sensitization of cells *in vitro* through the activation of complement beyond C1q. For the indirect AGT, erythrocytes should be incubated with appropriate sera or plasma, usually at 37°C. for 15 to 30 minutes. In both cases, erythrocytes should be washed at least four times to remove all unbound free globulins. The time and speed of centrifugation should be standardized using positive and negative controls. All negative tests should be confirmed by (1) reading under the microscope and (2) positive reaction with control cells coated with immunoglobulin or complement.

False Negative Antiglobulin Test (AGT). False negative reactions are usually derived from improper procedures or poor technique, which can be detected by the use of positive and negative controls as well as use of coated erythrocytes in all negative reactions. Common causes are (1) inadequate washing, (2) contamination with serum protein through dirty glassware or fingers, (3) failure to add AGS, (4) inadequate incubation or centrifugation, (5) elution of antibodies through excessive washing or high temperature, especially IgM antibodies, and (6) insufficient amount of serum for sensitization.

False Positive AGT. Common causes include (1) agglutination before the addition of AGS owing to strong cold agglutinins, polyagglutinable cells, prolonged incubation with enzyme treated cells, presence of metallic ions, polybrene, protamine, and use of a low ionic strength medium, which may induce non-specific agglutination; (2) presence of unexpected antibodies in AGS such as anti-species or anti-transferrin; and (3) overcentrifugation.

Sensitivity of AGT. Although the AGT is extremely sensitive, a negative test by no means excludes the presence of antibodies on erythrocytes. It is estimated that 100 to 500 IgG molecules bound on erythrocytes are required for detection by anti-globulin antibodies; a smaller number of IgG's bound on erythrocytes would give a negative reaction. AGS may be more potent against one or two subclasses of IgG but less potent for others; consequently, some antiglobulin sera may not be able to detect certain subclasses of antibodies on erythrocytes.

Applications of DAGT

INVESTIGATION OF AUTOANTIBODIES. The majority of warm autoantibodies are detectable by anti-IgG, while a small percentage are detected only with anti-C3d. Cold autoagglutinins are usually detectable by anti-C3d and rarely by anti-IgM.

ANTIBODIES INDUCED BY MEDICATION. Most are detectable by anti-IgG. Antibodies against a drug-protein complex usually fix complement on erythrocytes, which can then be detected by anti-C3b or anti-C3d.

HEMOLYTIC DISEASE OF THE NEWBORN. Only anti-IgG is needed.

INVESTIGATION OF A TRANSFUSION REACTION. Broad-spectrum AGS is usually used.

Applications of Indirect Antiglobulin Test (IAGT)

DETECTION AND IDENTIFICATION OF ERYTHROCYTE ANTIBODIES IN SERA. Anti-IgG and anti-C3d are recommended, although a broad-spectrum AGS may be sufficient for routine use. Anti-IgM and anti-IgA should be available in a reference laboratory.

TYPING OF ERYTHROCYTE ANTIGENS. Many antigens require specific antisera followed by the antiglobulin test; usually, only anti-IgG is required.

INCOMPATIBILITY TESTING. Broad-spectrum antiglobulin sera are generally used.

SPECIAL STUDIES. In addition to the antiglobulin consumption test and mixed agglutination reactions, AGS has been useful in the detection of antibodies against leukocytes and platelets.

Typing of erythrocyte antigens

Manual ABO and Rh_o Typing. Antisera, reagent red blood cells, and diluent controls are well standardized and readily available. ABO grouping includes cell (forward) and plasma or serum (reverse) grouping. Anti-A and anti-B are normally used for cell grouping. In addition, anti-A,B (from a group O person) is used to detect weak variants of A, and anti-A_1 is used to differentiate A_1 cells from A_2 cells. For serum typing, A_1 and B cells are normally used; A_2 cells may be used if anti-A_1 is suspected. While the results of red cell grouping are often clear-cut, the reactions of serum grouping may vary greatly in strength. An additional period of incubation or incubation at 4°C. may be required to demonstrate the presence of weak agglutinins. Group O cells are usually included for the antibody detection (screening) procedure. The room temperature results of these cells may be helpful when discrepancies with serum grouping arise.

For Rh_o typing, only anti-Rh_o(D) is required. Many laboratories also use anti-CD or anti-DE to supplement the typing. All Rh_o-negative tests should be followed by the antiglobulin test to detect D^u variants. When the DAGT is positive, saline-reacting anti-D should be used. Cells positive with anti-C or anti-E should not be considered Rh_o-positive. Since all anti-Rh_o sera contain a potentiating medium, a diluent control should be used rather than an albumin control.

Automated ABO and Rh_o Typing. Currently, a number of large blood centers use one of two types of machines: the continuous-flow system or the batch processing system.

The continuous-flow system (e.g., Technicon AutoAnalyzer) consists of a sampler, a proportioning pump, a manifold, a moving filter strip, and a vacuum pump. Plasma and cell aliquots are aspirated into the system through the sampler. Additional reagents, cells, and plasma are pumped into the manifold. After mixing and incubation, any aggregates formed decant out through the T-shaped decanter and deposit on the filter paper. Excess liquid is removed by the vacuum apparatus. The presence and absence of aggregates can be visualized on the filter paper. In addition to antisera and reagent red blood cells needed for cell and serum typing, Bromelin and PVP are usually used to enhance the reactivity. The presence of air bubbles in the system is essential to segregate the blood samples and to keep the system clean (Sturgeon, 1963). This system can also be used for automated reagin test (ART) (Schoeter, 1970) and, with modification, for antibody screening and identification (Lalezari, 1968; Lee, 1970). Modification of the AutoAnalyzer system to provide sample identification and printing capabilities by a computer is evolving.

The batch system (Groupamatic) consists of a sample identification device, aspirators, dilutors, a disc with 144 specially designed sample cups, a hydraulic transportation system, an agitator-centrifuge, photometers, and a computer. Twelve different tests can be carried out for each of 12 blood samples on one disc at one time. Each disc is transported from one station to the other for processing. Serologic reactivity is enhanced by agitation and centrifugation. Results are read by the colorimeters through cups with optically clear bottoms. The computer gathers the identification number and test results, makes an interpretation, and then prints out the final results (Matte, 1969).

Special Typings. Special typings are required in the following situations: (1) screening for compatible blood for recipients with irregular antibodies; (2) assisting in antibody identification; (3) determining zygosity of husbands of Rh_o-negative women; and (4) paternity testing or studies of twins. Special typing often requires several special antisera that are not standardized and may be very weak. These antisera should be tested with various techniques in order to determine which technique yields the best reaction. Then that particular technique should be adhered to strictly when using the antiserum. When many blood samples need to be screened, an AutoAnalyzer system is most helpful. Since some antigens have different frequencies among various ethnic groups, valuable time may be saved if selected blood samples are used. In larger blood centers, it is advisable to screen blood samples of all group O units for antigens such as D, Fy^a, Jk^a, K, or others to suit the local demand. It is of equal importance to freeze all units of erythrocytes with specific antibodies, as these units would be suitable for patients with the same antibody(ies).

Antibody detection (screening)

Reagent Red Blood Cells (RRBC). Many antibodies react more strongly with cells having a double dose (homozygous) of the same antigens than with those having only a single dose (heterozygous) of antigen. Since it is impossible to obtain cells having all desirable antigens in the homozygous state, two different sample cells (RRBC) are normally recommended for critical antibody screening. These two RRBC samples should be complementary (supplementary) to each other in terms of antigenic composition to provide most of the desirable antigens. When these two types of RRBC are pooled, 50 per cent of them should contain all the antigens reacting with all the so-called "clinically significant antibodies," such as Rh, Kell, Fy^a, Jk^a, S, s, and others. Selected types of cells may be included, such as I− and Le(a−b−), to meet local demands.

Procedures. Currently, none of the available techniques is capable of detecting all erythrocyte antibodies; it is unlikely that there will be such a technique in the future. It is also unfortunate that there is no general agreement about the so-called clinically significant antibodies. The best approach is to use at least two techniques for recipients and select the most practical one for blood donors.

Most laboratories use saline medium and room temperature incubation for 15 minutes, followed by centrifugation and reading. If results are negative, the tests are incubated at 37°C. for an additional 15 minutes, centrifuged, and read again. If these results are negative, the cells are washed four times with saline and antiglobulin serum is added. An additional set of tubes using a one-stage enzyme test or high-protein medium followed by the antiglobulin test is also used to complement the first technique. However, there are antibodies that may react only with the two-stage enzyme test plus antiglobulin test; others react only with an AutoAnalyzer system; and still others react only with the capillary methods. Only additional careful in-

Table 43–39. REACTIONS OF COMMON ERYTHROCYTE ANTIBODIES*

	ANTIBODY FOR	SALINE MEDIUM	ALBUMIN MEDIUM	ANTIGLOBULIN TEST	ENZYME TESTS	IN VITRO HEMOLYSIS	OPTIMAL C.° 4	24	37
Usually IgM	H, I	M	S	F	S	F	M	S	F
	i	M	S	F	S	S	M	S	F
	A, B, A,B	M	F	F	M	S	M	S	F
	Lu^a	M	S	F	F	N	M	S	M
	Lu^b	S	S	M	F	N	R	S	M
	M, N	M	S	S	F	N	M	M	F
	P$_1$	M	S	S	S	F	M	S	F
	PP$_1$P^k	M	M	M	M	M	S	M	M
	Le^a, Le^b	M	S	S	M	S	M	S	F
Usually IgG	S, s	S	S	M	S	N	F	S	M
	K, k, Js^a, Js^b	F	S	M	F	N	F	S	M
	C, D, E, c, e	S	S	M	M	N	F	S	M
	Fy^a, Fy^b	F	F	M	F	N	N	F	M
	Jk^a, Jk^b	F	S	M	M	F	N	S	M

M = Most (>20%), S = Some (5-20%), F = Few (1-5%), R = Rare (<1%), N = Not reported.

*LISS (low ionic strength saline solution) increases the rate of antibody association for weak IgG antibodies (Garratty, 1978; Moore, 1976; Hughes-Jones, 1964).

vestigation may resolve some of these unusual findings.

As reviewed previously, LISS appears to shorten the length of time required for antibody association with erythrocytes and enhances the sensitivity for low affinity antibodies (p. 1449).

The patterns of antibody reactions commonly encountered in hospital blood banks are listed in Table 43-39. Several comments can be made from the results of the antibody detection (screening) test.

1. IgM antibodies normally react in saline medium at room temperature or lower, while IgG antibodies react best at 37°C. by the antiglobulin test.
2. Antibodies of the P and Lewis systems may react with all techniques and under all conditions.
3. Albumin medium and enzyme tests are particularly useful for detecting Rh and Kidd antibodies.
4. The presence of hemolysis may normally exclude antibodies of Lutheran, MNSs, Kell, Duffy, and Rh systems.

Boral (1977), Mintz (1978), and Henry (1977) have reported on the safety of the type and screen as well as its use in terms of blood ordering strategy as a safe alternative to a two-unit crossmatch request for selected surgical procedures where the use of blood is unlikely or virtually nil.

Antibody identification

Using a Panel of Red Blood Cells. If we assume anti-D in the serum of Mrs. X, serum X would react with all D+ cells but would not react with D− cells. In other words, if another serum, Y, reacts similarly to that of serum X, we can assume that serum Y also contains anti-D. In order to accomplish this purpose, a panel of D+ and D− cells are required. Since each sample of erythrocytes possesses many other antigens in addition to D antigens, antibodies against other antigens can also be tentatively identified with the same panel of red blood cells. The following is a greatly simplified example:

CELLS IN A PANEL	KNOWN ANTIGENIC COMPOSITION					TEST SERUM	
	D	C	c	E	e	Y	Z
No. 1	+	+	+	−	−	+	−
No. 2	+	+	−	+	+	+	+
No. 3	+	−	+	−	+	+	−
No. 4	−	+	+	−	+	−	−
No. 5	−	+	−	−	+	−	−
No. 6	−	−	+	+	+	−	+

Serum Y, which reacts with 3 D+ cells but not with 3 D− cells, can be assumed to have anti-D; similarly, serum Z reacts with 2 E+ cells but not

with 4 E− cells. Can we then assume serum Z to contain anti-E? The fundamental question is: what is the chance that antigens other than E are also present in the 2 E+ cells but absent in 4 E− cells? One can also question what the chance is of antigens other than D being present in all 3 D+ cells but not in 3 D− cells. Thus, the number of different cells with known antigenic composition in a panel becomes a critical issue.

Fortunately, the chance of such a coincidence, as listed subsequently, can be estimated by Fisher's "exact method for 2 × 2 table" (Race, 1975).

TOTAL NUMBER OF TYPE OF CELLS IN A PANEL	PROBABILITY OF COINCIDENCE WITH NUMBER OF CELL SAMPLES THAT REACT POSITIVELY				
	1	2	3	4	5
6	1:6	1:15	1:20		
7	1:7	1:21	1:35		
8	1:8	1:28	1:56	1:70	
9	1:9	1:36	1:84	1:126	
10	1:10	1:45	1:120	1:210	1:252

Statistically, a chance of 1 in 20, or 5 per cent, is considered acceptable; a chance of less than 5 per cent is usually recommended (Mollison, 1972). From the listing, at least a total of seven cells with a minimum of two for each antigenic determinant is required to achieve such a statistic. In order to reduce the chance to less than 1 per cent for critical studies, a total of nine cells with a minimum of four for each antigenic determinant is needed.

For this reason, most of the commercially available panels consist of 8 to 10 reagent red blood cells. Since it is practically impossible to have four samples with the same determinant for each antigen, supplementary cells or panels should be available for a definitive study. In order to prepare a panel of cells capable of identifying many types of antibodies, each sample in the panel should be extensively typed for various known antigens.

The following simplified example is used to illustrate the identification of a single antibody.

CELLS IN A PANEL	KNOWN ANTIGENIC COMPOSITION									TEST SERUM	
	D	C	c	E	e	K	k	Fy^a	Fy^b	37°C.	AGT
No. 1	+	+	+	−	+	−	+	+	+	−	+
No. 2	+	+	−	−	+	−	+	+	−	−	+
No. 3	+	−	+	+	+	+	+	−	+	−	−
No. 4	−	+	+	−	+	+	+	−	+	−	−
No. 5	−	−	+	−	+	−	+	+	−	−	+
No. 6	−	−	+	+	−	−	+	−	+	−	−
No. 7	−	+	+	−	+	−	+	+	+	−	+
No. 8	−	−	+	−	+	−	+	−	+	−	−

Since the test serum reacts negatively with cell No. 3, one can rule out all antigens present on the

Table 43–40. AN EXAMPLE OF ANTIBODY IDENTIFICATION

MOUNT SINAI HOSPITAL MEDICAL CENTER

Name **Case #7 (Problem #82-73)**   Age **45**   Sex **F**   Date **8/18/1973**

Diagnosis **Pregnancy**   Previous Transfusion **None**   Date _____

Patient's Cell Type **O/DCCee**   Pregnancies **3**

Antibody _____

Rh-hr Code	D	C	C^w	E	e	f	V	M	N	S	s	Lu^a	Lu^b	P_1	Le^a	Le^b	K	k	Kp^a	Kp^b	Js^a	Js^b	Fy^a	Fy^b	Jk^a	Jk^b	Xg^a	Vial No.
r'r'	0	+	0	0	+	0	0	+	+	0	0	0	+	+	0	0	0	+	0	+	0	+	0	0	+	+	+	1
R₁R₁	+	+	+	0	+	0	0	0	+	0	+	0	+	+	+	0	0	+	0	+	0	+	+	0	+	+	0	2
R₁R₁	+	+	0	0	+	0	0	0	+	+	+	0	+	+	0	+	+	+	+	+	0	+	+	+	0	+	+	3
R₂'R₂	+	0	0	+	0	0	0	+	+	+	+	+	+	+	0	+	0	+	0	+	0	+	+	+	+	+	+	4
r"r"	0	0	0	+	0	0	+	+	0	+	+	0	+	+	0	+	0	+	0	+	0	+	0	+	0	+	+	5
rr	0	0	0	0	+	+	0	+	+	+	+	0	+	+	0	+	0	+	0	+	0	+	0	0	+	0	0	6
rr	0	0	0	0	+	+	0	+	+	+	+	0	+	0	+	0	0	+	0	+	0	+	0	+	0	+	+	7
R_ZR₁	+	0	0	0	+	+	0	+	+	0	0	0	+	+	0	+	+	+	0	+	0	+	+	+	0	+	+	8
r_yr_y	0	+	0	+	0	0	0	0	0	+	+	0	+	+	0	0	0	+	0	+	0	+	0	0	0	+	+	9
	+	+	0	+	+	0		0	+	0	+	0	+	0	0	0	0	+	0	+	0	+	+	+	+	+	+	10
PATIENT	+	+	0	0	+	0	0																					
R₁R₁	+	+	0	0	+	0	0	0	+	+	+	0	+	+	0	0	+	+	0	+	0	+	+	0	0	+	+	I
R₂R₂	+	0	0	+	0	0	0	0	+	+	+	0	+	+	+	0	0	+	0	+	0	+	0	+	+	+	+	II

VIAL NUMBER	1	2	3	4	5	6	7	8	9	10	I	II	AUTO
I. Saline: 4°C.													
a. Immediate Spin	2+	0	0	2+	4+	2+	2+	2+	4+	0	2+	0	0
b. Room temp.—30 min	+w	0	0	+w	2+	+w	+w	+w	2+	0	+w	0	0
c. 37°C.—30 min	1+	0	0	1+	2+	1+	1+	1+	2+	0	1+	0	0
d. Saline 37°C. plus antiglobulin	0	0	0	1+	1+	1+	1+	1+	0	0	0	1+	0
II. Albumin:													
a. Immediate Spin	0	0	0	0	+w	0	0	0	+w	0	0	0	
b. 37°C.—30 min	0	0	0	+w	+w	+w	+w	+w	0	0	0	+w	0
c. 37°C. plus antiglobulin	0	0	0	2+	2+	2+	2+	2+	0	0	0	2+	0
III. Enzyme (Cysteine Papain)													
a. 37°C.—30 min	0	0	0	+w	+w	+w	+w	+w	0	0	0	+w	0
b. 37°C. plus antiglobulin	0	0	0	2+	2+	2+	2+	2+	0	0	0	2+	0

No. 3 cell except C and Fy^a; with No. 4 cell, the antigen C is excluded; with No. 6 and No. 8, Fy^a remains unexcluded. One can, then, tentatively identify the presence of anti-Fy^a in the test serum with a chance of coincidence of $1:70$ or 1.5 per cent.

Table 43-40 shows an actual antibody identification sample. Several conclusions can be drawn from the results.

1. Since the auto control is negative, the serum contains no autoantibodies.
2. Since panel cells No. 2, No. 3, and No. 10 reacted negatively with the test serum, antibodies against antigens on those cells can be excluded (crossed-out), with only antibodies for c, f, V, M, Lu^a, and Js^a remaining unexcluded.
3. From the pattern of reactions, at least two antibodies may be involved; one reacts best at 4°C. while the other reacts by antiglobulin test.
4. Anti-M would react similarly to the pattern presented. Positive reactions are seen with 7 M+ cells but not with 3 M− cells, with the strongest being the two homozygous M cells (No. 5 and No. 10).
5. Anti-c would react more strongly with AGT, and reactions with 5 c+ cells but not with 5 c− cells are seen.
6. However, co-existence of antibodies against f, V, Lu^a, and Js^a cannot be excluded. Anti-Lu^a was excluded when the test serum did not agglutinate M−, c−, Lu(a+) cells. Anti-Js^a was excluded when the test serum did not agglutinate M−, c−, Js(a+) cells. Serum absorbed with M−, cDE cells was no longer reactive with f+ or V+ cells; the presence of anti-f and anti-V was ruled out.
7. The presence of anti-M and anti-c was confirmed by absorption and elution.
8. Cells of the patient were M− and c−, compatible with the presence of allo-anti-c and anti-M.
9. While anti-M is likely naturally occurring, previous pregnancies may be responsible for development of anti-c.
10. Although this serum contains only two antibodies, a considerable amount of work has to be done in order to establish unequivocally the antibodies identified. Not infrequently, co-existing antiodies cannot be ruled out because of the presence of several antibodies and the lack of cells of proper antigenic composition for such a discriminatory study.

Absorption. Absorption is a process used to remove or neutralize antibodies in sera. It can be accomplished by using (1) washed erythrocytes, (2) enzyme-treated erythrocytes, (3) formalinized erythrocytes, (4) stromata, or (5) soluble antigens (also known as neutralization). Each type of antigenic material has its advantages and disadvantages with its specific applications. The antigenic composition of the material used for absorption must be known and selected for a particular purpose.

The absorption temperature and time depend a great deal on the nature of the antibodies being absorbed. In general, the lower the ratio of antibody to antigen, the higher the efficiency of absorption. Agitation during the absorption period is always helpful.

Absorption has the following applications:
1. To confirm the specificity of an antibody, such as saliva with H or Le^a substance for anti-H and anti-Le^a, milk with I substance for anti-I, hydatid cyst fluid with P_1 substance for anti-P_1, urine with Sd^a substance for anti-Sd^a, and plasma with Ch^a substance for anti-Ch^a.
2. To remove cold or warm autoagglutinins for the evaluation of the possible presence of an alloantibody or antibodies. Cells from the patient are most useful, provided the patient has received no transfusions recently. Enzyme treatment of these cells is usually very effective.
3. To remove unwanted antibodies such as anti-A, anti-B, or others to prepare reagent antisera. Stromata and formalinized cells may be useful for this purpose in that hemolysis is avoided during the absorption procedure.
4. To remove a single antibody from a serum with multiple antibodies by the use of cells with appropriate antigens to assure the identity of the antibodies.
5. To sensitize cells for subsequent elution studies.

Elution. Elution is a process used to remove antibodies bound to erythrocytes. First, one must be certain that there are antibodies on the erythrocytes; this is usually ascertained with a positive antiglobulin test. Second, one must be certain that there are no unbound antibodies in the suspending medium. This is accomplished by checking the last saline fluid washing with appropriate cells reacting with the expected antibody. Eluates are usually made in saline and should be prepared and tested on the same day. When storage is anticipated, the eluate should be prepared in AB serum or 6 per cent albumin and kept at −20°C. or lower.

Elution can be accomplished in one of three ways: (1) By heating at 56° to 60°C. for 10 minutes with frequent agitation. Separation is accomplished by centrifugation in cups with prewarmed water to hold the test tubes. This procedure is most effective for IgM antibodies. (2) By the addition of 2 volumes of ether and 1 volume of saline to 1 volume of washed packed erythrocytes followed by inserting a stopper and shaking vigorously for 1 minute. The tube is centrifuged and the ether is removed by aspiration. Evaporation of residual ether is accomplished by placing the tube in a warm water bath. This procedure is useful for eluting IgG antibodies. (3) Other methods of elution, such as repeated freezing and thawing or use of ethyl alcohol (Weiner, 1957), or digitonin (Kochwa, 1964) may have specific applications and are being used in some laboratories.

4

Elution has the following applications:

1. To confirm the presence of a single antibody in the presence of several antibodies suggested by the use of a panel of red blood cells.
2. To determine the specificity of antibodies bound to erythrocytes, such as in cases of autoimmune hemolytic anemia, hemolytic disease of the newborn, possible transfusion reaction, and antibodies induced by medication.
3. To prepare a small amount of monospecific antibody by separation from other unwanted antibodies, such as anti-A, anti-B, and other irregular antibodies, which interfere with the monospecific antibody in special typings.
4. To demonstrate the presence of subgroups of A such as A_x, A_m, and A_{el}. Cells of these subgroups may not be agglutinated by anti-A or anti-A,B, but they will absorb large quantities of anti-A, and anti-A can then be eluted. This procedure confirms the presence of A antigen on these cells.
5. To prepare cells free of attached antibodies for additional studies, such as proper typing, which can then be carried out even by an antiglobulin test if required (partial elution).

Elution of antibodies can also be accomplished in an AutoAnalyzer system to characterize antibodies in a different manner (Lalezari, 1971). By increasing the temperature of the water bathing the coils containing sensitized erythrocytes, antibodies gradually elute from these cells. The temperature at which elution begins and at which complete elution takes place may be used to characterize a given antibody. For example, one might elute an anti-M between 21° and 35°C., while an anti-S may be eluted between 30° and 49°C.

Other Helpful Means for Antibody Identification. By use of a panel of cells, absorption and elution may identify most antibodies but may not do so in some other instances. Table 43-41 lists some of the antibodies that require the use of cells of a special type for their identification. It should be emphasized that the typing and DAGT of patient's cells is of particular importance to evaluate the presence of one or more alloantibodies. Least incompatible blood can be successfully used in patients with autoantibodies, but this procedure must not be used for patients with alloantibodies. Some antibodies listed in Table 43-39 are uncommon but are seen in many laboratories. The list may serve as a check when unusual antibodies are encountered.

Absorption removes specific antibodies but may also remove non-specific antibodies (no homologous antigens of the erythrocytes used for absorption). This is known as the Matuhasi-Ogata phenomenon.

Eluates may require concentration before use. Excessive amounts of fluid can be removed by either vacuum evaporation or by dialysis against macromolecular concentration media, such as Carbowax* or Lyphogel†.

It becomes obvious that a large collection of different antisera with different specificities and of erythrocytes with various types of antigenic composition is essential in order to complete a more complicated antibody identification. Antisera aliquots can be kept in a frozen state. Special reagent red blood cells can also be kept in a frozen state either at −20°C. or in liquid nitrogen. To store erythrocytes at −20°C., increasing concentration of glycerin, from 4 to 8 per cent, and then to 16 per cent is required to be equalized with the cells. Before use, decreasing concentration of glycerol, 16 per cent, 8 per cent, and then 4 per cent, is required to process the cells prior to suspension in saline.

*Union Carbide, New York, New York.
†Gelman, Ann Arbor, Michigan.

Table 43-41. ANTIBODIES NOT IDENTIFIABLE WITH USUAL PANEL OF CELLS*

| ANTIBODY FOR | ERYTHROCYTES USED FOR DETECTION | | | |
	Own	Type O	Donor	Specially Selected
Auto: warm	+	+	+	Rh_{null}, LW−, D− −, U−
cold	+	+	+	A_1, O_h, p, i
Very frequent	−	+	+	U−, Lan−, Vel−, . .
Very infrequent	−	−	+	Husband, child, Wr^a, Di^a, Co^b. . .
Compound (Rh system)	−	+	+	ce, CE, Ce, cE, ce^s, (r^G for anti-G)
Complex (2 systems)	−	+	+	HI, Le^{bH}
Multiple	−	+	+	Positive for one antigen at one time
A or B	−	−	+	A or B but not O cells
Subtypes	−	+, −	+, −	A_1, M_1, Rh^b
Minus-minus phenotype	−	+, −	+, −	Fy(a−b−) for anti-Fy4, K_0 for anti-KL
Medicine, dye	+	−	+, −	Medicine or dye in the test system
Lactose	−	+	−	Preserved with or without lactose
Caprylate	−	+	+, −	Albumin with or without caprylate
Bromelin	−	+	−	Bromelin treated or untreated cells

* A positive reaction could also be due to presence of various types of polyagglutinable cells without specific antibody. Rouleaux must be excluded.

Many methods are available to preserve rare cells in liquid nitrogen. The method described by Behzad (1977) has been found to be uncomplicated and satisfactory.

PROCUREMENT, PREPARATION, PROCESSING, AND PRESERVATION OF BLOOD AND BLOOD COMPONENTS

PROCUREMENT OF BLOOD AND BLOOD COMPONENTS

Recruitment of blood donors

In recent years, two fundamental changes in donor recruitment have taken place. A shift from individual responsibility to community responsibility for blood replacement has occurred in some areas of our nation and from paid donors to voluntary donors throughout the United States.

For many years, motivation for blood donation has focused on individual responsibility to insure that present and future blood needs of the donor and/or his family are met. This approach may create a hardship for those who are not qualified for blood donation or for those who have no one else to donate for them. In addition, record keeping is required, which can increase the costs. Hence blood replacement as a community responsibility has become more acceptable. Motivation based on group or community responsibility has been successful in some countries and to a variable extent in this country. A pluralistic approach to donor recruitment embracing individual and community responsibility is favored by many, since it utilizes both forms of motivation that have been demonstrated to be effective. Indeed, there appears to be a need for both individual and/or community responsibility to provide an adequate blood supply in response to demands throughout the United States (geographically or regionally) and at all times throughout the year.

Based on present usage, if about 4 per cent of the population (approximately 10 million) donated one unit of blood each year, the nation's required blood needs would be met. However, a variable but significant percentage of blood donors donate two or more times per year. Organized institutions or groups are rich sources of qualified blood donors.

Voluntary donors are defined as blood donors who receive no direct monetary compensation, while paid donors receive such remuneration.

The seriousness of post-transfusion hepatitis has attracted a great deal of attention for the past 10 years. Sufficient evidence indicates that for the most part the chance of contracting hepatitis from blood obtained from paid donors is greater than from that obtained from voluntary donors. Results of testing for hepatitis B surface antigen support this view for hepatitis B. Similar findings are true for non-A, non-B hepatitis which is responsible for the majority of post-transfusion hepatitis. Since currently available tests can detect and prevent only about 20 per cent of transfusion-associated hepatitis (Prince, 1975), blood from voluntary donors is preferred.

It should be stressed, however, that not all blood from voluntary donors is free of hepatitis and not all blood from paid donors is infectious. However, elimination of paid donors with increasing use of voluntary blood appears to be a definite trend, and labeling the source of blood units accordingly as a paid donor has been required by the FDA (Food & Drug Administration) since May, 1978.

Selection of blood donors

In order to protect the donor as well as the recipient, each blood donor must be screened prior to each blood donation by medical history and limited physical examination on the day of donation. This is to insure that no harm will come to the donor by giving blood and that the transfused unit will not in any way harm the recipient (Technical Manual of AABB, 1977). Whenever a decision is made regarding acceptance or rejection of a blood donor, these two goals should be kept in mind, i.e., safety of donor and safety of patient.

Basic Qualifications
1. Age: Between the 21st and 66th birthday and between the 17th and 21st birthday depending on local law (age of majority) and consent of a guardian.
2. Body weight: 110 lb or more for 450 ($\pm$ 45) ml of blood collected in 63 ml of CPD anticoagulant plus up to 30 ml for additional tubes.
3. Temperature: Less than 37.5°C., or 99.5°F.
4. Pulse: Between 50-100 beats per minute, regular
5. Blood pressure: systolic between 90-180 mm Hg
   diastolic between 50-100 mm Hg
6. Minimum hemoglobin: 13.5 g/dl (male)
   12.5 g/dl (female)
   or Minimum hematocrit: 41% (male)
   38% (female)

Specific gravity   > 1.055 (male)
(copper sulfate often
used as a rapid   > 1.053 (female)
hemoglobin screen):

Deferment

1. Permanent: history of viral hepatitis, history of jaundice of unknown cause, the only donor implicated in post-transfusion hepatitis, malignant tumors, leukemia, convulsion after infancy, fainting spells, abnormal bleeding tendency, known positive HBsAg test, serious cardiopulmonary disease.
2. Temporary: conditions requiring rest or medication: cold, flu, diabetes, tuberculosis, syphilis, and other infections, and diseases of the heart, lungs, kidney, stomach, or liver.
3. For 3 years: After prior residence in areas endemic for malaria or after cessation of anti-malaria prophylaxis or therapy provided the donors have been asymptomatic in the interim.
4. For 1 year: Severe illness, therapeutic rabies vaccine.
5. For 6 months: close contact with viral hepatitis, tattoo, injection of blood or components, one of the donors implicated in post-transfusion hepatitis, major surgery, and travel to areas endemic for malaria without symptoms or suppressive medication.
6. For 2 months: German measles (rubella) vaccine.
7. For 8 weeks: previous blood donation.
8. For 6 weeks: after termination of pregnancy.
9. For 2 weeks: small pox, measles (rubeola), mumps, and yellow fever vaccines, oral polio vaccine, animal serum products.
10. For 72 hours: dental or minor surgery, hyposensitization injections for allergy, symptomatic bronchial asthma.
11. For 48 hours: plasmapheresis, aspirin consumption by donor who is to be the only source of platelets for a patient.
12. For 24 hours: other types of vaccines.

Other Important Considerations

1. Identification: Full name, address, telephone number, age, sex, race (helpful for special typing), and social security number or driver's license number are very helpful.
2. Consent: A written consent of the prospective donor is required.
3. Preparation before donation: Eat a regular meal, avoid fatty food, and no alcohol within 12 hours prior to donation.
4. Exceptions: Exceptions can be made by a physician, especially for therapeutic bleeding, autotransfusions, immunization and hyperimmunization, and especially rare blood donors.

Phlebotomy

1. Phlebotomists should be well-trained in aseptic techniques.
2. Materials used should be sterile (30 minutes at 121.5°C. by steam under pressure, or 2 hours at 170°C.). Disposable materials are preferred whenever feasible.
3. The donor blood bag, sample tube, and donor record should be properly identified and labeled before drawing blood.
4. The venipuncture site should be free of skin lesions of an infectious nature. Arms should also be inspected for needle marks, a sign of drug addiction.
5. Iodophor compounds (e.g., PVP-iodine or poloxamin-iodine complex) are preferred because they leave less odor and stain than does tincture of iodine. In addition, they do not cause skin reactions, and removal of iodine by additional washing is not required.
6. Plastic blood bags with additional satellite bags should be selected according to need. For instance, a single bag may be used for whole blood, double bags for red blood cell concentrates, triple bags for platelets or cryoprecipitate and quadruple bags for both platelets and cryoprecipitate from the same donation.
7. Each bag should be examined for defects and the anticoagulant inside inspected.
8. For a donor over 110 pounds, the amount of blood drawn should be 450 ± 45 ml for 63 ml of CPD, which is equivalent to 425 to 520 gm (weight of bag and anticoagulant not included).
9. A maximum of 30 ml in pilot sample is allowed for additional testing. Thorough mixing of the blood and anticoagulant in the bag and tubing is essential. Stripping the tubing several times before sealing is important.
10. After phlebotomy, establish that there is no leaking from the puncture site and that the donor is in satisfactory condition before leaving the room. A compress or adhesive bandage should be applied to the phlebotomy site.

Pheresis

Pheresis is a procedure in which blood is removed from a donor, separated, and a portion retained, with the remainder being returned (Technical Manual of AABB, 1977). The component removed may be plasma, platelets, or leukocytes, and the process is known respectively as plasmapheresis or cytapheresis, e.g., plateletpheresis or leukapheresis.

Pheresis donors should have the same general qualifications as whole blood donors. In addition, the body weight, total serum protein, platelet counts, and white blood cell counts should be monitored before and after the procedure whenever applicable or as indicated by the nature of the procedure. Usually not more than 15 per cent of the donor's blood volume should be extracorporeal at any time. Both the Code of Federal Regulations (640.2 and 640.6) and AABB Standards for Blood Banks and

Transfusion Services (1976) should be consulted for further details pertaining to pheresis procedures.

Plasmapheresis. Plasmapheresis may be performed for two reasons: (1) for collection of plasma for fractionation into therapeutic components such as plasma, cryoprecipitate, single donor fresh frozen plasma (FFP), and for plasma or derivatives such as albumin, gamma globulin, antihemophilic factor, and other factors (e.g., prothrombin complex, blood group typing sera) and (2) for therapeutic reasons (see p. 1483).

Technically, plasmapheresis is performed using manual bag systems or centrifugal separation devices (p. 1483). With the use of manual bag systems, usually 500 ml of blood is drawn from the donor, and after the plasma is removed following centrifugation, the erythrocytes are returned to donor. The process is usually repeated once more. Such a procedure may be repeated after 72 hours, but not more than four units (500 ml) of blood may be processed within seven days from the same blood donor. An eight-week interval is required for plasmapheresis following a whole blood donation. A plasmapheresis donor can donate a unit of whole blood 48 hours after the pheresis procedure.

Since the unit of blood is removed from the donor for centrifugation, proper identification of the unit is extremely important so that one avoids the reinfusion of the wrong unit of blood. Unit identification is usually done by a combination of a numerical system and either the donor's signature or a photo of the donor or both to insure that the donor receives back his own blood.

Plasma Exchange. Plasmapheresis can be carried out more effectively using equipment (centrifugal blood separation devices) designed primarily for plateletpheresis or leukapheresis. About 1000 to 2000 ml of plasma can be removed per hour with these devices; thus, they are suitable for plasma exchange purposes. Plasma exchange used mainly for therapeutic reasons is reviewed on page 1483.

Plateletpheresis. Plateletpheresis is aimed at harvesting several times (approximately 10) the number of platelets that can be derived from one unit of blood from a single donor. In this way, not only is the chance of transmitting hepatitis reduced, but also the selection of HLA-compatible platelets becomes possible for particular recipients who are refractory to transfusion of random platelets (see Chap. 41). Donors for plateletpheresis should have a minimal platelet count of $150,000/\mu l$ and should not take any aspirin for the previous 48 hours.

Six to eight units of platelets can be collected from a single donor by a manual technique, as in plasmapheresis. This technique requires several hours, but requires no special instruments.

A machine (Haemonetics Model 30)* has been developed to collect blood and anticoagulant into a centrifuge which separates whole blood into plasma, platelet, leukocyte, and erythrocyte fractions. From 400 to 700 ml of blood can be processed in each pass or batch depending on the size of the centrifuge bowl and the hematocrit of the donor. Normally six to eight passes can be processed in two to three hours. Approximately 6×10^{11} total platelets can usually be collected this way. In addition to a decrease in platelet count (between 40,000 and $90,000/\mu l$) the donor also loses about 350 ml of plasma and 25 to 30 ml of erythrocytes per donation (in addition to pilot sample).

Leukapheresis. Aggressive use of a large number of granulocytes has been successful in combating some infections unresponsive to antibiotics (Schiffer, 1974). Two types of procedures are currently available to harvest a large number of granulocytes: filtration technique and centrifugation technique.

In filtration leukapheresis, the calcium-dependent adhesion of granulocytes to nylon fibers is exploited. Granulocytes retained by the nylon filters can be eluted by flushing with a calcium-chelating citrated plasma. A continuous process is achieved by the use of a proportioning pump, and six to eight liters of blood can be pumped through the filters in a three- to four-hour donation period with a harvest of about 3×10^{10} granulocytes. A relatively large dose of heparin is used as the anticoagulant and protamine sulfate is sometimes used to neutralize the effect of heparin at the end of a run. Side effects of both chemicals cause concern for some investigators. The effectiveness of granulocytes eluted from nylon fibers is a controversial subject at the present time.

In centrifugation leukapheresis, two automated techniques are available. However, the manual pheresis method described previously for platelets is less than ideal to collect adequate numbers of granulocytes efficiently.

DISCONTINUOUS CENTRIFUGATION. Essentially this is the same technique as that used for plateletpheresis. A red blood cell sedimenting agent, hydroxyethyl starch, is used

---

*Haemonetics Corporation, Natick, Massachusetts 01760.

routinely to enhance erythrocyte-granulocyte separation.

CONTINUOUS CENTRIFUGATION.   Two rather expensive machines (IBM and AMINCO) are designed for this purpose. Blood is drawn continuously from a donor into a centrifuge-cell separator which isolates the leukocytes from other blood components. The leukocytes are retained, while the remainder is continuously returned to the donor through a second venipuncture. Again, hydroxyethyl starch is often used as a sedimenting agent.

The yield from centrifugation leukapheresis is less than from filtration leukapheresis, about 10^{10} leukocytes per run. Improved methods have been used to augment the yield by increasing the circulating leukocytes and by enhancing red cell sedimentation. Etiocholanolone (a steroid metabolite) causes a granulocytosis by stimulating release of mature granulocytes from the bone marrow, while dexamethasone (a corticosteroid) increases the circulating granulocytes by decreasing the accumulation of granulocytes in the marginal pool. Both drugs, when given to a donor, can double the yield of granulocytes.

Hydroxyethyl starch (HES), a glycopyranone, promotes erythrocyte rouleaux formation and allows clearer delineation of the white and red blood cell layers. The use of HES in all types of centrifugation leukaphereses can also double the yield of granulocytes. HES may improve the yield by sedimentation and thus make the procedure feasible in many small hospitals (Djerassi, 1977). The use of etiocholanolone or dexamethasone and HES increases the yield of leukocytes about sixfold and granulocytes six- to eightfold. These agents exhibit little if any adverse effect on the donor. The number of erythrocytes and the amount of plasma lost by the donor is comparable to that from plateletpheresis. The donor must be monitored before each donation. The postdonation leukocyte count is usually slightly increased. Transfusion of manually collected granulocytes from patients with untreated chronic myelogenous leukemia has achieved favorable clinical responses in many recipients (Freireich, 1964). This latter method, however, is no longer used.

Donor reactions

Common Blood Donor Reactions

1. Donor feels faint. Stop the blood donation and ask the donor to inhale aromatic spirits of ammonia.
2. Fainting, weakness, perspiration, pallor, un-consciousness, slow pulse rate, nausea, vomiting, low blood pressure. Stop the donation and place the donor's head in a low position. Be sure the donor has an adequate airway and apply cold compresses to forehead. If the needle is still in the donor's arm vein, the blood may be reinfused; otherwise, the needle should be removed.
3. Tetany or paresthesia and hyperventilation. Have the donor breathe several times into a paper bag.
4. Hematoma. Every effort should be made to prevent infiltration by inadvertent needle motion. Elevate the arm and apply compression locally, preferably cold.
5. Convulsions. Restrain the donor, remove the phlebotomy needle and use a tongue blade depressor or simple mouth airway to prevent biting. Maintain an adequate airway.

Reactions Observed During Pheresis

1. Chills. Cover the donor with a blanket and connect a blood warmer to the return channel.
2. Paresthesia and muscle cramping related to calcium binding by citrate (in centrifugal procedures). Slow the reinfusion and delay the next cycle until symptoms disappear.
3. Air embolus. Chest pain, shortness of breath, shock, pallor, sweating, mental confusion, and syncope. Although every effort should be made to prevent this from happening, if it does occur, place the donor on his left side with head down. Administer oxygen and transport promptly to an appropriate medical facility.
4. Sensitivity to heparin or protamine. Epistaxis or bleeding, chills, urticaria, or signs of anaphylactic shock. Discontinue infusion of heparin or protamine and treat anaphylaxis with epinephrine and steroids; transport promptly to an appropriate medical facility.
5. Bleeding from venipuncture site (heparinized donors). Remove needle if light pressure will not control it, then apply pressure and cold. If unusually troublesome, administer protamine.
6. Fever, chest pain, cough, shortness of breath, or other severe untoward reactions prompt stopping the procedure immediately for a physician's review and institution of appropriate measures.

Reactions 3, 4, and 6 are uncommon. However, adequate facilities should be available to handle all common reactions at the donor sites. A physician should be readily available to deal with reactions of pheresis donors.

PREPARATION OF BLOOD COMPONENTS

The development of plastic bags with integral tubing and of refrigerated centrifuges capable of handling large volumes at high speed makes possible splitting or separating a unit of whole blood into many components (red blood cells, platelets, cryoprecipitate, plasma, and leukocytes) and/or derivatives (plasma fraction subjected to physiochemical methods to generate albumin, coagulation concentrates such as antihemophilia factor (AHF), and prothrombin complex, plasma protein fraction (PPF), fibrinogen and immune globulins) for most appropriate effective and efficient hemotherapy. Thus, we are able to supply the exact components and/or derivatives to meet the needs of each patient and at the same time, to avoid certain elements in the blood that a patient should not receive.

Plastic bags.   Plastic bags are available in many forms, and each is designed for a specific purpose. When the unit is to be used as whole blood, a single bag is suitable. If packed red blood cells (red blood cells or erythrocyte concentrate) are to be prepared, double bags connected by integral tubing should be used. When the unit is to be used for preparation of platelet concentrate, a pack of triple bags is suitable. Special bags with multiple satellite bags are also available for pediatric patients and for frozen storage at ultra low temperatures. These bags are designed in such a way that transfer of the contents may be accomplished within a closed system to avoid contamination. Should a bag have to be entered for transfer purposes, sterile technique must be followed, and the contents of the bag used within 24 hours.

Segments of plastic tubing connected to the bag, which are used for testing, should have the same identification as the bag. Should the identification number be different from that on the bag, the segment closest to the bag with the same number as the other segments must not be removed.

Centrifugation

The outcome of centrifugation depends on two factors, the relative centrifugal force and the duration of centrifugation. The relative centrifugal force (RCF-g) is the product of $0.00001118 \times r \times N^2$, where r is the radius of the rotor in centimeters and N is the number of revolutions per minute. Since different rotors have different radii, different speeds are used to achieve the same RCF in different centrifuges (see Chap. 3). The following RCF/minutes combinations are useful in the preparation of blood components: 5000 g/5 min for preparation of erythrocyte or platelet concentrate; 4170 g/10 min for preparation of cryoprecipitate; 5000 g/7 min for preparation of leukocyte-poor erythrocytes or cell-free plasma. All three combinations are referred to as heavy spin; while 4170 g/2 minute for preparation of platelet-rich plasma is referred to as light spin. However centrifugation at 5000 g is known as a plasma heavy spin.

For preparation of a platelet concentrate, centrifugation is done at 22°C., while for all other blood components, centrifugation is carried out between 1 and 6°C. Balancing the material in opposite sides is important and can be easily done with rubber discs of different weights. A protective plastic bag is very useful. The ports and tubings attached to the bag should be protected from breakage. Manual braking which disturbs the final bag content of blood should be avoided. All safety precautions should also be observed.

Red blood cells (human).

Red blood cells are also known as packed cells. However, *erythrocyte concentrate* may be a more appropriate term. Blood should be drawn in a double bag. It can be prepared by transferring the plasma from the top of the unit to a satellite bag with the aid of a plasma expressor. The amount of plasma transferred to the satellite bag can be measured with a scale. Usually 225 ml of plasma is removed and the resultant erythrocyte concentrate has a hematocrit of about 70 per cent. When leukocyte-poor erythrocytes are needed (*vide infra*), the unit should be centrifuged and the buffy coat layer removed. The resultant erythrocyte concentrate would have a hematocrit of about 90 per cent and is also known as super-packed red blood cells. Erythrocyte concentrates can be prepared from whole blood at any time before the expiration date. If the unit has to be entered to remove the plasma, the cells must be used within 24 hours.

Washed red blood cells

Properly washed erythrocytes contain: (1) A small number of leukocytes and platelets, reducing the chance of HLA immunization (sensitization) and a febrile reaction. (2) Very few microaggregates. This may be important as a suitable preparation for patients with pulmonary dysfunction or those undergoing cardiopulmonary bypass or massive transfusion. (3) Trace amounts of plasma. Thus, they are virtually devoid of regular and irregular antibodies, including plasma proteins as well as anticoagulants or unwanted metabolites such as ammonia and lactate.

Erythrocytes can be washed by multiple batch processing through centrifugation and decanting of the supernatant fluid. It is more convenient but expensive to use machines designed for deglycerolization of frozen red blood cells. The efficiency of washing depends a great deal on the amount of fluid and the method used. Washed erythrocytes should be used within 24 hours, because they are prepared in an open system.

Leukocyte-poor red blood cells

The majority of febrile non-hemolytic transfusion reactions can be alleviated by transfusing leukocyte-poor erythrocytes (with less than 25 per cent of the original leukocytes).

Leukocyte-poor erythrocytes can be prepared by several techniques: (1) Double centrifugation: Light spin followed by a heavy spin with the bag in the inverted position. The supernatant from the light spin can be used to prepare platelet concentrate and fresh frozen plasma. After the heavy spin, only the lower 80 per cent of erythrocytes is used for transfusion. (2) Inverted centrifugation: One heavy spin is required, and again only the lower 80 per cent of erythrocytes is used for transfusion. (3) Filtration: Passing the blood through a nylon filter is an efficient method for removal of granulocytes. Only blood collected in heparin can be used for this procedure. It therefore is seldom used. The cotton filters used in Europe remove lymphocytes as well as granulocytes (Diepenhorst, 1975). Preparations made from the above three methods contain from 5 to 30 per cent of the leukocytes and platelets in the original blood. (4) Sedimentation with HES (Donner, 1975): This provides a 90 per cent yield of erythrocytes with only about 10 per cent of the original number of leukocytes or platelets. (5) Washing: Washing erythrocytes stored in the liquid or frozen state provides good recovery of erythrocytes with a low number of leukocytes and platelets. (6) Frozen deglycerolized red blood cells. The freeze-thaw and wash methodologies described below result in a product with the least content of plasma, platelets, and leukocytes. It is used when maximally leukocyte-poor red blood cells are needed.

Platelet concentrates

These have several characteristics and requirements. Single units are prepared from units of whole blood before refrigeration. Platelet-rich plasma is separated by a light spin from the erythrocytes. A platelet concentrate is then obtained by a heavy spin of the platelet-rich plasma. Centrifugation should be done at 22°C. The separation must be performed within four hours after the blood is drawn. Therefore, the plasma portion can be frozen and used as fresh frozen plasma. Between 30 and 50 ml of plasma should be left with the platelets when the concentrate is stored at 20 to 24°C. However, only 20 to 30 ml of plasma is required when the concentrate is stored at 1 to 6°C. A unit should contain more than 5.5×10^{10} platelets (75 per cent of units tested after storage for 72 hours at both temperatures). Multiple units of platelets from a single donor can be prepared by repeated bleeding using a manual method or an automated pheresis technique as described previously.

Fresh frozen plasma (FFP)

FFP can be prepared from a single heavy spin or from a double centrifugation to prepare platelet concentrate at the same time. Each unit contains about 225 ml of plasma. FFP should be frozen in a protective container within six hours after collection by placing it in a Dry Ice-alcohol bath or in a freezer at −30°C. or below. Bags should be frozen in a horizontal position and stored in a vertical position so that any inadvertent thawing will be apparent. When stored at −18°C. or less, the shelf-life is 12 months. When requested, FFP can be thawed with agitation in a 37°C. water bath and should be used within two hours.

Cryoprecipitate (Cryo) or cryoprecipitated anti-hemophilic factor (AHF)

Plasma should be separated from erythrocytes within four hours of collection by a heavy spin. The plasma should be frozen within two hours of separation (or six hours of collection) in a mechanical freezer at −30°C. or less or in a Dry Ice-alcohol (95 per cent) bath. Frozen plasma should then be thawed between 1 and 6°C. overnight in a refrigerator or more quickly in a water bath at 4°C. The AHF-poor plasma is separated from the cryoprecipitate after light centrifugation, leaving about 10 ml of plasma with the cryoprecipitate. The precipitate should be frozen within four hours and stored at −18°C. or below in such a manner that thawing will be apparent. A bag of cryoprecipitate should contain on the average about 80 to 100 units of AHF per unit. When stored at −18°C. or below, the shelf-life is 12 months. When requested, cryoprecipitate may be thawed in a 37°C. water bath and then should be maintained at room temperature and used as soon as possible or within six hours of thawing.

Other blood components

Single donor plasma stored at 1 to 6°C. may be used within 26 days after collection. If stored at −18°C., the shelf-life is five years. It is mainly used for fractionation purposes by specially equipped institutions. Plasma from which cryoprecipitate has been removed must be so designated.

Whole blood (human) with cryoprecipitate removed is occasionally used as is whole blood (human) with platelets removed.

PROCESSING AND DISTRIBUTION

Processing of blood

Tests for Each Unit of Blood or Blood Component

ABO and Rh_o TYPING. ABO grouping includes typing of cells (forward) and typing of serum or plasma (reverse). Anti-A,B should be included in cell typing to detect weak A variants, while A_2 cells should be included to confirm the presence of Anti-A_1 in the serum or reverse grouping. Typing for Rh_o should also include a diluent control or albumin control. Anti-DC or anti-DE may be included as a double check. Cells negative for anti-D must be examined by the antiglobulin test for the detection of the D^u variant. Manual methods are usually used for small number of donors, while automated procedures are usually used in large centers. Confirmation of all ABO and Rh_o negative types is required on receipt of whole blood or red blood cell-containing components from another institution.

ANTIBODY SCREENING (DETECTION). Emphasis on screening for irregular antibodies of donor blood has diminished in recent years for two reasons: (a) Antibodies other than anti-A or anti-B in donor's blood have not been reported to cause a hemolytic transfusion reaction (Mollison, 1972); (b) As erythrocyte concentrates are being widely used for transfusion, the antibodies in the remaining small amount of plasma become less significant.

In some countries, an acceptable practice is to pool plasma of several donors in a preliminary screening. Since only about 1 to 2 per cent of donor serum is expected to have irregular antibodies, the amount of antiglobulin serum used can then be greatly reduced. Since human body temperature is close to 37°C., testing of antibodies at room temperature or at 4°C. may not be a valid approach.

TEST FOR SYPHILIS. The wisdom of testing blood donors for syphilis by serologic methods has been questioned recently. If the donor has spirochetemia, serologic tests are usually negative, whereas, in the presence of anti-spirochetal antibodies, the donor blood is usually not infectious. VDRL or RPR tests are usually used for a small number of donors, while ART (automated reagin test) is usually used in large blood centers (see Chap. 54).

TESTS FOR HEPATITIS. Although viral hepatitis has been reviewed in Chapters 11 and 38, a brief review of testing is in order. Post-transfusion hepatitis has been found associated with type B (about 20 per cent), very rarely with type A, and the remaining with non-A and non-B. However, antigen or antibodies related to type A hepatitis can be demonstrated only in selected, specially equipped laboratories. Very little information is available for the non-A and non-B types of hepatitis. Type B hepatitis is caused by Dane particles which consist of DNA core and a protein coat. Anti-core antibodies and DNA polymerase can be demonstrated

during the acute stage of infection and occasionally post infection in selected laboratories. The protein outer coat has the same specificity as HBsAg (hepatitis B surface antigen). HBsAg itself is probably not infectious. HBsAg has several determinants: ayw1, ayw2, ayw3, ayw4, ayr, adw2, adw4, adr, adyw, and adyr. Only ad and ay can be determined easily for epidemiologic purposes. Persons with HBsAg are often positive for HBeAg or anti-HBe, which do not occur simultaneously. The presence of HBeAg may indicate infectivity, while the presence of anti-HBe indicates non-infectivity. More tests are available for HBsAg than perhaps for any other disease. Only the third generation tests are allowed for testing blood donors. Those tests capable of detecting all the antigens in the Bureau of Biologics (BoB) panel 2-C are qualified as third generation tests, i.e., RIA (radioimmunoassay), EIA (enzyme immunoassay), RPHA (reverse passive hemagglutination), and latex agglutination. All third generation tests are highly sensitive, but none of them is completely specific. Confirmatory tests such as neutralization are normally required. Third generation tests can detect a majority of donors who are capable of transmitting type B hepatitis. The fact that only about 20 per cent of post-transfusion hepatitis individuals are positive for HBsAg and that the percentage of reduction in post-transfusion hepatitis owing to testing is also about 20 per cent tends to support this conclusion (Prince, 1975; Barker, 1976).

Tests for selected components

Platelet Count. Platelet counts are used to establish the yield and proficiency of plateletpheresis. Occasional platelet counts from units of platelet concentrates are also required. The number of platelets in relation to the volume of plasma in the bag determines the pH and hence the viability of platelets. The pH of a platelet preparation must be 6.0 or greater at the time of expiration. The plasma-to-platelet count ratio, as well as storage temperatures, are important in this regard. Sterility should be checked periodically on expired units.

Leukocyte Count. A leukocyte count is useful in determining the yield and proficiency of a leukapheresis procedure. A differential count, including percentage of granulocytes, should also be done in order to derive an absolute granulocyte count.

HLA Typing. In recipients refractory to platelet transfusion, the use of HLA-compatible donors may be helpful (Chap. 41). The benefit of using HLA-compatible donors for granulocyte transfusion has not been well established (Schiffer, 1974). ABO matching, however, is important.

AHF Assay. Determination of AHF activity on selected units of cryoprecipitate is required. An average of 80 units of AHF (Factor VIII) per unit is required.

Total Protein. Determination of the donor's total serum protein is required for plasmapheresis programs.

4

Labeling of blood components

Each unit of blood or blood component should be labeled CORRECTLY AND CLEARLY with the nature of the contents in the bag and the date of expiration. Results of routine testing—ABO, Rh_o, antibody screening, and tests for syphilis and hepatitis—should also be included. Sufficient information should be on the unit so one can trace the donor and the institution where the unit was drawn and processed. With advances in computer technology, labels readable by a scanner as well as by the human eye have been proposed to reduce human transcription errors (Technical Manual of AABB, 1977, Chap. 6). In the United States, labels should satisfy the requirements set forth by the FDA (Food and Drug Administration) and the American Association of Blood Banks (AABB) or the Red Cross. For details, one should consult the most recent information from the Code of Federal Regulations, AABB Standards for Blood Banks and Transfusion Services, Technical Manual of AABB (1977), and Red Cross Blood Service Directives.

Shipping of blood components

All blood components are potentially hazardous and carry the possibility of transmitting hepatitis. Hence, they should be handled with meticulous care and respect. All components stored at 1 to 6°C. should be shipped with ice to insure a temperature of 1 to 10°C. Materials which melt at 10°C. may be used as monitoring devices. Platelet concentrates stored at 20 to 24°C. should be shipped at temperatures as close as possible to 22°C. Fresh frozen plasma and frozen erythrocytes stored at −80°C. should be shipped with Dry Ice. Frozen erythrocytes stored in liquid nitrogen (low glycerol technique) should be shipped in a liquid nitrogen container; however, this may be impractical for long-distance transportation.

Inventory control

Ideally, no blood or blood components should be allowed to outdate. Although this is impractical or even impossible in small hospitals, every effort should be made to reduce such waste. Effective inventory control and an efficient transportation system can be of great help to improve the shelf-life. Computerized inventory control was intensively investigated about 10 years ago without success, largely because of high cost hardware and inadequate technology at that time. With advances in telecommunication systems and reductions in the cost of data processing, there is no doubt that effective inventory control will soon be available in many hospitals. Several regional blood centers as well as regional associations of blood service units already provide such inventory control. The Red Cross Blood Program has such a computer facility in Washington, D.C., for its 57 blood programs. Like the National Clearinghouse programs of the AABB, such inventory control assists immeasurably in responding to local variations in blood supply and demand by facilitating shipments of blood to meet patient care requirements and reduce outdating of blood. Although accurate figures for the entire nation are not available, outdating of blood probably approaches 10 per cent. Most of the blood in the United States is transfused within the first two weeks of storage. Therefore, the recent extension of duration of preservation from 21 days with CPD to 35 days for CPD adenine may or may not have a significant impact on outdating of blood with associated waste of red blood cells.

PRESERVATION OF BLOOD COMPONENTS

Storage of erythrocytes in the liquid state

Criteria. Erythrocytes which are infused into a recipient must be viable and functioning properly. Viability can be measured by tagging the erythrocytes with ^{51}Cr and estimating the number of tagged cells remaining in circulation 24 hours after transfusion. The 70 per cent viability criterion was chosen as the minimal requirement for limiting the shelf-life to 21 days when erythrocytes are stored between 1 and 6°C. (Fig. 43-13). This type of assay requires the use of radioactive isotopes and has to be done *in vivo;* however, an alternative *in vitro* method has been found to approximate the survival rate by measuring the level of adenosine triphosphate (ATP) in erythrocytes. ATP plays an important role in the glycolytic process of the erythrocyte by providing 8000 calories/mole as energy when it is split into adenosine diphosphate or adenosine monophosphate. The percentage of ATP after different periods of storage shows excellent correlation with values obtained by the *in vivo* measurement (Table 43-42).

It is of equal importance that transfused erythrocytes function properly, i.e., release oxygen to the tissue cells. Recently, 2,3-DPG (diphosphoglycerate) has been shown to play an important role in erythrocyte capability of releasing oxygen (Fig.

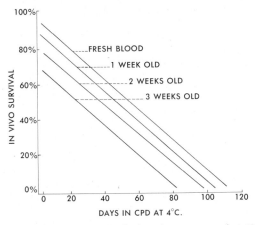

Figure 43–13. *In vivo* survival of erythrocytes stored at 4°C. (Modified from Huestis, 1976.)

28-4). 2,3-DPG is an intermediate metabolite in the glycolytic cycle of erythrocytes and has a strong affinity for hemoglobin; thus it promotes the release of oxygen from oxygenated hemoglobin (2,3-DPG + HbO_2→2,3-DPG · Hb + O_2). Consequently, the level of 2,3-DPG has become a useful index for measuring the function of erythrocytes. The 2,3-DPG level in ACD (acid-citrate-dextrose) blood begins to decrease after two days at 4°C., whereas in CPD (citrate-phosphate-dextrose) blood the decrease begins after one week. However, after transfusion, erythrocytes regenerate 2,3-DPG after three to eight hours, and normal levels are restored within 24 hours. The importance of 2,3-DPG levels is thus limited to those recipients who require oxygen supply urgently. Other criteria for successful preservation include a minimal accumulation of undesirable metabolites such as ammonia, plasma potassium, or acid equivalents (decrease in pH value). Some important changes in CPD blood are listed in Table 43-42.

Temperatures. The metabolic processes of erythrocytes are retarded at low temperatures. For liquid storage, 1° to 6°C. has been selected; for transportation 1° to 10°C. has been selected. For frozen storage, −65° to −95°C. for electric freezers and −150° to −196°C. for liquid nitrogen freezers have been designated.

Glycolytic metabolism is very slow between 1 and 6°C., practically at a standstill between −65° and −85°C., and virtually non-existent between −150° and −196°C.

Preservatives. The following are used for storage of erythrocytes in the liquid state (Table (43-43).

1. Heparin is an anticoagulant but not a preservative. Blood collected in heparin must be used within 48 hours and preferably within 24 hours. Heparin, which had been used for blood collected for cardiopulmonary bypass surgery and for exchange transfusion, is rarely used now except for removal of leukocytes by filtration leukapheresis. In addition to the short shelf-life of heparinized blood, heparin activates lipoprotein lipase, producing free fatty acids; these substances compete with bilirubin for binding sites on albumin. It also produces *in vivo* anticoagulation. These aspects should be taken into consideration when heparinized blood is used for exchange transfusion in newborns.

2. ACD (acid-citrate-destrose) has been the standard solution for collecting blood for transfusion since 1943 (Mollison, 1972). Citrate chelates calcium and serves as an anticoagulant, while dextrose provides the source of energy and citric acid gives the solution a pH of about 5 (at room temperature). After the addition of blood, the plasma-ACD mixture has a pH value of about 7.1 at room temperature and about 7.4 at 4°C. The composition of ACD is listed in Table 43-43.

3. CPD (citrate-phosphate-dextrose) has essentially replaced ACD in the past few years, at least in the United States. The presence of phosphate contributes to the adenosine phosphate pool and thus improves the viability of erythrocytes. CPD has a slightly higher pH than ACD (5.5 alone, 7.5 at

Table 43–42.   PRESERVATION OF BLOOD: IMPORTANT CHANGES IN STORED CPD BLOOD*

	DAYS OF STORAGE				
CHANGES	0	7	14	21	28
Percentage of viable cells (24 hr post-transfusion)	100	98	85	80	75
Percentage of ATP values	100	96	83	86	75
Percentage of 2,3-DPG values	100	99	80	44	35
Plasma pH (at 37°C.)	7.2	7.0	6.89	6.84	6.78
Plasma Na (mEq/l)	168	166	163	156	154
Plasma K (mEq/l)	3.9	11.9	17.2	21	22.5
Whole blood NH_3 (µg/dl)	282	300	447	500	705

*Condensed from Technical Manual of AABB, 1977.

Table 43-43. ANTICOAGULANTS FOR BLOOD COLLECTION

CONSTITUENT	HEPARIN	ACD FORMULA A	CPD	CPD ADENINE
Heparin sodium	75000 U	—	—	—
Sodium chloride to make	1000 ml	—	—	—
Trisodium citrate	—	22.0 g	26.3 g	26.3 g
Citric acid	—	8.0 g	3.27 g	3.27 g
Dextrose	—	24.5 g	25.5 g	31.9 g
NaH_2PO_4	—	—	2.22 g	2.22 g
Adenine	—	—	—	0.275 g
Water to make	—	1000 ml	1000 ml	1000 ml
Volume/100 ml blood	6 ml	15 ml	14 ml	14 ml

4°C. with blood) and thus maintains the 2,3-DPG level for about one week with a lesser decrease in pH at 4°C.

4. CPD-Adenine-One. (CPDA-1) The addition of 0.25 mmol/l adenine to the CPD solution as a preservative for blood collection can extend the shelf-life to at least 35 days. Adenine is required for the formation of ATP. CPD-adenine also maintains the 2,3-DPG level about as well as CPD does; CPD-adenine as a preservative has recently become available in the United States. It should be mentioned that the preservative ACD-adenine has been successfully used in Sweden for the past 10 years. Blood collected in CPD-adenine is currently not recommended for platelet collections, although it is likely to be soon.

5. Other Preservatives. The addition of inosine, pyruvate, ascorbate, and methylene blue to CPD-adenine is a subject of intensive study. Preliminary evidence indicates that it is possible to improve the normal, 2,3-DPG level to 170 per cent and to rejuvenate erythrocytes with low 2,3-DPG levels (Dawson, 1977; Valeri, 1972; Paniker, 1971).

Storage of erythrocytes in the frozen state (Lukomskyj, 1974)

Cryoprotectives. In order to keep erythrocytes in the frozen state, a cryoprotective agent must be added to prevent injury from freezing and thawing. There are two types of cryoprotectives, intracellular (penetrating) and extracellular (non-penetrating). Glycerol and DMSO(dimethyl sulphoxide) belong to the first category, while HES (hydroxyethyl starch) belong to the second. Currently only glycerol is used to keep erythrocytes in frozen state for hemotherapy. High concentrations of glycerol, about 40 to 47 per cent, are required for cells kept in an electric freezer, while low concentrations of glycerol, about 14 to 17 per cent, are required for cells kept in liquid nitrogen.

Glycerolization. Erythrocytes should be frozen within six days of collection. The unit should be equilibrated at room temperature with the plasma

Table 43-44. TWO TYPES OF PROCEDURES FOR FREEZING RED BLOOD CELLS

PROCEDURES	"HIGH GLYCEROL-SLOW FREEZE"		"LOW GLYCEROL-RAPID FREEZE"	
	Tullis-Meryman-Valeri (1970, 1972, 1973)	Huggins (1973)	Krijnen-Rowe (1964, 1968)	Åkerblom-Högman (1974)
Glycerol (w/v)				
Initial	57%	79%	35%	35%
Final	40%	47%	17.5%	14%
Stages	2	2	1	1
Storage				
At	−65°C. to −85°C.		−150°C. to −196°C.	
Freezer	Electric		Liquid Nitrogen	
Deglycerolization				
Number of solutions	3	4	2	2 3
Total volume in liters	2.5	6.6	1.5-2	1.2 3.6
Time in minutes	20 to 25	25 to 30	15 to 20	16 16
Methods of Washing				
Centrifugation	Yes	No	Yes	Yes
Agglomeration	No	Yes	No	Yes

removed prior to the addition of glycerol. The glycerol should be added slowly, with constant agitation to insure even and slow penetration of glycerol into the cells and to avoid a sudden change of osmotic pressure inside and outside the cells. After reaching equilibrium, the bag should be properly labeled and protected before being placed in a freezer. The excess glycerol may be removed to reduce space for storage and to improve the efficiency of deglycerolization. The exact procedure of glycerolization is determined by the method of storage and the techniques used for deglycerolization. Table 43-44 summarizes four protocols currently used for glycerolization of erythrocytes.

Deglycerolization. Erythrocytes to be deglycerolized should be thawed in a 37°C. water bath. Additional steps vary with the washing system in an institution. Table 43-45 summarizes the four systems used in the United States. While erythrocytes prepared by all protocols can be deglycerolized by centrifugation techniques, only erythrocytes glycerolized by the Huggins and Akerblom-Högman protocol can be deglycerolized by the agglomeration technique. It is important to remove glycerol slowly from the erythrocytes to avoid excessive hemolysis with a loss of cells. Incomplete removal of glycerol may be tested by measuring the intracellular glycerol concentration, by checking the freezing point (osmolality) of supernatant fluid, or simply by detecting presence of free hemoglobin when a few drops of washed erythrocytes are placed in a tube full of normal saline. Transfusion of erythrocytes with excessive glycerol may cause hemolysis *in vivo.*

Storage of platelets

Platelets can be stored at three different temperatures: (a) Between 20° and 24°C. Continuous gentle agitation is required for warm storage platelets. Excessive agitation may cause aggregation of platelets. Between 30 and 50 ml of plasma is required to keep the pH above 6 for the 72 hours of shelf-life. (b) Between 1° and 6°C. Only 20 to 30 ml of plasma is required and no agitation is necessary. Before use, platelets should be warmed to room temperature and resuspended. The increment in the platelet counts of the recipient is usually lower from platelets stored at 4°C. than those stored at 22°C. Some investigators believe that platelets stored at 4°C. may shorten the recipient's bleeding time more promptly. (c) At −80° to −150°C. Using DMSO as a cryoprotective, platelets can be kept either at −80°C. or at −150°C. Owing to the many steps involved, the recovery rate is somewhere between 20 and 30 per cent; hence, it is not yet practical for regular use.

Storage of other blood components

Fresh frozen plasma (FFP) and cryoprecipitate are stored at −18°C. for a period of one year. Freezers with temperatures lower than −18°C. preserve better the activity of the coagulation factors. Both products should be thawed in a 37°C. water bath and used as soon as possible, e.g., FFP within two hours and cryoprecipitate within six hours. Gentle agitation of FFP while thawing reasonably rapidly in a 37°C. water bath allows less fibrinogen to precipitate, since fibrinogen precipitates from plasma at about 13°C. Reagent lymphocytes can be stored in the frozen state. No clinical method is available for freezing leukocytes for transfusion purposes.

Other blood products such as albumin, gamma globulin, or Rh immune globulin are prepared and supplied mainly by commercial firms. Instructions for each derivative should be followed before use.

HEMOTHERAPY

SELECTION OF BLOOD COMPONENTS

Hemotherapy employs blood components (red blood cells, platelets, granulocytes, plasma, cyroprecipitate) and derivatives (al-

Table 43-45.   FOUR TYPES OF MACHINES FOR WASHING RED BLOOD CELLS

MACHINES	BLOOD PROCESSOR	CYTOGLOMERATOR	ELUTRAMATIC	CELL WASHER
Manufacturer	Haemonetics	Cryosan	Fenwal	IBM
Mode of Washing	Continuous	Batch	Continuous	Batch
Centrifugation	Yes	No	Yes	Yes
Agglomeration	No	Yes	No	No
Continuous-attention	No	Yes	No	No
Units washed at one time	1	5(WS 5) 1(WS 1)	2	1

Table 43-46. BLOOD COMPONENTS AND DERIVATIVES USED IN HEMOTHERAPY

BLOOD OR BLOOD COMPONENTS	QUANTITY	SHELF LIFE	INDICATIONS
Whole blood	450 ml blood 63 ml CPD 60 g hemoglobin 40% hematocrit	21 days at 4°C (CPD, ACD) 35 days at 4°C (CPD-Adenine)	Brisk active bleeding
Red blood cells (Erythrocyte concentrate)	280 ml volume 60 g hemoglobin 70% hematocrit	Same as whole blood (1 day if opened)	Anemias, slow blood loss
Washed red blood cells	250 ml volume 57 g hemoglobin 70% hematocrit	1 day (4°C.)	Prevention of febrile non-hemolytic transfusion reaction. Prevent HLA and protein sensitization.
Frozen-thawed red blood cells (washed)	250 ml volume 54 g hemoglobin 60% hematocrit	3 years in freezer 1 day after washing	Supply of rare blood, autotransfusion, inventory control. Prevention of HLA and protein immunization as well as febrile nonhemolytic transfusion reaction.
Platelet concentrate	30–50 ml 20–30 ml 5.5×10^{10}	3 days (22°C.) 3 days (4°C.)	Hemorrhage, quantitative or qualitive platelet disorder.
Plateletpheresis	350 ml 5×10^{11}	1 day (22°C.) or (4°C.)	HLA-compatible recipient possible.*
Granulocyte concentrate pheresis	400 ml 2×10^{10}	Should be transfused immediately (4°C.)	Infections unresponsive to antibiotics in granulocytopenic patients
Fresh frozen plasma	225 ml 13 g protein	1 year (−18°C.)	Supply coagulation factors, maintain blood volume, supply plasma for exchange transfusion.
Cryoprecipitate	10 ml 80 AHF units	1 year (−18°C.)	Supply factor VIII and fibrinogen (hemophilia A, Von Willebrand's disease, and hypofibrinogenemia)
Factor VIII concentrate (lyophilized)	Up to 1000 units	2 years (2-8°C.)	Hemophiliacs
Factor IX concentrate (lyophilized Factors II, VII, IX, X)	500 ml	Up to 2 years (2-8°C.)	Factor IX deficiency (Hemophilia B)
†Albumin 5% 25%	250–500 ml 50–100 ml	3 years below 30°C.	Hypovolemia, burns, for binding bilirubin Cerebral edema, hypoalbuminemia
Plasma protein fraction 5%	250–500 ml	3 years below 30°C.	Hypovolemic shock, hypoproteinemia
Immune serum globulin	2–10 ml	3 years (2-8°C.)	Prevent and modify type A hepatitis and certain other infections. Prophylactic use in patients with hypogammaglobulinemia
Anti-Rh$_0$ (D) immune globulin	300 μg	1½ years (2-8°C.)	Prevent Rh$_0$ (D) immunization (e.g., postpartum or postabortion and after inadvertent transfusion of Rh$_0$ (D)-positive red blood cell–containing components to an Rh$_0$ (D)-negative person.

*With less exposure to hepatitis and red cell antigen.
†Practically no risk of hepatitis.

bumin, plasma protein fraction, Factor VIII concentrate, prothrombin complex* concentrate, and immune serum globulin) for treating patients. Blood transfusions may greatly benefit patients, but certain risks are also involved, such as transmission of infection, immunization (sensitization) to foreign antigens, and the possibility of a transfusion reaction. The physician must weigh the expected benefits against the potential danger before requesting blood for his patient. The following are useful recommendations:

a. Don't order a blood transfusion unless it is definitely indicated. Avoid "cosmetic" transfusions.

b. When a transfusion is indicated, use as little blood as possible. The incidence of hepatitis and other complications increases proportionately with the number of units transfused. Although demand for the "one unit transfusion" has been questioned, there are times when it is more appropriate to transfuse one unit than two.

c. Transfuse only the components needed by the patient, reducing complications due to unwanted components in whole blood and saving the other components for other recipients. Common blood components and derivatives with quantity expected from each unit, shelf-life (preservation or storage interval), and main indications are listed in Table 43-46. The values are approximate and may vary from unit to unit.

Some blood components are not listed in Table 43-46. For instance, leukocyte-poor blood has been largely replaced by thawed frozen or washed erythrocytes, which offer many additional theoretical advantages. Single-donor plasma has essentially been replaced by fresh frozen plasma or albumin preparations. Quite often, patients may need platelets and granulocytes; combined pheresis can harvest both at the same time.

The risk of transmitting hepatitis is a serious consideration. Albumin, immune serum globulin, and anti-$Rh_o(D)$ immune globulin are practically hepatitis free. Commercial fibrinogen and Factor II, VII, IX, and X preparations, which carry a high incidence of transmitting hepatitis, are not recommended. Cryoprecipitate can be used as a substitute for fibrinogen, and FFP can be substituted for Factors II, VII, IX, and X. All other blood components can transmit

hepatitis; furthermore, washed erythrocytes (fresh or frozen) are believed to have less risk of hepatitis because of the dilution factor.

In summary, indications for transfusion of blood components and derivatives embrace the following:

1. Volume replacement for acute blood loss, i.e., hemorrhage, trauma, burns.
2. Red blood cell mass deficiency (chronic anemia with symptoms).
3. Coagulation factor deficiencies.
4. Leukocyte or platelet defect or decreased number.
5. Cardiopulmonary bypass (open heart surgery).
6. Exchange transfusion.

d. The selection of blood components or derivatives for various clinical conditions is dependent on the judgment of the clinician to provide for the needs of each patient. However, according to current knowledge, some general guidelines can be made, as summarized in Table 43-47. A number of clinical conditions which may not need any blood components or derivatives but which require the assistance of blood bank personnel are listed in Table 43-48.

e. It is important to request blood for transfusion well in advance so that appropriate components can be prepared and tests can be performed properly. Table 43-49 lists the approximate time required for pretransfusion examination and preparation.

f. Consider autotransfusion for elective surgery, especially for female children and women in child-bearing age groups and for patients requiring blood from rare donors.

Whole blood transfusion

Indications. Whole blood transfusion is rarely indicated except in cases of active bleeding that cannot be stopped immediately and in exchange transfusions.

Limitations. When whole blood is stored at 4°C., the majority of granulocytes lose their phagocytic activity in three days, and practically all phagocytic activity is lost after four days. The number of granulocytes in one unit of blood (approximately 2.5×10^9) is too small to be of therapeutic value, even when all are alive and functioning. Whole blood cannot provide any meaningful number of granulocytes even when the blood is fresh.

Platelets in whole blood lose most of their viability after 12 hours, and almost all viabil-

---

*Factor IX

Table 43–47. BLOOD COMPONENTS AND DERIVATIVES RECOMMENDED FOR
VARIOUS CLINICAL CONDITIONS

CLINICAL CONDITIONS	PREPARATION(S) RECOMMENDED AND COMMENTS
Active bleeding	Whole blood, less than three days old, if possible, for massive bleeding; red blood cells* or erythrocyte concentrate (EC)* and fresh frozen plasma (FFP) plus platelets can also be used.
Anemia: Transient Aplastic	Red blood cells (RBC) or EC within 7 days to reduce frequency of transfusion and exogenous iron.
Routine surgery	Whole blood, RBC,* or EC* of any age; fresh whole blood for unusual or massive bleeding; RBC, FFP, and platelets in lieu of fresh whole blood.
Cardiopulmonary bypass	Fresh RBC and non-colloid solution, washed RBC and colloid solution, fresh whole blood.
Repeated febrile/allergic transfusion reactions	Washed frozen or fresh erythrocytes; leukocyte-poor blood for febrile reaction.
Intrauterine transfusion	Washed erythrocytes (erythrocytes without lymphocytes).
Exchange transfusion for newborn	Fresh whole blood for Rh_0 sensitization. EC of mother's group + FFP (child's group) for ABO sensitization; albumin may replace FFP.
Hemodialysis, renal or hepatic failure	Frozen-thawed RBC or washed erythrocytes, red blood cell concentrate.
Anti-IgA requiring transfusion	Washed erythrocytes, frozen-thawed preferred; blood from IgA deficient donors.
Thrombocytopenia with hemorrhage or impending hemorrhage	Platelet concentrate (PC), HLA compatible in refractory patients.
Granulocytopenia with infection or impending infections	Granulocyte concentrate for antibiotic refractory cases.
Agammaglobulinemia or preventing hepatitis A	Immune serum globulin, recommended for laboratory accidental needle sticks.
Hemophilia or von Willebrand's disease	Cryoprecipitate or AHF concentrate (not in von Willebrand's disease).
Afibrinogenemia or hypofibrinogenemia	Cryoprecipitate, FFP, no commercial concentrate available.
Other coagulopathy	FFP or FFP deficient in Factor VIII.
Shock without hemorrhage	Albumin, colloid or non-colloid solutions.
Cerebral edema	25% albumin.
Prevention of Rh_0 sensitization	Anti-Rh_0 (D) immune globulin for Rh_0 (D)-negative women in pregnancy or after accidental transfusion with Rh_0 (D)-positive blood.

*The terms *erythrocyte concentrate* (EC) and *red blood cells* (RBC) are used interchangeably.

Table 43–48. THERAPEUTIC PROCEDURES RELATED TO
BLOOD BANK

CLINICAL CONDITIONS	PROCEDURES USED AND COMMENTS
Elective surgery, rare blood type, many antibodies	Autotransfusion of liquid or frozen stored blood Avoids many other complications
Polycythemia, hemosiderosis	Therapeutic phlebotomy to reduce viscosity or exogenous iron
Macroglobinemia, undesirable elements in plasma	Plasmapheresis or plasma exchange to reduce viscosity or harmful agents in plasma
Selected types of leukemia	Leukapheresis (in experimental stages only)
Aplastic bone marrow	Bone marrow transplantation requires HLA compatible donors
End-stage renal disease	Kidney transplantation requires HLA- and ABO-compatible donors

Table 43–49. APPROXIMATE TIME REQUIRED FOR PREPARING FOR A BLOOD TRANSFUSION*

PROCEDURES	TIME IN MINUTES
1. Collecting the blood specimen	10
2. ABO and Rh_0 typing	10
3. ABO and Rh_0 typing plus antibody screening	45
4. Typing, antibody screening, and crossmatching	60
5. Antibody identification, additional	60+ (up to several days)
6. Fresh frozen plasma, thawing and testing	40
7. Cryoprecipitate, thawing and testing	20
8. Washing erythrocytes	45
9. Thawing and washing of frozen erythrocytes	60

*Excluding pick-up and delivery.

ity is lost in 24 hours. Whole blood is thus not a reliable or effective substitute for platelets.

There are changes in plasma proteins in stored blood. The half-life of Factors V, VIII, and XI is about one week. Therefore, whole blood is not the best substitute for these three factors.

When whole blood is used for transfusion, only ABO type-specific blood should be used; otherwise, strong anti-A or anti-B in donor's blood plasma can cause a severe hemolytic transfusion reaction.

Since whole blood cannot be relied upon to provide meaningful numbers of platelets, granulocytes, or coagulation factors, the major consideration is erythrocyte storage. The survival rate of erythrocytes stored in CPD at 4°C. for one week is about 98 per cent, and their 2,3-DPG level is about 99 per cent, both of which are essentially the same as in one- to two-day-old blood. The accumulation of metabolites or change in pH is also minimal. Thus, one can define fresh blood as blood less than seven days old. However, the *in vivo* survival rate decreases as the duration of storage of erythrocytes at 4°C. increases (Fig. 43–13). This fact should be taken into consideration for those patients with aplastic anemia, sickle cell anemia, thalassemia and other chronic anemias, who require repeated transfusions. The use of fresh red cells will reduce the number of transfusions and, hence, decrease the chance of hemosiderosis.

Massive transfusions

For patients with severe trauma or burns, and those requiring cardiac and vascular surgery or exchange transfusions, the amount of blood transfused may approach or exceed the recipient's blood volume. The following factors should be taken into consideration:

a. For active bleeding, whole blood is preferred. However, red blood cells (erythrocyte concentrate) and fresh frozen plasma (FFP) are excellent substitutes.

b. A large-bore needle or even a catheter may be required to increase the rate of infusion.

c. A blood warmer is usually required.

d. For extreme emergencies, ABO type-specific blood should be infused without crossmatching; however, O Rh_0-negative blood may be given (sometimes even O Rh_0-positive may be necessary) with crossmatching performed after the transfusion. Oberman (1978) has proposed the feasibility of a modified crossmatch.

e. The platelet count may drop sharply to 40,000 to 70,000/μl. However, replacement with platelets may not be required until the count is below 15,000/μl, although bleeding time may be prolonged below 100,000/μl.

f. Two units of FFP are recommended for every 10 units of stored blood infused.

g. There is no evidence that citrate and potassium in stored blood create a serious problem in massive transfusion. One ampule of sodium bicarbonate (44.5 mEq) for every 5 units of blood is recommended by some physicians (Greenwalt, 1977, p. 13).

h. Filters designed to retain microaggregates are recommended except in cases where the infusion rate must be fast, and when either fresh whole blood (as a source of viable platelets) or platelet concentrates are to be infused. Such filters should be changed after every 2 to 3 units infused to prevent reduction in flow rate and saturation of filter with particles. Table 43–50 shows sev-

Table 43–50. FILTERS FOR INFUSION OF BLOOD AND BLOOD COMPONENTS

BLOOD FILTERS	PORE SIZE	FILTER MATERIAL	USE	CONTRAINDICATIONS
Standard				
Fenwal STD Blood Filter (large and reg. size surface area)	170 μ	Lexan plastic nylon mesh	All blood components	None
McGaw STD Blood Filter	170 μ	Nylon mesh	All blood components	None
Special				
Fenwal 4C2100	170 μ	Nylon mesh with smaller "dead" space	Fresh whole blood, platelets, AHF, cryoprecipitate	
Microaggregate (Micropore)				
Pall 40 μ Ultipor Disposable Blood Filter (Pall Corp., Glen Cove, Long Island, N.Y.)	40 μ	Pleated polyester mesh	Essentially all blood components (see contraindications) and where massive transfusions are indicated or after third unit infused within a 24-hour period.	Do not use for platelet concentrates or fresh whole blood infusions.
Bentley Disposable Blood Filter (PF127, Bentley Lab., Inc., Irvine, Cal.)	27 μ	Polyester urethane foam		
Swank In-Line Blood Filter (IL-200 Pioneer Filters, Inc., Beaverton, Ore.)	20 μ	Dacron wool		
Fenwal Microaggregate Blood Filter (Fenwal Lab., Morton Grove, Ill.) 4C2423 or 4C2131 (with tubing)	20 μ	Polyester non-woven fiber		
Intersept Blood Filter (Johnson & Johnson Co., New Brunswick, N.J.)	20 μ	Woven Dacron mesh		

eral filters used with infusion sets for blood and blood components.

Autologous transfusion

The only 100 per cent compatible blood is one's own blood or blood from an identical twin. Receiving one's own blood is known as autologous transfusion (versus homologous transfusion—receiving blood from others). In an autologous transfusion, the problem of introducing foreign antigens, antibodies, or infectious or toxic agents is eliminated. Multiple phlebotomies usually stimulate erythrocyte production; the resultant mild anemia is thought to improve capillary blood flow.

Autologous transfusions can be achieved by (a) predeposit, (b) intraoperative deposit, or (c) intraoperative salvage.

Predeposit. A patient can donate several units of blood, which can be stored at 4°C. or in the frozen state for future use such as elective surgery or for unexpected needs. This type of practice is particularly suitable for patients with multiple antibodies or for those who require rare blood types or have religious beliefs prohibiting acceptance of homologous blood. Individuals at risk for a nuclear accident with excessive radiation exposure should also consider the feasibility of such frozen storage of their own red blood cells.

The candidate should be in good health with a hemoglobin of at least 11 g/dl. While age and body weight can differ from the requirements for routine blood donation, the amount of anticoagulant in the bag must be adjusted according to the amount of blood drawn. Since only three days after donation are required to reestablish the original volume (often 24 hours is sufficient), one donation every four days is acceptable. Thus, at least four units could be available for 21-day storage. The unit should be processed routinely, and crossmatching is recommended as a check for unit identification. Unit identification should be done as in a manual pheresis procedure to insure against the error of misidentification. In case there is an unexpected delay in surgery, the unit can be re-infused and another unit drawn to avoid outdating. However, this so-called "leapfrog" technique may be too involved to be of any practical benefit.

Intraoperative Deposit. This is known as hemodilution. Phlebotomy is performed immediately after induction of anesthesia. Lost blood volume is replaced with either saline, lactated Ringer's solution, or serum albumin. Hemodilution has been widely used in cardiopulmonary bypass. With this procedure, proportionately fewer erythrocytes are lost per volume of blood shed during surgery and less homologous blood replacement is required.

Intraoperative Salvage. In many types of surgery, such as for a ruptured ectopic pregnancy, chest and abdominal trauma, neurosurgery, and joint surgery, large volumes of blood may be recovered and given back to the patient. To avoid microaggregates, tissue fragments and clots, the blood must be filtered and preferably washed before reinfusion to the patient. This procedure should not be used in patients with malignancy, contaminated wounds, severe hepatitis, renal failure, or a coagulopathy. The theoretical risk of disseminated intravascular coagulation from red cell fragments is reduced by using appropriate microaggregate filters (Table 43–50).

Transfusion of red blood cells

Indications. In chronic anemia, patients may have a hemoglobin as low as 4 g/dl without symptoms. On the other hand, virtually no surgeon is willing to accept a patient for major surgery with a hemoglobin below 8 g/dl except under special conditions. In a newborn child, a hemoglobin level of 14 g/dl is considered anemic. An average adult can afford to lose up to one liter of blood and have it replaced with a crystalloid or colloid solution (Table 43–51), while a loss of 2 liters of blood may be critical to life. These are only general guidelines to orient blood bankers. Each patient's particular condition must be judged by his own physician.

Conventional erythrocyte concentrates with 60 to 70 per cent hematocrits are satisfactory in most conditions; those with about 90 per cent hematocrit are difficult to infuse and are suitable only under selected conditions where blood volume is a critical issue. For minimizing febrile transfusion reactions, leukocyte-poor erythrocytes have essentially been replaced by frozen-thawed or washed erythrocytes whenever feasible.

Freezing and Washing. The use of frozen washed erythrocytes increased fivefold from less than 1000 in 1970 to 5000 in the 1975 in the American Red Cross system (Meryman, 1975). However, when medical conditions are analyzed for its usage, over 90 per cent of frozen-thawed erythrocytes were used for conditions not necessarily requiring frozen cells (Fig. 43–14). In other words, the same benefit at less cost could probably have been achieved by washing alone in the majority of these cases.

It should be stressed that the frozen state does not reduce the infectivity of type B viral hepatitis, but that dilution does (Barker, 1970). In their classic experiment, high concentrations (10^{-4} to 10^6) of infectious agents (in the frozen state for years) produced clinical hepatitis in volunteers, lower concentrations (10^{-5} to 10^{-7}) produced antigenemia (HBsAg +), while very low blood concentrations (10^{-8}) produced neither hepatitis nor antigenemia. It should be mentioned further that the titer of HBsAg may not be parallel to the assumed infectious agent—Dane particles. Washing with large amounts of fluid dilutes infectious agents; although it may not completely prevent the infection, it appears to reduce the severity as reported in chimpanzees (Alter, 1978). For reducing the infectivity of viral hepatitis, washing is obviously the main factor. From an economic point of view, washing

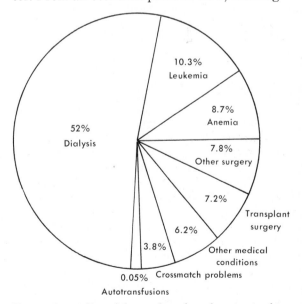

Figure 43–14. Use of frozen thawed erythrocytes in the American Red Cross System, 1974. (Data from Meryman, 1975.)

Table 43–51. PLASMA EXPANDERS DERIVED FROM BLOOD

	FRESH FROZEN PLASMA	5 PER CENT ALBUMIN	25 PER CENT SALT-POOR ALBUMIN	PLASMA PROTEIN FRACTION
Unit volume	230 ml	250 ml	50 ml	250 ml
Protein content	16 g+	12.5 g	12.5 g	12.5 g
Protein concentration	7 g/dl+	5 g/dl	25 g/dl	5 g/dl
Sodium (mEq/l)	128+	100–160	100–160	130–160
Approximate cost/unit (1978)	$15.00	$35.00	$35.00	$35.00
Cost/ml	$ .06	$ .14	$ .70	$ .14
Cost/g protein	$ .93	$ 2.80	$ 2.80	$ 2.80
*Relative hepatitis risk/unit	2	3	3	3

+Represents estimates.
*1 = Greater than whole blood.
  2 = Same as whole blood.
  3 = Less than whole blood (approaches zero risk).

erythrocytes costs much less than washing frozen erythrocytes. In addition to reducing the incidence of hepatitis, febrile and urticarial reactions may be minimized with washed erythrocytes. For patients with anti-IgA, washed erythrocytes or compatible blood from an IgA-deficient donor should be used. In at least one case, frozen-thawed washed erythrocytes worked better than washed erythrocytes as transmembranous passage of glycerol may completely remove the IgA on the surface of erythrocytes (Miller, 1975).

Compatibility. ABO compatibility is an absolute requirement in erythrocyte transfusion. The majority of fatal transfusion reactions are due to ABO incompatibility. Group O erythrocytes can be used in the form of erythrocyte concentrate for other groups, and group A or B can be used for an AB recipient when group-specific blood is not available (Table 43–51). Since the $Rh_o(D)$ antigen is very antigenic, one should use erythrocytes which are $Rh_o(D)$-specific. While $Rh_o(D)$-negative cells can be used for Rh_o-positive recipients, the reverse is true only in emergency situations (Table 43-52). If the recipient is a female of child-bearing age, $Rh_o(D)$ immune globulin (RIG) can be used to prevent immunization (300 μg for each 15 ml of erythrocytes). Hence, large volumes of RIG are required to prevent immunization to only one unit of $Rh_o(D)$-positive blood. Matching Rh antigens other than D is impractical at the present time. However, should the patient have or have had IgG irregular antibodies against antigens such as K, Fy^a, Jk^a, c, or E, erythrocytes negative for such antigens should be used, even if these irregular antibodies are no longer in the patient's serum.

When a patient with group A_1 or A_1B blood has anti-HI active above room temperature, A_1 (or A_1B) erythrocytes should be used, as this antibody has been known to cause rapid destruction of incompatible erythrocytes. When an A_2 or A_2B patient has anti-A_1 active at 37°C., A_2 erythrocytes should be transfused (Mollison, 1972); frozen-thawed group O erythrocytes may also be used when A_2 erythrocytes are not available; this is especially true when additional irregular antibodies are present, e.g., anti-M.

Post-transfusion Increment of Hemoglobin. The post-transfusion increment of hemoglobin is inversely related to the blood volume of the patient and directly related to the volume of red blood cells transfused. The popular guideline that one unit of blood will increase the recipient's hemoglobin by about 1 g/dl should be qualified in two ways: it is applicable only for recipients who weigh about 100 lb and for erythrocyte concentrate (not whole blood). The example on the opposite page may illustrate this point:

Table 43–52. ABO AND Rh_0 COMPATIBILITY IN BLOOD TRANSFUSION

BLOOD TYPE OF RECIPIENT	BLOOD TYPE OF DONOR					
	O	A	B	AB	D–	D+
O	Yes	No	No	No		
A	S	Yes	No	No		
B	S	No	Yes	No		
AB	S	S	S	Yes		
D–					Yes	E
D+					Yes	Yes

S = substitute as erythrocyte concentrates without high titer anti-A or anti-B or in form of washed erythrocytes.
E = only under extreme emergency conditions, especially if the recipient is a young female.

	BLOOD VOLUME*		HEMOGLOBIN		
	ml	Increment (%)	g/dl	Total (g)	Increment (g/dl)
Pretransfusion					
Recipient No. 1, 100 lb	3200		10	320	
No. 2, 150 lb	4800		10	480	
Whole blood (WB)	510		14	63	
Erythrocyte concentrate (EC)	280		22.5	63	
Post-transfusion					
Recipient No. 1 infused with WB	3710	16	10.3	383	0.3
EC	3480	9	11	383	1
No. 2 infused with WB	5310	11	10.2	543	0.2
EC	5080	6	10.7	543	0.7

*Recipient's blood volume is estimated by body weight in lb $\times$ 32.

The patient's blood volume (approximately 8 per cent of body weight of an adult) after hemotherapy will usually return to pretransfusion values, so that the hematocrit rise with EC (erythrocyte concentrate) and WB (whole blood) will ultimately be the same.

Platelet transfusion

Effective platelet transfusion became practical when platelet concentrates could be stored for 72 hours and a large number of platelets could be harvested from a single donor. Platelet transfusion has successfully prevented death from hemorrhage in many leukemic patients. In general, platelet transfusion is useful in thrombocytopenia due to poor production (leukemia or aplastic anemia) and in patients with platelet dysfunction. Platelets are less effective in idiopathic thrombocytopenia and in hypersplenic thrombocytopenia. Platelets are ineffective and may be harmful in (1) disseminated intravascular coagulation (prior to heparinization) and (2) thrombotic thrombocytopenic purpura.

Whenever feasible, ABO-compatible platelets should be used, although, ABO-incompatible platelets are effective. However, the presence of strong anti-A or anti-B in large volumes (300 to 350 ml) of plasma may cause positive direct antiglobulin test and shortened red cell survival (including a hemolytic transfusion reaction) and therefore cannot be ignored. Hence, plasma compatibility is more important than erythrocyte compatibility in platelet transfusion therapy if the platelets are relatively free of red blood cells. Rh_o antigen is an important consideration only for the female recipient of child-bearing age or where

the number of transfused Rh_o-positive erythrocytes is large. In such cases, anti-Rh_o immune globulin may be used concurrently to prevent immunization. In patients refractory to platelet transfusion, HLA-compatible donors should be used.

Patients undergoing major surgery with a platelet count of 30,000/μl seldom bleed; furthermore, bedridden patients seldom bleed with platelet counts of 10,000/μl. Therefore, to prepare a patient for major surgery, the patient should have a platelet count above 30,000, perhaps 50,000/μl. For patients with platelet counts below 20,000/μl, preventive platelet transfusion has been found very useful.

Guidelines for matching and volume considerations for infusion warrant further consideration. Rh_o compatibility is of primary importance for young females who have child-bearing potential. Rh_o incompatibility will not influence the platelet response and Rh-positive platelets will not harm an Rh-negative recipient. There is a small risk of developing anti-Rh_o(D), which is harmless except during pregnancy with an Rh_o-positive fetus. Given the current inability to transfuse *all* Rh_o-negative recipients with Rh_o-negative platelets, Rh_o-negative platelets should be reserved when possible for this group whose immunization to the Rh_o(D) antigen would have the most impact.

Pooling of platelets of different ABO groups has certain theoretical disadvantages (soluble antigen-antibody complexes may induce platelet clumping) and therefore should be avoided.

We use the following guidelines for platelet matching:
1. A or AB platelets should be given to group A or AB patients if available.

2. Any group platelets can be given to O patients.
3. Although B platelets are preferable, supply situations often dictate that any platelets may be given to a B recipient. Alternatively, plateletpheresis of a B donor can be performed.
4. Rh_o-negative female patients under 40 will be given Rh_o-negative platelets *if* available. If not available, the options are to order an Rh_o-negative pheresis collection, to give Rh_o-positive platelets, or to give Rh_o-positive platelets followed by Rh_o immune globulin. If Rh_o-negative platelets are not available, further medical consultation about the available options is in order. Rh_o-negative patients other than females under 40 may be given platelets without regard to Rh type.
5. Pooling platelets should be done only within ABO groups. If, for example, 5 "O" and 5 "B" platelets are available for a B recipient, two separate pools should be forwarded. Therefore, a single platelet order may consist of more than one bag.

There will be occasions when these guidelines cannot be followed, mainly because of an inability to supply the needed product. Consultation with the transfusion service physician experienced in hemotherapy is necessary in these cases to determine the most appropriate course of action.

When volume involved is of clinical concern, the platelet order should be reduced or the daily dose divided into two or more transfusion episodes. In addition, pheresis platelet concentrates can be utilized. They provide the equivalent of 10 units of platelets in a 250 to 300 ml volume. Since they outdate in 24 hours, they must be used promptly.

One unit of platelet concentrate usually contains more than 5.5×10^{10} platelets. When a unit is transfused into a recipient with a blood volume of 5,500 ($5.5 \times 10^6/\mu l$ of blood) the increment is about $5.5 \times 10^{10}/5.5 \times 10^6 = 10,000/\mu l$. In practice, only about half of the expected number is demonstrated one hour after transfusion. As a rough guide, one unit of platelet concentrate would produce an increment of $10,000/\mu l$ in a 100-pound patient. The remaining platelets may be retained by the spleen or used up at the bleeding sites. The consumption of platelets is usually increased if the patient has a fever, sepsis, or splenomegaly. For an average adult bleeding case, 4 to 8 units of random donor platelets is a reasonable quantity to transfuse initially. If the platelet increment is not adequate, this process may be repeated every 6 to 8 hours until the bleeding stops. Chills and febrile reactions are common in patients receiving repeated platelet transfusions and are related to immunization through previous platelet or leukocyte transfusions. These symptoms can be relieved by an injection of meperidine hydrochloride or by pretreatment with corticosteroids.

Granulocyte transfusion

Before platelet transfusions became a routine procedure, many leukemic patients died from hemorrhage. Although hemorrhage can now be largely controlled by platelet transfusion, the aggressive use of chemotherapy and radiation often leads to severe infections in leukemic patients. By repeated transfusions of large numbers of granulocytes, some of these infections unresponsive to antibiotics can be brought under control.

When the absolute granulocyte count is below $500/\mu l$, the patient's chance of contracting infection is great, and with counts of $100/\mu l$ or below, infection is almost inevitable. In granulocytopenic patients with sepsis refractory to antibiotic therapy, granulocyte transfusion is indicated. Herzig (1977) has reported granulocyte transfusion for gram-negative septicemia to be effective in a controlled clinical study. For those patients with a count less than $100/\mu l$, preventive granulocyte transfusion has been recommended, although the prophylactic use of granulocytes has not yet been demonstrated to be effective in most clinical situations. However, Clift (1978) has reported granulocyte transfusion to be effective for prevention of infection in patients receiving bone marrow transplants. Alavi (1977) has reviewed the use of granulocyte transfusion for infection in acute leukemia.

Since the half-life of granulocytes in the circulation is only about 6 to 8 hours, the therapeutic effect may not be obtained unless a minimum of 10^{10} granulocytes are transfused daily to an average adult for at least four to five days. A significant rise in circulating granulocyte level post-transfusion is usually not observed. ABO-compatible granulocytes appear to be essential for a successful therapeutic response, while the importance of HLA compatibility remains unclear. Because preformed leukoagglutinins in the recipient's plasma have been found in some studies

(Herzig, 1975) to result in negligible intravascular recovery of transfused granulocytes, a crossmatch for leukoagglutinating antibodies has been used by some investigators to exclude donor-recipient pairs.

Granulocytes should be transfused as soon as possible after collection; arbitrarily we have used six hours as a cut-off time with storage at room temperature. Granulocytes should be infused via a standard administration set, ordinarily over three to four hours to minimize reactions. Careful observation of the patient by nursing personnel, with a physician readily available for reactions, is necessary. Granulocyte counts should be performed immediately after completion of transfusion, at which time a small (200 to 2000/μl) increment should be observed. When such is not observed, patient and product factors causing such failure should be investigated. The presence of an increment more than 12 hours after transfusion suggests endogenous production due to bone marrow recovery rather than successful transfusion.

Granulocyte transfusion is often accompanied by chills and fever and sometimes by severe hypotension. These reactions can be minimized by giving no more than 10^{10} cells/hour and by administering to the patient meperidine hydrochloride (25 to 50 mg parenterally to an adult) or protecting him with corticosteroids (e.g., Solu-Cortef IV prior to infusion). Less commonly, pulmonary reactions (dyspnea, cough, cyanosis, pulmonary infiltrates) may be observed; these are attributed to leukocyte adherence or clumping in pulmonary capillaries. Other reactions can also occur, e.g., urticaria, bacterial contamination causing sepsis, hemolytic reactions due to incompatible red blood cells in the granulocyte concentrate, hepatitis, and delayed graft-versus-host disease.

Transfusion of plasma components and/or derivatives

Fresh Frozen Plasma (FFP). FFP is indicated in patients with hypovolemia and/or a deficiency in coagulation factors (see Chap. 33). FFP is often used to treat shock and to supplement massive transfusions and exchange transfusions. FFP has the risk of transmitting viral hepatitis and requires 20 minutes or more for thawing. If Factor VIII has been removed in the preparation of cryoprecipitate, the unit should be so labeled.

Cryoprecipitate (Cryo). Cryoprecipitate is indicated in patients with Factor VIII deficiency, such as hemophiliacs and those with von Willebrand's disease, as well as patients with hypofibrinogenemia from various causes. The potency of each unit of cryo varies greatly, but the average value must be 80 units of Factor VIII (the majority range from 60 to 120 units). Lyophilized AHF concentrate, which may contain up to 1000 units/vial, is available and is suitable when many units are required to prevent or to stop hemorrhage. The lyophilized form does not require a freezer for storage but has a greater risk of transmitting hepatitis and may contain strong anti-A and anti-B.

About a 30 per cent Factor VIII activity level is required for major surgery. Since the half-life *in vivo* is about 12 hours, a level of 50 to 60 per cent may be required several hours before the surgery. If a patient has only a 20 per cent activity and a 60 per cent activity is desirable, then the increase is 60 per cent minus 20 per cent = 40 per cent. If the patient is about 50 kg in weight, the plasma volume should be approximately 50 × 40 = 2000 ml, and the total number of units required would be 2000 × 40 per cent = 800 units. If the activity of each bag is roughly 100 units, then 8 bags of cryo are required. As a rough guide, one bag of cryo with about 100 units of AHF activity will increase the AHF activity about 5 per cent in a 100-lb. recipient. In the case of a patient with inhibitors to AHF who is hemorrhaging, larger doses may have to be tried. If unsuccessful, plasma exchange (e.g., therapeutic plasmapheresis) or other experimental therapy may be attempted to remove the AHF inhibitor.

Since many factors are involved, namely, actual blood volume, activity in each bag, and response of the patient, this type of estimation is only approximate. Determination of AHF activity post transfusion or a bleeding time in von Willebrand's patients is the best guide for the amount of cryo required.

Albumin. Albumin is probably the most widely used plasma derivative (Tullis, 1977). It is indicated in patients with hypovolemia, especially in shock, with severe burns, with cerebral edema, and with hyperbilirubinemia. Albumin preparations that have been heated at 60°C. for 10 hours have no risk of transmitting hepatitis. Since albumin is readily available, it is often used for treatment of shock. Albumin contains 96 per cent albumin and is available in 5 per cent and 25 per cent solutions. Plasma protein fraction (PPF), which contains 83 per cent albumin and 17 per cent globulin, is available in 5 per cent preparations (Table 43–51).

Plasma albumin with a half-life of about 17 days represents 50 to 60 per cent of circulating plasma protein and 80 per cent of plasma colloid osmotic pressure. Twenty-five grams (100 ml of a 25 per cent w/v solution) is the osmotic equivalent of 500 ml (2 units) of citrated plasma. It is also used to correct hypoproteinemia states with hypoalbuminemia secondary to (1) decreased or impaired protein intake, (2) excessive protein loss into gastrointestinal tract lumen or via kidneys, (3) decreased hepatic synthesis, (4) repeated removal of large amounts of transudates from peritoneal or pleural spaces, or (5) draining exudative wounds and transudation from large weeping surfaces, e.g., pemphigus or burns. In general, however, there is only mild improvement of patients with nephrotic syndrome and virtually none with protein-losing enteropathies after transfusion of albumin. Furthermore, albumin offers virtually no demonstrable value in the general supportive management of the hypoproteinemia of cirrhosis (Tullis, 1977).

Immune Serum Globulin (ISG). ISG is used to prevent or modify type A hepatitis and other infections. Since type A hepatitis can also be transmitted parenterally and since ISG may be effective in prevention of hepatitis B, ISG is recommended for accidental needle sticks in the laboratory. ISG is also used to supplement globulins in patients with hypogammaglobulinemia. ISG is available in a 16.5 per cent solution. It must be administered intramuscularly.

Specific Immunoglobulins. Anti-Rh_0(D) immunoglobulin (RIG) is widely used for the prevention of Rh_0(D) immunization in Rh_0-negative women with an Rh_0-positive baby or for those Rh_0-negative persons who have been accidentally transfused with Rh_0-positive erythrocytes or who have received Rh_0(D)-positive platelets. One vial contains 300 μg anti-Rh_0(D) and is recommended for 15 ml of packed erythrocytes or 30 ml of whole blood. Patients receiving multiple doses of anti-Rh_0(D) immunoglobulin may have a mild febrile reaction and a slight increase in bilirubin level. Additional discussion will be found in "Immunization Associated with Pregnancy" (p. 1501).

Specific anti-HBsAg hyperimmune serum is available, but its effectiveness in preventing or modifying type B hepatitis has not yet been fully established. It is believed to be useful in needle stick exposures to hepatitis B, but its use in other situations is less clearly indicated.

PRETRANSFUSION TESTING

Blood specimens from the recipient

1. The recipient must be positively identified by his or her first and last name plus hospital number or other available identifying number. This must correspond to the name on the wristband. In some hospitals, an additional wristband is used to identify the recipient from whom the blood has been drawn for compatibility testing.
2. Specimens must be labeled at the bedside with the full name of the patient, date, identification number, and the initials of the person drawing blood.
3. If the blood sample has to be drawn from intravenous (IV) tubing, it should be flushed with saline and the first 5 ml of blood discarded.
4. When additional transfusions are requested, a new specimen should be obtained at each 48-hour interval to identify an incompatibility from an antibody developed by an anamnestic response (see Chap. 34).
5. Hemolyzed blood samples should be avoided because they may mask hemolysis of donor erythrocytes in the crossmatch.
6. Normally a clotted specimen is used; however, if the patient has been heparinized, the blood specimen should be treated with protamine or glass beads to induce clotting.
7. The patient's erythrocytes may have to be washed if the patient has been receiving dextran or PVP or if there are protein abnormalities or strong cold agglutinins. It is good practice to wash red blood cells routinely before testing.
8. If the patient is going to be heparinized or receive PVP or dextran, a blood specimen should be drawn before such treatment.

ABO and Rh_0 typing, and antibody screening

ABO and Rh_0 typing should be done on every recipient before blood is issued. Under extreme emergency conditions we recommend ABO group-specific blood, but a physician may use O Rh_o-negative whole blood or preferably red blood cells (when there is inadequate time to determine ABO). The pretransfusion testing should then be completed subsequently as soon as possible (Oberman, 1978). ABO and Rh_o typing can be performed the same way as for blood donors. However, in this case the D^u test is less critical because the patient would receive Rh_o-negative blood.

Antibody detection or screening in patients is much more important than it is for donors because the patient has two to three liters of plasma, a much greater amount than that found in one unit of blood. Furthermore, weak reacting antibodies can become stronger after blood transfusion owing to a secondary (anamnestic) immune response. Antibody screening for patients must be done with two separate screening red blood cells in order to detect the commonly encountered and clinically significant antibodies (Boral, 1977). The antiglobulin test should be included routinely for antibody screening. An additional enzyme or albumin technique is commonly used. A negative antibody screening procedure does not exclude the presence of irregular antibodies in a patient's serum. For instance, low incidence and narrow thermal range cold antibodies may be missed (Oberman, 1978; Boral, 1977).

Many investigators do not believe that antibodies reacting at room temperature or below are clinically significant, provided that the patient is not under hypothermia or being transfused rapidly with cold blood (Giblett, 1977).

ABO and Rh_o typing and antibody detection (screening) should be done as early as possible, particularly for patients who are going to receive multiple transfusions. In this way, the blood bank can have sufficient time to identify the antibody, if present, and secure the special units of blood required. However, ABO and Rh_o typing with antibody screening may be used without crossmatch for patients who are undergoing the type of surgery which normally requires no blood transfusion. A list of such elective operative procedures and a strategy for ordering blood, which we have advocated and found both acceptable and cost efficient, are shown in Table 43-53.

If the patient's erythrocytes exhibit a positive direct antiglobulin (DAGT) test or if spontaneous agglutination in albumin occurs,

Table 43–53. PROCEDURES FOR WHICH BLOOD IS USUALLY CROSS-MATCHED BUT FOR WHICH TYPE AND SCREEN WOULD APPEAR ADEQUATE*

TYPE OF SURGERY	PROCEDURE
General	Cholecystectomy; exploratory laparotomy; thyroidectomy; parathyroidectomy; parotidectomy; colostomy; vein stripping
Gynecologic	Hysterectomy; uterine suspension; tuboplasty; ovarian wedge resection
Neurosurgery	Laminectomy; ventriculoperitoneal shunt
Orthopedic	Total knee; medial meniscectomy; leg amputation; arthroscopy; removal of hip pin
Otolaryngology	Transantral ethmoidectomy; Caldwell-Luc
Plastic	Reduction mammoplasty; skin flap; skin graft
Urologic	Transurethral resection of the prostate; pyelolithotomy; ureterolithotomy; cystotomy; transurethral resection of bladder tumor; fulguration of bleeding bladder tumor; orchiectomy; orchiopexy; ureteral reimplantation

*From Mintz, 1976.

partial elution at 45°C. may be attempted to remove some of the attached antibodies for successful phenotyping of the patient. The eluted antibodies should also be identified.

Compatibility testing

1. Compatibility testing in a real sense reveals only detectable incompatibility between the recipient and the donor. Except in identical twins and autologous transfusions, no blood can be 100 per cent compatible. Consequently, the term incompatibility testing may be more appropriate.

2. Compatibility testing or crossmatching consists of a major and a minor test.

3. The minor crossmatch is no longer used in many hospitals for erythrocyte transfusions because of the popular use of erythrocyte concentrates and routine antibody screening of donor blood. However, when a large volume of plasma is used, as may be the case with platelet or granulocyte pheresis concentrates or with fresh frozen plasma, es-

pecially for children, a minor crossmatch is desirable. Advocates of the minor crossmatch also point out that it confirms ABO typing, reflects a positive DAGT, and may permit recognition of a new blood group factor.

4. The minor crossmatch consists of testing the donor's plasma or serum against erythrocytes of the patient. As noted previously, it is useful to double check the ABO compatibility and occasionally to test for strong or hemolytic anti-A or anti-B (antibodies) in group O blood. The minor crossmatch may also reveal the presence of donor antibodies against low incidence antigens such as anti-C^W and anti-Wr^a.

5. The major crossmatch consists of testing the patient's serum or plasma against the donor's erythrocytes. Serum is normally preferable except under certain conditions where only plasma is available. In such cases, plasma can be converted into serum by the addition of calcium, thrombin, or glass beads. Patient's serum for crossmatch should not be inactivated.

6. It is recommended that donor erythrocytes be washed before testing. The possible presence of soluble antigens such as Le^a, Sd^a, and Ch^a, which may interfere with the testing, will then be minimized.

7. Segments from the blood bag are recommended rather than tubes attached to the bag as these segments are the true representative of the bag's contents.

8. The two-tube crossmatch is preferable to the one-tube crossmatch. In the former, one tube is incubated at room temperature in saline medium while the other is incubated at 37°C. in an albumin medium or with a one-stage enzyme technique. After 15 to 30 minutes incubation, the tubes are centrifuged and read. If negative, the second tube is converted to the antiglobulin test and read microscopically.

9. In an incompatible crossmatch, the presence of rouleaux should be ruled out before additional studies are conducted.

10. The autocontrol must be set up at the same time to differentiate alloantibodies from autoantibodies, a very important consideration in the selection of blood for transfusion.

11. When the autocontrol is negative, alloantibodies are suspected in an incompatible crossmatch. Anti-A_1 or anti-HI may be suspected if antibodies are reacting strongly at room temperature or below. Warm alloantibodies of many varieties may be suspected among those reacting strongly at 37°C. or with the antiglobulin test. They should be identified if possible before the patient receives any transfusions.

12. In emergency situations, random crossmatches may be performed at the same time as the antibody identification.

13. When the autocontrol is positive, autoantibodies or a positive antiglobulin test (often due to medication) should be suspected.

14. The possible presence of alloantibodies masked by autoantibodies should be ruled out before transfusion of a patient is attempted. This is best accomplished by autoabsorption when a sufficient number of erythrocytes is available. However, autoabsorption should be utilized only if the patient has not been transfused in the previous four months. Absorbed serum or specific eluates should be used for antibody identification or crossmatching.

15. Should the patient have previously identified antibodies, such as anti-K, anti-Fy^a, or anti-Jk^a, the compatible units should be typed for the specific antigen(s) to avoid a delayed transfusion reaction. Only units negative for the appropriate antigen should be used. This caution is not as necessary for ordinary room temperature or cold-reacting antibodies such as anti-Le^a, -Le^b, -P, -M, -N, or others.

16. Should the patient have autoantibodies without alloantibodies, transfusion of least incompatible units selected by titration crossmatch and reacting less strongly than the autocontrol may be attempted. Patients can usually tolerate such transfusions unless an underlying alloantibody is present but missed.

17. Patients with strong cold autoagglutinins should not be subjected to hypothermia, since this can induce a hemolytic transfusion reaction.

18. The compatibility test *in vivo* may be attempted under special conditions where patient requires blood in the presence of an incompatible crossmatch

and elucidation of the nature of the incompatibility has not been achieved or compatible blood cannot be found. Red cell survival studies using erythrocytes tagged with radioactive chromium (^{51}Cr) have been attempted in the more sophisticated hospitals.

For platelet concentrates that have a large volume of plasma when stored at room temperature, not only must volume be considered in terms of recipient's condition and blood volume, but ABO matching becomes more important for the plasma than the few red blood cells present; then anti-A is more important than anti-B.

INFUSION OF BLOOD COMPONENTS

Proper identification

Although a great deal of attention has been given to insure that a unit of blood is correctly identified, correct identification of a recipient has not been so emphasized. Before a unit of blood is transfused, many people are involved. Consequently, transcription error may occur in one of the many steps. The patient's full name, hospital number, and transfusion number (in some hospitals) must be clearly identified in each step of the transaction.

The majority of fatal transfusion reactions are due to *ABO INCOMPATIBILITY*. Therefore, ABO grouping of the patient from the correct specimen is of vital importance. In some hospitals, additional ABO grouping is done at the bedside and the patient is also checked by his or her ABO group. It should be re-emphasized that ABO compatibility is of utmost importance. The wrong patient may receive ABO-compatible blood, while the right patient cannot receive ABO-incompatible blood. This of course does not mean that the identification of the patient should be ignored. An identification of the patient by ABO group, especially as part of the armband, is highly recommended.

Before a unit of blood component is infused into the patient, the full name of the patient, identification code(s) identical to that on the transfusion request, the ABO group of the component, and Rh must be checked with that of the patient. In rare cases, under emergency conditions, Rh_o-positive blood can be given to an Rh_o-negative person (p. 1474).

Emergency situations (often in ER, OR, or intensive care units) are most commonly associated with a failure in proper identification. Personnel involved in blood specimen collection for crossmatching and in blood infusion must be particularly cautious at these times.

Conditions affecting the infusion of blood components

Intravenous Fluid. Only normal saline is suitable for use in blood transfusion. It is used to start the blood transfusion and can be used to dilute erythrocyte concentrates. Five per cent dextrose in water may cause red blood cell aggregation or hemolysis, while lactated Ringer's solution may cause clotting. Neither can or should replace normal saline. No medication should be added to or administered in the same line with blood or components. Blood components except platelets and thawed cryoprecipitate or fresh frozen plasma should be stored in a monitored blood bank refrigerator until immediately before transfusion. Therefore, one should not ask for a blood component from the blood bank until the infusion is underway or intravenous fluid has been started (Kienle, 1978).

Filters. Blood components should be transfused through a filter to eliminate infusion of fibrin clots and other particulate debris (see Table 43–50). Most standard blood and platelet transfusion sets have filters with a pore size of approximately 170 microns. Wide variations exist in the surface area of the filter and the arrangement of the filter and drip chamber. Under normal conditions one filter can be used for two to four units of blood; however, one must judge the condition of the filter and the total time involved and change the filter accordingly.

Microaggregates which form progressively in whole blood or packed red blood cells after one week of storage at 4°C. consist of platelets, cell fragments, and nuclei of granulocytes ranging from 13 to 100 μ in diameter. Although the effect of these microaggregates remains unsettled, no one believes that a recipient should receive a large number of microaggregates. Special filters with pore sizes between 20 and 40 μ for screening out particulate material have been developed (see Table 43–50).

Microaggregate filters are available in two basic types, using the adhesiveness of Dacron or Nylon fibers or the filtration effect of polyurethane foam or polyester mesh (see Table 43–50). There are filters using both fibers and mesh. The most effective filter is the Dacron

4

wool filter (Swank In-Line Blood Filter, IL-200 Pioneer Filters, Inc., Beaverton, Oregon) (Greenwalt, 1977; Solis, 1972) and the cotton wool filter (Diepenhorst, 1975). Microaggregate filters are recommended in cardiopulmonary bypass (to prevent cerebral embolism), in massive transfusions with blood more than one week old (large numbers of microaggregates), and in patients with pulmonary dysfunction. Microaggregate filters should not be used with platelet concentrates or fresh whole blood because viable platelets will be filtered out (excluded) from the infusion.

Blood Warmers. Rapid infusion of large volumes of cold blood may precipitate ventricular arrhythmia and even death of the patient (Dybkjaer, 1964). A blood warmer is recommended for patients receiving many units of cold blood in a short period of time, in exchange transfusions and transfusion of premature infants, and for patients with strong cold autoagglutinins. The temperature of the blood warmer should be maintained at about 37°C. No hemolysis or increase in plasma potassium level will result at this temperature; however, when the blood temperature exceeds 40°C., hemolysis may occur. We have found the Fenwal dry heat blood warmer (No. 4R4305) incorporating blood warming bag (4C2416) acceptable for precise regulation of blood temperature and flow rate. This system warms blood from 4°C. and maintains a range of 32 to 37°C. at flow rates up to 150 ml per minute. When more than 20 units of blood are transfused into a patient, in addition to a blood warmer, NaHCO₃ infusion may be used and may reduce the mortality (Howland, 1957). Warming the patient is recommended for those with cold agglutinin disease and in transfusion of patients with circulatory overload (dilation of peripheral blood vessels can accommodate over 200 ml of blood) (Mollison, 1972).

Speed of Infusion. In most administration sets, 15 drops equals 1 ml. At a rate of 60 drops/min, $60/15 \times 60 = 240$ ml of blood can be transfused in one hour. The duration of transfusion can thus be estimated by the rate of infusion. Under normal conditions for an average adult without cardiopulmonary dysfunction, one unit of blood should be infused within one to two hours (Boral, 1977). Blood transfusion should not be used to keep intravenous lines open, and extended time for infusions—unless critical for a patient with congestive heart failure—should be avoided. Blood is an ideal culture medium and when it warms up over several hours at room temperature while being infused may allow growth of bacteria that may enter the system during blood collection and/or infusion. In massive bleeding, the rate of infusion can be accelerated by the use of large needles at more than one site. In patients with severe anemia or heart failure, the rate of infusion should be reduced. The concurrent use of diuretics and/or digitalis may be useful. For the average size adult, furosemide, 20 to 40 mg intravenously for one to two units of red blood cells, has been most effective in our experience. However, it may be necessary to transfuse only half of one unit at one time. The remaining half should be stored in a blood bank refrigerator and used later within 24 hours. As a rule, during the first 15 minutes of transfusion, the rate of infusion should be slow in order to observe any patient reaction, especially when an incompatible or least incompatible unit is being transfused or when previous transfusion reactions have been reported. Careful observation of the patient and recording of vital signs immediately and after 15 minutes should preclude overlooking an early serious hemolytic transfusion reaction (Boral, 1977).

Monitoring the patient

Transfusion is a serious and potentially hazardous treatment. Reactions can be fatal if proper precautions are not observed. In the United States, any fatal transfusion reaction must be reported immediately (within 24 hours) to the Food and Drug Administration. Most transfusion reactions develop within 30 minutes of transfusion. If the patient is being monitored carefully by medical or nursing personnel, the majority of fatal transfusion reactions can be avoided by prompt, early, and appropriate action. A patient's vital signs should be taken and recorded immediately before the transfusion to serve as a baseline, then every 15 minutes after the beginning of the transfusion for at least three times, and at the end of the transfusion. When the patient is under general anesthesia, hypotension, hemoglobinuria, and unexplained oozing may be the only signs of a hemolytic transfusion reaction.

We have reported favorable experience with an outpatient transfusion clinic in a hospital based blood bank and transfusion service which is responsive to increasing demands for ambulatory medical care, as well as cost-effective and satisfying to patients (Boral, 1977).

THERAPEUTIC PHERESIS AND PLASMA EXCHANGE

Thomas A. Ruma, M.D.

Although the technique of plasmapheresis was first introduced in 1914, it did not gain widespread acceptance for nearly half a century. The current popularity can be attributed to technical advances that have overcome the problems of slow collection, processing, and storage.

Plasmapheresis may be performed for two reasons: first, for collection of plasma for fractionation into therapeutic components or derivatives or for production of various laboratory reagents, and second, for therapeutic reasons. Therapeutic pheresis or plasma exchange and its applications warrant further consideration.

Therapeutic plasmapheresis is a procedure in which whole blood is removed from a patient, plasma separated and removed, and the red blood cells alone, or in combination with other blood components, reinfused into the patient.

METHODS

Technically, plasmapheresis is performed using manual bag systems or centrifugal blood separation devices (NCI-IBM model 2990, Armonk, New York; Haemonetics, model 10, 30 or 50, Natick, Mass.; Aminco Cell Separator, American Instrument Company, Silver Spring, Maryland).

The advent of centrifugal blood separation systems allows removal of larger quantities of plasma and permits continuous and automatic return of red blood cells and other components to the patient (Pineda, 1977). In general, type-specific fresh frozen plasma (FFP) or albumin is used as replacement therapy for plasma removed.

APPLICATIONS

The ability to reconstruct or manipulate an abnormal circulating blood supply by means of plasmapheresis is a relatively new concept named "hemoengineering" (Pineda, 1977).

Currently, therapeutic plasmapheresis is performed to remove specific toxic or disease-causing substances from the plasma of patients. These "substances" consist of specific antibodies in excess, antigen-antibody complexes, or toxic metabolites. Table 43-54 outlines the therapeutic application of pheresis and plasma exchange. Many of these are experimental treatment modalities.

The most common role for therapeutic plasmapheresis is adjunctive therapy in diseases caused or complicated by circulating antibodies in excess. This is probably best exemplified by Waldenström's macroglobulinemia or multiple myeloma complicated by the hyperviscosity syndrome. In such patients immunosuppressive therapy alone is often not sufficient for removal of excess circulating antibody.

Hyperviscosity syndrome (HVS)

Viscosity is the property of fluids to resist flow. In protein solutions viscosity is influenced by the concentration and the intrinsic viscosity of the individual proteins in solution (Bloch, 1973). The intrinsic viscosity of the individual protein is determined by molecular size, weight, and shape of the molecule. This is exemplified by the fact that IgM is associated commonly with the hyperviscosity syndrome (HVS). The most likely explanation for this phenomenon is that the high molecular weight, unusual shape, and interaction of IgM with red blood cells cause RBC-IgM-RBC aggregates (rouleaux) in the circulation (Bloch, 1973). It should be noted that approximately 80 per cent of IgM is confined to the vascular space, compared with 40 per cent of IgG; hence, IgM can cause more of a viscosity problem if present in excess (Bloch, 1973). In fact, Waldenström's macroglobulinemia is the most common cause of HVS (85 to 90 per cent of cases of HVS). Multiple myeloma with IgA and IgG M-components accounts for the remainder of HVS caused by paraprotein.

Signs and Symptoms of HVS. Pathogenic factors causing signs and symptoms of HVS are multiple (McGrath, 1976). Increased serum viscosity and sluggish blood flow probably cause relative hypoxia in certain critical organs. Plasmapheresis has been shown to be effective in ameliorating many of these signs and symptoms.

Ocular manifestations vary from minor disturbances in vision to complete blindness. On fundoscopic examination, distention and tor-

Table 43–54. THERAPEUTIC APPLICATION OF PHERESIS AND PLASMA EXCHANGE*

ELEMENTS TO BE REMOVED	MEDICAL CONDITIONS
Excess: Erythrocytes	Polycythemia, hemosiderosis†
Leukocytes	Selected type of leukemias†
Platelets	Thrombocythemia†
Plasma protein	Waldenström's macroglobulinemia, multiple myeloma, IgM, IgG, IgA
Antibodies: To erythrocytes	High titer anti-D in pregnancy
	Against high incidence antigens
	Against multiple antigens
	Autoantibodies
To platelets	Idiopathic thrombocytopenia purpura
	No compatible platelet donor
To hemophilic Factor VIII	Hemophilia A with Factor VIII inhibitor
To basement membrane	Goodpasture's syndrome
To acetylcholine receptors	Myasthenia gravis
Complex with antigens	Systemic lupus erythematosus
	Thrombotic thrombocytopenic purpura
	Certain types of carcinomas
Microorganisms:	Septicemia uncontrollable by antibiotics or granulocyte transfusion
Toxin:	Acute hepatic necrosis

*To achieve symptomatic relief or to save patient's life during a critical period. (Courtesy of Dr. Chang Ling Lee.)
† Cytapheresis

tuosity of the retinal veins frequently present a beaded, "string of sausage" appearance. Flame-shaped hemorrhages, papilledema, and microaneurysms are other findings (Luxenborg, 1970). Hematologic manifestations include a mucocutaneous hemorrhagic tendency (e.g., gingival bleeding, epistaxis) and anemia secondary to decreased erythrocyte survival (Lackner, 1973; Cline, 1963). Neurologically, a spectrum from headaches to dizziness, stupor, or coma has been described. Cardiovascular manifestations due to hypervolemia (e.g., congestive heart failure) are rare. Subjective symptoms include weakness, malaise, and anorexia.

Laboratory Diagnosis of HVS. The diagnosis of HVS is made by appropriate clinical symptoms and signs, with evidence of increased serum viscosity. The viscosity of serum is compared to that of water at 37°C. (Ostwald Viscosimeter; Williams, 1977). The normal viscosity of serum relative to water is 1.4 to 1.8 (see Chap. 30, p. 1086). In general, serum viscosity levels between 2 and 4 rarely cause symptoms. A few patients with levels of 4 to 5 have symptoms, and most patients with levels of 5 to 8 are symptomatic. If serum viscosity levels are greater than 8, nearly all patients will have symptoms.

It should be noted, however, that the serum viscosity and associated clinical symptoms will vary from patient to patient, depending on the paraprotein, the cardiovascular status of the patient, and the hematocrit.

MISCELLANEOUS INDICATIONS FOR THERAPEUTIC PLASMAPHERESIS

Several other conditions have infrequently been managed by plasmapheresis to remove supposed detrimental antibodies in excess. In these conditions, the use of plasmapheresis represents an experimental therapeutic modality.

In hemophilia A patients refractory to Factor VIII concentrates because of a high titer factor VIII inhibitor, therapeutic plasmapheresis of the Factor VIII inhibitor has been of significant benefit and, on occasion, life saving (Edson, 1973). In autoimmune hemolytic anemia, circulating antibodies or antigen-antibody complexes capable of inflicting damage to red blood cells may be removed. Similarly, anti-$Rh_0(D)$ antibodies in severe Rh hemolytic disease of the newborn (HDN) have been removed from the mother's plasma with good clinical results.

Therapeutic plasmapheresis was performed on eight high-risk obstetric patients with a history of HDN (Graham-Pole, 1977). Phereses were performed before 28 weeks of gestation, when intrauterine transfusion is particularly hazardous. All eight patients had elevated amniotic fluid bilirubin levels as well as elevated $Rh_o(D)$ antibody titers. Therapeutic plasmapheresis reduced the amniotic fluid bilirubin and $Rh_o(D)$ antibody titers significantly in seven of the eight patients.

The removal of autoantibodies by therapeutic plasmapheresis has been attempted in idiopathic thrombocytopenic purpura (ITP) and recently in myasthenia gravis and Goodpasture's syndrome (Dau, 1977; Branda, 1975; Lockwood, 1976). In ITP, anti-platelet antibody or antigen-antibody complexes damaging to platelets can be removed. Antibodies to the acetylcholine receptors at the motor end plate of neuromuscular junctions have been implicated as the pathogenic factor in myasthenia gravis. It has recently been demonstrated that therapeutic plasmapheresis in conjunction with immunosuppressive therapy provides marked improvement compared to immunosuppressive therapy alone (Dau, 1977). Titers of antibody to acetylcholine receptors decreased to an average of 40 per cent of the initial titer after three plasmaphereses. In Goodpasture's syndrome removal of anti-glomerular basement membrane and anti-lung basement membrane antibodies is possible by therapeutic plasmapheresis.

Removal of antigen-antibody complexes in systemic lupus erythematosus has yielded variable clinical results (Moran, 1977; Jones, 1976). In thrombotic thrombocytopenic purpura (TTP), removal of either soluble immune complexes or some other circulating toxic substances may be the reason for remission in several cases described (Bukowski, 1977).

In the therapeutic approach to neoplastic disease, plasmapheresis may be of benefit in several ways. First, plasmapheresis may be used to remove specific or non-specific "blocking factors" interfering with chemotherapy and/or immunotherapy (e.g., blocking antibodies, antigen-antibody complexes, or other plasma proteins). It has been suggested that these "blocking factors" can obstruct or suppress normal host immunologic response by several mechanisms (Israel, 1976; 1977). Removal of these "blocking factors" by plasmapheresis and subsequent administration of immunotherapy has resulted in objective reduction of tumor size in several types of malignancy (Israel, 1977). Secondly, plasmapheresis may be of benefit in removing anti-platelet or anti-leukocyte antibodies that may arise in patients on chemotherapy who must receive repeated platelet and leukocyte transfusions (Branda, 1975). Therapeutic plasmapheresis can best be performed just prior to the needed platelet or leukocyte transfusions.

Therapeutic pheresis and plasma exchange for the removal of circulating toxic substances in acute hepatic failure has been studied (Buckner, 1973). In this limited study of four patients, with fulminant non-alcoholic liver necrosis and coma, three patients survived after intensive plasmapheresis.

COMPLICATIONS

Repeated plasmapheresis of normal donors at the rate of two units once or twice weekly (500 to 1000 ml plasma) produces a decrease in total serum protein during the initial six months (Friedman, 1975). This is mainly due to decreased immunoglobulins. However, the levels of immunoglobulins still remain in the normal range. With more intensive plasmapheresis and the use of centrifugal blood separators, thrombocytopenia may be a problem.

Immediate complications include transient hypotension, bradycardia, urticarial reactions, and hypocalcemia. The transient hypotension occurs most frequently at the end of the procedure and can be ameliorated with fluid replacement. The urticarial reactions and hypocalcemia are most likely due to allergens and CPD, respectively, contained in the replacement fresh frozen plasma. The development of viral hepatitis from the use of fresh frozen plasma as replacement therapy is another complication. The use of albumin or PPF as replacement therapy rather than the FFP decreases these complications but is more costly (see Table 43-51).

Prior to and following each pheresis session, several parameters have been monitored in studies using centrifugal blood separators (Israel, 1977) (Table 43-55).

Table 43-55. LABORATORY DETERMINATIONS COMMONLY MONITORED DURING PLASMAPHERESIS

CBC with differential white count
Platelet count
Serum calcium
Prothrombin time
Partial thromboplastin time
Serum viscosity
Serum electrolytes
Serum protein electrophoresis
Hepatitis B surface antigen (HBsAg)

SUMMARY

Since 1960 the use of therapeutic plasmapheresis has become diversified and intensified from its use in the hyperviscosity syndrome of Waldenström's macroglobulinemia to its exciting preliminary results in many other conditions. With the advent of centrifugal blood separators and the ability to reconstruct an abnormal circulating blood volume, physicians may be able to modify diseases associated with high levels of specific antibodies, antigen-antibody complexes, or toxic metabolites. The recent demonstration that therapeutic plasmapheresis in cancer patients may result in improved immune responsiveness and more effective immunotherapy will undoubtedly generate further interest and investigation (Israel, 1977).

Transfusion Reactions

Since the transfusion of blood is accompanied by significant morbidity and mortality estimated to be about 0.5 per cent of transfusions (with 6.5 million transfusions dispensed annually), a review of the untoward reactions to transfusion is warranted (Myhre, 1978).

Hemolytic transfusion reactions

Causes

1. The blood and recipient are mismatched, usually owing to clerical errors.
2. An incompatible crossmatch is missed by the technologist (much less often).
3. The crossmatch may be compatible under normal conditions but the patient has been subjected to hypothermia, activating potent cold agglutinins which lyse his own or transfused erythrocytes.
4. The antibody level of the recipient may be undetectable at the time of crossmatch but increases and becomes potent after the transfusion of erythrocytes with homologous antigens (anamnestic response) and hemolyzes the transfused cells. This is called a delayed hemolytic transfusion reaction because the shortened erythrocyte survival (hemolysis) follows the transfusion after a time interval of several days to two weeks. Such patients have most often received multiple transfusions, especially with trauma, but it may also occur in children with chronic anemia receiving intermittent hemotherapy.
5. Erythrocytes of the recipient may be defective, as in paroxysmal nocturnal hemoglobinuria; the erythrocytes hemolyze in the presence of complement in the transfused plasma.
6. The recipient may have a malfunctioning heart valve prosthesis causing hemolysis. Distilled water may enter the circulation as a result of irrigation of the bladder during prostate surgery. If the patient is also receiving a transfusion simultaneously, this may lead one to suspect erroneously a hemolytic transfusion reaction.
7. Erythrocytes of the patient may be hemolyzed by certain toxins such as those resulting from *Clostridium welchii* infection coincidental with transfusion.
8. Erythrocytes of the donor or patient may be defective in G6PD. If medication such as vitamin K, sulfonamide, or phenacetin is given, hemolysis may result.
9. Frozen-thawed erythrocytes, which may contain high levels of residual glycerol after inadequate washing, will hemolyze after being transfused.
10. The unit of blood may contain hemoglobin as a result of freezing (improper storage), contamination, or other mistreatment which may occur in collection, storage, and transportation.

Pathologic Physiology of Immune Hemolysis in Vivo.

Hemolytic reactions due to antigen-antibody reactions are designated immune hemolysis. Immune hemolysis *in vivo* is divided into two basic types (Table 43-56 and Fig. 43-15), intravascular and extravascular. Antibodies, such as anti-A, anti-B, anti-I, anti-Le^a, and anti-P+P$_1$, which can activate complement can cause intravascular hemolysis if sufficiently active *in vivo* at body temperature, i.e., wide thermal range. Symptoms such as flushing, pain at injection site, shock, and hypotension may be related to activation of complement and the subsequent release of histamine, serotonin, or kinins. Hemoglobin released from the lysed erythrocytes combines with haptoglobin and usually deposits in the liver, where it is subsequently split into iron and bilirubin. Since the amount of haptoglobin is limited, hemoglobin can also be handled in alternative ways. The heme released can combine with albumin to form methemalbumin or combine with hemopexin. It is then processed in the liver into bilirubin and free iron. In the laboratory, one can demonstrate the presence of free plasma hemoglobin (or in the urine when plasma level is above the renal threshold), a decrease in haptoglobin, hemopexin, and albumin binding capacity with an increase in lactate dehydrogenase, hemoglobinuria, hemosiderinuria, and a positive DAGT with a minor population of agglutinates. Serum bilirubin may be increased four to six hours later (Fig. 43-16).

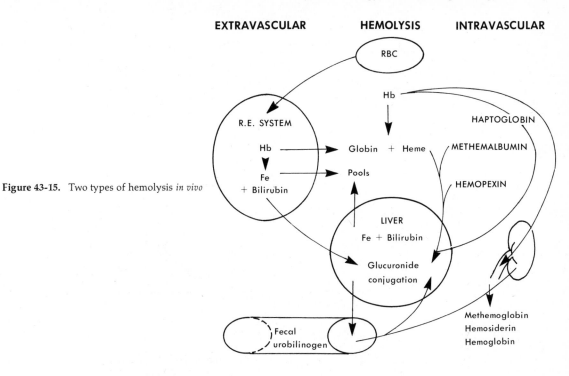

Figure 43-15. Two types of hemolysis *in vivo*

Most IgG antibody-coated erythrocytes are destroyed extravascularly, mainly through phagocytosis in the reticuloendothelial system of the spleen. Complement-coated erythrocytes are similarly destroyed, but primarily in the liver. Some IgG antibodies may activate complement *in vivo*, such as some anti-K, anti-Fy[a], and anti-Jk[a] and cause the complement and IgG-coated erythrocytes to be destroyed predominately in the liver. As stated previously, other IgG antibody-coated erythrocytes are destroyed primarily in the spleen (Mollison, 1972). Hemolytic transfusion reactions may not be evident until 7 to 10 days post transfusion. Anti-E and anti-c are not infrequent causes and anti-M, anti-Lu[a], anti-K, anti-Ce, anti-Jk[b], anti-Jk[a], anti-k, and anti-U have also been implicated (Mollison, 1972). Such delayed hemolytic transfusion reactions are often manifested solely or primarily by an unexplained post-transfusion decrease in hematocrit (Solanki, 1978). Pineda (1978) has reviewed the Mayo Clinic experience with 23 cases of delayed hemolytic transfusion reaction over a 10-year period. Death occurred in three patients and in one case hemolysis led to disseminated intravascular coagulation syndrome. Fever was the most

Figure 43-16. Laboratory findings in intravascular hemolysis. Positive direct antiglobulin test and presence of minor population of agglutinates are not listed. (Modified from Huestis, 1976.)

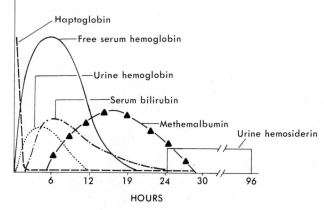

Table 43–56. MECHANISM OF IMMUNE HEMOLYTIC
TRANSFUSION REACTIONS

KEY FACTORS	POSSIBLE MECHANISM	LABORATORY FINDINGS	SYMPTOMS AND SIGNS
IgM antibodies	Primarily intravascular hemolysis (activation of complement)	Plasma Hgb ↑ Haptoglobin ↓ Hemopexin ↓ Methemalbumin ↑ Hemoglobinuria +	Chill, fever Hemoglobinuria* Oliguria
IgG antibodies	Primarily extravascular hemolysis (phagocytosis)	Direct AGT + Bilirubin ↑ (Liver function ↓) Hematocrit ↓	Anuria Jaundice
C3a C5a	Hemodynamic alternation	Histamine Serotonin Kinins	Flushing Pain Shock Hypotension*
Platelets Hageman factor	Disseminated intravascular coagulation	Coagulation factors ↓	Bleeding*

*Only signs under general anesthesia.

frequent presenting symptom in their series, and all but one demonstrated a positive DAGT.

Transfusion reactions related to leukocytes and platelets

Chills and fever are the most common symptoms of a transfusion reaction and are usually due to leukocytes contained in blood components. They are usually mild. However, since fever may be part of the symptomatology of a hemolytic transfusion reaction as well, chills and fever should be evaluated as a potential hemolytic transfusion reaction. Fever is more common in patients receiving granulocytes, particularly if prepared by filtration pheresis. Leukoagglutinins and cytotoxic antibodies can often be demonstrated in patients with febrile reactions; the use of leukocyte-poor blood or frozen-thawed red blood cells will usually alleviate these symptoms.

Immunization to HLA antigens and other white cell antigens seems to be the logical explanation for febrile reactions. Patients having repeated platelet transfusions also have a high incidence of febrile reactions. This fact tends to support the above assumption and indicates that platelet-poor erythrocytes may be just as important as leukocyte-poor preparations in preventing this type of reaction. Antipyretics, steroids, and meperidine may be used to relieve symptoms. Hypotension, dyspnea, and pulmonary infiltration have

also been related to the presence of leukocyte antibodies (Andrews, 1976) and may further complicate severe chill and fever reactions.

Transfusion reactions related to plasma proteins

1. The second most common transfusion reaction referred to as allergic is manifested by urticaria, which can be controlled by antihistamines. When unusually extensive or involving oral, pharyngeal, or laryngeal edema, it is also known as an anaphylactoid reaction.
2. The more severe anaphylactic reaction, characterized by dyspnea, hypotension, and flushing of skin, is rare following transfusion. It is also believed to be due to plasma protein hypersensitivity in the recipient.
3. Anti-IgA antibodies have been demonstrated in 86 per cent of subjects who have had anaphylactic or anaphylactoid reactions (Mollison, 1972). There is little evidence that other classes of immunoglobulins cause this type of reaction.
4. Patients lacking plasma IgA are at increased risk of forming anti-IgA antibodies and often have anti-IgA even without known stimulation. These persons should be transfused only with IgA-deficient blood or with frozen-thawed red blood cells or washed erythrocytes from normal donors. When Factor

VIII or fibrinogen is required for such patients, cryoprecipitate prepared from an IgA-deficient donor is indicated.

5. The anaphylactoid reaction is not uncommon following intramuscular injection of serum immune globulins that contain 95 per cent IgG but also a detectable amount of IgA.

6. Treatment of urticarial reactions: When urticaria is not extensive, the patient may be given diphenhydramine hydrochloride (Benadryl) intramuscularly or intravenously (10 to 50 mg for an adult). Prophylactic use of diphenhydramine hydrochloride (50 mg p.o. 1 hour in advance of hemotherapy) will prevent or ameliorate such an allergic reaction to blood or plasma in adult patients with a known history of such reactions. When the urticaria is under control, the transfusion may be resumed.

For more extensive urticaria or an anaphylactoid reaction, blood transfusion should be discontinued and more aggressive therapy begun in the form of Benadryl plus epinephrine and even steroids. Appropriate evaluation of such a patient for IgA status and other forms of hypersensitivity phenomena should be completed before resuming hemotherapy.

Other complications of blood transfusion

Circulatory Overload. A volume of 2 units of whole blood is more than 1 liter, which is about 20 to 25 per cent of the blood volume of an average-size person. Utilization of red blood cells as erythrocyte concentrate can deliver the same red cell mass in nearly half the volume. This should be considered carefully before a transfusion is attempted. Similar precautions should be followed with the use of albumin (each gram of albumin can retain about 20 ml of fluid in the circulatory system) as well as with infusions of a large volume of plasma, either fresh frozen or as suspension medium for large numbers of platelets (due to the plasma volume in platelet concentrates). Sudden increases in the blood volume may precipitate congestive heart failure, particularly in infants and in persons with chronic anemia with underlying heart disease or with renal failure. In such cases, slow infusion of erythrocyte concentrate is definitely recommended; concurrent use of diuretics (p. 1482),

and digitalis, and warming the patient may prevent circulatory overload.

Diseases Transmissible through Blood Transfusion

VIRAL HEPATITIS. Viral hepatitis is by far the most important disease transmitted through blood transfusion. The incidence varies with the source of blood donors, the number of units transfused, and the type of component used.

Accumulated evidence indicates that the incidence of hepatitis in recipients of voluntary blood is lower than that of paid donor blood. As expected, the incidence increases as the number of transfusions increases, such as in patients undergoing open-heart surgery or surgical burn therapy.

Among the various blood components, albumin and globulin preparations are free of agents causing hepatitis if properly prepared (heated at 60°C for 10 hours). Components or derivatives prepared from multiple donors have a higher incidence of causing hepatitis, especially those products such as fibrinogen and Factor II-VII-IX-X complex which have been prohibited in many hospitals. Fibrinogen has been removed from the market.

Among preparations from a single donor, the incidence varies with the amount of plasma in the preparation; the larger the amount of plasma, the greater the chance of hepatitis. Consequently, washed or frozen-thawed erythrocytes which contain only trace amounts of plasma have a minimal chance of transmitting hepatitis. Needless to say, the concentration of the infectious agents (not HBsAg) and the total amount of fluid used for washing play an important role in reducing infection. While the currently available tests for hepatitis are effective only in preventing about 20 per cent of post-transfusion hepatitis cases and while the effectiveness of hyperimmune anti-HBsAg globulin is not yet established, the best available means to reduce the incidence of post-transfusion hepatitis is to use volunteer blood donors as well as to avoid high-risk products, e.g., fibrinogen, pooled plasma, etc.

"POST-PERFUSION SYNDROME." A syndrome clinically resembling infectious mononucleosis may develop two to seven weeks after multiple transfusions, such as in open-heart surgery. There is serologic evidence to indicate that this syndrome is related to the transmission of cytomegalovirus. It is unrealistic to

4

test donor blood for cytomegalovirus as a preventive measure.

MALARIA. A total of 46 cases have been reported in the United States related to blood transfusion between 1958 and 1973 (Huestis, 1976, p. 276). Only two of the implicated donors had been away from an endemic area for malaria for more than three years. A careful history may help to reduce this complication. Current donor standards exclude donors likely to transmit malaria.

SYPHILIS. Spirochetes do not appear to survive in citrated blood at 4°C. for more than 72 hours. Very few cases have been reported following blood transfusion in recent years. When a unit with high-titer antispirochete antibodies is transfused, the recipient may become seropositive for a short time (Mollison, 1972, p. 613). For this reason, donors with a false positive serologic test for syphilis should not be utilized.

OTHER INFECTIONS. Isolated cases have been reported for brucellosis, filariasis, infectious mononucleosis, and toxoplasmosis following blood transfusion. They are extremely rare. Transmission of babesiosis is also a theoretical possibility.

Undesirable Rare Complications Other than Infections

1. Anticoagulants, especially citrate in high concentration, may produce muscle tremor and electrocardiographic changes. This is a rare complication of massive transfusion.
2. Excessive potassium, which increases in plasma of stored whole blood (approximately 1 mmol per liter per day after the first week, i.e., 23 mmol/liter at 21 days) when administered to patients with poor renal function may also produce EKG changes and be harmful.
3. Ammonia and lactic acid accumulated during storage require detoxification in the liver and excretion by the kidneys. Precautions should be taken in patients with hepatorenal deficiency to minimize the use of whole blood and transfuse red blood cells when necessary.
4. Microaggregates have been discussed previously under the use of filters (p. 1472). Bredenberg (1977) has reviewed the relationship between massive blood transfusions and the adult respiratory distress syndrome, noting that clinical evidence is remarkably limited and experimental data controversial.

5. Air embolism is extremely rare since the introduction of plastic bags without an air vent.
6. Hemosiderosis. Each unit of blood contains about 250 mg of iron, while the physiologic loss of iron is only 1 mg/day. Repeated transfusions introduce excessive amounts of exogenous iron which deposit in the reticuloendothelial system, a condition known as hemosiderosis. In the case of hypoplastic anemia requiring repeated blood transfusions (e.g., sickle cell anemia, thalassemia) fresher blood (less than 7 days of storage) should be used so that fewer transfusions are given to the same patient. In severe cases of hemosiderosis, therapeutic phlebotomy has been successful (Mollison, 1972, p. 616). More recently, iron chelating agents have been used in research protocols.

Investigation of transfusion reactions

Documentation. The physician in charge of the patient must be consulted to obtain as much information as possible to define the type of reaction and to guide the investigation. A useful check list is presented in Table 43-57.

Clerical Check. If the patient is suspected of having received the wrong unit of blood, the very first step is to check any possible clerical errors (Table 43-57).

Check the patient's full name, hospital number, transfusion number, and ABO group on the arm band against the information on the blood bag, crossmatching specimens, and blood bank records.

Laboratory Investigation (Table 43-58)

1. Routine tests for every transfusion reaction include (a) observation of any abnormal signs such as hemolysis, hemoglobinemia and/or hemoglobinuria, jaundice, poor clotting or bleeding, cloudy serum or plasma, or foul odor in blood specimens of the patient and the donor; (b) repeat of the ABO and Rh_o typing, direct antiglobulin test, and crossmatching.
2. Special tests are often required for selected cases, but each case should be dealt with individually to determine which additional tests are needed. The presence of strong or hemolytic donor plasma anti-A or anti-B should be ruled out first in a case of a hemolytic transfusion reaction. The presence of

Table 43-57.   INFORMATION ESSENTIAL TO AN INVESTIGATION OF TRANSFUSION REACTION

Patient's name_____ Age_____ Sex_____ Race_____

Admission No._____ Transfusion No._____ Rm No._____ Bed No._____

Physician's name_____ Diagnosis_____

Surgery_____ Hypothermia_____ Irrigation of bladder with_____

Medication: Penicillin_____ Glucose/water_____ Dextran_____ Vit. K_____ Alpha methyldopa_____

　　　　　　Others_____

Previous: Transfusions_____ Pregnancies_____ Allergy_____

Blood group: Patient_____ Donor (No._____) _____

Crossmatching: Major_____ Minor_____

Transfusion: Started_____ Stopped_____ ml infused_____

Pain_____ Dyspnea_____ Cyanosis_____ Vomiting_____ Urticaria_____ Chills_____ Others_____

	Before transfusion		During transfusion		
		15′	30′	60′	others
Temperature	_____	_____	_____	_____	_____
Pulse rate	_____	_____	_____	_____	_____
Blood pressure	_____	_____	_____	_____	_____

Under anesthesia: Untoward oozing_____ Tachycardia_____ Hypotension_____

Urine output_____ ml in_____ hours   Others_____

irregular antibodies in the patient, including those against leukocytes or platelets, should not be ignored.

In severe cases, it may be necessary to determine the extent of hemolysis as indicated by the presence of free hemoglobin in the plasma, ahaptoglobinemia, increase of methemalbumin, and bilirubin level (Fig. 43-16). Occasionally it may be necessary to check the extent of renal damage as indicated by serum urea and creatinine levels. If disseminated intravascular coagulation is suspected, a complete coagulation profile is warranted (see Chap. 33). If the

Table 43-58.   LABORATORY INVESTIGATION OF TRANSFUSION REACTIONS

	PATIENT'S BLOOD			DONOR'S BLOOD	
	Pretransfusion	Posttransfusion	URINE	Tube	Container
Routine for each case					
Abnormal signs: hemolysis, jaundice, not clotting, others	X	X	X		X
ABO and Rh$_0$ typing	X	X		X	X
Direct antiglobulin test	X	X			
Crossmatching	X	X		X	X
Whenever indicated					
Isoagglutinin titer/hemolysin	X			X	
Irregular antibodies	X	X		X	
Others		A, C	B		C

For A: 1. Free hemoglobin, haptoglobin, methemalbumin, hemopexin, bilirubin
　　　　2. Hemoglobin or hematocrit, differential count, white cell count
　　　　3. Platelet count, Factor VIII, fibrinogen, fibrin-split products
　　　　4. Urea, creatinine, and other indicators for renal function
　　　　5. IgA and anti-IgA, antileukocyte antibodies
　　　　6. G6PD
For B: Hemoglobinuria, hemosiderinuria, urobilinogen
For C: Smear and culture for microorganisms

reaction is of the anaphylactic type, determination of IgA and anti-IgA as well as anti-leukocyte antibodies may clarify the nature of the reaction. The possibility of G6PD deficiency and medication should be kept in mind. Microorganisms and bacterial toxins should not be forgotten. When deglycerolized erythrocytes are used, the presence of high residual glycerol may hemolyze the transfused erythrocytes.

HOSPITAL TRANSFUSION COMMMITTEE

Requirements

A transfusion committee is required in every hospital where a transfusion service exists. This is not only to observe government regulations and to meet the criteria of accreditation agencies but also to promote communication and to serve as an educational pivot among the various parties involved in blood transfusion practice. Such education can contribute to improved patient care through optimal hemotherapy.

Committee

All parties deeply involved in transfusion practice should be represented; namely, blood bank director, other physicians including surgeons, anesthesiologists, hematologists, nephrologists, nursing staff, and administrators. The chairman should be someone who uses blood extensively and is interested in transfusion problems. The committee should meet not less than once every three months. An example of a review form is shown in Table 43-59.

Activities

a. To assure adequate supplies of quality blood components and to maintain a cooperative relationship with the local supplier.
b. To establish transfusion policies and guidelines on the proper use of blood, blood components, and derivatives.
c. To prepare forms for adequate documentation of transfusion practice.
d. To review transfusion reactions and to improve the safety of blood transfusion.
e. To promote continuing education programs for various staff members and to inform them of any scientific advances or changes in regulatory policies.

IMMUNIZATION ASSOCIATED WITH PREGNANCY

MATERNAL IMMUNIZATION

With the exposure of the mother's immune apparatus to fetal blood, a maternal immune response with isoimmunization of fetus may ensue. The outcome of such isoimmunization may be hemolytic disease of the unborn or the newborn.

Table 43-59.   AN EXAMPLE OF A REVIEW FORM FOR TRANSFUSION COMMITTEE

BLOOD BANK AND TRANSFUSION SERVICE ANNUAL REPORT (1977)

	Medicine	Neuro-Surgery	Gyne-cology	Ortho-pedics	Pedi-atrics	Surgery	Open Heart	Urology	Otorhi-nolaryn-gology	Renal Trans-plant	Burns	Total
No. of units crossmatched	4009	1475	1125	1865	732	4255	4475	610	371	624	759	20300
No. of units transfused	2416	369	554	854	568	2020	2220	204	150	388	499	10242
Crossmatch/transfusion ratio (C/T)	1.6	4.0	2.0	2.2	1.3	2.1	2.0	3.0	2.5	1.6	1.5	2.0
Transfusion reactions												94
Allergic	7	2	1	3	10	9	6	1		1		40
Febrile	26	2	2	5		6	2			1		44
Hemolytic	1											1
Delayed												
Other	2		2			3		1	1			9

Factors affecting maternal immunization

Transplacental Hemorrhage (TPH). The presence of fetal erythrocytes in the mother's circulation can be demonstrated by the presence of erythrocytes containing fetal hemoglobin (Kliehauer, 1960) or by a positive D^u test in Rh_o negative(D−) mothers (Polesky, 1971). While neither of these two methods is very sensitive, they are the best available at the present time. Data from different laboratories indicate that TPH is negligible during the first and second trimesters; however, it may occur during the third trimester and is fairly common at the time of delivery.

Up to 50 per cent of D− mothers with a D+ fetus may have demonstrable fetal erythrocytes at the time of delivery. About 20 per cent of these women may have 0.1 ml or more of fetal red cells, 1 per cent may have 3 ml or more, and up to 0.3 per cent may have 15 ml or more (Mollison, 1972, p. 301). The minimal dose of D+ erythrocytes capable of inducing a primary immunization is probably less than 0.1 ml (Mollison, 1972, p. 308). As expected, caesarean section and manual removal of the placenta are often associated with a considerable increase in TPH. Amniocentesis also increases the risk of TPH.

Maternal-fetal bleeding has been demonstrated in D− infants whose blood contains D+ erythrocytes from the mother. This has been implicated in the development of anti-D in a D− person without known antigenic stimulation; however, such a hypothesis has not been well established (Jennings, 1976).

Responder and Non-responder. A successful immunization of D− mothers is dependent not only on the dosage of D+ erythrocytes, but also on the mother's ability to respond to D+ antigens. An immunized mother can be recognized by the presence of anti-D in her serum or by the shortened survival of injected D+ erythrocytes. About one third of D− persons are non-responders and fail to form anti-D despite repeated injections of D+ erythrocytes (Mollison, 1972, p. 285).

Antigens Responsible for Immunization. The mother must be negative for an antigen(s) which the fetus inherits from the father in order to be immunized. Although $Rh_o(D)$ antigen is by far the most important one involved in severe hemolytic disease of the newborn, other erythrocyte as well as leukocyte and platelet antigens can also induce maternal immunization by the formation of IgG antibodies. According to Giblett (1964), anti-D or anti-DC was found in 93 per cent of cases and anti-E, anti-c, or anti-Ce was found in 6 per cent of the cases. The remaining 1 per cent consisted of antibodies of other specificities. Anti-K, anti-k, anti-Fy^a, anti-Fy^b, anti-Kp^a, anti-Jk^a, anti-Jk^b, anti-M, anti-S, anti-s, anti-U, anti-Yt^a, anti-Di^a, anti-Di^b, anti-Co^a, anti-Wr^a, and many antibodies against low incidence antigens have been implicated in hemolytic disease of the newborn. In fact, many low incidence antigens were first recognized through the careful study of hemolytic disease of the newborn.

A or B antigens of the fetus can also immunize a group O mother, and the incidence is far greater than that induced by Rh antigens. However, clinically, the newborn presents a much milder disease and rarely requires the intensive treatment as in hemolytic disease of the newborn due to anti-D.

As early as 1943 Levine noted that ABO incompatibility between the mother and the fetus reduced the chance of Rh_o sensitization. His observation has been confirmed by many others. In general, Rh immunization occurs in only about half as many ABO-incompatible matings as ABO-compatible matings. Group O females offer stronger protection than those of other groups. For instance, in the mating of group B males with group O females, protection against Rh immunization was almost twice that found in the mating of group B males with group A females. The proportion of ABO compatible infants is approximately 0.8 (Mollison, 1972, p. 309).

The zygosity of the father of the infant also plays an important part in the immunization of the mother during subsequent pregnancies. If he is a homozygote, all their children are expected to be positive for that antigen; if he is a heterozygote, only 50 per cent of their children are expected to be positive when the mother is negative for that antigen. When zygosity is unknown, the gene frequency (approximately 0.6 for D) divided by phenotype frequency (approximately 0.84 for D), $0.6/0.84 = 0.71$, represents the chance that their children will be positive for that antigen (applied only to a two-allele system).

Thus, the chance for a $Rh_o(D)$-negative (−) woman (0.16) with a D+ husband (0.84) to be ABO compatible (0.8), to have a D+ fetus (0.71), to have sufficient transplacental hemorrhage to immunize the mother (0.2), and to be immunized again by a D+ fetus (0.71) is $0.16 \times 0.84 \times 0.8 \times 0.71 \times 0.2 \times 0.71 = 0.011$. In other words, about 1 per cent of all women (or 6 per cent of D− women), in the absence of suppressive therapy and pregnant for the second time, may have an affected infant. This figure is close to what has been observed clinically.

Previous Immunization. Except in rare instances, the infant from the first pregnancy is seldom affected. If it is affected, the disease is usually very mild. However, if the mother has been immunized previously either through pregnancies or transfusions, the immunizing dose may be very small and the immune response may be much greater than that found in the primary immunization. Hence, a history of previous transfusions or other possible sources of immunization, such as abortion, as well as other normal pregnancies, should be established in a prenatal work-up.

History of Affected Infant(s). Murray (1957) showed that the risk of stillbirth in an existing pregnancy is greatly influenced by the condition of previous infants at time of delivery. When previous infants were delivered without anemia or only mild anemia, the risk was below 7 per cent. Those with moderate anemia showed 20 per cent; with severe anemia, 55 per cent; with one stillbirth, 70 per cent; and with more than one stillbirth, 80 per cent.

Previous Treatment. The incidence of hemolytic disease of the newborn due to anti-D has been greatly reduced since the advent of suppressive treatment employing anti-D globulin or Rh_o immune globulin (IgG Rh_o antibodies).

Prenatal testing

Blood Specimen of the Mother

1. ABO and Rh_o typing of mother's blood should be done early in pregnancy.
2. Antibody screening (detection) should be performed not only against routine reagent red blood cells, but also against the erythrocytes of the father whenever feasible. If anti-D is present, repeated comparative titers should be performed to see whether there is any increase in titer. If no antibodies are detected, it is advisable to repeat screening of a patient's serum one month prior to delivery to assure that no unexpected antibodies have developed in the latter part of the pregnancy.
3. Proper antibody identification employing a panel of reagent red blood cells must be performed if the screening is positive.
4. A serologic test for syphilis and possibly

Table 43–60. LIKELIHOOD OF BEING HOMOZYGOUS FOR $Rh_0(D)$

PHENOTYPE	WHITES	BLACKS
Rh_0(Dce)	5%	48%
Rh_1rh(DCce)	10%	58%
Rh_2rh(DcEe)	10%	65%
Rh_1Rh_1(DCe)	95%	100%
Rh_2Rh_2(DcE)	92%	100%
Rh_1Rh_2(DCcEe)	96%	88%

Based on New York Population (Wiener, 1969).

one for hepatitis B antigen should also be performed, as both diseases may affect the fetus.

Blood Specimen of the Father

1. ABO grouping is useful information to predict the ABO group of the fetus and, hence, the chance of ABO compatibility with the mother.
2. Complete Rh phenotyping regardless of whether he is D + or D − is important. If he is D+, the chance for him to be a homozygote or heterozygote for D can be estimated as in Table 43-60.

If he is DccEe, or DccEE instead of DCcee, the chance of having a severely affected DccEe fetus is greater. If he is D−, other erythrocyte antigens may be inherited by the fetus and immunize the mother, especially E and c.

Hemolytic disease of the unborn

The passage of IgG Rh antibodies into the fetal circulation induces immune hemolysis and anemia in varying degrees of severity. In mild cases, the fetus can usually survive to term for natural delivery. In moderately severe cases, the fetus may live to near maturity and be delivered by early induction of labor, usually after 32 weeks of gestation. In very severe cases, the fetus may develop heart failure associated with other factors (anemia, asphyxia, and depressed serum protein concentration) with resulting massive edema and anasarca, known as "hydrops fetalis." Death *in utero* usually occurs in the latter instance. In a study of 1300 Rh-immunized women, the stillbirth rate was found to be approximately 12 per cent (Walker, 1956). In some cases with early diagnosis, the anemic fetus can be treated successfully by intrauterine transfusion. Repeated removal of antibodies from the mother's circulation by plasma exchange (Mollison, 1972, p. 642) has been attempted with successful results and may be used in selected cases. To establish the severity of disease in the affected fetus, the study of amniotic fluid described in Chapter 20 provides useful information.

Amniocentesis (see Chap. 20)

Transabdominal insertion of a needle into the amniotic cavity has long been used for injection of radiopaque material for amniography and for injection of hypertonic saline solution in order to terminate pregnancy. For the past decade, it has been widely used in prenatal diagnosis, assessment of fetal well-being or jeopardy, and prognosis of hemolytic disease of the newborn caused by Rh antibodies.

Indications

1. Serum AGT titer of anti-D of 16 or higher by antiglobulin test in a pregnant woman with a history of previous stillbirth due to Rh immunization.
2. Serum titer of anti-D of 32 or higher in a pregnant woman with history of previous child who received exchange transfusions.
3. Progressive rise of anti-D serum titer to 64 or higher in pregnant woman without history of affected fetus or child.

The initial amniocentesis is usually done between 24 and 28 weeks of gestation, or 6 to 8 weeks before gestational age of previous fetal loss caused by Rh immunization. Meaningful information usually requires at least two amniocenteses, at one to two weeks' interval, in order to confirm and compare the results of each tap.

The amniotic fluid should be protected against light, which affects the level of pigments. The fluid portion should be separated as soon as possible from cellular and other sediment. Turbid fluid should be clarified by high-speed centrifugation or by filtration before being tested (see Chap. 20).

Testing

BILIRUBIN PIGMENT. The level of bilirubinoid is by far the most important determination. The exact nature of this pigment and its pathway into the amniotic cavity are not yet known. Results of bilirubinoid determination provide a high degree of accuracy in predicting the outcome of the pregnancy in Rh immunization. Presence of bilirubin pigment leads to an abnormal elevation of optical density at 450 mμ in a spectrophotometric scan. The difference in optical density between baseline and peak of elevation is known as delta (Δ) O.D. The normal value of the Δ O.D. varies with gestational age; consequently, any value expressed must state the age of the fetus. As shown in Figures 43–17 and 20–4 (p. 697), Liley grouped all Δ O.D. values into three zones: Zone 1 requires immediate treatment with either exchange transfusion or the induction of labor. Zone 2 indicates a repeat analysis, while

4

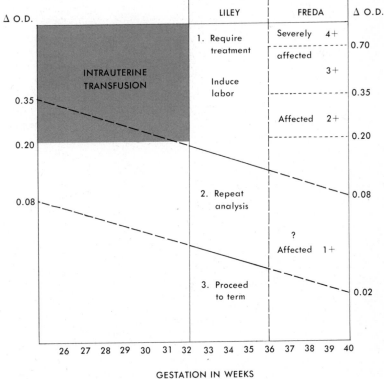

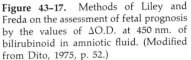

Figure 43–17. Methods of Liley and Freda on the assessment of fetal prognosis by the values of ΔO.D. at 450 nm. of bilirubinoid in amniotic fluid. (Modified from Dito, 1975, p. 52.)

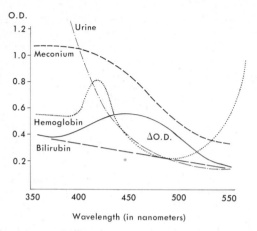

Figure 43-18. Differentiation of pigments commonly found in amniotic fluid by spectrophotometric scan.

Zone 3 can proceed to term. In the same figure, Freda grouped all Δ O.D. into four zones. Basically, the three upper zones (4+, 3+, 2+) are equivalent to Zone 1 of Liley, while the lower zone is equivalent to Liley's Zones 2 and 3.

Increased optical density in a spectrophotometric scan of amniotic fluid may be due to material other than bilirubin. Blood, which is present in various amounts in about 50 per cent of the taps, produces a peak at 415 mμ; meconium gives high Δ O.D. below 425 mμ; urine shows a very high Δ O.D. below 400 mμ. A mixture of blood and bilirubin pigment can be differentiated by repetition of the scan after extraction of bilirubin with chloroform (Figs. 43-18 and 20-10 (p. 700)).

MATURITY OF THE FETUS (see Chap. 20). As the fetus approaches maturity, the lecithin/sphingomyelin (L/S) ratio increases in value. An L/S ratio of 2 or greater suggests that pulmonary maturity is sufficient for extrauterine survival and one can anticipate no respiratory disease syndrome neonatally. L/S ratios between 1.5 and 1.9 indicate a transitional state of pulmonary maturity, and a mild respiratory disease syndrome may be expected. When L/S ratios are less than 1.5, severe respiratory disease syndrome is the usual outcome.

Creatinine concentration in amniotic fluid reflects the increase of fetal muscle mass and fetal glomerular filtration. A value of 2 mg/dl or greater indicates a sufficient fetal maturity. Other indices have also been used in selected laboratories (Dito, 1975—an excellent monograph on amniotic fluid which is recommended for additional information with our Chapter 20).

ANTI-D TITER. Comparison with the anti-D titer of the maternal serum has been reported to be useful as a prognostic index for viability of the fetus.

ABO TYPING. This can be done in three ways: (a) mixed agglutination of fetal epithelial cells using red blood cells of known group; (b) detection of soluble A, B, and H substances; or (c) direct erythrocyte typing, provided the red cells have been shown to be of fetal origin by means of the Kleihauer test. Rh typing and direct antiglobulin test can also be done with fetal red blood cells.

SEX DETERMINATION. Presence of sex chromatin (Barr body) in desquamated fetal cells indicates a female fetus.

Complications
1. Fetal or maternal bleeding and fetal death following amniocentesis have been reported.
2. Fetal-maternal hemorrhage, inducing additional immunization of the mother.
3. Infection, essentially preventable.

Intrauterine transfusion

Intrauterine transfusion was made possible on the basis of (1) absorption of functional red blood cells from the peritoneal cavity into the general circulation; and (2) ability of the fetus to swallow radiopaque material, permitting visualization of the fetal peritoneal cavity by radiographic amniography. It offers a means of correcting severe fetal anemia *in utero*, thus preventing development of hydrops fetalis. However, it should be applied only in critically selected cases following timely and accurate diagnosis.

Indications. The following factors must be considered in making the decision for intrauterine transfusion: (1) previous history of stillbirth or exchange transfusion due to Rh immunization; (2) comparison of gestational age of previous fetal loss (stillbirth) with weeks of gestation of the current pregnancy; intrauterine transfusion, as a rule, is given between 20 to 33 weeks of gestation; (3) anti-D titer of maternal serum and bilirubin level in the amniotic fluid; and (4) when amniography discloses definite signs of hydrops, this is considered a contraindication. In these considerations it is not enough simply to decide which fetuses need transfusion, but more important, which do not.

Selection of Blood. Group O Rh-negative packed red blood cells are generally used for intrauterine transfusion. Frozen red blood cells have also been recommended owing to the fact that the washing process used for removal of the cryoprotective agent also reduces the chance of (1) transmitting hepatitis, (2) potassium intoxication, and (3) graft-versus-host reaction because of removal of most immunocompetent leukocytes. Very recently, automated machines for obtaining washed fresh red blood cells with few leukocytes have become available; such fresh washed cells may be the choice for intrauterine transfusion. Radiation of the blood before infusion may be helpful in preventing a graft vs. host reaction. The recommended volume to be injected depends on the individual's peritoneal size such as the following: (Queenan, 1977)

Weeks of Gestation	20-22	23-24	25-26	27-29	30-31	32	33
Red blood cells (ml) (Hematocrit 70%)	20	30	35	40	50	60	70

During the initial transfusion, a self-retaining Teflon catheter is inserted to facilitate subsequent transfusions, which are usually repeated every two weeks until the infant can survive after delivery (more than 32 weeks of gestation).

Results.   The general survival rate of infants receiving intrauterine transfusion is about 30 per cent; in fetuses with some signs of hydrops, survival is less than 14 per cent, while it is 45 per cent in those without signs of hydrops (Queenan, 1977). However, the value of intra-uterine transfusion is doubtful in the presence of hydrops fetalis (Queenan, 1977).

Complications

FETAL.   The mortality related to the procedure is about 14 per cent. Since premature labor is a common complication, many instances of fetal loss result from prematurity and associated respiratory distress syndrome. Injury to various parts of the fetus is not uncommon. Potassium intoxication, serum hepatitis, and graft-versus-host reaction have been reported. Exposure to x-ray should be reduced to minimal amounts.

MATERNAL.   Infections may develop in about 10 per cent of women and bleeding in about 5 per cent (Queenan, 1977).

HEMOLYTIC DISEASE OF THE NEWBORN

Rh incompatibility

The exact mechanism by which IgG antibodies pass through the placenta is not yet known. Since other immunoglobulins of size comparable to IgG do not pass through the placenta, size is obviously not the only determining factor. All four subclasses of IgG are able to pass the placenta, although some IgG2 may fail to do so (see Table 43-8).

Anemia is probably the result of extravascular hemolysis. In a stillborn fetus, marked erythrophagocytosis is often found in the reticuloendothelial system, especially in the spleen. As a result of anemia, a large number of nucleated cells and reticulocytes can often be seen in the peripheral blood; hence, the term *erythroblastosis fetalis* has been used for this condition.

Before birth, the excessive amount of bilirubin (up to 22 mg/dl) derived from hemolysis is normally bound to albumin and then forms conjugated bilirubin in the mother's liver through the action of glucuronidase. In newborns, the glucuronidase levels in the liver are low and the amount of albumin is limited; therefore, a considerable amount of free (indirect) bilirubin accumulates. Free bilirubin has a high affinity for basal ganglia of the central nervous system and produces a yellow stain in brain tissue. Thus, the term *kernicterus* has been used to describe this condition. In severe cases, the infant becomes increasingly lethargic and exhibits opisthotonos and eventually respiratory failure, and death occurs. In milder cases, the infant may appear to be normal but may exhibit mental retardation later (Fig. 43-19).

According to the survey of Mollison (1951), when the bilirubin concentration in the plasma was 18 mg/dl or below, kernicterus was not observed. However, the incidence increased as bilirubin levels approached 19 mg/dl or higher. At a level of over 30 mg/dl, 8 out of 11 patients developed kernicterus. In many hospitals, a concentration of 16 mg/dl is used as the critical level to begin aggressive treatment regardless of the cause of the elevation. This lower level of bilirubin as a cut-off may be crucial and is attributed to variability in albumin binding capacity for bilirubin (measured by reserve albumin binding capacity), relative amount of free bilirubin in proportion to conjugated total serum bilirubin, and the possible existence of other facets of bilirubin transport and metabolism.

ABO incompatibility

ABO incompatibility is expected when the mother's blood is type O and the fetus has type A or B erythrocytes, or when the mother is A or B and the fetus is B or A, respectively. The theoretical chance of such combinations would be the mother's phenotype frequency multiplied by the gene frequency of the incompatible antigen, as follows:

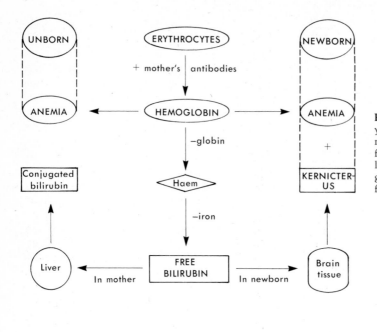

Figure 43-19. The effect of immune hemolysis in the unborn (anemia only) and in the newborn (anemia and kernicterus). This difference is due to the fact that the newborn's liver has insufficient glucuronidase to conjugate free bilirubin, which has a high affinity for brain tissue, thus producing kernicterus.

MATERNAL PHENOTYPE	PHENOTYPE FREQUENCY	FETAL PHENOTYPE	GENE FREQUENCY	CHANCE OF SUCH COMBINATION
O	0.44	A	0.27	0.12
O	0.44	B	0.07	0.03
A	0.44	B	0.07	0.03
B	0.1	A	0.27	0.03
Total Chance				0.21

Clinically, hemolytic disease of the newborn is usually found only in infants of group A or B with group O mothers. Infants with mild jaundice as a sign of ABO incompatibility have been observed in only about 1 in 150 births (Mollison, 1972, p. 663). Many factors could be involved in the finding of such a low incidence; the presence of A or B antigens in soluble form as well as in the tissues may spare the erythrocytes from being the only target. Qualitative and/or quantitative ABH modifications of fetal erythrocytes making such cells potentially less antigenic and the lack of well-defined criteria for making such a diagnosis may also play an important role.

Jaundice developing within 24 hours after birth is frequently associated with ABO incompatibility, and the term *icterus praecox* has been used for this syndrome. The presence of high titer immune anti-A or anti-B in the mother's serum does not indicate that the fetus or the infant is affected. The direct antiglobulin test of infant's erythrocytes is not always positive in spite of the fact that anti-A or anti-B may be recovered in the eluate of the infant's erythrocytes. Spherocytosis, reticulo-cytosis, and mild anemia are often encountered. In general, only rare cases are severe enough to require treatment. While hemolytic disease of the newborn due to Rh incompatibility is rarely seen in the firstborn, it is not unusual to have the firstborn affected by ABO incompatibility.

Diagnosis: Neonatal testing

Direct Antiglobulin Test. The direct antiglobulin test of the cord blood sample is usually strongly positive. However, the strength of this reaction is not correlated with the severity of the disease. An infant with a strongly reacting test may have very mild or no disease at all. When the test is weak, it may indicate the presence of antibodies other than anti-D, although the mother may be D−. In cases of ABO incompatibility, the eluate study of the cord blood cells is more useful than the direct antiglobulin test which is often weakly reactive or negative.

Hemoglobin Concentration. The normal concentration of cord and venous blood samples of newborns ranges from 15 g/dl to over 20 g/dl. When the hemoglobin values are around 14 g/dl, the infant may suffer from severe disease and even kernicterus. When the hemoglobin concentration is below 14 g/dl, the infant is usually affected; the lower the concentration, the more severely affected the in-

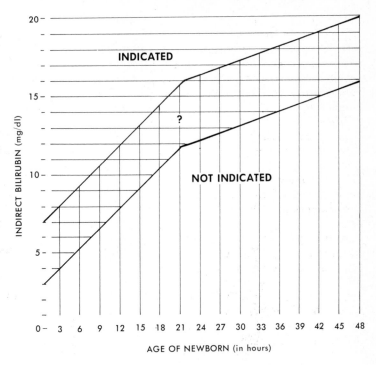

INDICATED

?

NOT INDICATED

INDIRECT BILIRUBIN (mg/dl)

20 –

15 –

10 –

5 –

0 –   3   6   9   12   15   18   21   24   27   30   33   36   39   42   45   48

AGE OF NEWBORN (in hours)

Figure 43-20. The use of the indirect bilirubin level of the newborn at different ages in hours as guide for exchange transfusion. (Adapted from Allen, 1957.)

fant and the greater the incidence of kernicterus and hydrops fetalis.

Bilirubin Concentration. The bilirubin concentration of the cord specimen is probably the best index for prognosis. The level of bilirubin represents the combined result of hemolysis and liver function of the infant. Normal cord total serum bilirubin values are between 1 and 3 mg/dl, and a cord value of 5 mg/dl is generally considered an indication for exchange transfusion. The significance of bilirubin level is closely related to the age of the infant. The recommendation made by Allen (1957) serves as a useful guide for the management of hemolytic disease of the newborn (Fig. 43-20).

Other Helpful Measurements and/or Examinations. Erythroblastemia and reticulocytosis are often found in $Rh_o(D)$ incompatibility, whereas spherocytosis is seen in ABO incompatibility. Hyperbilirubinemia from other causes may be found in newborns. Some examples would include prematurity with insufficient hepatic glucuronidase, congenital syphilis, hepatitis, cytomegalic inclusion disease, toxoplasmosis, other bacterial infections, G6PD deficiency, galactosemia, hereditary hemolytic anemia, or that associated with a diabetic mother. Appropriate determinations should be made to exclude such possibilities.

Management

In addition to exchange transfusion for hemolytic disease of the newborn secondary to blood group incompatibility, other clinical disorders of newborns may be treated as shown in Table 43-61.

Table 43-61. CLINICAL DISORDERS OF NEONATES TREATED WITH EXCHANGE TRANSFUSION*

1. Hemolytic disease of the newborn secondary to blood group incompatibility.
2. Neonatal hyperbilirubinemia resulting from
   a. hereditary red cell and bilirubin metabolism defects.
   b. hemorrhage into enclosed spaces.
   c. prematurity.
   d. hyaline membrane disease (Adamkin, 1977; Gottuso, 1976).
   e. intrauterine or neonatal infection (Phrod'hom, 1974).
3. Diffuse intravascular coagulation (DIC) secondary to abruptio placentae asphyxia, toxemia of pregnancy, sepsis, and generalized viral infections (Adamkin, 1977; Gross, 1971; Lascari, 1971).
4. Hypermagnesemia (Brandy, 1967).
5. Adenosine deaminase deficiency with severe combined immunodeficiency (Polmar, 1976).
6. Congenital isoimmune thrombocytopenia purpura (Adner, 1969).

*Modified from Kevy (1977) and others.

Rationale. The purpose of exchange transfusion is fourfold: (1) remove bilirubin to prevent injury to the brain tissue, (2) supply erythrocytes to correct the anemia, (3) remove erythrocytes coated with antibodies, and (4) remove free antibody which may cause additional hemolysis.

Indications. A bilirubin level above 5 mg/dl at birth, above 11.5 mg/dl 12 hours after birth, or above 16 mg/dl after 24 hours is definite indication for exchange transfusion. Hemoglobin concentrations below 14 mg/dl or prematurity of the newborn are two important factors and should be taken into consideration.

Blood to be Used. If the infant is affected by anti-Rh_o(D), ABO type- specific and Rh_o (D−) blood should be used. If the infant is affected by anti-A or anti-B, group O erythrocytes with A or B or AB plasma are recommended. If compatible blood cannot be found, incompatible blood can be used under emergency conditions. Blood of the mother without the plasma is a practical alternative. When whole blood is used, it is desirable to remove part of the plasma to reduce the side effects and to provide a higher hemoglobin concentration. Blood should be warmed before it is transfused, especially in the case of a premature baby.

Frozen-thawed red blood cells have also been advocated for exchange transfusion (Grajwer, 1976; Staples, 1976). In addition to excellent red cell recovery, including adequate levels of 2,3 diphosphoglycerate, there is decreased antigenic stimulation from leukocytes and platelets. Theoretically, lymphocytes transfused into a neonate might induce a graft-versus-host (GVH) disease (see Chap. 34); radiation of fresh blood before use has thus been proposed to destroy lymphocytes and minimize the likelihood of GVH disease (Kevy, 1977). Such red cell transfusions may be combined with albumin or FFP to enhance bilirubin binding and removal.

Compatibility testing for exchange transfusion can be done in three ways: The first choice is to use mother's serum against the donor's erythrocytes. The mother's serum is readily available and contains antibodies of higher titer than that in the infant's serum. However, the mother's serum may contain IgM antibodies such as anti-Le^a, anti-I, and anti-HI, which may confuse the crossmatching. The treatment of mother's serum with 2-mercaptoethanol before crossmatch may be necessary. Using the eluate from the cord erythrocytes is the second best choice; it is particularly useful when the mother's serum has IgM type of antibodies and blood specimen from the mother is not available, or the ABO group of the donor is not compatible with mother's serum. Finally, it may sometimes be necessary to use serum of the newborn.

At the end of the first exchange transfusion, a blood specimen should be saved for crossmatches in possible additional exchange transfusions; the mother's serum serves as a useful double check for compatibility.

About 90 ml of blood per pound (infant weight) is a useful guideline for determining the amount required for exchange transfusion. In case of technical difficulties, at least 60 ml/lb should be given in order to achieve beneficial effects. In infants with heart failure, a larger amount of blood could be withdrawn than the amount infused, but the exchange should be done slowly. To counteract the effect of citrate, 1 ml of a 10 per cent solution of calcium gluconate is usually given for each 100 ml of blood exchanged. To avoid the use of citrate, heparinized blood was commonly used; since heparinized blood has only a two-day shelf life, it is impractical to have it readily available. In addition, heparin activates lipase to produce fatty acids which compete with bilirubin for albumin, an obvious disadvantage, as well as result in systemic anticoagulation.

In order to reduce the amount of potassium, lactate, or ammonia in stored blood, fresher blood should always be used for exchange transfusion.

Effect of Exchange Transfusion. Hemoglobin concentration is increased. The level of bilirubin and antibodies is usually decreased, but to a much lesser extent because both components are also distributed extravascularly. In severe cases, a second or even a third exchange is required to lower the bilirubin level.

Exchange transfusion can be hazardous; toxic effects of the anticoagulant, high levels of potassium or ammonia, technical problems, and infections have been reported. In general, it is a safe and useful procedure and lives of many newborns have thus been saved.

Other Treatment. Phototherapy may reduce the bilirubin levels in serum by acceleration of bilirubin catabolism through the skin. This has proved to be helpful in mild cases. Phenobarbital, which induces the formation of glucuronidase in the liver, has been used to reduce the serum bilirubin level of the infants by giving it either to the mother prenatally or to the infant neonatally. Both types of treatment can be used to supplement but not replace exchange transfusion.

Prevention of Rh immunization

Rationale. It had been noted that when $Rh_o(D)$-negative volunteers were injected with D+ erythrocytes that had been coated *in vitro* with anti-D, they did not develop anti-D (Stern, 1961). When anti-D was administered to volunteers shortly after receiving D+ erythrocytes, the latter were removed rapidly from the circulation and no anti-D formed subsequently (Finn, 1961; Freda, 1964 and 1978). On the basis of these observations, immune anti-$Rh_o(D)$ has been used routinely to prevent Rh immunization of $Rh_o(D)$-negative mothers or other persons receiving D+ erythrocytes under various conditions. The exact mechanism of anti-$Rh_o(D)$ remains to be established.

Indications. $Rh_o(D)$ immune globulin is recommended for D− mothers without demonstrable anti-D in their plasma who deliver a D+ infant, or those who have had a miscarriage, abortion, ectopic pregnancy, or amniocentesis where the Rh of the fetus is unknown. It is also recommended for any women of childbearing age receiving D+ erythrocytes. Immune anti-D should not be given to a D+ person, to a D− person with anti-D, or to one who already has the potential of developing anti-D, such as one who has received transfusions of D+ erythrocytes within three months.

Dosage. Immune anti-D preparations in the United States contain about 300 μg of antibody/vial, which is sufficient to suppress antigenicity of about 15 ml of D+ erythrocytes (30 ml of blood). Since fetal maternal bleeding is seldom over 30 ml, one vial is adequate under normal conditions. When a larger amount of bleeding is suspected, the amount of fetal blood in the mother's circulation can be estimated by the fetal-maternal cell ratio using the acid elution technique. Taking all factors into consideration, a fetal-maternal cell ratio of 1:100 (1 per cent) in a 100 lb mother is equivalent to about 30 ml of fetal blood in the mother's circulation (slightly modified from Lee, 1976). Thus, regardless of any deviation from these two reference numbers, the number of vials of anti-D required can be readily calculated. For instance, if the

fetal-maternal cell ratio is 2 per cent and the mother is 150 lb, $2 \times 1.5 = 3$ vials would be needed. To insure complete protection, Walker recommends doubling the calculated dose (1977).

Since fetal-maternal hemorrhage happens also during pregnancy, investigators in Canada and Australia have been giving immune anti-D during the last trimester of pregnancy. The first injection is given during the 28th week of gestation and, in some cases, an additional injection is given sometime around the 33rd week of gestation. The results obtained seem better than those from their control groups (Davey, 1977; Bowman, 1976).

Administration. To test the mother's erythrocytes with immune anti-D prior to injection is not essential but is recommended for two purposes: to make sure that the mother is D− and to check for the possible presence of a large fetal maternal bleed, which would require an additional amount of immune anti-D. A large number of fetal cells in the mother's circulation can be revealed at the antiglobulin test phase (same as D^u test) in the form of a minor population of agglutinates. Should the D^u test be positive and the mother known to be D−, the fetal-maternal cell ratio could then be determined by the acid elution technique (Kliehauer, 1960) and the amount of immune anti-D adjusted according to the test results. Immune anti-D is normally given intramuscularly as soon as possible after delivery. However, beneficial effect has been observed even if it is administered after the recommended time limit of 72 hours under special situations. Mild local reactions at the injection site and a slight elevation in temperature are not infrequent. Fever, myalgia, lethargy, splenomegaly, and hyperbilirubinemia have been observed in persons receiving large doses of immune anti-D.

Specially prepared immune anti-D can be given intravenously, but this must be done slowly. This route is advisable for the recipient of a large dose. It not only relieves the painful effect of intramuscular injection but also provides a better clearance of D+ erythrocytes in the circulation (Mollison, 1972, p. 322).

After routine use of immune anti-D for D− mothers in the past decade, immunization to D antigen has been steadily decreasing. Morbidity and mortality of unborns (fetuses) or newborns due to Rh_o immunization have been greatly reduced. Exchange transfusion, a procedure which had been used very frequently for hemolytic disease of newborn, is now used only occasionally in many hospitals. Although the figures vary in different locations, the efficiency of immune anti-D in the prevention of Rh_o immunization is extremely high (Freda, 1978).

Since the discovery of Rh_o immunization in the early 1940's, diagnosis was advanced in the 1950's, effective management was achieved in the 1960's, and finally prevention became successful in the 1970's. The history of Rh_o immunization illustrates well the rapid achievements in the field of basic and applied immunohematology (Freda, 1978).

NEONATAL HEMOTHERAPY

Neonatology embraces the art and science of diagnosis and management of disorders of the newborn infant. Neonates are a special challenge to a blood transfusion service. Although exchange transfusions for hemolytic disease of newborn have diminished over the past decade, the volume of blood used by newborns in the United States remains essentially unchanged (Oski, 1977).

Normal blood volume for a neonate or newborn is approximately 10 per cent of body weight. A newborn weighing 1500 grams would have a blood volume of 150 ml, while a newborn of 1000 grams would have a blood volume of 100 ml. This relatively small blood volume makes the newborn liable to significant volume depletion after a minimal absolute amount of blood loss. For example, the loss of 10 ml in a 1000-gram infant with 100 ml blood volume would be equivalent to a loss of a full unit of blood, or 500 ml, in an adult. In other words, more than 10 to 20 ml of blood loss in such a small infant may result in incipient or overt shock associated with volume depletion.

Neonates are subjected to multiple laboratory measurements and examinations requiring blood collection, e.g., blood gases, chemical pathologic determinations, and hematologic measurements. When such measurements, even with microsampling techniques, are frequent, with blood loss in excess of 7 to 10 ml per day, a neonate's blood volume can be depleted rapidly. These losses and resulting iatrogenic anemia require blood replacement. Newborn infants may need minimal blood volume replacement therapy in the form of 7 to 10 ml or 10 to 20 ml blood transfusions per day to maintain their total blood volume. Neonates are also susceptible to hypovolemia from a variety of causes. Hence, the need for more frequent blood transfusions in neonatology today can be appreciated.

In addition to exchange transfusions for disorders shown in Table 43-61, blood transfusions in the newborn may be considered for the following:

1. Iatrogenic anemia.
2. Newborn infants requiring surgery for such entities as cardiac defects and necrotizing enterocolitis.
3. Many circumstances associated with infants born hypovolemic, usually identified in terms of obstetrical procedures or other factors associated with labor and delivery.
4. Respiratory distress syndrome and prematurity where blood transfusions, including exchange transfusions, may be beneficial.

The term infant has blood with an increased affinity for oxygen. The P_{50} gradually increases and the increase is related both to the concentration of fetal hemoglobin and to the concentration of 2,3-DPG (Delivoria-Papadopoulos, 1971, 1976). Infants with respiratory distress syndrome have a lower P_{50} than term infants or other infants without respiratory distress. This is primarily due to decreased intracellular 2,3-DPG, as shown in Figure 28-4 (p. 928).

Exchange transfusion is performed in anticipation that blood with less oxygen affinity (higher P_{50} and increased 2,3-DPG) will promote more release of oxygen to the tissues.

In the immediate post-transfusion period, the P_{50} of infused blood depends on the storage time and anticoagulant of the unit transfused (p. 1465).

Exchange transfusion has been shown to increase the survival of low birth weight infants and those with RDS, although the mechanism may be unrelated to tissue oxygenation (Delivoria-Papadopoulos, 1976; Gottuso, 1976). Arterial oxygen concentration rises shortly after exchange transfusion, and there may be an improvement in pulmonary ventilation and perfusion that is not related to the properties of the transfused erythrocytes.

Practical and safe approaches to transfusion of neonates include the following: (Kevy, 1977)

1. Collect a unit of blood into a CPD-quadruple donor pack. This can be aseptically separated into four units of 125 ml each. Each of these smaller units can then be further subdivided, provided that all the blood is utilized within 24 hours of the procedure. With this technique, the neonate need not be crossmatched more than once throughout a seven-

day period, during which time he can receive as many as 16 transfusions. Also, several infants may be crossmatched to a single donor unit, i.e., "cow" method.

2. Use of donor blood drawn to a volume of 225 ml into a CPD triple pack with an appropriate reduction of the anticoagulant volume. In this manner, the donor can again donate up to 225 ml within a few days.

3. Satellite bags attached to a small volume of packed red blood cells or whole blood.

4. Use of small aliquots of group O, RH-compatible frozen red blood cells (Staples, 1976).

Additional donor requirements for neonatal blood transfusion include freedom from sickle cell disease and glucose 6-phosphate deficiency in blacks, as well as direct antiglobulin, hemoglobin, hematocrit, and peripheral smear examination to exclude congenital erythrocytic abnormalities.

Some neonatal intensive care units have attempted to solve the problem of replacing blood in neonates with the so-called "walking donor" method. Traditionally, O negative hospital personnel volunteer a syringe-full of blood for injection into the neonatal patient. Oberman (1975) has summarized forcefully the disadvantages of the "walking donor" system:

1. Control of the blood transfusion is removed from the hospital transfusion service.

2. It is administratively difficult to maintain proper documentation of the source of blood in such programs.

3. In some instances, compatibility testing has been waived and hepatitis testing ignored.

4. The amount of heparin in the syringe may lead to inadvertent heparinization of the infant.

5. The hospital-based donor population has a higher incidence of hepatitis than the population at large.

Although we are opposed to a "walking donor" program, others believe that it is the most viable alternative in certain well-defined clinical situations. Hattersley (1976), for example, claims that the "walking donor" program may prove to be a useful "adjunct" to the intensive care nursery for premature infants with hyaline membrane disease requiring three or more transfusions.

4

REFERENCES

Åkerblom, O., and Högman, C. F.: Frozen blood, a method for low glycerol, liquid nitrogen freezing allowing different post-thaw deglycerolization procedures. Transfusion, *14*:16, 1974.

Alavi, J. B.: A randomized clinical trial of granulocyte transfusions for infection in acute leukemia. N. Engl. J. Med., *296*:706, 1977.

Allen, F. H., and Diamond, L. K.: Erythroblastosis fetalis. Boston, Little, Brown and Co, 1957.

Alter, H. J., Tabor, E., Meryman, H. T., Hoofnagle, J. H., Kahn, R. A., Holland, R. V., Gerety, R. J., and Barker, L. F.: Transmission of hepatitis B virus infection by transfusion of frozen-deglycerolized red blood cells. N. Engl. J. Med., *298*:637, 1978.

Andrews, A. T., Zmijewski, C. M., Bowman, H. S., and Reihart, J. K.: Transfusion reaction with pulmonary infiltration associated with HL-A-specific leukocyte antibodies, Am. J. Clin. Pathol., *66*:483–487, 1976.

Barker, L. F., Shulman, N. R., and Murray, R.: Transmission of serum hepatitis. J.A.M.A., *211*:1509, 1970.

Barker, L. F., and Purcell, R. H.: Hepatitis B virus. *In* Rose, N. R., and Friedman, H. (eds.): Manual of Clinical Immunology. Washington, D.C., American Society of Microbiology, 1976.

Behzad, O., and Lee, C. L.: A simple method for freezing reagent erythrocytes in liquid nitrogen. Transfusion, *17*:650, 1977.

Behzad, O., Lee, C. L., Gavin, J., and Marsh, W. L.: A new anti-erythrocyte antibody in the Duffy system: Anti-Fy⁴. Vox Sang., *24*:337, 1973.

Belzer, F. O., Kountz, S. L., and Perkins, H. A.: Red cell cold auto agglutinins as a cause of failure of renal allotransplantation. Transplantation, *11*:422, 1971.

Bird, G. W. G.: Lectins in blood banking: A brief review. Biotest Bulletin, *2*:2, 1976.

Bloch, K. J., and Maki, D. G.: Hyperviscosity syndromes associated with immunoglobulin abnormalities. Sem. Hemat., *10*:113, 1973.

Boral, L. I., Crowley, L. M., and Henry, J. B.: Adult outpatient transfusion clinic in a hospital-based blood bank. Transfusion, *17*:607, 1977.

Boral, L. I., and Henry, J. B.: The type and screen: A safe alternative and supplement in selected surgical procedures. Transfusion, *17*:163, 1977.

Bowman, J.: Winnipeg antenatal prophylaxis trial. *In* Scientific Symposium—Rh antibody mediated immunosuppression. Ortho Research Institute, Raritan, N.J., 1975.

Branda, R. F., Moldow, C. E., McCullough, J. J., and Jacob, H. S.: Plasma exchange in the treatment of immune disease. Transfusion, *15*:570, 1975.

Bredenberg, C. E.: Does a relationship exist between massive blood transfusions and the adult respiratory distress syndrome? If so, what are the best preventive measures? Vox Sang., *32*:211, 1977.

Buckner, C. D., Clift, R. D., Volwiler, W., Donohue, D. M., Burnell, J. M., Saunders, F. C., and Thomas, E. D.: Plasma exchange in patients with fulminant hepatic failure. Arch. Intern. Med., *132*:487, 1973.

Bukowski, R. M., King, J. W., and Hewlett, J. S.: Plasmapheresis in the treatment of thrombotic thrombocytopenic purpura. Blood *50*:413, 1977.

Cartron, J. P.: Diosynthese des antigenes de groupes sanguins humains. *In* Plenary Sessions Congress of the International Society of Blood Transfusion. Paris, 1978.

Clift, R. A., Sanders, J. E., Thomas, E. D., Williams, B., and Buckner, C. D.: Granulocyte transfusion for the prevention of infection in patients receiving bone marrow transplants. N. Engl. J. Med., *298*:1052, 1978.

Cline, M. J., Solomon, A., Barlin, N. I., and Fahey, J. L.: Anemia in macroglobulinemia. Am. J. Med., *34*:213, 1963.

Coombs, R. R. A., and Bedford, D.: The A and B antigens on human platelets demonstrated by means of mixed erythrocyte-platelet agglutination. Vox Sang., 5:11, 1955.

Coombs, R. R. A., Mourant, A. E., and Race, R. R.: A new test for the detection of weak and "incomplete" Rh agglutinins. Brit. J. Exp. Pathol., 26:225, 1945.

Dahr, W., Issitt, P. D., and Uhlenbruck, G.: New concepts of the MNSs blood group system. In Mohn, J. F., et al. (eds.): Human Blood Groups. Basel, Karger, 1976, pp. 197–205.

Dau, P. C., Lindstrom, J. M., Cassel, C. K., Denys, E. H., Shev, E. E., and Spitler, L. E.: Plasmapheresis and immunosuppressive drug therapy in myasthenia gravis. N. Engl. J. Med., 297:1134, 1977.

Davey, M. G.: Antenatal administration of anti-Rh: Australia 1969-1975. In Scientific Symposium—Rh antibody mediated immuno-suppression. Ortho Research Institute, Raritan N.J., 1976.

Davidsohn, I.: Immunohematology, a new branch of clinical pathology. Am. J. Clin. Pathol., 124:1333, 1349, 1954.

Dawson, R. B.: Blood storage XIII: 2,3-DPG maintenance for six weeks in a CPD-Adenine-Inosine preservative with and without methylene blue. Transfusion, 17:238, 1977.

Delivoria-Papadopoulos, M., Morris, G., III, Oski, F. A., Cohen, R., and O'Neal, P.: Exchange transfusion in the newborn infant with fresh and "old" blood: The role of storage on 2,3 diphosphoglycerate, hemoglobin-oxygen affinity, and oxygen release. J. Pediatr., 79:898, 1971.

Delivoria-Papadopoulos, M., Roncevic, N. P., and Oski, F. A.: Postnatal changes in oxygen transport of term, premature, and sick infants: The role of red cell 2,3-diphosphoglycerate and adult hemoglobin. Pediatr. Res., 5:235, 1971.

Delivoria-Papadopoulos, M., Miller, L. D., Forster, R. E., and Oski, F. A.: The role of exchange transfusion in the management of low-birth-weight infants with and without severe respiratory distress syndrome. I. Initial observations. J. Pediatr., 89:273, 1976.

Diepenhorst, P., and Engelfriet, C. P.: Removal of leukocytes from whole blood and erythrocyte suspensions by filtration through cotton wool. V. Results after transfusion of 1,820 units of filtered erythrocytes. Vox Sang., 29:15, 1975.

Dito, W. R., Patrick, C. W., and Shelly, J.: Clinical Pathologic Correlations in Amniotic Fluid. Chicago, American Society of Clinical Pathologists, 1975.

Djerassi, I.: Gravity Leucapheresis—A new method for collection of transfusable granulocytes. Exp. Hematol., 5:139, 1977.

Donahue, R. P., Bias, W. B., Renwick, J. H., et al.: Probably assignment of the Duffy blood group locus to chromosome 1 in man. Proc. Natl. Acad. Sci. USA, 61:949, 1968.

Donner, I., Moore, F. A., and Collins, F. A.: Efficacy of leukocyte-poor red blood cell suspensions prepared by sedimentation in hydroxyethyl starch. Transfusion, 15:439, 1975.

Dybkjaer, E., and Elkjaer, P.: The use of heated blood in massive blood replacement. Acta Anaesth. Scand., 8:271, 1964.

Edson, J. R., McArthur, J. R., Branda, R. F., McCullough, J. J., and Chou, S. N.: Successful management of a subdural hematoma in a hemophiliac with an anti-factor VIII antibody. Blood, 41:113, 1973.

Fearon, D. T., Daha, M. R., Weiler, J. M., and Austen, K. F.: Significance of the alternative complement pathway. In Pollack, W., Mollison, P. L., Reiss, A. M., Hammer, C., and Abramovitz, A. (eds.): An international symposium on "The nature and significance of complement activation." Ortho Diagnostics, Raritan, N.J., 1976.

Feizi, T., Kabat, E. A., Vicari, G., Anderson, B., and Marsh, W. L.: Immunochemical studies on blood groups. J. Immunol., 106:1578, 1971.

Finn, R., Clarke, C. A., Donahoe, W. T. A., McConnell, R. B., Sheppard, P. M., Lehane, D., and Kulke, W.: Experimental studies on the prevention of Rh hemolytic disease. Br. Med. J., 1:486, 1961.

Freda, V. J., Gorman, J. G., and Pollack, W.: Successful prevention of experimental Rh sensitization in man with an anti-Rh gamma$_2$-globulin antibody preparation: A preliminary report. Transfusion, 4:26, 1964.

Freda, V. J., Pollack, W., and Gorman, J. G.: Rh disease: How near the end? Hosp. Pract., 13:61, 1978.

Freireich, E. J., Levin, R. J., and Whang, J.: The function and fate of transfused leukocytes from donors with chronic myelocytic leukemia in leukopenic recipients. Ann. N.Y. Acad. Sci., 113:1081, 1964.

Friedman, B. A., Schork, M. A., Mocniak, J. L., and Oberman, H. A.: Short-term and long-term effects of plasmapheresis on serum proteins and immunoglobulins. Transfusion, 15:467, 1975.

Garratty, G.: The effects of storage and heparin on the activity of serum complement with particular reference to the detection of blood antibodies. Am. J. Clin. Pathol., 54:531, 1970.

Garratty, G.: Personal communication, 1978.

Giblett, E. R.: Blood group antibodies causing hemolytic diseases of the newborn. Clin. Obstet. Gynecol., 7:1044, 1964.

Giblett, E. R.: Blood group alloantibodies: An assessment of some laboratory practices. Transfusion, 17:299, 1977.

Gottuso, M. A., Williams, M. L., and Oski, F. A.: The role of exchange transfusions in the management of low birth-weight infants with and without severe respiratory distress syndrome. II. Further observations and studies of mechanisms of action. J. Pediatr., 89:279, 1976.

Graham-Pole, J., Barr, W., and Willoughby, M. L. N.: Continuous flow plasmapheresis in management of severe rhesus disease. Br. Med. J., 1:1185, 1977.

Grajwer, L. A., Pildes, R. S., Zarif, M., Ainis, H., Agrawai, B. L., and Patel, A.: Exchange transfusion in the neonate. A controlled study using frozen-stored erythrocytes resuspended in plasma. Am. J. Clin. Pathol., 66:117, 1976.

Greenwalt, T. J. (ed.): General principles of blood transfusion. Chicago, American Medical Association, 1977.

Gurner, B. W., and Coombs, R. R. A.: Examination of human leucocytes for the ABO, MN, Rh, Tj^a, Lutheran and Lewis systems of antigens by means of mixed erythrocyte-leucocyte agglutination. Vox Sang., 3:13, 1958.

Hattersley, P. G., Goetzman, B. W., Gross, S., and Blankenship, W. J.: A walking blood donor program for seriously ill premature infants. Transfusion, 16:366, 1976.

Henry, J. B., Mintz, P. D., and Webb, W.: Optimal blood ordering for elective surgery. J.A.M.A., 237:451, 1977.

Herzig, G. P., and Graw, R. G.: Granulocyte transfusion for bacterial infections. Prog. Hematol., 10:207, 1975.

Herzig, R. H., Herzig, G. P., Graw, R. G., Jr., Bull, M. I., and Kay, K. K.: Successful granulocyte transfusion for gram-negative septicemia. N. Engl. J. Med., 296:701, 1977.

Howell, E. D., and Perkins, H. A.: Anti-N-like antibodies in the sera of patients undergoing chronic hemodialysis. Vox Sang., 23:291, 1972.

Howland, W. S., Bellville, J. W., Zucker, M. B., Bryan, P., and Cliffton, E. E.: Massive blood replacement. V. Failure to observe citrate intoxication. Surg. Gynecol. Obstet., 105:529, 1957.

Huestis, D. W., Bove, J. R., and Bush, S.: Practical Blood Transfusion, 2nd ed., Boston, Little, Brown & Co., 1976.

Huggins, C. E.: Practical preservation of blood by freezing. *In* Red cell freezing. AABB, 1973, pp. 31–54.

Hughes-Jones, N. C., Gardner, B., and Telford, R.: The effects of pH and ionic strength on the reaction between anti-D and erythrocytes. Immunology, *7*:72, 1964.

Israel, L., Edelstein, R., Mannoni, P., and Radot, E.: Plasmapheresis and immunological control of cancer (Letter). Lancet, *2*:642, 1976.

Israel, L., Edelstein, R., Mannoni, P., Radot, E., and Greenspan, E. M.: Plasmapheresis in patients with disseminated cancer: Clinical results and correlation with changes in serum protein. Cancer, *40*:3146, 1977.

Issitt, P. D., and Issitt, C. H.: Applied Blood Group Serology, 2nd ed., Spectra Biologicals, Oxnard, Cal., 1975.

Jennings, E. R.: Maternal-fetal hemorrhage. *In* Scientific symposium—Rh antibody mediated immuno-suppression. Ortho Research Institute, Raritan, N.J., 1976.

Jones, J. V., Bucknall, R. C., Cumming, R. H., Asplin, C. M., Fraser, I. D., Bothamley, J., Davis, P., and Hamblin, T. J.: Plasmapheresis in the management of acute systemic lupus erythematosus. Lancet, *1*:709, 1976.

Kienle, P. C.: Methods of administration of blood and its components. Infusion, *2*:26, 1978.

Kevy, S. V.: Pediatric transfusion therapy. Technical Improvement Service, Number 29, Immunohematology. Chicago, American Society of Clinical Pathologists, 1977.

Kitagawa, S., Lee, C. L., and Behzad, O.: Antibody detection using plasma in place of serum. Transfusion, December, 1978.

Kleihauer, E., and Betke, K.: Praktische Anwendung des Nachweises von Hb F-haltigen Zellen in fixierten Blutausstrichen. Internist, *1*:292, 1960.

Kochwa, S., and Rosenfield, R.: Immunochemical studies of the Rh system. I. Isolation and characterization of antibodies. J. Immunol., *92*:682, 1964.

Kornstad, L., and Heisto, H.: The frequency of formation of Kell antibodies in recipients of Kell-positive blood. Proc. 6th Cong. Europ. Soc. Haemat. Copenhagen, 1957, p. 754.

Krijnen, H. W.: Glycerol treated human red cells frozen with liquid nitrogen Vox Sang., *9*:559, 1964.

Lackner, H.: Hemostatic abnormalities associated with dysproteinemias. Sem. Hematol., *10*:125, 1973.

Lalezari, P.: A new method for detection of red blood cell antibodies. Transfusion, *8*:372, 1968.

Lalezari, P., and Oberhardt, B.: Temperature gradient dissociation of red cell antigen-antibody complexes in the polybrene technique. Br. J. Haematol., *21*:131, 1971.

Landsteiner, K., and Van der Scheer, J.: Serological differentiation of steric isomers (antigens containing tartaric acids). J. Exp. Med., *50*:407, 1929.

Lapinski, F., Crowley, K. M., Merritt, C., and Henry, J. B.: Use of microplate in paternity testing. Am. J. Clin. Pathol., *70*:48, 1978.

Lee, C. L.: Estimation of fetal red cells in mother. N. Engl. J. Med., *295*:1080, 1976.

Lee, C. L., Behzad, O., Froker, A., and Mandin, B.: Identification of erythrocyte antibodies with an AutoAnalyzer. Adv. Automated Anal., *1*:317, 1970.

Levine, P.: Serological factors as possible causes in spontaneous abortions. J. Hered., *34*:71, 1943.

Lockwood, C. M., Pearson, T. A., Rees, A. J., Evans, D. J., Peters, D. K., and Wilson, C. B.: Immunosuppression and plasma exchange in the treatment of Goodpasture's syndrome. Lancet, *1*:711, 1976.

Löw, E., and Messeter, L.: Antiglobulin test in low-ionic strength salt solution for rapid antibody screening and crossmatching. Vox Sang., *26*:53, 1974.

Lukomskyj, L., and Lee, C. L.: Some aspects of frozen red blood cells. Med., *5*:42, 1974.

Luxenberg, M. N., and Mansolf, F. A.: Retinal circulation in the hyperviscosity syndrome. Am. J. Ophthalmol., *70*:588, 1970.

Marsh, W. L., Oyen, R., and Nichals, M. E.: Kx antigen; the McCleod phenotype and chromic granulomatous diseases: Further studies. Vox Sang., *31*:356, 1976.

Masouredis, S. P.: Quantitative and ultrastructural aspects of red cell membrane Rh antigens. *In* Henn, R. L. (ed.): A seminar on recent advances in immunohematology. Washington, D.C., AABB, 1973.

Matte, C.: Determination automatique des groupes sanguins realisation d'un appareil experimental. Rev. Fr. Transfus., *12*:213, 1969.

McGinniss, M. A.: The albumin agglutination phenomenon. *In* A seminar on problems encountered in pretransfusion tests. Washington, D.C., AABB, 1972.

McGrath, M. A., and Penny, R.: Paraproteinemia: Blood hyperviscosity and clinical manifestations. J. Clin. Invest., *58*:1155, 1976.

Meryman, H. T.: Preservation of blood by freezing. *In* Ikkala, E., and Nykanen, A. (eds.): Transfusion and immunology. Vammala, Vammalan Kirjapaino Oy, 1975.

Meryman, H. T., and Hornblower, M.: A method for freezing and washing red blood cells using a high glycerol concentration. Transfusion, *12*:145, 1972.

Miller M. V. (ed.): AABB Technical Manual, 7th ed., Washington, D.C., American Association of Blood Banks, 1977.

Miller, W. V., Holland, P. V., Sugarbaker, E., Strober, W., and Waldmann, T. A.: Anaphylactic reactions to IgA: A difficult transfusion problem. Amer. J. Clin. Pathol., *54*:618, 1975.

Miller, L. H., Mason, S. J., Dvorak, J. A., McGinniss, M. H., and Rothman, I. K.: Erythrocyte receptors for (*Plasmodium knowlesi*) malaria: Duffy blood group determinants. Science, *189*:561, 1975.

Mintz, P. D., Lauenstein, K., Hume, J., and Henry, J. B.: Expected hemotherapy in elective surgery: A follow up. J.A.M.A., *239*:623, 1978.

Mintz, P. D., Nordine, R. B., Henry, J. B., and Webb, W. R.: Expected hemotherapy in elective therapy. N.Y. J. Med., *76*:532, 1976.

Mollison, P. L.: Blood transfusion in clinical medicine. 5th ed. Oxford, Blackwell Scientific Publication, 1972.

Mollison, P. L., and Cutbush, M.: A method of measuring the severity of a series of cases of hemolytic diseases of the newborn. Blood, *6*:777, 1951.

Monaghan, W. P., Dickson, L. G., Moore, H. C., and Sipes, B. R.: A rapid compatibility test: The saline low-ionic crossmatch. Book of Abstracts, AABB, 30th Annual Meeting, November, 1977, p. 28.

Moore, H. C., and Mollison, P. L.: Use of a low-ionic strength medium in manual tests for antibody detection. Transfusion, *16*:291, 1976.

Moran, C. J., Parry, H. F., Mowbray, J., Richards, J. D. M., and Goldstone, A. H.: Plasmapheresis, in systemic lupus erythematosus. Br. Med. J., *1*:1573, 1977.

Mourant, A. E., Kopec, A. C., and Domaniewska-Sobczak, K.: The Distribution of the Human Blood Groups and Other Polymorphisms, 2nd ed. London, Oxford University Press, 1976.

Murray, W., Murray, S., and Russell, J. K.: Stillbirth due to haemolytic disease of the newborn. J. Obstet. Gynacol., *44*:573, 1957.

Myhre, B. A.: Antibody screening with the AutoAnalyzer using donor's plasma in place of sera. Am. J. Clin. Pathol., *58*:698, 1972.

Myhre, B., and Worthen, W.: Untoward response to blood transfusion. Lab. Med., *9*:29, 1978.

Oberman, H. A.: Replacement transfusion in the newborn infant: A commentary. J. Pediatr., *86*:586, 1975.

Oberman, H. A., Barnes, B. A., and Friedman, B. A.: The risk of abbreviating the major crossmatch in urgent or massive transfusion. Transfusion, *18*:137, 1978.

O'Neill, G. J., Yang, S. Y., Tegoli, J., Berger, R., and Dupont, B.: Chido and Rodgers blood groups are distinct antigenic components of complement C4. Fed. Proc., *37*:1269, 1977.

Oski, F. A.: Red cell transfusion and phlebotomy. *In* Nathan, D. G., and Oski, F. A., (eds.): Hematology of Infancy and Childhood. Philadelphia, W. B. Saunders Company, 1974.

Oski, F. A.: Personal communication, 1977.

Paniker, N. V., and Beutler, E.: Pyruvate effect in maintenance of ATP and 2,3-DPG of stored blood. J. Lab. Clin. Med., *78*:472, 1971.

Pineda, A. A., Brzica, S. M., Jr., and Taswell, H. F.: Continuous and semi-continuous-flow blood centrifugation systems: therapeutic applications, with plasma-, platelet, lympha- and eosinapheresis. Transfusion, *17*:407, 1977.

Pineda, A. A., Brzica, S. M., and Taswell, H. F.: Hemolytic transfusion reaction. Mayo Clin. Proc., *53*:378, 1978.

Pineda, A. A., Taswell, H. F., and Brzica, S. M., Jr.: Delayed hemolytic transfusion reactions: An immunologic hazard of blood transfusion. Transfusion, *18*:1, 1978.

Polesky, H. F., and Sebring, E. S.: Detection of fetal maternal hemorrhage: An evaluation of serological tests related to Rh$_o$(D) immune globulin (human). Transfusion, *11*:162, 1971.

Pollack, W., and Kochesky, R. J.: The importance of antibody concentration, binding constant and heterogeneity in the suppression of immunity to the Rh factor. Int. Arch Allergy, *38*:320, 1970.

Prince, A. M.: Post transfusion hepatitis: Etiology and prevention. *In* Ikkala, E., and Nykanen, A. (eds.): Transfusion and Immunology. Vammala, Vammalan Kirjapaino Oy, 1975.

Queenan, J. T.: Modern Management of the Rh Problem, 2nd ed., Hagerstown, Md., Hoeber Medical Division, Harper and Row, Publishers, 1977.

Race, R. R., and Sanger, R.: Blood group polymorphism. *In* Ikkala, E., and Nykanen, A. (eds.): Transfusion and Immunology. Vammala, Vammalan Kirjapaino Oy, 1975.

Race, R. R., and Sanger, R.: Blood Groups in Man, 6th ed. Oxford, Blackwell Scientific Publications, 1975.

Roitt, I.: Essential Immunology, 2nd ed. Oxford, Blackwell Scientific Publications, 1974.

Rosenfield, R. E., Haber, G. V., Schroder, R., and Ballard, R.: Problems in Rh typing as revealed by a single Negro family. Am. J. Hum. Genet., *12*:147, 1960.

Rowe, A. W., Eyster, E., and Kellner, A.: Liquid nitrogen preservation of red blood cells for transfusion, a low glycerol-rapid freeze procedure. Cryobiology, *5*:119, 1968.

Schiffer, C. A., and McCredie, K. B.: Cell component therapy for patients with cancer. *In* Dawson, R. B. (ed.): A technical workshop presented by committee on workshops of the American Association of Blood Banks, 1974.

Schoeter, A. L., Taswell, H. F., and Sweatt, M.: Adaption of the single-channel automated reagin test for syphilis to a multichannel automated blood grouping machine. *In* Advances in Automated Analysis. White Plains, NW Mediad, Inc., 1970, vol. 1, p. 265.

Solanki, D., and McCurdy, P. R.: Delayed hemolytic transfusion reactions. An often-missed entity. J.A.M.A., *239*:729, 1978.

Solis, R. T., and Gibbs, M. B.: Filtration of the micro-

aggregates in stored blood. Transfusion, *12*:245, 1972.

Staples, J. W., and Fritz, G. E.: Development and use of pediatric frozen red cell packs. Transfusion, *16*:566, 1976.

Sturgeon, P., Cedergre, B., and McQuiston, O.: Automation of blood typing procedures,. Vox Sang., *8*:438, 1963.

Springer, G. F., and Yang, H. J.: Isolation and partial characterization of blood Group M- and N-specific glycopeptides and oligosacchrides from human erythrocytes. Immunochemistry, *14*:497, 1977.

Stern, K., Goodman, H. S., and Berger, M.: Experimental isoimmunization to hemoantigens in man. J. Immunol., *87*:189, 1961.

Standards for Blood Banks and Transfusion Services, 8th ed. Washington, D.C., American Association of Blood Banks, 1976.

Technical Manual of the American Association of Blood Banks, 7th ed. Washington, D.C., American Association of Blood Banks, 1977.

Terrasaki, P.: Personal communication, 1977.

Treacy, M.: Is LISS bliss? Ortho Blood Lines, *2*:1, 1978. (Ortho Diagnostics, Raritan, N.J.)

Tullis, J. L.: Albumin. 1. Background and use. J.A.M.A., *237*:355, 1977.

Tullis, J. L.: Albumin. 2. Guidelines for clinical use. J.A.M.A., *237*:460, 1977.

Tullis, J. L., et al.: Advantages of the higher glycerol mechanical systems for red cell preservation, a 10 year study of stability and yield. *In* Spielman, W., and Seidl, S. (eds.): Modern problems of blood preservation. Stuttgart, Fischer Verlag, 1970, pp. 138-155.

Valeri, C. R.: Principles of cryobiology, high glycerol and storage at 80°C and low glycerol and storage at 150°C, Red cell freezing. AABB, 1-30, 1973.

Valeri, C. R., and Zaroulis, C. G.: Rejuvenation and freezing of outdated stored human red cells. N. Engl. J. Med., *187*:1307, 1972.

Walker, R. H.: Fetal-maternal hemorrhage. *In* Baer, D. M., (ed.): Blood banking for the hospital laboratory. State of the Art Discussion from the Technical Improvement Service. Chicago, American Society of Clinical Pathologists, 1977.

Walker, W., and Murray, S.: Haemolytic disease of the newborn as a family problem. Br. Med. J., *1*:187, 1956.

Watkins, W. M.: Blood group substances. Science, *152*:172, 1966.

Watkins, W. M., and Morgan, W. T. J.: Immunochemical observations on the human blood group P system. J. Immunogenet., *3*:15, 1976.

Westerveld, A., Jongsma, A. P. M., Meera, P., Khan, H., Van Someren, B., and Bootsma, D.: The assignment of the AK$_1$ ABO linkage group to human chromosome 9. Proc. Acad. Natl. Sci. USA., *73*:895, 1976.

Wiener, A. S.: Problems and pitfalls in blood grouping tests for non parentage. I. Distribution of the blood groups. Am. J. Clin. Pathol., *51*:9, 1969.

Wiener, A. S., and Gordon, E. B.: Repartition des facteurs de groupes sanguins dans un population de New York City, avec une etude speciale des agglutinogens rares. Rev. Haematol., *6*:45, 1951.

Wiener, W., and Vos, G. H.: Serology of acquired hemolytic anemias. Blood, *22*:606, 1963.

Wiener, W.: Eluting red-cell antibodies: A method and its application. Br. J. Haematol., *3*:276, 1957.

Williams, W. J.: Serum viscosity. *In* Williams, W. J., Beutler, E., Erslev, A. J., and Rundles, R. W. (ed.): Textbook of Hematology, 2nd ed. New York, McGraw-Hill Book Co., 1977.

44

LABORATORY EVALUATION OF DISPUTED PARENTAGE

Chang Ling Lee, M.D., and
John Bernard Henry, M.D.

4

BASIC INFORMATION FOR PATERNITY TESTING

COMMON DISPUTED PARENTAGE PROBLEMS

Disputed paternity is by far the most common issue in parentage problems. Traditionally, the emphasis has been placed on exclusion of paternity based on the result obtained from a "blood test." Quite often if the accused man is not excluded, the court rules that he must support the child. This practice has been altered slightly since 1975 when Congress passed a law (Pub. L. 93-647) requiring each state to develop an appropriate plan, in accordance with HEW standards, for the ascer-

tainment of paternity and for child support enforcement (Abbott, 1976).

This new ruling is aimed both at protecting the right of a child to have a father and at relieving the public of the burden of supporting illegitimate children. In spite of the common practice of birth control, more than 1,700,000 illegitimate children were born in the United States between 1966 and 1970 (Abbott, 1976). The present rate is probably much higher. Although "blood tests" cannot determine absolutely who is the father of a child, they yield the best scientific evidence available with present technology and have been used for this purpose in many European countries for several years.

Following passage of Pub. L. 93-647 in 1975,

the demand for paternity testing has been increasing steadily, in terms not only of the number of tests being done, but also of the quality of the tests. Since the judge's decision regarding child support relies heavily on the "blood test," the test results should be accurate and should provide the accused man a high per cent of exclusion. Then, if he is still not excluded, the judge can feel much more comfortable with a decision of requiring the alleged father to pay child support.

The second most common parentage problem involves immigration. An American citizen may want his or her parents or children who are not American citizens to become immigrants. "Blood tests" have been used to determine whether or not there is a false claim of kinship. At other times "blood tests" can be useful in child kidnapping cases and erroneous baby identification in a newborn nursery. Test results not only may exclude non-parents, but also may indicate the chances of parentage of those not excluded. In such cases, exclusion of both parents should be considered, since the mother cannot be assumed to be the true mother, a normal assumption in cases of paternity disputes.

While the "blood tests" have proved to be very useful in helping solve parentage problems, these tests have also contributed much to the understanding of population genetics, anthropology, and the differentiation of twins. For instance, in studying twins, the blood test results can show either dissimilar markers, indicating that the twins are dizygotic, or identical markers, indicating that the twins are probably monozygotic (Race, 1975). This same type of study can also be applied to the selection of donors for skin grafts or organ transplantation.

Many genetic markers used in paternity testing have been applied to the study of blood stains; hence "blood test" is one of the very important tools in crime detection laboratories. Culliford of Scotland Yard has published an excellent review on this subject (Culliford, 1971).

Numerous publications dealing with paternity problems are available. For basic information on erythrocyte antigens, *Blood Groups in Man* by Race and Sanger is most useful (Race, 1975). *Paternity Testing by Blood Grouping*, edited by Sussman (1976), and *Paternity Testing*, edited by Polesky (1975), supply much of the recent information on this subject. In addition to these, two recent publi-

cations in the Family Law Quarterly are helpful reviews (Abbott, 1976; Lee, 1975).

For frequencies of genetic markers for different ethnic groups, *The Distribution of the Human Blood Groups and other Polymorphisms* by Mourant, Kopec, and Domaniewska-Sobczak (1976) provides an excellent summary. In fact, most gene frequencies given in this chapter are taken from this book, which includes the largest studies on white and black populations in the United States. For a quick check on distribution of various genetic markers in different populations, Stedman's summary is also useful (Stedman, 1959).

LAW OF INHERITANCE, GENES, AND CHROMOSOMES

The so-called "blood test" used in disputed parentage problems is based on the existence of genetic markers in various blood components. Genetic markers in the established blood group systems have been shown to be inherited according to Mendel's law. By careful study of plants and insects, Mendel established three laws of inheritance: (1) unit inheritance: the unit of inheritance (gene) is transmitted through generations intact, (2) allelic segregation: a pair of genes is never found in the same gamete but always separate and pass to two different gametes, (3) independent assortment: different pairs of genes assort independently of each other.

The genes, which are the unit of inheritance containing the genetic information, are in fact double strands of deoxyribonucleic acid (DNA) consisting of phosphate, deoxyribose, adenine-thymidine, and guanine-cytosine. When the DNA undergoes replication, a complementary daughter strand is synthesized from each of the two strands. This single strand of DNA transmits the specific information to messenger ribonucleic acid (RNA), which consists of a single strand of phosphate, ribose, adenine-uracil, and guanine-cytosine. The messenger RNA then issues an order to the transfer RNA to collect all the required amino acids so that ribosomal RNA can synthesize a specific type of polypeptide chain. These polypeptides may possess enzymatic activity and act on a specific substrate or precursor which is then transformed into a recognizable genetic marker such as a blood group antigen.

Chromosomes, demonstrable during certain stages of cell division, consist mainly of DNA

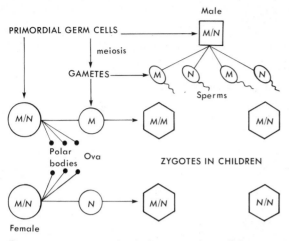

Figure 44–1. An example of inheritance of two allelic genes. During meiosis, each immature primordial germ cell with 46 chromosomes develops into gamete(s) with 23 chromosomes; 4 sperms in males, 1 ovum and 3 polar bodies in females. If *M* and *N* are allelic genes on a pair of chromosomes, each gamete can have only one of them, either *M* or *N*, but not both or neither. When an ovum is fertilized by a sperm in this example, the zygotes formed have 46 chromosomes again: 0.25 *M/M* homozygotes, 0.25 *N/N* homozygotes, and 0.50 *M/N* heterozygotes. Thus, a child always inherits half of a pair of genetic markers from the father and the other half from the mother; this constitutes the very basic principle of inheritance which is applied in the interpretation of paternity tests.

in their protein framework. The division of somatic cells is known as mitosis, whereas that of germ cells is meiosis. In meiosis, one ovum and three polar bodies are formed in females; whereas four spermatids are formed in males. Mature gametes, either ova or sperm, contain only half the number of chromosomes found in the primordial germ cells (Fig. 44–1).

In man, each somatic cell or primordial germ cell has 46 chromosomes, 22 pairs of autosomes, which are the same in both males and females, and one pair of sex chromosomes, XX in the female and XY in the male. The mature gametes, ova or sperm, contain only 23 chromosomes, i.e., half of the genetic information of the primordial cells. When an ovum is fertilized by a sperm, the new cell once again contains 46 chromosomes.

The 22 pairs of autosomes are numbered from 1 to 22, according to their structural differences. Each chromosome consists of a short "p" arm, a centromere, and a long "q" arm. With advances in cytogenetics, each arm has been further divided into regions and subregions. For instance, in chromosome No. 1,

the p arm can be divided into 3 regions and 11 subregions and the q arm into 4 regions and 13 subregions (McKusick, 1977) (see also Chap. 26, p. 814).

The genes governing many of the genetic markers have been assigned to a specific chromosome, and in some instances, even to a specific subregion (McKusick, 1977). Table 44–1 lists the known assignments of common human blood group genetic markers.

Since there are many genes on each chromosome, crossing over from one chromosome to the partner chromosome during meiosis is a normal process. Studying the recombinants often provides valuable information regarding the distance between two genes on a chromosome. If there is no crossing over between two or more genes, we can assume that these genes are linked to each other and can be treated as a gene complex, known as a haplotype, such as *MS*, *Ms*, *NS*, and *Ns*. On the other hand, if crossing over is quite frequent between two genes, they are not linked. If other evidence exists indicating that they are on the same chromosome, they may be referred to as syntenic, such as the genes governing the Rh and Duffy antigens. However, if one finds a small percentage of recombinants between two genes, one can assume that these genes are close to each other, such as HLA-A, -C, -B, -DR, and -D. The 1 per cent recombinant frequency is used to represent the distance between two closely linked genes and is known as a centimorgan, map unit, or cross over unit (see Chaps. 26 and 41).

Specific characteristics may be controlled either by two linked genes on the same chromosome, linked in coupling phase, or by two genes on the opposite sides of a pair of chromosomes, linked in repulsion phase. Only careful study of the family members can resolve these two types of linkages.

FAMILY GENETICS

Family studies are required to establish the nature of inheritance for any given marker. The results of these studies are often presented in pedigree charts using standard symbols (Fig. 44–2). The individual who was the first to be studied or who generated the study is known as the propositus or proband and is indicated on the chart by an arrow. The other individuals are often identified both by generation (Roman numerals) and position number

4

Table 44-1. ASSIGNMENT OF COMMON BLOOD GROUP
GENETIC MARKERS TO CHROMOSOME

COMMON BLOOD GROUP GENETIC MARKERS	CHROMOSOME NO. ASSIGNED TO						
Duffy, Rh, Scianna	1						
Chido, Rodgers, p		6					
ABO			9				
Xg							X
Phosphoglucomutase$_1$	1						
6-Phosphogluconate dehydrogenase	1						
Acid phosphatase	2						
Glyoxalase		6					
Adenylate kinase			9				
Esterase D				13			
Adenosine deaminase					20		
Glucose 6-phosphate dehydrogenase							X
HLA-A,C,B,D,DR		6					
Group-specific components	4						
Complement 2,4 Bf		6					
Haptoglobin-alpha						16	

Selected from the comprehensive listing by McKusick (1977) with a few minor
modifications.

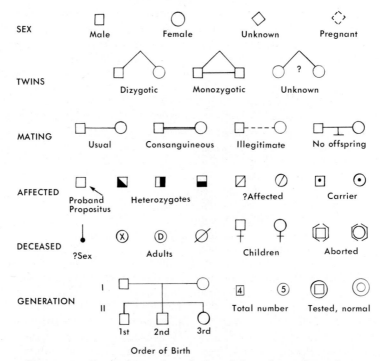

Figure 44-2. Terminology and standard symbols used in pedigree charts.

(Arabic numerals), e.g., II-3. However, such designations are frequently omitted from pedigree charts.

Inherited characteristics which appear in every generation are designated as dominant, whereas those which appear only among the siblings, usually one fourth of the sibs with consanguineous parents, are designated as recessive. When the characteristics appear with equal frequency in males and females, the governing genes are usually assumed to be autosomal. Sex-linked characteristics or traits are never transmitted directly from father to son, but rather from a father to daughters and then to their sons. Dominant sex-linked characteristics will then appear in either a 1:1 or a 2:1 ratio between females and males. On the other hand, recessive sex-linked characteristics appear much more frequently in males than in females.

ALLELES, GENOTYPES, AND PHENOTYPES

The location of a gene on a chromosome is designated as the locus. Alternate genes for the same locus are referred to as alleles. In some blood group systems, only two allelic genes are postulated, such as M and N in the MN system or Jk^a and Jk^b in the Kidd system; in others; three or more exist, such as O, A_1, A_2, and B in the ABO system and many in the HLA system.

Two identical genes at the same location on a pair of chromosomes are designated as homozygous, such as A_1/A_1, B/B, O/O, while two different genes are designated as heterozygous, such as A_1/A_2, A_1/O, A_2/O, B/O, A_1/B, and A_2/B (Fig. 44-3A) The gene governing Xg^a is on the X chromosome; thus males cannot have a pair. Therefore, the presence of Xg^a in the male is referred to as hemizygous. The expression of genes on a pair of chromosomes such as O/O, A_1/A_1, A_2/A_2, B/B, A/O, B/O, A/B, A_1/A_2, and A_2/B is known as genotype. Some genotypes such as A/B or M/N are known through direct demonstration of both antigens (gene products). Other genotypes, such as A_1/A_1, A_1/A_2, A_1/O, A_2/A_2, A_2/O, B/B, and B/O, can be determined only through studies of family members. When present with an A or B gene, the product of the O gene is not demonstrable by current techniques and consequently has been referred to as amorphic.

Since family members are not always

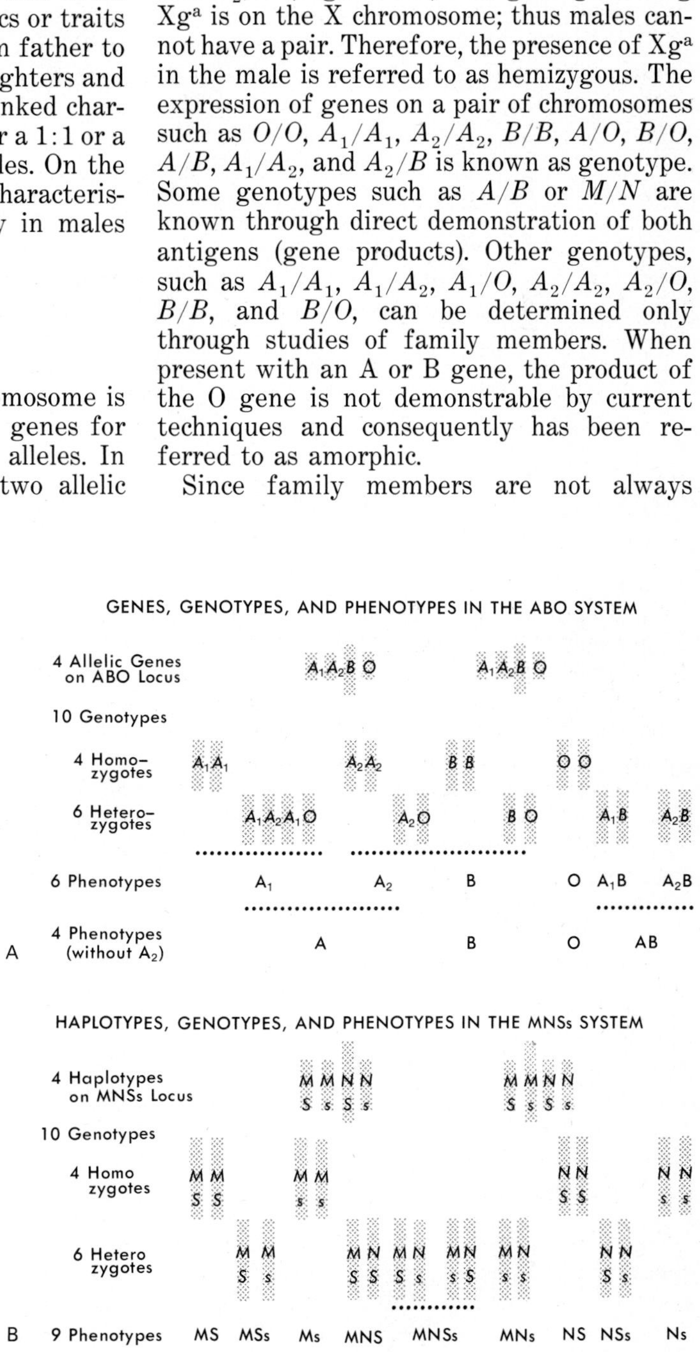

GENES, GENOTYPES, AND PHENOTYPES IN THE ABO SYSTEM

Figure 44-3. *A.* Relationship of genes, genotypes, and phenotypes of ABO blood group system. *B.* Relationship of genes, genotypes, and phenotypes of MNSs blood group system.

HAPLOTYPES, GENOTYPES, AND PHENOTYPES IN THE MNSs SYSTEM

available for study, it is not possible to express all genetic markers as genotypes. The term phenotype, denoting the types which are readily detected or observed, is more commonly used. Thus, the phenotype of A_1/A_1, A_1/A_2, and A_1/O is A_1 and that of B/B and B/O is B. As a result of this, there are 10 genotypes but only 6 phenotypes (A_1, A_2, B, O, A_1B, A_2B) in the ABO system (Fig. 44-3A). A similar relationship in the MN system is shown in Figure 44-3B.

Unfortunately, both alphameric and numeric notations have been used to express phenotypes. Alphameric notations include A, B, O, M, N, K+, k−, and Fy(a − b+). The numeric notations have been used when there are many antigens or new antigens in a system, such as Rh:1 (= positive for Rh1 antigen), Rh:−1 (= negative for Rh1 antigen), Rh:2, Rh:−3 . . . in the Rh system; K:1,−2, (= K + k−) in the Kell system; Lu:3, Lu:−4, Lu:−1 + 2(=Lu(a − b+)) in the Lutheran

system, and Fy: +1 − 2(=Fy(a + b−)) in the Duffy system.

Traditionally, genes, haplotypes, and genotypes are either italicized in printing such as *M*, *MS*, *Ms/Ns*, or underlined in typing with non-italicized type such as M, MS, Ms/Ns. Genotypes are expressed by using a slash to separate the two genes of a pair of chromosomes. An upper bar is used to denote the frequency in a given population; thus $\overline{M}$, $\overline{MS}$, and $\overline{MS/Ns}$ represent, respectively, the frequency of the genes *M*, *MS*, and *MS/Ns*, while $\overline{M}$, $\overline{N}$, and $\overline{MN}$ represent the frequency of the phenotype of M, N, and MN, respectively.

POPULATION GENETICS— FREQUENCIES OF GENES, GENOTYPES, AND PHENOTYPES

The relationship between different types of frequencies can be illustrated using the MN system as follows:

Frequency of genes	$\overline{M}$(0.51)	+	$\overline{N}$(0.49)	= 1	
Frequency of genotypes	$\overline{M}/\overline{M}$(0.32) +	$2\overline{M}/\overline{N}$(0.49) +	$\overline{N}/\overline{N}$(0.19)	= 1	
Frequency of phenotypes	$\overline{M}$(0.32)	+ $\overline{MN}$(0.49)	+ $\overline{N}$(0.19)	= 1	using anti-M and anti-N
	$\overline{M}$ + (0.81)	+	$\overline{M}$ − (0.19)	= 1	using anti-M only
	$\overline{N}$ − (0.32)	+	$\overline{N}$ + (0.68)	= 1	using anti-N only

Since both M and N are demonstrable and the genotypes are the same as the phenotypes, the estimation of gene frequency is an easy task which may be accomplished by taking the square root of the corresponding phenotype frequency. In cases where only anti-M serum is available, one estimates the gene frequency of *N* using the frequency of M negatives, and then obtains $\overline{M}$ by subtracting the frequency from unity (i.e., $1 - \overline{N}$).

From the example above, a general formula

can be derived. If p and q represent the frequency of two allelic genes, then $p + q = 1$, $(p + q)^2 = p^2 + 2pq + q^2 = 1$, where p^2 and q^2 represent the frequencies of homozygotes and $2pq$ that of heterozygotes. Since the value of q^2 is also known (frequency of the silent marker in a population), the value of q and of p can be easily solved. Using the same principle, frequency analysis of three allelic genes can be made as in the ABO system as follows:

Frequency of genes	p	+	q	+	r		= 1
Frequency of genotypes	$p^2 + 2pr$ +		$q^2 + 2qr$ +		r^2 +	2pq	= 1
Frequency of phenotype	$\overline{A}$ +		$\overline{B}$ +		$\overline{O}$ +	$\overline{AB}$	= 1

$r = \overline{O}^{1/2}$

$p = 1 - (q + r) = 1 - (q^2 + 2qr + r^2)^{1/2} = 1 - (\overline{B} + \overline{O})^{1/2}$

$q = 1 - (p + r) = 1 - (p^2 + 2pr + r^2)^{1/2} = 1 - (\overline{A} + \overline{O})^{1/2}$

The relationship between the frequencies of genotypes and phenotypes can now be visualized, and the calculation of the gene frequencies can be done by the formulas given. In

practice, since the sum of values of p, q, and r is seldom one because of sampling problems, adjustments should be made by the method published (Race, 1975).

The formula $p^2 + 2pq + q^2$ is generally known as the Hardy-Weinberg Law. It is a mathematical expression of the equilibrium of genetic markers within a population. Through random mating between various possible genotypes, the ratio between the homozygotes and heterozygotes remains constant from generation to generation. If M and N are two allelic genes with their frequencies being p and q respectively, the following relationship can be established.

Random : Father	M/M	M/M	M/M	M/N	M/N	M/N	N/N	N/N	N/N
	$\times$	$\times$	$\times$	$\times$	$\times$	$\times$	$\times$	$\times$	$\times$
Mating : Mother	M/M	M/N	N/N	M/M	M/N	N/N	M/M	M/N	N/N
	pp	pp	pp	2pq	2pq	2pq	qq	qq	qq
Frequency	$\times$	$\times$	$\times$	$\times$	$\times$	$\times$	$\times$	$\times$	$\times$
	pp	2pq	qq	pp	2pq	qq	pp	2pq	qq

Sum

$$pp(pp + 2pq + qq) + 2pq(pp + 2pq + qq) + qq(pp + 2pq + qq)$$
$$= (pp + 2pq + qq)(pp + 2pq + qq) = (p + q)^2(p^2 + 2pq + q^2)$$
$$= 1 \times (p^2 + 2pq + q^2) = p^2 + 2pq + q^2 \text{ (since p + q = 1)}$$

GENETIC MARKERS USEFUL FOR PATERNITY TESTING

BLOOD GROUP GENETIC MARKERS

Genetic markers are inherited characteristics that differentiate individuals from each other. They could be physical signs such as the color of skin and eyes or the type of hair, or they could be differences demonstrable in the various blood constituents. The value of the former is rather limited in resolving the disputed parentages, while the latter consists of many identifiable markers and has thus become the most useful tool in assisting the judge in making his final decision.

All genetic markers are controlled by genes located on a pair of chromosomes. At any one time, only two genes are involved in the formation of a specific characteristic. However, there may be additional alternative genes at the same locus of the pair of chromosomes. From the inheritance point of view, each parent can contribute only one of the two genes to the child. In other words, a child cannot inherit both genes from a single parent and none from the other.

Based on this principle, the following rules of inheritance can be stated:
1. A child cannot have a genetic marker which is absent in both parents.
2. A child must inherit one of a pair of genetic markers from each parent.
3. A child cannot have a pair of identical genetic markers (aa) unless both parents have the marker (a).
4. A child must have the genetic marker (a or b) which is present as an identical pair in one parent (aa or bb).

Based on these rules, four types of exclusion of paternity are possible:
1. The child has a genetic marker (such as blood group B) which is absent in the mother and cannot be demonstrated in the alleged father.
2. In a system with more than two genetic markers (as ABO), the child lacks both genetic markers (type O, absence of both A and B) which are demonstrated in the alleged father (type AB).
3. A child is homozygous for a genetic marker (such as E/E) which is not present in both parents.
4. A child lacks a genetic marker (M— negative), while the alleged father is homozygous for it (M/M).

The first two types of exclusion are based on the presence or absence of certain genetic markers demonstrable by direct examination and are known as *direct exclusion*. With extremely rare exceptions, these two types of exclusions can be accepted with great confidence.

The third and fourth types of exclusions, based on the inference of homozygous genotypes determined by a negative reaction in a particular test, are known as *indirect exclusion* and should be accepted with caution. The particular test should be repeated with the same and with different or alternative reagents, by a different technologist, or in a different laboratory. For some markers, zygosity may be determined by the use of the titration method or the study of family members. The use of other genetic markers may reveal additional exclusions.

Selection of genetic markers for paternity testing

Testing for all genetic markers demonstrable in the various constituents (cells and proteins) of blood is totally unrealistic.

There are far too many to make this approach practical and many are unsuitable for use in paternity testing. The guidelines discussed below should be taken into consideration before selecting particular genetic markers.

Inheritance. All markers used must follow the mendelian laws of inheritance as established through family studies and studies of population genetics.

Polymorphism. Genetic markers which exhibit wide variation in a given population are most useful for paternity testing. On the other hand, genetic markers of very high or very low frequency are of limited value in differentiating one individual from another. However, the latter markers are valuable in estimating the chance of paternity. If, for instance, the alleged father shares a very low incidence marker with the child, he is most likely the father of the child.

Practicality. The availability and reliability of the reagents as well as procedures are of great importance. The cost in relation to information provided should also be taken into consideration. However, compared with the cost to a falsely accused man for supporting a child, the fee for paternity testing is minimal.

Bearing in mind the criteria mentioned, five groups of genetic markers have been selected for discussion. These include erythrocyte antigens, erythrocyte enzymes, HLA antigens, serum proteins other than immunoglobulins, and immunoglobulins.

GENETIC MARKERS OF ERYTHROCYTE ANTIGENS

Erythrocyte antigens are by far the most popular and useful genetic markers for paternity testing. First, most technologists are familiar with the techniques for testing erythrocyte antigens; second, the reagents are standardized and most of them are readily available; third, a cumulative chance of exclusion of paternity of nearly 80 per cent can be achieved; and finally, it is the only group of

markers with which non-medical people have any familiarity.

On the other hand, erythrocyte antigens have been intensively studied and more variants have been reported. Interpretation of results is not always as clear-cut as once believed; however, if one is aware of these possible variants, additional tests can often be done to resolve the issue.

Table 44-2 lists the genetic markers of erythrocyte antigens that are currently being used for paternity testing. Gene frequencies (p) of whites and blacks for each marker are also listed; however, the phenotype frequencies ($\bar{P}$), which can be derived from the gene frequencies ($\bar{P} = 2p - p^2$), are omitted. Both types of frequencies are essential for calculating the chance of exclusion of paternity (included in the table) and also the chance of paternity.

The ABO system has been very well studied and the inheritance patterns well established. Reliable anti-A_1 is available and should be included for all group A or AB individuals. Since there is no specific antibody for the A_2 antigen, the genotype A_1/A_2 cannot be established without further studies of other family members. An A_1 infant less than 18 months old may be typed as A_2, since the A_1 antigen may not be well developed before that time. The A_3 subgroup is relatively rare and, like other low incidence antigens, greatly increases the chance of paternity when present in both the child and the alleged father. The A_x and A_m antigens are extremely rare and should not be considered in paternity exclusions. Other rare phenotypes include "Bombay," cis-AB, and acquired-B, all of which can be readily identified (Race, 1975).

The Rh system can provide as much as a 25 per cent chance of exclusion of paternity if anti-C, anti-c, and anti-E serums are included with the anti-D serum. The further addition of anti-e and anti-C^w, which are more expensive and more difficult to obtain, would increase the chance to 31 per cent. In cases involving blacks, the incorporation of anti-V and anti-e^s can be very informative, since they are polymorphic among blacks. In some cases, exclusion based on haplotypes may not be possible unless anti-ce(f) or anti-Ce(rh_i) is used to ascertain the genotype of the individuals. The possibility of gene suppression, weak variants, and deletions should also be considered before arriving at a final conclusion (p. 1529).

The MNSs system also provides a high per-

Table 44–2. GENE FREQUENCY OF ERYTHROCYTE ANTIGENS USED IN PATERNITY TESTING*

SYSTEM	GENETIC MARKERS	GENE FREQUENCY		CHANCE OF EXCLUSION/SYSTEM		PAGE(S) IN MOURANT, 1976
		Whites	Blacks	Whites	Blacks	
1. ABO	O	0.6602	0.7006			230
	A_1	0.2089	0.1161			
	A_2	0.0701	0.0585	18.5%	20.9%	
	B	0.0658	0.1248			
2. Rh	D	0.6652	0.7184			485,477
	C	0.4762	0.1345			
	C^w	0.0010				
	c	0.5138	0.8655			
	E	0.1510	0.2519			
	e	0.8490	0.7481			
	DCE	0.0017	0.0032			
	DCe	0.4603	0.1069			
	DC^we	0.0100				
	dCe	0.0142	0.0244			
	DcE	0.1348	0.0977	31.2%	31.4%	
	Dce	0.0297	0.5077			
	dcE	0.0145				
	dce	0.3348	0.2572			
	D^uce		0.0029			
3. MN	M	0.5536	0.4528	(18.6%)	(18.64%)	307,313
	N	0.4464	0.5472			
	S	0.3164	0.1582			
	s	0.6836	0.7281			
	S^u		0.1235			
	MS	0.2473	0.1028			
	Ms	0.3063	0.3500			
	NS	0.0691	0.0554			
	Ns	0.3773	0.3681	31.6%	27.9%	
	MS^u		0.0503			
	NS^u		0.0734			
4. Kell	K	0.0450	0.0038	4.1%	0.4%	532
	k	0.9550	0.9962			
5. Duffy	Fy^a	0.3858	0.0809			591,593
	Fy^b	0.6142	0.1564	18.1%	16.6%	
	Fy^4		0.7627			
6. Kidd	Jk^a	0.5360	0.7426	18.7%	15.5%	601
	Jk^b	0.4640	0.2574			
7. Lutheran	Lu^a	0.0335	0.0243	3.1%	2.3%	515
	Lu^b	0.9665	0.9757			
8. Xg	Xg^a	0.6709	0.5496	6.7%	8.3%	631
9. P_1	P_1	0.6537	0.2929	0.9%	7.0%	343
10. Secretor	Se	0.4957	0.4715	3.2%	3.7%	553,554
	Cumulative chance			78.8%	78.8%	

*Including also haplotype frequency.

centage of exclusion. If only anti-M and anti-N are used, the chance is approximately 18 per cent. The chance is increased to 24 per cent when anti-S is also used, and to 31 per cent if anti-s is included as well. When there is a possible indirect exclusion involving zygosity in the MN system, the presence of alternate alleles such as M^k, S^u, M^g, and N_2 should be taken into consideration; studying the dosage effect by titration may sometimes be helpful.

For example, if the child is typed as M+N−, while the alleged father is typed as M−N+, there seems to be an exclusion of paternity. However, should one also use anti-M^g for testing, one may find that the child is M/M^g and the alleged father is N/M^g. If this is indeed the case, not only is there no exclusion, but paternity is very likely. Since the incidence of M^g is less than 1 in 60,000, it is most unlikely that another man with the same marker (except possibly his brother) was involved with the same woman during that time period.

The S/S^u and s/S^u genotypes are not uncommon in blacks. Since there is no specific antiserum to detect the product of the S^u gene, exclusion based on the zygosity of S or s is not valid in blacks. The use of titrations to determine the dosage of the antigen (S or s), as well as studies of the family members of the alleged father, may shed some light on the matter but is not always conclusive. To date, all S^u/S^u, or U negative, individuals are also $S-s-$. However, the converse is not true, and the use of anti-U does not add any useful information. The use of anti-He, anti-Hu, and anti-M_1 may prove useful among blacks.

These rare possibilities do not affect direct exclusions in the MN system. If the child has a marker, whether it be M, N, S, or s, which is not found in either the mother or the alleged father, exclusion of paternity is valid, provided the test results are clear-cut and appropriate controls have been included. A second antiserum must also be included to confirm the results.

Although the Kell system contains numerous allelic antigens, its usefulness in paternity testing is somewhat limited, since most of the antigens are either of very high or very low incidence. However, anti-K provides a 3.7 per cent chance of exclusion in whites, and anti-Js^a approximately a 7.0 per cent chance in blacks. In considering indirect exclusions, the possibility of K_o or the McLeod phenotype should be kept in mind.

The Duffy system is considerably more helpful in paternity exclusion. Anti-Fy^a alone provides only approximately a 5.5 per cent chance of exclusion; however, if anti-Fy^b is added, the chance increases to over 18 per cent in whites. Since $Fy(a-b-)$ is common in blacks, indirect exclusions based on zygosity should not be considered in cases involving blacks; this situation may improve when anti-Fy4 becomes available.

The Kidd system offers more than an 18 per cent chance of exclusion in whites and nearly 16 per cent in blacks, if both anti-Jk^a and anti-Jk^b are used. The chance is reduced to 2.5 per cent if only anti-Jk^a is used. Unlike the Duffy system, the minus-minus phenotype is extremely rare.

Anti-Lu^a by itself offers a 2.9 per cent chance of exclusion. Since Lu^b is a high-inci-

dence antigen, testing with anti-Lu^b is unnecessary unless the individual(s) is $Lu(a+)$. The possibility of the rare "silent" allele Lu should be kept in mind when considering any indirect exclusions.

Anti-Xg^a is only useful in paternity exclusions if the child is a female. An $Xg(a+)$ male cannot have an $Xg(a-)$ daughter, if she is a normal XX; nor can a $Xg(a-)$ male have an $Xg(a+)$ daughter if the mother is also $Xg(a-)$.

P_1 should be used only as evidence for exclusion if the child is strongly P_1 positive and both the mother and the alleged father are P_1 negative. A weakly reactive P_1 antigen should not be considered as evidence for exclusion.

Collection of saliva for secretor studies is rather tedious, especially in children or infants; hence, secretor testing is rarely used for paternity studies.

Testing for the Lewis antigens is generally not recommended for use in paternity testing for several reasons. First, Le^a and Le^b are not alleles and must not be treated as such. Second, the Se gene is involved in the production of the antigens, thus complicating the interpretation, since secretor studies are not usually done concurrently. Third, the anti-Le^a and anti-Le^b serums are often unstable. Fourth, the antigen strength is variable during infancy and pregnancy and may be undetectable, causing false negative results. Finally, the Lewis antigens may not be basically erythrocyte antigens, but rather plasma antigens which are secondarily adsorbed onto red cells.

Other serums which may prove useful include anti-Di^a and anti-St^a for a Mongolian population. Anti-Do^a and anti-Do^b, when they become available, will offer an 18.5 per cent chance of exclusion.

GENETIC MARKERS OF ERTHROCYTE ENZYMES

Many red cell enzymes have been examined for polymorphism. While the majority of them show little variation in population studies, eight of them are suitable for paternity testing and are listed in Table 44-3. Four of the eight enzymes—ACP, ALT,* GLO, and PGM_1—offer a 13 to 18 per cent chance of

---

*Alanine aminotransferase, formerly known as glutamic pyruvate transaminase (GPT).

Table 44-3. USEFUL ERYTHROCYTE ENZYME GENETIC MARKERS FOR PATERNITY TESTING

| ERYTHROCYTE ENZYMES (ABBREVIATION) | FREQUENCY OF COMMON GENES | | | | CHANCE OF EXCLUSION OF PATERNITY | | KEY REFERENCE |
| | WHITES | | BLACKS | | | | |
	1	2	1	2	Whites	Blacks	
1. Phosphoglucomutase (PGM$_1$)	0.752	0.248	0.809	0.191	15.2%	13.1%	Giblett, 1969
2. Adenylate kinase (AK)	0.953	0.471	0.993	0.006	4.3%	.6%	Bowmann, 1976
3. 6-phosphogluconate dehydrogenase (6PGD)	0.976 (A)	0.024 (B)	0.965 (A)	0.035 (B)	2.3%	3.3%	Davidson, 1967
4. Adenosine deaminase (ADA)	0.952	0.048	0.979 0.005 (3)	0.016	4.3%	1.5%	Detter, 1970
5. Glyoxalase (GLO)	0.427	0.573			18.5%		Kompf, 1975
6. Esterase D (EsD)	0.902	0.098	0.902	0.098	8.1%	8.1%	Welch, 1975
7. Acid phosphatase (ACP)	0.394 (A) 0.060 (C)	0.547 (B)	0.250 (A) 0.014 (C)	0.720 (B)	27.1%	17.2%	Giblett, 1969
8. Alanine aminotransferase (ALT) or glutamic pyruvate transaminase (GPT)	0.523	0.472	0.814	0.179	18.6%	12.9%	Chen, 1972
Cumulative					66.3%	55.6%	

4

exclusion of paternity. The remaining four— EsD, AK, ADA, and 6-PGD—offer a 1 to 8 per cent chance of exclusion. The cumulative chance of exclusion for all eight is 66.3 per cent for whites, and 55.6 per cent for blacks.

Each of the eight enzymes has basically two common alleles (except ACP, which has three), designated either as 1 and 2 or as A and B, the products of which are demonstrable by electrophoresis. The phenotypes obtained, 1, 2-1, 2, or AA, AB, and BB, also represent the genotypes. Like the erythrocyte antigens, null types such as ACP_0, ALT_0 or GPT_0, ADA_0, and AK_0 have been reported, and uncommon alleles and variants have also been observed. Unless the results are clear-cut and appropriate controls tested simultaneously, conclusions should be drawn with great care.

Another enzyme, G6PD, can be useful for paternity testing in blacks. G6PD has two common alleles, Gd^A and Gd^B, with gene frequencies of 0.22 and 0.78, respectively. However, one should keep in mind that deficiencies of G6PD are not uncommon among blacks. Since these markers are located on the X chromosome, exclusions may be demonstrated in the female child only.

Other polymorphic enzymes are not as useful in paternity testing as those listed above.

For example, PGM$_3^1$ has a gene frequency of 0.74 in whites and 0.37 in blacks; however, demonstration of this enzyme requires preparation of a white cell lysate instead of a red cell lysate. PGM$_2$, peptidase A, and peptidase D have limited usefulness, as they exhibit only slight polymorphism in blacks.

GENETIC MARKERS OF HLA ANTIGENS

The only well-established leukocyte antigens are the HLA antigens (see Chap. 41). In 1977, antigens controlled by five loci, A, B, C, D, and DR, were described for the HLA system; a large number of specificities are recognized at each locus; 18 for A, 23 for B, 6 for C, 11 for D, and 7 for DR have been agreed upon by experts in this field. The use of 14 HLA-A and 15 HLA-B antiserums (as listed in Table 44-4) allows the determination of $14 \times 15 = 210$ haplotypes, $210 \times 211/2 = 22,155$ genotypes, and $(14 \times 15/2)(15 \times 16/2) = 12,600$ phenotypes. The 29 antisera offer a 60 to 84 per cent cumulative chance of direct exclusion. Thus, HLA antigens have become a powerful tool for studying parentage problems (Table 44-4).

At the present time, only direct exclusions

Table 44–4. GENE FREQUENCY (p) AND CHANCE OF EXCLUSION OF PATERNITY $(p(1 - p)^4)$ OF HLA ANTIGENS

SPECIFICITIES	CAUCASIAN		MONGOLIAN		AMER. INDIAN		AFRICA BLACK	
	p	$p(1-p)^4$	p	$p(1-p)^4$	p	$p(1-p)^4$	p	$p(1-p)^4$
HLA-A1	0.11	6.9%	0.02	1.8%	0.01	0.9%	0.05	4.2%
A2	0.24	8.0%	0.18	8.1%	0.48	3.5%	0.19	8.2%
A3	0.12	7.2%	0.01	0.9%	0.01	0.9%	0.08	5.7%
Aw23 : A9	0.03	2.7%	0.02	1.9%	0.00	0.0%	0.08	5.7%
Aw24 : A9	0.10	6.6%	0.34	6.5%	0.25	7.9%	0.05	4.2%
Aw25 : A10	0.01	0.9%	0.03	2.7%	0.00	0.0%	0.01	0.9%
Aw26 : A10	0.05	4.1%	0.07	5.2%	0.00	0.0%	0.07	5.2%
A11	0.09	6.2%	0.13	7.6%	0.01	0.9%	0.08	5.7%
A28	0.05	4.1%	0.02	1.9%	0.09	6.2%	0.09	6.2%
A29	0.02	1.9%	0.01	0.9%	0.00	0.0%	0.05	4.2%
Aw30	0.04	3.4%	0.02	1.9%	0.02	1.9%	0.16	8.0%
Aw31	0.01	0.9%	0.00	0.0%	0.09	6.2%	0.02	1.9%
Aw32	0.04	3.4%	0.00	0.0%	0.00	0.0%	0.04	3.4%
Aw33	0.04	3.4%	0.07	5.2%	0.04	3.4%	0.07	5.2%
Blank	0.04		0.06		0.02		0.02	
SUM FOR ALL HLA-A		59.7%		42.7%		31.8%		61.5%
HLA-B5	0.01	0.9%	0.09	6.2%	0.11	6.9%	0.08	5.7%
B7	0.11	6.9%	0.02	1.9%	0.01	0.9%	0.12	7.2%
B8	0.07	5.2%	0.01	0.9%	0.00	0.0%	0.04	.34%
B12	0.11	6.9%	0.03	2.7%	0.01	0.9%	0.12	7.2%
B13	0.02	1.9%	0.04	3.4%	0.00	0.0%	0.01	0.9%
B14	0.03	2.7%	0.00	0.0%	0.01	0.9%	0.03	2.7%
B18	0.07	5.2%	0.01	0.9%	0.01	0.9%	0.03	2.7%
B27	0.04	3.4%	0.04	3.4%	0.03	2.7%	0.00	0.0%
Bw15	0.07	5.2%	0.16	8.0%	0.15	7.8%	0.04	3.4%
Bw16	0.03	2.7%	0.05	4.2%	0.12	7.2%	0.01	0.9%
Bw17	0.06	4.7%	0.03	2.7%	0.01	0.9%	0.21	8.2%
Bw21	0.03	2.7%	0.00	0.0%	0.04	3.4%	0.01	0.9%
Bw22	0.02	1.9%	0.13	7.5%	0.00	0.0%	0.01	0.9%
Bw35	0.10	6.6%	0.06	4.7%	0.23	8.1%	0.06	4.7%
Bw40	0.05	4.2%	0.24	8.0%	0.16	8.0%	0.06	4.7%
Blank	0.11		0.12		0.16		0.15	
SUM FOR ALL HLA-B		61.1%		40.1%		41.4%		53.5%
CUMULATIVE FOR HLA-A AND HLA-B		84.3%		65.7%		60.0%		82.1%

The gene frequencies (p) were taken from Dausset (1973). The value for the chance of exclusion by each marker is estimated from the gene frequency (p) using the formula $p(1 - p)^4$. Cumulative chance of exclusion (CE) is derived by the formula $CE = 1 - (1 - CE_1)(1 - CE_2)$.

in this system can be considered with great confidence. Indirect exclusions are difficult to establish for several reasons. First, there is a lack of good monospecific antiserum. Second, a number of specificities show cross-reactions with antiserum of other known specificities. Third, there is a 1 to 2 per cent crossing-over rate for the HLA system as well as a known disequilibrium of haplotypes. Finally, the frequencies for many ethnic groups are not yet well established.

Testing the HLA antigens may also help greatly in the determination of the chance of paternity if the child and the alleged father share one or more low-frequency antigens or a low-frequency haplotype as revealed by the study of additional family members.

Additional information on HLA antigens is found in Chapter 41. Useful discussions of HLA antigens with regard to paternity testing are in the references (Jeannet, 1972; Mayr, 1971; Speiser, 1975; and Soulier, 1974).

Table 44–5. GENE FREQUENCY OF SERUM PROTEIN GENETIC MARKERS USED IN PATERNITY TESTING*

SERUM PROTEIN MARKER	COMMON ALLELES	GENE FREQUENCY		CHANCE OF EXCLUSION		PAGE IN REFERENCE (Mourant, 1976)
		White	Black	White	Black	
1. Haptoglobins	Hp¹	0.4169	0.5500	18.4%	18.6%	656
(Hp)	Hp²	0.5831	0.4500			
2. Group-specific	Gc¹	0.7155	0.8924			
components (Gc)	Gc²	0.2845	0.1076	16.2%	8.7%	692
3. Transferrin	Tf^B	0.0054	0.0000			
(Tf)	Tf^C	0.9939	0.9773	1%	2.2%	418
	Tf^D		0.0227			
4. Ceruloplasmin	Cp^A	0.0060	0.0519		4.2%	713
(Cp)	Cp^B	0.9940	0.9392			
5. Beta lipoprotein	Ag^x	0.2034	0.2705	13.6%	15.8%	697
(Ag)	Ag^y	0.7966	0.7295			
6. Beta lipoprotein	Lp^a	0.2183	0.1894	8.2%	8.2%	703
(Lp)						
7. Complement C3	C3^S	0.75	0.90	15.2%	8.2%	Alper, 1968
(C3)	C3^F	0.25	0.10			
8. Beta glycoprotein	Bf^S	0.709	0.437			
(Bf, glycine-rich)	Bf^F	0.278	0.512			
	Bf^{S1}	0.013		14.2%	24.2%	Alper, 1972
	Bf^{F1}		0.051			
Cumulative chance of exclusion				60.9%	66.5%	

*Excluding the immunoglobulins.

4

GENETIC MARKERS OF SERUM PROTEINS (EXCLUDING IMMUNOGLOBULINS)

Of the many proteins present in the serum, the genetic markers of haptoglobin (Hp), group-specific component (Gc), and immunoglobulins (Gm) are the ones most commonly tested. The Gm markers will be discussed subsequently. However, as shown in Table 44–5, there are many other serum proteins which are potentially useful for paternity testing, altogether providing over a 60 per cent chance of exclusion.

Multiple physiologic and pathologic conditions are known to affect the haptoglobin level and, hence, the phenotype determination. A null type, as well as many other variants, have been described. For more detailed information, Giblett (1969) should be consulted.

Group-specific component (Gc) is an alpha-2-globulin which has been extensively studied, especially with regard to the phenotype distribution patterns in various populations (Giblett, 1969).

Transferrin can be conveniently studied concurrently with Gc typing, and ceruloplasmin with haptoglobin typing; unfortunately, neither is very polymorphic. Conversely, two complement components C3 and Bf are highly polymorphic but are inconvenient to study because they are very unstable. Another protein which is highly polymorphic is alpha-1-acid glycoprotein; however, its inheritance has not yet been well established.

As for Ag and Lp, two beta lipoproteins which theoretically should be very useful, the lack of potent antiserum necessary for their demonstration precludes their wide application to paternity testing. Another antiserum, anti-Xm, detects an antigen controlled by Xm^a gene located on the X chromosome. The gene frequency of Xm^a is 0.3 for American white females and 0.36 for American black females. Theoretically it should be useful for paternity testing; however, good antisera are not yet available and the antigen may often be poorly developed in many young children.

GENETIC MARKERS OF IMMUNOGLOBULINS

In 1975, WHO sponsored a meeting of experts on genetic markers of immunoglobulins. These experts agreed upon 17 allotypes for the heavy chains of IgG, two of IgA, and three of

Table 44-6. IMMUNOGLOBULIN ALLOTYPES*

LOCATION	ALPHAMERIC	NUMERIC
IgG1	G1m(a)	G1m(1)
	(x)	(2)
	(f)	(3)
	(z)	(17)
IgG2	G2m(n)	G2m(23)
IgG3	G3m(b0)	G3m(11)
	(b1)	(5)
	(b3)	(13)
	(b4)	(14)
	(b5)	(10)
	(c3)	(6)
	(c5)	(24)
	(g)	(21)
	(u)	(26)
	(v)	(27)
	(s)	(15)
	(t)	(16)
IgA2	A2m(1)	A2m(1)
	A2m(2)	A2m(2)
κ chain	Km (1)	Km (1)
	(2)	(2)
	(3)	(3)

*World Health Organization, 1975.

kappa light chains (Table 44-6). In their recommendation, the number of the particular subclass is incorporated into the prefix such as G1m, G2m, G3m, and A2m. The allotypes of IgG can then be expressed either alphamerically, such as G1m(a), G1m(x), . . . or numerically, such as G1m(1), G1m(2) (Ceppellini, 1965).

Notations for phenotypes and genotypes were also suggested by the WHO committee as follows: (; between subclasses and . . for -n or -23)

	ALPHAMERIC	NUMERIC
PHENOTYPES	Gm(f;n;b1)	Gm(3;23;5)
	Gm(a,f,z;n;b1,g)	Gm(1,3,17;23;5,21)
	Gm(a,z;..;g)	Gm(1,3;..;21)
GENOTYPES	$Gm^{f;n;b1}/Gm^{g;n;b1}$	$Gm^{3;23;5}/Gm^{3;23;5}$
	$Gm^{a,z;..;g}/Gm^{f;n;b1}$	$Gm^{1,17;..;21}/Gm^{3;23;5}$
	$Gm^{a,z;..;g}/Gm^{a,z;..;g}$	$Gm^{1,17;..;21}/Gm^{1,17;..;21}$

The isoallotypes which behave as allotypic markers in one subclass, but as isoantigens in other subclasses, are expressed as follows:

	NOTATIONS	
Alphameric	Numeric	Previous
Na	N1	Non-a
Nb0	N11	Non-b0
Nb1	N5	Non-b1
Ng	N21	Non-g
N4a	N4a	Non-4a
N4b	N4b	Non-4b

Table 44-7 lists the genetic markers of immunoglobulins which either are currently being used in paternity testing or are potentially useful with the availability of proper reagents. Some markers are polymorphic only in selected ethnic groups; hence, their usefulness in paternity testing is restricted. This includes G1m(a) for whites, G3m(C3 or C5) for blacks, and G3m(s or t) for Japanese. The phenotype frequencies ($\bar{P}$) of each marker given for the white, black, Chinese, and Japanese ethnic groups were provided by Dr. M. Schanfield of the Milwaukee Blood Center, Wisconsin (1977). The gene frequency (p) of each marker was derived from the phenotype frequency using the formula $p = 1 - (1 - \bar{P})^{1/2}$.

The sum of the gene frequencies of each of four pairs of immunoglobulins, namely G1m(f) and G1m(z), G3m(bO) and G3m(g), A2m(1) and A2m(2), and Km(1) and Km(3), is close to 1.0, and only a very few persons have been found to be negative for both markers in a pair. Therefore, these markers can be treated as allelic, greatly increasing the chance of exclusion of paternity (Fudenberg 1978; Grubb 1970; van Loghem, 1975).

The chance of exclusion (CE) of paternity provided by each marker is estimated from the gene frequency (p), using $CE = p(1 - p)^4$. The sum of the chance of exclusion in the Gm system for the four ethnic groups is 0.317, 0.299, 0.222, and 0.407, respectively. Markers in the Am and Km systems are known to be allelic; the chance of exclusion can be estimated by the formula $CE = p(1 - p) \times (1 - p(1 - p))$. The cumulative chance of the three systems together can be obtained by the formula

$$1 - (1 - CEGm)(1 - CEAm)(1 - CEKm)$$

and they are 0.4, 0.51, 0.46, and 0.6, respectively, for whites, blacks, Chinese, and Japanese.

The haplotypes of Ig markers also show greater polymorphism in some ethnic groups than in others. Table 44-8 lists the most common haplotypes and their frequencies among whites, blacks, Chinese, and Japanese. These frequencies show that $Gm^{a,x,z;..;g}$ and $Gm^{a,z;..;g}$ are useful for paternity testing for whites,

ALLOTYPE OF	ISOANTIGEN OF
IgG1(f + a −)	IgG2,3
IgG3(b − f +)	IgG1,2
IgG3(b − f +)	IgG1,2
IgG3(b + g −)	IgG2
IgG4(4a + , 4b −)	IgG1,3
IgG4(4a −,4b +)	IgG2

Table 44-7. IMMUNOGLOBULIN GENETIC MARKERS FOR PATERNITY TESTING

COMMON IMMUNOGLOBULIN ALLOTYPES*	G1m f	G1m z	G1m x	G2m n	G3m b0	G3m g	OTHERS	Am 1	Am 2	Km 1	Km 3	CUMULATIVE CE
WHITE (Czechoslovakia)							G1m(a)					
A. Phenotype frequency	0.950	0.398	0.101	0.734	0.950	0.398	0.398	0.999	0.02	0.2	(0.99)	
B. Gene frequency	0.776	0.224	0.052	0.484	0.766	0.224	0.224	0.968	0.01	0.106	0.894	
C. CE: each marker	0.002	0.081	0.042	0.028	0.002	0.081	0.081	0.01	0.01	0.068		
each system				0.317					0.30		0.086	0.40
BLACK (Texas)							G3m(c3,c5)					
A. Phenotype frequency	0.241	0.983	0.060	0.210	0.997	0.120	0.326	0.586	0.872	0.51	(0.91)	
B. Gene frequency	0.129	0.870	0.030	0.112	0.938	0.062	0.179	0.358	0.642	0.30	0.70	
C. CE: each marker	0.074		0.027	0.069	0.002	0.048	0.081	0.061	0.010	0.072	0.006	
each system				0.299					0.177		0.166	0.51
CHINESE (San Francisco)												
A. Phenotype frequency	0.953	0.385	0.133	0.953	0.964	0.344		0.524	0.909	0.51	(0.91)	
B. Gene frequency	0.783	0.216	0.069	0.783	0.81	0.19		0.310	0.698	0.30	0.70	
C. CE: each marker	0.002	0.082	0.052	0.002	0.002	0.092		0.070	0.006	0.072	0.006	
each system				0.222					0.168		0.166	0.46
JAPANESE (San Francisco & Tokyo)							G3m(s,t)					
A. Phenotype frequency	0.279	0.977	0.279	0.278	0.654	0.830	0.454	0.780	0.718	0.50	(0.91)	
B. Gene frequency	0.151	0.849	0.151	0.151	0.41	0.59	0.261	0.531	0.469	0.30	0.70	
C. CE: each marker	0.078		0.078	0.078	0.078	0.017	0.078	0.026	0.037	0.072	0.006	
each system				0.407					0.187		0.166	0.60

A. Phenotype frequency ($\bar{P}$) Supplied by Dr. M. Schanfield (1977).

B. Gene frequency (p) estimated from the phenotype frequency $p = 1 - (1 - \bar{P})^{1/2}$.

C. CE = Chance of exclusion of paternity. Each marker: $CE = p(1 - p)^4$; Gm system: sum of CE of each marker; Am and Km systems: $CE = p(1 - p)(1 - p(1 - p))$ formula for two allelic markers.

*See text.

4

Table 44-8. FREQUENCIES OF COMMON GM HAPLOTYPES IN FOUR POPULATIONS*

HAPLOTYPES	WHITE	BLACK	CHINESE	JAPANESE
$Gm^{x,a,z;..;g}$	0.10	0.00	0.09	0.17
$Gm^{a,z;..;g}$	0.20	0.00	0.23	0.47
$Gm^{f;n;b0,b1}$	0.52	0.00	0.00	0.00
$Gm^{f;..;b0,b1}$	0.17	0.00	0.00	0.00
$Gm^{a,z;..;b0,b1}$	<0.01	0.55	<0.01	<0.01
$Gm^{a,z;..;b0,b1,c3,c5}$	<0.01	0.25	0.00	0.00
$Gm^{a,z;..;b0,s}$	0.00	0.12	0.00	0.00
$Gm^{a,z;..;b0,b1,c3}$	0.00	0.08	0.00	0.00
$Gm^{a,f;n;b0,b1}$	0.00	0.00	0.62	0.08
$Gm^{a,z;..;b0,s.t.}$	<0.01	0.00	0.06	0.28

*Taken from Dr. M. Schanfield (1977).

Chinese, and Japanese, but not for blacks, whereas $Gm^{f;n;b0}$ and $Gm^{g;..;b0}$ are basically markers for whites only. Similarly, $Gm^{a,z;..;b0}$ or $Gm^{a,z;..;b0,C3,C5}$ is for blacks, $Gm^{af;n;b0}$ is for Chinese, and $Gm^{a,z;..;b0,s,t}$ for Japanese.

Because of these racial variations, Gm typings can prove most useful in parentage problems involving individuals of different races. However, the estimated cross-over rate is 1 to 2 per cent, which should be considered before reporting exclusions based on haplotypes.

LABORATORY TESTING

PROPER IDENTIFICATION

Since proper identification of the individuals involved in a paternity case is of utmost importance, whenever feasible, all persons should be present at the same time to allow them to identify each other. Care should also be taken that the blood is drawn from the man identified as the alleged father and not from a male companion who might also be present.

Information kept in the records should include:

a. Name and location of the institution performing the testing.

b. Full name of each individual; identify the mother, the child, and the alleged father.

c. Age, sex, and race of each party, since they are pertinent in interpreting the results.

d. Address and telephone number (optional) of each party.

e. Signature of each adult and witness.

f. Thumb prints of the woman, the alleged father, and the child (foot prints if the child is less than one year old).

g. Initials of the person drawing the blood specimen.

In some laboratories, instant photographs are also being taken of all of the individuals. When this is done, each photograph should also bear the date and the signature of the person.

Whenever feasible, blood or saliva specimens should be obtained in duplicate so that any rechecking or duplicate testing can be done on a separate specimen. Whenever erythrocyte enzymes are being tested, a set of specimens must also be drawn in ACD or EDTA tubes. Another aliquot of specimen must also be collected if HLA testing is to be included. All tubes should be labeled with (1) the full name of the individual, (2) whether it is the mother or the alleged father or child, (3) the date drawn, and (4) the initials of the person drawing the specimens. The label should be marked in permanent ink and covered with transparent tape.

If the testing is not performed immediately, all specimens should be stored in a refrigerator, in a section with no other blood specimens. Any tubes or containers to be used for subsequent transfer of serum or cells must also be premarked with permanent ink.

GENERAL COMMENTS ON LABORATORY TESTING FOR GENETIC MARKERS

a. *Technologist(s):* Testing of the blood group genetic markers should be performed only by qualified technologists well trained in handling the various procedures involved, as well as any problems which might arise.

b. *Reagents:* As much as is possible, licensed or certified reagents should be used. The use of any other reagents is acceptable only if proper controls are tested simultaneously.

c. *Controls:* Both negative and positive controls must be run for each reagent being used on the day of testing.

d. *Specimens:* Blood samples of all individuals in each case should be tested at the same time, with the same reagent, and by the same technologist(s) whenever possible.

e. *Procedures:* Since many procedures and techniques are available for testing blood group genetic markers, only those mastered by the technologist(s) performing the testing should be used. All testing should be reproducible and yield clear-cut definitive results.

f. *Recording results:* Results should be recorded as they are read, with any changes initialed by the one making the correction. The strength of the reactions should also be recorded whenever applicable. The source and lot number of the reagents must be included with the test results. In dealing with electrophoresis or microtiter plates, some laboratories take photographs of the patterns and keep these as records.

g. *Repeating tests:* Any time a doubtful result or an exclusion is obtained, the test should be repeated using different/additional reagents and by a different technologist.

h. In addition to selection of examinations as well as methods, a physician with special competence should not only supervise testing and observe reactions, but also interpret results in a written format that is scientifically accurate and understood by other than medical personnel.

i. *Consultation:* In cases in which one laboratory encounters difficulty in testing or in interpretation, specimens may be mailed to a second laboratory which has more experience in dealing with the particular problem. Should the results disagree, a third laboratory should be consulted.

TYPING FOR ERYTHROCYTE ANTIGENS

General comments

The reagents and procedures used in paternity testing are essentially the same as those previously described in Chapter 43. The following comments are especially relevant to paternity testing.

Whenever possible, at least two and preferably three complete sets of antiserums of different lots and of different suppliers should be available for repeat or confirmatory testing. If feasible, anti-C^w, anti-f(ce), anti-rh_i(Ce), anti-V, anti-He, anti-M_1, anti-M^g, anti-Di^a, and anti-Js^a and their appropriate controls should also be available for supplemental testing as previously mentioned.

Reverse ABO grouping should include O cells, as well as A_1 and B cells. This is crucial in ruling out the possibility of the O_h phenotype, since these individuals have anti-H in their serum.

Although testing for hemagglutination is usually performed in test tubes, microtiter plates may be used if the technologist(s) is familiar with the technique (Lapinski, 1978). In fact, the possibility of introducing a human error may be reduced, since each well can be preassigned to a specific test and reactions photographed as a part of the record. The AutoAnalyzer, not currently available in most laboratories, has been used very successfully in paternity testing at the Charles Hymen Blood Center of Mount Sinai Hospital in Chicago (Fig. 44-4). In this way, a permanent recording can be kept. In the example shown, the child is positive for both A_1 and Fy^b, while the mother and the alleged father are negative for both, an apparent exclusion of paternity.

Determination of genotypes

Quite often it is necessary to determine the genotype of the individuals in order to interpret the results correctly. The probability of being homozygous or heterozygous for any given marker is easily derived from the known gene frequencies. More exact information can be obtained only from family studies, which are not always possible. However, two other approaches are possible: (1) the use of antiserums against compound antigens, such as anti-ce, anti-Ce, anti-CE, and anti-cE, and (2) the use of titration scores. An example of the latter follows.

| | DILUTIONS OF ANTISERUM | | | | | | | | ANTISERUM | TOTAL |
RBC'S	1:1	1:2	1:3	1:4	1:8	1:16	1:32	1:64	USED	SCORE
Mother (*C/c*)	4+	3+	2+	1+	+w	–	–	–	Anti-C	
	(10)	(8)	(5)	(3)	(1)					27
Child (*C/C?*)	4+	4+	3+	2+	2+	1+	–	–		
	(10)	(10)	(8)	(5)	(5)	(3)				41
Control (*C/C*)	4+	3+	3+	2+	2+	1+	–	–		
	(10)	(8)	(8)	(5)	(5)	(3)				39
Mother (*C/c*)	4+	3+	2+	1+	1+	–	–	–	Anti-c	
	(10)	(8)	(5)	(3)	(3)					29
Alleged father (*c/c?*)	4+	4+	4+	3+	3+	2+	1+	–		
	(10)	(10)	(10)	(8)	(8)	(5)	(3)			54
Control (*c/c*)	4+	4+	3+	3+	2+	2+	1+	–		
	(10)	(10)	(8)	(8)	(5)	(5)	(3)			49

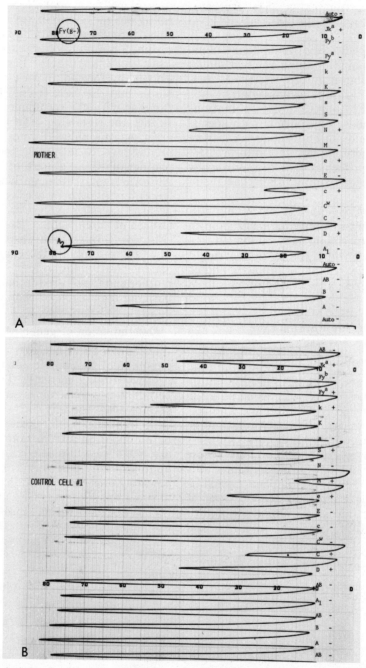

Figure 44-4. Recorded results of erythrocyte antigen phenotyping through the use of an Auto-Analyzer. Positive results are identified by a transmittance (%T) less than 70 per cent. *A*, Specimen of the mother typed as A2,Fy(a—). *B*, Control cell, No. 1.

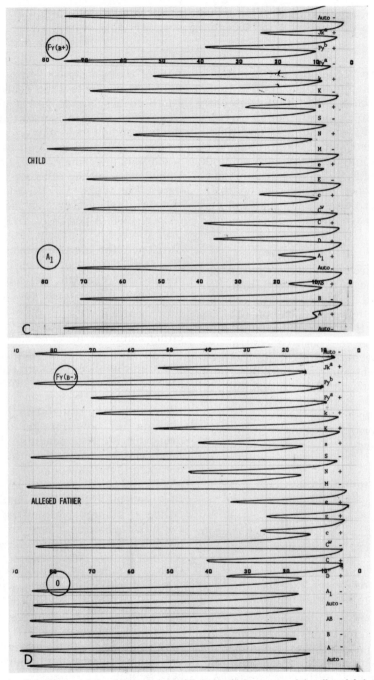

Figure 44-4. *Continued.* *C,* Specimen of the child typed as A1,Fy(a−). *D,* Specimen of the alleged father typed as O,Fy(a+).

	CONTROLS		TESTS		
Tube No.	1	2	3	4	5
Anti-H lectin	Yes	Yes	Yes	Yes	Yes
Saline or saliva	Saline	H	Mother	Child	Alleged father
O RBC's	Yes	Yes	Yes	Yes	Yes
Hemagglutination	2+	-	2+	-	2+
Interpretation	--OK--		Non-secretor	Secretor	Non-secretor

Interpretation. The mother, being C/c, serves as a double control. The child is apparently C/C, and the alleged father apparently c/c; therefore, the alleged father is excluded from paternity, if both the child and the alleged father are negative for C^w. It should be noted that for some antigens, such as M, N, M^g, s, c, C^w, e, and E, their dosage can often be determined if properly prepared monospecific antiserum is used. Other antigens may or may not show any dosage effect.

Secretor studies

The saliva collected should be boiled and filtered before use. Anti-H lectin from *Ulex europeaeus* should be diluted to give less than a 2+ reaction with O cells. A sample of saliva known to contain H substance should be tested simultaneously as the positive control. Although it is unnecessary to test for the presence of A or B substance merely to determine the secretor status, antiserums and controls should be prepared in the same way as anti-H if this testing is to be done. An example of an exclusion of paternity based on secretor studies is shown above.

TESTING OF ERYTHROCYTE ENZYMES

Owing to the diversity of procedures for testing each enzyme, readers should consult the original publications listed in Table 44-3.

TYPING OF SERUM PROTEINS (EXCLUDING IMMUNOGLOBULINS)

Both immunologic and electrophoretic techniques can be used for typing genetic markers in serum proteins. Although immunologic methods have been used for testing Gc, Ag, Lp, Xm, and Ig, potent antiserums for Gc, Ag, Lp, and Xm are not readily available. Testing for Ig will be discussed subsequently.

Electrophoresis seems to be the method of choice for typing Gc, Hp, Tf, Ce, C3, and Bf. Acrylamide gel is generally used for the first four of these, whereas agarose seems to produce better results when dealing with C3 and Bf. Both acrylamide and agarose produce a sieve effect, allowing separation of the components based on molecular sizes as well as electrophoretic mobility, and providing better resolution and superior results to those obtained with either cellulose acetate or filter paper. For typing C3, Bf, and ceruloplasmin, the original articles should be consulted (Alper, 1968; Alper, 1972; Dykes, 1976).

A number of different protocols have been developed for electrophoresis typing of Gc, Hp, and Tf, most of which give satisfactory results. For example, gel concentration may vary from 5.5 to 7 per cent acrylamide, the buffer system may be either continuous or discontinuous, and the electrophoresis may be either columnar (disc) or slab. There are also many types of power supplies and electrophoresis chambers commercially available. In general, vertical electrophoresis is preferred, since cooling of the system is easier. It is possible to read the transferrin, haptoglobin, and albumin in the same gel used for typing group-specific components (Gc). However, much clearer, more distinct results may be obtained if the haptoglobin is bound to hemoglobin and electrophoresed separately. For details, consult Dykes, 1975 and Polesky, 1975.

Just as a number of protocols are available for electrophoresis, there are several stains available for serum protein. Amido black, a commonly used stain, has the disadvantage that it requires destaining the background before the protein bands can be read. On the other hand, Coomasie blue, which also stains the protein bands, requires no destaining (Diezel, 1972). When weak Hp_1 bands are encountered, Lueco-Malachite green (0.1 gm/dl in 5 per cent acetic acid) has been found to be very helpful.

TYPING OF IMMUNOGLOBULINS

Testing genetic markers of immunoglobulins is based on the principles of passive hemagglutination inhibition. Serum containing antibodies which agglutinate red cells coated with specific Ig markers is incubated with the test serum. The coated red cells are then added to the system. If the test serum contains the specific Ig marker, inhibition of the agglutinator antibody will occur, and the red cells will show no agglutination. If the test serum does not contain the specific marker, there will be no inhibition and the red cells will be agglutinated. Because of the small volume of reagents which are required, microtiter plates with V-shaped wells have been found to be well suited to this test. The following reagents are essential for typing of immunoglobulins (Schanfield, 1975).

Agglutinators. Sera containing antibodies against specific Gm, Am, or Km markers are referred to as agglutinators. These antibodies are often of the IgM class and are often found in persons without any known sensitization to serum proteins. They may be used for testing only after the specificity of the antibodies has been confirmed, preferably by a WHO-sponsored reference laboratory, using a panel of erythrocytes coated with Ig markers of known specificities. Most of these sera require centrifugation to remove particles, as well as testing to determine the dilution necessary to obtain optimal results in any given test system.

Coating Agents. Theoretically, any serum containing antibodies with any specificity could be used if the Ig marker is known. It would be pas-

sively attached to erythrocytes by a binding agent such as chromium chloride. However, in practice, an incomplete anti-D of known Ig markers is used to coat $Rh_o(D)$-positive cells. Quite often, one anti-D serum may have several Ig specificities, such as $G1m^a$, $G1m^x$, and $G1m^z$. Thus, the same coated cells may be used for testing all three markers. Each of the anti-D serums used should be diluted in such a way as to give optimal results.

Erythrocytes for Coating. When anti-D sera are used as the coating agents, group O DCe or DCE cells are normally selected. Cells from an Oriental donor seem to work better than those from Caucasian donors. If possible, cells from the same donor should be used each time to assure consistent coating by the anti-D. Erythrocytes are coated as follows:

1. Wash the selected cells three times with saline.
2. Mix one drop of the washed packed cells with 0.1 ml of the diluted anti-D.
3. Incubate at 37°C. for one hour.
4. Wash three times with saline.
5. Prepare a 0.2 per cent cell suspension.

Inhibitors. Control serums of known Ig types for each marker tested should be used to insure that the inhibitor system is functioning properly. In typing immunoglobulins, it is essential that the appropriate controls be included with each run and that the results of these controls are as expected. If they are not, the test results are invalid.

Materials, Reagents, and Reactions	CONTROLS			Test	
	Agglutinator	Inhibitor	Test Serum		
Tube (well) No.	1	2	3	4	
Agglutinator for Glm(x)	Yes	Yes		Yes	
RBC's coated with Glm(x)	Yes	Yes	Yes	Yes	
Saline	Yes		Yes		
Inhibitor with Glm(x)		Yes			
Test serum			Yes	Yes	
Agglutination	Yes	No	No	Yes	No
Inhibition				No	Yes
Test	...... Controls O.K. = test valid			Negative	Positive

Tube (well) Nos. 1 and 2 are essentially the positive and negative controls for the Gm factors, while tube (well) No. 3 is essentially the serum control. The serum control must be included to ascertain whether or not the patient has antibodies either to the Gm markers or to the erythrocyte antigens. If this tube (well) shows agglutination, the testing is invalid. In such a case, the test serum should either be absorbed to remove the antibodies or be heated at 70°C. for 10 minutes to inactivate the antibodies. An example of a protocol using the microtiter plate follows.

1. Add 1 drop of saline, inhibitor, or test serum (dilute 1:10 or 1:20) to each well.
2. Add 1 drop of the appropriate agglutinator to wells in columns 1 to 8, and 1 drop of saline to wells in columns 9 to 12.
3. Add 1 drop of coated RBC's to the appropriate wells.
4. Incubate at room temperature for 30 to 60 minutes.
5. Centrifuge the plates in special carriers at 1000 rpm for 60 seconds (Sorval GLC-1) or equivalent.

6. Place the plates in holders at a 60 degree angle to the horizontal for 20 minutes.
7. Read by checking for either (1) agglutination—solid button or (2) inhibition—long uniform stream from the center (no agglutination).

		AGGLUTINATOR FOR						RBC'S COATED WITH*				
		Glm				G3m	Km		Glm		G3m	Km	
		a	x	f	z	g	1	3	axz	f	g	1	3
		1	2	3	4	5	6	7	8	9	10	11	12
Saline control	A	+	+	+	+	+	+	+	−	−	−	−	−
Inhibitor control	B	−	−	−	−	−	−	−	−	−	−	−	−
Mother's serum	C	+	+	+	−	+	+	−	−	−	−	−	−
Child's serum	D	−	−	+	−	−	+	−	−	−	−	−	−
Alleged father's (All. F.) serum	E	+	+	+	−	+	−	+	−	−	−	−	−

READING.   ○ = + = agglutination = no inhibition = no marker in the serum
◊ = − = no agglutination = inhibition = marker in the serum

A valid test 1. Serum controls (RBC's coated with markers*) should be negative.
2. Saline controls should all be positive.
3. Inhibitor controls should all be negative.

INTERPRETATION.

Mother Gm(a−x−f−z+;g−)   Km(1−3+)
Child Gm(a+x+f−z+;g+)   Km(1−3+)
All. F. Gm(a−x−f−z+;g−)   Km(1+3−)

The alleged father is excluded from paternity by the markers underlined above.

EVALUATION OF TEST RESULTS

CRITERIA FOR EXCLUSION OF PATERNITY

One Genetic Marker (P). If the child is positive for a given genetic marker and both the mother and the alleged father are negative for the marker, then the alleged father is excluded from paternity. Exceptions to this type of an exclusion are extremely rare. This type of exclusion usually occurs (1) in a system in which the allelic marker is either unknown or not demonstrable, such as P_1, Xg^a, Se, $Rh_o(D)$, Glm(a), and Glm(x); (2) in a system with two allelic markers when only one is being tested for, such as K, Fy^a, Jk^a, Lu^a, and Km(1); and (3) in a system with a relatively high frequency of recombinants, such as the HLA-A and HLA-B markers.

Two Allelic Markers (P,Q). Exclusion of paternity can be concluded in each of the four combinations shown below. An example of each is included in parentheses.

	MOTHER	CHILD	ALLEGED FATHER
1.	P−Q+(M−)	P+Q+(M+)	P−Q+(M−)
2.	P+Q−(N−)	P+Q+(N+)	P+Q−(N−)
3.	any	P+Q−(M/M)	P−Q+(N/N)
4.	any	P−Q+(N/N)	P+Q−(M/M)

In combinations 1 and 2, only one marker is involved as is described in the above section, whereas in combinations 3 and 4, the interpretation is based upon zygosity. Whenever this type of exclusion is being considered, possible variants must be kept in mind. Exclusions of this type are normally seen with the following allelic markers: M-N, S-s, C-c, E-e, K-k, Fy^a-Fy^b, Jk^a-Jk^b, Lu^a-Lu^b, PGM_1^1-PGM_1^2, AK^1-AK^2, ADA^1-ADA^2, $6PGD^A$-$6PGD^B$, GLO^1-GLO^2, EsD^1-EsD^2, GPT^1-GPT^2, Hp^1-Hp^2, Gc^1-Gc^2, $C3^1$-$C3^2$, Ag^x-Ag^y, G1m(f)-G1m(z), and Km(1)-Km(3).

More Than Two Allelic Markers (P,Q,R). Exclusion of paternity can also be obtained from combination of markers as shown below.

	MOTHER	CHILD	ALLEGED FATHER
	any	P−Q−R+	P+Q+R−
e.g.		Fy(a−b−4+)	Fy(a+b+4−)
		A−B−H+(0)	A+B+H−(AB)

In the ACP (acid phosphatase) system, all three of the common markers are demonstrable by electrophoresis. The presence of any two of these markers in the child, both of which are absent in the alleged father, constitutes an exclusion of paternity.

Genetic Markers on the X Chromosome. G6PD (for the black population only) and Xg^a

can provide exclusion of paternity only if the child is a female, as in combinations 1 and 2 shown in the example below. In combination 3 of this example, the mother is excluded.

MOTHER	CHILD	ALLEGED FATHER
(1) Xg(a−)	fem. Xg(a+)	Xg(a−)
(2) any	fem. Xg(a−)	Xg(a+)
(3) Xg(a−)	male Xg(a+)	any

Haplotypes. This type of exclusion can be concluded when (1) more than one child is being tested, (2) the frequency of certain haplotypes is known for a given population, (3) special antiserums for complex antigens are used, and (4) family members are studied. Examples of each of these cases are shown below.

	MOTHER	CHILD		ALL. FATHER	COMMENTS
		No. 1	No. 2		
(1) Phenotype	MNs	MSs	Ms	MNSs	
Possible		*MS/Ms*	*Ms/Ms*	*MS/Ns*	Can't have child No. 2
genotypes		*MS/Ms*	*Ms/Ms*	*Ms/NS*	Can't have child No. 1
(2) Phenotype	K+k+	K+k+		K−k+	
	Js(a+b+)	Js(a+b+)		Js(a−b+)	
	Kp(a−b+)	Kp(a−b+)		Js(a−b+)	
Possible	*KJs^{b}Kp^b/*	*KJs^{b}Kp^b/*		*kJs^{b}Kp^b/*	Exclusion
genotypes	*kJs^{a}Kp^b*	*kJs^{a}Kp^b*		*kJs^{b}Kp^b*	No apparent exclusion,
	*KJs^{a}Kp^b/	*KJs^{b}Kp^b/*		*kJs^{b}Kp^b/*	but **KJs^{a}Kp^b* has never
	kJs^{b}Kp^b	*kJs^{b}Kp^b*		*kJs^{b}Kp^b*	been reported.
(3) Phenotype	DCe	DCce		DCcEe	No exclusion
Possible	*DCe/DCe*	*DCe/dce*		*DCE/dce*	(0.2 per cent chance
genotype		*(Dce)*		*(Dce)*	if anti-f +)
		dCe/Dce		*dCe/DcE*	Would have maternal
					exclusion
				DCe/DcE	Exclusion
				(dcE)	(99.8 per cent chance
					if anti-f −)

(4) In case No. 3, if the alleged father's father and mother were typed, and the father found to be CDe and the mother to be cDE, exclusion of paternity could be concluded without the aid of the anti-f, since the son (alleged father) would have to be *CDe/cDE*.

Exclusion in the HLA system based on haplotypes should be reported with great caution, since the frequency of recombination is rather high and there is also a large problem with cross-reactivity in this system. The same precautions should also be kept in mind with the Gm system, since it too has a relatively high recombination frequency (Table 44-8).

When reporting exclusions in the ABO, MNSs, or Rh systems, the following considerations should also be kept in mind.

ABO Systems. Since both the O and A$_2$ markers are essentially amorphs by testing, exclusion of paternity can be reported only in specific combinations. For convenience, Table 44-9 lists the phenotypes of various mother-child combinations in conjunction with that of the alleged father which would constitute an exclusion.

MNSs and Rh Systems. When considering possible exclusion based on haplotypes, the MNSs system is relatively straightforward as long as possible variants have been excluded. On the other hand, this is not true of the Rh system. To facilitate the interpretations of the test results for these two systems, Tables 44-10 and 44-11 have been constructed. They show the various mother-child combinations and the phenotypes of the alleged father which would give exclusion of paternity.

VARIANTS IN HUMAN BLOOD GROUP GENETIC MARKERS

The Null or Minus-Minus Phenotypes. Below is a tabular review of the minus-minus phenotypes that have been reported for the blood group antigens, the red cell enzymes, and the serum proteins. The excellent review of this subject by Allen (1976) should be consulted for additional information.

Table 44-9.   PHENOTYPES OF ALLEGED FATHER EXCLUDED FROM PATERNITY FOR VARIOUS MOTHER-CHILD COMBINATIONS*

PHENOTYPES OF MOTHER	PHENOTYPES OF CHILD					
	O	A_1	A_2	B	A_1B	A_2B
O	A_1B, A_2B	O, A_2, B, A_2B	O, B, A_1B	O, A_1, A_2	em	em
A_1	A_1B, A_2B	None	A_1B	O, A_1, A_2	O, A_1, A_2	O, A_1, A_2
A_2	A_1B, A_2B	O, A_2, B	A_1B	O, A_1, A_2	em	O, A_1, A_2
B	A_1B, A_2B	O, A_2, B, A_2B	O, B, A_1B	None	O, A_2, B, A_2B	O, B, A_1B
A_1B	em	None	em	None	O, A_2	O, B, A_1B
A_2B	em	O, A_2, B, A_2B	A_1B	None	O, A_2, B, A_2B	O

*By the use of anti-A, anti-A_1, and anti-B serums. em = Exclusion of maternity.

Table 44-10.   PHENOTYPES OF ALLEGED FATHER EXCLUDED FROM PATERNITY FOR VARIOUS MOTHER-CHILD COMBINATIONS*

PHENOTYPES OF MOTHER	PHENOTYPES OF CHILD								
	1 MS	2 Ms	3 MSs	4 NS	5 Ns	6 NSs	7 MNS	8 MNs	9 MNSs
1. MS	2, 4, 5 6, 8	em	1, 4, 5 6, 7	em	em	em	1, 2, 3 5, 8	em	1, 2, 3 4, 7
2. Ms	em	1, 4, 5 6, 7	2, 4, 5 6, 8	em	em	em	em	1, 2, 3 4, 7	1, 2, 3 5, 8
3. MSs	1, 4, 5 6, 7	2, 4, 5 6, 7	4, 5, 6	em	em	em	1, 2, 3 5, 8	1, 2, 3 5, 8	1, 2, 3
4. NS	em	em	em	1, 2, 3 5, 8	em	1, 2, 3 4, 7	2, 4, 5 6, 8	em	1, 4, 5 6, 7
5. Ns	em	em	em	em	1, 2, 3 4, 7	1, 2, 3 5, 7	em	1, 4, 5 6, 7	2, 4, 5 6, 8
6. NSs	em	em	em	1, 2, 3 4, 7	1, 2, 3 4, 7	1, 2, 3	2, 4, 5 6, 8	1, 4, 5 6, 7	4, 5, 6
7. MNS	2, 4, 5 6, 8	em	1, 4, 5 6, 7	1, 2, 3 5, 8	em	1, 2, 3 4, 7	2, 5, 8	em	1, 4, 7
8. MNs	em	1, 4, 5 6, 7	2, 4, 5 6, 8	em	1, 2, 3 4, 7	1, 2, 3 5, 8	em	1, 4, 7	1, 5, 8
9. MNSs	2, 4, 5 6, 8	1, 4, 5 6, 7	4, 5, 6	1, 2, 3 5, 8	1, 2, 3 4, 7	1, 2, 3	2, 5, 8	1, 4, 7	None

*By the use of anti-M, anti-N, anti-S, and anti-s serums. em = Exclusion of maternity.

Table 44-11. PHENOTYPES OF ALLEGED FATHER EXCLUDED FROM PATERNITY FOR VARIOUS MOTHER-CHILD COMBINATIONS*

PHENOTYPES OF MOTHER	PHENOTYPES OF CHILD											
	1 dce	2 dCe	3 dcEe	4 Dce	5 DCce	6 DCCe	7 DCcEe	8 DC^we	9 DC^wCe	10 DC^wEe	11 DcEe	12 DcEE
1. rh	6, 7, 9 10, 12	all but 2, 6, 7	all but 3, 7, 12	all but 4, 5, 11	all but 5, 6, 7, 9	em	em	all but 8, 9, 10	em	em	all but 7, 11, 12	em
2. rhrh'	6, 7, 9 10, 12	9, 10, 12	all but 3, 7, 12	all but 4, 5, 11	all but 5, 6, 7, 9	all but 5, 6, 7, 9	all but 7, 11, 12	all but 8, 9, 10	em	em	all but 7, 11, 12	em
3. rhrh''	6, 7, 9 10, 12	all but 2, 6, 7	6, 9, 10	all but 4, 5, 11	all but 5, 6, 7, 9	em	all but 5, 6, 7, 9	all but 8, 9, 10	em	em	all but 7, 11, 12	all but 7, 11, 12
4. Rh_0rh	6, 7, 9 10, 12	all but 2, 6, 7	all but 3, 7, 12	6, 7, 9 10, 12	all but 5, 6, 7, 9	em	em	all but 8, 9, 10	em	em	all but 7, 11, 12	em
5. Rh_1rh Rh_1Rh_0	6, 7, 9 10, 12	all but 2, 6, 7	all but 3, 7, 12	6, 7, 9 10, 12	10, 12	all but 2, 5, 6, 7, 9	all but 3, 7, 12	all but 8, 9, 10	all but 8, 9, 10	em	all but 7, 11, 12	em
6. Rh_1Rh_1 Rh_1rh' Rh_1rh'	em	6, 7, 9 10, 12	em	em	6, 7, 9 10, 12	all but 2, 5, 6, 7, 9	all but 3, 7, 12	em	all but 8, 9, 10	em	em	em
7. Rh_2Rh_2 Rh_2rh'' $rh'Rh_2$	em	6, 7, 9 10, 12	6, 7, 9 10, 12	em	6, 7, 9 10, 12	all but 2, 5, 6, 7, 9	1, 4, 8	em	all but 8, 9, 10	all but 8, 9, 10	6, 7, 9 10, 12	all but 3, 7, 11, 12
8. Rh_1^wrh	6, 7, 9 10, 12	all but 2, 6, 7	all but 3, 7, 12	all but 4, 5, 11	all but 5, 6, 7, 9	em	em	6, 7, 12	all but 5, 6, 7, 9	all but 7, 11, 12	all but 8, 9, 10	all but 7, 11, 12
9. $Rh_1^wRh_1$	em	em	em	em	6, 7, 9 10, 12	all but 5, 6, 7, 9	all but 3, 7, 11, 12	6, 7, 9 10, 12	1, 2, 3, 4 11, 12	all but 7, 11, 12	em	em
10. $Rh_1^wRh_2$	em	em	em	em	em	em	all but 5, 6, 7, 9	6, 7, 9 10, 12	all but 5, 6, 7, 9	1, 2, 3, 4 5, 6	6, 7, 9 10, 12	all but 3, 7, 11, 12
11. Rh_2rh Rh_2Rh_0	6, 7, 9 10, 12	all but 2, 6, 7	all but 3, 7, 12	6, 7, 9 10, 12	all but 5, 6, 7, 9	em	all but 2, 5, 6, 7, 9	all but 8, 9, 10	em	all but 8, 9, 10	6, 9	all but 3, 7, 11, 12
12. Rh_2Rh_2 Rh_2rh''	em	all but 2, 6, 7	6, 7, 9 10, 12	em	em	em	all but 2, 5, 6, 7, 9	em	em	all but 8, 9, 10	6, 7, 9 10, 12	all but 3, 7, 11, 12

* Determined by anti-Rh_0(D), anti-rh'(C), anti-rh^{w1}(C^w), anti-hr'(c), anti-rh''(E), and anti-hr''(e) serums. em = Exclusion of maternity. Phenotypes and their genotypes with frequency below 0.1 percent are not considered in the exclusion.

SYSTEM	PHENOTYPES		SYSTEM	PHENOTYPES
ABO	$A-B-H+(O)$		P	p
	$A-B-H-$ (Bombay, $O_h{}^A$, $O_h{}^B$)		Kell	K_o
MNSs	$M-N-$ (En(a−))			
	$S-s-(S^u)$		Acid phosphatase	ACP_0
	$M-N-S-s-(M^k)$		Adenylate kinase	AK_0
Rh	$E-e-(D--, DC^w-, Dc-)$		Alanine aminotrans-	
	$D-C-c-E-e-(Rh_{null}, ---/---)$		ferase	ALT_0(GPT)
Duffy	Fy(a−b−)		Haptoglobin	Hp_0
Kidd	Jk(a−b−)		Complement	$C3_0$
Lutheran	Lu(a−b−)		Group specific	
Wright	Wr(a−b−, En(a−))		component	Gc_0
Colton	Co(a−b−)		Transferrin	Tf_0
Scianna	Sc(−1−2)			
Lewis	Le(a−b−)			

All of the phenotypes listed in the above table can be considered rare under normal circumstances except as follows: First, group O is fairly common in many populations. Second, Fy(a−b−) and Le(a−b−) are fairly common in the black populations, although they are considered rare in Caucasians. Similarly, the p phenotype is not uncommon in northern Sweden.

Two mechanisms have been postulated to explain the existence of these null phenotypes. The hypotheses are based on the assumption that at least two genes are required for the production of detectable genetic markers, the regulator and the structural gene. The purpose of the regulator gene is to produce or transform a precursor substance into a product on which the structural gene can act, thus producing a detectable genetic marker. Either of these two genes can be partially or totally non-functional, resulting in the null or minus-minus phenotype.

If the regulator gene is absent, not functioning properly, or being suppressed, there is no precursor substance being formed for the structural gene to act upon, with the end result of an incomplete or non-detectable genetic marker. In this case, the normal structural gene can be passed to the child. If the child then inherits a normal regulator gene from the other parent, a normal genetic marker will be produced. The Bombay phenotype, some of the Rh nulls, and the McLeod phenotype can all be explained by this hypothesis. In the ABO system, the H substance has been shown to be the precursor of A and B substances. Thus, in the Bombay type, the regulator H gene is absent, while the A or B structural gene capable of transforming precursor H substance to A or B substance is normal (Fig. 44-5A); in a group O person, both the A and B genes are absent (Fig. 44-5B). At the present time, no such biochemical evidence is available for other null phenotypes. There is, however, evidence to indicate that the regulator gene for the McLeod phenotype is located on the X chromosome. This type of abnormal-

ABSENCE OF A REGULATOR GENE H GOVERNING THE FORMATION OF PRECURSOR SUBSTANCE H. A SILENT GENE h IS ASSIGNED TO THE SAME LOCUS

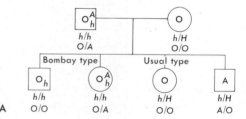

ABSENCE OF A STRUCTURAL GENE A OR B GOVERNING THE FORMATION OF A OR B. AN AMORPHIC O GENE IS ASSIGNED TO THE SAME LOCUS

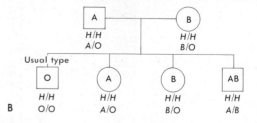

Figure 44-5. Explanations of the formation of two types of Group O: *A*, Absence of regulator gene. *B*, Absence of structural gene.

ity is the rare exception to the direct exclusion, since it is possible for two seemingly group O individuals to have a group A or B child, just as it is possible for two Rh null individuals to have a child with normal Rh antigens.

A second mechanism by which minus-minus or null phenotypes can be produced is an absence or a malfunction of the structural gene. This is the case in phenotypes such as D--, DC^w-, and Dc-, where neither of the normal alleles E or e is expressed. If this defect were affecting only one of the two genes, the result would be a phenotype which appeared homozygous for the allele able to be expressed. An example of this would be $E/-$ or $e/-$, which would be interpreted as EE or ee, respectively. These possibilities are what render an indirect exclusion less reliable than a direct exclusion.

A third possibility which should be kept in mind as an explanation for other null phenotypes is the presence of an alternate allele that results in an end product for which no antiserum is currently available. The recent demonstration of anti-Fy4 has shown that the majority of the blacks who are Fy(a−b−) are Fy^4/Fy^4, and that those who type as Fy(a−b+) or Fy(a+b−) are in actuality Fy^b/Fy^4 or Fy^a/Fy^4 and not necessarily Fy^b/Fy^b or Fy^a/Fy^a, as was generally assumed. Therefore, exclusion of paternity in blacks based on zygosity in the Duffy system is not valid. However, the Fy(a−b−) phenotype is extremely rare in Caucasians.

Similarly, one must remember that uncommon but demonstrable alleles also exist in other systems, such as C^w and e^s in the Rh system and M^g in the MNSs system. A person could be C/C^w and not C/C, E/e^s and not E/E, or N/M^g and not N/N, etc. In these cases, exclusion of paternity cannot be concluded unless these uncommon alternate markers have been tested for and ruled out as possibilities.

Crossing Over. Although several cases of crossing over in the MNSs system and one case in the Rh system have been reported, the incidence of such an occurrence is extremely rare and need not affect the interpretation of paternity testing in most instances. In the HLA and the Gm systems, the rate of crossing over is estimated between 1 and 2 per cent, allowing much less confidence to be placed in an indirect exclusion.

Trans- or Cis- Effects. When C is present in trans-position (located on the other chromosome of the pair), the Rh$_o$(D) antigen is often typed as D^u, as in the genotype D^uCe/dCe. Thus, when the haplotype D^uCe is passed to a child who may inherit dce or other haplotypes without the C from the other parent, the child will be typed as Dce, not D^{u}ce. Both A and B genes can be inherited as one unit on the same chromosome, known as cis-AB. About a dozen or so cases of this have been reported in the literature. In this rare exception, an AB parent may have an O child, normally considered as an exclusion of maternity or paternity. This variant can be recognized by both the weakness of the B antigen and a weak anti-B present in the serum.

Mutation. Theoretically, the presence of a genetic marker in the child not found in both parents can be explained on the basis of mutation. However, the mutation rate in man has been estimated as close to one in a million, and no convincing example of a mutation involved in paternity testing has ever been found (Race, 1975).

Physiologic Variations. Many genetic markers are known to be poorly developed during infancy, such as A$_1$, I, P$_1$, Le^b, Xg^a, Lu^a, Gm, and Hp. Some of these markers are not fully developed until as late as 6 to 18 months of age. Other antigens such as D^u, C^u, E^u, c^v, e^i, M$_2$, and N$_2$ are expressed only very weakly in adults. It is not unusual, therefore, that these weak antigens may react with some antiserum and not with others of the same specificity; antiserums specific for these weak antigens are unknown. Another consideration is the presence of mother's IgG in the infant's circulation. Thus, the results of a Gm typing of a young infant should be interpreted with caution.

Pathologic Variations. In addition to the physiologic variations discussed in the previous paragraph, it is necessary to remember that certain pathologic variations do occur that also influence test results. For instance, any conditions which result in hemolysis *in vivo* will lower the haptoglobin level significantly. Both the Gm and Km typings would be affected if the patient had abnormal immunoglobulin levels, such as agammaglobulinemia. Persons with abnormal markers in the Kell system, such as the McLeod phenotype, may have chronic granulomatous disease and/or acanthocytosis. Rh$_{null}$ persons may have a compensated hemolytic anemia and have demonstrable stomatocytosis when a peripheral

4

smear is reviewed. Adenocarcinoma of the upper gastrointestinal tract is often associated with an excess production of group-specific substance which may interfere with ABO grouping results. Bacterial infections of the large intestine may lead to persons having an acquired B antigen. Other conditions, such as intrauterine transfusions, bone marrow transplantation, or recent blood transfusions could lead to blood group chimerism.

CHANCE OF EXCLUSION OF PATERNITY

If a man is not excluded from paternity by the "blood test," the court usually rules that he must pay child support. Thus, he should have the right to ask how good the "blood test" is with regard to excluding a falsely accused man. In other words, the chance of exclusion provided by the "blood test" becomes a very relevant issue (Jancik, 1952).

The chance of exclusion of paternity by a "blood test" depends on

a. the type of genetic markers used.
b. the number of systems and the number of genetic markers in each system tested.
c. the genetic pattern of a given mother-child combination.

The type of genetic markers

The ability of a genetic marker to provide an exclusion depends on the gene frequency of that marker in a given population and the existence of a demonstrable allelic marker. For example, let P and Q be the two genetic markers with gene frequencies of p and q respectively, where $p + q = 1$. The following two formulas can then be derived:

(1) If only anti-P serum is used for the testing, the only exclusion possible is when the child is positive for P and both the mother and the alleged father are negative for P.

Then, $\quad p$ = chance of the child being $P+$

$(1 - p)^2$ or q^2 = chance of the mother *or* the alleged father being $P-$

$q^2 \times q^2 = q^4$ = chance of both the mother and the alleged father being $P-$

$p \times q^4 = pq^4$ = chance of exclusion (CE) with anti-P

Similarly, p^4q = chance of exclusion with anti-Q

(2) When anti-P and anti-Q serums are both available, the chance of exclusion would be as follows:

MOTHER	CHILD	ALLEGED FATHER	CHANCE OF EXCLUSION
$P - (= q^2)$	$P + (= p)$	$p - (= q^2)$	$q^2 \times p \times q^2 = pq^2$
$Q - (= p^2)$	$Q + (= q)$	$Q - (= p^2)$	$p^2 \times q \times p^2 = p^4q$
any	$P + Q - (\bar{P}/\bar{P}, = p^2)$	$P - Q + (\bar{Q}/\bar{Q}, = q^2)$	$p^2 \times q^2 \quad = p^2q^2$
any	$P - Q + (Q/Q, = q^2)$	$P + Q - (\bar{P}/\bar{P}, = p^2)$	$q^2 \times p^2 \quad = p^2q^2$

Sum of chances $= pq^4 + p^4q + 2p^2q^2 = pq(p^3 + q^3 + 2pq)$
$\qquad = pq((p + q)(p^2 - pq + q^2) + 2qp)$
$\qquad = pq(1)((p^2 + 2pq + q^2 - 3pq) + 2pq)$
$\qquad = pq(1)(((p + q)^2 - 3pq) + 2pq) = pq(1)(1 - pq)$
$\qquad = \underline{pq(1 - pq)}$ with anti-P and anti-Q serums

---

Example: Let M be the P marker and N be the Q marker, then $p = 0.5656$ and $q = 0.4344$.

Chance of exclusion with anti-M
anti-M $= pq^4 = 0.5656 \times 0.4344^4 = 2\%$
anti-N $= p^4q = 0.5656^4 \times 0.4344 = 4.5\%$
anti-M and anti-N
$\qquad = pq(1 - pq)$
$\qquad = 0.5656 \times 0.4344\,(1 - 0.5656 \times 0.4344)$
$\qquad = 18.5\%$

Thus, it is clear that the chance of exclusion obtained when a pair of antisera are used is much greater than that obtained from each antiserum alone. The chance of exclusion in a system with more than two allelic markers is even greater.

The maximal chance of exclusion obtainable with one antiserum is about 8.19 per cent; this is the maximal value of pq^4 when $p = 0.2$; i.e., the gene frequency is 0.2 and the phenotype frequency is close to 0.36. The maximal chance of exclusion obtainable with a pair of antisera is 0.1875; this is the maximal value of $pq(1 - pq)$ when $p = 0.5$; i.e., the gene frequency of the marker is close to 0.5 or the phenotype frequency is near 0.75.

Table 44–12. CHANCE OF EXCLUSION OF PATERNITY BY GENETIC MARKERS OF FOUR MAJOR BLOOD GROUP COMPONENTS

	WHITES	BLACKS
Erythrocyte antigens	78.8%	78.8%
Erythrocyte enzymes	66.3%	55.6%
HLA antigens	84.3%	82.1%
Serum proteins	77.0%	84.0%
Cumulative chance	99.7%	99.7%

Cumulative chance of exclusion

Since genetic markers in one system are independent of those in other systems, a man could be excluded concurrently by markers in more than one system. However, since a man needs to be excluded from paternity only once, the cumulative chance is not equal to the sum of those individual systems, but can be calculated as shown below.

If CE1 and CE2 are the chances of exclusion of two systems, the chance of being excluded by both systems would be CE1 $\times$ CE2. The cumulative chance is then CE1 + CE2 − (CE1 $\times$ CE2).

Example: In the ABO system, CE1 = 0.185; in the MNSs system, CE2 = 0.316

Cumulative chance
= 0.185 + 0.316 − (0.185 $\times$ 0.316)
= 0.442   or   44%

Since CE1 + CE2 − (CE1 $\times$ CE2) = 1 − (1 − CE1)(1 − CE2), as shown by the example, CE = 1 − (1 − 0.184)(1 − 0.316) = 0.442 = 44 per cent, the formula can be extended to estimate the cumulative CE of more than two systems; i.e.,

CE = 1 − (1 − CE1)(1 − CE2)
                  (1 − CE3) .... (1 − CEn)

The cumulative chance of exclusion of the erythrocyte antigens, the erythrocyte enzymes, the HLA antigens, and the serum proteins previously discussed, as well as the combinations of four groups, is listed in Table 44–12.

The Number of Markers and Systems Tested. The larger the number of systems or genetic markers tested, the greater the cumulative chance of exclusion. However, the cumulative chance slowly reaches a plateau, and from the cost-effectiveness point of view, the slight increase may not be worth the additional effort and cost. In fact, if one used only 18 markers in 5 systems of erythrocyte antigens, a total of 10 genetic markers in 3 systems of serum proteins, the cumulative chance of exclusion would be 88.1 per cent for a Caucasian population, as shown below.

		CHANCE OF EXCLUSION	
SYSTEM	MARKERS	Individual	Cumulative
ABO	A_1, A_2, B, O	0.185	
MNSs	M, N, S, s	0.316	0.443
Rh	D, C, C^w, c, E, e	0.312	0.614
Duffy	Fy^a, Fy^b	0.181	0.686
Kidd	Jk^a, Jk^b	0.187	0.745
Hp	Hp^1, Hp^2	0.184	0.798
Gc	Gc^1, Gc^2	0.162	0.826
Gm	a, f, z; n; g, bO	0.317	0.881

For this reason, each laboratory may select a combination of certain markers of its choice to provide a high rate of exclusion while reflecting local conditions of the laboratory and interests of the professional staff. The number of genetic markers tested within each system will also affect the rate of exclusion, as illustrated by the following example:

LABORATORY	ABO	MNSs	Rh	CHANCE OF EXCLUSION
No. 1	A, B, O	M, N	D	0.33
No. 2	A_1, A_2, B, O	M, N, S	D, C, E, c	0.547
No. 3	A_1, A_2, B, O	M, N, S, s	D, C, C^w, c, E, e	0.614

Each laboratory uses the same three ABO, MN, and Rh systems, yet because of the difference in the number of genetic markers tested, the rate of exclusion can vary from 0.33 to 0.614.

The Genetic Pattern of a Given Mother-Child Combination. The chance of exclusion is calculated on the basis of the normal frequencies of the genetic markers in a given population. It will also vary depending on the genetic pattern of the mother-child combination. For instance, if a child has a few relatively low incidence markers, such as B, E, and K, and the mother lacks all three, the alleged father must have all three or he would be excluded. The chance of a Caucasian male having all three markers is $0.11 \times 0.08 \times 0.3 = 0.00264$, or less than 3 in 1000. This also means that if only these markers were examined, 99.7 per cent of Caucasian males could be excluded from the paternity of this child. On the other hand, if both the mother and the child are heterozygotes for many common genetic markers, such as A/O, M/N, S/s, CDe/cde, K/k, Fy^a/Fy^b, Jk^a/Jk^b . . . , very few males could be excluded from paternity even though many more genetic markers are being tested (p. 1538).

With the current technology, it is not difficult to test for genetic markers that would provide at least a 70 per cent chance of exclusion of paternity for a falsely accused man. With some additional effort, a 90 per cent chance of exclusion can be reached.

CHANCE OF PATERNITY (LIKELIHOOD OF PATERNITY)

It is a generally accepted philosophy that not even the mother can be sure who the father of the child is when there is more than one man involved during the conception period. However, if the child and the alleged father share one marker of very low incidence or a few uncommon markers, the chance of finding another male of the same genetic make-up approaches one in a thousand or one in a million; unless he has a brother of the same genetic pattern who was also involved with the woman during the designated time period, he is most likely the father of the child.

In court, the judge often seeks a decision based on the majority of evidence rather than absolute evidence, which is usually unavailable. Consequently, he could theoretically arrive at a decision based on 51 per cent of the evidence being positive and the other 49 per cent being negative. This principle can be applied as follows: if a man is not excluded from paternity and the chances of his being the father are 95 per cent in favor and 5 per cent against, the difference is statistically significant. For this reason, estimation of the chance of paternity has been used for years in some European countries as a basis for judging child support cases. It should be noted that the legislation of Pub. L. 93-647 asks for the *ascertainment* of paternity, not the exclusion of paternity.

When a man is not excluded from paternity, it does not in any way imply that he is automatically assumed to be the father of the child. This can be proven mathematically as follows. If p is the gene frequency of a given marker, it is also the chance for him to be the father. The phenotype frequency of the marker would be $2p - p^2$ (positive for that marker), which is also the chance for him not to be excluded. Since p is always a fraction of 1, p will always be greater than p^2, and $2p - p^2$ greater than p. The following examples also illustrate these conclusions.

If an alleged father is group A_1 while the child is group O, he is not excluded from paternity. However, he has approximately a 20 per cent chance of being A_1/A_1 or A_1/A_2 rather than A_1/O, both of which would exclude him. If the child were an A_1B instead, he would have approximately a 40 per cent chance of not passing the A_1 marker to the child, although he still could not be excluded. The odds are even closer in the Kell system; if the alleged father is $K+$ and the child is $K-$ and the mother is $K-$, he has only a 51 per cent chance of being the father and a 49 per cent chance of not being the father. Thus, the term "non-exclusion" must clearly be differentiated from the term "chance of paternity."

Estimating the chance of paternity can be approached in two different ways. The first approach is based on the cumulative chance of exclusion for the test systems used. For instance, if the test systems used provide a high cumulative chance of exclusion, such as 95 per cent, and he is not excluded, the odds in favor of his being the father are 95 per cent:5 per cent. On the other hand, if the test systems used provide only a 70 per cent cumulative chance of exclusion, and he is not excluded, the odds are only 70 per cent:30 per cent, a value of little statistical significance. Since very few laboratories perform sufficient tests to yield a 95 per cent chance of exclusion, this particular approach would not be suitable for most laboratories at the present time. In addition, this approach is theoretically unsound in that the calculated chance of exclusion based on random phenotype frequencies does not take into consideration the genetic pattern of a given mother-child pair.

A second approach to estimating the chance of paternity is based on analysis of the genetic patterns of a given mother-child pair; in this way, one compares the pattern of genetic markers of the alleged father with that needed to be the father of the child. Since this approach does not rely so heavily on the particular test system involved, it is obviously preferable.

Many complicated formulas have been developed to estimate the chance of paternity; but all of them revolve around the same principle, *the chance that a single sperm of the accused man carries all the necessary genetic markers required to be the father in a given mother-child pair.* For this reason, it is possible to estimate the chance of paternity based on common logic without complicating the calculation with extraneous theorems and equations. The following method is currently being used at our institutions. Note that the same example is used throughout the procedure for continuity.

Establish the Genetic Markers Required for the Father of a Given Mother-Child Pair. For instance, if the child is positive for the B, E, and K markers and the mother is negative for all three markers, then the alleged father must be positive for all three markers; otherwise, he is excluded from paternity.

Find the Gene Frequency (p) of the Genetic Markers in Question. From Table 44-2, the gene (not phenotype) frequency of B, E, and K among Caucasians is 0.066, 0.16, and 0.045, respectively. The product of these, 0.00048, would be the chance of a sperm or gamete of a white man carrying all three of these genes. For example, if the alleged father were merely a random man who had been falsely accused, his chance of having all three of these markers would be about 5 in 10,000 or 1 in 2,000. Therefore, this is also the chance of a non-father or a random man in the same population. It should be mentioned here that a non-father or a random man is one who could have been involved with the woman, but who has not been tested.

Find the Chance of the Alleged Father Passing the Three Markers to His Children Under the Following Conditions. (1) If the zygosity of the three markers is known:

All homozygous, B/B, E/E, and K/K; 100 per cent of his children would be $B+$, $E+$, and $K+$; the chance of paternity would then be $1 \times 1 \times 1 = 1$ or 100 per cent.

All heterozygous, B/O, E/e, and K/k; 50 per cent of his children would be $B+$, $E+$, or $K+$;

the chance of paternity for all three would be $0.5 \times 0.5 \times 0.5 = 0.125$ or 12.5 per cent. With a mixture such as B/B, E/e, K/k, the chance would be $1 \times 0.5 \times 0.5 = 0.25$ or 25 per cent.

(2) If the zygosity of a marker is unknown, the chance of passing the marker can be estimated by the gene frequencies (p for the dominant gene and q for the silent gene) using the formula $(p + q)/(p + 2q)$ or $1/(2 - p)$ when $p + q = 1$. Thus, when the gene frequency of $O = 0.66$, the chance of a B person to pass a B gene $= (0.066 + 0.66)/(0.066 + 0.66 \times 2) = 0.52$ or 52%.

The chance of an E+ person to pass an E gene
$$= 1/(2 - 0.16) = 0.54 \text{ or } 54\%.$$

The chance of a K+ person to pass a K gene
$$= 1/(2 - 0.045) = 0.51 \text{ or } 51\%.$$

The combined chance is then $0.52 \times 0.54 \times 0.51 = 0.14$ or 14%

Note: The formula $(p + q)/(p + 2q) = (p^2 + (\frac{1}{2} \times 2pq))/(p^2 + 2pq)$.

$$p^2 = 100\% \text{ of all homozygotes}$$
$$\tfrac{1}{2} \times 2pq = 50\% \text{ of all heterozygotes}$$

$p^2 + 2pq$ = homozygotes + heterozygotes (phenotype frequency) = $\bar{M}$ (in Table 44-13)
When $p + q = 1$, then $q = 1 - p$; $(p + q)/(p + 2q) = 1/(p + 2 - 2p) = 1/(2 - p)$

Total Chance of Paternity. In the previous discussions, the mother was always negative for the marker. When the mother is positive for the marker under consideration, the following situations should be considered.

1. If the mother is a homozygote, the child must also be positive for that marker. The allelic marker of the child must then come from the father. Likewise, if the father is a homozygote, the allelic marker must come from the mother. If the child is homozygous, both parents must have the marker. Therefore, whenever any one of the three is a homozygote, the chance is predetermined and need not be calculated.

2. If both the mother and the child are heterozygotes in a two-allelic gene system, the total chance for the non-father or the alleged father of any genotypes would be 0.5. This relationship can be shown as follows:

4

FROM THE MOTHER		ALLELIC GENE	CHANCE FOR NON-FATHER	CHANCE FOR ALLEGED FATHER		
Gene	Chance			P/P	P/Q	Q/Q
P	0.5	Q	1 − p	0	0.5	1
Q	0.5	P	p	1	0.5	0
Total			1	1	1	1

The total chance in each case is $0.5 \times 1 = 0.5$.

This means that when the mother and the child are both heterozygotes, every man in the same population has an equal chance of being the father; thus, for practical purposes, these markers can be disregarded in estimating the chance of paternity.

3. If the zygosity of the marker involved is unknown, such as group B in the previous example, the total chance of paternity can be calculated in the following way:

EXPECTED FROM THE MOTHER		GENE FROM THE FATHER	CHANCE TO PROVIDE THE REQUIRED GENE		
Gene	Chance		Random Man	Group B Man	Group O Man
B	0.52	B or O	$0.07 + 0.66 = 0.73$	1	1
O	0.48	B only	0.07	0.52	0

The total chance of paternity can be estimated as follows:

A random man
$0.52 \times 0.73 + 0.48 \times 0.07 =$
$$0.38 + 0.03 = 0.41$$
A Group B man
$0.52 \times 1 + 0.47 \times 0.52 = 0.52 + 0.24 = 0.76$
A group O man
$0.52 \times 1 + 0.47 \times 0 = 0.52 + 0 = 0.52$

Paternity Index. The chance of paternity is inversely related to the number of genetic markers tested; in other words, the larger the number, the smaller the chance of paternity. Consequently, the chance of paternity by it-self has little meaning, just as if one would say 100 in money without specifying whether it is dollars or cents. Therefore, the chance of paternity of a non-father or a random man (Y) is used as a unit of measurement or reference to evaluate the chance of paternity of the alleged father (X). This value, X/Y, is known as the "Paternity Index" (PI) (Hennigson, 1968), and means essentially the same as the *ratio* or the *odds* for the person being the father. The relationship between the different types of paternity indices is shown in Tables 44–13 and 44–14. It is possible to determine the paternity index for each marker and use the product of the individual indices as the total index; however,

Table 44-13. CHANCE OF PATERNITY (CP) AND PATERNITY INDEX (PI)

	PHENOTYPE	GENOTYPE	CP	PI (= X/Y)
Non-father (random man)	Unknown	Unknown	p (Y)	1
	(not tested)		(reference)	
Alleged father	M+	Homozygote	1	1/p
	M+	Heterozygote	0.5 (X)	½/p
	M+	Unknown*	$p/\bar{M}$ (= 1/(2 − p))	$1/\bar{M}$

M = marker with gene frequency p and phenotype frequency $\bar{M}$. Mother M− and Child M+.
CP = Chance of a sperm to pass the required gene to the child.
*For 2 allelic markers only, when p + q < 1, the formula (p + q)/(p + 2q) should be used.

Table 44-14. TOTAL CHANCE OF PATERNITY

CHANCE TO PASS THE GENE(S) BY	IN CONDITION		TOTAL CHANCE OF PATERNITY
	A	B	
The mother	$1/(2 - p) = s$	$1 - s$	
A random man	1	p	$s \times 1 + p(1 - s) = s + p - sp$
Alleged father, M+	1	s	$s \times 1 + s(1 - s) = 2s - s^2$
Alleged father, M−	1	0	$s \times 1 + 0(1 - s) = s$

Paternity index: M+, $(2s - s^2)/(s + p + sp)$; M−, $s/(s + p + sp)$

Mother and child, both M+, zygosity unknown, two conditions possible:
  A. Mother passes the M, the father could be M+ or M−.
  B. Mother passes the non-M, the father must pass the M.

it is much simpler to obtain the product of the chances of paternity for each marker of the alleged father (X) and then divide this by the product of the gene frequencies of the non-father (Y), since this second method contains many 1's and 0.5's as the X value.

For the example used above the paternity index would be:

If the alleged father is homozygous for all three markers:

$$1 : 0.00048 = 2083$$

If the alleged father is heterozygous for all three markers:

$$0.125 : 0.00048 = 260$$

If the zygosity for all three markers is unknown:

$$0.14 : 0.00048 = 292$$

An index of 19:1 or greater is considered statistically significant. Of course, the court may have to balance this with other information in making the final decision.

For convenience, the chance of paternity and paternity indexes for the alleged father of different ABO groups against various mother-child genetic patterns are listed in Table 44-15.

Using the same principle, general formulas can be derived for only one of the two allelic markers being tested and the mother and the child are both positive for marker but zygosity is unknown (Table 44-16). Some useful values for the estimation of paternity are summarized in Tables 44-17, 44-18, and 44-19.

Plausibility of Paternity (W). The term plausibility of paternity (W) is used to indicate the relative chance of paternity and is calculated by using the Essen-Möller equation, $W = X/(X + Y)$, where X = the chance of paternity of the alleged father and Y = the chance of paternity of the non-father (Hummel, 1972). Since these X and Y values are essentially the same as those used in the formula for calculating the Paternity Index, it is not difficult to see that

$$W = X(X + Y) = (X/Y)/((X + Y)/Y)$$
$$= (X/Y)/(X/Y + 1)$$
$$= PI/(PI + 1)$$
$$\text{Conversely, } PI = W(1 - W)$$

Since $W = X/(X + Y)$, or $1/(1 + Y/X)$, this equation can also be expressed as $1/(1 + Y_1/X_1 \cdot Y_2/X_2 \cdot Y_3/X_3 \cdot Y_n/X_n)$ to cover many genetic markers.

Interpretation of Paternity Index (PI) and Plausibility of Paternity (W)

Before the small electronic calculators became widely available, Hummel, with the aid of a computer, prepared a set of tables which would simplify calculation by avoiding a great

PI	W	CHANCE OF PATERNITY
—	—	
≥ 399	99.80–99.90	Practically proved
≥ 99	99.1 –99.75	Extremely likely
≥ 19	95 –99	Very likely
≥ 9	90 –95	Likely
≥ 4	80 –90	Hint
≥ 2.3	70 –80	Merely suggestive
> 1.2	50 –70	On the positive side
< 1	< 50	On the negative side

(*Text continued on p. 1544*)

Table 44–15. CHANCE OF PATERNITY/PATERNITY INDEX OF ALLEGED FATHER OF VARIOUS ABO PHENOTYPES AGAINST VARIOUS MOTHER-CHILD GENETIC PATTERNS

WHITE POPULATION

PHENOTYPE OF THE mother	child	GENE OF THE CHILD FROM mother	father	Random Man (Y)	Alleged Father (X), Phenotype — O	A₁	A₂	B	A₁B	A₂B
O, A₁, A₂, B	O	O	O	0.66 / 1	1 / 1.5	0.4 / 0.6	0.47 / 0.71	0.47 / 0.71	0 / 0	0 / 0
O, A₂, B	A₁, A₁B	O, A₂, B	A₁	0.2 / 1	0 / 0	0.56 / 2.8	0 / 0	0 / 0	0.5 / 2.5	0 / 0
O, B, B	A₂, A₂B	O, B	A₂	0.07 / 1	0 / 0	0.04 / 0.6	0.53 / 7.6	0 / 0	0 / 0	0.5 / 7.1
O, A₁, A₂ / A₁ / A₂	B, A₁B, A₂B	O, A₁, A₂	B	0.07 / 1	0 / 0	0 / 0	0 / 0	0.53 / 7.6	0.5 / 7.1	0.5 / 7.1
A₁	A₁	A₁ 0.56, A₂ 0.04, O 0.4	A₁, A₂, O 0.93; A₁ 0.2; A₁ 0.2	0.61 / 1	0.56 / 0.9	0.81 / 1.3	0.56 / 0.9	0.26 / 0.4	0.5 / 0.8	0.28 / 0.5
A₂	A₂	A₂ 0.53, O 0.47	A₂, O 0.73; A₂ 0.07	0.42 / 1	0.53 / 1.3	0.25 / 0.6	0.78 / 1.9	0.21 / 0.5	0 / 0	0.5 / 0.12
A₁	A₂	A₂ 0.09, O 0.91	A₂, O 0.73; A₂ 0.07	0.13 / 1	0.09 / 0.7	0.08 / 0.6	0.57 / 4.4	0.04 / 0.3	0 / 0	0.49 / 3.8
B	B	B 0.53, O 0.47	B, O 0.73; B 0.07	0.42 / 1	0.53 / 1.3	0.21 / 0.5	0.20 / 0.5	0.78 / 1.9	0.5 / 1.2	0.5 / 1.2

Header note: CHANCE OF PATERNITY/PATERNITY INDEX (X/Y). Each alleged-father cell shows chance of paternity (upper) / paternity index (lower).

Table 44–15. CHANCE OF PATERNITY/PATERNITY INDEX OF ALLEGED FATHER OF VARIOUS ABO PHENOTYPES AGAINST VARIOUS MOTHER-CHILD GENETIC PATTERNS (*continued*)

BLACK POPULATION

PHENOTYPE OF THE		GENE OF THE CHILD FROM		Random Man (Y)	CHANCE OF PATERNITY/PATERNITY INDEX (X/Y) Alleged Father (X), Phenotype					
mother	child	mother	father		O	A_1	A_2	B	A_1B	A_2B
O, A_1 A_2, B	O	O	O	0.7 / 1	1 / 1.4	0.43 / 0.6	0.46 / 0.7	0.45 / 0.6	0 / 0	0 / 0
O, A_2 B	A_1 A_1B	O, A_2 B	A_1	0.12 / 1	0 / 0	0.53 / 4.4	0 / 0	0 / 0	0.5 / 4.2	0 / 0
O, B B	A_2 A_2B	O B	A_2	0.06 / 1	0 / 0	0.04 / 0.67	0.53 / 9	0 / 0	0 / 0	0.5 / 8.3
O, A_1, A_2 A_1 A_2	B A_1B A_2B	O A_1 A_2	B	0.13 / 1	0 / 0	0 / 0	0 / 0	0.55 / 4.2	0.5 / 3.9	0.5 / 3.9
A_1	A_1	A_1 0.53 A_2 0.04 O 0.43	A_1, A_2, O 0.88 A_1 0.12 A_1 0.12	0.52 / 1	0.53 / 1	0.78 / 1.5	0.53 / 1	0.24 / 0.5	0.5 / 1	0.27 / 0.5
A_2	A_2	A_2 0.54 O 0.46	A_2, O 0.76 A_2 0.06	0.44 / 1	0.54 / 1.2	0.27 / 0.6	0.79 / 1.8	0.24 / 5.5	0 / 0	0.5 / 1.1
A_1	A_2	A_2 0.09 O 0.91	A_2, O 0.76 A_2 0.06	0.12 / 1	0.09 / 0.8	0.04 / 0.3	0.58 / 4.8	0.04 / 0.3	0 / 0	0.5 / 4.2
B	B	B 0.55 O 0.45	B, O 0.83 B 0.13	0.52 / 1	0.55 / 1	0.24 / 0.5	0.23 / 0.4	0.80 / 1.5	0.5 / 1	0.5 / 1

4

Table 44–16. CHANCE OF PATERNITY OF RANDOM MAN (Y) AND ALLEGED FATHER (X) AND PATERNITY INDEX (X/Y) WHEN ONLY ONE GENETIC MARKER IS BEING TESTED

Each cell gives the chance (upper value) and the paternity index (lower, italic value).

MARKER TESTED	PHENOTYPE OF Mother	PHENOTYPE OF Child	GENE OF THE CHILD FROM Mother	GENE OF THE CHILD FROM Father	WHITES Y ?	WHITES X +	WHITES X −	BLACKS Y ?	BLACKS X +	BLACKS X −
P_1	−	+	Non-P_1	P_1	0.65 / 1	0.74 / 1.1	0 / 0	0.29 / 1	0.59 / 2	0 / 0
	− +	−	Non-P_1	Non-P_1	0.35 / 1	0.26 / 0.7	1 / 2.9	0.71 / 1	0.41 / 0.6	1 / 1.6
	+	+	P_1 / Non-P_1	P_1, Non-P_1 / P_1	0.91 / 1	0.93 / 1	0.74 / 0.8	0.71 / 1	0.83 / 1.2	0.59 / 0.8
Se	−	+	se	Se	0.5 / 1	0.67 / 1.3	0 / 0	0.47 / 1	0.65 / 1.4	0 / 0
	− +	−	se	se	0.5 / 1	0.33 / 0.7	1 / 2	0.53 / 1	0.35 / 0.7	1 / 2
	+	+	Se / Se	Se, se / Se	0.83 / 1	0.88 / 1	0.67 / 0.8	0.81 / 1	0.88 / 1	0.65 / 0.8
Xg^a	−	+	Xg	Xg^a	0.33 / 1	0.5 / 1.5	0 / 0	0.28 / 1	0.5 / 1.8	0 / 0
	− +	−	Xg	Xg	0.17 / 1	0 / 0	0.5 / 3	0.22 / 1	0 / 0	0.5 / 2.3
	+	+	Xg^a / Xg	Xg^a, Xg / Xg^a	0.46 / 1	0.5 / 1	0.38 / 0.8	0.44 / 1	0.5 / 1.1	0.35 / 0.8
Fy^a	−	+	Non-a	a	0.39 / 1	0.62 / 1.5	0 / 0	0.08 / 1	0.52 / 6.5	0 / 0
	− +	−	Non-a	Non-a	0.61 / 1	0.38 / 0.6	1 / 1.7	0.92 / 1	0.48 / 0.5	1 / 1
	+	+	a / Non-a	a, Non-a / a	0.77 / 1	0.86 / 1.1	0.62 / 0.8	0.56 / 1	0.77 / 1.4	0.52 / 1

? = not tested; + = positive; − = negative

Table 44–16. CHANCE OF PATERNITY OF RANDOM MAN (Y) AND ALLEGED FATHER (X) AND PATERNITY INDEX (X/Y) WHEN ONLY ONE GENETIC MARKER IS BEING TESTED (*continued*)

MARKER TESTED	PHENOTYPE OF — Mother	PHENOTYPE OF — Child	GENE OF THE CHILD FROM — Mother	GENE OF THE CHILD FROM — Father	WHITES Y ?	WHITES X +	WHITES X −	BLACKS Y ?	BLACKS X +	BLACKS X −
Jk^a	−	+	Non-a	a	0.54 / *1*	0.68 / *1.2*	0 / *0*	0.74 / *1*	0.8 / *1.1*	0 / *0*
	−/+	−	Non-a	Non-a	0.46 / *1*	0.32 / *0.7*	1 / *2*	0.26 / *1*	0.2 / *0.8*	1 / *0.4*
	+	+	a / Non-a	a, Non-a / a	0.85 / *1*	0.90 / *1*	0.68 / *0.8*	0.94 / *1*	0.96 / *1*	0.8 / *0.8*
Glm^a	−	+	Non-a	a	0.22 / *1*	0.56 / *2.5*	0 / *0*	0.87 / *1*	0.89 / *1*	0 / *0*
	−/+	−	Non-a	Non-a	0.78 / *1*	0.44 / *0.5*	1 / *1.2*	0.13 / *1*	0.11 / *0.9*	1 / *0.8*
	+	+	a / Non-a	a, Non-a / a	0.66 / *1*	0.81 / *1.2*	0.56 / *0.9*	0.99 / *1*	0.99 / *1*	0.89 / *0.9*
Glm^x	−	+	Non-x	x	0.05 / *1*	0.51 / *10*	0 / *0*	0.07 / *1*	0.53 / *7.4*	0 / *0*
	−/+	−	Non-x	Non-x	0.95 / *1*	0.49 / *0.5*	1 / *1*	0.93 / *1*	0.48 / *0.5*	1 / *1*
	+	+	x / Non-x	x, Non-x / x	0.54 / *1*	0.76 / *1.4*	0.51 / *1*	0.56 / *1*	0.77 / *1.4*	0.56 / *1*
Km^1	−	+	Non-1	1	0.11 / *1*	0.52 / *5*	0 / *0*	0.3 / *1*	0.58 / *2*	0 / *0*
	−/+	−	Non-1	Non-1	0.89 / *1*	0.48 / *0.5*	1 / *1.1*	0.7 / *1*	0.42 / *0.6*	1 / *1.6*
	+	+	1 / Non-1	1, Non-1 / 1	0.57 / *1*	0.77 / *1.3*	0.52 / *1*	0.7 / *1*	0.82 / *1.2*	0.58 / *0.8*

4

Table 44-17. SOME USEFUL VALUES FOR THE ESTIMATION OF CHANCE OF PATERNITY

GENE OR HAPLOTYPE	FREQUENCY (p) White	FREQUENCY (p) Black	CHANCE* White	CHANCE* Black	GENE OR HAPLOTYPE	FREQUENCY (p) White	FREQUENCY (p) Black	CHANCE* White	CHANCE* Black
O	0.66	0.70			PGM^1	0.75	0.81		
A_1	0.20	0.12	0.56	0.53	AK^1	0.97	0.99		
A_2	0.07	0.06	0.52	0.52	ADA^1	0.95	0.98		
B	0.07	0.13	0.52	0.54	$6PGD^A$	0.98	0.96		
					AcP^A	0.39	0.25		
MS	0.25	0.10			AcP^B	0.55	0.72		
Ms	0.31	0.35			AcP^C	0.06	0.014		
NS	0.07	0.06			GPT^1	0.52	0.81		
Ns	0.38	0.37			EsD^1	0.90	0.90		
MS^u		0.05			GLO^1	0.43			
NS^u		0.07			Gc^1	0.72	0.89		
DCE	0.002	0.003			HP^1	0.42	0.55		
DCe	0.460	0.108	0.97	0.85	Tf^c	0.994	0.977		
DC^we	0.01								
dCe	0.014	0.024			Gm^a	0.224	0.87	0.56	0.89
DcE	0.135	0.098	0.91	1.00	Gm^x	0.052	0.069	0.51	0.52
Dce	0.030	0.508	0.52	0.75	Km^1	0.106	0.300	0.52	0.59
dcE	0.015				$Gm^{f;bo}$	0.69	0.00		
dce	0.335	0.257			$Gm^{a,z;g}$	0.30	0.00		
D^uce		0.003			$Gm^{a,z;bo}$	0.01	1.00		
K	0.05	<0.01	0.51						
Js^a		0.104		0.53					
Fy^a	0.39	0.08	0.62	0.52					
Fy^b	0.61	0.16	0.72	0.54					
Fy		0.76							
Jk^a	0.54	0.74	0.69	0.79					
Lu^a	0.03	0.02	0.51	0.51					
P_1	0.65	0.29	0.74	0.59					
Xg^a (female)	0.67	0.55	0.76	0.69					
Xg^a (male)	0.34	0.28	0.5	0.5					
Se	0.50	0.47	0.67	0.65					

*Chance of a parent with the specific marker but of unknown genotype to pass that marker to the children = $(p + q)/(p + 2q)$, when q is the gene frequency of the silent or untested allelic marker.

deal of multiplication and division (Hummel, 1972). Unfortunately, his publications offer no explanation regarding how those values were derived; consequently, one has to depend solely on his many tables in obtaining an answer, and has to limit the estimation to those markers having particular gene frequencies listed.

Two examples, taken from the literature, are included to illustrate the relationship of

Table 44-18. CHANCE OF PASSING THE MARKER IN A PHENOTYPE WITH THREE OR MORE MARKERS

PHENOTYPE	MARKER	CHANCE OF PASSING MARKER White	CHANCE OF PASSING MARKER Black	PHENOTYPE	MARKER	CHANCE OF PASSING MARKER White	CHANCE OF PASSING MARKER Black
A	A_1	0.56	0.53	MNSs	MS or Ns	0.81	0.64
	A_2	0.04	0.04		Ms or NS	0.19	0.36
	O	0.40	0.43	DCce	DCe	0.5	0.435
DCcEe	DCe	0.4815	0.343		dce	0.46	0.145
	DcE	0.447	0.421		Dce	0.04	0.355
	dCe	0.0135	0.078		dCe	0.0015	0.065
	dcE	0.048	0.000	DcEe	DcE	0.495	0.5
	Dce	0.0005	0.053		dce	0.455	0.168
	dce	0.0045	0.026		Dce	0.045	0.332
	DCE	0.005	0.079		dcE	0.005	

Table 44-19. TOTAL CHANCE OF PASSING THE MARKER WHEN MOTHER AND CHILD HAVE THE SAME MARKER

PHENOTYPE OF						TOTAL CHANCE OF PATERNITY									
						White					Black				
Mother	Child	Alleged father				Y	X				Y	X			
		1	2	3	4		1	2	3	4		1	2	3	4
P+	P+	P+	P−			0.91	0.93	0.74			0.71	0.83	0.59		
Xg(a+)	Xg(a+)	Xg(a+)	Xg(a−)			0.46	0.50	0.38			0.44	0.50	0.35		
A_1	A_1	A_1	A_2	B	0	0.61	0.81	0.56	0.26	0.56	0.52	0.78	0.53	0.24	0.53
A_2	A_2	A_1	A_2	B	0	0.42	0.25	0.78	0.21	0.53	0.44	0.27	0.79	0.24	0.54
B	B	A_1	A_2	B	0	0.42	0.21	0.20	0.73	0.53	0.52	0.24	0.23	0.80	0.55
DCe	DCe	DCe	dCe			0.47	1.00	0.015			0.13	0.98			
DcE	DcE	DcE	dcE			0.14	0.99	0.045			0.10	1.00			
Dce	Dce	Dce	dce			0.23	0.77	0.24			0.71	0.94	0.125		

the various ways of expressing the same data (Tables 44-20 and 44-21). The principle behind each method is essentially the same. Having the final result expressed as a ratio or paternity index is preferable, since (1) it is comprehensible by most people, (2) it can be derived readily from the gene frequency of each genetic marker, and (3) it can also be utilized in directly comparing two or more men involved in the same case.

Table 44-20. AN EXAMPLE ILLUSTRATING THE PRINCIPLE OF THE ESTIMATION OF THE CHANCE OF PATERNITY

| PHENOTYPE* OF | | | GENE REQUIRED TO BE THE FATHER | CHANCE OF PATERNITY | | |
Mother	Child	Alleged Father		Non-father(Y)*	Alleged Father(X)	Log(Y/X) + 10*
O	A	A_1	A_1	0.2274	0.57†	9.6006
MS	MNS	NSs	NS	0.0748	0.5	9.1749
k	k	k	k	0.9607	1	9.9826
Fy(a−)	Fy(a−)	Fy(a−)	Fy^{-a}	0.5857	1	9.7677
cde	cde	CcDee	cde	0.4089	0.4789‡	9.9314
Hp2−2	Hp1−2	Hp1−1	Hp^1	0.3765	1	9.5758
Gc1−1	Gc1−1	Gc1−1	Gc^1	0.7175	1	9.8558
Gm(−1−2)	Gm(1,2)	Gm(1,2)	$Gm^{1,2}$	0.0979	0.5257§	9.2700
Km(−1)	Km(−1)	Km(−1)	Km^{-1}	0.9348	1	9.9707
AcPAB	AcPAB	AcPAB	AcP^B	0.9353	1	9.9710
$PGM_1$1−2	$PGM_1$1−1	$PGM_1$1−1	PGM_1^1	0.7720	1	9.8876
			Product:	0.00006986	0.0718	Sum: 106.9881
			RATIO	(1) :	(1028)	−100.0000
						6.9881

*From Hummel, 1971.

Value of individual X: 1 for homozygote, ½ for heterozygote

zygosity unknown: 100% of homozygotes + 50% of heterozygotes (or 1/(2−p), p = gene frequency).

† Group A_1 person: 14% homozygotes, 86% heterozygotes, $0.14 \times 1 + 0.86 \times \frac{1}{2} = 0.57$.

‡ A CcDee phenotype person: 0.8578 would be CDe/cde, $0.8578 \times \frac{1}{2} = 0.4789$.

§ A Glm(1,2) person: 0.0979/0.1862 (= 1/(2−0.0979), phenotype frequency) = 0.5257.

Paternity index(PI) = X/Y = 0.0718/0.00006986 = 1028

Plausibility of paternity(W) = X/(X + Y) = 0.0718/(0.0718 + 0.00006986) = 99.9%

= PI/(PI + 1) = 1028(1028 + 1) = 99.9%

Check: Log(Y/X) + 10 = 6.9881, Log(Y/X) = 6.9881 − 10 = −3.0119

Y/X = 0.000973, X/Y = 1/0.000973 = 1028, 1028/(1028 + 1) = 99.9%

The value of W, 99.9% is identical to that found in Hummel, (1971), Table III, p. 89.

Comment: From this example, it is obvious that one can obtain the same answer without depending on logarithm or specific tables. At the same time, one can add any genetic markers of known gene frequency to the calculation.

Table 44–21. AN EXAMPLE ILLUSTRATING THE PRINCIPLE OF THE ESTIMATION OF THE CHANCE OF PATERNITY

PHENOTYPE* OF			GENE REQUIRED TO BE THE FATHER	CHANCE OF PATERNITY		
Mother	Child	Alleged Father		Non-Father (Y)†	Alleged Father (X)	Log(Y/X) + 10*
A_1	A_1	A_1	A_1 or A_2, 0	0.6228‡	0.8151‡	9.8831
cDe	cDe	CcDe	cde	0.4089	0.5	9.9127
MN	N	MN	N	0.4469	0.5	9.9512
K−	K+	K+	K	0.0393	0.51§	8.8865
Fy(a−)	Fy(a+)	Fy(a+)	Fy^a	0.4143	0.6306§	9.8176
			Product:	0.001853	0.0655	Sum: 48.4695
			RATIO	(1) :	(35)	−40
						8.4695

* Abbott, 1976.

† Hummel, 1971.

‡ Group A_1 persons: 0.14 are A_1/A_1, 0.86 are $A_1/0$ (or A_1A_2)

Chance of passing A_1 gene, $0.14 \times 1 + 0.86 \times \frac{1}{2} = 0.57$

Chance of passing 0 or A_2 gene $1 − 0.57 = 0.43$

GENE FROM THE MOTHER	CHANCE OF PATERNITY	
	Non-father (Y)	Alleged father (X)
A_1(0.57)	(without B gene) $0.9211 \times 0.57 = 0.5250$	$0.57 \times 1 = 0.57$
0 or A_2(0.43)	(with A_1 gene) $0.2274 \times 0.43 = \underline{0.0978}$	$0.43 \times 0.57 = \underline{0.2451}$
Total	0.6228	0.8151

§ Chance of passing a marker if zygosity unknown = gene fre./phenotype fre.

A K+ person: $0.0379/0.077 = 0.5100$; A Fy(a‡) person: $0.4143/0.657 = 0.6306$

Paternity index(PI) = X/Y = $0.0655/0.0001853 = 35$

Plausibility of paternity(W) = X/(X + Y) = $0.0655/(0.0655 + 0.0001853) = 97\%$

Check: Log(Y/X) = $8.4695 − 10 = −1.5305$, Y/X = 0.02948, X/Y = $1/0.02948 = \underline{35}$

W = PI/(PI + 1) = $35/36 = 97\%$

Comment: This example shows that in a system with amorphic markers such as 0 and A_2, the chance of paternity should be evaluated slightly differently from those having two dominant alleles. As in the previous sample, this one also demonstrates that the ratio and the paternity index, as well as the plausibility of paternity, can be derived by using common logic.

A third example is also included to show the way in which the test results are used to calculate the chance of paternity as it is done at our institution (Table 44-22).

LEGAL ASPECTS OF PATERNITY

The legal aspects of paternity testing fall into three categories: (a) medical malpractice, (b) evidence, and (c) confidentiality.

Medical malpractice

The basis for a medical malpractice suit could be the possibility of improper testing or a failure to exclude an alleged father; however, it is impossible to be 100 per cent accurate in dealing with any biologic system. A person's duty is always to use reasonable care to avoid any mistakes; consequently, a breach of this duty may be the proximal cause of damage and liability. This type of suit must be filed within one year according to the statute of limitations.

Evidence

Written laboratory reports are usually acceptable in court and the presence of an expert witness is unnecessary. This written report must, however, include all records and interpretations of the test results. It should also be noted that often the court will accept only positive evidence, such as an exclusion of paternity, considering no exclusion as a negative finding. However, estimating the chance of paternity may, at some time in the future, change this practice.

Table 44–22. ESTIMATING THE CHANCE OF PATERNITY

GENETIC MARKER SYSTEM EXAMINED	PHENOTYPE OF			MARKER REQUIRED TO BE THE FATHER	CHANCE OF PASSING THE REQUIRED GENETIC MARKER	
	Mother	Child	Alleged Father		Non-father (Y)	Alleged Father (X)
ABO	O	B‡	B‡	B	0.07	0.52*
MN	MNs	MS	MSs	MS	0.25	0.5
Rh	dce	DCce	DCe	DCe	0.46	0.97*
Kell	K−k+	K−k+	K−k+	k	0.96	1
Duffy	a+b+	a+b+	a+b+	Fy^a or Fy^b	0.5†	0.5†
Kidd	a+b−	a+b+	a−b+	Jk^b	0.46	1
P	P_1+	P_1+	P_1+	P_1	0.91‡	0.93‡
Xg	a−	a+	a+	Xg^a	0.33§	0.5§
PGM_1	1−2	1−2	1−1	$PGM_1{}^1$	0.5†	0.5†
AK	1−1	1−1	1−1	AK^A	0.95	1
6PGD	AA	AA	AA	$6PGD^A$	0.98	1
ADA	1−2	1−2	1−2	ADA^1, ADA^2	0.5†	0.5†
GLO	1−1	1−2	2−2	GLO^2	0.57	1
ACP	BB	BB	AB	ACP^B	0.55	0.5
EsD	1−1	1−1	1−1	EsD^1	0.90	1
ALT	1−2	1−1	1−2	ALT^1	0.52	0.5
Gc	1−2	1−1	1−1	Gc^1	0.72	1
Tf	C	C	C	Tf^C	0.99	1
Hp	1−2	1−1	1−2	Hp^1	0.42	0.5
Gm	f;b0	f;b0	a,f;b0	$Gm^{f;b0}$	0.69	0.5
Km	1−, 3+	1−, 3+	1−, 3+	Km^3	0.89	1
				Product:	0.000003351	0.0001773746
				RATIO:	1	53

Y values: gene frequency (p) of the required marker of U.S. whites
X values: 1 for homozygote, ½ for heterozygote, (p + q)/(p + 2q) = s for zygosity unknown*
Total chance of paternity (mother has the marker)   Non-father   Alleged father

$$0.5 \qquad\qquad 0.5$$
$$s + p - sp \qquad 2s - s^2$$

*q = Gene frequency of the allelic marker of p, silent or untested; when p + q = 1, $\dfrac{p + q}{p + 2q} = \dfrac{1}{2 - p}$

†Mother and child, both heterozygotes
‡Zygosity unknown
§Adjusted for having boys

Confidentiality

As in all reports of this type, the records of the test results and the parties involved are considered confidential information. In our institution, forms are included which state to whom the reports are to be sent. These are entered in the records, in the presence of both parties involved, before the blood specimens are drawn. It is also a good policy not to give out results over the telephone, since there is no way of positively identifying the one to whom you are speaking.

Examples of reporting forms currently in use are available upon request to the authors.

REFERENCES

Abbott, J.P., Sell, K.W., Krause, H.D., Miali, J.B., Jennings, E.R., and Rettberg, W.A.H. Joint AMA-ABA guidelines: Present status of serologic testing in problems of disputed parentage. Fam. Law. Q. *9*:3, 1976.

Allen, F.H.: Null types of the human erythrocyte blood groups. *Am. J. Clin. Pathol.*, *66*:467, 1976.

Alper, C.A., Boenisch, T., and Watson, L.: Genetic polymorphisms in human glycine-rich beta-glycoprotein. J. Exp. Med., *135*:68, 1972.

Alper, C.A., and Propp, R.P.: Genetic polymorphism of the third component of human complement (C′3). J. Clin. Invest., *47*:2181, 1968.

Bowman, J.E., Frischer, H., Ajmar, F., Carson, P.E., and Gower, M.L.: Population family and biochemical investigation of human adenylate kinase polymorphism. Nature, *214*:1156, 1976.

Ceppellini, R., et al.: Notation for genetic factors of human immunoglobulins. Bull. W.H.O., *33*:447, 1965.

Chen, S., Giblett, E.R., and Anderson, J.E.: Genetics of glutamic pyruvate transaminase; its inheritance, common and rare variants, population distribution and differences in catalytic activity. Ann. Hum. Genet., *35*:401, 1972.

Culliford, B.J.: The examination and typing of blood stains in the crime laboratory. Washington, D.C., U.S. Government Printing Office, 1971.

Dausset, J., and Colombani, J.: Histocompatibility Testing, 1972, 1973. Baltimore, Williams and Wilkins Co., 1973.

Davidson, R.G.: Electrophoresis variants of human 6-phosphogluconate dehydrogenase: Population and family studies and description of a new variant. Ann. Hum. Genet., *30*:355, 1967.

Detter, J.C., Stamatoyannopoulos, G., Giblett, E.R., and Motulsky, A.G.: Adenosine deaminase: Racial distribution and report of a new phenotype. J. Med. Genet., *7*:356, 1970.

Diezel, V.: An improved procedure for protein staining in polyacrylamide gels with a new type of Coomassie brilliant blue. Analyt. Biochem., *48*:617, 1972.

Dykes, D.: Serum proteins and erythrocyte enzymes in paternity testing. *In* A Seminar On Polymorphisms in Human Blood. Washington, D.C., AABB, pp. 27-42, 1975.

Dykes, D.D., and Polesky, H.F.: The usefulness of serum protein and erythrocyte polymorphisms in paternity testing. Am. J. Clin. Pathol., *65*:6982, 1976.

Fudenberg, H.H., Pink, J.R.L., Stites, D.C., and Wang, A.C.: Basic Immunogenetics. New York, Oxford University Press, 1978.

Giblett, E.R.: Genetic Markers in Human Blood. Philadelphia, F.A. Davis Company, 1969.

Giblett, E.R., and Scott, N.M.: Red cell acid phosphatase: Racial distribution and report of a new phenotype. Am. J. Hum. Genet., *17*:425, 1965.

Grubb, R.: The Genetic Markers of Human Immunoglobulins. New York, Springer-Verlag Company, 1970.

Hennigsen, K.: On the application of blood tests to legal cases of disputed paternity. Rev. Transfusion, *12*:137, 1968.

Hummel, K., Ihm, P., Schmidt, V., and Wallisser, G.: Biostatistical opinion of parentage. Based upon the results of blood group tests. Vol. 1 Table—part 1, 1971; Vol 2. Table—part 2, 1972.

Jancik, W.E., and Speiser, P.: Calculated Values of Probability of Paternity Exclusion: Based on the hereditary blood factors of the erythrocytes of mother and child. Vienna, Springer-Verlag, 1952.

Jeannet, M., Hassig, A., and Bernheim, J.: Use of the HLA-A antigen system in disputed paternity cases. Vox Sang., *23*:197, 1972.

Kompf, P., Bissbort, S., Gussmann, H., and Hiller, H.: Red cell glyoxalase I (E.C.:4.4.1.5): Formal genetics and line age relations. Hum. Gen., *28*:249, 1975.

Lapinski, F.L., Crowley, K.M., Merritt, C., and Henry, J.B.: Use of microplate in paternity testing. Am. J. Clin. Pathol., *70*(Oct.), 1978.

Lee, C.L.: Current status of paternity testing. Fam. Law. Q., *9*:615, 1975.

Mayr, W.R.: Die genetik des HL-A systems. Populations and Familienuntersuchungen unter besonder Berucksichtigung der Paternitatsserologie. Humangenetik, *12*:195, 1971.

McKusick, V.A., and Ruddle, F.H.: The status of the gene map of the human chromosome. Science, *196*:390, 1977.

Mourant, A.E., Kopec, A.C., and Domaniewska-Sobczak, K.: The Distribution of the Human Blood Groups and Other Polymorphisms, 2nd ed. London, Oxford University Press, 1976.

Polesky, H.F.: Paternity Testing. Chicago, American Society of Clinical Pathologists, 1975.

Polesky, H.F., Rokala, D., and Hoff, T.: Serum Proteins in Paternity Testing. Chicago, American Society of Clinical Pathology, 1975.

Race, R.R., and Sanger, R.: Blood Groups in Man, 6th ed. Oxford Blackwell Scientific, 1975.

Schanfield, M.S.: Personal communication, 1977.

Schanfield, M.S., Polesky, H.F. and Sebring, E.S.: Gm and inv Typing in Paternity Testing. Chicago, American Society of Clinical Pathologists, 1975.

Speiser, P.: Das HL-A system in Paternitatsprozess mit Berucksichtigung des Beweiswertes. Wien. Klin. Wochenschr. *87*:321, 1975.

Soulier, J.P., Prou-Wartelle, O. and Muller, J.Y.: Paternity research using HL-A system. Haematologia (Budapest), *8*:249, 1974.

Stedman, R.: Human population frequencies in twelve blood grouping systems. J. Forensic. Sci. Soc., *12*:379, 1959.

Sussman, L.N.: Paternity testing by blood grouping, 2nd ed. Springfield, Ill., Charles C Thomas, Publisher, 1976.

van Loghem, E.: Polymorphism of immunoglobulins. *In* Ikkala, E., and Nykanen (eds.): Tranfusion and Immunology. Vammala, Vammalan Kirjapaino Oy, 1975.

Welch, S.G.: Red cell esterase D in studies of paternity cases in the United Kingdom. Vox Sang., *28*:366, 1975.

Part 5

MEDICAL MICROBIOLOGY

Edited by John A. Washington, II, M.D.,
and John Bernard Henry, M.D.

45

MEDICAL MICROBIOLOGY

John A. Washington II, M.D.

The laboratory diagnosis of an infectious disease is contingent upon prior determination of a differential diagnosis on the basis of the patient's history and physical examination, a consideration of those organisms most likely to have caused the disease, and the selection of those tests and procedures that are most likely to lead to the organism's detection and identification by means of microscopic examination, cultures, or immunologic techniques. Because infectious diseases may involve any body surface, system, and organ and because infectious diseases may be due to a wide variety of microorganisms, including bacteria, fungi, parasites, and viruses, selection of the proper specimen for the laboratory to examine is a critical but often neglected component of the diagnostic process.

The specimen for examination should be representative of the disease process and should be adequate in quantity for complete examination. It should be collected in such a way as to avoid contamination with the microflora that is indigenous to the skin and mucous membranes. Invasive techniques, such as transtracheal or suprapubic aspiration, may be required to obviate contamination of specimens by indigenous microflora. Specimens should, in general, be forwarded promptly to the laboratory for processing so that fastidious organisms do not perish or are not overgrown during storage. In some cases, special provisions may have to be made to ensure survival of organisms, such as the use of transport media or anaerobic containment. Recommendations regarding specimen selection, collection, and transport are made in the chapters that follow according to categories of etiologic agents causing infectious diseases.

In many instances, close cooperation between the microbiologist and histopathologist is essential for establishing the diagnosis of an infectious disease. Material removed surgically is obtained at considerable expense and some risk to the patient, and every effort should be made to ensure that it is examined microbiologically and histologically as carefully and completely as possible. Histologic examination shows whether the lesion is malignant or inflammatory and, if the latter, whether it is suppurative or granulomatous. Often, the material's histopathology will suggest a microbial etiology other than that originally suspected and additional special stains, cultures, and immunologic studies must be performed. Multiple specimens should be obtained from a large lesion and when several lesions are present. Tissue should be minced with sterile scissors and ground with a sterile abrasive, such as alundum, for microbiologic studies. Residual tissue should be stored at 5°C. for at least two weeks, pending the results of initial microbiologic and histopathologic examination, in case further studies are indicated.

The value of postmortem bacteriology is limited because of the poor correlation between ante- and postmortem culture results and because of the frequency of positive cultures and their lack of correlation with clinical or autopsy evidence of infectious disease. Because of the selectivity of the procedures used for their isolation and identification, mycobacteria, fungi, and viruses should be sought only when their presence was suspected clinically ante mortem or considered likely on the basis of postmortem findings.

Not all laboratories provide the same microbiologic services. The variety and extent of services provided by a laboratory depend on multiple factors, including the size of inpatient and outpatient facilities served, the interests and expertise of those directing and supervising the laboratory, the availability of

5

tests and procedures in nearby or distant reference laboratories, and the cost-effectiveness of each procedure as determined by the clinical need and justification for its performance on-site, its test volume and cost, and the laboratory's ability to maintain its proficiency in performing the test. Basic bacteriologic procedures, such as preparing Gram's stained smears and inoculating media, are required of nearly all hospital laboratories. Whether or not specimens are examined for the presence of mycobacteria, fungi, viruses, and parasites and the extent of identification of microorganisms must be determined by each laboratory director on the basis of factors mentioned above.

Many specialized microbiologic services are provided by city, state, and regional laboratories and by other reference laboratories (DORA File, 1977). Shipment of specimens to these laboratories must comply with Public Health Service regulations (Huffaker, 1974). Services are also provided by the Center for Disease Control (CDC), Atlanta, Georgia; however, the Center's primary responsibility is to serve as a resource for state and regional laboratories, and physicians seeking CDC assistance should do so through their own state health departments. Specific notations are made in the text of subsequent chapters when direct consultation with CDC is recommended. *In vitro* diagnostic reference products are available from the Biologic Products Division of CDC to other federal agencies; international, state, regional, and local public health agencies; public health service grantees when the products are required by their grants; commercial producers of *in vitro* diagnostic products for use in evaluating production lots;

collaborating researchers; and when there is a public health need for diagnostic products that can neither be purchased nor prepared in non-commercial laboratories.

In the chapters that follow, emphasis has been placed on specimen requirements, organism descriptions, and interpretation of findings. Detailed descriptions of techniques, stains, reagents, media, and methods of identification of organisms have not been included, since there are several excellent published books and manuals covering these aspects of medical microbiology. These resources are listed as general references at the end of each chapter. When a procedure considered to be particularly important and useful could not be located in the general references, citation of the specific reference describing the procedure was added.

In conclusion, there is no area of the clinical laboratory except microbiology in which the sources and varieties of specimens are so diverse; the process of selection, collection, and transport of the specimen so important; and the communication between physician and laboratory personnel so essential to the diagnosis of a disease. The laboratory needs to know what disease and etiologic agent are suspected. The laboratory requires a properly selected and collected specimen. An understanding by the clinician of the pathogenetic properties of microorganisms is essential for the correct interpretation of the laboratory's findings. The mere isolation of an organism or the demonstration of an immunologic response to a particular microbial antigen does not always constitute definitive evidence of its role in causing disease.

REFERENCES

Directory of Rare Analyses (DORA). Clin. Chem., *23*:323, 1977.

Huffaker, R. H. (ed.): Collection, handling and shipment of microbiological specimens. U.S. Department of Health, Education, and Welfare. Public Health Service. Atlanta, Ga., Center for Disease Control (DHEW Publication No. [CDC] 75-8263), 1974.

46

MICROBIOLOGY: SPACE, EQUIPMENT, MATERIALS, AND TECHNIQUES

Thomas L. Gavan, M.D.

SPACE

GENERAL LABORATORY DESIGN AND PLANNING

The approach to designing a laboratory has been to allocate space on the basis of a certain number of square feet per hospital bed, number of anticipated patient days, number of anticipated employees, or some other similar rule of thumb (see Chap. 58). The "appropriate" number of square feet to be allocated is thus usually determined by surveying the average amount of space in a number of existing laboratories and then to relate this space to the other denominator parameters. For example, Bartlett (1974) surveyed 86 community hospital laboratories and found an average of 120 net sq. ft.* per employee with a range from 40 to 350 net sq. ft. for the microbiology

laboratory. He observed that although personnel gradually accommodate to increasingly crowded conditions, activities are significantly encumbered below 75 sq. ft. per worker, and this, therefore, should be considered a minimum.

Of all the parameters, determining space requirements by the number of workers is the best, since this can be directly related to the nature and volume of the work to be accomplished.

Although this approach may lead to a feeling of security by copying from others, the end result is not innovative and old errors may be repeated. To design, construct, or remodel a laboratory of a certain size, because other hospitals of similar bed capacity have laboratories that size is potentially wasteful.

The first consideration in designing any facility is a determination of exactly what is to be accomplished within the facility. This requires the participation of the laboratory director and cannot be the responsibility of architects or administrators. The active par-

---

*Net square feet is usable space. This excludes walls, corridors, elevators, utilities, and staircases and is obtained by measuring the inside dimensions of a room, including space occupied by benches and equipment.

ticipation of the individual with professional knowledge of the laboratory's intended and projected function is essential. This may extend to consideration of the efficient and economical use of a community's resources through cooperation between facilities to avoid unnecessary duplication. A functional plan for the current and anticipated activities of the laboratory must be developed. Once this has been determined, a competent architect experienced in laboratory design will have little difficulty in designing the physical facilities needed to accomplish the task (see Chap. 58).

Clinical laboratory work loads have been increasing steadily in recent years at an average rate of 10 to 15 per cent per year. Microbiology laboratories share in this growth at a rate which is close to this average. In contrast to the chemistry and hematology laboratories, microbiology has not yet felt any significant impact from automation. When volume increases, the number of workers must also increase if the quality of the work performed is to be maintained. This situation may change somewhat in the future, since a number of automated or semiautomated pieces of equipment are being developed which may find their place in the laboratory. Recently, there has been an increased number of miniaturized products available which replace bulky individual tubes of differential media and thus save valuable bench and incubator space.

A laboratory designed today should be prepared to accommodate a 100 to 200 per cent increase in volume during a 10-year period. This can be accomplished in three ways: (1) the original facility must be designed with the reserve built in at the start, (2) the original facility must be designed to be expandable, or (3) the extra work load must be handled elsewhere. Thomas (1977) has developed an excellent manual concerned with laboratory design and planning.

MICROBIOLOGY LABORATORY PLANNING

The degree of sophistication and the extent and volume of procedures to be performed must be determined, as this will dictate the number of workers and the size and design of the laboratory.

Some consideration should be given to the location of microbiologic function within the laboratory area in general. Local statutes and safety codes regarding venting must be met. The laboratory should be located in close proximity to central glassware washing and sterilization facilities, unless the laboratory is of sufficient size to warrant having these functions within its own area. The location should be some distance from the main entrance to the general laboratory area to limit the amount of traffic.

An enclosed room provides greater safety than an open one in the event of accident with aerosolizable materials, and it is strongly recommended that another enclosed room be available within the laboratory for handling more highly infectious materials. This space will usually be devoted to mycology and mycobacteriology, but it should be accessible to other sections of the laboratory and available for their use. It should be equipped with a biologic safety cabinet.

The following functions in a microbiology laboratory should be considered:

1. Specimen handling, including initial culturing and subculturing.
2. Isolation facilities
3. Staining and microscopy
4. Media preparation
5. Fluorescent microscopy
6. Instrumentation
7. Disposal of contaminated items

Specimen Handling. This includes the receiving area for specimens, as well as the area where initial inoculation procedures are performed and subsequent identification and antimicrobial susceptibility testing is carried out. This type of work is best performed at "sit down" benches where tedious hand work can be done in greater comfort. If standing-height benches must be used, appropriate stools with footrests are necessary. Benches must contain drawers for storage. It is extremely important to provide each technologist in the bacteriology laboratory with an adequate amount of bench top area. Petri dishes, racks of tubes, worksheets, and report forms require considerable space. The technologist must have these items at hand and still have space to carry out necessary manipulations. At least four linear feet of bench top should be provided for each bacteriologic work station. Refrigerators and incubation facilities should be close at hand. These may be the "walk in" type in larger laboratories or of the "reach in" type. Gas outlets are necessary for each work station. Space must be available for tanks of gas for the CO_2 incubator or anaerobic chamber or glove box. Air and vacuum sources, although convenient, are not necessary at every work station.

Isolation Facilities. This area should be completely enclosed and away from the work flow of the remainder of the laboratory. It should be independent of the other work areas so that infectious materials can be brought in and confined. Ventilation should be such that the room is at a negative pressure relative to the rest of the laboratory. Equipment should include a biologic safety cabinet with proper filtration and exhaust. Gas, water, electrical outlets, and vacuum should be available.

Staining and Microscopy. Microscopic work is tedious and technologist comfort is important. Benches should be of the sit-down type and provide ample surface area for microscopes, lamps, slide trays, writing materials, and accessories for microscopy. Adequate space and drawers or overhead shelves must be provided for storage of supplies. Gas and electricity are required. The staining sink should be conveniently located and equipped with a staining rack and tap that can accommodate a length of tubing for use in rinsing slides. A vacuum breaker is required over all taps where the water source can be extended below the overflow point of the sink, as in this case.

Media Preparation. Several points must be considered in planning this area: (1) storage of materials, (2) preparation of media, (3) sterilization, (4) storage and/or transport of media, and (5) quality control. The area must be as free from traffic flow as possible and at the same time be located near the point of media usage, as well as glass washing and sterilization. In this area stand-up benches are preferred. If the media preparation laboratory is located remotely from the point of media usage, space and facilities must be provided for packaging the final product, for refrigerated storage and/or transport. Adequate storage of finished media must be provided to quarantine newly manufactured media until it has been appropriately quality controlled and declared ready for use. Leg room at standing benches is not required and these benches should be used to the fullest for storage. Autoclaves and hot air ovens must be nearby. Ventilation and heat and humidity control are extremely important in these areas. This laboratory should be provided with full bench util-

ities: at least one sink (preferably double), gas, electricity, vacuum, and air outlets. Distilled water in large volume is required either by piping in distilled water or by providing a still on site. If water is piped in, additional demineralization may be required if the central distilled water is not of sufficient purity. Appropriate refrigerated storage is required. Carts for transportation of media and supplies must be provided and space must be available for their use and storage.

Fluorescent Microscopy. In addition to the requirements for microscopy, this area must be enclosed and completely free of light. If preparative procedures are also to be carried out in this area, there should be standing benches, a sink, storage areas, refrigeration, and incubation facilities. Gas and electric outlets are necessary.

Instrumentation. New instruments are becoming available or are under development for use in microbiology; some thought should be given to providing space for future equipment. Factors to be considered are the bench top space required, floor space for free-standing components (e.g., teleprinters), power requirements (e.g., voltage and current stability for computers), and integration with work flow. Some of these instruments include (1) bacterial detection devices, radiometric or impedance, (2) turbidity measuring equipment for dilution and standardization, (3) colony counting apparatus, (4) antimicrobial susceptibility testing devices, e.g., nephelometric, turbidometric, microdilution, (5) gas chromotography, and (6) automated identification systems.

Disposal of Contaminated Materials. All contaminated materials must be disposed of in a manner that prevents dissemination of microorganisms. This is best accomplished by providing adequate autoclaving facilities within or very close to the laboratory. This area should be small and easily cleaned and disinfected. Garbage cans with autoclavable plastic bag liners should be provided for disposal of Petri dishes and other disposable contaminated items. Reusable materials are placed in pans or other containers for disinfection as discarded. These should be autoclaved before washing. Disposables in plastic bags may be autoclaved or incinerated in an incinerator approved for disposal of microbiologic wastes. The disposal area should be isolated from the general laboratory work flow.

5

EQUIPMENT

The microbiology laboratory has not yet achieved the degree of sophistication in automated or semiautomated equipment that has been witnessed in clinical chemistry or hematology laboratories. Nevertheless, a number of items of electrical, mechanical, and optical equipment are required for the laboratory to function efficiently. In large part, the amount and complexity of this equipment will be dependent upon the size and range of services offered by the laboratory. Much microbiology laboratory equipment is concerned with maintaining optimal environmental conditions for the growth or maintenance of microorganisms. This includes temperature- and atmosphere-controlled devices. Several semiautomated devices have appeared and are now being sold for use in microbiology laboratories. These include instruments for performing antimicrobial susceptibility tests (e.g., Autobac 1, Pfizer Diagnostics), for monitoring cultures of blood (e.g., BACTEC, Johnston Laboratories, Inc.) and a variety of devices for partially automating various processes in media preparation and distribution. Several additional instruments are currently under development, and within the next five years microbiology should begin to experience a phase of rapid growth in the application of automation or mechanization to bacterial isolation and identification.

The following is a brief description of the essential items of equipment which should be found in nearly all clinical microbiology laboratories, regardless of size. Descriptions of currently available apparatus for semiautomated antimicrobial susceptibility testing will be found in Chapter 55.

MICROSCOPES

The compound binocular microscope is an essential piece of apparatus in every microbiology laboratory. However, for routine use in the examination of Gram's stained smears, wet mounts, and similar microbiologic preparations, an elaborate and expensive instrument is not required. The basic microscope should have the following features: low power (10×, 16 mm), high dry (45×, 4 mm), and oil immersion (95×, 1.9 mm) achromatic objectives; a pair of 8× or 10× wide field and high eye point (for those who wear eye glasses) oculars; a mechanical stage; achromatic condenser with substage rack and pinion with condenser centering screws; and a good light

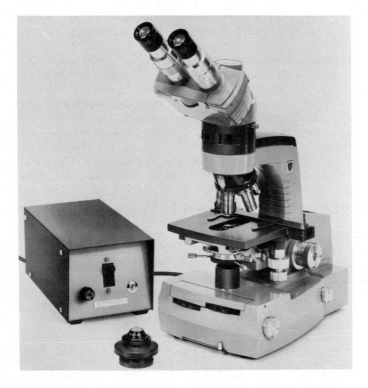

Figure 46–1. Fluorescence microscope with power supply. (Courtesy of American Optical Co., Buffalo, New York.)

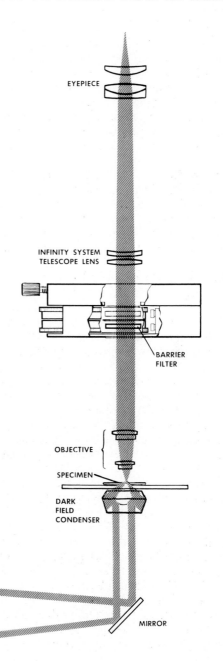

source, either internal or external. It is desirable to have at least one microscope in the laboratory equipped with a dual viewing head so that two observers can be accommodated simultaneously. This is particularly important in teaching situations and when consulting with clinicians. The "routine" microscope is probably the most abused piece of equipment in any laboratory. It is essential that all users be familiar with the mechanical and optical principles and also with the routine cleaning and maintenance procedures required. All microscope manufacturers provide detailed instructions in the operator's manual.

For darkfield microscopy, the basic microscope can be fitted with a darkfield condenser and, if oil immersion examinations are to be made, a funnel stop for the oil immersion objective. For most routine purposes the funnel stop is adequate and a special objective with an adjustable diaphragm is not required.

Although many observations of colonial morphology can be made with a simple or compound hand lens, a low power dissecting or stereoscopic microscope is useful when examining very small colonies and doing subcultures. An instrument that can be illuminated from above and/or below is desirable. Paired 10× oculars and objectives to yield an image of magnification from 10× to 30× are satisfactory.

Attachments are available that will convert the routine light microscope for use with phase or fluorescence microscopy. A special condenser and phase objectives are necessary for phase microscopy, and filter systems, a darkfield condenser, and ultraviolet light source for fluorescence microscopy. If either of these systems of microscopy is used, it is recommended that a microscope be dedicated to this work to avoid the problems of set up, alignment, and adjustment associated with frequent conversion.

For fluorescent antibody work, the standard microscope equipped with glass optics is generally satisfactory (Fig. 46-1). The microscope should be equipped with a darkfield condenser (Fig. 46-2). If one expects to deal with weakly fluorescing materials, a monocular head is preferred over a binocular head. Appropriate exciter and barrier filters are accommodated below the condenser and in the oculars. The

Figure 46-2. Path of light in fluorescence microscopy. (Courtesy of American Optical Company, Buffalo, New York.)

ultraviolet light source is usually a high pressure mercury arc lamp, such as the Osram HBO-200.* Lower power mercury arcs are also available, as are halogen quartz lamps. Care should be taken to assure that these lower output lamps will provide sufficient ultraviolet light for the type of studies to be carried out. Special exciter filters and barrier filters may be required.

INCUBATORS

Maintenance of a constant temperature environment is necessary for optimum bacterial growth. Incubators vary widely in size from small desk or shelf models to large walk-in units. Incubator types include gravity convection, forced air, carbon dioxide, and anaerobic. Although most incubators are electrically heated, gas or oil can be alternative sources of energy.

When purchasing an incubator, several items in the specifications in addition to capacity should be considered. These include temperature range, temperature sensitivity (e.g., maximum deviation from a mean equilibrium temperature), temperature uniformity (e.g., average deviation from the mean of temperatures taken at many locations within the incubator chamber), and recovery time. Most incubator manufacturers provide these figures in their catalogs. In general, larger incubators show smaller temperature fluctuations when the door is opened; therefore, the largest model that can be accommodated is preferred. Water-jacketed incubators provide for more closely controlled temperature sensitivity and uniformity because heat is radiated from at least five walls of the unit rather than from a heating element in the bottom of the unit as in the gravity convection type. Uniformity and sensitivity are improved in forced air incubators where a fan or blower circulates the warm air. One should be aware that forced air units may exert an extra dehydrating effect on the contents of the incubator, and special attention should be given to providing adequate humidification. For general bacteriologic purposes, incubators can be set between 35 and 37°C. Most clinically important bacteria grow as well at 35°C. as at 37°C.; therefore, many laboratories set the temperature at this point. A rise of 2 to 3 degrees from 35°C. is tolerable, whereas this same increase from

*Available from Scientific Products, McGaw Park, Illinois.

37°C. can be deleterious to some organisms. The temperature sensitivity for routine use can be ±1°C. Humidification of incubators is frequently neglected; adequate amounts of water should be maintained in humidification pans. The relative humidity when monitored should be 40 to 70 per cent.

Temperatures other than 35°C. may be required. For example, 42 to 45°C. is helpful for determining growth characteristics of certain mycobacteria and streptococci and 30°C. for growth of leptospirae and fungi. When 22°C. incubation ("room temperature") is required, a special incubator incorporating cooling and heating elements is needed. This usually has a temperature range from 10°C. to 50°C.

So-called anaerobic incubators will generally reduce and maintain oxygen and free air to approximately 1.5 per cent. This is not adequate for the growth of clinically important anaerobes. Chambers designed specifically for anaerobic work should be used. Many are large enough to accommodate a small standard incubator inside. Alternatively, the entire chamber can be heated with a thermostatically controlled heater, although temperature fluctuations and uniformity will not be as satisfactory as with a standard incubator.

Certain safety features may be included with some incubators; these include recording thermometers and thermostatically controlled safety switches with alarms that will cut off electricity to the heating elements if the interior rises above a preset level.

WATERBATHS

The temperature of the contents of test tubes or flasks placed in a waterbath will reach the desired temperature more rapidly than if placed in an incubator. These units are, therefore, useful for short-term incubation, such as preparing cultures of organisms to be tested for antimicrobial susceptibility. All waterbaths are equipped with thermostatic controls which can maintain the temperature to within ±0.5°C. of the desired value. To improve temperature uniformity throughout the bath, stirrers or other circulators may be included. Lids should be used to prevent excessive heat loss and evaporation. Distilled or deionized water must be used routinely to avoid mineral deposits on the interior walls and racks.

If care is not taken to change the water and clean the interior frequently, waterbaths can become the source for contamination in the laboratory. Many *Pseudomonas* species can be cultured from waterbaths not subjected to a regular cleaning schedule.

To avoid some of the problems inherent in immersing tubes in a liquid bath, a number of dry block heaters (e.g., Marsters incubator, Clay Adams) are available. These can be obtained with blocks that accommodate a variety of tube sizes, and temperatures can be set as close as $\pm 0.1°$C. over a range from ambient temperature to 125°C. Although these units may be more convenient in many applications, they lack the versatility of a waterbath in accommodating odd-shaped or oversized vessels.

REFRIGERATORS AND FREEZERS

The temperature requirements for storage of perishable media, reagents, antisera, antibiotic discs, stock solutions, and some stock cultures demand a variety of refrigeration equipment. The small laboratory may find a good quality household refrigerator with deep freezing compartment satisfactory, but in general it is recommended that separate units be purchased.

Refrigerators vary in size from compact desktop or under-the-counter models to large walk-in units. The former are convenient for use in specimen receiving and initial processing areas. Specimens can be delivered directly to the refrigerator and then removed by the technologist when he or she is ready to initiate processing.

Ordinary household refrigerators or freezers should never be used for storage of combustible, volatile materials such as ether. If these substances are to be stored at reduced temperatures, special explosion-proof units must be used. These are specially constructed so that there are no interior wiring components, no metal-to-metal contacts anywhere in the chamber, and thermostats, switches, relays, and compressors are totally enclosed. These units are usually approved by Underwriters Laboratories or a similar agency as meeting OSHA requirements for safe storage of highly volatile materials. Failure to observe this precaution can result in serious injury and property damage.

Care should be taken when selecting a self-defrosting refrigerator or freezer. Some materials that require frozen storage have melting points in the range of $-10°$ to $-5°$C.

During the defrost cycle these units may have temperature fluctuations which cause these materials to thaw. This is particularly true when very small volumes of the material are involved, such as in the case of microdilution antimicrobial susceptibility testing materials. Here, 0.1 ml of dilute antimicrobial agents is distributed in the wells of a microdilution tray; these agents may be thus subjected to repeated freeze-thaw cycles which will promote their deterioration. A consistent temperature below $-15°$C. is required. For laboratory purposes, freezers or freezing compartments in refrigerators should be capable of operation at temperatures between $-15°$ and $-25°$C.

For storage of materials or specimens that require temperatures less than $-25°$C., mechanical ultra low temperature freezers are required. These specially constructed and designed units are available in either chest or upright models. Upright units usually have a series of separate smaller interior compartments, each with a door closed to minimize temperature fluctuation when the main door is opened. Chest type units with top opening doors are not as subject to this problem. The temperature range of ultra freezers generally extends to $-70°$C. and in some models to as low as $-100°$C.

There are two alternatives to the mechanical ultra low temperature freezer, the dry ice chest and the liquid nitrogen refrigerator. Both of these units are independent of the electrical mains and thus not subject to power or mechanical failure. However, they require a reliable and constant supply of dry ice or liquid nitrogen. Dry ice chests can accommodate nearly every type of material that can be stored in the ultra low temperature freezer. The liquid nitrogen refrigerator can usually handle materials that can be stored in small cryogenic vials. Liquid nitrogen storage of important stock cultures is convenient; a 30-liter tank requires refilling approximately once every 1 to 3 weeks depending on the number of times the unit is opened.

Refrigerator and freezer temperatures should be monitored at least daily. Ultra low temperature freezers usually are equipped with continuous temperature chart recorders. All refrigerators or freezers containing materials that would constitute a serious loss in the event of a power failure should be equipped with an alarm, preferably wired to sound in a location where a fully instructed and responsible staff is present 24 hours a day (e.g., security office, power house, etc.), as well as in the laboratory. If this is not possible, then security guards should be alerted to respond to such alarms when making rounds at night. Full instructions for action to be taken in the event of an alarm should be posted on the equipment itself.

AUTOCLAVES

Moist heat in the form of steam is the most frequently used method of sterilization in the clinical microbiology laboratory. Steam is used under increased pressure, at ambient atmospheric pressure (tyndallization with flowing steam), or under pressure mixed with air (inspissation). All these processes can be carried out in an autoclave, although laboratories producing large volumes of media requiring inspissation will use equipment specifically designed for this purpose.

Autoclaves are available in a variety of sizes and styles with horizontal or vertical chambers, manual or automatic controls, jacketed or unjacketed, and with or without self-contained steam generators. Although autoclaves with completely automatic controls are convenient, they are considerably more expensive ($2000 to $4000) than manually operated models. Operator attention throughout the entire sterilization cycle is required if manual controls are selected. Rectangular chambers allow a more efficient utilization of the available space, but care must be taken not to overload the autoclave. This may disturb the flow of steam or impede the discharge of air. Autoclaves should be equipped with a pressure gauge, preferably with a chart recorder. Steam jacketed gravity displacement autoclaves must be equipped with a thermometer (or automatic control) in the exhaust line.

It is extremely important that all air be exhausted from the autoclave chamber by the flowing steam. In the presence of air, a lower temperature will result at a given pressure. Air can also settle to the bottom of the chamber, further contributing to an irregular distribution of the internal temperature. Therefore, it is essential that all air be discharged and the exhaust valve be closed only when the exhaust temperature reaches 121°C. and the temperature of steam is at 15 pounds per square inch pressure. Timing of sterilization normally begins at this point.

Operators must be thoroughly familiar with the specific autoclave being used. Manufactur-

ers give detailed instructions for the use of their equipment and these should be rigidly followed. The efficiency of sterilization should be monitored by the use of biologic indicators as described in Chapter 56 (p. 1941).

CENTRIFUGES

Two general types of centrifuges are available, angle head and horizontal head (Chap. 3). In the angle head, tubes are held in a fixed position at an angle of 30 to 50°. The horizontal head has cups held by trunnion rings. The cups and their contents assume a horizontal position as the head is rotated. The angle centrifuge can attain a greater rotational speed, but sediments are deposited near the side of the tube. Larger units of either type have changeable heads and/or cups to accommodate a variety of containers. For microbiologic work, it is important that centrifuges used with materials containing pathogenic organisms be equipped with aerosol-free sealed cups.

Centrifuges must be properly balanced before starting. Cups and trunnion rings are sold in balanced sets, usually with the weight marked. Marking matched sets with distinctive colors will aid operators in properly setting up the centrifuge for a run. Lack of attention to balancing will lead to tube breakage as well as serious damage to the centrifuge.

In most laboratories a small table-top centrifuge accommodating 10 to 12 15-ml tubes, and a larger floor model taking tubes or bottles with 50-ml capacity, should be adequate.

Many procedures specify the centrifugal force required. Each laboratory centrifuge should be calibrated so that these forces can be reproducibly obtained. Facilities should be available for determining the number of revolutions per minute (rpm) developed at various speed control settings. Some larger centrifuges are or may be equipped with direct reading tachometers for this purpose. Various portable tachometers are also available (Chap. 3). Some of these must be used with the centrifuge lid open; this is a source of danger to the operator and special care must be taken. In addition, speeds may be different between lid-up and lid-down conditions. Tachometers that can be used with closed lids are preferred.

The relative centrifugal force (RCF) or g is expressed by the following formula: $RCF(g) = 1.118 \times 10^{-5} \times R \times N^2$, where R is the rotational radius (distance in cm from the center of the centrifuge axis to the end of the centrifuge tube) and N is the rotational speed (rpm). At least 3000 RCF(g) is required to sediment bacteria within a reasonable time period, depending on the suspending medium and its cellular content. A force of 10,000 RCF(g) is required to sediment haemophili in 10 minutes.

MICROBIOLOGIC SAFETY CABINETS

Microbiologic procedures with mycobacteria must be carried out in an appropriate microbiologic safety cabinet. It should also be used for any other work which involves airborne infectious material, e.g., *Brucella, Francisella tularensis*, Q fever, respiratory viruses, or arboviruses. It is highly desirable to conduct all initial processing of clinical specimens in a safety cabinet, since at this point the least is known of the bacterial content of the specimen. Any procedure that may involve the generation of aerosols of infected materials (e.g., tissue grinding) should be carried out in the safety cabinet.

For most clinical laboratory purposes a class II open-fronted or "half barrier" cabinet is adequate. A class III enclosed or "full barrier" cabinet equipped with gloves is recommended for handling extremely hazardous materials or when performing procedures that may create aerosols.

Modern safety cabinets in general utilize vertical laminar air flow designs and provide a highly protective air curtain across the open face of the hood. This in turn permits a high face velocity or rate of air flow through the working face of the cabinet from the outside room air. In some models the face velocity is as much as 170 and 200 feet per minute. The exhaust system is equipped with either a high efficiency particulate air (HEPA) filter or an incinerator unit. The simplest is the HEPA filter. This provides 99.9 per cent filtration of particles 0.30 μ or larger. The exhaust from a properly designed HEPA filter system may be safely discharged into the room or discharge duct system. Consult the manufacturer of the cabinet to be installed regarding specific venting requirements. The average useful life expectancy of HEPA filters in continuous use is two to three years. When filters are changed, the cleaning and disinfection procedures recommended by the cabinet's manufacturer must be carefully followed.

Horizontal laminar air flow cabinets with open faces are designed for maintaining the sterility of the working field and offer no protection to the operator. These are suitable for handling tissue cultures, sterile product preparations, and sterility testing procedures, and for subculturing blood cultures in the routine clinical laboratory.

EQUIPMENT MAINTENANCE

Every component of every instrument or piece of equipment deteriorates with use; therefore, complete quality control in any laboratory must include a regular preventive maintenance program. A written procedure based on the equipment manufacturer's recommendations must be set up for each item, and each maintenance or function check, defects detected, and corrective measures taken must be recorded, dated, and initialed. For convenience in recording observations, a maintenance manual should be attached to or located near the specific item of equipment.

The following are examples of maintenance procedures adapted from the Standards for Accreditation of the College of American Pathologists (1974) for equipment in the microbiology laboratory. These and other appropriate procedures as recommended by the equipment manufacturer should be carried out according to a regularly scheduled program.

Balances. All balances, but particularly analytical balances, must be protected against temperature variation, vibration, and humidity. Knife edges must be smooth and pans scrupulously clean. National Bureau of Standards Class S weights should be used to check the accuracy of analytical balances periodically.

pH Meter. A manual describing the proper handling and care of electrodes and preparation, standardization, and operation of the pH meter must be readily available at the bench. Individuals using this equipment must be familiar with the maintenance of electrodes and proper preparation of buffers for calibration. The operator must be constantly alert for deviation from linearity owing to amplifier failure.

Automated Equipment. Automated equipment must be maintained according to the manufacturer's instructions and recommendations. These must be dated, initialed, and maintenance records kept on file to verify constant surveillance.

Centrifuges. Each centrifuge must be kept in proper mechanical condition by regular lubrication, changing of brakes and brushes, and detection and replacement of worn bearings. Instructions should be posted at each centrifuge specifying the proper method of balancing and appropriate speed. A tachometer should be available and the actual revolutions per minute at each setting determined initially and verified frequently.

Incubators. Incubators of acceptable quality and adequate capacity must be used. The temperature of operation must be checked and recorded daily. Incubators should be kept clean and uncluttered. Servicing of circulating fans, temperature, humidity, and CO_2 controls should be included in maintenance procedures. Maintenance records of incubators in microbiology should include evidence of surveillance for contamination and should specify the frequency and nature of decontamination procedures.

Autoclaves. Autoclaves must have accurate temperature and pressure gauges for control of sterilization procedures. Records should verify the operating efficiency of autoclaves as checked by biologic controls and heat-sensitive indicator methods.

Waterbaths and Dry Heat Blocks. Water baths and dry heat blocks must be kept scrupulously clean and must have an accurate thermometer to monitor temperature range and stability. Thermometers in dry heat blocks should be immersed in a non-volatile liquid.

Refrigerators. All refrigerators must be maintained in proper working order with regular inspection and maintenance schedules for compressor and fan. The temperature should be determined daily to confirm proper operating conditions. If cultures or specimens for culture are stored in a refrigerator, there should be specified procedures for periodic documentation. The storage of food and other extraneous items in laboratory refrigerators is not condoned.

Hot Air Ovens. Hot air ovens must be kept clean and in good operating condition. Operating temperatures of ovens should be checked periodically to confirm the adequacy of automatic thermostatic control.

Microscopes. Microscopes must be clean. Objectives and oculars should be protected against scratching, etching, and cracking. Solvents should be applied to objectives sparingly and with caution. Mechanical stages should be properly adjusted and lubricated. Condensers should be easily adjusted, free from scratches, and clean. Light sources must be of sufficient intensity to provide adequate, adjustable illumination. Cleaning and maintenance of special types of microscopes should be performed regularly according to manufacturer's instructions. Complete dismantling and cleaning of microscopes is usually beyond the capability of hospital maintenance personnel, and yearly maintenance should be arranged with one of many companies specializing in this service.

MATERIALS

CULTURE MEDIA

Choice of Media. One of the problems in all laboratories is the choice of media for particular purposes. Practically, it is desirable to limit the number of media and to choose those that offer the greatest usefulness. Once media are chosen, it is important that the technologist become thoroughly familiar with each. This is best accomplished by constant use and careful observation. Changes in media should be made when improved formulas become available, but should be done with care. Cultures on the new medium should be run alongside the old for a time to decide whether the new medium offers advantages.

Media may be divided into the following categories: isolation media, enrichment media, maintenance media, identifying or differentiating media (such as carbohydrate fermentation, hemolysis, or indole production), and media for storage of microorganisms.

Isolation media are used to streak out specimens, such as urine or feces. They may be used for general isolation or for the selective isolation of a particular organism or group of organisms. To be used for general isolation, a medium must be capable of supporting a large variety of pathogenic and non-pathogenic bacteria. Blood and chocolate agar are such media widely used in routine isolation work. Special media are designed for isolation of certain bacteria when their presence is suspected; they may be used by larger laboratories, but for most laboratories blood and chocolate agar, used either under ambient atmospheric conditions or in the CO_2 jar or incubator, should serve very well. These general isolation media are satisfactory with such specimens as spinal fluid, urine, and throat swabs in which the number of types of bacteria is not excessive, but when one deals with fecal cultures, it becomes necessary to use selective media.

Selective media incorporate substances inhibitory to propagation of one group of bacteria but allow other groups to grow. Thus, for enteric culture, media routinely used contain certain dyes and other ingredients, which inhibit gram-positive organisms and allow the gram-negative enteric bacilli to propagate. If, on the other hand, one wishes to isolate staphylococci in enteric work, one can incorporate substances, such as phenylethyl alcohol or certain antibiotics in blood agar, which inhibit the gram-negative bacilli.

Enrichment media may be used to good advantage, particularly in enteric cultures. Such media are designed to enhance the propagation of certain organisms without favoring others. They are routinely used in the isolation of *Salmonella* from feces.

Identification media are of various types and range from the fluid base with specific carbohydrates added, through semisolid motility media and urea media for aid in identifying members of the genus *Proteus*, to the more complex media, such as triple sugar iron or lysine iron agar medium, for aid in differentiation among the Enterobacteriaceae.

Maintenance media may be of various types. Infusion broth is satisfactory for many of the less fastidious organisms, as are infusion agar slants or semisolid preparations. For some organisms one needs an enriched medium, and blood or chocolate agar slants can be used. Certain organisms, e.g., *Streptococcus pneumoniae*, produce considerable amounts of acid from dextrose and tend to autolyze. In these cases a medium with only a little fermentable carbohydrate is advisable, or the culture may be lost. In general, cultures are best maintained by lyophilization, freezing at $-70°C.$, or storage in liquid nitrogen.

Aside from these general statements, the experienced bacteriologist must be guided in the choice of media for use in any instance by the type of specimen, the nature of the suspected clinical condition, and the results of a preliminary examination of the specimen, such as a Gram's stain.

Subsequent chapters will deal with the specifics of specimen collection, initial processing, and methods of cultivation of various microorganisms.

Preparation of Media. The preparation of bacteriologic culture media has undergone a dramatic change in the last 10 to 15 years. In the past, laboratories prepared all their own culture media, normally from the basic ingredients or from commercially available dehydrated materials. Now, many of these laboratories purchase ready-to-use commercially prepared media. The choice of preparing media in-house or purchasing prepared media or a combination of both must be made. Factors that need to be considered include availability of space, personnel, and equipment, volume and variety of media required, availability and usefulness of commercial identification kits (e.g., API-20E Analytab Products Inc.; Enterotube, Roche Diagnostics; r/b system, Corning Diagnostics; etc.).

The responsibility for quality control of prepared media is shared to a great extent with the manufacturer. This, however, does not relieve the users of all responsibility for quality control; sterility testing, as well as performance testing, should be carried out in the laboratory to verify that the media perform as intended, especially after prolonged transportation and storage. When the laboratory makes its own media, it assumes full responsibility for its performance and must pay careful attention to the quality of the basic ingredients, correct formulation of the media, accuracy in preparation, adequate sterilization, proper packaging, and protection from contamination, dehydration, or excess moisture during storage. Whether in-house prepared media will be of higher quality than that produced commercially will depend greatly on the laboratory's ability to adhere to these basic principles.

The principles of preparing, dispensing, and sterilizing media are essentially the same, whether one uses the dehydrated form or starts from the beginning and adds the various ingredients separately. All the basic media contain a peptone and certain salts to which may be added growth-promoting substances or agar, depending on the need. Since numerous peptones of superior quality are now available commercially, it is no longer necessary to prepare infusions and extracts.

A number of variables enter into the preparation of microbiologic culture media from dehydrated materials. If these are not rigidly controlled, the finished product will not be likely to give satisfactory performance. Careful consideration of and adherence to the principles outlined here will be of great assistance to any laboratory choosing to enter into or continue media manufacture in house. Powers (1975) lists the following factors that may contribute to unsatisfactory media.

5

1. Incorrect weighing of dry material through human error or the use of a faulty balance.

2. Use of dry material taken from previously opened bottles which may have deteriorated from exposure to heat, moisture, oxidation, or other environmental factors.

3. Incorrect measurement of water, or the use of tap water or water from a malfunctioning still or deionizing resin column. Water should generally meet the requirements of the United States Pharmacopeia (USP) for purified water or be of proven microbiologic quality.

4. Use of unclean containers or glassware, especially those contaminated with detergent or other chemicals. The use of metal containers other than stainless steel (e.g., copper or zinc) must not be employed, since these may contaminate media with bactericidal substances.

5. Incomplete mixing or incomplete solution resulting in failure to prepare a homogeneous medium. This may produce stiff medium in some plates and soft medium in others.

6. Overheating occurring during preparation and sterilization or resulting from being held too long in the molten state before dispensing into plates, tubes, or bottles. This can result in loss of productivity through hydrolysis of agar, caramelization of carbohydrates, lowering of pH, increase in inhibitory action, loss of dye content in selective or differential media, and formation of precipitates. Generally, tubed media not containing heat-labile or heat-coagulable ingredients may be melted once.

7. Improper determination of pH resulting in the addition of too much acid or alkali. The pH of a medium should be determined when the medium has cooled to room temperature. The pH meter electrodes should be in contact with the solidified agar medium, which may be removed from the plate or tube, placed in a beaker, and macerated. Additional water should not be added. Surface electrodes are available for some models of pH meters. These can be used to determine the pH for the contact surface of plated media and may more accurately reflect the conditions to be encountered by bacteria inoculated on that surface.

8. Improper addition or incorporation of unsatisfactory supplements or enrichments, such as contaminated blood, etc., or addition of supplements at the wrong temperature, possibly causing alteration of the supplements if the temperature is too high or gelation of media before proper mixing if too cold.

9. Failure of the laboratory to subject samples of the finished media to quality control procedures with stabilized cultures before the media are used.

Sterilization of Media. Sterilization of most bacteriologic culture media can be accomplished by autoclaving at 121°C. for 15 minutes. For volumes larger than 500 ml, 20 to 30 minutes or more may be required. If the autoclave chamber is overloaded, sterilization may not take place. There must be sufficient space for the steam to circulate freely about the material being sterilized. Test tubes should be standing in racks with screw caps loosened.

Some media require different pressures for various lengths of time. It is important that media not be over-sterilized and thus exposed to prolonged heating. Media containing heat-stable carbohydrates are best autoclaved at temperatures not exceeding 116° to 118°C. Heat-labile carbohydrates should preferably be sterilized by filtration and added aseptically to the autoclaved, cooled basal medium. When the sterilization time is up, the steam supply should be shut off and the pressure allowed to drop slowly. The media are removed when the chamber temperature has dropped to 80°C. and the pressure is equal to that outside.

For media that cannot tolerate temperatures above 100°C., two alternative methods of heat sterilization may be used, flowing steam and inspissation. For example, selenite F broth should not be autoclaved, but tubes should be exposed to flowing steam for 30 minutes. This method of sterilization is accomplished in the autoclave by introducing steam into the chamber with the exhaust valve left open. Sometimes, with a manually controlled autoclave, the incoming steam pressure is so high that pressure builds up with a resultant rise in temperature above 100°C. In that case the autoclave door can be left ajar, or the steam supply can be turned down. The manufacturer's specific instructions must be followed. To insure that spores are killed, the technique of tyndallization or fractional sterilization should be followed. The medium is exposed to flowing steam for 30 minutes on each of three successive days. Between these periods the medium is kept at room temperature to allow spores that were not killed to germinate. The resulting vegetative cells are then killed by the subsequent flowing steam exposures.

Media containing coagulable protein, such as egg or serum, must be sterilized by inspissation. In this process, air is deliberately not exhausted from the autoclave chamber; this results in a temperature at 15 pounds pressure that ranges from 75 to 85°C. Again, the autoclave manufacturer's instructions must be followed in setting up the autoclave for this method. If the laboratory produces its own egg-containing media in large volumes, an inspissator designed for this purpose should be obtained.

Sterilization by means of a filter should be used for those media or additives which will be adversely affected by the heat produced by any of the previously mentioned sterilization methods or if the flowing steam or inspissation methods cannot be accomplished with the existing autoclave. These include ascitic fluid, blood serum, certain carbohydrates, and urea. The most commonly used filters are the Seitz* and the membrane filters (Millipore Corporation or Gelman Company). The membrane filter is preferable to the Seitz filter because it is less absorptive. A full line of filter sterilizing accessories is distributed by the membrane filter manufacturers for use with their products. Of particular convenience to the small laboratory is the Swinnex (Millipore Corporation) filter holder. This is attached to any syringe with Luer fittings and is useful in sterilizing small volumes of solutions, reagents, or media. These units are available assembled, prepackaged, sterile, and disposable after use, or can be obtained as reusable units. The material to be sterilized is drawn into the syringe, a sterile Swinnex filter unit installed, a sterile needle attached to the output end of the filter, and the material forced through the filter by pressure on the syringe plunger. Membrane filters may be used as obtained from the manufacturer for bacteriologic purposes. However, these filters may contain up to 2 to 3 per cent of their dry weight as detergents. This may have an adverse effect on tissue culture media. For such work membrane filters should be washed prior to use, or detergent-free filters should be obtained from the manufacturer.

Dispensing Media. The methods of dispensing the dissolved and/or sterilized media into tubes or flasks depends on the type of medium and the purpose for which it is to be used. Fluid media (e.g., infusion broth) may be pipetted into tubes before sterilization by

*Available from Scientific Products, McGaw Park, Illinois.

using a serologic pipette or an automatic pipette calibrated to deliver the desired amount. It is not necessary to use sterile tubes for this purpose, although at times this has considerable advantage, especially in handling material that needs to be inspissated. One may use specially constructed flasks with delivery tubes at the bottom to which is attached a standard glass filling device.

Media containing sufficient agar to be solid on cooling (1.5 per cent or more) are used ordinarily for agar slants or Petri dishes. For slants the medium is dispensed into test tubes, autoclaved in the vertical position, and then cooled in a slanted position. The amount of medium per tube is determined by the length of slant and butt desired. To pour Petri plates, the agar medium must first be sterilized in flasks or tubes and then poured to a depth of about 3 mm into sterile plates. The melted agar is cooled to 47 to 52°C. before pouring the plates to prevent condensation of moisture on the walls of the container. Semisolid media (0.1 to 0.5 per cent agar) are tubed and sterilized in the same manner as fluid media.

For carbohydrate fermentation tests, it is necessary to use a base medium free of carbohydrate to which the desired carbohydrate, such as dextrose or maltose, is then added to produce a 0.5 to 1.0 per cent concentration. It is convenient to add the desired carbohydrate aseptically (in a filtered 10 to 20 per cent solution) to a previously sterilized base medium. Such base media containing an indicator (bromthymol blue, bromcresol purple, or phenol red) are readily available. The indicator changes color when acid is produced by bacteria or fungi.

Sterile discs of dehydrated fermentation media are now available; when added aseptically to tubes with sterile distilled water, they provide a medium for fermentation tests. There are also discs containing various carbohydrates that may be added to a suitable base in the same manner or may be placed on agar plates. These materials seem ideally suited for use in smaller laboratories. When using these discs, the use of control organisms to demonstrate that appropriate reactions are produced is essential.

To detect gas production, one can place an inverted vial or Durham tube (3 by 20 mm) in the medium. When autoclaved, this vial fills with medium. Gas production is indicated when a bubble of gas appears in the vial after bacterial propagation. If one uses semisolid agar (0.3 to 0.5 per cent agar), the vial is unnecessary because gas production will be revealed by bubbles in the medium.

Preparation of Blood and Chocolate Agar. Media containing whole blood are the most commonly employed in the diagnostic laboratory. The type of blood, the agar base, and the technique of preparation are very important for the proper isolation of microorganisms.

There seems to be general agreement that defibrinated sheep blood is the most desirable for use in making blood and chocolate agar. The advantages of sheep blood are consistency in hemolysis with streptococci, staphylococci, *Listeria*, etc., and its ability to support propagation of a wide variety of organisms. Also, *Haemophilus haemolyticus*, the colonies of which resemble beta-hemolytic streptococci, is inhibited. Sheep or human blood should not be used in blood agar intended to demonstrate the characteristic hemolytic patterns of various *Haemophilus* species, since these bloods contain heat-labile inhibitors of *H. influenzae*.

The blood should not be more than a few days old and is preferably defibrinated. If the blood is too old, the red blood cells are likely to be fragile and may hemolyze, making the blood agar unsuitable for use. There are several good blood agar bases that can be obtained commercially.

To make blood agar, the sterile blood agar base contained in a flask is melted in a boiling water-bath and cooled to 47 to 52°C. Blood near the same temperature as the agar is then added to the melted agar (5 ml of blood per 100 ml of medium) and thoroughly mixed by rotating the flask. If a heated magnetic stirrer is available, cool blood from the refrigerator may be used. Place the magnetic stirring bar in the flask before autoclaving. After the basal medium is cooled to the proper temperature, place on the heating surface and start the stirrer. Distribute blood down the sides of the flask as usual. Do not overheat. After it is mixed, the agar is carefully poured into sterile Petri dishes to a depth of one-eighth to one-fourth inch. The depth to which the plate is poured is of considerable importance, since one is often interested in the presence or absence of hemolysis. If the agar is too thick, the hemolysis may be missed. Too vigorous shaking should be avoided, since air bubbles may make the agar rough. Air bubbles that do appear in the plates may be removed by passing a Bunsen flame quickly over the surface before the agar has set. Some workers prefer to place a layer of plain agar over the bottom of the plate and superimpose a thin layer of 10 per cent blood agar over this.

To make chocolate agar, the flask containing the medium with blood added is placed in a water bath at 80°C. and shaken gently until it has attained a definite chocolate color. This usually takes about 5 minutes. Excessive heating should be avoided. The agar should then be cooled to 47 to 52°C.; supplements such as IsoVitaleX* or various antibiotics,

---
*Bioquest, Cockeysville, Md.

such as bacitracin, are added, if desired, and poured into Petri dishes.

Blood and chocolate agar plates can be stored in the refrigerator for several days, but should not be used if there is evidence of excessive drying or if the blood has darkened or otherwise changed its appearance. A sample from each batch of blood and chocolate agar plates should be incubated overnight and checked for sterility before use.

Storage of Media. Prepared commercial media are packaged in a manner to maximize shelf life, and current FDA regulations require that an expiration date be included in the labeling. Plated media are sealed in airtight plastic sleeves and tubed media have tightly fitting screw caps. Storage time and temperatures recommended by the manufacturer should be followed.

Most media prepared in-house should be stored in the refrigerator to minimize dehydration and deterioration of labile components. Plates should be stored in sealed metal containers with tight-fitting lids or sealed in plastic bags. Under these conditions, plates can be stored for 3 to 4 weeks. If not so protected, plates should be kept under refrigeration for not more than two weeks. Tubed media with loose-fitting cotton plugs and metal or plastic enclosures should not be stored longer than two weeks even when refrigerated. If screw cap tubes are used, media can be stored under refrigeration, or, with some media, at room temperature for as much as six months. Tables 56-2 and 56-3 list storage conditions for a variety of plated and tubed media (p. 1947).

REAGENTS

Included in this category are chemical reagents, immunodiagnostic antisera and antigens, and reagent-impregnated paper discs or strips. Stains are covered separately. Except for certain chemical reagents and buffers prepared in the laboratory, most of these reagents will be obtained commercially ready for use.

Chemical Reagents. Chemicals must be purchased from reputable sources and be of approved quality. All bottles should be dated upon receipt and again when they are opened. Chemicals should be obtained in small quantities to assure freshness and stability. All reagents must be carefully prepared and their containers dated with the date of preparation and an expiration date. The initials of the person preparing the reagent should also be included. It is good practice to assign a lot number to each batch of reagent prepared and to record the lot or control numbers of all the chemical(s) used in the preparation of the reagent. This will facilitate trouble-shooting should problems arise. Most reagents can be stored in tightly closed opaque or amber bottles at room temperature. Some reagents, such as coagulase plasma and H_2O_2, must be stored in the refrigerator.

Reagent-impregnated Paper Discs and Strips. Discs and strips are stored in tightly sealed containers with a desiccant usually supplied by the manufacturer. The date of receipt and lot number should be noted on the label. Antimicrobial susceptibility testing discs, especially those of the penicillin family, should be stored at $-14°C.$ or less. Working supplies can be stored in the refrigerator at 2 to 8°C. Other discs and strips containing reagents such as bacitracin, optochin, or X and V factor for bacterial differentiation can be stored at 4 to 8°C. These reagents all have expiration dates included in their labeling. These dates should be adhered to rigidly.

Antisera. All antisera should be dated when received and when reconstituted. The labeled expiration date must be observed. Rehydration and storage conditions of the manufacturer must be followed. Each time an antiserum is used it should be visually inspected and discarded as unsatisfactory if turbidity or precipitate is seen.

TECHNIQUES

STAINS

The examination of specimens received in the microbiology laboratory involves two general types of procedure. First, they may be examined by direct smear, stained or unstained, and, second, they may be cultured on appropriate media.

When certain specimens are submitted for bacteriologic or mycologic examination, properly prepared and stained preparations may give excellent leads as to what media to inoculate or what further examination can be done. A preliminary report on such observations may, as in the case of spinal fluid, urethral smears, and sputum, be of great value to the physician in the management of the patient and/or interpretation of the culture results.

Clean slides must be used to make smears, and the slide must be marked adequately for identification and for delineation of the area in which the smear is to be placed. A slide may be divided into several sections with a marking pencil and several smears placed on the same slide, provided they are to be stained identically.

One or two inoculating loopfuls of the material to be smeared are spread evenly over the designated area of the slide and allowed to dry. The dried smear is then passed rapidly through a flame to heat-fix the material to the slide.

Several staining procedures are used in bacteriologic work, the most common and useful being Gram's stain or one of its many modifications. Loefflers' methylene blue, the acid-fast stain, spore stains, capsule stains, and flagella stains may be useful for special purposes. Organisms of known staining characteristics should be included as a staining control.

Gram's staining is most likely to yield valuable information and should be done in all cases when staining is indicated. It is also used routinely for the examination of cultures to determine purity, and for purposes of identification. Two of the best modifications of Gram's stain follow:

Hucker's modification of Gram's stain

Solutions
1. Ammonium oxalate crystal violet
   SOLUTION A

Crystal violet (certified)	2 g
Ethyl alcohol (95 per cent)	20 ml

   SOLUTION B

Ammonium oxalate	0.8 g
Distilled water	80 ml

Mix solution A and B, store for 24 hours and filter through paper.
2. Iodine solution (mordant)

Iodine	1 g
Potassium iodide	2 g
Distilled water	300 ml

Grind iodine and potassium iodide in mortar, adding water a few milliliters at a time until dissolved. Store in dark bottle.
3. Counterstain

Safranine 0 (2.5 per cent solution in 95 per cent ethyl alcohol)	10 ml
Distilled water	100 ml

Procedure. After the smear has been dried and heat-fixed, proceed as follows:
1. Stain smears 1 minute with the crystal violet solution.
2. Wash briefly in tap water.
3. Add iodine solution and let stand for 1 minute.
4. Wash in tap water.
5. Decolorize until the solvent flows colorlessly from the slide. Wash briefly with acetone, or a mixture of equal parts of acetone and alcohol.
6. Counterstain 10 seconds with safranine.
7. Wash in tap water.

Results. Gram-positive organisms stain blue; gram-negative, red.

Burke's modification

This modification of Gram's stain has the advantage that all solutions are aqueous and the decolorization is more vigorous, resulting in easier differentiation of the organisms in thick preparation.

Solutions

1. Alkaline crystal violet
SOLUTION A

Crystal violet	1	g
Distilled water	100	ml

SOLUTION B

NaHCO$_3$	5	g
Distilled water	100	ml

Add merthiolate (1:20,000)

2. Iodine solution

Iodine	1	g
KI (potassium iodide)	2	g
Distilled water	200	ml

3. Decolorizing solution

Ether	1 volume
Acetone	3 volumes

4. Counterstain

Safranine 0 (85 per cent dye content)	0.5	g
Distilled water	100	ml

Procedure

1. Flood slide with Solution A. Then add 3 to 5 drops of solution B, depending on the size of the flooded area, and allow to stand 1 minute. Wash well with water.
2. Cover with iodine solution and let stand 1 minute or longer.
3. Rinse with water.
4. Decolorize at once with the ether-acetone mixture, adding it to the slide drop by drop until no more color comes off in the drippings. Care must be taken to avoid excessive decolorization.
5. Wash with water.
6. Counterstain 10 to 15 seconds with the safranine 0.
7. Wash in tap water.
8. Dry and examine.

Results. Gram-positive organisms stain blue; gram-negative, red.

Acid-fast stain
(Ziehl-Neelsen for mycobacteria)

Solutions

CARBOL FUCHSIN STAIN

Basic fuchsin	0.3 g
Ethyl alcohol, 95 per cent	10.0 ml
Phenol, melted crystals	5.0 ml
Distilled water	95.0 ml

Dissolve the basic fuchsin in the alcohol; the phenol in the water. Mix the two solutions. Let stand for several days before use.

ACID ALCOHOL

Ethyl alcohol, 95 per cent	97 ml
Hydrochloric acid, concentrated	3 ml

METHYLENE BLUE COUNTERSTAIN

Methylene blue	0.3 g
Distilled water	100.0 ml

Procedure. Flood entire slide with carbolfuchsin and heat slowly to the steaming point. Use low or intermittent heat to maintain steaming for 3 to 5 minutes. Cool. Wash briefly with tap water and decolorize with acid alcohol until no more stain comes off. Wash with tap water and counterstain for 20 to 30 seconds. Wash, dry, and examine. Acid-fast organisms are red; the background and non-acid-fast organisms are blue.

Acid-fast stain (Truant's auramine-rhodamine stain for mycobacteria)

Solutions

SOLUTION A (FLUORESCENT DYES)

Auramine 0 Cl 41000	1.50 g
Rhodamine B Cl 479	0.75 g
Glycerol	75.00 ml
Phenol	10.00 ml
Distilled water	50.00 ml

Combine dyes with phenol and 25 ml of water and mix well. Add the remainder of the water and the glycerol, and mix well. Clarify by filtration through glass wool. The solution may be stored for several months at 4°C. or at room temperature.

SOLUTION B (DECOLORIZER)

Acid alcohol, 0.5 per cent HCl in 70 per cent ethyl alcohol

SOLUTION C (COUNTERSTAIN)

Potassium permanganate, 0.5 per cent aqueous solution

Procedure

1. Prepare slides and fix with heat.
2. Stain for 15 minutes at room temperature or at 37°C.
3. Rinse with distilled water.
4. Decolorize for 2 to 3 minutes; then rinse thoroughly with distilled water.
5. Flood smear with counterstain for 2 to 4 minutes. Longer exposure results in loss of brilliance. The "counterstain" renders tissue and debris nonfluorescent.
6. Rinse, dry, and examine.

Spore stain (Schaeffer and Fulton's method)

Malachite green (5 per cent) in distilled water. When freshly prepared allow to stand one-half hour and filter.
Safranine (0.5 per cent) in distilled water.
Flood the fixed smear with malachite green and steam gently over the flame for one-half minute. Wash thoroughly with water. Stain with safranine for one-half minute. Wash, blot, dry, and examine. Spores stain green; bacilli, red.

Spore stain (Bartholomew and Mittwer's method)

Procedure

1. Fix the smear by passing it through flame.

2. Stain 10 minutes with saturated aqueous malachite green (approx. 7.6 per cent) without heat.

3. Rinse about 10 seconds with tap water.

4. Counterstain 15 seconds in 0.25 per cent aqueous safranine.

5. Rinse and dry.

Result. Spores stain green; rest of cell, red.

Capsule stain (Hiss)

Solution

Basic fuchsin (90 per cent dye content)	0.15 to 0.3 g
Crystal violet (85 per cent dye content)	0.05 to 0.1 g
Distilled water	100 ml

Procedure

1. Grow organisms in ascitic fluid or serum medium, or mix with drop of serum and prepare smears from this mixture.

2. Dry smears in air and fix with heat.

3. Stain with one of the above solutions a few seconds by gently heating until stain rises.

4. Wash with 20 per cent aqueous $CuSo_4 \cdot 5 H_2O$.

5. Blot dry and examine.

Result. Capsules stain faint blue; cells, dark purple.

Capsule stain (Muir's method)

Mordant

Tannic acid	2 parts
Saturated aqueous solution of mercuric chloride	2 parts
Saturated aqueous solution of potassium alum	5 parts

Procedure

1. Prepare an even, thin film of the bacteria. Allow to dry with heating. Cover the film or smear with a strip of filter paper cut to the shape and size of the slide and flood with Ziehl-Neelsen carbolfuchsin. Warm with a flame until it just steams for 30 seconds.

2. Rinse gently with alcohol, then with water.

3. Add the mordant for 15 to 30 seconds and wash well with water.

4. Decolorize with alcohol until faintly pink.

5. Wash with water.

6. Counterstain with methylene blue for 30 seconds.

7. Allow to dry in air and examine.

Result. Cells are stained red and capsule is stained blue.

Flagella stain (Leifson)

Solution

$KAl(SO_4)_2 \cdot 12 H_2O$ or $NH_4Al(SO_4)_2 \cdot 12 H_2O$ saturated aqueous solution	20 ml
Tannic acid (20 per cent aqueous)	10 ml

Distilled water	40 ml
Ethyl alcohol, 95 per cent	15 ml
Basic fuchsin* (saturated solution in 96 per cent ethyl alcohol)	3 ml

Mix ingredients in order named. Keep in tightly stoppered bottle.

Procedure

1. Prepare slides by cleaning in dichromate cleaning solution, wash in water, rinse in alcohol, wipe with clean piece of cheesecloth. Pass slides through a flame several times.

2. Flood slides with solution and allow to stand 10 minutes at room temperature in warm weather or in an incubator in cold weather.

3. Wash with tap water.

4. Dry and examine.

Result. Flagella are stained red, except with those bacteria that have extremely delicate flagella.

Stain for spirochetes (Fontana)

Preparation of Ammoniacal Silver Nitrate. Dissolve 5 g of $AgNO_3$ in 100 ml of distilled water. Remove a few milliliters, and to the rest of the solution add drop by drop a concentrated ammonia solution until the precipitate which forms redissolves. Then add drop by drop enough $AgNO_3$ solution to produce a slight cloud which persists after shaking. The solution should remain in good condition for several months.

Staining Schedule

1. Prepare smear, and fix with heat.

2. Pour on a solution of 5 per cent tannic acid in 1 per cent phenol, and allow to steam 30 seconds.

3. Wash 30 seconds in running water.

4. Cover with a drop of the above ammoniacal silver nitrate, heat gently over a flame, and allow it to stand 20 to 30 seconds after steaming begins.

5. Wash in tap water.

6. Blot dry, and examine.

FLUORESCENCE MICROSCOPY

The development of techniques for conjugating antibodies with fluorescein and the application of these techniques to identification of specific microorganisms introduced a valuable tool in the microbiology laboratory. Thus, it is desirable at this point to describe a broad outline of fluorescent antibody (FA) techniques. In some cases, FA techniques completely replace time-consuming cultural methods; in other cases preliminary identification of microorganisms may be followed by cultural confirmation. It is probable that FA techniques will replace some of the older serologic methods of making final identification of bacteria. There are now available commercially such reagents for the identification of

*This stain is available commercially in powder form (Harleco, Gibbstown, N.J.).

Streptococcus pyogenes and *Neisseria gonorrhoeae*. A great deal of investigative work is in progress in various laboratories which will no doubt elucidate the role that FA techniques may play in clinical microbiologic work. Clinical microbiologists should be prepared to adapt proven methods to their routine procedures at the earliest possible moment, since FA techniques can offer the opportunity to speed up microbiologic diagnosis.

The basic principle on which FA techniques depend is the nature of the combination of specific antibody with antigen (Chap. 35). In the direct method the antibody coats the antigen (e.g., bacteria and protozoa) and cannot easily be removed. If such an antibody has been rendered fluorescent by conjugation with fluorescein and all the non-antibody globulin is removed by washing, all that remains is that which is attached to the antigen. Thus, if the antigen is a bacterial cell and is viewed with an appropriate optical system, the fluorescent outline of the bacterial cell can be seen easily. The specificity of the test, as in any serologic procedure, depends on the purity of the antibody in the conjugated serum. To produce such a specific serum, one can immunize an appropriate animal with an organism (antigen) and absorb the serum to remove all but the specific, identifying antibody. For example, an animal may be given a series of inoculations with a suspension of *Streptococcus pyogenes*, and by appropriate absorption the cross-reacting antibodies can be removed. The absorbed serum then contains specific streptococcal group A antibodies and, when conjugated with fluorescein, can be used to identify these organisms in smears.

An indirect FA technique may also be used. The basic principle of this method is as follows: the specific antiserum is not labeled with fluorescein and is allowed to react with the antigen, and the non-antibody globulin is washed off. If one is using a rabbit antiserum, the antigen is now coated with rabbit serum globulin. Treatment of this preparation with fluorescein-labeled anti-rabbit globulin results in a specific combination of this labeled antibody with the rabbit globulin already specifically attached to the antigen. When the antibody globulin is washed off, the antigen now can be seen as in the case of the direct technique. This indirect method has the advantage of reducing the number of labeled antisera needed, since, if all diagnostic antisera were produced in the rabbit, one would need only a fluorescein-labeled anti-rabbit globulin. Such a serum can be produced by inoculation of rabbit globulin into a sheep or other suitable animal. The indirect technique can be used for detecting antibody in the serum of patients by combining such serum with specific organisms, such as *Toxoplasma*, and then using a fluorescein-labeled anti-human globulin serum.

An inhibition method has also been used for the purpose of checking the specificity of the reactions with a given antigen-antibody system. There is also a complement staining method which, although rather complex, may be quite useful in certain types of work. As FA work progresses, the new applications of this technique that will no doubt evolve will mean possible changes and refinements of present techniques. Detection of antigen in tissues has been reported as well as the successful demonstration of antibody. A rapid method for detecting human influenza virus infection utilizing nasal smears has been described. Fluorescent antibody studies have been extended to include members of the following genera of bacteria: *Leptospira*, *Haemophilus*, *Streptococcus*, *Salmonella*, *Treponema*, *Pasteurella*, *Yersinia*, *Escherichia*, and many others. The technique has also been used in the detection of numerous viruses, fungi, and protozoa. These cited cases represent but a few adaptations of fluorescence microscopy as a tool for studying and identifying microorganisms (see Fig. 47-1.)

BASIC CULTURE TECHNIQUES

The most frequently used item of equipment in the bacteriology laboratory is the inoculating loop. This can be made of platinum wire, nichrome wire, or other similar material, and inserted in a holder. One should also have a straight wire for stab inoculations and for picking isolated colonies from streaked plates. Numerous types, most of which are satisfactory, are available at low cost from commercial sources.

The inoculation of bacteria from specimens submitted to the laboratory is almost invariably accomplished by streaking on the surface of an agar plate. The purpose of streaking is to spread an inoculum to insure the appearance of isolated colonies on incubation. Most such isolated colonies will be pure cultures of an organism and may be picked for the next step—identification. The characteristics and the cellular morphology will also assist in final

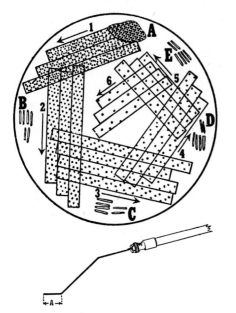

Figure 46–3. Method of streaking a plate so as to secure well-isolated colonies. The original material is deposited at *A*. The wire is afterward sterilized in the Bunsen flame. The material is then streaked with the flat part of the wire at 1, 2, 3, 4, 5, and 6, the wire being thrust into the agar to remove excess organisms, as at *B, C, D,* and *E,* after each series of parallel strokings. Isolated colonies are almost invariably found at the areas numbered 4, 5, and 6. The wire used in streaking is shown below the plate. The flat portion at *A* is brought into contact with the agar from tip to "heel." (From Frobisher, M., Jr.: Fundamentals of Bacteriology, 4th edition.)

identification. It is, therefore, imperative that a suitable streaking technique be used.

A recommended technique is as follows: with a sterile inoculating loop place two loopfuls of the material near the edge of the plate. The loop should then be sterilized in the flame and allowed to cool. It should then be applied to the material on the plate and streaked, using a gentle pressure in the manner illustrated in Figure 46–3.

The streaked plates are incubated in an inverted position, media side up, at 35°C. and examined at 24- and 48-hour intervals. The various colonies should be observed carefully and individual ones picked for Gram's stain and for transfer to appropriate media for further study. Picking of colonies may be done with a loop, but it is better to use a straight wire, especially if the colonies are close together. It is essential that Gram's stains be done on all colonies to study staining characteristics, morphology, and purity.

Pour plates are sometimes used on certain types of specimens, e.g., urine or blood. The pour plate is made by placing a measured amount of the material in a sterile Petri plate and pouring in melted agar (cooled to 50°C.). The plate is then rotated to mix the material thoroughly throughout the me-

dium. After solidifying at room temperature the plate is inverted, incubated at 35°C., and examined for colonies. This technique has the advantage of giving quantitative bacterial counts. For heavily contaminated specimens, dilution must be done before inoculation.

Agar slants are used frequently for maintenance of cultures or for certain biochemical studies. The slant is inoculated from a colony picked from a plate or from a broth culture. A loop is used to transfer the inoculum to the slant and is streaked over the entire slant. Slants are used only with pure cultures and not for isolation. It is sometimes necessary to stab into the butt of a slant, as with triple sugar iron agar. This is done with a straight wire, stabbing carefully in a straight line into the center of the tube. The stab should never be made completely to the bottom of the tube. Slants are examined after 24 hours and 48 hours of incubation, and Gram's stains are made to check purity of the culture.

Semisolid media are used for motility or biochemical studies and are stabbed with a straight wire. The stab is not extended to the bottom of the tube. Motility is read by examining for migration of growth away from the stab line; thus, it is important that the stab be made with care.

Broth media (e.g., infusion and extract media) are used for maintenance of cultures and other studies (such as carbohydrate fermentation). They are inoculated by transfer from colonies or other growth with a loop or wire. Propagation of bacteria in such media is indicated by the development of cloudiness. It is important to ascertain growth in fermentation media, since failure of growth results in no change of the indicator and may lead to false negative interpretation. Gram's stains should be done on all broth cultures to determine the purity of the culture and to make sure no contamination has occurred.

For short-term storage of cultures one should use broth or agar slant cultures, since Petri dishes tend to dry out unless sealed with a rubber or plastic band.

BASIC ANAEROBIC TECHNIQUES

The specimen is the most important factor in proper anaerobic culturing. Without an adequately collected and properly transported specimen, the finest laboratory will not successfully isolate fastidious strictly anaerobic bacteria. Education of clinicians is necessary if quality work is to be done. Details of specimen collection, transport, and processing are found in Chapter 47.

In the laboratory the methods to be used will depend greatly on the training and experience of personnel, as well as on the equip-

5

ment and space available. Regardless of the methods used, the simple Gram's stain of the original specimen is important. Because anaerobes frequently exhibit a characteristic morphology, a preliminary indication of their presence can be immediately ascertained.

The three basic approaches to anaerobic culturing are (1) the roll tube and prereduced media technique, (2) the anaerobic chamber, and (3) direct plating with incubation in anaerobic jars. Any one method or a combination of these methods, if carried out properly, can be expected to yield satisfactory results with clinical materials.

The roll tube technique advocated by the Anaerobe Laboratory at Virginia Polytechnic Institute (1975) requires special training and equipment: the anaerobic culturing apparatus and special prereduced anaerobically sterilized media. The apparatus and many of the media are available commercially. With this method roll tubes with agar coating the walls are used for the isolation of colonies from specimens. Each tube contains an atmosphere devoid of significant amounts of oxygen, and in effect is a miniature anaerobic chamber. The specially designed apparatus that is required ensures that the tubes can be inoculated in a manner to prevent the entrance of air. Identification of isolates thus obtained is determined by use of prereduced biochemical differential media in conjunction with gas chromatography.

Direct plating techniques are carried out as with routine aerobic bacteriology. Fresh enriched media in plates may be inoculated and immediately placed into anaerobic jars (Fig. 46-4). Selective media may also be used, such as phenylethyl alcohol blood agar, to isolate gram-positive organisms and kanamycin-vancomycin blood agar for anaerobic gram-negatives. An enriched liquid medium, such as chopped meat glucose broth, should also be inoculated. Thioglycollate medium, although capable of supporting the growth of many anaerobes, is not a good general purpose medium.

An anaerobic glove box or chamber can be

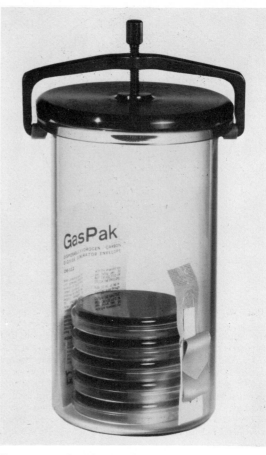

Figure 46-4. GasPak anaerobic system. (Courtesy of Bioquest, Cockeysville, Maryland.)

used as an alternative to the anaerobic jars. The specimens can be introduced through the air lock and the entire process carried out within the chamber where an anaerobic atmosphere is maintained.

As a rule, anaerobic incubation periods are longer than those required for qualitative organisms. At least two days are recommended. If roll tubes or the anaerobic chamber is used, plates may be examined at 24 hours without exposing the developing colonies to an oxygen-containing atmosphere. This is not possible with anaerobic jars.

REFERENCES

Bartlett, R. C.: Medical Microbiology: Quality Cost and Clinical Relevance. New York, John Wiley & Sons, Inc., 1974.

Collins, C. H., and Lynne, P. M.: Microbiological Methods, 4th ed. London, Butterworths, 1976.

Holdeman, L. V., and Moore, W. E. C.: Anaerobe Labora-

tory Manual, Blacksburg, Va., Virginia Polytechnic Institute and State University, 1975.

Lennette, E. H., Spaulding, E. H., Truant, J. P. (eds.): Manual of Clinical Microbiology, 2nd ed. Washington, D.C., American Society for Microbiology, 1974.

Power, D.: Quality control of commercially prepared bacteriological media. *In* Prier, J. E., et al. (eds.): Quality Control in Microbiology. Baltimore, University Park Press, 1975, pp. 47–54.

Prier, J. E., Bartola, J. T., and Friedman, J. (eds.): Quality Control in Microbiology. Baltimore, University Park Press, 1975.

Standards for Accreditation of Medical Laboratories. Chicago, College of American Pathologists, 1974.

Stewart, J. A.: Methods of Media Preparation for the Biological Sciences. Springfield, Ill., Charles C Thomas, Publisher, 1974.

Thomas, R. G., De Lashmutt, R. E., Beautyman, W., Garikes, A., and Mennich, D.: Manual for Laboratory Planning and Design. Chicago, College of American Pathologists, 1977.

Vera, H. D.: Quality control in diagnostic microbiology. Health Lab Sci., 8:176, 1971.

5

47

MEDICAL BACTERIOLOGY

John A. Washington II, M.D.

SPECIMEN SELECTION AND
COLLECTION
    Blood
    Sterile Body Fluids
    Tissue
    Eye
    Respiratory Tract
    Genitourinary Tract
    Feces
PROCESSING
    Smears
    Media
    Incubation
    Examination of Cultures

MEDICALLY IMPORTANT BACTERIA
    Pyogenic Cocci
    Coryneform and Related Bacteria
    Aerobic Spore-forming Bacilli
    Gram-negative Aerobic and
        Facultatively Anaerobic Rods
    Oxidase-positive Glucose Fermenters of
        Medical Significance
    Glucose Oxidizers
    Gram-negative Aerobic and
        Facultatively Anaerobic Rods
        Requiring Special Growth Factors or
        Conditions
    Anaerobic Bacteria

An understanding of the locations, varieties, and roles of the bacterial flora indigenous to the skin and mucous membranes is essential to the proper selection and collection of material for cultures and to the interpretation of the results of cultures. The isolation and identification by the laboratory of a large number of bacteria from a specimen contaminated

Table 47–1. BACTERIA COMMONLY FOUND ON HEALTHY HUMAN BODY SURFACES*

BACTERIA	SKIN	CONJUNCTIVA	UPPER RESPIRATORY TRACT	MOUTH	LOWER INTESTINE	GENITOURINARY TRACT external genitalia	anterior urethra	vagina
Aerobic and facultatively anaerobic								
Staphylococci	+	+	+	+	±	+	+ +	+
Streptococci								
viridans	±	±	+	+ +	+	+	±	+
group A			±	±				
group D			±	+	+	+	+	+
S. pneumoniae		±	+	+				
Neisseriae		±	±	+			+	±
Corynebacteria	+	+	+ +	+	+	+	+	+
Haemophili		±	+	+				
Enterobacteriaceae			±	±	+ +	+	+	±
Anaerobic								
Clostridia				±	+ +		±	±
Propionibacteria	+ +		+	±	±		±	
Actinomycetes			+	+	±			
Lactobacilli				+	+		±	+ +
Bifidobacteria				+	+ +			+ +
Bacteroides			+	+ +	+ +	+	+	+
Fusobacteria			+	+ +	+	+	+	±
Cocci								
gram-positive	+		+	+ +	+ +	+	±	+
gram-negative			+	+ +	+		±	+

*Adapted from Rosebury, 1962, and Sutter, 1975. ±, irregular; +, common; + +, prominent.

with indigenous flora is extraordinarily time-consuming and defies rational interpretation and therapy. The complexity of the problem posed by indigenous flora can best be illustrated in Table 47–1, in which are listed those bacteria commonly encountered on healthy human body surfaces. The magnitude of the problem can best be illustrated by the fact that the number of bacteria on some areas of the skin, in the mouth, and in the descending colon may reach 10^6 organisms/sq. cm, 10^9 organisms/ml, and 10^{11} organisms/g, respectively.

A specimen for bacterial culture that has been contaminated with indigenous flora has limited utility unless only specific organisms, e.g., group A streptococci in the throat, are being sought or certain precautions are taken.

These precautions include disinfection of the area through which the specimen is aspirated or passes, as with a phlebotomy for blood culture or collection of a clean-voided midstream specimen for urine culture; bypassing the area, as with a transtracheal aspiration of lower respiratory secretions or with a suprapubic aspiration for bladder urine; or quantitation to establish the probability of disease, e.g., significant bacteriuria. Given these precautionary steps, the laboratory needs to define specimen requirements and instructions for microbiologic examination. A suggested list of instructions is shown in Table 47–2.

Having established these general guidelines, the next and probably more difficult step for the laboratory is to define criteria for re-

Table 47–2. INSTRUCTIONS FOR SPECIMEN COLLECTION AND TRANSPORT FOR BACTERIOLOGIC CULTURE

SPECIMEN	CONTAINER OR TRANSPORT DEVICE	VOLUME (ml)	OTHER CONSIDERATIONS
Blood			
Bacteria	Vacuum blood culture bottles containing liquid medium with SPS	Adults: 10 ml/100 ml bottle Infants: 1–3 ml/100 ml bottle	A minimum of 2 separate collections per 24 hr period is required; more than 3 per 24 hr period are rarely needed and will be collected only following consultation with laboratory consultant.
Brucella, Neisseriae	Castaneda bottle containing biphasic medium without SPS	10 ml/bottle	As for bacteria.
Catheters	Sterile, screw-capped or anaerobe tube	–	Disinfect surrounding entry site, remove catheter, and aseptically clip off tip into tube.
Exudates			
Transudate, drainages, ulcers	Swab or sterile, screwcapped tube	–	Such specimens are rarely suitable for anaerobic culture.
Eye	See "Other Considerations"	–	Cultures of patients with conjunctivitis are rarely useful. With corneal lesions swab material and scrapings should be applied directly to slides for smears and to media for culture.
Fecal material	Screw-capped jar	–	Freshly passed or collected material recommended. Transport medium should be used when delay anticipated.
Fluids			
Cerebrospinal	Sterile, screw-capped tube	1–5	Must be delivered to laboratory *immediately;* refrigeration of fluid may be deleterious to survival of certain bacteria.
Other (e.g., synovial, pleural, peritoneal)	Anaerobe vial	1–5	Collect with sterile needle and syringe; expel air bubbles before injection into vial.
Genitourinary			
For *Neisseria gonorrhoeae*	Swab or modified Thayer-Martin agar (e.g., JEMBEC)	–	*Women:* Cervix—moisten speculum with water before inserting into vagina; insert swab into cervical canal. Anal canal—insert swab approximately 2 cm and move from side to side to sample crypts. Urethra or vagina—cultures indicated when cervical not possible. *Men:* Urethra—swab may be used when a discharge is present; otherwise, a sterile bacteriologic loop is inserted to obtain scrapings for smear and culture. Anal canal—as for women.

Table 47–2. INSTRUCTIONS FOR SPECIMEN COLLECTION AND
TRANSPORT FOR BACTERIOLOGIC CULTURE (continued)

SPECIMEN	CONTAINER OR TRANSPORT DEVICE	VOLUME (ml)	OTHER CONSIDERATIONS
Cervix, vagina for other bacteria	Swab	–	These specimens are unsuitable for anaerobic culture.
Urine			
midstream or catheterized	Sterile, screw-capped tube or jar	1–10	Specimen should be delivered to the laboratory immediately or, if delay (>1 h) is anticipated, refrigerated during transport.
suprapubic aspirate	Anaerobe tube	1–10	Collect with sterile needle and syringe; expel air bubbles before injection into tube. This is the *only* type of urine specimen that is acceptable for anaerobic culture.
Abscess, wound	Anaerobe vial	–	Collect with sterile needle and syringe; expel air bubbles before injection into vial.
Respiratory tract		–	
Nasopharynx	Flexible wire calcium alginate-tipped swab		Useful for detecting carrier states of *Neisseria meningitidis, Corynebacterium diphtheriae,* and *Bordetella pertussis,* although nasopharyngeal aspirate with soft rubber catheter is better for detecting *B. pertussis.*
Throat	Swab	–	Tonsillar areas, pharynx, and areas of purulence, ulceration, inflammation, or capsule formation must be swabbed with minimal oral contamination. Ordinarily, cultures for group A streptococci suffice; however, the laboratory must be notified when diphtheria, pertussis, or gonococcal infection is suspected clinically so that appropriate selective media can be inoculated.
Sputum	Sterile, screw-capped jar	–	Submit fresh specimen resulting from deep cough as soon after collection as possible. Specimens with >25 squamous epithelial cells/lpf are not acceptable for culture.
Transtracheal aspirate	Anaerobe vial	–	Collect with sterile needle and syringe or in trap; expel air bubbles before injection into vial.
Bronchial washings	Sterile, screw-capped vial	–	These specimens are unsuitable for anaerobic culture.
Tissue	Sterile, screw-capped jar or anaerobe tube	–	Samples representative of disease process must be submitted.

jection of certain requests for bacteriologic studies. Obvious criteria include discrepancies between patient identification data on the request form and on the specimen container or the absence of identification data on a container that arrives in the laboratory separated from a request form. Although erroneous reports are certainly intolerable, pinning the diagnosis of gonorrhea, tuberculosis, or hepatitis on the wrong patient has social and epidemiologic connotations of incredible magnitude. Dried-out specimens on swabs or swab specimens accompanied by requests for bacterial, mycobacterial, fungal, and viral cultures are clearly unacceptable unless it is simply impossible to obtain additional material. Under such circumstances the report should certainly bear the message that the specimen was unsatisfactory. Leaking containers bearing normally sterile body fluids should be reported as such.

SPECIMEN SELECTION AND COLLECTION

BLOOD

The indications for obtaining blood cultures are manifold but are basically the occurrence of a sudden relative change in pulse rate and temperature, with or without chills, prostration, and hypotension; a history of mild, intermittent, and persistent fever in association with a heart murmur; and generally any time sepsis is suspected. Bacteremia is generally intermittent, with the notable exception of that associated with endocarditis; therefore, it is imperative that more than one set of cultures be performed. Because bacteria indigenous to the skin can be associated with infectious processes of prosthetic material, careful antisepsis of the phlebotomy site with iodine or an iodophor is essential, as is the collection of more than one set of blood cultures. In nearly all cases of endocarditis two sets of blood cultures are sufficient to isolate the etiologic agent; in other types of bacteremias three sets, collected separately, usually suffice. The collection of a single set of blood cultures only is clearly unacceptable, and the laboratory should establish a policy that a minimum of two sets within a 24-hour interval be required. Conversely, the collection of more than three sets of cultures within this time interval is rarely indicated and should be performed only following consultation with the laboratory director.

Because the order of magnitude of bacteremia is very low in adults, the isolation rates of bacteria from blood are directly related to the volume of blood cultured. It is recommended, therefore, that between 20 and 30 ml of blood be collected for each set of cultures. In infants the order of magnitude of bacteremia is considerably greater so that between 1 and 3 ml of blood should be adequate for each set of cultures. The volume of blood and the number of blood culture sets collected are independent variables reflecting the low order of magnitude of bacteremia on the one hand and its intermittency on the other.

Ordinarily, blood is inoculated at the bedside directly into bottles containing media; alternatively, it can be transported to the laboratory in a sterile tube containing sodium polyanethol-sulfonate (SPS) and then inoculated into bottles containing media. It is suggested that the blood be diluted at least 10 per cent vol/vol in liquid medium; therefore, 20 or 30 ml of blood should be inoculated into two or three bottles, respectively, containing 100 ml of medium apiece. A suitable medium is soybean-casein digest (e.g., Tryptic soy, Difco Laboratories, Detroit, Mich.; Trypticase soy, BioQuest, Cockeysville, Md.), but brain-heart infusion broth appears to represent a satisfactory alternative. In most cases media with lower oxidation-reduction potentials (E_h) do not provide better recovery of anaerobes than do commercially prepared vacuum blood culture bottles containing soybean-casein digest

or brain-heart infusion broth; however, this equivalency in performance may vary according to the manufacturer of the bottled media. Certainly, media with low E_h values, such as Thiol and thioglycollate broths, should not be relied upon exclusively for blood cultures, since they are distinctly inferior to other media for recovering pseudomonads and yeasts. Among commercially produced blood culture bottles, those containing 100 ml of media are preferred.

Whether or not media made hypertonic by the addition of sucrose yield higher isolation rates than nonhypertonic media remains a controversial issue. In my own studies such media have clearly not been advantageous; however, the value of hypertonicity may be medium- or even system-dependent. Similarly, the potential advantages of prereduced anaerobically sterilized (PRAS) blood culture bottles may be medium- and system-dependent. In my own experience, PRAS bottles have provided no more frequent isolation of anaerobic bacteria than the conventional vacuum blood culture bottle.

With the exception of cases of suspected meningo- or gonococcemia, blood should be anticoagulated with sodium polyanetholsulfonate (SPS), either in its transport tube or in the blood culture medium itself. Concentrations of SPS ranging from 0.025 to 0.05 per cent are satisfactory. SPS also possesses antiphagocytic and anticomplementary properties, and it inactivates aminoglycosidic antibiotics. Concerns about its use in blood culture media because of its inhibitory effects on *Peptostreptococcus anaerobius* have proved to be more theoretical than real in clinical trials, and the use of another polyanion, sodium amylosulfate (SAS), has proved to be less efficacious than SPS because of its greater turbidity and apparent inhibitory effects on gram-negative bacilli and *Staphylococcus aureus*. SPS is inhibitory against some strains of *Neisseria meningitidis* and *N. gonorrhoeae;* therefore, blood from patients with suspected sepsis due to these species should be inoculated either into media without SPS or into media containing added (1.2 per cent) gelatin along with SPS (Eng, 1977).

The value of adding penicillinase to blood culture media is uncertain; however, it is probably worthwhile when patients are receiving penicillins parenterally at the time the blood is collected.

Blood cultures should be incubated at 35°C.

In a two or three vacuum bottle system, one should be incubated unvented while the other bottle(s) should be transiently vented prior to incubation. This procedure is necessary because of the mutually incompatible atmospheric requirements of anaerobes on the one hand and *Pseudomonas* and yeasts on the other. These requirements exist despite the recommended routine use of subcultures. Most commercially produced vacuum bottles contain CO_2 so that it is not necessary to add this gas to them.

Cultures should be incubated for a minimum of seven days prior to their being discarded as negative. In special circumstances, e.g., patients suspected of having endocarditis with negative cultures, incubation should be prolonged for two or three weeks. In my opinion, cultures should be incubated routinely for two weeks in referral centers.

Bottles should be examined macroscopically later in the day on which they were inoculated and daily thereafter for evidence of turbidity, hemolysis, gaseousness, and colony formation. In the presence of any of these signs, subcultures should be made to media appropriate to the isolation of the organism seen in a Gram's stained smear of the medium. Subcultures should routinely include a blood agar plate to be incubated anaerobically. Nearly 10 per cent of bacteremias are polymicrobial so that suitable differential media should be used for subcultures. In the absence of macroscopic evidence of growth, each bottle should be routinely subcultured later in the day on which it was inoculated and after 48 hours of incubation by withdrawing an aliquot of the blood-broth mixture through the rubber stopper with a sterile needle and syringe and inoculating the mixture onto a quadrant of chocolate blood agar plate that is incubated at 35°C. in 5 to 10 per cent CO_2 for 48 hours. Neither additional subcultures nor routine anaerobic subcultures are necessary.

Unless isolated from multiple cultures, the isolation of *Bacillus*, *Corynebacterium*, *Propionibacterium*, and *Staphylococcus epidermidis* represents contamination; however, because of the fact that these organisms commonly cause infections of prosthetic material, e.g., valves, joints, and shunts, their presence in blood cultures should not be casually dismissed or ignored prior to discussing the findings with the patient's physician. All other positive blood cultures should be reported promptly by phone to a physician as soon as the results of Gram's stained smears become available. Isolates should undergo antimicrobial susceptibility testing as expeditiously as possible so that appropriate adjustments in the antibiotic regimen can be made.

Several newer systems have become available or are being evaluated for the detection of bacteremia. Essentially, these approaches can be placed into two categories. In the first category are systems that concentrate microorganisms by filtration, usually following red cell lysis by one of several methods, or by centrifugation. Neither of these systems has yet proved to be practical in the clinical laboratory.

In the second category are systems that detect the presence of bacteria in blood cultures by physicochemical means. One example of such a system is the radiometric technique wherein actively growing bacteria metabolize various substrates labeled with ^{14}C to $^{14}CO_2$, the evolution of which is monitored by a suitable detection device. This system (BACTEC) is available commercially. One of this system's advantages is that a certain number of positive cultures are detected sooner than by conventional methods; however, there are disadvantages that must be recognized. These include the small volume of blood cultured, the equipment's expense, the use and disposal of radioisotopes, the somewhat lower recovery rates of haemophili, Enterobacteriaceae, and anaerobic bacteria, and the substantial rate of false positives. Furthermore, radiometric techniques do not obviate the necessity of performing routine subcultures.

Another example of a physicochemical technique used to detect the presence of bacteria in blood is that of monitoring changes in electrical impedance of broth cultures. Although an apparatus (Bactometer) capable of measuring impedance in bacterial cultures is commercially available, blood culture bottles to which the electrodes can be conveniently attached are not. Also, the numbers of bacteria that are needed to cause detectable changes in impedance are of the order of magnitude that cause visible turbidity. Nonetheless, should it become possible to attach electrodes easily and economically to culture bottles, impedance may provide a convenient system for monitoring large numbers of cultures without actually having to inspect them on a daily basis.

Undoubtedly, new systems will be developed in the future to facilitate the detection of bacteremia and, perhaps, fungemia. Each will require critical evaluation and documentation of efficacy by carefully controlled studies comparing their efficacy with established, conventional methods.

STERILE BODY FLUIDS

CEREBROSPINAL

Meningitis is a medical emergency requiring early therapy to prevent death or serious neurologic sequelae. In childhood and particularly in infancy its diagnosis may be delayed or missed because signs of meningeal irritation are often absent and the findings are vague and non-specific. Children between the ages of six months and one year are at greatest risk, with the majority of cases occurring during the first five years. Beyond the neonatal period of life when gram-negative bacilli and group B streptococci are the principal etiologic agents, *Haemophilus influenzae*, *Streptococcus pneumoniae*, and *Neisseria meningitidis* are the predominant causes of acute bacterial meningitis.

Although partial therapy prior to hospital admission of patients with meningitis does modify the cerebrospinal fluid findings somewhat, the differences between the laboratory findings in this population and those in a previously untreated population are not statistically significant (Feigin, 1976a). In some situations in which the initial puncture yields normal results a second one may be required for proper diagnosis and therapy.

As for the collection of blood for culture, careful skin antisepsis is mandatory in preparation for a lumbar puncture. Since bacteremia is frequently associated with meningitis, cultures of blood should be made. Moreover, since the number of bacteria present in infected cerebrospinal fluid may be as few as 10/ml, it is important to provide the laboratory with an adequate ("as much as possible") volume for culture. This is even more important in cases of suspected mycobacterial or fungal meningitis in which the numbers of organisms are frequently few.

Specimens for microbiologic examination should be placed into sterile, screwcapped, and airtight tubes. It behooves the laboratory to examine specimen tubes included in lumbar puncture trays for sterility, the absence of stainable microorganisms, and the adequacy of the seal formed by the cap. It is our practice to select randomly on a regular basis a few tubes from different lots of lumbar puncture trays, fill them partially with filter-sterilized cerebrospinal fluid, and have them sent from a nurses' station to the laboratory by conventional means for processing as a simulated specimen bearing deceased patients' names and registration numbers. By this means, all of the parameters that have been mentioned are tested, in addition to our laboratory's ability to process the specimen aseptically.

Cerebrospinal fluid should be transported to the laboratory promptly without refrigeration because of the sensitivity of *Haemophilus influenzae* and *Neisseria meningitidis* to prolonged transportation and temperature variations. Fluid should be examined microscopically by preparing a Gram's stained smear of spun sediment. Bearing in mind the fact that one organism will be seen per oil immersion field ($\times 1000$) when there are 10^5/ml and that concentrations of organisms below this level occur frequently, prolonged examinations of multiple fields in stained smears are required. When organisms resembling *Haemophilus*, *Neisseria*, or *Streptococcus* are seen, their identity can be confirmed rapidly by performing a quellung test or by examining smears by fluorescent antibody techniques. Reports of the accuracy of the Gram's stained smear vary but range from 60 to 80 per cent.

In recent years two rapid diagnostic techniques have received increasing attention. These techniques include the detection by countercurrent immunoelectrophoresis (CIE) of specific polysaccharide antigens in cerebrospinal fluid, blood, and urine (Feigin, 1976b) and the detection of endotoxin in cerebrospinal fluid in gram-negative bacterial meningitis by the limulus lysate test (Nachum, 1973). These tests are usually unaffected by prior partial therapy and may, therefore, be helpful when bacterial meningitis is suspected on the basis of clinical and laboratory data other than cultures. Their speed of performance makes them a useful adjunct to the Gram's stained smear.

The principle of CIE is that a negatively charged bacterial antigen and a neutral or slightly charged antibody are placed in two opposed wells on an agarose-coated slide. Although the two will migrate slowly toward one another in alkaline (pH 8.2 to 8.6) media, electrophoresis causes the antigen to move rapidly towards the positive electrode. The antibody moves rapidly in the opposite direction be-

5

cause of the normal flow of buffer from the positive to the negative electrode. The two enter a zone of reaction and, if they combine into an antigen-antibody complex, form a precipitin line between the two wells.

With cerebrospinal fluid from a patient suspected of having meningitis serving as the antigen, electrophoresis is carried out with the following: *Haemophilus influenzae* type b antiserum, polyvalent pneumococcal antiserum, and *Neisseria meningitidis* antisera (poly A-D, poly X-Z). Because pneumococcal types VII and XIV are neutral and do not migrate toward the positive electrode, it is necessary to incorporate a sulfonated derivative of phenylboronic acid in the buffer system to ensure their detection (Anhalt, 1975). In suspected neonatal meningitis, streptococcal group B antiserum is included. Of note is the fact that *Neisseria meningitidis* group B antiserum will react with the Kl antigen of *Escherichia coli*, which is a frequent cause of neonatal meningitis.

The principle of the limulus lysate test is that a lysate prepared from amebocytes of the horseshoe crab, *Limulus polyphemus*, undergoes gelation when exposed to endotoxin. The assay of cerebrospinal fluid is rapid and provides a high level of sensitivity in the diagnosis of meningitis due to *Neisseria meningitidis*, *Haemophilus influenzae*, and other gram-negative bacteria.

Because of the small numbers of organisms that may be present in cerebrospinal fluid, some method of concentration prior to culture is usually performed. In many laboratories centrifugation at 2500 rpm for 15 minutes is used. This procedure is probably effective when there are numerous leukocytes present; however, in some cases the cell counts may be normal, especially early in the course of meningitis, and a force of 10,000 g may be required to sediment bacteria. It is our practice, therefore, to concentrate the specimen by filtering it through a 0.45 μm membrane filter contained in a sterile, disposable unit (Swinnex, Millipore Corporation) and then to remove the filter and apply it directly to the surface of chocolate blood agar for culture (Washington, 1974).

Other fluids require no special instruction or precautions except for the use of careful aseptic technique in their collection and processing. Although anticoagulation of joint and pleural fluids may be desirable, it should be pointed out that heparin usually contains the preservative, benzyl alcohol, that may adversely affect the recovery of microorganisms.

TISSUE

SURGICAL

Whereas specimens such as blood and cerebrospinal fluid usually reflect medically urgent situations, those obtained surgically are done so at great expense and at considerable risk to the patient. It therefore behooves the surgeon to obtain an amount of material that is adequate both for histopathologic and for microbiologic examination. Swabs are obviously rarely adequate for this purpose. The histopathology of the lesion may not only serve to differentiate between infection and malignancy but also can help to distinguish between a suppurative and a granulomatous process. In some cases special stains are helpful in establishing the etiology of the process. In chronic lesions the differential diagnosis includes disease due to actinomycetes, brucellae, mycobacteria, and fungi, any one of which may be present only in small numbers, again emphasizing the need for obtaining adequate samples for examination.

Biopsies of ulcers and curettings of sinus tracts should be obtained to recover organisms that might be present only in the ulcer or sinus tract wall. Cultures of the drainage from such lesions are apt to be contaminated with flora indigenous to the skin or adjacent mucous membranes or with secondary invaders. Aspirations of closed abscesses are preferable to obtaining material on a swab after such lesions have been opened. Local anesthetics may be necessary for the collection of specimens; however, it must be remembered that these agents possess antimicrobial activity (Schmidt, 1970).

Tissue obtained surgically for culture should be placed into a sterile, wide-mouthed, screw-capped jar. Pus should be injected into an anaerobe vial for transport to the laboratory, or it can be sent in the syringe into which it was aspirated by plugging the needle with a sterile rubber stopper. When an abscess cavity is opened and drained, a portion of its wall should also be submitted for culture. If several abscesses are present, portions of each should be removed for culture. As a general rule, tissue should be bisected aseptically by the surgeon in the operating room and material representative of the pathologic process submitted for both histopathologic and microbiologic examination. Good communication between histopathologist and microbiologist is important, especially in cases with fever of unknown origin for which an exploratory laparotomy is being done and multiple biopsies are taken. The tendency is to send most of the material to the pathologist and a small portion of it or even a swab to the microbiologist and to request smears and cultures for bacteria, mycobacteria, fungi, and perhaps even viruses. This approach is clearly one that the laboratory cannot meet and represents a tremendous injustice to the patient.

Tissue received by the laboratory should be examined and its characteristics described on a work card before processing. It should then be finely minced with sterile scissors into a mortar where it is mixed with a sterile abrasive (alundum) in broth and ground with a pestle to render a 20 per cent suspension. This suspension is most conveniently transferred into a sterile dropper bottle that can be used to inoculate all of the necessary culture media and is then stored under refrigeration for at least two weeks before being discarded. We use the histopathology to determine what cultures should be made of each specimen we receive and perform special stains when necessary to try to elucidate the etiology of an infectious process. Our approach to tissue microbiology has been outlined elsewhere (Brewer, 1976).

POSTMORTEM

The value of postmortem bacteriology is limited. Most studies have demonstrated that cultures performed on a single organ obtained postmortem rarely, if ever, provide sufficient information to determine the significance of a positive culture, even in the presence of histologic evidence of infection; that, in selected cases, postmortem cultures of multiple organs may be of value in identifying the etiologic agent of an infectious process, especially in cases of well-recognized clinical entities caused by a single organism or in cases of overwhelming sepsis; and that human tissues are not necessarily sterile at any given time (Wilson, 1972). A high percentage of postmortem bacterial cultures of lung, liver, and spleen from patients without apparent infection are positive. Routine postmortem cultures of any kind should be discouraged and should

be reserved for selected cases in which a closed lesion or space can be sampled aseptically or in which material from multiple organs can be obtained.

EYE

Microbiologic studies of the eye in patients with conjunctivitis are of limited utility in establishing the etiologic diagnosis in many cases and are, therefore, probably seldom warranted. The most important step in the management of bacterial corneal ulcers, however, is prompt and meticulous laboratory investigation (Jones, 1973). Because of the small amount of material that can be obtained for culture, the laboratory should have certain materials available for the ophthalmologist to use. These are sterile calcium alginate, cotton, or dacron-tipped swabs, a Kimura platinum spatula, glass microscopic slides, an alcohol lamp, and media including chocolate blood agar, fluid thioglycollate, Sabouraud dextrose agar, and Lowenstein-Jensen agar. The procedure for laboratory investigation of a corneal ulcer is to obtain material from the conjunctivae with a swab which is used to inoculate a chocolate blood agar plate and a Sabouraud dextrose agar, to anesthetize the cornea with proparacaine hydrochloride, and then to scrape the ulcer with the spatula to obtain material for smears and cultures (Jones, 1973). The slides are used for preparing Gram's stained smears and potassium hydroxide (KOH) preparations. Other slides may be used for acid-fast smears or for staining with Gomori methenamine silver for fungi. Corneal scrapings are spot inoculated onto chocolate blood agar and Sabouraud dextrose agar and into fluid thioglycollate medium. Lowenstein-Jensen agar can be inoculated in cases of suspected mycobacterial disease.

Although some ophthalmologists may have the interest, facilities, and expertise to perform these studies themselves, in most cases it will be necessary for the laboratory to carry them out. We have assembled the required materials into a kit and arranged to have a technologist available to take it to the ophthalmologist and to provide instructions for its use when a request for cultures of a corneal ulcer is received. Because of the need for prompt laboratory investigation of the lesions and the limited amount of material available

5

for examination, close cooperation between the ophthalmologist and the laboratory in these cases is imperative.

RESPIRATORY TRACT

EAR

Since the organisms associated with acute otitis media have been quite consistent and limited to only a few species, there is little reason in uncomplicated cases to perform tympanocentesis in order to obtain material for culture. In patients with severe pain and bulging tympanic membranes and in those who have impaired host defenses or fail to respond to therapy, tympanocentesis and culture are probably indicated. The correlation between cultures of the middle ear and of the nasopharynx is sufficiently poor that there is little reason to culture the latter site. In most cases the etiologic agent is *Streptococcus pneumoniae, S. pyogenes,* or *Haemophilus influenzae;* however, in neonates it is more frequently *Staphylococcus aureus, Escherichia coli,* or *Klebsiella pneumoniae,* and in chronic infections *Staphylococcus aureus* and *Pseudomonas aeruginosa* are predominant.

NASOPHARYNX

Nasal cultures are frequently performed to detect carrier states of *Staphylococcus aureus,* a procedure which is seldom indicated, however, because of the high incidence of carriers in the normal population and especially among hospital personnel and because of the generally poor correlation between phage types found in the nose and those isolated from wound infections. Phage typing of staphylococci is performed in a small number of medical centers and at the Center for Disease Control, but generally only in epidemic situations.

Nasopharyngeal swabs may be used for the detection of carriers of *Streptococcus pyogenes, Corynebacterium diphtheriae, Bordetella pertussis,* and *Neisseria meningitidis.* They may also be used to aid in the diagnosis of pneumonia in infants and small children unable to expectorate a sputum specimen. A flexible wire Dacron, calcium alginate, or cotton-tipped swab should be passed gently through the nose into the nasopharynx and rotated to obtain material for culture. In clinically suspected cases of pertussis it is preferable to aspirate material from the nasopharynx by using a suction catheter (16 in. No. 8 French) attached to a syringe.

Those bacteria that produce pharyngitis are *Streptococcus pyogenes* (or group A), *Neisseria gonorrhoeae, Corynebacterium diphtheriae,* and *Bordetella pertussis.* As has already been stated, nasopharyngeal aspirates represent the specimen of choice in cases with suspected pertussis. A swab of the membrane itself should be taken in cases of suspected diphtheria. Otherwise, an attempt should be made to swab with minimal oral contamination the posterior pharynx, the tonsils or tonsillar pillars, and any areas of purulence, exudation, or ulceration. The laboratory must be notified when gonorrhea, diphtheria, or pertussis is suspected so that cultures with suitable selective media are performed; otherwise, the laboratory is unlikely to recognize these pathogens or even be able to find them if a delayed request is made for their cultivation. In cases of suspected diphtheria, smears can be prepared for staining with Loeffler alkaline methylene blue to determine whether or not typical coryneform bacteria containing metachromatic granules are present. Pertussis may be rapidly diagnosed in many cases by staining smears directly with fluorescein-conjugated anti-*Bordetella pertussis* antiserum. Swabs from patients with suspected meningococcal carrier state or gonococcal pharyngitis are best inoculated directly onto modified Thayer-Martin agar that has been brought to room temperature prior to its use. Whether contained in a Transgrow bottle or in a biologic environmental chamber (JEMBEC), this medium should be incubated overnight prior to its shipment to the laboratory.

The diagnosis of group A streptococcal pharyngitis is often made in the office bacteriology laboratory. Certain precautions should be observed in these instances to ensure that the diagnosis of this disease is accurately made. First, a diagnosis of streptococcal pharyngitis cannot be made reliably on clinical grounds alone and, therefore, requires that a throat culture be made. Second, the posterior pharynx, tonsils, or tonsillar pillars, and any areas of purulence, inflammation, or ulceration should be cultured, since sampling does affect the outcome of cultures. Third, the swab is used to inoculate a soybean-casein digest agar containing 5 per cent sheep blood. Such plates are available from a variety of commercial sources, but they must be stored in sealed plastic wrappers or bags under refrigeration to prevent deterioration. Their performance must be controlled by inoculation of each lot on a regular basis with a known group A streptococcus. Fourth, the area of primary inoculation must be streaked out for isolation with a sterile wire loop, and the surface of the agar must be stabbed in several areas to ensure detection of strains producing oxygen-sensitive hemolysin only. Fifth, the bacitracin disc test for presumptive identification of group A streptococci is unreliable when it is placed directly onto the primary plate and should be performed only with a purified subculture. Finally, the blood agar plates should be incubated at 35°C. for 18 to 24 hours in an atmosphere of room air to minimize growth of β-hemolytic streptococci belonging to Lancefield groups other than A. Cultures that are negative after 24 hours of incubation should probably be reincubated for an additional day before being discarded as negative.

SPUTUM

Bacterial cultures of sputum represent a major problem because they are commonly collected carelessly, frequently are more representative of saliva than of lower respiratory secretions, usually contain large numbers of bacteria indigenous to the oral cavity, and in seriously ill hospitalized patients often contain gram-negative bacilli that have colonized the oropharynx shortly after hospitalization. Such cultures lack sensitivity and specificity and are, therefore, difficult to interpret. At the very least, the laboratory should impose a microscopic screening procedure for specimens submitted for culture in which the relative numbers of leukocytes, macrophages, and squamous epithelial cells can be assessed. In our laboratory, specimens with fewer than 25 white blood cells or macrophages per low power field ($\times 100$) do not get cultured unless there are fewer than 25 squamous epithelial cells per low power field. Specimens with more than 25 squamous epithelial cells per low power field are rejected for culture. A report as to the unsatisfactory nature of the specimen and a request for another specimen is made both by phone and in writing. For those specimens deemed acceptable for culture, a report of the Gram's stained smear is issued stating the morphology of those organisms observed and their relative numbers (e.g., gram-positive cocci resembling pneumococci—many) and the relative numbers of

white blood cells (> 25/lpf = many, < 25/lpf = few) and squamous epithelial cells (> 25/lpf = many, < 25/lpf = few).

In years past, attempts were made to quantify bacterial isolates from sputum following its digestion on the principle that those organisms present in large numbers ($> 10^5$/ml) were more likely to be significant than were those present in small numbers; however, these results have been of little clinical value and have correlated poorly with the results of transtracheal aspiration.

In the patient with serious pulmonary infection and with multiple potentially pathogenic bacteria in cultures of sputum, it may then be necessary to consider performing bronchoscopy with aspiration or biopsy, transtracheal aspiration, thoracentesis, transthoracic needle biopsy, or open lung biopsy to establish the diagnosis. It must be pointed out that although fiberoptic bronchoscopy represents a major technical advance for those involved in the diagnosis of pulmonary disease, inner channel aspirates have been found to be contaminated with oropharyngeal flora and do not, therefore, reliably reflect the bacteriology of the lower respiratory tract (Bartlett, 1976). While associated with certain definite risks, transtracheal aspiration can generally be done safely by a person experienced in its performance. Indications for its performance include cases of suspected anaerobic or gram-negative pneumonia or cases from whom an adequate expectorated sample cannot be obtained. Transthoracic needle aspiration may provide more valuable information than transtracheal aspiration but is probably associated with a higher frequency of complications.

GENITOURINARY TRACT

GENITAL

The bacteria most commonly found to be associated with sexually transmitted disease are *Neisseria gonorrhoeae* and *Chlamydia trachomatis*, the latter of which will be dealt with in another chapter in this section. It is not possible to distinguish on the basis of clinical signs and symptoms between urethritis due to these organisms. Cultures must be made; however, since the isolation of chlamydiae requires the use of cell culture techniques, most laboratories are unable to detect them.

In the male, Gram's stained smears of urethral exudates are both sensitive and specific in establishing the diagnosis of gonorrhea. In males with negative smears, cultures should be made. In the female, Gram's stained smears of vaginal or cervical smears lack sensitivity and specificity and are definitely *not* recommended as a means of establishing or ruling out the diagnosis of gonorrhea. Urethral exudate or scrapings obtained with a small, smooth platinum wire loop should be obtained routinely from males suspected of having gonorrhea. However, since gonococcal pharyngitis and proctitis are not uncommon manifestations of the disease in those practicing fellatio or homosexuality, cultures of the throat or of the anal crypts may also be indicated. In the female, cultures of the cervical os and of the anal crypts should be performed routinely. Adequate visualization of the cervix must be obtained by means of a speculum lubricated with water. Swabs should be inoculated directly onto either Thayer-Martin or modified Thayer-Martin agar which has been prewarmed to room temperature. Thayer-Martin agar plates may be used, provided they can be placed shortly thereafter into an environment with increased CO_2. A candle extinction jar method is quite satisfactory for this purpose. Alternatively, the swab may be inoculated onto modified Thayer-Martin agar in a bottle containing CO_2 (Transgrow) or in a rectangular dish to which a CO_2-generating tablet is added and which is then placed into a ziplock bag (JEMBEC). Despite the slightly greater inconvenience of the latter system over the former for the person inoculating the culture, I prefer JEMBEC because one can ensure that CO_2 will be present in the system and because its agar surface is much more visible than it is in the Transgrow bottle. Cultures that are mailed into the laboratory for processing must first be incubated overnight; otherwise, a significant number of cultures will fail to become positive.

A rare form of sexually transmitted disease in the United States is chancroid, which is caused by *Haemophilus ducreyi*. Cultivation of this organism is difficult and requires inoculation of material from the lesion into rabbit or human serum for growth. Gram's stained smears of freshly expressed exudate from the edges of the lesion will often display pairs and short chains of gram-negative coccobacilli, while in cultures tangled chains and long parallel rows of bacilli are more frequently seen.

The presence of other bacteria in cultures of the urethra and vagina is of questionable clinical significance because of the enormous variety of flora indigenous to these sites. The role of *Haemophilus vaginalis* (or *Corynebacterium vaginale*) in causing vaginitis is as confusing as its taxonomy and nomenclature. Although its inoculation into the vagina of asymptomatic volunteers has produced disease, its presence in vaginal cultures of many asymptomatic females beclouds the issue.

Because of its prominence in causing neonatal meningitis, there has been much interest lately in identifying vaginal carriers of group B streptococci; however, there is as yet no consensus about the clinical management of this problem in pregnant females.

Anaerobic bacteria play a prominent role in severe infections of the female genital tract, including pelvic abscesses, septic abortions, puerperal sepsis, tubo-ovarian abscess, and endometritis. Because of the large number and variety of anaerobes in the vagina, cultures of material draining into the vagina are rarely of value in establishing the etiology of the infection. Attempts should be made to aspirate closed lesions with a sterile needle and syringe or to aspirate endometrial material with a needle or syringe or catheter following careful disinfection of the vagina and cervix. Since it is difficult to disinfect the cervical os, some have devised systems whereby sterile catheters or swabs can be inserted into the uterine cavity through the lumen of a larger catheter placed in the cervical canal. Culdocentesis has also been successfully used for obtaining material for culture. Pus obtained surgically from pelvic infections should always be placed into an anaerobic vial for transport and cultured for anaerobes.

URINARY

There are three categories of urinary specimens that may be collected for bacterial culture. The most frequently submitted one is the clean-voided midstream specimen. This approach should be used whenever possible, since it is relatively easy and can be taught to ambulatory patients and paramedical personnel, is safe, and, when properly performed, provides accurate results in the great majority of instances. The major problem with the procedure in hospitals is that it is often carelessly carried out by the least trained and motivated aide, and the specimen is rarely transported to the laboratory as soon as it should be. To reiterate a point that has already been made several times, the vagina and urethra harbor indigenous bacterial flora that can multiply rapidly in urine stored at room temperature and produce spurious results in cultures. Every effort should be made to obtain a properly collected clean-voided midstream specimen by procedures described elsewhere in detail (Kunin, 1974). This effort will result in a very low incidence of contaminated cultures and produce results that are interpretable. Unfortunately, this objective is not easily done, and it is desirable, particularly in larger hospitals, to train a team of paramedical personnel to collect all urine specimens for cultures. This responsibility may be one of several duties assigned to this team, the other responsibilities of which may include urinary catheter care and replacement. This basic concept has already been implemented in many hospitals in the form of intravenous catheter and phlebotomy teams. Because of the improved quality and reliability of specimens collected in this manner, multiple cultures are not required in a vain attempt to determine which of several organisms appears most consistently in the largest numbers and is likely (by default) to represent the real pathogen. The value of a properly collected specimen, therefore, more than offsets the costs of multiple poorly collected ones, not to mention the fact that the patient's management is more likely to be appropriate.

The second category of urinary specimen is the suprapubic aspiration, the indications for which include the collection of urine from infants and small children, adults in whom cultures of repeated clean-voided specimens have yielded equivocal results, and patients with suspected anaerobic bacteriuria. Bacteriuria due to anaerobes is rare and may be suspected when negative cultures of specimens with positive Gram's stained smears occur. In such cases the only acceptable specimen for anaerobic culture is that aspirated suprapubically.

The third category of specimen is that obtained by instrumentation, most commonly catheterization or cystoscopy. Although there are many indications for catheterization, the insertion of a catheter for the sole purpose of collecting urine for culture is discouraged because of the risk of development of bacteriuria associated with the procedure. This risk has been reported to be in the vicinity of 1 per cent in healthy ambulatory men and women and as high as 20 per cent when performed in women during labor. In patients with chronic indwelling catheters the urine should be collected by needle aspiration through a disinfected portion of the wall of the catheter and *not* from the drainage bag or by disconnecting the catheter from the collection tube.

Urine should be cultured within two hours of its collection or refrigerated during storage. Either of these precautions will help to ensure the accuracy of the results of quantitative cultures. Because of the difficulties encountered in getting specimens to the laboratory promptly, some have resorted to the direct inoculation of microcultures at the time the specimen is collected.

The simplest and most rapid method for detecting significant bacteriuria is to examine microscopically ($\times 1000$) a Gram's stained smear of well-mixed, uncentrifuged urine. The presence of at least two bacteria per high power field correlates with the presence of significant bacteriuria in over 90 per cent of instances in experienced hands. An alternative procedure is to examine a wet mount, with or without methylene blue, of centrifuged urinary sediment with the high-dry objective ($\times 400$) under reduced light.

Quantitative cultures of urine should always be performed by inoculating a measured volume of urine into molten agar which is mixed and poured into a Petri dish or onto the surface of agar in a Petri dish. For practical purposes, the calibrated loop (0.001 or 0.01 ml) streak-plate technique is most rapid and convenient.

Quantitation is the essential parameter used for determining the presence of significant bacteriuria. Colony counts of 10^5/ml or greater are indicative of infection, while those exceeding 10^4/ml are indicative of probable infection. Colony counts between 10^3 and 10^4/ml indicate probable contamination, while fewer colonies are considered to represent contaminants. Obviously, if the specimen was improperly collected and transported to the laboratory, these interpretative criteria become less reliable. Low colony counts that are clinically significant may occur in urine from patients receiving antimicrobial therapy, or those with an obstructed ureter or with infections due to fastidious organisms (e.g., anaerobes). Colony counts may be reduced slightly by hydration. As a rule, the presence of an organism in any quantity in urine obtained by suprapubic aspiration is significant. Because of the importance of quantitation in urine

5

bacteriology, cultures of urine in liquid media or of urinary sediment are unsuitable procedures yielding uninterpretable results.

There are a variety of commercially prepared microculture techniques for detecting bacteriuria (Kunin, 1974). These devices have their greatest utility in screening programs, in office practice, and in reducing numbers of contaminants resulting from delays in transporting urine specimens from the ward to the laboratory. A number of chemical screening methods have also been described; however, they tend to have less sensitivity and specificity than do the microbiologic methods.

FECES

Our concepts about the etiology of diarrhea have changed drastically in the past few years. Salmonellae, shigellae, *Vibrio cholerae*, *Staphylococcus aureus*, clostridia, and certain serotypes of *Escherichia coli* comprised the list of enteric pathogens for many years. The etiology of most cases of diarrheal disease remained obscure. The importance of enterotoxigenic and invasive strains of *E. coli* has only been recognized for a few years, as has the lack of correlation between these two pathogenic properties and serotypes of *E. coli* called "enteropathogenic." Other bacteria are now recognized as causing diarrhea (Table 47–3). To complicate the picture further, reovirus-like and parvovirus-like agents have been clearly associated in recent years with diarrhea.

Table 47–3. PATHOGENIC MECHANISMS OF BACTERIA CAUSING DIARRHEA*

MECHANISMS	ORGANISMS
Preformed toxins	*Staphylococcus aureus* (enterotoxins A, B)
	Clostridium botulinum A, B, E
Enterotoxins following colonization	*Vibrio cholerae*
	Escherichia coli
	Bacillus
	Clostridium perfringens A
	Shigella dysenteriae 1
	Aeromonas hydrophila (?)
Invasiveness	Salmonella
	Shigella
	Escherichia coli
	Staphylococcus aureus
	Vibrio parahaemolyticus
	Yersinia enterocolitica (?)

* Adapted from Donta, 1975.

Despite all of these advances in our understanding of diarrheal disease, the clinical laboratory is pretty well limited to the diagnosis of salmonellosis and shigellosis because the techniques used to determine enterotoxigenicity and invasiveness are complex and time consuming. The heat-labile enterotoxin of *Vibrio cholerae* and of some strains of *E. coli* induces morphologic changes in adrenal tumor or Chinese hamster ovary cells. The procedure is not difficult for laboratories experienced in cell culture technique; however, there are few such clinical laboratories around. The heat-stable enterotoxin produced by some strains of *E. coli* cannot be detected by an in vitro system. Its detection, as well as that of invasiveness by other strains of *E. coli*, requires animal inoculation.

Because most bacterial diarrheas are self-limited, stool cultures are generally limited to cases with severe diarrhea requiring hospitalization, persistent or recurrent diarrhea, and a dysentery-like clinical presentation.

Microscopic examination of diarrheal stool may be helpful in certain circumstances. In patients with suspected staphylococcal enterocolitis, an uncommon entity today, the finding of large numbers of gram-positive cocci resembling staphylococci is virtually diagnostic and may expedite the initiation of appropriate therapy. A methylene blue stain for leukocytes may be helpful in differentiating invasive and enterotoxigenic causes of diarrhea (Harris, 1972).

In the evaluation of a patient with diarrhea, a history of recent dietary intake and travel should be elicited. *Vibrio cholerae* has been encountered in patients who have recently travelled or resided in areas in which disease due to this organism is endemic. Disease due to *Vibrio parahaemolyticus* has been clearly associated with the ingestion of raw or incompletely cooked seafood or shellfish. Most laboratories do not inoculate media suitable for the isolation of vibrios unless specifically requested to do so.

In view of what has been stated about the lack of correlation between enterotoxigenicity or invasiveness and "enteropathogenic" serotypes of *Escherichia coli*, laboratories should no longer screen rectal swabs or stool material from infants for these organisms. Although most invasive strains of *E. coli* belong to a few serotypes, they are different from those that were formerly classified as "enteropathogenic." Although enterotoxigenicity is determined by a plasmid that is transferable by means of conjugation to other strains, it does nonetheless appear that this property may be limited to a relatively small number of serotypes which, however, do not correspond to the "enteropathogenic" serotypes identifiable with currently available methodology. One additional consideration is that it now appears that the capability of enterotoxigenic strains to produce disease may be related to another plasmid-determined property, a colonization factor. This subject is an area of intense interest and research so that further data will surely be forthcoming. It seems likely that other in vitro systems for detecting heat-labile toxin will become available in the near future.

Invasive forms of *Escherichia coli* diarrhea have thus far been rare. Enterotoxigenic forms of *E. coli* are frequent causes of travellers' diarrhea; however, their frequency of distribution in the United States remains unclear. Shigellosis and salmonellosis are global in distribution with the former being most common in young children and the latter affecting all age groups. Yersiniosis is common in Scandinavian countries and has only rarely been recognized in this country. Diarrhea due to enterotoxigenic strains of *Bacillus cereus* or *B. subtilis* is common in Eastern Europe and is but rarely recognized in the United States. Enterotoxigenic strains of *Aeromonas hydrophila* have been reported from Asian countries but have not yet been confirmed as enterotoxigenic here.

PROCESSING

Each laboratory must organize the processing of its specimens so that none of the efforts devoted to their proper selection, collection, and transport are wasted. Certain specimens, such as cerebrospinal fluid, must be processed immediately, since the results of stained smears or of counterimmunoelectrophoresis can have a major impact on therapy. Other specimens with lower orders of priority can be processed as time becomes available, provided that suitable steps are taken to ensure their integrity during periods of temporary storage. Small numbers of bacteria in urine do proliferate just as rapidly on a laboratory bench as at a nursing station unless refrigerated! Stained smears of medically urgent specimens should be prepared, examined, and reported as quickly as possible. Requests for additional material or for specimens to replace unsuitable ones must be made quickly, as should the notification of specimen rejection. In other words, the laboratory must establish a system of priorities based not only upon the urgency with which results are expected but also upon the feasibility of obtaining suitable material before therapy is instituted.

SMEARS

The laboratory should institute a system for routinely examining stained smears of certain types of specimens. Usually sterile body fluids, pus, urine, and material from wounds should be examined microscopically on a regular basis, primarily to provide preliminary results for clinical purposes and secondarily as a quality control measure. One should ordinarily expect to culture bacteria compatible morphologically with those observed in the stained smear.

Great care must be taken in preparing Gram's stained smears to prevent distortion of the organisms and to ensure accuracy of the staining reactions. A thin smear of an aliquot of the specimen that is representative of the infectious process should be prepared on a clean microscopic slide, allowed to dry, gently heat fixed, and then stained. Since 10^5 organisms/ml must be present for there to be at least one per oil immersion field ($\times 1000$), most normally sterile body fluids must be examined microscopically for 15 to 30 minutes in order to detect small numbers of organisms. The relative numbers of white blood cells and squamous epithelial cells per low power field are useful in assessing the quality of certain specimens, e.g., sputa, wounds. Technologists should be encouraged to be as descriptive in their interpretation of Gram's stained smears as possible. Reporting that gram-positive cocci occur in pairs that resemble pneumococci can be very helpful. Pleomorphic gram-negative bacilli usually represent anaerobes and may be presumptively reported as such. Obviously, the reliability of such reports will be directly re-

5

lated to the experience and expertise of the technologist.

A Gram's stained smear of a drop of well-mixed uncentrifuged urine will provide a rapid and accurate determination of whether or not significant bacteriuria ($\geq 10^5$ colonies/ml) is present. The drop of urine should be placed on a clean microscopic slide, allowing it to dry without spreading, and then heat fixing and staining it. The finding of at least two bacteria per oil immersion field ($\times 1000$) is indicative of significant bacteriuria, and the smear should, therefore, be reported as positive. Fewer than two bacteria per field consti-

tute a borderline finding, while no bacteria per field should be reported as negative.

Another technique for examining bacteria is with fluorescent antibody microscopy. Although it is useful in examining specimens directly for the presence of *Bordetella pertussis*, *Listeria monocytogenes*, brucellae, and *Yersinia pestis*, its more common applications are for the detection of group A streptococci in throat swabs, either after a short period of incubation of the swab in broth or after the growth of β-hemolytic streptococci on blood agar, for the rapid presumptive identification of organisms resembling *Haemophilus influ-*

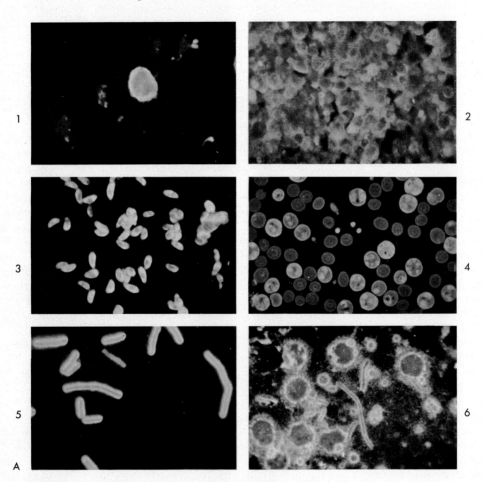

Figure 47-1. *A*, Fluorescent antibody staining* of microorganisms. *1, Entamoeba histolytica* in dried smear from culture ($\times 1050$). *2, Toxoplasma gondii* in spleen of infected mouse. Tissue fixed in alcoholacetic acid and embedded in paraffin ($\times 1050$). *3, Toxoplasma gondii* in peritoneal exudate of infected mouse ($\times 1050$). *4, Plasmodium berghei*, a parasite of rodents, as seen in rat blood during preliminary studies of human malaria. *5, Bacillus anthracis* is an impression smear from the liver of a mouse. Homologous antibody was prepared by injecting whole encapsulated antigen. Note both encapsulated and stripped forms ($\times 600$). *6, Pasteurella pestis* in smear of fluid aspirated from bubo of a fatal case of plague. Homologous antibody prepared by injecting whole-cell antigen. Note bizarre forms of plague bacilli and specifically stained soluble antigen surrounding tissue cells ($\times 1050$). (From W. B. Cherry, M. Goldman, and T. R. Carski: Fluorescent Antibody Techniques. U.S. Department of Health, Education, and Welfare, 1960).

*By the direct method.

(*Figure 47-1 continued on the opposite page.*)

enzae, Streptococcus pneumoniae, and *Neisseria meningitidis* seen in Gram's stained smears of cerebrospinal fluid; and for rapid identification of colonies resembling *Neisseria gonorrhoeae* growing on Thayer-Martin agar. Examples of fluorescent antibody staining of various microorganisms are seen in Figure 47–1. The sensitivity and specificity of this technique varies according to the conjugate and whether it is used for the direct or indirect fluorescent antibody stain. For example, direct staining of cervical or vaginal material for *N. gonorrhoeae* has in many instances lacked sensitivity and specificity; however, fluorescent antibody staining of colonies suspected of being *N. gonorrhoeae* has been reported to be sensitive and specific.

MEDIA

Media should be selected carefully to provide the optimal conditions for growth of pathogens commonly encountered in a particular site or type of specimen. Consideration must be given to special growth requirements of bacteria associated with a particular type of infection or to the necessity of selecting out

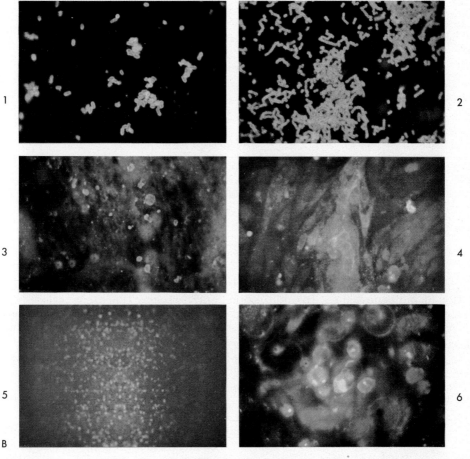

Figure 47–1. Continued. *B,* Fluorescent antibody staining* of microorganisms. *1, Escherichia coli* in feces from a case of infantile diarrhea. Stained with pooled antibodies for enteropathogenic types of *E. coli* (×600). *2,* Group B streptococci in pure culture (×600). *3,* Rabies virus in impression smear of the brain of a mouse infected with street virus. Note the large aggregates of stained antigen (Negri bodies) and the numerous smaller particles that stain (×210). *4,* Simian foamy agent in a culture of monkey-kidney tissue on a coverslip. Two days after inoculation. Note stained antigen in nuclei of the multinucleated cells whose formation was induced by the infection (×210). *5, Rickettsia prowazekii* (epidemic typhus) in a smear of egg yolk sac. Stained with homologous antibody (×210). *6,* Polio virus type I in monkey-kidney tissue cultures, 12 hours post-inoculation. Stained by complement method, using antipolio monkey serum and guinea pig complement followed by labeled anti–guinea pig complement (×210). (From W. B. Cherry, M. Goldman, and T. R. Carski: Fluorescent Antibody Techniques. U.S. Department of Health, Education, and Welfare, 1960.)

*By the direct method except for polio virus in 6.

Table 47-4. GUIDELINES FOR MEDIA SELECTION FOR VARIOUS SPECIMENS*

SPECIMEN	MEDIA FOR RECOVERY OF AEROBIC AND FACULTATIVELY ANAEROBIC BACTERIA						MEDIA FOR RECOVERY OF ANAEROBIC BACTERIA†			
	Suppl thiogly	BA	EMB	CNA	CBA	HE, GN	BA	BA K-V	PEA	Suppl thiogly
Fluids										
cerebrospinal	X	X			X					
abdominal	X	X	X	X			X	X	X	X
pleural	X	X	X	X	X		X	X	X	X
synovial	X	X	X	X	X		X	X	X	X
Wound										
swab	X	X	X	X						
aspirate	X	X	X	X			X	X	X	X
Tissue	X	X	X	X			X	X	X	X
Respiratory tract										
throat		X								
sputum		X	X		X					
transtracheal aspirate	X	X	X	X	X		X	X	X	X
bronchial washings	X	X	X	X	X					
Genitourinary										
cervix, vagina		X	X	X	X‡					
uterus, cul-de-sac	X	X	X	X	X		X	X	X	X
prostate	X	X	X	X	X					
urethra					X‡					
urine										
clean-voided		X	X							
suprapubic aspirate	X	X	X				X	X	X	X
Fecal material		X	X			X				

*Abbreviations: Suppl thiogly = fluid thioglycollate + 10% rabbit serum; BA = blood agar; EMB = eosin methylene blue; CNA = colistin-nalidixic acid blood agar; CBA = chocolate blood agar; HE = Hektoen enteric agar; GN = enrichment broth; K-V = kanamycin-vancomycin; PEA = phenylethyl alcohol blood agar.

†Only for specimens from suitable source and received in anaerobe vial.

‡Modified Thayer-Martin agar.

certain pathogenic bacteria from a mixed population of indigenous flora. In addition to the standard nutrient broth or agar media, therefore, one will often also inoculate differential or selective media. Guidelines for the selection of media to be used with different types of specimens are shown in Table 47-4. For each medium shown there are acceptable alternatives and, obviously, the list of potential types of specimens is far from complete.

INCUBATION

Bacterial cultures are generally incubated at 35°C. and examined initially after 18 to 24 hours of incubation. Added CO_2 in concentrations of 5 to 10 per cent enhances the growth of many bacteria and should be used whenever feasible. Exceptions to this recommendation are those cultures on differential and selective media in which pH alteration is used to differentiate colony types (e.g., xylose-lysine-deoxycholate [XLD] agar, Hektoen enteric [HE] agar). CO_2 is either essential or stimulatory to the growth of certain bacteria, e.g., Neisseria gonorrhoeae, Haemophilus influenzae. A variety of relatively inexpensive methods for CO_2 incubation can be devised (Washington, 1974), and there is an extensive line of CO_2 incubators on the market today.

Certain types of specimens should probably be stored following their inoculation onto culture media in case additional studies become necessary. Of greatest importance are tissues removed surgically, cerebrospinal and other normally sterile body fluids, foreign objects, intravascular cannulae, and prosthetic materials. Many laboratories store other types of specimens overnight under refrigeration in case of a mix-up or other problem requiring repetition of the culture. In many such instances, however, requesting another specimen is preferable to reculturing an old specimen.

ANAEROBIC INCUBATION SYSTEMS

Specimens submitted from appropriate sources and in proper containers for anaerobic culture should be processed expeditiously (Fig. 47–2), although it now appears that clinically significant anaerobes in large volumes of pus or in anaerobe transport vials do survive for 24 hours without difficulty. It is probably important, however, for media that has already been inoculated to be incubated anaerobically or to be placed into a CO_2 flush jar for storage until it can be transferred into an anaerobic incubation system.

There are three types of anaerobic culture systems in use in clinical laboratories today. The most convenient and widely used is the anaerobic jar (GasPak, BioQuest, Cockeysville, Md.) in which water is added to a CO_2 and H_2 generator package and O_2 is catalytically con-

verted with H_2 to water with palladium-coated alumina pellets contained in a lid chamber. There are also evacuation-replacement jars on the market; however, these are somewhat less convenient for routine use in the clinical laboratory. Since the majority of clinically significant anaerobic bacteria require at least 48 hours for growth, it is recommended that jars be opened and plates be examined initially only after this period of incubation, a constraint which represents the jar system's major disadvantage.

A second anaerobic system is the roll tube technique (Hungate, 1969), in which prereduced anaerobically sterilized (PRAS) medium is distributed under anaerobic conditions as a thin layer around the internal surface of test tubes. Air is excluded from the tube during inoculation and subculture by displacement with an oxygen-free gas, such as CO_2, and by keeping it stoppered at all other times. This method has been adapted for clinical laboratory purposes by the Anaerobe Laboratory at the Virginia Polytechnic Institute. The ad-

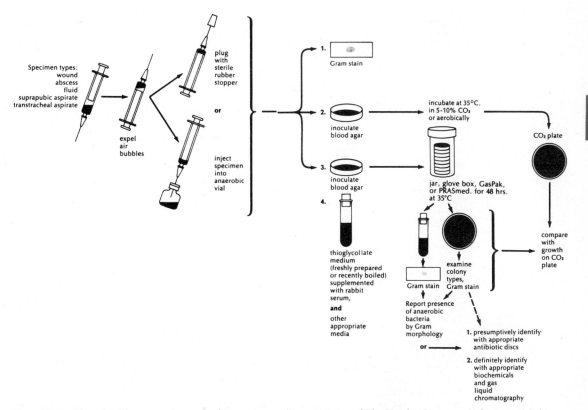

Figure 47–2. Flow chart for processing anaerobic specimens. (By permission of The Upjohn Company, Kalamazoo, Michigan, and J. A. Washington and L. LeBeau.)

vantages of this approach are that each tube becomes its own incubation system and each tube can be examined without disturbing the anaerobic conditions within. Its disadvantages are that the tubes are more cumbersome and time-consuming to work with and the colonial morphology may be less distinct on the agar layer within the tube than on agar plates.

The third approach to anaerobic culture is the anaerobic glove box or chamber which consists of a large, clear plastic, airtight bag filled with an oxygen-free gas mixture of nitrogen, hydrogen, and carbon dioxide (Aranki, 1969). Specimens, plates, and tubes are introduced into or removed from the chamber through a gas interchange lock. Anaerobiasis in the chamber is maintained by palladium catalysts and the hydrogen gas in the chamber. All manipulations within the chamber are done with neoprene gloves sealed to the chamber wall. The chamber can function as its own incubation system by placing heating units in it. Alternatively, incubators can be placed into the chamber; however, they occupy a lot of space and are less desirable than the units which heat the whole chamber. Like the roll tube, the chamber permits examination of cultures at any time without interruption of anaerobiasis. In contrast to the roll tube, conventional isolation and subculture techniques are used. The chamber itself requires a substantial amount of space.

Each of the three anaerobe systems has its advantages and disadvantages, but they are all equally effective for isolating clinically significant anaerobic bacteria from specimens. The selection of one of these systems for routine purposes depends upon many factors ranging from economics to technical. In our own laboratory a combination of jars and the anaerobic chamber has been found to be the most practical and efficient approach. Freshly plated specimens are incubated initially in jars and transferred after overnight incubation into the chamber in which they are first examined. Subcultures of colonies on agar at this time are made for purposes of purification or identification. All plates are then incubated for an additional 24 hours before preliminary reports are issued. By this means, the mandatory 48-hour delay in examining plates imposed by use of the jar method alone is obvi-

Table 47-5. DURATION OF INCUBATION AND FREQUENCY OF EXAMINATION OF CULTURES

TYPE OF CULTURE	INCUBATION TIME BEFORE NEGATIVE CULTURE REPORT (DAYS)	FREQUENCY OF EXAMINATION
Blood	14	daily for 7d and after 14d
Fluids	7*	daily
Abscesses, wounds	7*	daily
Tissue	7*	daily
Respiratory tract		
throat	2	daily
sputum	1	once
transtracheal aspirate	7*	daily
bronchial washings	7*	daily
Genitourinary		
cervix, vagina	2	daily
uterus, cul-de-sac	7*	daily
prostate	2	daily
urethra	2	daily
urine	1	once
Fecal material	1†	once
Anaerobic	7*	daily
Brucella	30	3 × weekly
Actinomyces	21	1 × weekly

*Plates are discarded after 48 h, but tubes with supplemented fluid thioglycollate are kept for time specified in column.

†Initial cultures and subcultures of enrichment broth are examined after 18 to 24 h for presence of lactose-negative colonies; if none are present, the cultures are reported as negative for salmonellae and shigellae.

ated and all work with positive cultures can begin in an anaerobic environment. It is important to re-emphasize, however, the necessity of incubating cultures for at least 48 hours, since many anaerobic bacteria will not be evident after only 24 hours of incubation.

EXAMINATION OF CULTURES

All bacterial cultures should be examined routinely after 18 to 24 hours of incubation. The suggested duration of incubation and frequency of examination of different types of cultures are listed in Table 47-5. In general, cultures of normally sterile body fluids, wounds, abscesses, tissues, and anaerobic cultures are retained for one week, although in most instances the plates are discarded in 48 hours and only the broth cultures are reincubated for the longer period of time. Stool cultures and subcultures are each examined for the presence of lactose-negative colonies and are discarded if none are present. Urine cultures that have no growth or only a few colonies after 18 to 24 hours of incubation are discarded as being negative. Throat cultures are examined for the presence of β-hemolytic streptococci after 18 to 24 hours of incubation; if none are present, the cultures are reincubated for another day. Identification procedures for colonies in sputum cultures can begin after a day's incubation with no added incubation being necessary.

With positive cultures it is a good idea to develop a system of preliminary reports, since identification procedures may take as long as several days to complete. Although the timing of a preliminary report will vary according to the type of culture performed and the importance of the bacteria isolated, it is a good general rule to issue a preliminary report within the first 48 hours after receipt of the specimen. In some cases this report can be sooner and in some (e.g., blood, cerebrospinal fluid) it should be by phone as soon as any information becomes available.

MEDICALLY IMPORTANT BACTERIA

PYOGENIC COCCI

GRAM-POSITIVE

Staphylococcus (Baird-Parker, 1974)

Definitions and Characteristics. Staphylococci are catalase-positive spherical cocci, often appearing in grape-like clusters in stained smears. They grow well on any peptone-containing nutrient medium under aerobic and anaerobic conditions and may produce hemolysis of various species of animal blood and yellow or orange pigment on agar. Growth of staphylococci is readily detected on blood agar plates or in various types of nutrient broths. A selective medium for the isolation of *Staphylococcus aureus* is one containing 7.5 to 10 per cent NaCl with mannitol.

Staphylococci have generally been distinguished from micrococci on the basis of their ability to produce acid anaerobically from glucose; however, this test has been difficult to interpret in some people's hands and criticized by others as providing an indistinct division between the two genera. Other test systems have, therefore, been described that are based on the ability of staphylococci to produce acid aerobically from glycerol in the presence of 0.4 μg/ml of erythromycin and on their sensitivity to lysostaphin (Schleifer, 1975). These tests provide more clearcut separation of the genera, are simpler to perform, and yield more rapid results than those dependent upon the production of acid from glucose under anaerobic conditions.

Staphylococcus aureus is differentiated from other species of staphylococci principally by its production of coagulases. Two antigenically distinct forms of coagulase have been recognized, one being bound to the cell wall and the other being released by or free from the cell wall. Although its mechanism has not been completely elucidated, it is thought that a plasma factor or coagulase-reacting factor reacts with cell-bound coagulase to form a coagulase-thrombin complex which, in turn, acts upon fibrinogen to form a fibrin clot. Cell-bound coagulase is called clumping factor by some and forms the basis of the slide coagulase test. Cell-free or unbound coagulase appears to form a complex with prothrombin to give a thrombin-like product. This form of coagulase serves as the basis for the tube co-agulase test. Human and rabbit plasmas have been shown to be suitable for both of these tests; however, the appropriate dilution of plasmas must be determined for the optimal detection of coagulase, since their perform-ance is affected by the presence of inhibitory and accessory factors. Under these circum-stances it is more practical to use plasma pre-pared commercially for coagulase testing. Provided that a very dense, homogeneous bac-terial suspension is mixed with a loopful of reconstituted rabbit plasma, clumping should be observed in nearly 99 per cent of instances with *Staphylococcus aureus*. Inoculation of a few colonies of *S. aureus* into a tube contain-ing 0.5 ml of the same reconstituted rabbit plasma should produce a clot in over 99 per cent of instances and in nearly all cases within a four-hour period of incubation. The utiliza-tion of human plasma from normal, healthy donors requires careful quality control and titration to determine the dilution most suita-ble for routine use. The arbitrary selection of a specific dilution of donor plasma for routine purposes will result in a serious loss of sensi-tivity and of specificity in either coagulase test.

Pathogenesis and Virulence Factors. Most strains of *Staphylococcus aureus* produce α-, β-, and δ-toxins and a variety of other extracellular proteins, including leukocidin, urease, lipase, gelatinase, and phosphatase. Whereas the α-, β-, and δ-toxins are hemolytic, only the α- and β-toxins are considered to exert lethal and dermonecrotic activities. An epidermolytic toxin, which can be separated from the β-, α-, and δ-hemolysins, has been identified among phage group II staphylococci as the cause of the scalded skin syndrome. Otherwise, the roles of each of these toxins in the pathogenicity of staphylococci are unclear because of often contradictory data. Some staphylococci produce enterotoxins that pro-duce vomiting and diarrhea. Five such entero-toxins have been identified thus far from strains of *S. aureus;* however, enterotoxin production by rare strains of coagulase-nega-tive staphylococci has been reported.

Factors of importance in the development of infections due to *S. aureus* include breaks in the continuity and integrity of mucosal and cutaneous surfaces, the presence of foreign bodies or implants, prior viral diseases, ante-cedent antimicrobial therapy, and underlying diseases with defects in cellular or humoral immunity. *S. aureus* may be present among the indigenous flora of the skin, eye, upper respiratory tract, gastrointestinal tract, ure-thra, and vagina. Infection may, therefore, arise from an endogenous or an exogenous source, involve local sites, spread contiguously, or invade the bloodstream with, possibly, the development of metastatic sites of infection (Fig. 47-3). Staphylococcal food poisoning, characterized by the occurrence of vomiting and diarrhea between one and six hours fol-lowing ingestion of food containing entero-toxins, is not at all uncommon, although its true incidence is poorly defined, since it is not a reportable disease. Staphylococcal enterocoli-tis, often following prolonged preoperative intestinal antisepsis, is a disease characterized by high fever, profuse diarrhea, and hypoten-sion but is rarely seen today for reasons that are not entirely known.

Infections due to *Staphylococcus epider-midis* usually occur in patients with foreign bodies and especially in those with implanted prosthetic valves, joints, and shunts. The pathogenicity of micrococci is uncertain owing to a great extent to problems associated with their identification.

Laboratory Diagnosis. The observation microscopically of typical rounded, gram-posi-tive cocci in clusters in smears of material taken from previously unopened or drained lesions is indicative of staphylococcal infec-tion. Care should be taken in the interpreta-tion of Gram's stained smears when only sin-gle or paired organisms are seen because of their possible confusion with pneumococci and streptococci. The finding of myriads of gram-positive cocci resembling staphylococci and numerous leukocytes in the diarrheal stool of a patient who has undergone prolonged intesti-nal antisepsis prior to surgery is most sugges-tive of staphylococcal enterocolitis and re-quires immediate notification of the clinician responsible for the case.

In addition to collecting material from the infected lesion for smear and culture, consid-eration should be given in more seriously ill patients to performing blood cultures.

It is recommended that a slide coagulase test be performed initially, provided there is a sufficient number of colonies available to pre-pare a dense emulsion. The formation of clumping within 30 seconds is sufficient for the identification of *Staphylococcus aureus*. In the absence of clumping within 30 seconds or if only a few isolated staphylococcal colonies are

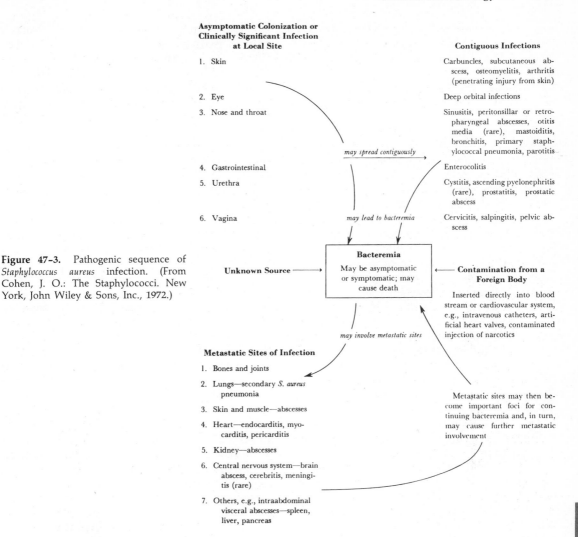

Figure 47-3. Pathogenic sequence of *Staphylococcus aureus* infection. (From Cohen, J. O.: The Staphylococci. New York, John Wiley & Sons, Inc., 1972.)

Asymptomatic Colonization or Clinically Significant Infection at Local Site

1. Skin

2. Eye

3. Nose and throat

4. Gastrointestinal

5. Urethra

6. Vagina

may spread contiguously

may lead to bacteremia

Contiguous Infections

Carbuncles, subcutaneous abscess, osteomyelitis, arthritis (penetrating injury from skin)

Deep orbital infections

Sinusitis, peritonsillar or retropharyngeal abscesses, otitis media (rare), mastoiditis, bronchitis, primary staphylococcal pneumonia, parotitis

Enterocolitis

Cystitis, ascending pyelonephritis (rare), prostatitis, prostatic abscess

Cervicitis, salpingitis, pelvic abscess

Unknown Source ⟶

Bacteremia
May be asymptomatic or symptomatic; may cause death

⟵ **Contamination from a Foreign Body**

Inserted directly into blood stream or cardiovascular system, e.g., intravenous catheters, artificial heart valves, contaminated injection of narcotics

may involve metastatic sites

Metastatic Sites of Infection

1. Bones and joints

2. Lungs—secondary *S. aureus* pneumonia

3. Skin and muscle—abscesses

4. Heart—endocarditis, myocarditis, pericarditis

5. Kidney—abscesses

6. Central nervous system—brain abscess, cerebritis, meningitis (rare)

7. Others, e.g., intraabdominal visceral abscesses—spleen, liver, pancreas

Metastatic sites may then become important foci for continuing bacteremia and, in turn, may cause further metastatic involvement

5

present, several colonies should be transferred with a wire loop into a tube containing 0.5 ml of plasma that is incubated at 35°C. for four hours and then examined for clot formation. If no clot has formed, the tube should be reincubated and re-examined after a total of 20 hours of incubation. Examination of the test after only four hours of incubation is necessary because the vast majority of isolates of *S. aureus* will produce a clot within this time interval and because some strains produce a fibrinolysin that can lyse the clot and thereby produce a false-negative reaction if the test is only observed after 20 hours of incubation. Although many species of coagulase-negative staphylococci have been proposed, their taxonomy and nomenclature have not yet been firmly established. Until they are, it is probably sufficient for the clinical laboratory to call these *Staphylococcus epidermidis*.

Staphylococci may be classified on the basis of their susceptibility to different bacteriophages. This classification is used for epidemiologic purposes in attempting to identify common source infections. Bacteriophage typing is generally available only through reference laboratories.

Antimicrobial Susceptibility. Whereas most staphylococci associated with community-acquired infections used to be susceptible to penicillin and most of those associated with nosocomially acquired infections were resistant to penicillin, this difference between susceptibility of strains according to their mode of acquisition has largely disappeared. It therefore behooves the laboratory to perform antimicrobial susceptibility tests. Penicillin, if the organism is susceptible to it, remains the antibiotic of choice in the therapy of staphylococcal infections. Methicillin resistance occurs in 5 to 20 per cent of isolates of *Staphylococcus epidermidis* but has remained rare among isolates of *S. aureus*, except in a few focal outbreaks, in the United States.

Penicillin resistance (minimal inhibitory concentration $\geq 0.2\,\mu g/ml$) is due to the production of a β-lactamase (penicillinase) associated with a plasmid in staphylococci. Methicillin resistance, on the other hand, is not related to a plasmid, and its mechanism remains unclear. Plasmid-related resistance of staphylococci to aminoglycosides, especially gentamicin, is being reported, albeit infrequently as yet. Staphylococci are generally quite susceptible in vitro to cephalosporins, erythromycin, chloramphenicol, and the lincomycins.

Prevention.   A variety of measures have been attempted to prevent staphylococcal disease. Various types of vaccines have been tried with conflicting results in the literature. Clinical laboratories are often requested to prepare autogenous vaccines; however, this practice is being discouraged because of the unstandardized nature of such vaccines, the existence of federal regulations surrounding the preparation of vaccines, and the absence of objective, carefully controlled trials substantiating their efficacy.

In some instances the application of bacterial interference has been successful in eliminating a virulent strain of *S. aureus* by replacing it with a less virulent strain (502A). Occasional reports of disease associated with *S. aureus* 502A have served to limit the use of this technique.

In the hospital the most successful means of prevention of staphylococcal disease has been careful surveillance and infection control measures, including the appropriate type of isolation of infected patients and the use of suitable control measures. Containment and the proper disposal of infected materials, implementation of methods to prevent cross-contamination, institution of standardized antiseptic techniques, and improved operating room design represent some of the measures that have been used to prevent the spread of staphylococcal infections. These measures notwithstanding, the marked decline in the incidence of infections due to *S. aureus* of phage type 80/81, so prevalent and devastating in the 1950's, remains an enigma.

Streptococcus

Definitions and Characteristics.   Streptococci are catalase-negative, gram-positive, spherical, ovoid, or lancet-shaped cocci often seen in pairs or chains. Their minimal nutritional requirements are rather complex, with considerable interspecies variability. They are facultatively anaerobic. Some strains require added CO_2 for their initial isolation but may lose this requirement in subcultures. These CO_2-dependent strains have often been called "microaerophilic"; however, use of this term should probably be discouraged because of its imprecision and the fact that most such strains can be classified into recognized species.

Streptococci can be broadly classified according to at least three schemes that unfortunately overlap and are, therefore, potentially confusing. One scheme places the streptococci into physiologic divisions: pyogenic, viridans, lactic, and enterococcal. In another they are categorized according to serologically active carbohydrates ("C" substance) into Lancefield groups. In the third scheme they are categorized according to their hemolytic reactions. Those strains that completely hemolyze the red cells about their colonies are called β-hemolytic, those that produce partial hemolysis are α-hemolytic, and those that do not hemolyze at all are γ-hemolytic. Four examples of the overlapping nature of these three schemes are given. A gamma-hemolytic *Streptococcus* may belong serologically to Lancefield's group D and physiologically be an enterococcus. Alpha hemolytic strains are generally non-groupable serologically but physiologically represent viridans streptococci. β-Hemolytic streptococci belong to a Lancefield's group and are pyogenic. Group D streptococci are usually γ-hemolytic but may be α- or β-hemolytic.

Each of these schemes for classifying streptococci serves a useful purpose so that it is generally not possible to eliminate any one of them completely. From the clinical standpoint, the separation of streptococci isolated from the blood of patients with subacute bacterial endocarditis into the physiologic divisions of viridans or enterococcus is of considerable importance in determining both the selection and the duration of antimicrobial therapy. The patient with viridans streptococcal endocarditis requires but two weeks of intramuscularly administered penicillin and aminoglycoside, while the patient with enterococcal group D streptococcal endocarditis requires three or four weeks of intravenously administered penicillin with intramuscularly administered aminoglycoside. Although the role of β-hemolytic streptococci belonging to Lancefield groups other than A in producing pharyngitis remains controversial, some physicians do advocate short-term penicillin therapy in these cases. Be that as it may, it is essential for the laboratory to distinguish between group A streptococci and those belonging to other Lancefield groups in throat cultures, since the therapy in cases with group A streptococcal pharyngitis is directed toward the prevention of non-suppurative sequelae and must be of longer duration.

From the laboratory's point of view, the hemolytic reactions on blood agar produced by streptococci represent a useful point of departure for purposes of classification (Table 47-6). It should be emphasized that there is not universal agreement on this classification but that it represents one proposed by Facklam (1977) at the Center for Disease Control, Atlanta, Ga., that has proved to be workable in my laboratory for the past several years. The methodology employed for classifying streptococci will be outlined in the section on laboratory diagnosis. It should be pointed out that most group D streptococci are not β-hemolytic and that this reaction is generally limited to a small percentage of isolates of *Streptococcus faecalis* and of *S. faecium*. These represent

Table 47-6. CLASSIFICATION OF STREPTOCOCCI*

HEMOLYTIC REACTION	GROUP	SPECIES
β	A	*S. pyogenes*
	B	*S. agalactiae*
	C	*S. equisimilis*
		S. zooepidemicus
		S. equi
	D	*S. faecalis*
	F	*S. anginosus*
	G	unnamed
	E,L,M,P,U	-
α or γ	D	*S. faecalis*
		S. faecium
		S. bovis
		S. equinus
	F	*S. anginosus*
	none of above	*S. pneumoniae*
		S. mutans
		S. sanguis
		S. mitis
		S. salivarius
		S. MG
		S. uberis
		S. acidominimus
		S. morbillorum

*Based on Facklam, 1977.

enterococcal group D streptococci, while *S. bovis* and *S. equinus* are non-enterococcal group D streptococci. The species designation for pneumococci, formerly called *Diplococcus pneumoniae*, is now *S. pneumoniae*. Commonly included among the viridans streptococci are *S. mutans, S. sanguis, S. mitis, S. salivarius,* and *S. MG*.

Group A streptococci may be typed according to their M and T protein antigens, the former of which represent essential virulence factors and convey type-specific immunity and the latter of which are unrelated to virulence and do not stimulate formation of protective antibodies. M antigens are often undetectable in unselected collections of group A streptococci; therefore, typing by the T agglutination system is also usually performed. Pneumococci are typable into more than 80 antigenic types on the basis of their capsular polysaccharide.

Pathogenesis and Virulence Factors. Group A streptococci elaborate more than 20 distinct exotoxins, including streptolysins O and S, which are hemolytic; erythrogenic toxin, which produces the rash in scarlet fever; streptokinase, which is fibrinolytic; hyaluronidase, which is a spreading factor; and diphosphopyridine nucleotidase, which is cardiotoxic. The M protein inhibits phagocytosis. The pneumococcal capsule inhibits or prevents phagocytosis.

The common clinical manifestations of streptococcal diseases and their pathogenesis are listed in Table 47-7.

Laboratory Diagnosis. The diagnosis of streptococcal pharyngitis requires laboratory confirmation because the clinical parameters typically associated with the disease are highly variable and lack specificity. The diagnosis is complicated by the fact that only half of the children with pharyngitis and with throat cultures positive for group A streptococci demonstrate an antibody response and do, therefore, have true streptococcal infection. The remaining children represent carriers, often with antibody titers indicative of previous infections with pharyngitis due to other causes. Since, however, the demonstration of antibody response is only helpful retrospectively, the throat culture remains for all practical purposes the most frequently relied upon diagnostic test. The laboratory is frequently under pressure from the child's attending physician and he or she, in turn, from the child's parents to produce a rapid result, despite the fact that a delay in the initiation

Table 47-7. COMMON CLINICAL MANIFESTATIONS AND
PATHOGENESIS OF STREPTOCOCCAL DISEASE

DISEASE	RESERVOIR	ETIOLOGY
Group A		
Local and invasive forms		
pharyngitis	open lesions, normal skin, upper	intimate contact, minor trauma,
skin and soft tissue infections	respiratory tract, perianal area;	insect bites, scratching; surgery,
superficial pyodermas	?domestic animals, fomites, in-	burns, wounds
deeper skin and soft tissue	sect vectors	
erysipelas		
omphalitis		
septicemia		
Poststreptococcal diseases		
rheumatic fever	-	?autoimmunity, cross-reactivity be-
acute glomerulonephritis	-	tween streptococcal components
		and mammalian tissue
Group B		
neonatal sepsis and meningitis	upper respiratory tract, vagina,	?
	nosocomial	
Group D		
endocarditis	oral cavity, intestinal tract, vagina	instrumentation of oral cavity and
urinary tract infection		urinary tract resulting in tran-
intra-abdominal, pelvic abscess		sient bacteremia; abdominal or
		pelvic surgery; pre-existing val-
		vular disease, prosthetic valve.
Viridans streptococci		
endocarditis		
intra-abdominal, pelvic, pulmonary,		(as for group D)
brain abscess		
Streptococcus pneumoniae		
pneumonia	upper respiratory tract	prior viral infection of upper or
sinusitis		lower respiratory tract, respira-
otitis		tory tract injury, pulmonary con-
mastoiditis		gestion, malnutrition, debility,
meningitis		sickle cell disease

of therapy for a few days does not significantly alter the risk of developing non-suppurative sequelae and does not appreciably
change the course of the disease. It therefore
behooves the laboratory to perform throat cultures properly and to provide accurate results.

The posterior pharynx, tonsillar pillars or
tonsils, and areas of exudation, inflammation,
or ulceration should be swabbed vigorously
with minimal oral contamination. Group A
streptococci on a swab in transport medium,
e.g., Stuart's, will survive at room temperature
for at least five days and usually longer. The
swab should be inoculated onto a quarter to a
third of a Petri dish containing 5% sheep
blood. A wire loop is then used to streak the
inoculum for isolation over the remaining agar
surface and for stabbing the surface of the
agar in areas of the heaviest and lightest inocula. Cultures should be incubated for 18 to 24
hours at 35°C. in an atmosphere of room air.
The presence of added CO_2 or anaerobiasis
does not enhance the recovery of group A

streptococci but does increase significantly the
recovery of non-group A β-hemolytic streptococci. As has already been mentioned, the role
of non-group A β-hemolytic streptococci in
producing pharyngitis has not been clearly
established; however, pharyngitis associated
with the isolation of these groups of streptococci is usually treated, if at all, with short
term (3 to 5 days) antimicrobial therapy in
contrast to that associated with group A
streptococci in which therapy is given for 10
days, primarily to prevent the potential non-
suppurative complications of group A streptococcal infection. Be that as it may, incubation
of agar plates in an atmosphere of room air
does improve the specificity of throat cultures
for group A streptococci.

Presumptive identification of group A
streptococci by the bacitracin differentiation
disc test is best accomplished with a pure subculture of β-hemolytic colonies, since the direct application of the disc to the primary
culture plate provides unreliable results. The

incidence of isolation of group A streptococci and the proportion of β-hemolytic streptococci representing group A varies seasonally in many parts of the country. In our laboratory the proportion representing group A has varied from 25 to nearly 70 per cent, with the greatest proportion occurring during the winter and spring months. Nearly 10 per cent of non-group A β-hemolytic streptococci will be inhibited by bacitracin, while fewer than 1 per cent of group A strains will fail to be inhibited. It is for these reasons that bacitracin differentiation is considered to be a test for presumptive identification of group A streptococci.

Other presumptive grouping tests for streptococci include those for determining the hydrolysis of sodium hippurate and the hydrolysis of esculin in the presence of 40 per cent bile (Table 47-8). In contrast to bacitracin differentiation, the bile-esculin test is highly sensitive and specific for group D streptococci. This is important because some strains of enterococcal group D streptococci hydrolyze hippurate, a reaction which is otherwise very sensitive and specific for group B. Bile-esculin positive strains can be further subdivided into enterococcal and non-enterococcal group D streptococci by determining their ability to grow in 6.5 per cent NaCl. A simple and reliable presumptive test for identifying group B streptococci is the CAMP reaction, which is a lytic phenomenon that occurs when group B streptococci are grown in the presence of β-toxin-producing staphylococci (Darling, 1975).

Definitive grouping of streptococci is usually performed by serologic means. The group-specific "C" substance can be extracted from cells by acid treatment, autoclaving, or enzymatic action. The extract and antiserum usually are combined in a capillary tube, and a white, flocculent precipitate forms at the antigen-antibody interface when the two are homologous. Counterimmunoelectrophoresis with and without (Hill, 1975) extraction procedures have also been successfully used for grouping streptococci and are both rapid and accurate. Protein A containing stabilized staphylococci coated with group-specific antibody have provided another rapid and accurate approach to grouping (Christensen, 1973; Edwards, 1974).

Immunofluorescence has been used for identifying group A and group B streptococci. With group A streptococci both direct and indirect techniques have been used. In the former a throat swab is incubated in Todd-Hewitt broth for between two and four hours, and a smear of spun sediment is stained with fluorescein-labeled anti-group A streptococcal reagent. This test is rapid, sensitive, and specific. In approximately 5 per cent of instances cultures will be positive and smears negative; the converse occurs in less than 1 per cent of instances. Fluorescent microscopy (indirect) of smears of isolated β-hemolytic colonies stained with group-specific fluorescein-labeled conjugate is a rapid, sensitive, and specific method for identifying group A and group B streptococci. For group A streptococci this approach is somewhat more economical in its use of labeled conjugate than performing direct fluorescent microscopy of smears of all throat swabs received in the laboratory.

Table 47-8. PRESUMPTIVE TESTS FOR GROUPING STREPTOCOCCI

TEST	A	B	D enterococcal	D non-enterococcal
Bacitracin inhibition*	+	−	−	−
Hippurate hydrolysis†	−	+	−	−
Esculin hydrolysis in presence of 40% bile	−	−	+	+
Growth in 6.5% NaCl	−	−	+	−

* Approximately 10% of non-group A β-hemolytic streptococci are inhibited by bacitracin.

† Some enterococci hydrolyze hippurate; therefore, hippurate-positive streptococci should have a negative bile-esculin reaction before being reported as belonging to group B.

Identification of groups other than A, B, and D is not necessary for routine clinical purposes. The majority will be streptococci belonging to Lancefield groups C, F, and G.

The identification of α- and γ-hemolytic streptococci has been discussed by Facklam (1977). For practical purposes, it is important to identify the group D streptococci, and it is helpful to distinguish between enterococcal and non-enterococcal strains, especially when they are isolated from the blood. It is also important to identify *Streptococcus pneumoniae*. This may be readily accomplished by use of a disc containing ethyl hydrocupreine hydrochloride (optochin) or of a bile solubility test with 10 per cent sodium deoxycholate. In the former test an inhibitory zone of at least 18 mm is indicative of susceptibility and that the organism is a pneumococcus. Direct application of 10 per cent deoxycholate solution will produce lysis of α-hemolytic colonies which are pneumococci. In clinical practice it is seldom necessary to provide further identification of the α- and γ- or viridans streptococci, and it is satisfactory to report them according to their hemolytic reactions or as viridans streptococci.

Antimicrobial Susceptibility. β-Hemolytic streptococci are inhibited by 0.005 to 0.01 μg/ml of penicillin with the exceptions of group B streptococci, which require up to eight times as much penicillin for inhibition, and enterococcal group D streptococci, which require 0.8 to 6.25 μg/ml for inhibition and nearly none of which are killed by as much as 100 μg/ml. At any rate, susceptibility testing with penicillin of group A streptococci isolated from patients with persistent or recurrent infection is not indicated. Among other orally administered antibiotics, resistance of group A streptococci to erythromycin and cephalexin is rare, but to the tetracyclines it is relatively frequent (10 to 30 per cent), so that susceptibility testing of isolates from penicillin allergic patients is indicated.

Although there have been isolated reports of diminished susceptibility of pneumococci to penicillin (0.1 to 0.5 μg/ml) in the United States, Australia, and New Guinea and of penicillin resistance in South Africa, the incidence of such strains remains so extremely low that routine susceptibility testing of pneumococci with penicillin is not warranted at this time. As with the group A streptococci, however, erythromycin resistance occurs rarely and tetracycline resistance not infrequently in pneumococci.

One of the best examples of the requirement for combined antimicrobial therapy is provided by the enterococcal group D streptococci which are not killed by high concentrations of penicillins or aminoglycosides and which cause endocarditis that cannot be cured by either of these classes of antibiotics alone. Combinations of a penicillin and an aminoglycoside are synergistic both *in vitro* and *in vivo* against these organisms. Although usually very susceptible to penicillin, the viridans streptococci are also synergistically affected by a combination of an aminoglycoside and penicillin. Susceptibility testing of some viridans streptococci can be difficult because of their fastidious nature and their requirement for CO_2.

Prevention and Control. Much thought has been devoted to the detection of streptococcal pharyngitis and to the prevention of its non-suppurative sequelae without, however, the achievement of a totally satisfactory solution. Many of the problems precluding satisfactory solution have been reviewed by Wannamaker (1972). Among these is the fact that group A streptococci account for but a small proportion of all respiratory illnesses and for approximately a third of acute pharyngitides. Many from whom group A streptococci are isolated are carriers and do not represent true infections. Acute nephritis is often not prevented by early treatment of pharyngitis and is clearly related to infection with a nephritogenic strain. Finally, approximately a third of children developing rheumatic fever give no antecedent history of upper respiratory tract infection. The value, therefore, of massive community or statewide programs of culturing all sore throats in school children and requiring treatment of all from whom group A streptococci were recovered remains unclear and requires futher objective study.

There is general agreement on the need for a streptococcal vaccine to protect against acute nephritis and rheumatic fever in high risk groups; however, much work and many problems remain in this area. Type-specific and polyvalent pneumococcal vaccines have been evaluated successfully in clinical trials; however, geographic and temporal variations in the incidence of pneumococcal infections and types, as well as the identification and vaccination of high-risk populations, pose significant problems in vaccine use.

GRAM-NEGATIVE

Neisseria and Branhamella

Definitions and Characteristics. These genera are non-motile, catalase-, and oxidase-positive, aerobic gram-negative cocci which are often arranged in pairs with flattened adjacent surfaces. The genus *Branhamella* was separated from the neisseriae on the basis of differences in DNA base composition. It consists of the species *Branhamella catarrhalis*, although it has been proposed that *Neisseria caviae* and *Neisseria ovis* also be placed in the genus *Branhamella*. Recognized species of *Neisseria* are *N. meningitidis, N. gonorrhoeae, N. sicca, N. subflava, N. flavescens,* and *N. mucosa.*

Closely resembling *Neisseria* and *Branhamella* are the genera *Moraxella* and *Acinetobacter,* which can produce rods, however, in contrast to *Neisseria* and *Branhamella,* which produce only cocci. These rod forms, sometimes referred to as coccobacillary, will be considered in a later section dealing with non-fermenting gram-negative bacilli.

With the exception of *Acinetobacter,* all of these organisms are somewhat fastidious in their growth requirements, requiring in some instances the addition of blood, serum, cholesterol, or oleic acid to the medium to counteract growth inhibitors. Gonococci and meningococci generally require prompt incubation in CO_2 for growth; however, this requirement is strain-dependent, varies with the phase of the organism's growth curve, and is often lost in subcultures. Gonococci and meningococci are not inhibited by the presence of vancomycin or lincomycin, colistin, and nystatin, a characteristic that is particularly useful in their selective isolation from specimens contaminated with other bacteria.

Pathogenesis and Virulence Factors. Although opportunistic infections due to species of *Branhamella* and of *Neisseria* other than *N. gonorrhoeae* and *N. meningitidis* have occasionally been reported in compromised hosts, these species are generally non-pathogenic. The pathogenesis and clinical manifestations of meningococcal and gonococcal diseases differ considerably and will, therefore, be considered separately.

Meningococci may colonize the mucous membranes of the upper respiratory tract, an event that is usually followed in 7 to 10 days by the formation of bactericidal and hemagglutinating antibodies which, however, may not eliminate the carrier state but which convey group-specific immunity. In a few cases, however, disease results shortly after colonization, most frequently in the form of meningococcemia and meningitis (Figure 47-4). The organism also has a tendency to invade serous membranes and joint tissues with the development of pleuritis, pericarditis, and arthritis. Carriage of meningococci in the nasopharynx is not uncommon; however, a direct correlation between carrier rates and incidence of meningococcal disease has not been established, with the possible exception of members of large households or households with an infant or childhood case during epidemics of meningococcal disease. Meningococci have also been isolated from genital sources, where their clinical significance remains uncertain but where they may be readily misidentified as gonococci unless appropriate tests for distinguishing these two species are carried out.

The principal virulence factor of meningo-

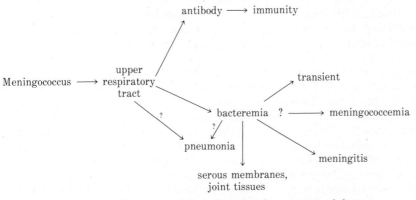

Figure 47-4. Pathogenesis and clinical aspects of meningococcal disease.

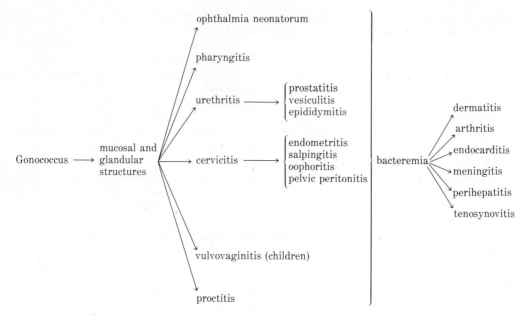

Figure 47–5. Pathogenesis and clinical manifestations of gonococcal disease.

cocci is a lipopolysaccharide-endotoxin complex, which in experimental animals activates the clotting cascade, depositing fibrin in small vessels, producing hemorrhage in the adrenals and other organs, and altering peripheral vascular resistance, leading to shock and death.

The pathogenesis and clinical manifestations of gonococcal infections differ somewhat from those of the meningococci (Figure 47–5). Pathogenic types (1 and 2) of *Neisseria gonorrhoeae* adhere by means of pili, which nonpathogenic types (3 and 4) lack, to various human cells. These pili, which represent one of the principal virulence factors of the gonococcus, also may inhibit phagocytosis, are antigenically heterogeneous, and stimulate strain-specific antibody formation. Other possible virulence factors of *N. gonorrhoeae* are less clearly defined at this time.

Laboratory Diagnosis. The single most important element in the laboratory diagnosis of meningo- and gonococcal diseases is the specimen, its proper selection, collection, and transport to the laboratory. These points have already been discussed elsewhere but bear re-emphasis. The pathogenic species are sensitive to drying and extremes of temperature, and material should be cultured promptly for their recovery. They are mesophilic and grow poorly, if at all, at room temperature. Many require prompt incubation in CO_2 (2 to 18 per cent) for primary isolation. Media containing

chocolatized blood are commonly used for cultures and should contain antibiotics, i.e., vancomycin or lincomycin, as well as colistin, nystatin, and trimethoprim, if the specimen is contaminated with indigenous flora. Direct inoculation of specimens "at the bedside" is, therefore, often performed. This can be accomplished in several ways: the inoculation of Thayer-Martin medium with prompt incubation at 35°C. in CO_2, most frequently a candle jar; or the inoculation of modified Thayer-Martin medium in a bottle or chamber containing CO_2 (Transgrow) or in which CO_2 can be generated from a citric acid-bicarbonate tablet (JEMBEC). If any of these culture systems must be mailed to a reference laboratory for processing, they must first be incubated overnight to ensure growth of the organisms.

Cerebrospinal fluid from patients with bacterial meningitis should be rapidly transported to the laboratory for culture and must not be stored under refrigeration under any circumstances. Synovial and pericardial fluids should also be handled expeditiously. In these cases contamination of the specimen with indigenous flora is rarely a problem and selective media, such as Thayer-Martin, need not be used; however, chocolatized blood agar supplemented with yeast extract should be used not only for the recovery of meningococci but also for that of other pathogenic bacteria which can cause infection of these sites.

Table 47-9. DIFFERENTIATION OF SPECIES OF *NEISSERIA* AND *BRANHAMELLA**

	N. GONORRHOEAE	N. MENINGITIDIS	N. LACTAMICA†	N. SICCA	N. SUBFLAVA	N. FLAVESCENS	N. MUCOSA	B. CATARRHALIS
growth								
Thayer-Martin medium	+	+	+	−	−	−	−·	−
nutrient agar, 25C	−	−	d	d	d	+	+	+
oxidase	+	+	+	+	+	+	+	+
β-galactosidase	−	−	+	−	−	−	−	−
reduction of nitrate	−	−	−	−	−	−	+	+
production of acid from								
glucose	+	+	+	+	+	−	+	−
maltose	−	+	+	+	+	−	+	−
lactose	−	−	+	−	−	−	−	−
sucrose	−	−	−	+	v	−	+	−
fructose	−	−	−	+	v	−	+	−

*+, ≥90% of strains positive; −, ≥90% of strains negative; d, some strains positive and others negative; v, inconstant reaction within strain.
†Species incertae sedis.

Characteristics that may be useful in differentiating the species of *Neisseria* and *Branhamella* are listed in Table 47-9. The isolation from a genital source of oxidase-positive gram-negative diplococci from Thayer-Martin medium constitutes presumptive identification of *Neisseria gonorrhoeae*. Confirmatory tests are, however, recommended because of the occasional isolation of *N. meningitidis* and *N. lactamicus* from such sources. In cultures of the oropharynx carriage of these other two species is more frequent so that confirmatory tests must always be made with oxidase-positive gram-negative diplococci isolated from these sources on Thayer-Martin medium. As a rule, confirmatory tests may be limited to those for detecting the production of β-galactosidase and of acid from glucose, maltose, and sucrose. Immunofluorescence of colonies of *N. gonorrhoeae* is sufficiently specific to be used for the identification of this species.

Many approaches to determining acid production from carbohydrate by neisseriae have been described, reflecting the occasional occurrence of problems with the customarily recommended cystine tryptophan agar (CTA) medium. One method which has proved to be far more satisfactory in our hands is that prescribed by Flynn (1972) in which carbohydrates (1 per cent) are added to GC medium base supplemented with ferric nitrate, L-glutamine, and phenol red.

Antimicrobial Susceptibility. Meningococci have remained susceptible to the penicillins and chloramphenicol to date, so that determining their susceptibility to these agents for therapeutic reasons is seldom necessary. Testing the inhibitory activity of sulfonamides, however, is indicated at the present time because of the proven efficacy of sulfonamides in eradicating the carriage of susceptible strains (minimal inhibitory concentration ≤ 10 μg/ml) from close contacts. Currently, 23 per cent of case isolates from the United States are resistant to sulfonamides (Center for Disease Control, 1976). All are susceptible to rifampin, the agent recommended in the United States for prophylaxis among household contacts unless susceptibility to sulfonamides is demonstrated. One problem, however, with the use of rifampin is the emergence of resistant meningococci. Some experts, therefore, prefer a plan of careful observation of contacts of cases with sulfonamide-resistant meningococcal disease.

Despite the fact that the concentrations of penicillin required to inhibit gonococci have increased somewhat in recent years, leading to recommendations that probenecid and increased dosages of penicillin be administered, outright penicillin resistance of gonococci due to β-lactamase was not reported until 1976. The prevalence of these strains is unknown, but they can be rapidly detected by testing for the presence of β-lactamase by any one of several acidimetric or iodometric methods. In the United States gonococci have remained susceptible to spectinomycin and tetracycline, which are the recommended alternatives to the penicillins in the treatment of gonorrhea.

Prevention. Polysaccharide vaccines against *Neisseria meningitidis* serogroups A and C have been licensed in this country and may be of value for travellers in countries known to have epidemic meningococcal disease, as an adjunct to antibiotic prophylaxis in household contacts of patients with meningococcal disease, and in populations at risk in epidemic situations. A satisfactory serogroup B vaccine has not been developed. Antibiotic prophylaxis should be limited to household contacts and those who have had contact with patients' oral secretions. Rifampin, 600 mg q12h for 2 days, is the drug of choice currently unless susceptibility to sulfonamides can be demonstrated. Some, as has already been pointed out, prefer to observe contacts carefully when sulfonamide resistance is demonstrated. One of the most common dilemmas occurring in laboratories is the isolation and identification of meningococci from throat swabs taken from patients with pharyngitis who coincidentally are carriers of this organism. Since reporting such findings is rarely of any clinical value and usually creates considerable consternation, it is recommended that the species designation of neisseriae from throat cultures not be reported unless (1) it is requested for purposes of identifying carriers or (2) it is *Neisseria gonorrhoeae*, the isolation of which is virtually always of clinical importance. To re-emphasize a point made earlier, when specific requests are made for culture of meningococci and gonococci, the specimen should be inoculated onto modified Thayer-Martin medium.

The use of pre-exposure antibiotics to prevent gonococcal disease is discouraged because of the potential risks of sensitization and the emergence of resistant strains. The sole exception to this rule is the application of silver nitrate solution or antibiotic ointment to the eyes of newborns to prevent gonococcal ophthalmia.

CORYNEFORM AND RELATED BACTERIA

The term coryneform has been used to describe gram-positive, non-spore-forming, non-filamentous rods which may exhibit pleomorphic morphology. In its broadest sense, the term might include *Actinomyces*, *Propionibacterium*, *Mycobacterium*, and *Nocardia*, as well as *Corynebacterium*, *Listeria*, and *Erysipelothrix;* however, taxonomists disagree as to the proper limits of the term. For purposes of simplicity of organization in this book, the term will be limited to *Corynebacterium*, *Listeria*, and *Erysipelothrix*. No endorsement, implied or otherwise, is intended by this approach.

Corynebacterium

Definitions and Characteristics. The corynebacteria or "diphtheroids," as they are sometimes called, are widely distributed in nature and on the mucous membranes and skin of man and animals. Most species are rarely pathogenic in humans, with the notable exceptions of *Corynebacterium diphtheriae* and its closely related species or varieties, *C. diphtheriae* var. *ulcerans* and *C. pseudotuberculosis*. *C. pyogenes* and *C. haemolyticum* have been associated with diseases in humans; however, other than in their microscopic morphology, they share few characteristics in common with *C. diphtheriae*, and their taxonomic status remains uncertain at this time. Other species of *Corynebacterium* have been clearly associated with infections of implanted prosthetic materials, e.g., heart valves, cerebrospinal fluid shunts, joints, have caused subacute bacterial endocarditis, and have been involved in a variety of opportunistic infections. Their etiologic role in causing such infections is established with considerable difficulty and often only after their repeated isolation from a particular source.

Pathogenesis and Virulence. Lysogenic strains of *Corynebacterium diphtheriae* harboring prophages carrying the *TOX+* gene excrete a toxin which enters the body of susceptible persons through lesions in epithelial surfaces or by attachment to and transport into epithelial cells, whence it is transported via the blood and lymphatics to a variety of organs, including the heart, kidneys, liver, pancreas, lungs, and peripheral nervous system. The exotoxin is a protein with a molecular weight of about 62,000, 25 ng of which injected subcutaneously will kill a 250 g guinea pig in four or five days. The organisms and their exotoxin produce a serum exudate and cellular infiltrate of the mucous membrane in the pharynx, leading to formation of a grayish pseudomembrane. Although toxin production and pathogenicity are often considered to be synonymous, pseudomembranes may form in persons infected with non-toxigenic strains. Extension of the pseudomembrane superiorly into the nasopharynx or inferiorly into the larynx may be so marked as to produce respiratory obstruction. Although *C. diphtheriae* infections of other parts of the body do occur, the most frequent ones observed in the United States today are those of the skin.

Transmission of *C. diphtheriae* is by droplet nuclei from the respiratory tract or by contact from cutaneous foci of infection.

Laboratory Diagnosis. Because of the relative rarity of diphtheria in the United States today, the diagnosis may be overlooked clinically and the laboratory may easily fail to recognize its causative agent in cultures. A tentative diagnosis must always be provided to the laboratory so that the specimen will be inoculated onto suitable media for isolation of the organism. Cystine-tellurite (CT) blood agar is the preferred medium for isolation of the organism, while the more nutritionally deficient Loeffler's (coagulated serum) or Pai's (coagulated egg) medium is more useful for microscopic morphology. The cells are often pleomorphic in appearance, are characteristically arranged side by side in palisade formation, and frequently display metachromatic granules. On CT medium colonies of *C. diphtheriae* are grayish black after 48 hours of incubation. Three colony types can be encountered: *gravis,* which are large, flat, dark gray, and have irregular edges with radial striations; *mitis,* which are black, convex, and moist; and *intermedius,* which are quite small and black.

Strains of corynebacteria can be speciated with biochemical tests (Table 47-10), but it is necessary to establish the virulence of isolates suspected of being *C. diphtheriae* by determining whether or not they produce exotoxin. This can be done by inoculating a broth culture subcutaneously into two guinea pigs, one of which has received diphtheria antitoxin intraperitoneally two hours previously. The unprotected guinea pig will die within one to four days if the inoculated strain was toxigenic. Alternatively, the elaboration of toxin may be detected *in vitro* by streaking the culture to be tested at right angles to a paper strip impregnated with antitoxin and embedded in agar and observing the formation of precipitin lines at 45 degree angles to the paper strip. Many modifications of this test have been described resulting from the failure of toxigenic strains to produce precipitin lines or from the formation of non-specific lines by nontoxigenic strains. The potency of the antitoxin, the inoculum size, the type of enrichment serum, and the duration of incubation all affect the outcome of this test.

The classification of the oral and skin corynebacteria or diphtheroids is difficult and confusing. Multiple approaches have been proposed and are based on characteristics such as oleate dependence, fluorescence, nitrate reduction, urease activity, and carbohydrate fermentations. Published fermentation reactions are highly variable, often conflicting, and reflect, among other things, the organisms' growth characteristics and whether or not the basal medium has been supplemented with serum or a source of oleate, e.g., Tween-80.

Antimicrobial Susceptibility. Although antitoxin remains the only specific method of treatment of diphtheria, antibiotics are administered to patients with disease and to asymptomatic carriers of toxigenic strains. *Corynebacterium diphtheriae* is usually inhibited by ≤ 0.5 µg/ml of penicillin, ≤ 0.05 µg/ml of erythromycin, and ≤ 0.3 µg/ml of clindamycin. Because of its activity and because it is well tolerated, erythromycin is often used for this purpose; however, benzathine penicillin may be useful in instances in which patient cooperation is suspect. Because of its potential side effects, clindamycin is not the agent of choice in such cases.

The antimicrobial susceptibilities of other species of corynebacteria or diphtheroids are far less predictable. They are, however, often resistant to the penicillins and cephalosporins,

Table 47-10. DIFFERENTIAL CHARACTERISTICS OF SOME SPECIES WITHIN THE GENUS *CORYNEBACTERIUM**

TEST	C. DIPHTHERIAE	C. ULCERANS	C. PSEUDOTUBERCULOSIS	C. XEROSIS	C. PSEUDODIPHTHERITICUM	C. HAEMOLYTICUM	C. PYOGENES
catalase	+	+	+	+	+	−	−
hemolysis	+	+	+	−	−	+	+
gelatinase	−	+	d	−	−	−	+
urease	−	+	d	−	+	−	−
NO$_3$ reduction	+	−	d	+	+	−	−
sucrose fermentation	−	−	d	+	−	d	+

*d = variable.

variably susceptible to most other antibiotics, and almost uniformly susceptible to vancomycin. The therapy of infections due to these organisms is often complicated by the presence of compromised host defenses and of implanted prosthetic materials.

Prevention. The methods of prevention of diseases due to corynebacteria are almost exclusively those directed against diphtheria and include active and passive immunization programs with supplemental antibiotics to eliminate the carrier state of toxigenic strains during epidemics. Immunity can be determined by the Schick test in which a small amount of toxin is injected intradermally on one forearm and toxoid into the other. The absence of erythema, induration, and necrosis 120 hours later in either forearm is indicative of immunity.

Listeria

Definitions and Characteristics. The pathogenic species for man, *Listeria monocytogenes*, is most successfully isolated from tissue by culture of finely ground material, since it is frequently present within cells. Fluids and swabs are directly plated on conventional bacteriologic media. The organism's growth is optimal at temperatures of 30 to 37°C.; however, growth does occur between 3 and 45°C. and does, in fact, appear to be enhanced in some instances after storage of the specimen under refrigeration. It is, therefore, recommended that material from patients with suspected listeriosis be stored under refrigeration and that, if their initial cultures are negative, they be recultured at regular intervals over a period of three months.

L. monocytogenes is a facultatively anaerobic, catalase- and Voges-Proskauer-positive, gram-positive, non-spore-forming, non-acid-fast organism which may appear coccoid, coccobacillary, or bacillary microscopically. Rods may arrange themselves into palisades with V and Y forms typical of other coryneform bacteria. A narrow zone of β-hemolysis is produced on blood agar by fresh isolates. A characteristic tumbling motility occurs at room temperature but rarely at 35°C. This same temperature-dependent motility is also noted in semisolid media.

Pathogenesis and Virulence. *L. monocytogenes* is a rare or rarely recognized cause of meningitis and septicemia, predominantly in newborns, although it has a predilection for causing serious disease in patients with lymphoproliferative disorders. Cases of brain abscess, endocarditis, oculoglandular fever, pneumonia, urethritis, infectious mononucleosis-like disease, and habitual abortion have been associated with *Listeria*. A number of cases of *Listeria* sepsis and meningitis in renal transplant recipients have been described.

Intraperitoneal injection of the organism is fatal to rabbits and mice, with autopsy findings of foci of necrosis in the liver, spleen, lungs, adrenals, tonsils, and intestinal tract. The inflammatory infiltrate is predominantly mononuclear. The organism is an intracellular parasite, like tubercle bacilli, salmonellae, and brucellae; however, relatively little is known about its mechanisms of pathogenicity. Its hemolysin is lethal when injected into mice and may function by disrupting membranes. Its mode of transmission has not yet been clearly established.

Laboratory Diagnosis. Since listeriosis is a rare disease, it is rarely suspected clinically and the organism is often disregarded in the laboratory as being a diphtheroid or *Corynebacterium*, which it resembles microscopically. The isolation, especially from cerebrospinal fluid or blood, of small grayish-blue colonies surrounded by a narrow zone of β-hemolysis on blood agar should make one think of *L. monocytogenes* and lead one to perform a test for motility at 20°C. It does produce catalase and acid from glucose, trehalose, and salicin. A rapid presumptive diagnosis can also be made by fluorescent microscopy.

The organism is often stated to be easily confused with *Erysipelothrix rhusiopathiae*; however, there are several distinguishing characteristics between these two species (Table 47-11).

Antimicrobial Susceptibility. *L. monocytogenes* is usually inhibited by $\leq 0.5 \, \mu g/ml$ of penicillin or ampicillin, $\leq 6 \, \mu g/ml$ of chlor-

Table 47-11. DIFFERENTIAL CHARACTERISTICS OF *LISTERIA MONOCYTOGENES* AND *ERYSIPELOTHRIX RHUSIOPATHIAE*

TEST	L. MONOCYTOGENES	E. RHUSIOPATHIAE
β-hemolysis	+	−
growth at 4°C.	+	−
catalase	+	−
motility	+	−
esculin hydrolysis	+	−
gluconate utilization	+	−
Voges-Proskauer	+	−

amphenicol, $\leq 4 \mu g/ml$ of tetracycline, ≤ 16 $\mu g/ml$ of kanamycin, and $\leq 4 \mu g/ml$ of genta-micin. Considerably higher concentrations of these antimicrobial agents are required for bactericidal activity, although substantially increased killing has been demonstrated in studies with combinations of penicillin or am-picillin with an aminoglycoside. Ampicillin, alone or in combination with an aminoglyco-side, has been used successfully in the treat-ment of infections due to *Listeria monocyto-genes*.

Erysipelothrix rhusiopathiae

Definitions and Characteristics. *Ery-sipelothrix* is a catalase-negative, non-spore-forming, non-motile, facultatively anaerobic gram-positive bacillus which has a world-wide distribution. Cells from smooth phase colonies are small, straight, or slightly curved rods, while those from rough colonies are long and filamentous.

Pathogenesis and Virulence. *Erysipelo-thrix* infection is usually transmitted to man from animals by means of skin wounds pro-duced with contaminated objects or in contact with blood, flesh, viscera, or feces of infected animals. The organism can be present in many species of mammals, birds, and fish; however, its most important animal reservoir is in do-mestic swine in which it can produce acute, subacute, subclinical, and chronic infection. Erysipeloid is principally an occupational dis-ease of individuals in contact with animals and their products or by-products and wastes. The most common form of erysipeloid is a local cutaneous infection manifested by pain, swel-ling, and a cutaneous eruption characterized by a slowly progressive, slightly elevated, vio-laceous zone around the site of inoculation. The swelling and erythema migrate peripher-ally and the lesion involutes without desqua-mation. Systemic disease is rare, but numer-ous single cases of septicemia and endocarditis have been reported. Also rarely reported have been cases of arthritis and brain abscess.

Laboratory Diagnosis. Since positive cul-tures infrequently result from swab specimens of a local cutaneous lesion, biopsy or tissue aspirates represent the specimens of choice and should be placed into an infusion broth containing 1 per cent glucose followed by sub-culture onto blood agar. *Erysipelothrix* is rap-idly fatal to mice when injected intraperi-toneally and can be isolated in pure culture from the heart blood. Conventional blood cul-ture media are suitable for its isolation from blood.

Erysipelothrix is oxidase- and catalase-neg-ative. Characteristically, it produces H_2S in triple sugar iron agar (TSIA). It is non-motile, does not reduce nitrates to nitrite, and fer-ments glucose and lactose. It can be readily distinguished from *Listeria* (Table 47-11).

Antimicrobial Susceptibility. *Erysipelo-thrix* is susceptible to the penicillins, cephalo-sporins, erythromycin, clindamycin, chloram-phenicol, and tetracyclines but resistant to sulfonamides and aminoglycosides.

Prevention. Preventive measures include an awareness on the part of those occupation-ally or recreationally (e.g., hunters) exposed to infected animals and their observance of sim-ple hygienic practices; rodent control; and regular disinfection of fish tanks. Immuniza-tion is ineffective.

AEROBIC SPORE-FORMING BACILLI

Bacillus

Definitions and Characteristics. The cells of members of this genus are strictly aerobic or facultatively anaerobic, rod-shaped, spore-forming, gram-positive, and catalase-positive. With the notable exception of the anthrax bacillus, they are usually motile by means of lateral or peritrichous flagella. Some strains will stain gram-negatively and because of their variable oxidase reactions are con-fused with gram-negative bacilli. The most reliable diagnostic characteristic of the genus is spore formation which occurs optimally and on a variety of media under aerobic conditions at 25 to 30°C. In Gram's stained smears endo-spores are detectable by the presence of un-stained defects or holes within the cell. The spores themselves can be stained by any one of several methods.

Pathogenesis and Virulence Factors. Of the 22 distinct species of *Bacillus*, *Bacillus anthracis* is the only one that is uniformly and highly pathogenic. Great care must be exer-cised when handling material suspected of harboring this species. Work should be per-formed in biologic safety cabinets by gloved, gowned, masked, and immunized personnel; work surfaces must be disinfected with 5 per cent hypochlorite or 5 per cent phenol; and all supplies, materials, and equipment must be decontaminated. Animals should be inoculated only by properly attired and immunized personnel, should be housed separately, and should be autoclaved and incinerated after death.

There are three forms of anthrax which are recognized: cutaneous, inhalation, and intestinal. In its cutaneous form, anthrax produces a small, red, macular lesion that progresses on to a vesicle and finally necrosis with formation of a characteristic black eschar. Regional lymphadenopathy and septicemia may occur. The mortality in untreated cases with this form of disease is approximately 20 per cent. Inhalation of anthrax spores can lead to acute bronchopneumonia, mediastinitis, and septicemia. The mortality in recognized cases with this form of disease is nearly 100 per cent. Intestinal anthrax follows the ingestion of contaminated food and is manifested by nausea, vomiting, and diarrhea. In some cases there is gastrointestinal bleeding, followed by prostration, shock, and death. Septicemia can occur in all three forms of anthrax and may lead to a fatal purulent meningitis.

A major factor in the organism's pathogenic capabilities is its glutamyl polypeptide capsule that inhibits phagocytosis but antibodies to which are not protective against the disease. A complex toxin with three components is responsible for the signs and symptoms of anthrax.

Man becomes infected with anthrax by contact with and inhalation or ingestion of infected animals, their carcasses, or their by-products. Cattle, sheep, horses, and goats are the animals most frequently infected and provide a ready source of vegetative organisms which sporulate and perpetuate the environmental contamination.

Although usually saprophytic, other species of *Bacillus* have been recognized as causing disease. *B. cereus* has been associated with eye and ear infections, pneumonias, post-traumatic wound infections, septicemias, and endocarditis. Patients with pneumonias and septicemias are often immunosuppressed.

Acute diarrheal disease due to *B. cereus* has been reported in the European literature for many years but has been scarcely recognized in this country. The organism is widely distributed in foods, ordinarily in low numbers; however, it can reproduce rapidly to levels as high as 10^7 to 10^8/g of food. This almost invariably results from bulk preparation of foods followed by storage at room temperature with or without modest reheating prior to their being served. An illness characterized mostly by vomiting has been described in association with the consumption of cooked rice in Chinese restaurants. Illness in either case follows a brief incubation period of less than 18 hours. Diarrhea is due to an enterotoxin similar in activity to that of *Vibrio cholerae* and *Escherichia coli* which produces fluid accumulation in the rabbit ileal loop preparation. Other cytotoxic products of *Bacillus* have precluded use of tissue cultures for detection of the enterotoxin.

Laboratory Diagnosis. Swabs of the vesicles and under the edge of the eschar in the cutaneous form of anthrax should be taken for smear and culture. Sputum in the inhalation form should be collected for smear and culture. Cultures of stool should be made in the intestinal form. Smears and cultures should be made of cerebrospinal fluid in suspected meningitis. In the septicemic stage, cultures of blood should be prepared.

The finding of large, boxcar-shaped, gram-positive cells in smears of any of these specimens should suggest the diagnosis. Fluorescent microscopy, available in some state health laboratories and at the Center for Disease Control, can provide a rapid presumptive diagnosis. Cultures can be made on blood agar or, in the case of blood cultures, in conventional blood culture media.

Colonies of *B. anthracis* are usually flat, with an irregular margin ("Medusa head"), appear off-white with a ground glass surface, and are non-hemolytic. When touched with an inoculating loop, the colonies are tenacious and will stand up like beaten egg white. Anthrax bacilli are non-motile in either a hanging drop test or in semisolid media. Both *B. anthracis* and *B. cereus* ferment glucose, maltose, and sucrose and produce a positive Voges-Proskauer reaction. Other distinguishing features of *B. anthracis* are listed in Table 47–12.

Virulence tests may be performed by inoculating mice with either 0.2 ml subcutaneously or 0.5 ml intraperitoneally of a barely turbid saline suspension prepared from colonies on agar. A broth culture should not be used for virulence testing because of the toxigenic products formed in broth by other *Bacillus* species. The mice will die in 24 to 72 hours, and the organisms can be demonstrated in smears and cultures of heart blood, liver, and spleen.

Table 47–12. DIFFERENTIAL CHARACTERISTICS OF *BACILLUS ANTHRACIS* AND *BACILLUS CEREUS*

TEST	B. ANTHRACIS	B. CEREUS
hemolysis	−	+
motility	−	+
capsulation	+	−
fluorescent antibody	+	−
animal pathogenicity	+	−
gelatin liquefaction	−,(+)*	+
lecithinase	−	+
peptonization of milk	−	+
salicin, acid	−,(+)*	+

*(+) = delayed reaction.

The detection of enterotoxin-producing strains of *B. cereus* depends upon the injection of sterile culture filtrates into the rabbit ileal loop preparation with resulting fluid accumulation. It is uncertain at this time how closely the *Bacillus* enterotoxin resembles that of *Vibrio cholerae* and *Escherichia coli;* however, the elaboration of other toxins that are cytotoxic to tissue culture interfere with the use of this enterotoxin detection method.

Antimicrobial Susceptibility. Although susceptible to a variety of agents, the antibiotic therapy of anthrax has centered on the use of penicillin with or without streptomycin. Both of these agents are highly active against *B. anthracis;* however, some strains do elaborate a β-lactamase.

The antimicrobial susceptibility of other species of *Bacillus* to the penicillins and cephalosporins is highly variable. Most strains are, however, inhibited by tetracycline, aminoglycosides, and chloramphenicol at low concentrations.

Prevention. Prevention of anthrax in humans ideally depends upon its control in animals. Prompt diagnosis of sick animals, their isolation and therapy, and cremation of carcasses are indicated when sporadic outbreaks occur. In enzootic areas vaccination with non-encapsulated spore preparations are used. Occupationally exposed persons should also be immunized.

Acute diarrheal disease due to *B. cereus* may be prevented by properly cooking and refrigerating foods prepared in bulk to prevent proliferation of vegetative forms of the bacteria and formation of the enterotoxin.

GRAM-NEGATIVE AEROBIC AND FACULTATIVELY ANAEROBIC RODS

For strictly functional reasons the laboratory classifies these organisms according to their manner of utilization of glucose (Fig. 47–6) and whether or not special growth factors or conditions are required (Table 47–13).

ENTEROBACTERIACEAE

Definitions and Characteristics. The Enterobacteriaceae are aerobic and facultatively anaerobic, non–spore-forming, non-motile or peritrichously flagellated, oxidase-negative gram-negative bacilli which produce acid fermentatively from glucose and reduce ni-

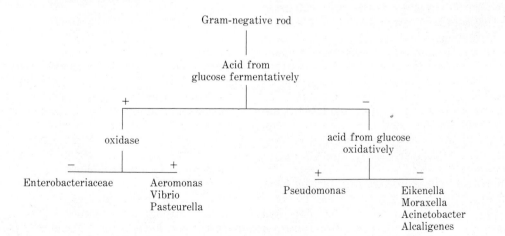

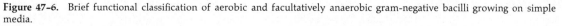

Figure 47–6. Brief functional classification of aerobic and facultatively anaerobic gram-negative bacilli growing on simple media.

Table 47–13. CLINICALLY IMPORTANT AEROBIC AND FACULTATIVELY ANAEROBIC GRAM-NEGATIVE BACILLI REQUIRING SPECIAL GROWTH FACTORS OR CONDITIONS

Brucella
Bordetella
Haemophilus
Eikenella
Actinobacillus
Cardiobacterium
Francisella

Table 47–14. NOMENCLATURE OF THE FAMILY ENTEROBACTERIACEAE*

TRIBE	GENUS	SPECIES
Escherichieae	Escherichia	E. coli
	Shigella	S. dysenteriae
		S. flexneri
		S. boydii
		S. sonnei
Edwardsielleae	Edwardsiella	E. tarda
Salmonelleae	Salmonella	S. choleraesuis
		S. typhi
		S. enteritidis
	Arizona	A. hinshawii
	Citrobacter	C. freundii
		C. diversus
Klebsielleae	Klebsiella	K. pneumoniae
		K. ozaenae
		K. rhinoscleromatis
	Enterobacter	E. cloacae
		E. aerogenes
		E. hafniae
		E. agglomerans
	Serratia	S. marcescens
		S. liquefaciens
		S. rubidaea
Proteeae	Proteus	P. vulgaris
		P. mirabilis
		P. morganii
		P. rettgeri
	Providencia	P. alcalifaciens
		P. stuartii
Yersinieae	Yersinia	Y. pestis
		Y. pseudotuberculosis
		Y. enterocolitica
Erwinieae	Erwinia	E. amylovora
	Pectobacterium	P. carotovorum

*From Washington, J. A., II: Laboratory approaches to the identification of Enterobacteriaceae. Hum. Pathol., 7:151-159, 1976.

trates to nitrites. Their classification is reasonably simple and straightforward, although there are differences between that used in the eighth edition of Bergey's Manual (Buchanan, 1974) and that commonly used in the United States (Table 47–14) which is based largely on the work of Edwards (1972) and subsequent publications and recommendations by Ewing, as described in some detail in the Manual of Clinical Microbiology (1974).

Pathogenesis and Virulence Factors. Endotoxins which are present within the cell walls of the Enterobacteriaceae, as well as other gram-negative bacilli, are responsible for the most part for the morbidity and mortality resulting from infections associated with these bacteria, the most common manifestations of which are listed in Table 47–15. Endotoxins consist of lipid and polysaccharide moieties with small amounts of amino acids. They may produce fever, granulocytosis, thrombocytopenia, disseminated intravascular coagulation, and activation of both the classic and alternate complement pathways (Elin, 1976). Endotoxin shock is the result of gram-negative septicemia with endotoxemia reacting with leukocytes, platelets, complement, and other serum proteins to increase the blood levels of proteolytic enzymes and vasoactive substances and resulting in pooling of blood, increased peripheral vasoconstriction, and diminution in cardiac output. Endotoxin also has effects on the endocrine, reticuloendothelial, and immunologic systems, as well as on metabolism of carbohydrates, lipids, proteins, and minerals.

There are three recognized pathogenetic mechanisms of bacterial diarrheas of acute onset (Table 47–3), and those related to invasiveness and enterotoxin production following colonization are germane to the Enterobacteriaceae. Two types of enterotoxin have been found to be elaborated by *Escherichia coli:* a heat-stable toxin which is non-antigenic and is detectable primarily by quantitation of fluid accumulation in the gastrointestinal tract of infant mice and a heat-labile toxin which is antigenic and is detectable primarily by quantitation of fluid accumulation in the rabbit ileal loop or by morphologic alterations in mouse adrenal tumor or Chinese hamster ovary cells in tissue cultures.

Other pathogenetic factors of the Enterobacteriaceae include the capsule of *Klebsiella pneumoniae,* which, like that of the pneumococcus, inhibits phagocytosis, and the Vi anti-

Table 47-15. FREQUENT MANIFESTATIONS OF
DISEASES ASSOCIATED WITH THE ENTEROBACTERIACEAE

GENUS	FREQUENT MANIFESTATIONS
Escherichia	bacteriuria, septicemia, diarrhea
Shigella	diarrhea
Edwardsiella	diarrhea, wound infection, septicemia, meningitis
Salmonella	
S. choleraesuis	septicemia
S. typhi	enteric fever
S. enteritidis	diarrhea
Klebsiella	bacteriuria, pneumonia, septicemia
Enterobacter	bacteriuria, wound infection (especially post-traumatic), septicemia
Serratia	bacteriuria, wound infection, pneumonia, septicemia
Proteus	bacteriuria, septicemia
Providenica	bacteriuria
Yersinia	
Y. pestis	plague
Y. pseudotuberculosis⎱ *Y. enterocolitica* ⎰	mesenteric adenitis, diarrhea
Erwinia ⎱ *Pectobacterium* ⎰	post-traumatic wound infection

gen of *Salmonella typhi*, which may interfere with intracellular killing of this organism.

The distribution of species of Enterobacteriaceae encountered in various diseases varies considerably. In the urinary tract those most frequently isolated are *Escherichia coli*, *Proteus mirabilis*, and *Klebsiella pneumoniae*. *Providencia* occurs almost exclusively in the urinary tract and most frequently in patients with chronic indwelling catheters. Gram-negative pneumonias associated with the Enterobacteriaceae are most frequently due to *K. pneumoniae*. Gram-negative bacteremias related to the Enterobacteriaceae are most frequently due to *Escherichia coli*, *Klebsiella pneumoniae*, and *Proteus mirabilis*. Infections acquired in the hospital are apt to be due to the more highly resistant groups, such as *Citrobacter*, *Enterobacter*, *Serratia*, and species of *Proteus* other than *P. mirabilis*. Shigellae are but rarely isolated from sources other than the gastrointestinal tract, while salmonellae are not infrequently isolated from other sources, such as urine or blood.

Laboratory Diagnosis. The isolation of gram-negative bacilli, including the Enterobacteriaceae, is greatly facilitated by and in some instances requires the use of differential and selective media (Table 47-16). Eosin methylene blue (EMB) and MacConkey agar can be used interchangeably as differential media, as can xylose-lysine-desoxycholate (XLD) and Hektoen enteric (HE) agar as selective media for salmonellae and shigellae. Both XLD and HE are superior to Salmonella-Shigella (SS) agar for the isolation of enteric pathogens. Bismuth sulfite (BS) is especially useful for the detection of salmonellae in endemics or epidemics.

For specimens other than feces a differential medium should usually be inoculated in addition to a non-inhibitory, general-purpose nutrient agar medium, e.g., soybean-casein digest agar with 5 per cent sheep blood. For fecal specimens a differential medium and a selective medium should be inoculated, as well as an enrichment medium, such as selenite-F or gram-negative (GN) broth. With cultures of specimens other than feces, portions of colonies with distinct colonial morphologies should be inoculated into identification media. With cultures of feces, it is necessary only to identify colorless colonies on EMB or MacConkey agar (red on XLD and green to blue-green on HE). Salmonellae will often produce colonies with black centers owing to their production of H_2S.

Innumerable schemes based on the use of conventional biochemical media and of a variety of diagnostic kits have been described for the identification of the Enterobacteriaceae (Washington, 1976). It is beyond the scope of this chapter to describe them all, and the reader is referred to the laboratory procedure

Table 47-16. ENTERIC DIFFERENTIAL AND SELECTIVE MEDIA

MEDIUM	GRAM-POSITIVE BACTERIOSTATIC AGENT	FERMENTABLE CARBOHYDRATE	INDICATOR	COLONY COLOR		CATEGORY*
				Fermenter	Non-fermenter	
eosin methylene blue (EMB)	eosin Y methylene blue	lactose†	eosin Y methylene blue	red or black with sheen	colorless	D
MacConkey	crystal violet bile salts	lactose	neutral red	red	colorless	D
xylose-lysine-desoxy-cholate (XLD)	bile salts	xylose lactose sucrose	phenol red	yellow	red	S
Hektoen enteric (HE)	bile salts	salicin lactose sucrose	bromothymol blue	yellow-orange	green, blue-green	S
Salmonella-shigella (SS)	bile salts	lactose	neutral red	red	colorless	S
bismuth sulfite (BS)	brilliant green	glucose	bismuth sulfite	‡	‡	S
thiosulfate citrate bile salts sucrose (TCBS)§	bile salts citrate pH 8.6	sucrose	thymol blue bromothymol blue	yellow	colorless	S

*D = differential, S = selective.
†Levine's formulation.
‡H₂S-producing salmonellae have black colonies.
§Used for isolation of vibrios.

manuals listed in the general references or to the manuals prepared by the diagnostic kit manufacturers for more specific details. Most laboratories inoculate an initial series of tests usually including lysine and ornithine decarboxylases, deaminase, indole, citrate, urease, hydrogen sulfide, and motility. Additional tests are required for more specific identification of isolates. The selection and number of additional tests are predicated on factors including cost, interest, and skill. Precision increases with the number of tests performed but the advantages of performing an increasing number of tests can be offset by practicality and the skill of the technologists doing the work. A series of 20 tests, for example, to identify a gram-negative bacillus, colonies of which produce a green metallic sheen on EMB agar, is carrying precision to the point of absurdity, since a positive rapid indole test will provide the identification of *Escherichia coli* with equivalent precision in skilled hands. Even in unskilled hands the appropriate reactions in a series of five or six tests will provide the same level of precision in identifying this species under the conditions described above. Performing a sufficient number of tests to speciate an organism precisely often has little clinical value. Variabilities in individual biochemical test reactions, moreover, reduce the reliability of applying biotypes to epidemiologic investigation.

Table 47-17. DIFFERENTIAL CHARACTERISTICS OF TRIBES OF ENTEROBACTERIACEAE*

TEST	ESCHERICHIEAE	EDWARDSIELLEAE	SALMONELLEAE	KLEBSIELLEAE	PROTEEAE	YERSINIEAE	ERWINIEAE
H₂S (TSI)	−	+	+	−	+ or −	−	−
urease	−	−	−	+ or −	+ or −	+ or −	−
indole	+ or −	+	− or +	− or +	+ or −	− or +	− or +
methyl red	+	+	+	−	+	+	−
Voges-Proskauer	−	−	−	+	−	−	− or +
citrate	−	−	+	+	+	−	+ or −
malonate	−	−	+ or −	+ or −	−	−	−
deaminase	−	−	−	−	+	−	−

*Symbols: +, ≥90% positive within 48 h; −, ≤90% negative within 48 h; (+), positive reaction in 3 or more days; + or −, most strains positive; − or +, most strains negative; + or (+), most reactions positive within 48 h but some delayed; d, different reactions, +, (+), or −.

There are a variety of diagnostic kits on the market today for identifying the Enterobacteriaceae. Most of these or modifications thereof have published records of accuracy so that a laboratory's selection of any one of them for routine purposes can be based on personal preference and cost. All should be used according to their manufacturers' recommendations.

The Enterobacteriaceae can be broadly classified according to their reactions in a few selected tests (Table 47-17). Additional tests are required for generic or species identification.

Escherichieae

Members of this tribe have a mixed acid fermentation pattern and are, therefore, methyl red-positive and Voges-Proskauer-negative. They neither utilize citrate nor hydrolyze urea. Differential characteristics of *Escherichia*, *Shigella*, and *Edwardsiella* are listed in Table 47-18.

H₂S, urease, or citrate positive variants which resemble *Escherichia coli* in every other respect have been rarely isolated from clinical specimens.

In the past it was customary to determine whether or not *E. coli* isolated from fecal material from infants belonged to an "enteropathogenic" serotype. Although epidemiologically associated with newborn nursery outbreaks of diarrhea, strains belonging to these serotypes have been found not to elaborate enterotoxin or to invade. Routine serotyping of strains isolated from fecal material of infants is, therefore, unnecessary and should not be done. Testing for agglutination in serogroups A, B, C, or D of a suspension of colonies suspected of representing *Shigella* should be performed.

Edwardsielleae

Edwardsiella tarda closely resembles *Escherichia coli* biochemically except that it produces H₂S, does not utilize acetate, and fails to ferment mannitol (Table 47-18).

Salmonelleae

The species designations of the salmonellae remain in a state of some controversy. Classically, each new serotype has been given a new species designation, more recently derived from the town, region, or country of origin, e.g., *Salmonella minnesota*. With over 1500 serotypes already described, this system of nomenclature has been confusing and has been largely supplanted in this country by the recognition of only three species (Ewing, 1972): *S. choleraesuis*, *S. typhi*, and *S. enteritidis* (Table 47-19). All salmonellae, with the exceptions of those representing the first two species, are thereby considered to be serotypes or bioserotypes of *S. enteritidis* and are given infrasubspecific designations, e.g., *S. enteritidis* ser Typhimurium.

It is perhaps reasonable at this point to review several factors that are germane to grouping and typing of the Enterobacteriaceae in general and the salmonellae in particular. Grouping is based upon the slow and granular agglutinability of the "O" antigens, which are heat-stable, somatic antigens with intergeneric cross-reactivity, antibodies to which are frequently of the IgM class. They are predominantly lipopolysaccharide in content. The "H" antigen is the heat-labile, flagellar, protein antigen, antibodies to which are predominantly IgG and agglutination with which is rapid and fluffy. This antigen provides type-specificity to a strain. The "Vi" antigen is a heat-labile, surface or capsular, principally polysaccharide antigen which is generally associated with virulence and the presence of which is usually determined with isolates suspected of representing *S. typhi*.

Complete characterization of serotypes of salmonellae is impractical except in certain reference laboratories. It is, however, practical for clinical laboratories to test isolates for

Table 47-18. DIFFERENTIAL CHARACTERISTICS OF ESCHERICHIEAE AND EDWARDSIELLEAE*

TEST	ESCHERICHIA	SHIGELLA†	EDWARDSIELLA
gas from glucose	+	−	+
H₂S (TSI)	−	−	+
indole	+	− or +	+
decarboxylase			
lysine	d	−	+
ornithine	d	− or +	(+)
acid from			
lactose	+	−	−
mannitol	+	+ or −	−
salicin	d	−	−
sucrose	d	−	−
sodium acetate	+ or (+)	−	−
motility	+ or −	−	+

*Symbols: See Table 47-17.

†*Shigella sonnei* ferments lactose and sucrose slowly and usually decarboxylates ornithine promptly.

5

Table 47-19. DIFFERENTIAL CHARACTERISTICS OF THE TRIBE SALMONELLEAE*

TEST	SALMONELLA			Arizona hinshawii	CITROBACTER	
	S. choleraesuis	S. typhi	S. enteritidis		C. freundii	C. diversus
β-galactosidase	−	−	−	+	+ or −	+
H₂S	+ or −	+ (weak)	+	+	+ or −	−
urease	−	−	−	−	d	d
indole	−	−	−	−	−	+
citrate	(+)	−	+ or (+)	+	+	+
decarboxylase						
lysine	+	+	+	+	−	−
ornithine	+	−	+	+	d	+
arginine dihydrolase	(+)	d	+ or (+)	(+) or +	d	+ or (+)
malonate	−	−	−	+	d	+ or −
dulcitol	d	− or (+)	+	−	d	+ or −

*Symbols: See Table 47-17.

agglutination in the more commonly encountered group-specific antisera (A through E), as well as in a polyvalent grouping antiserum and Vi antiserum. Strains should then be submitted to a reference laboratory, usually a state health department laboratory, for serotyping for epidemiologic purposes.

Arizona hinshawii, as it is recognized in this country, has been designated *S. arizonae* in the latest edition of Bergey's Manual (1974). Biologically, biochemically, and serologically, it does closely resemble the salmonellae but can be readily distinguished from them in the laboratory (Table 47-19).

Although two species of *Citrobacter*, *C. freundii* and *C. diversus*, are currently recognized in the United States, the situation internationally remains confusing. Without appearing to endorse any particular nomenclature, it is probably important to recognize the species designations which do appear in

publications, as well as their similarities and dissimilarities (Table 47-20). Certain antimicrobial susceptibility patterns of *C. freundii* and *C. diversus* are sufficiently characteristic to be helpful in their differentiation, the former being resistant and the latter nearly always susceptible to cephalothin and the former being susceptible and the latter resistant to carbenicillin. Since approximately 20 per cent of isolates of *C. freundii* fail to produce H₂S in TSI, these other characteristics can be helpful in its identification.

Klebsielleae

The species of *Klebsiella* are uniformly non-motile and fail to produce ornithine decarboxylase. Nearly all clinical isolates are *K. pneumoniae* with only rare isolations of *K. ozaenae*. *K. rhinoscleromatis* is hardly ever encountered in the United States. The differ-

Table 47-20. DIFFERENTIAL CHARACTERISTICS AND NOMENCLATURE OF *CITROBACTER*

TEST	CITROBACTER		CITROBACTER INTERMEDIUM		
			(BIOTYPE A)	(BIOTYPE B)	
	FREUNDII	DIVERSUS	Levinea amalonatica	Citrobacter koseri	Levinea malonatica
H₂S	+ or −	−	−	−	−
urease	d	d	+	+ or −	+ or −
indole	−	+	+	+	+
lysine decarboxylase	−	−	−	−	−
arginine dihydrolase	d	+ or (+)	+	+	+
malonate	d	+ or −	−	+	+
adonitol	−	+	−	+	+
KCN	+	−	+	+ or −	+ or −

*Symbols: See Table 47-17.

Table 47-21. DIFFERENTIAL CHARACTERISTICS
OF THE *KLEBSIELLA* SPECIES*

TEST	K. PNEUMONIAE	K. OZAENAE	K. RHINOSCLEROMATIS
urease	+	d	−
indole	− or +	−	−
methyl red	− or +	+	+
Voges-Proskauer	+	−	−
citrate	+	d	−
malonate	+	−	+ or −
lysine decarboxylase	+	− or +	−

*Symbols: See Table 47-17.

Table 47-22. DIFFERENTIAL CHARACTERISTICS OF THE *ENTEROBACTER* SPECIES*

TEST	E. CLOACAE	E. AEROGENES	E. HAFNIAE	E. AGGLOMERANS
urease	+ or −	−	−	d
indole	−	−	−	− or +
methyl red (35°C.)	−	−	+ or −	− or +
Voges-Proskauer (35°C.)	+	+	+ or −	+ or −
citrate	+	+	(+) or −	d
malonate	+ or −	+ or −	+ or −	+ or −
decarboxylase				
lysine	−	+	+	−
ornithine	+	+	+	−
arginine dihydrolase	+	−	−	−
phenylalanine deaminase	−	−	−	− or +
gelatin liquefaction (22°C.)	(+)	(+) or −	−	d
adonitol (acid)	− or +	+	−	−
inositol (acid)	d	+	−	d

*Symbols: See Table 47-17.

5

Table 47-23. DIFFERENTIAL CHARACTERISTICS
OF *SERRATIA* SPECIES*

TEST	S. MARCESCENS	S. LIQUEFACIENS	S. RUBIDAEA
urease	d	d	d
indole	−	−	−
methyl red (35°C.)	− or +	+ or − †	− or +
Voges-Proskauer (35°C.)	+	− or + †	+
citrate	+	+	+ or (+)
malonate	−	−	+ or −
decarboxylase			
lysine	+	+ or (+)	+ or (+)
ornithine	+	+	−
arabinose (acid)	−	+	+
raffinose (acid)	−	+	+
sorbitol (acid)	+	+	−
lactose (acid)	−	d	+

*Symbols: See Table 47-17.
†Reactions reversed at 22°C.

ential characteristics of the three species are listed in Table 47–21.

The species of *Enterobacter* are nearly always motile and usually produce ornithine decarboxylase, with the notable exception of *E. agglomerans*, which has no decarboxylase or dihydrolase activity and most colonies of which develop a distinctive yellow pigment within a few days after isolation (Table 47–22). *Serratia*, formerly recognized only when it produced a characteristic red pigment, consists of three species (Table 47–23). It is now known that fewer than 10 per cent of isolates produce pigment on conventional isolation media and that their detection hinges on the use of suitable biochemical tests. *Serratia marcescens* accounts for over 90 per cent of the species isolated.

Proteeae

The Proteeae are characterized by their ability to deaminate amino acids, of which phenylalanine and lysine are the most frequently tested in the clinical laboratory. Deamination by *Proteus morganii* in lysine iron agar may be delayed beyond the first 18 to 24 hours of incubation. Other characteristics are listed in Table 47–24. Swarming and the production of H_2S are often seen with *P. vulgaris* and *P. mirabilis*. The production of urease by *P. rettgeri* may be weak or delayed, reflecting the fact that this is an inducible enzyme synthesized specifically in the presence of urea, so that the differentiation between this species

and *Providencia stuartii* may pose some difficulty.

Yersinieae

Members of the genus *Yersinia* share many characteristics with the Enterobacteriaceae, fermenting glucose, reducing nitrates to nitrites, utilizing carbohydrates fermentatively, being oxidase-negative, and bearing peritrichous flagella. Differential characteristics of the species of *Yersinia* are listed in Table 47–25.

Material and cultures suspected of harboring *Y. pestis* should be handled very cautiously, since the organism is highly infective. It grows optimally at 27 to 28°C. Its characteristic bipolar staining is more apt to be seen in smears of clinical material than of cultures. Definitive tests for identification of the species include agglutination and immunofluorescence with specific antiserum, lysis by specific bacteriophage, and animal virulence studies.

The other species of *Yersinia* are rarely isolated or recognized in the United States. Their presence should be suspected any time a lactose- and H_2S-negative, urease-positive gram-negative bacillus which is motile at room temperature is isolated. They may be isolated from a variety of sources including mesenteric nodes, serous effusions, and feces. Antibodies can be demonstrated as a result of diseases due to *Y. enterocolitica;* however, cross-reactivity with other organisms and particularly with *Brucella abortus* limits the

Table 47–24. DIFFERENTIAL CHARACTERISTICS OF THE PROTEEAE*

| TEST | PROTEUS | | | | PROVIDENCIA | |
	P. vulgaris	P. mirabilis	P. morganii	P. rettgeri	P. alcalifaciens	P. stuartii
H_2S	+	+	−	−	−	−
urease	+	+	+	+	−	−
indole	+	−	+	+	+	+
citrate	− or +	+ or −	−	+	+	+
ornithine decarboxylase	−	+	+	−	−	−
phenylalanine deaminase	+	+	+	+	+	+
acid from						
adonitol	−	−	−	d	+	− or +
esculin	d	−	−	d	−	−
inositol	−	−	−	+	−	+
maltose	+	−	−	−	−	−
mannitol	−	−	−	+ or −	−	d

*Symbols: See Table 47–17.

Table 47-25. DIFFERENTIAL CHARACTERISTICS
OF THE YERSINIEAE*

TEST	Y. PESTIS	Y. PSEUDOTUBERCULOSIS	Y. ENTEROCOLITICA
H_2S	−	−	−
urease	−	+	+
indole	−	−	d
methyl red	+	+	+
Voges-Proskauer			
22°C.	−	−	+ or −
35°C.	−	−	−
citrate	−	−	−
ornithine decarboxylase	−	−	+
phenylalanine deaminase	−	−	−
β-galactosidase	+	+	+
acid from			
lactose	−	−	−
sucrose	−	−	+
rhamnose	−	+	−
salicin	+	+	−
adonitol	−	+ or −	
motility			
22°C.	−	+	+
35°C.	−	−	−

*Symbols: See Table 47-17.

usefulness of this determination as a diagnostic tool, and the test is not generally available in the United States.

Erwinieae

The taxonomy and nomenclature of the genera *Erwinia* and *Pectobacterium* remain unsettled. These organisms are primarily plant pathogens that can be saprophytic and rarely cause disease in man.

Antimicrobial Susceptibility. The susceptibility of the Enterobacteriaceae to various antimicrobial agents is highly variable. As

Table 47-26. MECHANISMS OF ENZYMATIC
INACTIVATION OF ANTIBIOTICS
BY GRAM-NEGATIVE BACILLI

ENZYME	SUBSTRATE
β-lactamases	penicillins, cephalosporins
acetyltransferases	chloramphenicol gentamicins tobramycin kanamycin amikacin
phosphotransferase	kanamycin neomycin
adenylyltransferases	gentamicins tobramycin kanamycin amikacin

a rule, therefore, clinically significant isolates require susceptibility testing to assist in their proper therapy. The frequency with which chromosome- and plasmid-mediated resistance is encountered, particularly in organisms responsible for hospital-acquired infections, further diminishes the predictability of susceptibility of a given species to a particular antibiotic. For example, the vast majority of *Klebsiella pneumoniae* isolated from the Mayo Clinic and its affiliated hospitals during 1976 were susceptible to cephalothin and all were susceptible to gentamicin; yet, outbreaks of infections due to cephalothin- and gentamicin-resistant strains of this species have been encountered in other hospitals.

Antibiotic resistance by the Enterobacteriaceae can be related to enzymatic inactivation (Table 47-26), to altered permeability of components of the cell wall, to an altered structural target, to an altered metabolic pathway bypassing a reaction inhibited by the drug, or to alteration of an enzyme which remains functional but is less affected by the drug.

Despite all of the foregoing discussion, it is possible to make some generalizations about the activity of antimicrobial agents against the more frequently isolated groups of Enterobacteriaceae (Table 47-27). It should be noted that these data show no agent to be uniformly active against any group of organisms, that they represent one major medical institution's

5

Table 47-27. ACTIVITY OF VARIOUS ANTIMICROBIAL AGENTS
AGAINST FREQUENTLY ISOLATED ENTEROBACTERIACEAE*

	ESCHERICHIA COLI	KLEBSIELLA	ENTEROBACTER	SERRATIA	PROTEUS MIRABILIS	PROTEUS (INDOLE +)	PROVIDENCIA
Amikacin	+++	+++	+++	+++	+++	+++	+++
Ampicillin	+++	+	+	0	+++	0	+
Carbenicillin	+++	+	+++	++	+++	+++	+++
Cephalothin	+++	+++	0	0	+++	0	+
Chloramphenicol	+++	++	++	+	+++	++	++
Kanamycin	+++	+++	+++	+++	+++	+++	+++
Gentamicin	+++	+++	+++	+++	+++	+++	+++
Tetracycline	++	++	+++	+	+	++	+
Nalidixic acid	+++	+++	+++	++	+++	+++	+++
Nitrofurantoin	+++	+++	++	+	+	+	+

*Mayo Clinic and affiliated hospitals, 1976. Symbols: + + + +, uniformly active; + + +, highly active; + +, moderately active; +, poorly active; 0, inactive.

experience in one year, and that they do not reflect the existence of any isolated hospital epidemic of infections due to resistant organisms, e.g., gentamicin-resistant *Klebsiella pneumoniae* or *Serratia marcescens*. As has already been mentioned, such focal outbreaks in hospitals are being reported around the world.

Specific comments regarding the antimicrobial susceptibility and therapy of certain diseases due to the Enterobacteriaceae should be made.

Although usually susceptible to a variety of antimicrobial agents, non-typhoidal, uncomplicated enteric infections due to salmonellae are generally not treated with antibiotics, since there are data demonstrating that such therapy may actually prolong the carrier state. Infections due to susceptible strains of *Salmonella typhi* are preferentially treated with chloramphenicol, despite this organisms's susceptibility to other agents. Therapy with amoxicillin, ampicillin, or cotrimoxazole should be used in instances of chloramphenicol resistance.

It is desirable to treat patients with shigellosis in order to eliminate shedding of the organism in feces as rapidly as possible; however, the frequency of resistance of shigellae to ampicillin and other antimicrobial agents in several parts of the United States has forced some modifications in this practice. While ampicillin remains the drug of choice for the treatment of susceptible strains, cotrimoxazole appears to be a satisfactory alternative for ampicillin-resistant strains.

Prevention. The prevention of infections due to the Enterobacteriaceae is closely allied with infection control in hospitals, a topic covered in considerable detail in Chapter 57.

OXIDASE-POSITIVE GLUCOSE FERMENTERS OF MEDICAL SIGNIFICANCE

Vibrio

Definitions and Characteristics. Vibrios are facultatively anaerobic, oxidase-positive, short, curved, or straight gram-negative bacilli which are usually motile by means of polar flagella, ferment carbohydrates, and reduce nitrates to nitrites. Two recognized species are medically important: *V. cholerae* and *V. parahaemolyticus*. The second species consists of two biotypes: 1 (parahaemolyticus) and 2 (alginolyticus), the latter of which is sometimes identified as a distinct species, *V. alginolyticus*. Other less well characterized and unnamed halophilic vibrios ("non-cholera," "related") are also medically important. *Campylobacter fetus*, formerly *V. fetus*, is more appropriately considered as an anaerobe.

Pathogenesis and Virulence Factors. Cholera manifests itself by massive intestinal fluid loss secondary to stimulation of the adenyl cyclase system of cells in the small intestine with production of cyclic AMP. In this respect the enterotoxin acts in a manner similar to that of the heat-labile toxin of *Escherichia coli*. The mechanism of pathogenicity of *V. parahaemolyticus* appears to be related to invasiveness rather than to enterotoxin production. This halophilic organism is widely distributed in marine environments and has been found to contaminate fish and shellfish. Outbreaks of acute diarrheal disease following ingestion of contaminated food have been especially common in Japan but have also occurred in this and other countries. Wound infections and septicemias have been associated with non-cholera halophilic vibrios. *Campylobacter fetus* has been associated with septicemia, subacute bacterial endocarditis, septic arthritis, meningitis, and a variety of other infections.

Laboratory Diagnosis. Laboratories in the United States are unaccustomed to isolating vibrios from fecal material. Nonetheless, because cholera is pandemic in many other countries, its importation by travellers into western countries does occur. Moreover, the increasing recognition of *V. parahaemolyticus* in countries other than Japan means that laboratories in the United States should be familiar with the techniques required for the isolation and identification of vibrios. Obviously, the laboratory must be informed that infection due to *V. cholerae* or *V. parahaemolyticus* is suspected on the basis of travel or dietary history so that the appropriate media can be inoculated. These include a non-selective taurocholate gelatin agar (TGA) and a selective agar, such as thiosulfate-citrate bile salts (TCBS). TCBS should not be autoclaved, and its final pH should be 8.4. An enrichment broth, such as alkaline peptone water, should also be inoculated and subcultured in 6 to 8 hours to a second set of TGA and TCBS plates. Colonies which are surrounded by cloudy zones on TGA (due to gelatinase activity) and yellow colonies on TCBS (due to sucrose fermentation) should be selected for further study with biochemical and serologic tests. The vibrios can be differentiated among themselves and from other enteric gram-negative bacilli according to reactions listed in Table 47-28. It may be necessary to carry out biochemical testing of the halophilic vibrios in media supplemented with 1 to 3 per cent NaCl. If triple sugar iron agar (TSIA) and lysine iron agar (LIA) are inoculated for screening purposes, their reactions will be acid slant/acid butt with no gas (A/A-) or H_2S and alkaline slant/alkaline butt (K/K), respectively. Agglutination of a saline suspension of the organism by polyvalent antiserum against *V. cholerae* should occur within a minute if the organism is present.

The distinction between the two biotypes of *V. parahaemolyticus*, parahaemolyticus and alginolyticus, is based on the latter's ability to ferment sucrose and to form acetylmethylcarbinol (Voges-Proskauer reaction positive).

Antimicrobial Susceptibility. *V. cholerae* and the non-cholera halophilic vibrios are susceptible to a variety of agents, including

5

Table 47-28. DIFFERENTIAL CHARACTERISTICS OF ENTERIC GRAM-NEGATIVE BACILLI*

TEST	VIBRIOS			Aero-monas	Plesi-omonas	Pseu-domonas	Entero-bacteriaceae
	V. cholerae	V. para-haemolyticus	Non-cholera				
flagella	polar	polar	polar	polar	polar	polar	peritrichous
oxidase	+	+	+	+	+	+	−
gelatinase	+	+	+	+	+	−	d
urease	−	−	−	−	−	−	d
decarboxylase							
lysine	+	+	+	−	+	d	d
ornithine	+	+	+ or (+)	−	+	−	d
arginine dihydrolase	−	−	−	+	+	d	d
carbohydrate							
metabolism (O/F)	F	F	F	F	F	0	F
acid fermentatively from							
lactose	(+)	−	+	d	+ or (+)	−	d
mannitol	+	+	+ or −	+	−	−	d
salicin	−	− or (+)	+	d	− or +	−	d
sucrose	+	−	−	d	−	−	d
growth in nutrient broth†							
without NaCl	+	−	−				
with 6% NaCl	d	+	+				
with 7% NaCl	d	+	−				

*Symbols: See Table 47-17.
†Reactions given for vibrios only.

tetracyclines, chloramphenicol, ampicillin, cephalosporins, and trimethoprim/sulfamethoxazole. *V. parahaemolyticus* is resistant to the penicillins but is otherwise susceptible to the other agents which are active against *V. cholerae.*

Prevention. The primary means of transmission of cholera is contaminated water. Otherwise, the disease itself is not particularly communicable, provided that thorough handwashing and careful handling of patients' excreta are properly enforced. Simple enteric precautions in any general hospital should be adequate. Although the risk of contracting the disease is small, travelers to infected areas should be vaccinated, preferably within two months of their travel to such areas. Two vaccinations at one week's to one month's interval are recommended. Booster vaccinations should be given every three to six months if periods of exposure continue.

Aeromonas

Definitions and Characteristics. Members of this genus are facultatively anaerobic, oxidase- and catalase-positive, rod-shaped gram-negative bacilli that are motile by means of polar flagella and form acids from carbohydrates by respiratory and fermentative metabolism. There are three species: *A. hydrophila*, *A. punctata*, and *A. salmonicida*. Another species, formerly *A. shigelloides*, is now classified as *Plesiomonas.*

Pathogenesis and Virulence Factors. *Aeromonas* has been isolated from tap water, rivers, soil, marine animals, and various foods. It has been isolated from feces of healthy persons and from patients with diarrheal disease of otherwise unexplained origin. Its role in producing diarrheal disease is possibly related to the production of an enterotoxin by some strains. A hemolysin and a cytopathic factor have also been described.

Aeromonas may cause infection of traumatically acquired wounds which are contaminated with soil or water. It may also cause septicemia in patients with acute leukemia.

Laboratory Diagnosis. The isolation of a fermenting, oxidase-positive, gram-negative bacillus should suggest strongly the possibility of *Aeromonas*. It grows readily on conventional laboratory media and produces colonies that resemble those of *Pseudomonas*, have a greenish ground glass appearance, and give off a fruity odor. They can be distinuished readily

from *Pseudomonas* and from the Enterobacteriaceae (Table 47-28).

Antimicrobial Susceptibility. *Aeromonas* is susceptible to the aminoglycosides, chloramphenicol, and tetracyclines but produces a β-lactamase mediating resistance to the penicillins and cephalosporins. *Aeromonas* has been found to maintain R plasmids of both the Enterobacteriaceae and *Pseudomonas.*

Pasteurella

Definitions and Characteristics. The pasteurellae are facultatively anaerobic, oxidase- and catalase-positive, non-motile gram-negative bacteria that may range morphologically from coccobacilli to long filamentous rods. Four species are recognized: *P. multocida*, *P. pneumotropica*, *P. haemolytica*, and *P. ureae.*

Pathogenesis and Virulence Factors. Encapsulated strains are usually pathogenic for mice, and virulence has been found to be enhanced by free iron in various forms. The cell wall contains endotoxin but no exotoxin has been identified.

The pasteurellae are indigenous to many animals and are isolated frequently from wounds resulting from animal bites or scratches. Local infections can become systemic, and there have been a number of reports of septicemia, osteomyelitis, and meningitis. Pasteurellae have been associated with respiratory tract infections, including sinusitis, peritonsillar abscess, mastoiditis, pulmonary abscess, pneumonia, empyema, bronchitis, and bronchiectasis, usually in patients wih chronic pulmonary disease.

Laboratory Diagnosis. Pasteurellae grow well on blood agar but are, with the exception of *P. haemolytica*, unable to grow on gramnegative differential agar media, such as eosin methylene blue (EMB) or MacConkey agar. The finding of a gram-negative bacillus that grows on blood agar only and is oxidase- and indole-positive and ONPG negative, strongly constitutes presumptive evidence for the isolation of *P. multocida*, the most frequently encountered species.

Antimicrobial Susceptibility. Characteristic of *P. multocida* is its susceptibility to penicillin G. Other agents with excellent activity *in vitro* against the organism include the cephalosporins and tetracyclines.

Prevention and Control. Primary attention should be devoted to proper wound care

Table 47-29. DIFFERENTIAL CHARACTERISTICS OF
PSEUDOMONADS ISOLATED FROM CLINICAL MATERIAL*

TEST	P. AERUGINOSA	P. FLUO-RESCENS GRP.	P. MALTO-PHILIA	P. STUTZERI	P. CEPACIA	P. ALCA-LIGENES	P. DIMINUTA	P. MALLEI	P. PSEUDO-MALLEI	P. PUTRE-FACIENS
oxidase	+	+	−	+	+	+	+	+	+	+
decarboxylase										
lysine	−	−	+	−	+	−	−	−	−	−
ornithine	−	−	−	−	− or +	−	−	−	−	+
arginine dihydrolase	+	+	−	−	−	−	−	+	+	−
acid (oxidatively) from										
glucose	+	+	+ or (+)	+	+	−	−	+	+	d
maltose	−	+ or −	+	+	+	−	−	(+)	+	d
xylose	+	+	+ or −	+	+	−	−	−	+	−
denitrification	+	−	−	+	−	−	−	−	+	−
deoxyribonuclease	− or +	−	+	−	−	−	+	−	−	+
citrate, Simmons	+	+	− or +	+	+	+ or −	−	−	+	− or +
fluorescein	+	+	−	−	−	−	−	−	−	−
pyocyanin	+	−	−	−	−	−	−	−	−	−
growth at 42°C.	+	−	+	+	+ or −	+ or −	+	−	+	+
flagella (No.)	1	>1	>1	1	>1	1	1	0	>1	1

*Symbols: See Table 47-17.

with close observation of those secondary to animal bites. The value of penicillin G as prophylaxis is uncertain.

GLUCOSE OXIDIZERS

Pseudomonas

Definitions and Characteristics. Pseudomonads are strictly aerobic, catalase-positive, usually oxidase-positive gram-negative bacilli whose metabolism is respiratory and never fermentative and whose motility is by polar flagella. At least 29 species have been well characterized; however, only those deemed to be medically important will be considered here (Table 47-29). Other species have occasionally been isolated from clinical material and have been reported as causes of opportunistic infection. *P. testosteroni* and *P. acidovorans* have been included by some into the species *Comamonas terrigena*, which resembles *P. diminuta* and *P. alcalifaciens* except that it does not produce deoxyribonuclease and usually has two to four polar flagella.

Because of the fact that the pseudomonads are very adaptable and can use a large number of organic compounds for growth, they are essentially free-living and can be found in a tremendous variety of habitats (Table 47-30). Moreover, they are more resistant to antiseptic agents and disinfectants than most vegetative forms of bacteria.

Pathogenesis and Virulence Factors. The species causing the greatest morbidity and mortality today is *P. aeruginosa*. As has

Table 47-30. RESERVOIRS AND CLINICAL MANIFESTATIONS OF CERTAIN PSEUDOMONADS

SPECIES	RESERVOIRS	CLINICAL MANIFESTATIONS
P. aeruginosa	soil, floors, sinks, baths, soaps, benzalkonium chloride, humidifiers, respirators, utensils, vases, salads, and other items used or present in hospitals; skin, feces	wound infection, bacteriuria, pneumonia, bacteremia, and other opportunistic infections; chronic otitis media, ophthalmic infection
P. fluorescens	soils, floors, baths, sinks, respirators, soaps, contaminated blood or blood products	rarely, causes opportunistic infection
P. maltophilia *P. stutzeri*	ubiquitous (water, sewage, soil, raw milk, lower animals)	rarely, causes opportunistic infection
P. cepacia	water, soil, respirators, detergents, lubricants	wound infection, foot rot, pneumonitis, bacteremia, endocarditis, bacteriuria
P. pseudomallei	soil and water in endemic areas	melioidosis
P. mallei	warm-blooded animals	glanders

already been stated, it is nearly ubiquitous in the hospital environment, existing almost anywhere there is any moisture. The organism is more resistant than most vegetative bacteria to many disinfectants and antimicrobial agents. Although it produces a variety of enzymes and toxins, in addition to slime and endotoxin, the mechanisms by which *P. aeruginosa* produces disease remain unclear. Its surface polysaccharide is released from cells multiplying in vitro, as are small amounts of endotoxin. It produces an elastase that inactivates components of complement, thereby inhibiting to some degree opsonization and the inflammatory response and perhaps contributing to its invasiveness. Hemolysins and exotoxins from *P. aeruginosa* have also been identified. The organism produces infection in patients with burn, traumatic, and operative wounds; following urinary tract manipulation; in patients with diseases of the hematopoietic, reticuloendothelial, and lymphoid systems; and in those with impaired cellular or humoral defenses. Pulmonary infection occurs commonly in patients with cystic fibrosis. The mortality rate is highest in severely leukopenic (<1000 PMN/cu mm) patients.

P. pseudomallei is endemic in Southeast Asia, where asymptomatic or subclinical infection is frequent. A pulmonary form resembling tuberculosis or a mycotic infection occurs less frequently and has a relatively good prognosis. Its septicemic form is highly lethal.

P. mallei causes glanders, which may present as an acute fulminating and frequently fatal septicemic form, as an acute pneumonia with or without septicemia, as an acute or chronic suppurative infection, as a latent infection with eventual acute manifestations of the disease, or in an occult form with encapsulated nodules in various organs and especially the lungs.

Other species of *Pseudomonas*, although often isolated from clinical specimens, are only occasionally involved in disease (Table 47-30).

Laboratory Diagnosis. The presence of *P. aeruginosa* in cultures can often be suspected because of its musty odor, the rough or ground glass appearance of its colonies, and the presence of pigment or metallic sheen in its colonies. Its identification can be made easily with a positive oxidase reaction, an alkaline slant/neutral butt reaction in triple sugar iron agar (TSIA), and the formation of sheen and/or pigment on the slants of TSIA and Pseudomonas P agar. If all of these reactions do not occur, additional tests should be performed (Table 47-29). Tests of carbohydrate utilization should be carried out in O-F basal medium which contains a minimal quantity of peptone and a relatively large quantity of carbohydrate and which will provide detection of the very small quantities of acid formed by this group of bacteria. Reactions are usually complete within 48 hours but may require as long as seven days in some instances.

There are numerous as yet unnamed groups of organisms resembling *Pseudomonas* that are classified according to a numerical designation (Manual of Clinical Microbiology, 1974). Their clinical significance, as well as their taxonomy and nomenclature, remains obscure.

Antimicrobial Susceptibility. As a general rule, *P. aeruginosa* is susceptible to gentamicin, tobramycin, and amikacin. Most isolates are also susceptible to carbenicillin. Hospital epidemics of strains resistant to gentamicin have, however, occurred owing to aminoglycoside acetylating and, less often, adenylylating enzymes. Tobramycin resistance due to such enzymes is being reported, as is amikacin resistance due to an acetyltransferase. Carbenicillin and ticarcillin resistance may also occur, owing to R plasmid mediated β-lactamase.

The susceptibility of other species of *Pseudomonas* varies considerably. Kanamycin, which is essentially inactive against *P. aeruginosa*, inhibits most strains of *P. stutzeri* and the *P. fluorescens* group. *P. cepacia* is usually resistant to aminoglycosides but is often susceptible to chloramphenicol and trimethoprim/sulfamethoxazole. Many isolates of *P. maltophilia* are resistant to aminoglycosides, but they are more frequently inhibited by gentamicin than by amikacin or tobramycin.

P. pseudomallei is usually susceptible to tetracycline, chloramphenicol, sulfonamides, and trimethoprim/sulfamethoxazole but not to penicillins, cephalosporins, polymyxins, or aminoglycosides. Antimicrobial susceptibility data on *P. mallei* are limited owing to the eradication of glanders in many parts of the world; however, sulfonamides have generally been considered to represent the agents of choice in the treatment of the disease.

Prevention and Control. With the exceptions of *P. pseudomallei* and *P. mallei*, prevention of disease due to pseudomonads is highly dependent upon hospital infection control and surveillance programs.

Acinetobacter

Definitions and Characteristics. Organisms in this genus are rod-shaped, sometimes nearly spherical, non-motile, oxidase-negative, strictly aerobic, and gram-negative. Their metabolism is oxidative and those which form acid from carbohydrates do so by oxidation of aldehyde groups to produce aldobionic acids. Such organisms lack β-galactosidase and are, therefore, ONPG negative.

The taxonomy and nomenclature of these organisms has been in a state of turmoil for years. Acid-producing strains have been known as *Bacterium anitratum* and *Herellea vaginicola* and non-acid-producing strains as *Mima polymorpha*. The tribe Mimeae has, however, lost its standing in nomenclature, and both acid- and non-acid-producing strains are currently called *Acinetobacter calcoaceticus*. Some, however, recognize two varieties, *anitratum* and *lwoffi*, the former to include acid-producing and the latter to include non-acid-producing strains.

Pathogenesis and Virulence Factors. *Acinetobacter* is commonly found in soil and water and uncommonly found on the skin and mucous membranes of healthy people. Little is known about virulence factors in this group of organisms, but they do appear to form small amounts of endotoxin. Although usually non-pathogenic, they have been associated with a wide variety of diseases, including septicemia, bacteriuria, pneumonia, and abscesses. They are frequently encountered in mixed cultures of wounds or respiratory tract material without any clear-cut relationship with disease.

Laboratory Diagnosis. *Acinetobacter* can be distinguished readily from the pseudomonads on the basis of its lack of motility, inability to reduce nitrates, and its negative oxidase reaction. The ability by some strains to oxidize various carbohydrates and 10 per cent lactose agar slants provides ready identification of *A. calcoaceticus* var. *anitratus* (Table 47–31); however, non-acid-forming strains var. *lwoffi* require differentiation from the similarly inactive moraxellae (Table 47–31).

Antimicrobial Susceptibility. *Acinetobacter* is susceptible to aminoglycosides, including kanamycin, gentamicin, tobramycin, and amikacin. It is moderately susceptible to tetracycline but usually quite susceptible to minocycline. Most strains are inhibited by nalidixic acid. Other antimicrobial agents are usually inactive.

GRAM-NEGATIVE AEROBIC AND FACULTATIVELY ANAEROBIC RODS REQUIRING SPECIAL GROWTH FACTORS OR CONDITIONS (Table 47–13)

Brucella

Definitions and Characteristics. Brucellae are small, gram-negative coccobacilli, non-motile, strictly aerobic, catalase- and usually oxidase-positive rods. Growth is often en-

Table 47–31. DIFFERENTIAL CHARACTERISTICS OF
ACINETOBACTER AND *MORAXELLA**

	A. CALCOACETICUS		
TEST	var. anitratrum	var. lwoffi	MORAXELLA
oxidase	−	−	+
nitrate reduction	−	−	d
carbohydrate metabolism	oxidative	inactive	inactive
acid from			
dextrose	+	−	−
maltose	(+) or −	−	−
xylose	+	−	−
acid on 10% lactose slant	+	−	−
phenylalanine deaminase	−	−	d
citrate utilization	+	+	d
urease	(+) or −	(+) or −	d
penicillin	resistant	resistant	originally susceptible

*Symbols: See Table 47–17.

hanced by the presence of 5 to 10 per cent CO_2. Although growth may occur on ordinary media, it is usually optimal on a soybean-casein digest agar (trypticase soy, tryptic soy, tryptone soya, etc.) or in its liquid counterpart. Of the recognized species, *B. melitensis, B. abortus, B. suis,* and *B. canis* are those of medical importance in man.

Pathogenesis and Virulence Factors. The preferential hosts for brucellae are sheep and goats for *B. melitensis,* cattle for *B. abortus,* swine for *B. suis,* and dogs for *B. canis;* however, each species may occasionally infect other animals. Infection is acquired by man by direct contact with infected material, including animal carcasses, fetal membranes, vaginal discharges, fetuses, skin or mucous membranes, as well as by ingestion of unpasteurized milk or milk products from infected animals. Local lymphadenopathy often occurs with dissemination and secondary localization in the reticuloendothelial system and formation of granulomas in the spleen, bone, genitourinary tract, lungs, and soft tissues. Organisms may be seen within phagocytes.

Signs and symptoms are often variable and non-specific with chills, fever, sweats, and anorexia occurring frequently. The fever is characteristically diurnal ("undulant"). Diagnosis of the disease beyond the acute bacteremic phase is difficult to establish.

The most common sources of infection in the United States in recent years are cattle and swine, and the majority of reported cases of brucellosis are in individuals working in packing plants. Infections due to *B. canis* have been acquired predominantly by contact with infected dogs or by accidental exposure to cultures of the organism in laboratories.

Laboratory Diagnosis. Blood cultures in a biphasic bottle (Castaneda technique) containing soybean-casein digest medium have been shown to be highly effective in detecting the presence of bacteremia in the early stages of brucellosis. Other normally sterile body fluids should be concentrated by filtration through a 0.45 µm membrane filter which is then placed onto a soybean-casein digest blood agar plate for culture. Tissue should be minced and then ground with a sterile abrasive in broth to produce a 20 per cent suspension which is then inoculated onto the appropriate medium. Specimens contaminated with other bacteria should be inoculated onto the more selective "W" or Wisconsin medium (Washington, 1974). Guinea pig inoculations subcutaneously or intraperitoneally may also be helpful. Cultures should be incubated in an atmosphere containing 5 to 10 per cent CO_2 and should be retained for three or four weeks before being discarded as negative. Blood cultures in Castaneda bottles should be tipped twice weekly so that the blood-broth mixture flows over the agar surface.

Smears of specimens may be examined by the fluorescent antibody technique, as may colonies suspected of being *Brucella* which have grown in cultures. Colonies appear slowly and may initially be very small and difficult to see. The advantage of a biphasic medium for blood cultures is that it obviates the need for routine subcultures, a step that is otherwise quite important because of the lack of turbidity usually imparted to broth by *Brucella*.

Urease activity is manifested rapidly by *B. suis* and slowly or not at all by *B. melitensis* and *B. abortus*. *B. canis* shares some characteristics with *B. suis* so that its standing as a separate species is provisional. Dye inhibition tests with basic fuchsin and thionin are usually used in the identification process (Table 47–32). As has already been mentioned, the serologic confirmation at the genus level can be made with fluorescein-conjugated antiserum. Monospecific antisera can be used to distinguish between the *B. abortus-B. suis* complex and *B. melitensis;* however, such antisera are not widely available.

The diagnosis of brucellosis is often made

Table 47–32.   DIFFERENTIAL CHARACTERISTICS OF SPECIES OF *BRUCELLA**

| | | | | GROWTH ON | | |
| | | | | basic fuschsin | thionin | |
SPECIES	CO₂ REQUIRED	H₂S	UREASE	1:50,000	1:25,000	1:50,000
B. melitensis	−	−	− or (+)	+	−	+
B. abortus	d	+	(+) or −	+	−	+
B. suis	−	+ or −	+	− or +	+	+
B. canis	−	−	+	−	+	+

*Symbols: See Table 47–17.

serologically. A minimum titer of 1:160 in a standard tube agglutination test should lead one to suspect the diagnosis; however, evidence of recent brucellosis can be accepted only when a fourfold or greater rise in titer occurs during the first month or two of illness. Inhibitory prozones can occur in patients with titers as high as 1:640 so that all sera from patients with suspected disease should be diluted to at least 1:1280. Cross-reactivity with *Francisella tularensis* and with *Vibrio cholerae*, including cholera vaccination, occurs. The tube agglutination test is very sensitive and yields the most standardized results, in contrast to the more rapid slide agglutination tests which may give both falsely positive and falsely negative results.

Antimicrobial Susceptibility. The drugs of choice in the treatment of brucellosis are tetracycline or, secondarily, chloramphenicol with or without streptomycin. In general, relapse rates have been lower in patients receiving combinations including streptomycin.

Prevention and Control. Since the major reservoirs of brucellae are livestock and milk and meat, eradication programs have been oriented to breaking the chain of infection and have included immunization, testing and disposal of infected animals, and pasteurization of milk and its by-products.

Bordetella

Definitions and Characteristics. Bordetellae are strictly aerobic, non-fermentative, minute coccobacilli requiring nicotinic acid, cysteine, and usually methionine but not hemin (X factor) or coenzyme I (V factor) for growth. Excess fatty acids are formed during growth and are inhibitory to further growth so that blood, charcoal, starch, or ion-exchange resins must be added to the medium to act as an adsorbent. Phase variation from smooth virulent strains to rough avirulent strains occurs after cultivation on artificial media.

Pathogenesis and Virulence Factors. The proposed pathogenetic sequence of infection due to *Bordetella pertussis* has been reviewed extensively by Olson (1975). The organism attaches to the ciliated epithelium of the respiratory tract, multiplies, and releases toxins with a variety of proposed effects which result, though not necessarily in sequence, in inflammation and epithelial necrosis, leukocytosis and lymphocytosis, accumulation of secretions, cough, and ultimately bronchopneu-

monia, hypoxic episodes, and encephalopathy. *B. pertussis* contains a protective antigen which when combined with antibody abolishes its infectivity. It appears, however, that both cellular and humoral immunity are needed to eradicate the organism.

B. parapertussis may infrequently cause a pertussis-like illness. *B. bronchiseptica*, on the other hand, is isolated from humans after contact with guinea pigs, rabbits, dogs, cats, and rodents in which it may represent a component of their indigenous flora or it may actually cause disease. Its role in causing human infection is much less clearcut.

Laboratory Diagnosis. The rate of isolation of *B. pertussis* from patients declines with the duration of illness. Normal healthy individuals are not carriers of the organism so that its isolation always represents disease.

The most commonly recommended specimen is the nasopharyngeal swab; however, nasopharyngeal aspirates with a soft rubber catheter have provided higher rates of isolation in some peoples' hands. In general, swabs or aspirates should be inoculated onto suitable media, e.g., charcoal or Bordet-Gengou agar, as quickly as possible; however, Stuart's transport medium has been found to be satisfactory for storage purposes for up to 24 hours. Other suitable transport media have been described but are less widely available. Swabs or aspirates may be inoculated onto charcoal agar slants for mailing purposes.

Direct examination of smears stained with fluorescein-conjugated *B. pertussis* antiserum represents a rapid diagnostic test. Cultures are recommended, however, because a low rate of falsely positive and falsely negative smears does occur.

Specimens should be inoculated onto Bordet-Gengou or charcoal agar with added (20 per cent) rabbit, sheep, or horse blood. One plate with and one without antibiotic should be used. Although penicillin (0.5 U/ml) is most frequently used, overgrowth by indigenous flora is better prevented by cephalexin (40 μg/ml), which has a broader spectrum of activity than penicillin. The cultures should be incubated at 36° C. and examined daily for up to six days.

Colonies suspected of representing *B. pertussis* can be presumptively identified by examining a smear stained with fluorescein-labeled specific antiserum. *B. pertussis* is rather inactive and will not grow on blood-free media, usually requires three to four days to grow on charcoal or Bordet-Gengou agar, and does not reduce nitrates, produce urease, or utilize citrate. *B. parapertussis* will grow on blood-free media, grows rapidly on charcoal or Bordet-Gengou agar, utilizes citrate, produces urease, but does not reduce nitrates. *B. bronchiseptica* is the most active of the three and grows readily on conventional nutrient media, reduces nitrates, utilizes citrate, and rapidly ($\leq$4h) hydrolyzes urea.

Antimicrobial Susceptibility. Antimicrobial agents probably play no role in the therapy of pertussis but do render negative nasopharyngeal cultures within one or two days which may prevent bacterial complications in patients with the disease and may be effective in preventing spread of the disease to nonimmune contacts. Although several groups of agents are active in vitro against *B. pertussis*, erythromycin has been the only one consistently shown to be rapidly effective in vivo.

Prevention and Control. Vaccination represents the most effective means of control of pertussis in children, and current recommendations are to begin immunization at two months of age and to restrict it to the first six years because of the risks of neurologic complications. Workers in the health care fields probably should, however, also be immunized because of their greater risk of exposure and acquisition of the disease.

Haemophilus

Definitions and Characteristics. Members of the genus are small gram-negative rods or coccobacilli with a requirement for haemin or other porphyrins (X factor) and/or nicotinamide adenine di- or trinucleotides (V factor). The medically important species, as classified by Kilian (1976), are listed in Table 47-33. *Haemophilus parahaemolyticus* is not listed because it loses its hemolytic property rapidly in subcultures and becomes indistinguishable from *H. parainfluenzae*. *H. aegyptius* is omitted because of its close similarity to *H. influenzae* and doubts among taxonomists about the justification for differentiating these two species. *H. vaginalis* is also omitted, since there is general agreement that it does not belong in the genus. A proposal has been made to reclassify it as *Corynebacterium vaginale*, but its taxonomic position remains unsettled.

Pathogenesis and Virulence Factors. The virulence factors of species of *Haemo-*

philus are as yet poorly understood. Endotoxin is not produced by *H. influenzae*, and this species is rapidly killed once ingested by macrophages unless antibody, complement, or the phagocytes are deficient. The role of antibodies in immunity is also poorly understood. Antibodies develop with age, presumably following natural infection with *H. influenzae* or with cross-reacting antigenic organisms, so that most persons older than 15 years have antibodies. Which antibody and what level of that antibody are protective remain unknown.

Most *Haemophilus* species are indigenous to the upper respiratory tract and the oral cavity, and the encapsulated strains of *H. influenzae*, particularly those belonging to group B, are most often responsible for diseases due to *Haemophilus*, including meningitis, bacteremia, endocarditis, epiglottitis, otitis, conjunctivitis, and pneumonia. *H. parainfluenzae* has been associated with meningitis, while it, *H. paraphrophilus*, and *H. aphrophilus* have been associated with subacute bacterial endocarditis. *H. ducreyi* is responsible for chancroid. The clinical significance of *H. vaginalis* is, not unlike its taxonomy, confusing. There appears to be little doubt about its ability to produce vaginitis when introduced experimentally into the vaginas of normal, healthy women; however, its isolation from vaginal cultures of a quarter to a third of asymptomatic women poses a puzzling dilemma.

Laboratory Diagnosis. The isolation of *Haemophilus* usually requires the presence of haemin (X factor) and/or nicotinamide adenine nucleotides (V factor) in the culture medium. The former is most frequently supplied by the incorporation of heat-lysed ("chocolatized") blood cells in agar, although it may also be provided by whole human, horse, or rabbit blood cells. The V factor is commonly supplied either by the incorporation of yeast extract or other appropriate supplements in the medium or by a *Staphylococcus* which is streaked across the agar surface and about which satellite colonies of V-dependent strains of *Haemophilus* grow. The differential characteristics of members of this genus are listed in Table 47-33.

The requirements for X and V factors are determined by placing paper discs or strips impregnated with each and with both factors onto a soybean-casein digest agar surface that has been streaked with the test strain. There are a number of difficulties posed by this approach. First of all, carry-over of haemin from

Table 47–33. DIFFERENTIAL CHARACTERISTICS OF MEDICALLY IMPORTANT
HAEMOPHILUS SPECIES*

SPECIES	TESTS					
	δ-ALA† Utilization	V-Factor Requirement	Indole	Urease	Ornithine Decarboxylase	CO_2 Enhancement
H. influenzae						
biotype I	−	+	+	+	+	−
II	−	+	+	+	−	−
III	−	+	−	+	−	−
IV	−	+	−	+	+	−
V	−	+	+	−	+	−
H. haemolyticus	−	+	d	+	−	−
H. ducreyi	−	−	−	−	−	−
H. parainfluenzae		+				−
biotype I	+	+	−	−	+	−
II	+	+	−	+	+	−
III	+	+	−	+	−	d
H. paraphrophilus	+	+	−	−	−	d
H. aphrophilus	+	−	−	−	−	d

* Adapted from Kilian, 1976. Symbols: See Table 47–17.
† δ-aminolevulinic acid.

the original isolation plate is almost unavoidable so that growth of an X- and V-dependent strain, such as *H. influenzae*, about the V strip or disc may occur, leading to an erroneous identification of *H. parainfluenzae* or *H. paraphrophilus*. One way of minimizing this transfer of haemin is to place a colony of the test strain into 1 to 2 ml of soybean-casein broth, mix the suspension thoroughly, and then use a swab to inoculate the surface of the agar on which the X and V factor requirements are to be tested. Despite this precaution, traces of haemin may still be transferred and lead to an erroneous test result. Therefore, although X factor is commonly listed among tests required to identify haemophili, it is suggested that a different test system be used for separating V-dependent species from the others. One such test which is simple and very reliable was described by Kilian (1974) and determines the ability of V-dependent species to use δ-aminolevulinic acid in the biosynthesis of porphobilinogen and porphyrins. The formation of porphobilinogen can be detected by adding Kovac's reagent to the reaction mixture and observing the development of a red color in the aqueous phase. Alternatively, the formation of porphyrins in the reaction mixture can be demonstrated by red fluorescence under a Wood's lamp. Haemolytic properties of human isolates of haemophili can be determined on rabbit or horse blood agar;

however, neither taxonomic nor clinical considerations justify the performance of this test.

H. aphrophilus must often be distinguished from species such as *Actinobacillus actinomycetemcomitans*, *Cardiobacterium hominis*, and *Eikenella corrodens* (Table 47–34), all of which have been associated with subacute bacterial endocarditis.

The cultivation of *H. ducreyi* from chancroid lesions has not been terribly satisfactory. A Gram's stained smear of material from the lesion may be helpful if gram-negative bacilli in pairs or in rows ("schools of fish") are seen. Material may be inoculated into fresh, heat-inactivated serum which is incubated at 35°C. for several days. Smears of the culture are made regularly and examined microscopically for the appearance of gram-negative bacilli in chains and rows.

H. vaginalis may be detected microscopically in either wet mounts or in Gram's stained smears by the finding of "clue cells," which are finely granulated epithelial cells surrounded by masses of small, pleomorphic gram-negative bacilli. Media containing proteose peptone No. 3, e.g., Casman agar and proteose peptone-starch-dextrose agar (PSD), have most often been used for isolation of this species. Columbia CNA (colistin, 10 μg/ml; nalidixic acid, 15 μg/ml) agar has been found to be useful as a selective medium for *H. vaginalis*. The

Table 47–34. DIFFERENTIAL CHARACTERISTICS OF *HAEMOPHILUS APHROPHILUS,*
ACTINOBACILLUS ACTINOMYCETEMCOMITANS, CARDIOBACTERIUM HOMINIS,
AND *EIKENELLA CORRODENS**

TEST	H. APHROPHILUS	A. ACTINOMYCETEMCOMITANS	C. HOMINIS	E. CORRODENS
oxidase	−	−	+	+
catalase	−	+	−	−
δ-ALA utilization†	+	+	+	+
V-requirement	−	−	−	−
indole	−	−	+	−
urease	−	−	−	−
lysine decarboxylase	−	−	−	+
ornithine decarboxylase	−	−	−	+
acid from				
glucose	+	+	+	−
sucrose	+	−	+	−
lactose	+	−	−	−
mannitol	−	+	d	−
xylose	−	d	−	−

*Symbols: See Table 47–17.
†δ-aminolevulinic acid.

organism is catalase- and oxidase-negative and ferments dextrose, maltose, and levulose but not sucrose. Nitrates are not reduced, and indole is not formed.

The presence of typable strains of *H. influenzae* in smears can be rapidly confirmed microscopically by fluorescent antibody methods. They can also be detected rapidly in normally sterile body fluids, such as cerebrospinal or synovial fluid, by counterimmunoelectrophoresis (CIE). While fluorescent microscopy is usually reserved for situations in which organisms are seen in Gram's stained smears and rapid confirmation of their identity is sought, CIE is useful for screening the fluid directly for bacterial antigen in the absence of visible organisms in the smear. Another rapid detection method is to test the agglutinability of protein A-rich staphylococci coated with *H. influenzae* antiserum in the presence of soluble bacterial antigen in body fluids (Suksanong, 1977).

Antimicrobial Susceptibility. Since approximately 5 per cent of clinical isolates of *H. influenzae* are resistant to ampicillin because of β-lactamase production, it is now necessary for the susceptibility of isolates from normally sterile body fluids or spaces to be tested. A variety of rapid acidimetric and iodometric tests for determining the elaboration of β-lactamase by bacteria have been described (see Chap. 55) and usually suffice for clinical purposes. Although a few cases of infections due to chloramphenicol-resistant

H. influenzae have been reported, chloramphenicol, either alone or in combination with ampicillin, is recommended for the initial therapy of patients with diseases suspected to be due to haemophili. With β-lactamase-negative strains ampicillin remains the drug of choice. With the exceptions of several newer cephalosporins, including cefamandole, cefoxitin, and cefuroxime, most antibiotics in this class are not particularly active against haemophili.

Eikenella

Definitions and Characteristics. Formerly classified as *Bacteroides corrodens,* the "corroding bacilli" that are facultatively anaerobic have been assigned to the species *Eikenella corrodens.* Strictly anaerobic corroding bacilli, which differ in several important respects from the facultatively anaerobic bacilli, remain classified as *Bacteroides corrodens.* Strains of *E. corrodens* are the same as King's subgroup Hb-1. They are oxidase-positive, catalase-negative, non-fermentative gram-negative bacilli, colonies of which may corrode or pit agar. Growth is enhanced by 5 to 10 per cent CO_2 and usually requires the presence of haemin (X factor) in the medium.

Pathogenesis and Virulence Factors. Little is known about factors contributing to the organism's virulence, and it has a low level of pathogenicity for animals. *Eikenella* resides predominantly in the nasopharynx and is isolated frequently from the upper respiratory tract. It has been recovered from abscesses and other types of infections in almost any site, may invade the bloodstream, and may cause endocarditis. Infections are usually mixed.

Laboratory Diagnosis. The most striking feature of *Eikenella* in cultures is its ability to pit the agar; however, pitting does not occur with all strains. The colonies appear slowly and are generally small (0.5 to 1.0 mm in diameter). It must usually be distinguished from other fastidious, slowly growing gram-negative bacilli (Table 47-34).

Antimicrobial Susceptibility. *Eikenella* is susceptible to the penicillins and chloramphenicol. Its susceptibility to aminoglycosides is variable, but it is resistant to clindamycin.

Actinobacillus actinomycetemcomitans

Definitions and Characteristics. Other than the sesquipedalian character of its name, this organism currently occupies an uncertain taxonomic position. It is small, coccoid to bacillary in shape microscopically, grows aerobically and somewhat better in CO_2 and anaerobically, and may grow in broth in the form of small granules adhering to the walls of the tube. Colonies on blood agar appear slowly and are small.

Pathogenesis and Virulence Factors. *Actinobacillus actinomycetemcomitans* has a low level of pathogenicity. It derives its name from its frequent association with actinomycotic lesions. In recent years, however, it has most frequently been reported as a cause of subacute bacterial endocarditis.

Laboratory Diagnosis. The most frequently reported source of the organism in recent years is in blood cultures from patients with endocarditis. It appears to grow slowly in most currently used blood culture media. It must be differentiated from other slowly growing, somewhat fastidious gram-negative bacilli (Table 47-34).

Antimicrobial Susceptibility. Although not consistently susceptible to the penicillins, ampicillin alone has been successfully employed in the treatment of a number of reported cases. Ampicillin and streptomycin have been found to be bactericidal but not synergistic against the organism and have also been used in the therapy of endocarditis associated with it. Other active antimicrobial agents include the tetracyclines and chloramphenicol.

Cardiobacterium hominis

Definitions and Characteristics. *Cardiobacterium*, formerly "Group II-D," is a pleomorphic, facultatively anaerobic, fermentative, oxidase- and indole-positive gram-negative bacillus that is antigenically unrelated to the Brucellaceae. Microscopically, the cells may occur in pairs, short chains, tear-drop shapes, rosette clusters, or in filamentous forms. The ends of the cells may be bulbous and may retain crystal violet. Sudanophilic bodies and metachromatic inclusions are demonstrable.

Pathogenesis and Virulence Factors. Pathogenicity tests in laboratory animals have been negative. All recorded cases of human infection with *Cardiobacterium* had endocarditis nearly always superimposed on pre-existing valvular malformation or disease.

Laboratory Diagnosis. The organism grows slowly in blood cultures, usually requiring at least 5 to 7 days of incubation for its detection. In a recent case at the Mayo Clinic the organism required between 12 and 23 days of incubation. Colonies are small on blood agar. The organism grows well on soybean-casein digest agar with and without added blood in an atmosphere of increased CO_2 or high humidity. It can be distinguished from other slowly growing fastidious gram-negative bacilli by the reactions listed in Table 47-34.

Antimicrobial Susceptibility. *Cardiobacterium* is susceptible to the penicillins, cephalosporins, aminoglycosides, tetracyclines, and chloramphenicol.

Calymmatobacterium granulomatis

Description and Characteristics. Previously known as *Donovania granulomatis*, *Calymmatobacterium* is a gram-negative, nonmotile, encapsulated, pleomorphic rod that may be cultured in yolk sacs or on fresh egg yolk medium. The organism possesses antigenic determinants similar to those of *Klebsiella*, leading some authors to classify it among the Enterobacteriaceae.

Pathogenesis and Virulence Factors. The organism does not produce disease in animals. In humans it causes granuloma inguinale characterized by ulcerogranulomatous lesions of the skin and mucosa of the genital and inguinal areas.

Laboratory Diagnosis. A fragment of tissue removed from the margin of an ulcer is pressed and rubbed against a glass slide and stained with Wright's or Giemsa's stain. The finding of small, straight or curved, pleomorphic rods with rounded ends and characteristic polar granules giving a safety pin appearance within mononuclear cells is the most effective way of establishing the diagnosis.

Antimicrobial Susceptibility. The tetracyclines, erythromycin, ampicillin, and chloramphenicol are active against *Calymmatobacterium*. Resistance may develop to streptomycin.

Streptobacillus moniliformis

Description and Characteristics. *Streptobacillus* is a facultatively anaerobic, fermentative, non-encapsulated, and non-motile gram-negative rod, frequently in chains and filaments, and often with a series of oval to elongated bulbous swellings giving a string-of-beads appearance. Blood, serum, or ascitic fluid is needed for growth in agar or broth. The microscopic morphology varies with time, being more homogeneously filamentous in young cultures and becoming fragmented into irregular coccobacilli with age. L-phase colonies may occur spontaneously on agar, have a "fried egg" appearance, become stabilized if penicillin is incorporated in the medium, and are indistinguishable from L-phase colonies of other bacteria and from mycoplasmas.

Pathogenesis and Virulence Factors. *Streptobacillus* occurs as indigenous flora in the upper respiratory tract of wild and laboratory rodents. Infection (Haverhill disease) in humans follows rodent bites, ingestion of contaminated food, or traumatic injury. Local lymphangitis and lymphadenitis may develop up to three weeks later, followed by the onset of fever, chills, malaise, and later by a general morbilliform maculopapular or petechial rash. Some patients develop a migratory polyarthritis. Endocarditis has been reported.

The histopathology is non-specific and demonstrates a chronic inflammatory reaction.

Laboratory Diagnosis. Sedimented red blood cells can be used to prepare pour plates by adding them to molten heart infusion (HI) agar supplemented with yeast extract. Red cells and sterile body fluids can also be plated on HI agar supplemented with yeast extract and with heat-inactivated sterile horse serum. Normally sterile body fluids should be examined microscopically after staining with Gram's and Giemsa's stains. Material should

also be inoculated into HI broth containing the supplements described above.

The identification of *Streptobacillus* is rather complex. Colonies in broth form as fluff balls, while those on agar are small and slightly translucent to opaque with a slightly irregular edge. L-phase variants may form on agar. Subcultures are made from broth with pipets or by agar block transfers. Biochemical tests must be performed in HI agar or broth supplemented with yeast extract and horse serum.

Antimicrobial Susceptibility. Penicillin alone and in combination with streptomycin is active against *Streptobacillus*.

Prevention and Control. Since 10 to 65 per cent of rats are infected with the organism, their control and precautions against bites represent the only effective methods of control of the disease.

Francisella

Definitions and Characteristics. Formerly classified as *Pasteurella tularensis*, *Francisella tularensis* is a very small, strictly aerobic, coccoid to pleomorphic rod-shaped, gram-negative bacillus which requires cystine or cysteine for its growth. Faint bipolar staining occurs with aniline dyes.

Pathogenesis and Virulence Factors. Virulence appears to be related to a smooth colonial morphology. Repeated subcultures result in an alteration from smooth to rough colonies with a concomitant loss of virulence. Highly virulent strains for humans have citrulline ureidase activity and ferment glycerol and are most often associated with tickborne disease in rabbits. Toxins have not been recognized.

Tularemia may manifest itself after an incubation period of one to 10 days in various forms. Headache, fever, chills, vomiting, and myalgias characteristically occur at the onset. In the ulceroglandular type of disease, lymphadenitis and lymphadenopathy occur in the region draining the primary lesion. The lesion is initially papular and later ulcerative. A variation of this form of disease, the oculoglandular type, is characterized by inflammation of the conjunctiva and usually a papule of the lower lid with lymphadenitis of the preauricular, parotid, submaxillary, and anterior cervical nodes. An ingestion form of tularemia is characterized by ulcerative lesions of the mouth, throat, and upper gastrointestinal tract. Pneumonia may result from inhalation or secondary to bacteremia from another focus of infection.

Tularemia should be suspected in anyone who has been in an endemic area, has had contact with wild animals or livestock, has been engaged in farming operations, has drunk impure water, or has been exposed to cultures or infected animals in the laboratory. Trappers, hunters, fur and meat industry workers, agricultural workers, and laboratory personnel are at greatest risk. Because of its protean manifestations, tularemia is readily confused with many other diseases, such as brucellosis, anthrax, sporotrichosis, typhoid fever, tuberculosis, histoplasmosis, and syphilis.

Laboratory Diagnosis. Material suitable for examination includes fluid or curettings from the primary lesion, aspirates of enlarged regional nodes, sputum, pharyngeal washes, and gastric aspirates. Microscopic examination of clinical material or of colonies stained with specific fluorescein-labeled conjugate constitutes the most rapid and reliable means of identifying *Francisella*. Cultures may be made on glucose-cysteine agar supplemented with 5 per cent defibrinated rabbit blood. If the clinical material is contaminated with other bacteria, 1 ml each of penicillin, 100,000 U/ml; polymyxin B, 100,000 U/ml; and cycloheximide, 0.1 mg/ml, should be included in each liter of medium. Special care must be exercised in handling infected material to prevent aerosolization or direct contact with the skin. Cultures are incubated at $35°C$. in an environment with or without added CO_2. Colonies usually appear within 24 hours and their identification may be confirmed by slide agglutination or immunofluorescence with specific antiserum.

The diagnosis can also be established serologically. Agglutination titers as low as 1:40 in the absence of previous disease are diagnostic and may rise within the first three weeks to levels of 1:640 or greater. Brucella agglutinins may also rise non-specifically but usually to a significantly lower level.

Antimicrobial Susceptibility. Streptomycin is bactericidal while the tetracyclines and chloramphenicol are bacteriostatic to *Francisella*. Since relapses are not infrequent after treatment with these bacteriostatic agents, streptomycin is the agent of choice.

Prevention and Control. The most common methods of acquiring tularemia are insect bites by bloodsucking arthropods and contact with or ingestion and inhalation of infected material. A variety of vertebrates and invertebrates have been reported to be infected with *Francisella*, the most frequent mammalian species of which are rabbits, beavers, muskrats, voles, and sheep. Vectors include ticks, deerflies, and mosquitoes. Preventive measures, therefore, have been directed toward increasing public awareness, developing protective measures for persons at risk, decreasing the vector population, and controlling vertebrate sources.

ANAEROBIC BACTERIA

It is important to re-emphasize that anaerobes represent a major component of the indigenous flora of the skin and mucous membranes and, therefore, that their isolation and identification should be contingent upon the proper selection and collection of specimens, as well as upon their proper transport to the laboratory. Anaerobic infections are frequently mixed, consisting either of several species of anaerobes or of anaerobes with facultatively anaerobic bacteria. Mixed cultures commonly consist of an average of two facultatively anaerobic and three anaerobic species. The first task, therefore, in examining an anaerobic culture is to separate facultatively anaerobic from anaerobic bacteria by subculturing each distinct morphologic type of colony onto blood agar plates to be incubated for 48 hours in air and in CO_2. Concurrently, each colony type is subcultured into thioglycollate broth supplemented with hemin and vitamin K_1. The morphology, presence of pigment, hemolytic properties, and microscopic characteristics of anaerobic colonies are recorded. With experience, the more commonly isolated anaerobes can often be recognized on the basis of their colonial and microscopic morphologies and presumptively identified on the basis of a few additional tests, including their susceptibility to certain antibiotics. Definitive identification is based upon biochemical reactions, physiologic and genetic characteristics, and pathogenicity and toxin neutralization tests.

The extent to which anaerobes are identified varies according to the facilities and expertise available, the interest of the laboratory personnel and clinical staff, and the clinical utility of the information available from the laboratory. In a small hospital laboratory, preliminary information based on colonial and microscopic morphology and aerotolerance studies is probably adequate. Presumptive identification based on morphology, antibiotic susceptibility patterns, and a few other tests should be adequate for most clinical purposes. Definitive identification of isolates on a routine basis is probably unnecessary except in large reference laboratories or for investigational purposes.

Definitions and Characteristics. The term *anaerobe* can be defined, according to Finegold (1977), as a bacterium that requires an atmosphere with reduced oxygen tension for its growth and that fails to grow on the surface of solid media in an atmosphere of room air with 10 per cent CO_2. A facultatively anaerobic bacterium will grow in either the presence or absence of room air. The term *microaerophile* has not been strictly defined and is commonly applied to bacteria, usually streptococci, that grow only or preferentially in an atmosphere with reduced oxygen and with increased carbon dioxide. Whether or not the so-called microaerophilic or air-tolerant streptococci should be classified as anaerobes or as viridans streptococci remains unsettled (Facklam, 1977).

The major groups of an aerobic bacteria which are encountered in clinical infections are listed in Table 47-35. Many additional species representing indigenous flora in humans and occasionally associated with disease are known.

Pathogenesis and Virulence Factors. Little is known about the factors responsible for the pathogenic and virulence properties of most anaerobes other than the histotoxic clostridia. Endotoxic, proteolytic, and heparinase activity have been identified among the Bacteroidaceae. In pure culture, however, these organisms do not produce disease in experimental animals and do so only when inoculated with other anaerobes or with facultatively anaerobic bacteria. The clostridia, on the other hand, elaborate potent exotoxins,

Table 47–35. MEDICALLY IMPORTANT ANAEROBIC BACTERIA*

DESCRIPTION	GENUS	SPECIES
Gram-positive bacilli, spore-forming	Clostridium	C. perfringens
		C. ramosum
		C. septicum
		C. novyi
		C. histolyticum
		C. sporogenes
		C. sordellii
Gram-positive bacilli, non–spore-forming	Actinomyces	A. israelii
	Arachnia	A. propionica
	Eubacterium	E. lentum
		E. limosum
		E. alactolyticum
	Bifidobacterium	B. eriksonii
	Propionibacterium	P. acnes
	Lactobacillus	L. catenaforme
Gram-positive cocci	Peptococcus	P. magnus
		P. asaccharolyticus
		P. prevotii
	Peptostreptococcus	P. anaerobius
		P. intermedius
		P. micros
Gram-negative cocci	Veillonella	V. parvula
Gram-negative bacilli	Bacteroides	B. fragilis
		B. melaninogenicus
	Fusobacterium	F. nucleatum
		F. necrophorum
		F. varium
		F. mortiferum
	Campylobacter	C. fetus

*Adapted from Finegold, 1977.

including lethal and necrotizing toxins, hemolysins, lecithinases, gelatinases, hyaluronidases, and so on.

While clostridial infection may be either exogenous or endogenous in origin, disease due to the other anaerobes usually originates endogenously from the normal indigenous anaerobic flora of a contiguous mucous membrane, the integrity of which has been disrupted by surgery, instrumentation, trauma, or malignancy. Essential to the establishment of anaerobes in the infectious process is a decrease in the oxidation-reduction potential (E_h) of the area, which may result from a failure of its blood supply or from the presence or multiplication of other bacteria at the site.

Much of the older literature on anaerobic infections dealt almost exclusively with the histotoxic clostridial infections and with the clostridial intoxications, tetanus and botulism. Although these infections and intoxications are unquestionably of major medical importance, the role of other anaerobes in causing cellulitis and myonecrosis has been recognized only relatively recently.

Most isolates of *Clostridium perfringens* in hospital practice today are the result of simple contamination of a wound. In such instances, the clostridia may multiply in cellular debris, a hematoma, or necrotic tissue without observable clinical symptomatology. Anaerobic cellulitis is a necrotizing process of the soft tissues. Its onset is gradual, but it can progress rapidly and extensively. Gas is produced; however, the process typically does not involve muscle. In addition to or instead of clostridia, the bacteriology of anaerobic cellulitis may involve anaerobic cocci and anaerobic gram-negative bacilli.

In contrast to anaerobic cellulitis, gas gangrene or clostridial myonecrosis is an acute and rapidly progressive invasive process producing marked changes in muscles. Distinguishing between anaerobic cellulitis and gas gangrene is critical in order to avoid performing unnecessarily aggressive and mutilating surgery in the former condition.

The histotoxic clostridia associated with gas gangrene include *C. perfringens, C. novyi, C. septicum, C. histolyticum, C. sporogenes,* and *C. bifermentans.* While *C. perfringens* has been the species most frequently involved in most reports of gas gangrene, the prevalence of the other species in this process has varied widely.

Tetanus and botulism are described as intoxications rather than infections because their manifestations are related to the elaboration of potent neurotoxins. Botulism is most frequently related to the ingestion of home-processed foods which have been improperly preserved or canned; however, sporadic outbreaks of the disease have been related to commercially processed food and to wounds infected with the organism. The incubation period for botulism is short, and signs and symptoms usually occur between 18 and 36 hours following ingestion of contaminated food. Of the seven antigenic types of botulinum toxin known, type A is the most common, followed by types B, E, and F in cases of food poisoning in North America. The toxin is absorbed from the intestinal tract and, rarely, from an infected wound and attaches ultimately to motor nerve terminals, thereby preventing acetylcholine release at the nerve endings.

Tetanus typically occurs in non-immunized persons within the first two weeks following a traumatically acquired puncture, laceration, or abrasion. Cases have been reported to occur postoperatively; following dental work, childbirth, and abortion; or in association with stasis and decubitus ulcers. The toxin, tetanospasmin, is transported to gangliosides in the central nervous system via the lymphatics and blood stream and by migration through the perineural spaces of peripheral nerves.

As has already been mentioned, other anaerobic bacteria, particularly the anaerobic cocci and gram-negative bacilli, have been associated with anaerobic cellulitis in addition to or instead of the histotoxic clostridial species. These organisms are part of the indigenous flora of the mucous membranes of the oral cavity and of the gastrointestinal and genitourinary tracts. As such, they are encountered in aspiration pneumonias, lung abscesses, empyemas, intra-abdominal infections and abscesses, pelvic abscesses, brain abscesses, and bacteremias. Anaerobic intra-abdominal infections commonly follow abdominal and especially colon surgery and are most frequently associated with *Bacteroides fragilis.* Clinically significant anaerobic bacteremias are also most frequently due to this species.

Laboratory Diagnosis. Although the extent of identification of anaerobes may vary considerably, certain basic and simple grouping procedures can be performed with a pure culture or subculture of an anaerobic organism: Gram's stained smear, motility, and an-

Table 47-36. GROUP IDENTIFICATION FROM PRELIMINARY TESTS*

| GROUP | GRAM REACTION | SPORES | ANTIBIOTIC DISC IDENTIFICATION | | | | | | LECITHINASE | LIPASE | NAGLER· | INDOLE | CATALASE | MOTILITY |
			C 10 µg	E 60 µg	K 1000 µg	P 2 U	R 15 µg	V 5 µg						
Gram-positive cocci	+	−	R			S		S	−	−	−	V	V	−
Gram-negative cocci	−	−	S			S		R	−	−	−	−	V	−
B. fragilis	−	−	R	S	R	R^S	S	R	−	−	−	V	V	−
*B. melaninogenicus—*oralis-ochraceus group	−	−	V	S	R	S	S	V	−	V	−	V	−	−
B. corrodens	−	−	S	S	S	S	S	R	−	−	−	−	−	−
*F. mortiferum—*varium group	−	−	S	R	S	S^R	R	R	−	−	−	V	−	−
Certain other *Fusobacterium* sp.	−	−	S	S^R	S	S	S	R	−	V	−	V	−	−
Certain GPNSB†	+	−	R			S^R		S^R	−	−	−	V	V	−
Clostridium sp.—α-toxin producers	+	+	R			S^R		V	+	−	+	V	−	V
Certain other *Clostridium* sp.	+	+	R			S^R		S^R	V	V	−	V	−	V

*Reproduced by permission from Sutter, 1975.

†Gram-positive, non-spore-forming bacilli
+ = positive or present
− = negative or absent
V = variable
C = colistin   E = erythromycin   K = kanamycin

S = sensitive, zones ≥ 10 mm
R = resistant, zones < 10 mm
S^R = usually sensitive, sometimes resistant
R^S = usually resistant, sometimes sensitive
P = penicillin   R = rifampin   V = vancomycin

tibiotic disc identification (Table 47-36). It should be pointed out that the antibiotic content in each of the discs differs from that of discs used in the standard antimicrobial susceptibility test. Anaerobic gram-negative bacilli that are not inhibited in thioglycollate medium (without glucose or indicator) containing 20 per cent oxgall (bile) and 0.1 per cent deoxycholate and that are susceptible to erythromycin and rifampin (Table 47-36) may be presumptively identified as *Bacteroides fragilis*. Colonies suspected of representing *B. fragilis* can also be rapidly and presumptively identified in smears stained with fluorescein-labeled specific antiserum. *Bacteroides melaninogenicus* can be identified by the formation of black or reddish-brown colonies which fluoresce red under ultraviolet light after a few days of incubation. Colonies of *Bacteroides corrodens* erode or pit agar after a few days of incubation. *Fusobacterium nucleatum* has a distinct microscopic morphology.

Propionibacterium acnes is catalase-positive and indole-positive and is the only non-spore-forming gram-positive bacillus that can be reliably identified without further tests. *Clostridium perfringens* usually produces a characteristic double zone of hemolysis and produces lecithinase on egg yolk agar.

Much can, therefore, be done to group the anaerobic bacteria with a few simple tests. Definitive identification requires the performance of many additional tests (Table 47-37), including gas-liquid chromatography for end-product analysis. Details of test reactions and endpoint analysis are available in the anaerobic bacteriology manuals of Sutter (1975) and of Holdeman (1977).

Table 47–37. TESTS REQUIRED FOR IDENTIFICATION OF ANAEROBES*

	NON-SPORULATING GRAM-NEGATIVE BACILLI	ANAEROBIC COCCI	CLOSTRIDIUM	NON-SPORULATING GRAM-POSITIVE BACILLI†
Motility	X		X	X
Indole	X	X	X	X
Nitrate	X	X		X
Esculin	X	X		X
Gelatin	X	X	X	X
Bile + DOC	X			
Catalase		X		X
Antibiotic suscept.	X	X‡		
EYA (Nagler lec., lip.)			X	
Spores			X	X
Starch			X	X
Urease			X	
GC, ether, meth.	X§	X	X¶	X
Carbohydrate fermentation				
Glucose	X	X	X	X
Levulose	X	X		
Lactose	X	X	X	X
Mannose	X			
Rhamnose	X			
Trehalose	X			X
Mannitol	X		X	X
Maltose		X	X	X
Sucrose		X		X
Cellobiose		X		X
Arabinose				X
Erythritol				X
Inositol				X
Raffinose				X
Sorbitol				X

*Reproduced by permission from Rosenblatt, 1976. Abbreviations: DOC = sodium deoxycholate; lec. = lecithinase; lip. = lipase; GC = gas chromatography; meth. = methylated; lac. = lactate; thr. = threonine; prop. = propionate.

†Check aerotolerance by subculturing in air and 5 per cent carbon dioxide.

‡Col, PCN, VM only.

§Not done on easily identified *Bacteroides melaninogenicus* and *Bacteroides fragilis*.

¶Not necessary for α-toxin producers.

Because of their rapid progression and considerable morbidity and mortality, the initial diagnosis and management of diseases due to the clostridia must be based upon their clinical presentation and manifestations. In some patients with tetanus, no primary wound is evident. When a wound is present, organisms typical of *Clostridium tetani* are seldom seen in stained smears even though they may be recovered from cultures. Moreover, because of this organism's widespread distribution in nature, its isolation from a wound is not necessarily indicative of the diagnosis of tetanus. Laboratory confirmation of botulism requires detection of the toxin in serum, wounds, gastric contents, feces, or the food suspected of causing the disease. Procedures for extracting the toxin and for performing mouse neutralization tests are complex; therefore, it is suggested that the appropriate materials be referred to the Center for Disease Control, Atlanta, Ga., for examination. Telephone consultation should be made in such instances to ensure that the requisite specimens are properly collected and transported to the Center and that the appropriate authorities are alerted about the situation.

In cases with suspected anaerobic cellulitis or gas gangrene, the laboratory can be helpful by examining exudate or tissue microscopically. The finding of numerous, large, "boxcar" shaped, gram-positive bacilli provides presumptive confirmation of the diagnosis. Stained smears may also be diagnostic of anaerobic streptococcal myositis. Cultures of exudate, tissue, and blood should also be performed. Once again, the level or extent of identification varies considerably among laboratories; however, *Clostridium perfringens* may be easily identified by its Gram's stained morphology, the production of double zones of hemolysis on blood agar, and a positive Nagler reaction on egg yolk agar.

Antimicrobial Susceptibility. With the notable exception of *Bacteroides fragilis*, the anaerobic bacteria are usually susceptible to the penicillins and cephalosporins. *B. fragilis* is inhibited *in vitro* by high concentrations of the penicillins and cephalosporins. Nearly all anaerobes are susceptible to clindamycin, chloramphenicol, and metronidazole. For the past several years most anaerobes have been resistant to tetracycline. Although its analogs, minocycline and doxycycline, are more active, significant numbers of anaerobes remain resistant to them. Resistance to clindamycin by rare strains of *B. fragilis* and species of clostridia other than *C. perfringens* has been reported by some investigators.

By and large, the lack of a standardized disc diffusion susceptibility testing method for anaerobes and the largely predictable nature of their susceptibility to various agents obviate the necessity for performing susceptibility tests on a routine basis. Testing should be reserved, therefore, for problem cases. Larger laboratories should regularly monitor the susceptibility of clinically significant anaerobes in order to determine whether or not any significant alterations are occurring.

Prevention and Control. The prevention and control of anaerobic infections remains most effectively directed against the histotoxic clostridial infections and the clostridial intoxications in which debridement, wound care, immunization, and care in food handling play important roles.

Immunization with tetanus toxoid remains the most effective means of prevention of tetanus itself. Guidelines for tetanus prophylaxis

Table 47-38. GUIDE TO TETANUS PROPHYLAXIS IN WOUND MANAGEMENT*

TETANUS IMMUNIZATION (DOSES)	CLEAN, MINOR WOUNDS		ALL OTHER WOUNDS	
	Td	TIG	Td	TIG
uncertain	yes	no	yes	yes
0-1	yes	no	yes	yes
2	yes	no	yes	no†
≥3	no‡	no	no§	no

*Based on Recommendation of the Public Health Service Advisory Committee on Immunization Practices, June, 1972. Symbols: Td = Tetanus and diphtheria toxoids, adult type; TIG = tetanus immune globulin (human).

†Unless wound is more than 24h old.

‡Unless more than 10 years have elapsed since last dose.

§Unless more than 5 years have elapsed since last dose.

in wound management are listed in Table 47-38. The prevention of botulism hinges on the use of proper canning techniques, both commercially and in the home. In suspected cases consultation and laboratory assistance are available on a 24-hour basis at the Center for Disease Control, Atlanta, Ga. A trivalent ABE antitoxin (Connaught) is also available through the Center.

The prevention of gas gangrene hinges on prompt surgical wound care, including thorough debridement. Antibiotics appear to play an important ancillary role to surgery in the management of traumatically acquired wounds. The therapy of gas gangrene is also largely surgical. As in prevention, antimicrobial therapy is also important. Of less certain value in the treatment of gas gangrene are antitoxin and hyperbaric oxygen.

Since other anaerobic infections are largely of endogenous origin, prevention is more difficult to accomplish. Perioperative antibiotic therapy in preparation for colon surgery and for pelvic surgery has been shown in controlled trials to reduce the incidence of postoperative infections which are due for the most part to anaerobes.

GENERAL REFERENCES

Buchanan, R. E., and Gibbons, N. E. (eds.): Bergey's Manual of Determinative Bacteriology, 8th ed. Baltimore, Williams and Wilkins Co., 1974.

Cohen, J. O. (ed.): The Staphylococci. New York, John Wiley and Sons, Inc., 1972.

Edwards, P. R., and Ewing, W. H.: Identification of Enterobacteriaceae, 3rd ed. Minneapolis, Burgess Publishing Co., 1972.

Finegold, S. M.: Anaerobic Bacteria in Human Disease. New York, Academic Press, Inc., 1977.

Hoeprich, P. D.: Infectious Diseases, 2nd ed. Hagerstown, Md., Harper and Row, Publishers, 1977.

Holdeman, L. V., Cato, E. P., and Moore, W. E. C.: Anaerobe Laboratory Manual, 4th ed. Blacksburg, Va., Virginia Polytechnic Institute and State University, 1977.

Hubbert, W. T., McCulloch, W. F., and Schnurrenberger, P. R. (ed.): Diseases Transmitted from Animals to Man, 6th ed. Springfield, Ill., Charles C Thomas, Publisher, 1975.

Lennette, E. H., Spaulding, E. H., and Truant, J. P. (eds.): Manual of Clinical Microbiology, 2nd ed. Washington, D. C., American Society for Microbiology, 1974.

Sutter, V. L., Vargo, V. L., and Finegold, S. M.: Wadsworth Anaerobic Bacteriology Manual, 2nd ed. Los Angeles, Cal. Regents of the University of California, 1975.

Top, F. H., Sr., and Wehrle, P. F.: Communicable and Infectious Diseases. St. Louis, The C. V. Mosby Co., 1972.

Wannamaker, L. W., and Matsen, J. M. (eds.): Streptococci and Streptococcal Diseases: Recognition, Understanding, and Management. New York, Academic Press, Inc., 1972.

Washington, J. A., II (ed.): Laboratory Procedures in Clinical Microbiology. Boston, Little, Brown and Company, 1974.

Youmans, G. P., Paterson, P. Y., and Sommers, H. M.: The Biologic and Clinical Basis of Infectious Diseases. Philadelphia, W. B. Saunders Company, 1975.

SPECIFIC REFERENCES

Anhalt, J. P., and Yu, P. K. W.: Counterimmunoelectrophoresis of pneumococcal antigens: Improved sensitivity for the detection of types VII and XIV. J. Clin. Microbiol. 2:510, 1975.

Aranki, A., Syed, S. A., Kenney, E. B., and Freter, R.: Isolation of anaerobic bacteria from human gingiva and mouse cecum by means of a simplified glove box procedure. Appl. Microbiol., 17:568, 1969.

Baird-Parker, A. C.: Micrococcaceae. In Buchanan, R. E., and Gibbons, N. E. (eds.): Bergey's Manual of Determinative Bacteriology, 8th ed. Baltimore, Williams and Wilkins Co., 1974, pp. 478-490.

Bartlett, J. G., Alexander, J., Mayhew, J., Sullivan-Sigler, N., and Gorbach, S. L.: Should fiberoptic bronchoscopy aspirates be cultured? Am. Rev. Resp. Dis., 114:73, 1976.

Brewer, N. S., and Weed, L. A.: Diagnostic tissue microbiology methods. Hum. Pathol., 7:141, 1976.

Center for Disease Control: Morbidity and Mortality Weekly Report, 24:455, 1976.

Christensen, P., Kahlmeter, G., Jonsson, S., and Kronvall, G.: New method for the serological grouping of streptococci with specific antibodies adsorbed to protein A-containing staphylococci. Infect. Immunity, 7:881, 1973.

Darling, C. L.: Standardization and evaluation of the CAMP reaction for the prompt, presumptive identification of Streptococcus agalactiae (Lancefield group B) in clinical material. J. Clin. Microbiol., 1:171, 1975.

Donta, S. T.: Changing concepts of infectious diarrheas. Geriatrics, 30:123, 1975.

Edwards, E. A., and Larson, G. L.: New method of grouping beta-hemolytic streptococci directly on sheep blood agar plates by coagglutination of specifically sensitized protein A-containing staphylococci. Appl. Microbiol., 28:972, 1974.

Elin, R. J., and Wolff, S. M.: Biology of endotoxin. Ann. Rev. Med., 27:127, 1976.

Eng, J., and Holten, E.: Gelatin neutralization of the inhibitory effect of sodium polyanethol sulfonate on Neisseria meningitidis in blood culture media. J. Clin. Microbiol., 6:1, 1977.

Ewing, W H.: The nomenclature of Salmonella, its usage, and definitions for the three species. Can. J. Microbiol., 18:1629, 1972.

Facklam, R. R.: Physiological differentiation of viridans streptococci. J. Clin. Microbiol., 5:184, 1977.

Feigin, R. D., and Dodge, P. R.: Bacterial meningitis; newer concepts of pathophysiology and neurologic sequelae. Pediatr. Clin. North Am., 23:541, 1976a.

Feigin, R. D., Wong, M., Shackelford, P. G., Stechenberg,

B. W., Dunkle, L. M., and Kaplan, S.: Countercurrent immunoelectrophoresis of urine as well as of CSF and blood for diagnosis of bacterial meningitis. J. Pediatr., 89:773, 1976b.

Flynn, J., and Waitkins, S. A.: A serum-free medium for testing fermentation reactions in Neisseria gonorrhoeae. J. Clin. Pathol., 25:525, 1972.

Harris, J. C., DuPont, H. L., and Hornick, R. B.: Fecal leukocytes in diarrheal illness. Ann. Intern. Med., 76:697, 1972.

Hill, H. R., Riter, M. E., Menge, S. K., Johnson, D. R., and Matsen, J. M.: Rapid identification of group B streptococci by counterimmunoelectrophoresis. J. Clin. Microbiol., 1:188, 1975.

Hungate, R. E.: A roll tube method for cultivation of strict anaerobes. In Norris, J. R., and Ribbons, D. W. (eds.): Methods in Microbiology, vol. 3B. New York, Academic Press, Inc., 1969, pp. 117-132.

Jones, D. B.: Early diagnosis and therapy of bacterial corneal ulcers. Int. Ophthalmol. Clin., 13:1, 1973.

Kilian, M.: A rapid method for the differentiation of Haemophilus strains. Acta Pathol. Microbiol. Scand., 82(B):835, 1974.

Kilian, M.: A taxonomic study of the genus Haemophilus, with the proposal of a new species. J. Gen. Microbiol., 93:9, 1976.

Kunin, C. M.: Detection, Prevention and Management of Urinary Tract Infections, 2nd ed. Philadelphia, Lea and Febiger, 1974.

Nachum, R., Lipsey, A., and Siegel, S. E.: Rapid detection of gram-negative bacterial meningitis by the limulus lysate test. N. Engl. J. Med., 289:931, 1973.

Olson, L. C.: Pertussis. Medicine, 54:427, 1975.

Rosenblatt, J. E.: Isolation and identification of anaerobic bacteria. Hum. Pathol., 7:177, 1976.

Rosebury, T.: Microorganisms Indigenous to Man. New York, McGraw-Hill Book Co., Inc., 1962.

Schleifer, K. H., and Kloos, W. E.: A simple test system for the separation of staphylococci from micrococci. J. Clin. Microbiol., 1:337, 1975.

Schmidt, R. M., and Rosenkranz, H. S.: Antimicrobial activity of local anesthetics: Lidocaine and procaine. J. Infect. Dis., 121:597, 1970.

Shulman, J. A., and Nahmias, A. J.: Staphylococcal infections: Clinical aspects. In Cohen, J. O. (ed.): The Staphylococci. New York, John Wiley and Sons, Inc., 1972, pp. 457-481.

Suksanong, M., and Dajani, A. S.: Detection of Haemophilus influenzae type b antigens in body fluids, using specific antibody-coated staphylococci. J. Clin. Microbiol., 5:81, 1977.

5

Sutter, V. L., Vargo, V. L., and Finegold, S. M.: Wadsworth Anaerobic Bacteriology Manual. Los Angeles, Cal., Regents of the University of California, 1975.

Wannamaker, L. W.: Perplexity and precision in the diagnosis of streptococcal pharyngitis. Am. J. Dis. Child., *124*:352, 1972.

Washington, J. A., II: The Detection of Septicemia. Boca Raton, Florida, CRC Press Inc., 1978.

Washington, J. A., II: Laboratory approaches to the identification of Enterobacteriaceae. Hum. Pathol., *7*:151, 1976.

Washington, J. A., II (ed.): Laboratory Procedures in Clinical Microbiology. Boston, Little, Brown and Co., 1974.

Wilson, W. R., Dolan, C. T., Washington, J. A., II, Brown, A. L., Jr., and Ritts, R. E., Jr.: Clinical significance of postmortem cultures. Arch. Pathol., *94*:244, 1972.

MYCOBACTERIAL DISEASES

Herbert M. Sommers, M.D.

Before the introduction of streptomycin, the diagnosis of tuberculosis was often made on the basis of clinical symptoms, including cough, weight loss, and night sweats, an abnormal chest x-ray, and the finding of acid-fast bacilli in the sputum. Cultures were not always obtained, as there was little to be gained by recovering the organism. Therapy for all forms of mycobacterial disease was essentially the same and was based on putting the patient and the diseased organ at rest.

With introduction of streptomycin, it soon became apparent that resistance could develop rapidly, but to be able to detect resistance it was necessary to recover the organism. As more and more cultures were taken, improvements were made in both digestion and concentration procedures and culture media. Many of the cultures yielded "atypical" strains in that they were acid-fast but had colonial and/or other characteristics that differentiated them from *Mycobacterium tuberculosis.* As more and more of these atypical strains were isolated, many were found to have similar characteristics and have subsequently been classified in well-defined species. Not surprisingly, the control of tuberculosis has resulted in a relative increase in patients with disease from mycobacterial species other than *M. tuberculosis.*

SPECIMEN COLLECTION AND PREPARATION

Specimens from patients with tuberculosis usually contain mixed bacterial flora. The successful recovery of mycobacteria depends on properly collected specimens and on suppression of contaminating bacteria that might otherwise overgrow the mycobacteria. Therefore, methods for the collection of specimens should be directed toward minimizing the number of contaminating bacteria.

Sputum specimens containing *Mycobacterium tuberculosis* show faster growth with fewer contaminants when collected early in the morning with an ultrasonic or similar nebulizing device. Although it has been reported that pooled 24-hour sputum collections will yield more positive cultures than early morning specimens (Krasnow, 1969), growth is usually slower and the contamination rate is significantly higher in sputum pools (Kestle, 1967). Depending on whether there is minimal or advanced disease, there will be intermittent or continual shedding of tubercle bacilli. A minimum of three and not more than five early morning specimens will usually be sufficient to identify the patient with active disease (Krasnow, 1969).

Single clean-voided specimens collected

early in the morning are preferred for the diagnosis of urinary tract tuberculosis. Three to five specimens are usually sufficient. Although 24-hour urine collections can be obtained, some laboratory workers believe tubercle bacilli can suffer irreversible injury with prolonged exposure to urine.

Cerebrospinal fluid should be inoculated to Middlebrook 7H9 broth or other types of noninhibitory culture media after centrifugation.

If a pellicle is present in the cerebrospinal fluid, divide it into pieces for inoculation to several different types of culture media, saving a small fragment for an acid-fast stain. Portions of tissue from surgical biopsies or autopsies should be cut into small fragments and then either ground in a mortar and pestle with sterile sand or alundum powder or homogenized with a ground glass or Teflon homogenizer. The homogenized tissue should be inoculated to both selective and non-inhibitory culture media to provide optimal growth and control of contaminating bacteria.

Recovery of mycobacteria from a suspected tuberculous draining sinus is best from exudate or biopsies. Swabs taken from sinuses should be placed directly on culture media or in broth. Growth of mycobacteria from swab specimens is often inhibited by the hydrophobic nature of the lipid-containing mycobacterial cell wall, the mycobacteria preferring the interstices of the swab to the water-containing culture medium. Under these conditions growth of contaminating bacteria often masks the presence of mycobacteria.

Gastric washings are obtained at considerable discomfort to the patient and are frequently contaminated with commensal mycobacteria. Therefore, this method of specimen collection should be reserved for clinical situations in which more suitable specimens cannot be obtained. The frequent occurrence of commensal mycobacteria renders direct staining procedures of questionable value and necessitates complete identification of mycobacteria isolated. When required, specimens should be collected after an overnight fast and promptly neutralized.

DIGESTION AND CONCENTRATION

The isolation of mycobacteria from sputum and other clinical specimens poses a problem for the laboratory. The doubling time for *Mycobacterium tuberculosis* is approximately 20 to 22 hours, while other types of bacteria that can be present in the specimen may have doubling times of only 40 to 60 minutes. This disproportionate rate of growth between the two types of microorganisms can result in the accumulation of metabolic waste products from the rapidly growing bacteria and thereby make the culture medium unsatisfactory for the growth of mycobacteria. Therefore, the successful isolation of mycobacteria is dependent upon selective suppression of non-mycobacterial contaminating bacteria.

The high lipid content of mycobacterial cell walls makes them more resistant than contaminating bacteria to killing by strong acid and alkaline solutions. Specimens submitted for culture of mycobacteria which originate from sites normally colonized with other organisms are first treated with a chemical decontaminating agent to reduce bacterial overgrowth and liquefy mucus in order to facilitate concentration by centrifugation. After a carefully timed exposure during mechanical shaking, the acid or alkaline solution is neutralized and then centrifuged at 2000 g for 30 minutes to concentrate the mycobacteria. The relative centrifugal force (RCF) should be as high as possible, as the lipid content of the mycobacterial cell wall provides a buoyant effect to tubercle bacilli, making their specific gravity close to unity. This makes selective sedimentation of mycobacteria in a thick, viscous sputum specimen difficult.

In the past, decontaminating solutions were often so strong that if exposure times were not carefully controlled, large numbers of mycobacteria were either killed or so seriously injured that they did not grow or grew only very slowly. Decreasing the strength of decontamination solutions has resulted in the improved survival and recovery of mycobacteria but frequently at the price of a higher incidence of culture contamination. Exposure of specimens to strong decontaminating agents, such as 4 per cent NaOH, 5 per cent oxalic acid, and 3 per cent NaOH, must be carefully timed to prevent excessive chemical injury. Neutralization of a strong decontaminating solution requires an equally strong acid or alkaline solution, but often titration to a neutral endpoint is incomplete, with the specimen concentrate remaining either strongly alkaline or acid. Although the culture medium can act as a buffer for a moderate pH shift, an inadequately neutralized specimen can destroy the culture medium and prevent growth of any mycobacteria present. The use of decontaminating agents milder than 4 per cent NaOH or 5 per cent oxalic acid, such as trisodium phosphate (TSP) or TSP with benzalkonium chloride (Zephiran), has become an alternative in some laboratories. Specimens containing large numbers of *M. tuberculosis* can withstand the action of these agents for periods of time as long as 16 to 24 hours and still grow out as positive cultures. All specimens treated with TSP-benzalkonium chloride should be inoculated to egg-base culture media to neutralize the growth inhibition characteristics of benzalkonium choride. The concentrate can also be neutralized by adding lecithin if it is to be inoculated to agar-base media (Runyon, 1974).

In response to the increased need to recover mycobacteria for susceptibility testing, Kubica (1963) developed a concentrating solution containing 2 per cent NaOH and N-acetyl-L-cysteine (NALC). NALC is a mucolytic agent that can liquefy mucus by splitting disulfide bonds. It does not have any antibacterial activity. Mild decontamination is effected by 2 per cent NaOH, and with the mucus liquefied, the mycobacteria are sedimented by centrifugation. Occasionally the concentration of NaOH has to be increased to 3 per cent during periods of warm weather or for specimens from patients with large pulmonary cavities associated with persistent non-mycobacterial contamination. One advantage of the NALC decontamination procedure is neutralization of the specimen by the addition of a large volume of a slightly acid, pH 6.8 phosphate buffer. The use of the buffer makes strong pH shifts less likely and, in addition, acts as a "wash" during centrifugation, diluting any toxic substances as well as decreasing the specific gravity of the specimen to make sedimentation of mycobacteria more effective. Following centrifugation, the sediment is resuspended in 0.2 per cent bovine albumin, which has a buffering and detoxifying effect on the sedimented concentrate. A second mucolytic agent, also very useful for concentrating mycobacteria, is dithiothreitol. Dithiothreitol (Sputolysin) is similar in action to NALC, splitting disulfide bonds to liquefy mucin (Shah, 1966). Cetyl-pyridium chloride with NaCl has recently been shown to be an effective decontaminating agent for specimens transported through the mail. Mycobacteria have withstood transit times of eight days without significant loss of viability (Smithwick, 1975b).

Table 48-1 lists decontamination and concentration agents. The selection of one or more agents by a laboratory will depend on the number and types of specimens it receives

Table 48–1. AGENTS FOR DIGESTION AND CONCENTRATION OF SPECIMENS CONTAINING MYCOBACTERIA

	COMMENTS
N-acetyl-L-cysteine (NALC) + 2% NaOH	Mild decontamination solution with mucolytic agent—NALC—to free mycobacteria entrapped in mucus. NaOH may have to be increased to 3% to control contamination on occasion. NALC should be discarded after 24 to 48 hours.
Dithiothreitol (Sputolysin, Calbiochem, La Jolla, Cal.) + 2% NaOH*	Very effective mucolytic agent used with 2% NaOH. Reagent more expensive than NALC, but has the same advantages as NALC.
13% Trisodium phosphate + benzalkonium chloride (Zephiran)	Preferred by laboratories that cannot always control time of exposure to decontamination solution. Benzalkonium chloride should be neutralized with lecithin if not inoculated to egg base culture medium.
1% Cetyl-pyridium chloride + 2% NaCL†	Effective as a decontamination solution for sputum specimens mailed from outpatient clinics. *M. tuberculosis* has survived 8-day transit without significant loss of viability.
4% NaOH	Traditional decontamination and concentration solution. Time of exposure must be carefully controlled. 4% NaOH will effect mucolytic action to promote concentration by centrifugation.
4% Sulfuric acid	The use of 4% sulfuric acid when decontaminating urine specimens has improved recovery for many laboratories.
5% Oxalic acid	Most useful in the processing of specimens that contain *Pseudomonas aeruginosa* as a contaminant.

*(See Shah, 1966)
†(See Smithwick, 1975b)

5

and the time and technical staff available to process the specimens. The decontaminating procedures useful in laboratories receiving specimens from hospitalized patients may differ from those serving outpatient clinics. The specimens from some patients may require the use of different types of decontaminating agents if persistent contamination occurs; e.g., specimens containing *Pseudomonas aeruginosa* may survive 2 per cent NaOH-NALC and require concentration with 5 per cent oxalic acid.

CULTURE MEDIA

Culture media for mycobacteria can be classified as those solidified from coagulated eggs—"egg-base media"; those solidified with agar—"agar-base media"; liquid media; and media containing antimicrobial agents—"selective media."

Early attempts to recover mycobacteria by culture were only partially successful until a medium solidified with coagulated eggs was used. A large number of "egg-base" media have been developed, each differing slightly from the others. Most egg-base media are composed of varying combinations of whole eggs, potato flour, salts, and glycerol. Egg-base media are solidified by heating to 85 to 90°C. for 30 to 45 minutes (inspissation). Contaminating bacteria, particularly gram-positive bacteria, are controlled in part by the addition to the medium of aniline dyes such as crystal violet and malachite green. The concentration of aniline dye in a medium is im-portant, as slight increases over the specified amount can result in significant inhibition of mycobacterial growth.

Egg-base culture media

Numerous types of egg-base culture media have been described and are currently in use. The most commonly used egg-base medium for primary isolation of mycobacteria is Lowenstein-Jensen (see Table 48-2). Petragnani medium is more inhibitory and should be reserved for specimens known to contain large numbers of contaminants. A less inhibitory egg-base medium is the American Thoracic Society (ATS) medium. ATS is particularly helpful in the primary isolation of mycobacteria from specimens not likely to be contaminated, e.g., cerebrospinal fluid, pleural fluid, tissue biopsies, etc.

Agar-base culture media

During the 1950's Cohen and Middlebrook developed a series of mycobacterial culture media. These media were synthesized from salts, a series of organic compounds, glycerol, and albumin. Agar containing Middlebrook media is transparent and when scanned with a dissecting microscope can yield growth of *M. tuberculosis* after 12 to 14 instead of 18 to 24 days incubation. Middlebrook 7H9 broth is a popular liquid culture medium, and both 7H10 and 7H11 agar are widely used for primary isolation and susceptibility testing. The 7H11 medium differs from 7H10 only by the addition of 0.1 per cent casein hydrolysate which was found to improve the rate and amount of growth of mycobacteria resistant to isoniazid

Table 48–2.   NON-SELECTIVE MYCOBACTERIAL ISOLATION MEDIA

MEDIUM	COMPONENTS	INHIBITORY AGENT
Lowenstein-Jensen	Coagulated whole eggs, defined salts, glycerol, potato flour	0.025 g/100 ml malachite green
Petragnani	Coagulated whole eggs, egg yolks, whole milk, potato, potato flour, glycerol	0.052 g/100 ml malachite green
American Thoracic Society Medium	Coagulated fresh egg yolks, potato flour, glycerol	0.02 g/100 ml malachite green
Middlebrook 7H10	Defined salts, vitamins, co-factors oleic acid, albumin, catalase, glycerol, dextrose	0.0025 g/100 ml malachite green
Middlebrook 7H11	Defined salts, vitamins, co-factors oleic acid, albumin, catalase, glycerol, 0.1% casein hydrolysate	0.0025 g/100 ml malachite green

(Cohn, 1968). Both 7H10 and 7H11 contain malachite green but in much smaller quantities than in egg-base media. Although most culture media will yield more and larger colonies of mycobacteria when incubated in 5 to 10 per cent CO_2, the Middlebrook media must be incubated in CO_2 for recovery of equivalent numbers and size of colonies.

Agar media may be used in slanted culture tubes or poured in whole or divided Petri plates. The use of Petri plates permits the use of microscopy for early detection of growth and observation of colonial morphology, and facilitates the isolation of individual colonies. Some commercially available 7H11 medium has been modified to increase the amount of malachite green. Although the increased content of aniline dye retards growth of contaminating bacteria, it can also inhibit the growth of mycobacteria.

Exposure of 7H10 to strong light or storage of the media at 4°C. for more than four weeks can be associated with deterioration and release of formaldehyde. The presence of formaldehyde results in a very inhibitory medium with little or no growth of mycobacteria (Miliner, 1969).

Both Middlebrook 7H10 and 7H11 can be used for mycobacterial drug susceptibility testing, although 7H11 is preferred. Incorporation of antimycobacterial agents into the medium after sterilization and just before it solidifies reduces the loss of drug activity that can occur with some agents during the long heating period used in preparing inspissated egg-based media. The components of

non-selective culture media are listed in Table 48-2.

Selective culture media

Mycobacterial culture media containing antimicrobial agents to suppress bacterial and fungal contamination have been used for many years. Although certain antimicrobial agents will reduce bacterial contamination, they can also exert a significant growth inhibition on mycobacteria as well. Despite the inhibition of growth of some mycobacterial species, the use of selective culture media can result in greatly improved recovery of mycobacteria. The name and components of several selective culture media are listed in Table 48-3.

One of the more commonly used selective culture media was developed by Gruft, who added penicillin, nalidixic acid, and RNA to Lowenstein-Jensen medium (Gruft, 1971). Subsequently, it was found that a medium containing cycloheximide, lincomycin, and nalidixic acid was also effective in the control of fungal and bacterial contaminants (Petran, 1971). By varying the amount of each of these three agents, the medium could be prepared in either a Lowenstein-Jensen or 7H10 base (Table 48-3).

The culture medium Selective 7H11 is a modification of an oleic acid agar medium first described by Mitchison. It contains four antimicrobial agents and was originally developed to be used for sputum specimens without exposure to a decontaminating agent. McClatchey (1976) suggested that the carbeni-

5

Table 48-3. SELECTIVE MYCOBACTERIAL ISOLATION MEDIA

MEDIUM	COMPONENTS			INHIBITORY AGENTS
Gruft modification of Lowenstein-Jensen	Coagulated whole eggs, defined salts, glycerol, potato flour, RNA—17mg/100 ml	0.025	g/100 ml	malachite green
		50	units per ml	penicillin
		35	µg per ml	nalidixic acid
Mycobactosel Lowenstein-Jensen	Coagulated whole eggs, defined salts, glycerol, potato flour	0.025	g/100 ml	malachite green
		400	µg/ml	cycloheximide
		2	µg/ml	lincomycin
		35	µg/ml	nalidixic acid
Middlebrook 7H10	Defined salts, vitamins, co-factors, oleic acid, albumin, catalase, glycerol, and dextrose	0.0025	g/100 ml	malachite green
		360	µg/ml	cycloheximide
		2	µg/ml	lincomycin
		20	µg/ml	nalidixic acid
Selective 7H11 (Mitchison's medium)	Defined salts, vitamins, co-factors, oleic acid, albumin, catalase, glycerol, dextrose, and casein hydrolysate	50	µg/ml	carbenicillin
		10	µg/ml	amphotericin B
		200	units/ml	polymyxin B
		20	µg/ml	trimethoprim lactate

cillin be reduced from 100 to 50 μg/ml and that 7H11 medium be used instead of oleic acid agar, calling this modification Selective 7H11. Several reports comparing Selective 7H11 medium with Lowenstein-Jensen and 7H11 have shown a distinct increase in recovery of mycobacteria when used with the NALC-2 per cent NaOH decontamination and concentration procedure.

STAINING FOR ACID-FAST BACILLI

The lipid-containing cell walls of mycobacteria have a unique characteristic in binding carbolfuchsin stain so tightly that it resists destaining with strong decolorizing agents such as alcohols and strong acids. This "acid-fast" staining reaction of mycobacteria, along with their unique beaded and slightly curved shape, is a valuable aid in the early detection of infection and monitoring of therapy. The finding of acid-fast bacilli in the sputum, combined with a history of cough, weight loss, and a chest x-ray showing a pulmonary infiltrate, is considered presumptive evidence of active tuberculosis and is sufficient to initiate therapy.

It has been estimated that there must be 10,000 acid-fast bacilli per milliliter of sputum to be detected by microscopy. Patients with extensive disease will shed large numbers of mycobacteria and show a good correlation between a positive smear and a positive culture. In patients with minimal or less advanced disease, the correlation of positive smears to positive cultures may be only 60 to 70 per cent.

Acid-fast stains performed on a weekly basis are also useful in following the response of patients to drug therapy. After drugs are started, cultures will become negative before smears, indicating that the bacilli are injured sufficiently to prevent replication but not to the point of preventing binding of the stain. With continued drug treatment, more organisms are killed and fewer shed, so that following the number of stainable organisms in the sputum during treatment can provide an early objective measure of response. *It should be noted that not all stainable organisms are viable.* Should the number of organisms fail to decrease after therapy is started, the possibility of drug resistance must be considered. Additional cultures should be taken and drug susceptibility studies obtained.

Two types of acid-fast stains are frequently used:

1. The carbolfuchsin stains, so called because of the reagent formed by mixing the stain fuchsin with the disinfectant phenol (carbolic acid). Two procedures using carbolfuchsin stains are in common use:
   a. the Ziehl-Neelsen, or "hot stain"
   b. the Kinyoun or "cold stain"
2. The fluorochrome dye, auramine 0, sometimes used in combination with a second fluorochrome stain, rhodamine.

Both stains bind to mycolic acid in the mycobacterial cell wall. Because of the small size of the organism and the low contrast in the color of the organism and the bright background, smears stained by carbolfuchsin must be scanned with the 100$\times$ oil immersion objective, thereby restricting the area of a slide that can be viewed in a given period of time. In comparison, smears stained with auramine 0 can be scanned using a 25$\times$ objective. Fluorochrome-stained mycobacteria appear bright yellow against a dark background obtained by counterstaining with potassium permanganate, thereby permitting the slide to be scanned under the lower magnification without losing sensitivity. The sharp visual contrast between the brightly colored mycobacteria and the dark background offers a distinct advantage in scanning a much larger area of the slide during the same time necessary for looking at the carbolfuchsin stain. For this reason, the fluorochrome stain will often result in the detection of mycobacteria in smaller numbers per slide than when using a carbolfuchsin stain. Fluorochrome-stained smears require a strong blue light source for illumination, either a 200 watt mercury vapor burner or a strong blue light source with a fluorescein isothiocyanate (FITC) filter. Modifications of the auramine fluorochrome staining procedure include the addition of rhodamine to give a more golden appearance to the mycobacteria or the use of acridine orange (Runyon, 1974; Vestal, 1975) as a counterstain to stain the background red to orange.

Enthusiasm for the carbolfuchsin and fluorochrome staining methods varies between laboratories, with different workers strongly partial to one method or the other. Specificity for mycobacteria seems to be the same for both, with the exception of a series of 15 strains of *Mycobacterium fortuitum*, in which 5 of the 15 did not stain with auramine but all 15 stained with carbolfuchsin (Joseph, 1967). Reports differ as to which of the two types of stain will bind to non-viable bacilli for the longest period of time. These differences probably reflect the care devoted to staining and microscopy by individual laboratories. As mentioned above, when using the auramine stain, a significantly larger area of the smear can be scanned in the same period of time used to scan a carbolfuchsin-stained smear. For this reason the fluorochrome stain offers the possibility of greater sensitivity. Because some workers are still hesitant to give up carbolfuchsin stains, some laboratories scan smears by the fluorochrome method and then confirm positive slides by destaining and restaining with a carbolfuchsin stain. Once laboratory workers have become familiar with the auramine stain, they usually prefer the fluorochrome method to carbolfuchsin stains.

Reports from examination of smears should provide some quantitation of the number of organisms present on a smear, inasmuch as there can be a relationship to the number of acid-fast bacilli present and the degree of activity of the disease. The American Lung Association recommends the following method:

NUMBER OF BACILLI	REPORT
0	No acid-fast bacilli found
1-2 in entire smear	Report number found and request additional specimens
3-9 in entire smear	Rare or +
10 or more in entire smear	Few or + +
1 or more per field	Numerous or + + +

The use of the sputum smear as a screening procedure for the diagnosis of pulmonary tuberculosis has recently been criticized following the finding by several large laboratories that up to 55 per cent of specimens that had positive smears failed to grow in culture. A review of the clinical symptoms and chest x-rays of many of these patients failed to show supporting clinical evidence for tuberculosis. The point has been made that as the incidence of tuberculosis decreases, the predictive value of a positive smear will also decline. When carried to the extreme, if there were no tuberculosis, 100 per cent of the positive smears would be false positives (Boyd, 1975; Pollock, 1977). As techniques for detecting mycobacteria become more sensitive, the finding of commensal mycobacteria that may be more susceptible than *M. tuberculosis* to the decontamination and concentrating procedures will result in a higher incidence of positive smears and negative cultures. Important factors in the predictive value of the smear include the presence or absence of abnormal findings on a chest x-ray, the clinical history, the patient's symptoms, and the number of bacilli present on a slide, with a correlation between increasing numbers of bacilli and the incidence of active infection.

The similarities and differences between the Ziehl-Neelsen, Kinyoun, and fluorochrome stains are listed in Table 48–4. For further details on preparing and interpreting these stains, please consult Runyon (1974), Vestal (1975), and Smithwick (1975a). It should be remembered that the auramine and auramine-rhodamine fluorochrome stains are not fluorescent antigen-antibody reactions. Fluorescent tagged antibodies, which are useful for the identification of individual species of mycobacteria, have been described but are not in widespread use nor are they commercially available.

INCUBATION OF CULTURES

Most mycobacteria show growth stimulation when incubated in an atmosphere of increased concentration of carbon dioxide. Studies have

Table 48–4. COMPARISON OF THE COMPONENTS OF ACID-FAST STAINS

ZIEHL-NEELSEN	KINYOUN'S "COLD" STAIN	AURAMINE FLUOROCHROME
Carbol-fuchsin: 3.0 g of basic fuchsin in 10.0 ml of 90–95% ethanol dissolved in 90 ml of 5% aqueous solution of phenol.	*Carbol-fuchsin:* 4.0 g of basic fuchsin in 20 ml of 90–95% ethanol added to 100 ml of a 9% aqueous solution of phenol.	*Phenolic auramine:* 0.1 g auramine 0 in 10 ml of 90–95% ethanol added to 3 g of phenol in 87.0 ml of distilled water.
Acid-alcohol: 3.0 ml of concentrated HCl in 97.0 ml of 90–95% ethanol.	*Acid-alcohol:* 3 ml of concentrated HCl in 97.0 ml of 90–95% ethanol.	*Acid-alcohol:* 0.5 ml of concentrated HCl in 100 ml of 70% alcohol.
Methylene blue counterstain: 0.3 mg of methylene blue chloride in 100 ml of distilled water.	*Methylene blue counterstain:* 0.3 mg of methylene blue chloride in 100 ml of distilled water.	*Potassium permanganate counterstain:* 0.5 g potassium permanganate in 100 ml of distilled water.

suggested that the optimal concentration of CO_2 is between 8 and 12 per cent. Increased CO_2 tension is a requirement for the proper use of 7H10, 7H11, and selective 7H11 culture media, and will also improve the number and size of colonies of mycobacteria on egg-base culture media. Candle extinction jars are not acceptable for this purpose, which is best served by a CO_2 incubator. The CO_2 concentration in the incubator should be monitored and recorded in the quality control chart on a daily basis.

M. tuberculosis will grow most rapidly when cultures are incubated at 37°C. In contrast, *M. marinum* and *M. ulcerans*, organisms causing disease of the skin, should be incubated at 30 to 32°C. for optimal recovery. Incubation of cultures at 37°C. for the recovery of *M. marinum* or *ulcerans* will greatly delay or even prevent their growth. Similarly, cultures containing *M. xenopi* will show optimal growth and recovery when incubated at 42°C. If incubators for 30 to 32°C. are not available, cultures from skin infections or other sources thought to contain *M. marinum* can be placed in a temperature-monitored box or container at 24°C., away from heating or cooling air currents. A 42°C. incubator can be shared with other sections of the laboratory. Incubation of cultures at this temperature can offer a valuable identification characteristic for bacteria (*Pseudomonas aeruginosa*) as well as for mycobacteria.

IDENTIFICATION

Laboratories receiving only occasional clinical specimens for mycobacteria may find the technical effort required to maintain competence for all services in the mycobacterial laboratory to be expensive and not cost effective. Other laboratories will find the number of specimens and patients seen in their institution require complete identification as well as susceptibility testing of all mycobacterial isolates. In order to help each laboratory decide how far it should go in establishing mycobacterial services, the College of American Pathologists has suggested four "Extents" of service. A similiar list of "Levels of Proficiency" has subsequently been suggested by the American Thoracic Society. When these two lists are compared (Table 48-5), the similarities are readily apparent.

Inasmuch as *Mycobacterium tuberculosis* is the most common cause of mycobacterial disease in man, most laboratories will want to be able to identify this organism. The recommended procedures for the identification of *M. tuberculosis* are:

1. The determination of rate of growth and the optimal temperature for isolation.
2. photoreactivity.
3. niacin accumulation.
4. reduction of nitrates to nitrites.
5. catalase production—heat stable and semiquantitative.

Table 48-5. SUGGESTED LIMITS OF MYCOBACTERIOLOGICAL SERVICES

EXTENTS OF SERVICE COLLEGE OF AMERICAN PATHOLOGISTS	AREAS OF PROFICIENCY AMERICAN THORACIC SOCIETY
1. No mycobacteriologic procedures performed. 2. Acid-fast stain of exudates, effusions, and body fluids, etc., with inoculation and referring of cultures to reference laboratories for further identification. 3. Isolation of mycobacteria; identification of *Mycobacterium tuberculosis* and preliminary identification of the atypical forms such as photochromogens, scotochromogens, non-photochromogens, and rapid growers. Drug susceptibility testing may or may not be performed. 4. Definitive identification of mycobacteria isolated to the extent required to establish a correct clinical diagnosis and to aid in the selection of safe and effective therapy. Drug susceptibility testing may or may not be performed.	1. Collection and transportation of specimens; preparation and examination of smears for acid-fast bacilli. 2. Detection, isolation, and identification of *Mycobacterium tuberculosis*. 3. Determination of drug susceptibility of mycobacteria. 4. Identification of mycobacteria other than *M. tuberculosis*.

Table 48-6.   IDENTIFICATION CHARACTERISTICS OF MYCOBACTERIA

ORGANISM	OPTIMUM ISOLATION TEMPERATURE AND RATE OF GROWTH	PIGMENTATION GROWTH IN: Light	Dark	NIACIN TEST	NITRATE REDUCTION	CATALASE Semi-quantitative[1]	pH 7.0 68°C	TWEEN 80 HYDROLYSIS 10 DAYS	ARYLSUL-FATASE 3 DAYS	UREASE	RESISTANCE TO T₂H 1 µg/ml	GROWTH ON 5% NaCl	IRON UPTAKE
M. tuberculosis	37°C. 12-25 days	buff	buff	+	3-5+	<40[2]	-	∓	-	+	+	-	-
M. africanum	37°C. 31-42	buff	buff	V	V	<20	-	-	-		+	-	-
M. bovis	37°C. 24-40	buff	buff	V	-	<20	-	-	-	+	-	-	-
M. ulcerans	32°C. 28-60	buff	buff	-	-	>50	+	-	-		+		
M. kansasii	37°C. 10-20	yellow	buff	-	1-5+	>50	+	+[3]	-	+	+	-	-
M. marinum	31-32°C. 5-14	yellow	buff	V	-	<40	∓	+	∓	+	+	-	-
M. simiae	37°C. 7-14	yellow[4]	buff	+	∓	>50	+	-	-	+	+	-	
M. szulgai	37°C. 12-25	yellow to orange	yellow—37°C buff—25°C.	-	+	>50	+	∓	∓	+	+	-	-
M. scrofulaceum	37°C. 10+	yellow	yellow	-	-	>50	+	-	-	+	+	-	-
M. gordonae	37°C. 10+	yellow to orange	yellow	-	-	>50	+	+	-	-	+	-	-
M. flavescens	37°C. 7-10	yellow	yellow	-	+	>50	+	+	-	+	+	+	-
M. xenopi	42°C. 14-28	yellow	yellow	-	-	<40	+	-	±	-	+	-	-
M. intracellulare-avium complex	37°C. 10-21	buff to pale yellow	buff to pale yellow	-	-	<40	-	-	-	-	+	-	-
M. gastri	37°C. 10-21	buff	buff	-	-	<40	-	+	-	+	+	-	-
M. terrae complex	37°C. 10-21	buff	buff	-	1-5+	>50	+	+	-	-	+	-	-
M. triviale	37°C. 10-21	buff	buff	-	1-5+	>50	+	+	∓	+	+	+	+
M. fortuitum	37°C. 3-5	buff	buff	-	2-5+	>50	+	±	+	+	+	+	+
M. chelonei ss borstelense	37°C. 3-5	buff	buff	V	-	>50	+	-	+	+	+	-	-
ss abscessus	37°C. 3-5	buff	buff	V	-	>50	+	-	+	+	+	+	-
M. smegmatis	37°C. 3-5	buff to yellow	buff to yellow	-	1-5+	>50	±	+	-		+	+	+

Key to results: + = 84% of strains +; ± = 50-84%; ∓ = 16-49%; − = 16% of strains +; V = variable; blank spaces = little or no data.
[1] Numbers indicate millimeters of bubbles.
[2] INH = resistant strains may be negative.
[3] Positive (most) in 24-48 hours.
[4] Photochromogenicity unstable with repeated subcultures.
From Sommers, H. M.: The identification of mycobacteria. In Baer, D. M. (ed.): *Technical Improvement Service Number 28* (Chicago: American Society of Clinical Pathologists, 1977). Used by permission.

6. growth inhibition by thiophene-2-carboxylic acid hydrazide (T_2H).

The details for determining these characteristics are available in standard laboratory manuals and will not be repeated here (Runyon, 1974; Vestal, 1975; David, 1976). Although it is not always necessary to determine growth inhibition by T_2H on all isolates of *M. tuberculosis*, similarities between certain strains of the Bacille-Calmette-Guerin (BCG) mutants of *M. bovis* and *M. tuberculosis* can best be resolved by this characteristic. *M. bovis* is inhibited by 1 to 5 $\mu g/ml$ of T_2H, while *M. tuberculosis* is not. The increased use of BCG in the immunotherapy of malignant melanoma with subsequent isolation of the organism from regional lymph nodes and other clinical specimens has made the need to distinguish between these two species a more common problem today than in the recent past.

Identification of the other species of the clinically significant mycobacteria can be accomplished by use of the characteristics listed in Table 48-6. It can be seen that with the addition of the Tween 80 hydrolysis, urease, and three-day arylsulfatase tests, most species can be identified or placed in clinically relevant species complexes. Laboratories interested in developing special competence in the speciation of mycobacteria should consult more detailed manuals (Runyon, 1974; Vestal, 1975; David, 1976; Sommers, 1977).

CLASSIFICATION OF MYCOBACTERIA

As more cultures were made and increasing numbers of "atypical" mycobacteria isolated, there was a need for some form of classification of these organisms. In 1954, after studying a series of these "atypical" strains, Timpe proposed a classification of four groups of organisms based on (1) the rate of growth at 37°C, and (2) the presence or absence of pigmented colonies when grown in the dark and then exposed to light. Runyon (1959) further refined this classification, which is summarized briefly here:

I. Group I organisms are characterized by the ability to make a yellow carotene pigment when viable mycobacteria are exposed to a strong light. Because they make pigment only when exposed to light, these organisms are called photochromogens. Photochromogenic mycobacteria include *M. kansasii*, *M. simiae*, and *M. marinum*.

II. Group II mycobacteria produce bright yellow pigmented colonies when grown either in the light or the dark, although in some species of *M. scrofulaceum* the pigment may be intensified on exposure to light. This group of organisms is called "scotochromogens" for their characteristic to generate pigment in the dark. Species in the Group II scotochromogens include *M. scrofulaceum*, *M. gordonae*, and *M. flavescens*.

III. Runyon's third group of mycobacteria include a number of species, some producing small amounts of pale yellow pigment. Exposure of these organisms to bright light does not intensify the color, and hence they are designated "non-photochromogens." Species in this group include members of the *M. avium-intracellulare* complex, *M. gastri*, and a group of organisms showing little or no pathogenicity for man termed the *M. terrae-nonchromogenicum-triviale* complex.

IV. The last of Runyon's four groups of atypical mycobacteria are characterized by the ability to grow more rapidly than the other three groups, often showing mature colonies in three to five days. These organisms are called "rapid growers." While some species of the "rapid growers" show an intense yellow pigmentation, the two species that are known to cause infection in man, *M. fortuitum* and *M. chelonei*, are non-pigmented.

Although Runyon's classification was helpful in organizing many of the "atypical" mycobacterial isolates into some form or order, it has become apparent that it is now necessary to speciate all isolates to determine their clinical significance and to avoid the confusion and misunderstanding that can occur with the terms photochromogen, scotochromogen, etc. The need for speciation of isolates rather than use of the Runyon group designation can be illustrated by *M. szulgai*, a mycobacterial species recently recognized to be associated with disease in humans. *M. szulgai* is scotochromogenic when incubated at 37°C. but photochromogenic when grown at 22 to 24°C. In contrast to most scotochromogenic mycobacteria, *M. szulgai* has been found to be associated with active, progressive disease in almost all instances (Davidson, 1976). Identification to species can help to either establish or exclude the role of the isolate in causing infection.

CLINICAL SIGNIFICANCE OF MYCOBACTERIAL SPECIES

Mycobacterium tuberculosis

The clinical significance of the different mycobacterial species in infection in humans depends in large part on the state of the host's immune system. *Mycobacterium tuberculosis* is the most common cause of pulmonary tuberculosis and remains the most virulent of all mycobacterial species. The disease is highly contagious and with the diagnosis of a new case of tuberculosis, careful investigation of close family contacts usually reveals additional cases of active disease. Although the disease may involve all susceptible individuals, there appears to be higher incidence of infection among disadvantaged minorities than in middle or upper class groups. This is considered likely because of the increased incidence of crowded housing and the possibility of nutritional deprivation. Outbreaks frequently involve multiple members of closed population groups, such as teachers and students in classrooms, sailors on ships, and family units living in limited housing. Such outbreaks are all too common and have established the value of intensive epidemiologic investigations in patients with newly recognized infections.

Mycobacterium bovis

Infection with *M. bovis* in the United States today is uncommon, owing in large part to the highly effective campaign to control tuberculosis in dairy herds and mandatory pasteurization of milk. Recently the use of a mutant strain of *M. bovis*, Bacille-Calmette-Guerin (BCG), in the immunotherapy of malignant melanoma has resulted in occasional isolates from regional lymph nodes or other sites of dissemination. Laboratories should be able to identify *M. bovis*, as a clinical history is not always available.

In contrast to the other mycobacterial species, *M. bovis* does not show growth stimulation with added glycerol, and, in fact, may be inhibited. Such specimens should be inoculated to media without added glycerol, such as 7H10 or 7H11, prepared by the processing laboratory. Petragnani medium contains a lower glycerol content than most other egg-base media and will show preferential recovery of some strains of *M. bovis* and BCG.

Disease from mycobacteria other than *M. tuberculosis* is becoming more apparent clinically, probably not on an absolute basis, but rather as a reflection of decreasing incidence of infection of *M. tuberculosis* and the improvement in the sensitivity of detection and identification of other mycobacterial species.

Mycobacterium ulcerans

M. ulcerans, the cause of "Buruli ulcer," is a very slowly growing, non-pigmented organism responsible for chronic skin ulcers in patients living in the tropics. The incidence of the disease in the United States is very low and infection seen here was usually acquired in the tropics (Tsang, 1975). The ulcers are indolent and may progress to significant destruction of skin and underlying tissue (Conner, 1966). Primary recovery of the organism on culture is difficult but works best when incubated at 30 to 33°C. A culture may take as long as six to nine months to become positive. Incubation at 37°C. may delay or prevent isolation.

Mycobacterium kansasii

Clinical infection from *M. kansasii* may occur in all age groups and at any site in the body. In contrast to *M. tuberculosis*, pulmonary disease from *M. kansasii* is not highly contagious, with only rare reports of infection in more than one member of a family. In one epidemiologic study, pulmonary disease from *M. kansasii* was most frequently seen in middle-aged white males living in middle-class residential neighborhoods (Lichtenstein, 1965). This is in sharp contrast to infection from *M. tuberculosis*, in which many of the patients live in crowded slum housing. The lack of communicability and the predominance of middle-aged males, as well as abnormal pulmonary function studies in patients with *M. kansasii* infection (Ahn, 1976), have suggested that disease with this organism may be an opportunistic infection. Disseminated infection occurs infrequently and is usually associated with some defect in host defense. Clinically, isolates of *M. kansasii* exhibiting a strong catalase reaction are more frequently associated with pathogenicity than those showing only a weak reaction (Wayne, 1962). *M. kansasii* infections will usually respond to therapy with three or more antituberculous drugs, despite *in vitro* resistance to low levels of INH, ethambutol, and frequently other primary antituberculous drugs (Harris, 1975).

5

The organism has been noted to cause infection in a number of patients with renal homografts, and can present as a cellulitis in patients on active immunosuppressive therapy (Fraser, 1975). A switch to alternate day corticosteroid therapy modified the host inflammatory response from cellulitis to a more characteristic granulomatous tissue reaction. Disseminated infection from *M. kansasii* is usually associated with either an underlying defect in the host defense mechanism or active immunosuppression (Fraser, 1975).

Mycobacterium marinum

M. marinum, formerly known as *M. balnei*, is a photoreactive mycobacterium growing best at 30 to 33°C. and is usually associated with chronic ulcerating granulomas of the skin. The organism can live in fresh or salt water, and infections are usually associated with minor trauma to the skin before or during immersion in water. Infections following skin abrasions in swimming pools ("swimming pool granulomas") have been reported (Schaefer, 1961), as well as infections in patients who are scratched on the hand or arm while caring for fish in aquariums (Heineman, 1972). Recovery of the organism by culture can be rapid (7 to 12 days) when incubated at skin temperature, 30 to 33°C. Growth is slow when incubated at 37°C.

Mycobacterium simiae

M. simiae was first described in 1965 during an investigation of spontaneous mycobacterial disease of monkeys (Karassova, 1965). Subsequently the organism was isolated from humans. In 1971, similar bacteria were isolated from the sputum of 35 patients in Havana (Valdivia, 1971). Studies by agglutination antibodies and immunodiffusion have shown the two organisms to have identical surface antigens. The name *Mycobacterium simiae* has been proposed, as it has precedence over *Mycobacterium habana* (Weiszfeiler, 1976).

Mycobacterium simiae has been recovered from a number of patients, but in only a few has it been shown to be associated with a granulomatous tissue reaction. The organism is resistant to many of the standard antimycobacterial drugs *in vitro*. Association of the organism in infection of monkeys and the appearance of disease in humans caring for monkeys raises certain epidemiologic questions.

Mycobacterium szulgai

Mycobacterium szulgai is a scotochromogenic mycobacterium when incubated at 37°C. and photochromogenic when grown at 24°C. It was first recognized because of its unique pattern of cell wall lipids demonstrated by thin-layer chromotography (Marks, 1972).

M. szulgai is known to cause granulomatous infection in the lung, lymph nodes, olecranal bursae, and palmar tendon sheaths (Davidson, 1976).

Most isolates have been recovered from patients who have had active infection. Patients who repeatedly yield scotochromogenic mycobacteria on culture and show evidence of active or progressive infection should be considered to have infection with *M. szulgai* until proven otherwise.

Mycobacterium szulgai is more susceptible to rifampin, ethionamide, ethambutol, and a higher concentration of isoniazid than other scotochromogens (Davidson, 1976). Seroagglutination and agglutination-absorption tests are specific and provide one means of identification (Schaefer, 1973).

Mycobacterium scrofulaceum

M. scrofulaceum (*M. marianum*) is a scotochromogenic mycobacterium widely distributed in the environment. Although it has been recovered from more than half of a series of soil specimens, the serotypes were different from those associated with human disease so that the source of the organism in human disease is not readily apparent (Wolinsky, 1968). The high incidence of skin sensitivity to PPD prepared from the Gause strain (PPD-G) of this organism suggests that it is widely available in our environment, although the incidence of clinical infection is low. *M. scrofulaceum* is one of the most common causes of cervical lymphadenitis in children ("scrofula") (Prissick, 1957). In contrast, scrofula in adults is usually due to *M. tuberculosis*. *M. scrofulaceum* is known to colonize old tuberculous cavities, but in such patients it is not thought to be clinically significant. Primary pulmonary disease with *M. scrofulaceum* occurs, but it is distinctly uncommon. The organism can sometimes be isolated from the sputum of patients with carcinoma of the lung or patients with other chronic pulmonary disease. When this occurs, it is usually not associated with a granulomatous inflammatory response and may represent commensal colonization.

Mycobacterium xenopi

First described in 1959 by Schwabacher, who cultured it from a skin lesion of the South African toad *Xenopus laevis*, *M. xenopi* has been found to cause pulmonary disease in England, France, and the United States. It has been shown to colonize the hot water systems of hospitals in the United States (Bullin, 1970; and Gross, 1976) and Britain. Although Gross isolated *M. xenopi* at least three or more times from each of 105 patients, pulmonary disease could be attributed to the organism in only 11. It is important to differentiate the organism from the similar-appearing *Mycobacterium intracellularae* or scotochromogenic mycobacteria, as *M. xenopi* is much more responsive to drug therapy.

Mycobacterium intracellulare

M. intracellulare ("Battey bacillus") is very closely related to *M. avium*. Differentiation between the two and a series of closely related organisms can be difficult and may not be clinically significant. With this in mind, the term *M. avium-intracellulare* complex has been proposed to emphasize the similarities and the differences in this group of organisms.

For many years the organism causing disease of this type was called the "Battey bacillus" for the Battey State Hospital in Rome, Georgia. Like *M. kansasii*, *M. avium-intracellulare* causes disease more frequently in middle-aged men than in other groups. Quite often, patients with infection from *M. avium-intracellulare* have evidence of an underlying chronic pulmonary disease (Ahn, 1976). Infections with *M. avium-intracellulare* are not highly contagious, and infection in more than one member of a family is distinctly uncommon.

Infection with *M. avium-intracellulare* is usually seen in the lung, although other sites may be involved and disseminated infection has been reported. In contrast to infection with many of the other species of mycobacteria, *M. avium-intracellulare* causes an indolent, chronic infection that is particularly difficult to treat. Therapy with 3-4 and 5-6 drugs may be only partially successful, with slowly progressive disease resulting (Dutt, 1977). Surgical resection combined with aggressive drug therapy has provided the best clinical results.

Mycobacterium fortuitum and Mycobacterium chelonei

Both *Mycobacterium fortuitum* and *M. chelonei* are closely related members of Runyon's group IV rapidly growing mycobacteria. Because of similarities between the two species, both in the cultural characteristics and in the type of disease caused in humans, it has been proposed that the term *M. fortuitum-chelonei* complex be used instead of the individual species. *M. fortuitum* can be differentiated from *M. chelonei* without difficulty by nitroreductase activity, and the two subspecies of *M. chelonei*, *M. chelonei* ss *borstelense* and *M. chelonei* ss *abscessus*, can be separated by the ability of the latter to grow on Lowenstein-Jensen medium containing 5 per cent NaCl. Of the two subspecies of *M. chelonei*, *M. chelonei* ss *abscessus* is more often associated with disease. Few, if any, infections are documented as having been caused by *M. chelonei* ss *borstelense*.

Infections from the *Mycobacterium fortuitum-chelonei* complex organisms usually involve the skin or epidermal derivatives. Skin abscesses resulting from vaccinations have been reported (Borghans, 1973), and eye infections, usually involving the cornea, have been described following trauma (Zimmerman, 1969).

Members of the *Mycobacterium fortuitum-chelonei* complex can be recovered from sputum, frequently without evidence of pulmonary disease, but lung infections do occur and when present are a difficult therapeutic problem. Most of the antimycobacterial drugs in current use are not effective against the *M. fortuitum-chelonei* complex. More recently, *M. fortuitum* has been found as a postoperative infectious complication of cardiac valve replacement. Contamination from porcine valves has been documented, resulting in a myocardial abscess (Levy, 1977).

Non-pathogenic mycobacteria

Mycobacterium gordonae ("tap-water bacillus," *M. aquae*) is a scotochromogenic myco-

5

bacterium that has not been clearly shown to be the cause of disease in humans. *M. gordonae* can colonize water taps and stills and, like *M. xenopi*, offers a challenge to the laboratory to determine its clinical significance. *M. gordonae* should be distinguished from *M. scrofulaceum* and *M. xenopi*, both of which are more likely to be the cause of active infection. Similarly, *M. flavescens* is not known to cause disease and should be identified to differentiate it from one of the more pathogenic scotochromogenic mycobacteria.

Non-pathogenic mycobacterial species in the non-photochromogenic Runyon group III, include *Mycobacterium gastri* and a poorly defined group termed the *M. terrae-non-chromogenicum-triviali* complex. It is generally believed that this group of organisms is without pathogenic potential unless there has been some serious defect in the patient's host defense mechanisms.

With the exception of *Mycobacterium fortuitum* and *M. chelonei*, very few, if any, mycobacteria of group IV cause clinical disease in humans. Most rapidly growing mycobacteria are pigmented yellow with the exception of *M. fortuitum* and *M. chelonei*. Both species are buff in color.

SUSCEPTIBILITY TESTING OF MYCOBACTERIA

Random drug resistance in mycobacteria is independent of exposure to the agent. The frequency of drug-resistant mutants in a culture of tubercle bacilli has been estimated to be between 1 in 10^5 to 10^7 bacteria for isoniazid and 1 in 10^6 to 10^8 for streptomycin. If two drugs, isoniazid and streptomycin, are both given, the incidence of resistance will be the product of the two separately, or 1 of every 10^{15} organisms. The importance of the incidence of spontaneously resistant mutants becomes apparent when it is known that patients with an open pulmonary cavity may have a total bacillary population of 10^7 to 10^9 bacteria. If such patients are treated with a single antituberculous agent, their cultures will soon be populated only with resistant organisms and treatment will fail. For this reason, patients with tuberculosis must be treated with two or preferably three drugs. Failure to take all drugs may lead to the rapid emergence of drug-resistant tubercle bacilli. Clinically, it has been found that if more

than 1 per cent of a patient's tubercle bacilli are resistant to a drug *in vitro*, therapy with that drug will not be effective *in vivo*. Therefore, the susceptibility test must determine the *number* of bacilli susceptible and resistant. The inoculum should be adjusted so that the number of naturally resistant mutants will not mislead the laboratory worker to interpret the culture as resistant. At the same time, there must be a sufficiently dilute inoculum so that the incidence of drug resistance in the range of 1 per cent can be determined. For optimal results, such an inoculum will result in 100 to 300 colony-forming units on each quadrant of a four quadrant Petri plate. Because it is difficult to standardize an inoculum of mycobacteria, particularly *M. tuberculosis*, it is usually necessary to inoculate two sets of susceptibility test plates, the first with a 10^{-2} or 10^{-3} dilution of a barely turbid broth culture and the second set with a 100-fold dilution of the inoculum used for the first set. This procedure is known as the proportional susceptibility testing method.

Eleven drugs are used in the treatment of tuberculosis. Five are considered "primary" and include streptomycin, isoniazid, para-aminosalicylic acid, rifampin, and ethambutol, while the remaining six, ethionamide, capreomycin, kanamycin, cycloserine, viomycin, and pyrazinamide are considered secondary and used only when resistance develops to the primary drugs. The suggested concentrations of the drugs used for mycobacterial susceptibility testing are listed in Table 48-7.

The test is performed in plastic Petri plates divided into four quadrants. Five milliliters of agar are placed in each quadrant. The medium in the first quadrant does not contain any

Table 48-7. *IN VITRO* CONCENTRATIONS OF ANTIMYCOBACTERIAL AGENTS USED IN SUSCEPTIBILITY TESTING

	CONCENTRATION ($\mu g/ml$)
Isoniazid	0.2/1.0
Streptomycin	2.0/10.0
Para-aminosalicylic acid	2.0/10.0
Ethambutol	7.5/15.0
Rifampin	1.0/5.0
Ethionamide	10.0/15.0
Cycloserine	20.0/30.0
Capreomycin	5.0
Kanamycin	6.0/12.0
Viomycin	10.0/15.0
Pyrazinamide	50.0

Table 48-8. DISTRIBUTION OF DRUG-CONTAINING DISCS
FOR SUSCEPTIBILITY TESTS*

PLATE NO.	QUADRANT NO.	AMOUNT OF DRUG PER DISC (μg)	FINAL DRUG CONCENTRATION (μg/ml)
1	I Control #1	–	0
	II Isoniazid	1	0.2
	III Isoniazid	5	1.0
	IV Rifampin	5	1.0
2	I Streptomycin	10	2.0
	II Streptomycin	50	10.0
	III Ethambutol	25	5.0†
	IV Ethambutol	50	10.0†
3	I Para-aminosalicylic acid	10	2.0
	II Para-aminosalicylic acid	50	10.0
	III Control #2	–	0
	IV -	–	–

*Reproduced with permission of Kubica, G. P., et al.: Laboratory services for mycobacterial diseases. Am. Rev. Resp. Dis., *112*:773, 1975.

†Improved correlation with clinical response has been noted with ethambutol concentrations of 7.5 and 15 μg/ml. These can be achieved by using 1½ 25 μg discs in each quadrant for the 7.5 μg/ml concentration and a 25 and 50 μg disc for the 15 μg/ml concentration.

antimycobacterial agent and acts as a growth control. The other three quadrants contain dilutions of the drugs to be tested. Although drugs have been incorporated in inspissated egg-base media in the past, most laboratories now prefer using either 7H11 or 7H10 as a base medium, adding the drugs after cooling the agar to 45°C. Adding the drugs to the agar medium after autoclaving decreases the loss of activity that can occur in egg-base medium during inspissation. An additional loss of drug activity may occur in egg-base media with binding of some agents to egg albumin and other proteins.

A simplified method for preparing drug susceptibility plates has been developed which does not require weighing and dilution of each drug, and which uses filter paper discs containing the primary antituberculous drugs. Discs are available from microbiologic supply sources. With this method, preparation of drug-containing media is facilitated by placing a drug-containing disc in one quadrant of the plate and adding 5 ml of 7H10 or 7H11 agar which diffuses into the medium and results in the recommended concentration of drug to be tested. Since each disc is marked with the name and concentration of drug it contains, labeling errors are eliminated, as well as errors that can occur in weighing, dilution, and measuring of drug solutions (Wayne,

1966). Recent results have suggested that a better correlation with the clinical response to ethambutol has been noted with concentrations of 7.5 and 15.0 μg/ml rather than 5 and 10 μg/ml (McClatchy, 1977). A suggested schedule for the use of drug-containing paper discs is given in Table 48-8.

To perform the test, susceptibility plates are inoculated with three drops in each quadrant of a 10^{-2} and 10^{-4} dilution of a barely turbid broth culture. Plates are incubated in CO_2 at 37°C. and interpreted at between two and three weeks. Incubation of ethambutol-containing media for more than three weeks may result in the appearance of microcolonies following the inactivation of the drug. Interpretation of the inoculated plates should include either an estimate or a direct count of the total number of colonies on the control and drug-containing media. All colonies, even those showing inhibition of growth on drug-containing media, should be counted and related to the number of colonies on the control quadrant. Since the control quadrant should contain the same number of colonies inoculated to the test quadrants, the percentage of resistant colonies can be readily calculated from the two sets of plates inoculated with dilutions of organisms 100-fold apart.

The *direct mycobacterial susceptibility* test is inoculated from digested and concentrated sputum found to be positive for acid-fast bacilli. The *indirect susceptibility test* is inoculated from colonies isolated from a primary culture. The direct test will usually give good results only if large numbers of mycobacteria are present in the specimen. The advantage of the direct susceptibility test is an earlier report (three to four weeks) in contrast to the indirect test, which may take up to six to eight weeks. The disadvantage of the direct susceptibility test is that it usually requires a large number of mycobacteria for successful growth and is often overgrown by large numbers of contaminating bacteria.

Susceptibility studies are not indicated for all mycobacterial isolates, as the incidence of primary drug resistance (defined as a drug-resistant organism isolated from a previously untreated patient) is less than 3 to 5 per cent. Even if primary resistance to one drug is present, treatment with the recommended triple drug therapy will provide coverage. Susceptibility tests should be routinely performed on mycobacterial isolates from patients who have shown relapse while on drug therapy. The probability of induced resistance in this group of patients is high. Other indications for performing antimycobacterial drug susceptibility tests are given in Table 48-9. If susceptibility tests are not performed on isolates obtained from patients previously seen by a laboratory, at least one culture should be saved for six months or a year should the patient not

Table 48-9. INDICATIONS FOR SUSCEPTIBILITY STUDIES FOR MYCOBACTERIA ISOLATES *

1. May not be indicated for previously untreated patients.
2. Should be obtained under the following conditions:
   A. Sputum-positive patients who have had previous chemotherapy (relapsed or retreatment cases).
   B. Patients on therapy whose sputum reverts to positive.
   C. Patients whose sputum smears do not convert to negative within two to three months of treatment.
   D. Patients whose cultures do not convert to negative within four to six months of treatment.
   E. Patients with increasing numbers of tubercle bacilli seen in smears after an initial decrease.
   F. Patients with mycobacterial infections other than *Mycobacterium tuberculosis*.
   G. Patients suspected of having primary resistance:
      (1) Tuberculosis patients who have lived abroad.
      (2) Persons possibly infected by patients with drug-resistant tuberculosis.

---

* Adapted from Pennsylvania State Public Health Laboratories, and McClatchy, J. K.: personal communication.

respond to therapy. Controls for mycobacterial susceptibility studies should be run with each set of test cultures and include both susceptible and resistant, as well as intermediately susceptible, strains, e.g., *M. kansasii* resistant to 0.2 µg/ml of isoniazid but susceptible to 1.0 µg/ml. Further details for determining antimycobacterial drug susceptibility tests can be found in Runyon, 1974; Vestal, 1975; Kubica, 1975; and McClatchy, 1977.

REFERENCES

Ahn, C. H., Nash, D. R., and Hurst, G. A.: Ventilatory defects in atypical mycobacteriosis. A comparison study with tuberculosis. Am. Rev. Resp. Dis., *113*:273, 1976.

Borghans, S. G. A., and Stanford, J. L.: *Mycobacterium chelonei* in abscesses after injection of Diphtheria-pertussis-tetanus-poliovaccine. Am. Rev. Resp. Dis., *107*:1, 1973.

Boyd, J. C., and Marr, J. J.: Decreasing reliability of acid-fast smear techniques for detection of tuberculosis. Ann. Intern. Med., *82*:489, 1975.

Bullin, C. H., and Tanner, E. I.: Isolation of *Mycobacterium xenopei* from water taps. J. Hyg. (Camb.), *68*:97, 1970.

Cohn, M. L., Waggoner, R. F., and McClatchy, J. K.: The 7H11 medium for the culture of mycobacteria. Am. Rev. Resp. Dis., *98*:295, 1968.

Conner, D. H., and Lunn, H. F.: Buruli ulceration. Arch. Pathol., *81*:183, 1966.

David, H. C.: Bacteriology of the Mycobacterioses. U.S. Dept. Health, Education and Welfare, Public Health Service Publication No. (CDC) 76-8316.

Davidson, P. T.: *Mycobacterium szulgai*. A new pathogen causing infection of the lung. Chest, *69*:799, 1976.

Dutt, A. K., and Stead, W. W.: Results of treatment of patients infected with *M. intracellulare*. Am. Rev. Resp. Dis., *115* (Suppl.):396, 1977.

Fraser, D. W., Buxton, A. E., et al.: Disseminated *Mycobacterium kansasii* infection presenting as cellulitis in a recipient of a renal homograph. Am. Rev. Resp. Dis., *112*:125, 1975.

Gross, W., Hawkins, J. E., and Murphy, D. B.: Water as a source of contamination. Amer. Rev. Resp. Dis., *113* (Part 2):78, 1976.

Gruft, H.: Isolation of acid-fast bacilli from contaminated specimens. Health Lab. Sci., *8*:79, 1971.

Harris, G. D., Johanson, W. G., and Nicholson, D. P.: Response to chemotherapy of pulmonary disease due to *Mycobacterium kansasii*. Am. Rev. Resp. Dis., *112*:31, 1975.

Heineman, H. S., Spitzer, S., and Pianphongsant, T.: Fish tank granuloma. A hobby hazard. Arch. Intern. Med., *130*:121, 1972.

Joseph, S. W.: Lack of auramine-rhodamine fluorescence of Runyon Group IV mycobacteria. Am. Rev. Resp. Dis., *95*:114, 1967.

Karassova, V., Weissfeiler, J., and Krasznay, E.: Occurrence of atypical mycobacteria in *Macacus rhesus*. Acta Microbiol. Acad. Sci. Hung., *12*:275, 1965.

Kestle, D. G., and Kubica, G P.: Sputum collection for cultivation of mycobacteria. An early morning specimen or the 24- to 74-hour pool? Am. J. Clin. Pathol., *48*:347, 1967.

Krasnow, I., and Wayne, L. G.: Comparison of methods for tuberculosis bacteriology. App. Microbiol., *18*:915, 1969.

Kubica, G. P., Dye, W. E., et al.: Sputum digestion and decontamination with N-acetyl-L-cysteine-sodium hydroxide for culture of mycobacteria. Am. Rev. Resp. Dis., *87*:775, 1963.

Kubica, G. P., Gross, W. M., et al.: Laboratory services for mycobacterial diseases. Am. Rev. Resp. Dis., *112*:883, 1975.

Levy, C. Curtin, J. A., et al.: *Mycobacterium chelonei* infection of porcine heart valves. N. Engl. J. Med., *297*:667, 1977.

Lichtenstein, M. R., Takimura, Y., and Thompson, J. R.: Photochromogenic mycobacteria pulmonary infection in a group of hospitalized patients in Chicago. II. Demographic studios. Am. Rev. Resp. Dis., *91*:592, 1965.

Marks, S., and Jenkins, P. A.: *Mycobacterium szulgai*—a new pathogen. Tubercle, *53*:210, 1972.

McClatchy, J. K., Waggoner, R. F., Kanes, W., et al.: Isolation of mycobacteria from clinical specimens by use of Selective 7H11 medium. Am. J. Clin. Pathol., *65*: 412, 1976.

McClatchy, J. K.: Susceptibility testing of mycobacteria. *In* Baer, D. M. (ed.): Technical Improvement Service. Chicago, Commission on Continuing Education, American Society of Clinical Pathologists, No. 29, 1977.

Miliner, R. A., Stottmeir, K. D., and Kubica, G. P.: Formaldehyde: A photothermal activated toxic substance produced in Middlebrook 7H10 medium. Am. Rev. Resp. Dis., *99*:603, 1969.

Petran, E. I., and Vera, H. D.: Media for selective isolation of mycobacteria. Health Lab. Sci., *8*:225, 1971.

Pollock, H. M., and Wieman, E. J.: Smear results in the diagnosis of mycobacterioses using blue light fluorescence microscopy. J. Clin. Microbiol., *5*:329, 1977.

Prissick, F. H., and Masson, A. M.: Yellow-pigmented pathogenic mycobacteria from cervical lymphadenitis. Can. J. Microbiol., *3*:91, 1957.

Runyon, E. H.: Anonymous mycobacteria in pulmonary disease. Med. Clin. North Am., *43*:273, 1959.

Runyon, E. H., Karlson, A. G., et al.: Mycobacterium. *In* Lennette, E. H., Spaulding, E. H., and Truant, J. P. (eds.): Manual of Clinical Microbiology, 2nd ed. Washington, D.C., American Society for Microbiology, 1974, p. 148.

Schaefer, W. B., and Davis, C. L.: A bacteriologic and histopathologic study of skin granuloma due to *Mycobacterium balnei*. Am. Rev. Resp. Dis., *84*:837, 1961.

Schaefer, W. B., Wolinsky, E., Jenkins, P. A., and

Marks, J.: *Mycobacterium szulgai*—a new pathogen. Serologic identification and report of five new cases. Am. Rev. Resp. Dis., *108*:1320, 1973.

Schwabacher, H.: A strain of mycobacterium isolated from skin lesions of a coldblooded animal, *Xenopus laevis*, and its relation to atypical acid-fast bacilli occurring in man. J. Hyg., (Camb.), *57*:57, 1959.

Shah, R. R., and Dye, W. E.: The use of dithiothreitol to replace N-acetyl-L-cysteine for routine sputum digestion-decontamination for the culture of mycobacteria. Am. Rev. Resp. Dis., *94*:454, 1966.

Smithwick, R. W.: Laboratory Manual for Acid-fast Microscopy. U.S. Dept. Health, Education and Welfare, Public Health Service Center for Disease Control, Mycobacterial Reference Section, Atlanta, Ga., 1975a.

Smithwick, R. W., Stratigos, C. B., and David, H. L.: Use of cetylpyridium chloride and sodium chloride for the decontamination of sputum specimens that are transported to the laboratory for the isolation of *Mycobacterium tuberculosis*. J. Clin. Microbiol., *1*:411, 1975b.

Sommers, H. M.: The identification of mycobacteria. *In* Baer, D. M. (ed.): Technical Improvement Service. Chicago, Commission on Continuing Education, American Society of Clinical Pathologists, No., 28,1977, p. 1.

Timpe, A., and Runyon, E. H.: The relationship of "atypical" acid-fast bacteria to human disease. J. Lab. Clin. Med., *44*:202, 1954.

Tsang, A. Y., and Farber, E. R.: The primary isolation of *Mycobacterium ulcerans*. Am. J. Clin. Pathol., *59*:688, 1973.

Valdivia, A., Mendez, J. S., and Font, M. S.: *Mycobacterium habana:* Probable nueva especie dentro de las micobacterias no classificadas. Bol. Hig. Epidemiol. Habana, *9*:65, 1971.

Vestal, A. L.: Procedures for the Isolation and Identification of Mycobacteria. U.S. Dept. Health, Education and Welfare, Public Health Service Publication No., (CDC) 75-8230, 1975.

Wayne, L. G.: Two varieties of *Mycobacterium kansasii* with different clinical significance. Am. Rev. Resp. Dis., *86*:651, 1962.

Wayne, L. G., and Krasnow, I.: Preparation of tuberculosis drug susceptibility testing media using drug impregnated discs. Tech. Bull. Reg. Med. Tech., *36*:5 7, 1966.

Weiszfeiler, J. G., and Karczag, E.: Synonymy of *Mycobacterium simiae* Krasseva et al. 1965 and *Mycobacterium habana* Valdivia et al. 1971. Int. J. Syst. Bacteriol., *26*:474, 1976.

Wolinsky, E., and Rynearson, T. K.: Mycobacteria in soil and their relation to disease-associated strains. Am. Rev. Resp. Dis., *97*:1032, 1968.

Zimmerman, L. E., Turner, L., and McTigue, J. W.: *Mycobacterium fortuitum* infection of the cornea. Arch. Ophthalmol., *82*:596, 1969.

5

49

SPIROCHETES AND SPIRAL BACTERIA

Richard T. Kelly, M.D.

TREPONEMA
    Syphilis
    Yaws and Pinta
BORRELIA

Relapsing Fever
Fusospirochetal Infection
LEPTOSPIRA
SPIRILLUM

Spirochetes are motile, spiral-shaped organisms that divide by binary fission. Organisms pathogenic for man are found in three genera: Treponema, Borrelia, and Leptospira. Most of the spirochetes are so narrow that they cannot be visualized by conventional microscopy when stained with common bacteriologic stains. Special staining methods by which the width of the organisms is increased by the deposition of metallic salts allow visualization with the ordinary light microscope. Spirochetes are easily seen with darkfield microscopy, and this technique is usually employed when screening clinical specimens or evaluating cultures.

All pathogenic treponemes are morphologically indistinguishable from one another as well as from some non-pathogenic organisms. Because of this and the inability to cultivate any pathogenic treponemes *in vitro*, great care is required in interpreting clinical specimens. In addition to being morphologically identical, the three species of treponemes are immunologically identical. Thus, an individual with yaws or pinta has reactive serologic tests for syphilis. All treponemal infections respond to penicillin therapy. The amount and duration of antibiotic therapy varies with the stage of disease (Hoeprich, 1977).

TREPONEMA

Treponemes are considered to be anaerobic microorganisms. Several non-pathogenic treponemes can be cultivated, but only under anaerobic conditions. Although pathogenic treponemes have not been cultured *in vitro*, survival studies (based on retention of motility) have shown that survival is greatly prolonged when the microorganisms are incubated in an oxygen-free environment and in the presence of reducing agents.

SYPHILIS

The etiologic agent of syphilis, *Treponema pallidum*, is a thin, spiral-shaped organism measuring 6 to 15 μ in length but only 0.2 μ in width (Fig. 49-1). The spirals vary in number from 4 to 14 and are rather uniform in appearance when compared with those of certain saprophytic organisms.

Following World War II, the reported incidence of early syphilis in the United States declined each year until 1958, when the rate once again began to progressively rise. In 1976, the incidence of primary and secondary syphilis declined slightly compared to 1975. Whether this represents the beginning of a significant downward trend remains to be de-

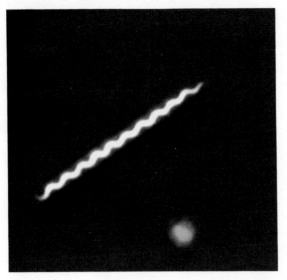

Figure 49–1. *Treponema pallidum,* dark field preparation ×3500.

termined. At present, syphilis is the third most common of the specified reportable infectious diseases in the United States (MMWR, 1977).

Syphilis is usually acquired by the venereal route. After a variable incubation period of 10 days to several months, the primary lesion or chancre appears. This begins as a small, usually solitary nodule that with enlargement and subsequent necrosis of the overlying epithelium results in the formation of a relatively painless ulcer. In contrast to other bacterial infections of the skin, pus is usually absent unless the lesion has become secondarily infected with other bacteria. Lesions are most frequently seen on the external genitalia; however, in women lesions may occur in the vagina and cervix. Chancres heal spontaneously without specific therapy. The systemic nature of the disease becomes apparent six to eight weeks after the appearance of the initial chancre when a generalized rash involving both skin and mucous membranes occurs. During this secondary phase of syphilis, there may also be involvement of the central nervous system, eyes, bones and liver. After a period of weeks to months, the lesions of secondary syphilis resolve spontaneously and the individual enters the latent phase of the disease. In latent syphilis, serologic tests for syphilis are reactive but clinical signs or symptoms are absent. Approximately one third of individu-

als with untreated latent syphilis will subsequently develop signs of tertiary syphilis—gummas, cardiovascular syphilis, or neurosyphilis.

Gummas are localized areas of granulomatous inflammation which may be found in any organ or tissue in the body. The gumma varies in size from microscopic up to 10 cm in diameter. On histologic examination, the lesions are found to be composed of caseous material surrounded by lymphocytes, plasma cells, and areas of perivascular inflammation. Spirochetes are rarely seen in the lesions, and it is therefore believed that gummas result from tissue hypersensitivity.

The basic lesion in cardiovascular syphilis is aortitis, which results from necrosis of the media secondary to endarteritis of the vasa vasorum of the vessel wall. This may lead to (1) narrowing of the coronary ostia, which is manifested clinically as angina pectoris, (2) dilatation of the aortic commissure and thickening of the valve leaflets, resulting in aortic regurgitation, or (3) aneurysm formation, most frequently of the ascending aorta, due to destruction of the elastic fibers in the wall and fibrosis.

The manifestations of neurosyphilis are highly variable and depend on whether involvement is predominantly meningovascular or parenchymatous. Tabes dorsalis results from degeneration of dorsal roots and columns at the lumbosacral and lower thoracic levels of the spinal cord. In paresis, the brain is shrunken and there is dilatation of the lateral ventricles. Silver impregnation staining techniques will demonstrate *Treponema pallidum* in the brain tissue. In neurosyphilis, the cerebrospinal fluid is reactive for reagin antibody. In addition, the cerebrospinal fluid has an increased cell count (over 4 lymphocytes per cu mm) and protein is elevated above 40 mg per 100 ml.

After the eighteenth week of pregnancy, an infected pregnant woman with early or early latent syphilis will transmit treponemes to the fetus with resultant infection. This may result in stillbirth or congenital syphilis. A diagnosis of congenital syphilis can be readily made in the newborn if treponemes can be demonstrated in mucus from the nasopharynx or lesions. Because of transplacental transfer of maternal antibodies, serologic tests for syphilis in the newborn must be carefully evaluated. Serologic tests for syphilis are covered in Chapter 54.

5

A diagnosis of syphilis and its stage is determined by evaluating three factors: (1) clinical findings, (2) demonstration of spirochetes in clinical specimens, and (3) presence of antibodies in blood or cerebrospinal fluid.

The demonstration of typical, motile treponemes by darkfield microscopy in properly prepared specimens is diagnostic in primary and secondary syphilis. Particular care is required in obtaining specimens from the mouth and oropharynx because of the presence of non-pathogenic treponemes that occur as part of the normal flora. Surgical gloves should be worn to protect the examiner from possible infection when obtaining specimens for darkfield microscopy. Lesions to be sampled are repeatedly cleansed with saline-soaked gauze sponges after removal of any surface crusts and then dried with a dry gauze sponge. The surface of the lesions is then abraded with a dry sponge or swab until bleeding occurs. Excess blood is removed with a sponge until a serous exudate is observed. Pressure applied to the base of the lesion is helpful in increasing the volume of exudate. A coverslip is touched to the surface of the lesion to pick up the exudate and is then inverted onto a microscope slide. The edges of the coverslip should be sealed with Vaspar or lanolin to prevent evaporation and contact with oxygen in the air. As rapidly as possible, preparations are examined with the darkfield microscope at a magnification of about $450\times$. Erythrocytes are invariably present and serve as a convenient guide to measuring the length of observed organisms. The length of *Treponema pallidum* averages one to two times the diameter of the red cell. The coils of *Treponema pallidum* are uniform and rather tightly wound when compared with those of saprophytic organisms. Marked directional motility is not seen with pathogenic treponema but may be seen in non-pathogenic organisms. If many bacteria other than spirochetes are present, it may indicate that the site was not sufficiently cleansed before sampling, or the lesions may be due to a different infectious process.

YAWS AND PINTA

The etiologic agents of yaws, *Treponema pertenue*, and pinta, *Treponema carateum*, are morphologically and immunologically identical to *Treponema pallidum*. Yaws is a disease of skin and bone affecting primarily children in tropical and subtropical countries. The initial lesion or mother yaw develops three to four weeks after exposure. This begins as an erythematous nodule and subsequently ulcerates. Disseminated secondary lesions of a similar nature develop six weeks to three months after the initial lesion and may continue for months to years. Tertiary lesions consisting of gummatous lesions of skin and bone do occur, but visceral lesions are rare. Pinta is found primarily in children in Central and South America. It affects only the skin and initially is manifested as red and blue lesions that later become depigmented. Both yaws and pinta are acquired by contact with infected persons; it is also possible that flies serve as vectors of transmission. Diagnosis is established by darkfield microscopy of material from suspect lesions.

BORRELIA

Borreliae are loosely coiled, spiral-shaped organisms that measure 10 to 20 μ in length and 0.2 to 0.4 μ in width. In contrast to other spirochetes, borreliae can be visualized by staining with aniline dyes (Fig. 49-2). A number of borrelia species have been successfully grown *in vitro* in complex enriched media.

RELAPSING FEVER

Two varieties of relapsing fever based on the arthropod vector transmitting the disease are recognized (Felsenfeld, 1971). *Borrelia recurrentis* is the sole etiologic agent of louse-borne relapsing fever and is transmitted from man to man by the human body louse, *Pediculus humanus*. Tick-borne relapsing fever is caused by a variety of different species of borrelia, each of which is transmitted by and named for the species of Ornithodoros tick that acts as vector for the organisms. Rodents serve as natural reservoirs for tick-borne borreliae, and, in addition, borreliae are transmitted transovarianly in the tick, thus increasing the number of infected ticks. In the United States, the principal species of tick-borne borreliae are *B. hermsi*, *B. turicatae*, and *B. parkeri*.

Relapsing fever develops 2 to 15 days after infected lice are crushed during scratching or following the bite of an infected tick. It is a septicemic illness and is characterized by high fever and prostration that persist for three to seven days. An afebrile interval of days to

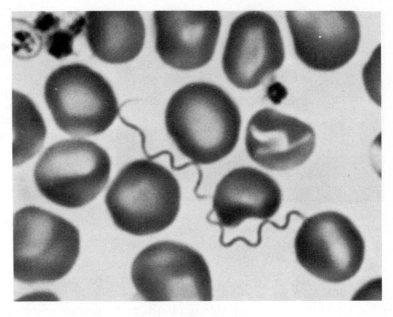

Figure 49-2. *Borrelia hermsi* in blood, Giemsa stain ×3500.

weeks then occurs followed by relapse. In untreated individuals, the number of sequential relapses may be as high as five. During the acute phases of the disease, borreliae can be seen in blood smears stained by the Wright or Giemsa method, or in darkfield preparations of wet mounts. During afebrile periods, the number of organisms present may be inadequate for microscopic detection, and animal inoculation or cultures may be necessary to recover borreliae. Young mice are inoculated intraperitoneally with 1 ml of citrated blood. At daily intervals, the tips of the tails are snipped with scissors to obtain a drop of blood that is either smeared and stained or examined by darkfield microscopy. Borreliae will not grow in conventional blood culture media and until recently could not be cultured *in vitro*. Complex media have been developed that permit isolation and growth of a number of species, including those found in the United States (Kelly, 1976).

Because of the lack of commercially obtainable reagents, serologic methods are not helpful in establishing a diagnosis of relapsing fever.

Relapsing fever responds well to treatment with a number of antibiotics. Tetracycline therapy is frequently employed.

FUSOSPIROCHETAL INFECTION

In acute necrotizing ulcerative gingivitis (trenchmouth, *Vincent's angina*), a number of species of anaerobic bacteria have been implicated as etiologic agents. Fusobacteria, bacteroides, and various spirochetes including *Borrelia* (*Treponema*) *vincenti* have been isolated or observed in smears. The various anaerobes apparently act synergistically in the pathogenesis of the disease process. The diagnosis is established by examining Gram's stains of smears from clinical infection that will demonstrate fusiform bacteria and numerous spirochetes. Penicillin or tetracycline therapy is effective.

LEPTOSPIRA

Leptospires are 6 to 20 μ long but only 0.1 μ wide. The organisms usually have hooked ends and are tightly coiled (Fig. 49-3). Two species of leptospires are recognized. *Leptospira biflexa* is a saprophyte found in fresh water. Over 100 different serotypes of the pathogenic species, *Leptospira interrogans*, are known. Human infections are most commonly due to organisms in the canicola, icterohaemorrhagiae, pomona, and autumnalis serogroups. Many different mammals serve as reservoir hosts for leptospira. Organisms are localized in the kidneys of chronically infected animals and are passed in the urine. Human infection results from contact with animal urine or water which has been contaminated with urine. Leptospirosis develops after an incubation period of 10 to 12 days. The signs and

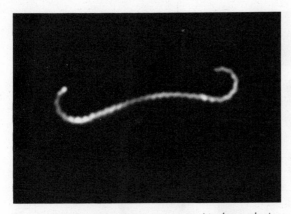

Figure 49–3. *Leptospira interrogans,* serovar *icterohaemorrhagiae,* dark field preparation × 4000.

symptoms vary from a mild fever to severe illness, including jaundice, kidney failure, and meningitis.

Leptospirosis is an uncommon disease with only 73 cases being reported in the United States during the year 1976. Because of this and the relative non-specificity of clinical symptoms, a diagnosis of leptospirosis may at times be difficult to establish. Although frequently requested by clinicians, darkfield examination of blood for the presence of leptospires is unreliable because of the presence of artifacts that may resemble leptospires. During the first week of illness, leptospira may be cultured from the blood. Urine cultures are more likely to be positive in the second week of illness, and organisms may be seen in darkfield preparations of urine. Special culture techniques and enriched media are required for recovery of leptospira from clinical specimens. Fletcher's or Stuart's medium containing 10 per cent heat-inactivated rabbit serum is inoculated with one or two drops of blood and incubated at 30°C. (Alexander, 1974). The incorporation of 5-fluorouracil, 200 μg/ml, in media for urine cultures inhibits the growth of contaminating bacteria but does not affect growth of leptospira. Because of the presence of possible inhibitory substances in urine, it is advisable to inoculate tubes of media with one or two drops of urine diluted 1 to 10 as well as undiluted urine. Cultures should be examined weekly by darkfield microscopy for six weeks before discarding as negative.

Serologic tests are very helpful in establishing a diagnosis of leptospirosis, particularly when cultures are negative. Agglutination tests using as antigen commercially available suspensions of pooled, killed leptospires will show rising titers by the second or third week of illness.

Although penicillin and other antibiotics inhibit the growth of leptospira *in vitro,* treatment of clinical cases with antibiotics does not appreciably alter the course of the disease (Stoenner, 1976).

SPIRILLUM

Spirillum minor is the only species pathogenic for man in the genus *Spirillum.* This spiral-shaped, gram-negative organism contains bipolar flagella and measures 0.5 μ in width and 1.7 to 5.0 μ in length. *Spirillum minor* and *Streptobacillus moniliformis* are both etiologic agents of rat-bite fever. The disease that occurs in man following exposure to *Spirillum minor* is termed sodoku and develops approximately two weeks after being bitten by a rat, mouse, or other rodent, or by rodent-eating animals such as cats. Sodoku is more common in Asia, and cases in the United States are quite rare. *Spirillum minor* has not been successfully grown *in vitro* and diagnosis is dependent on demonstrating organisms in clinical specimens or by animal inoculation. Sodoku responds to penicillin or tetracycline therapy (Bulger, 1977).

REFERENCES

Alexander, A. D.: Leptospira. *In* Lennette, E. H., Spaulding, E. H., and Truant, J. P.: Manual of Clinical Microbiology, 2nd ed. Washington, American Society for Microbiology, 1974, p. 347.

Bulger, R. H.: Rat-bite fever. *In* Conn, H. R. (ed.): Current Therapy. Philadelphia, W. B. Saunders Company, 1977, p. 64.

Center for Disease Control: Reported morbidity and mortality in the United States. Morbidity and Mortality Weekly Report, 25:2, 1977.

Felsenfeld, O.: Borreliae. St. Louis, Warren H. Green Publishing Co., 1971.

Hoeprich, P. D. (ed.): Infectious Diseases. Hagerstown, Md., Harper and Row, Publishers, Inc., 1977, pp. 517 and 823.

Kelly, R. T.: Cultivation and physiology of relapsing fever borreliae. *In* Johnson, R. C. (ed.): The Biology of Parasitic Spirochetes. New York, Academic Press, Inc., 1976, p. 87.

Stoenner, H. G.: Treatment and control of leptospirosis. *In* Johnson, R. C. (ed.): The Biology of Parasitic Spirochetes. New York, Academic Press, Inc., 1976, p. 375.

50

CLINICAL AND LABORATORY DIAGNOSIS OF MYCOTIC DISEASE

Elmer W. Koneman, M.D.,
and Glenn D. Roberts, Ph.D.

5

Interest in medical mycology has been on the upswing in the United States for the past decade. To some degree, attention to medical mycology has been a necessity because of the dramatic increase in the number of compromised patients who are receiving long-term courses of broad-spectrum antibiotics, corticosteroids, antimetabolites, or anticancer drugs or who are undergoing complex surgical procedures that require intensive postoperative life support. General improvement in medical care has led to a large population of individuals who are living to an older age with chronic diseases, such as diabetes mellitus, but who also are more susceptible to opportunistic fungal infections.

To a greater extent, however, this resurgent interest in mycology reflects a new discovery among general microbiologists and medical technologists that the study of mycology is innately fascinating. To a large degree, this has been brought about through the circulation of unknown fungal samples to clinical laboratories participating in various survey and proficiency test programs where technologists have the opportunity to study fungal species not frequently encountered in routine practice. The development of practical identification schema that have recently been published in the literature and discussed in detail in mycology workshops throughout the country has served to remove some of the fear of approaching a subject that until recently was considered difficult and obscure.

Although this laboratory enthusiasm has to some extent had its effect in improving the diagnosis of mycotic disease, many primary care practitioners are still woefully lacking in their understanding of the basic principles of clinical mycology and how to properly approach a patient with potential fungal disease. There is a great need to increase physician awareness of the various clinical signs and symptoms of mycotic disease and of how to properly collect specimens and have them transported to the laboratory. Clinical pathologists, microbiologists, and medical technologists have a unique opportunity, even an obligation, to participate frequently in infectious disease conferences, grand rounds, and other teaching activities in which the clinical and laboratory diagnosis of mycotic disease can be openly discussed.

Therefore, the approach to the discussion of mycotic diseases in this chapter will take a somewhat different turn from the presentations in most current textbooks. The discussion will follow a natural sequence paralleling the manner in which the diagnosis of fungal disease is made in actual clinical practice.

There are three major areas of diagnostic activity, as outlined in Figure 50-1.

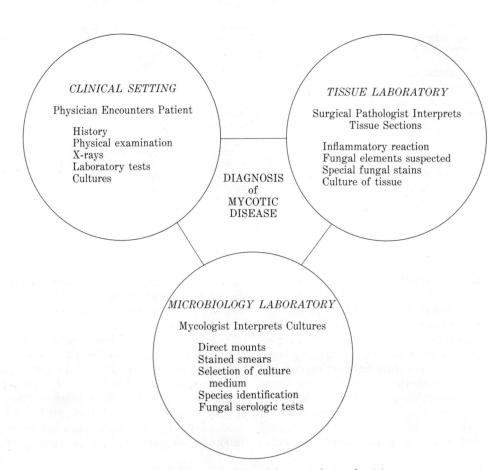

Figure 50-1. Diagnosis of fungal disease: spheres of activity.

CLINICAL SETTING

Physician Encounters Patient

History
Physical examination
X-rays
Laboratory tests
Cultures

TISSUE LABORATORY

Surgical Pathologist Interprets
Tissue Sections

Inflammatory reaction
Fungal elements suspected
Special fungal stains
Culture of tissue

DIAGNOSIS
of
MYCOTIC
DISEASE

MICROBIOLOGY LABORATORY

Mycologist Interprets Cultures

Direct mounts
Stained smears
Selection of culture
    medium
Species identification
Fungal serologic tests

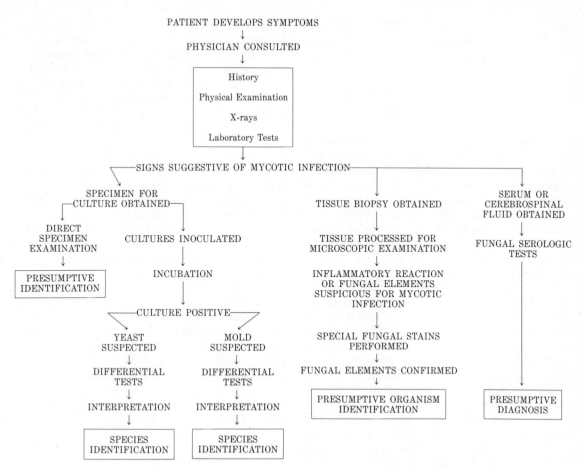

Figure 50-2. Algorithm for approach to diagnosis of fungal disease.

1. *The Clinical Setting.*

The physician encounters a patient with certain symptomatology, takes a history, performs a physical examination, requests x-rays and diagnostic laboratory tests, and obtains an appropriate culture.

2. *The Tissue Laboratory.*

The surgical pathologist examines tissues submitted to the laboratory, prepares tissue sections, and examines them microscopically for characteristic tissue reactions and fungal elements. Special stains may be required. Portions of tissue are submitted for culture.

3. *The Microbiology Laboratory.*

The microbiologist or mycologist processes and interprets cultures and makes a final species identification of any fungal organisms recovered.

The effectiveness with which any given patient with potential mycotic disease is evalu-

ated and properly treated is dependent upon how well the communications are maintained among these three activities. If the physician is not alert to leading signs and symptoms of fungal infection or fails to obtain proper specimens, perhaps sending them to the laboratory in improper containers or fixed in formalin; if the surgical pathologist fails to recognize tissue reactions or the presence of structures suspicious for fungal infection or does not submit a portion of the tissue for culture; or if the mycologist fails to prepare direct mounts or stained smears or does not select appropriate culture media for the recovery of certain species of fungi, either by omission or because he was not informed of the physician's clinical impression, the ability to make a final diagnosis may be lost or severely compromised.

Figure 50-2 is an algorithm serving to illustrate the clinical and laboratory approach to the diagnosis of mycotic disease and also to outline the subsequent discussion in this chapter.

CLINICAL PRESENTATION OF MYCOTIC DISEASE

The time-honored taxonomy of the mycoses, based on clinical presentation of fungal diseases—namely (1) superficial mycoses, (2) subcutaneous mycoses, and (3) disseminated (deep-seated) mycoses—must now be viewed from a somewhat different perspective. The many situations in which host defenses are now compromised, as discussed above, has made the practical implementation of this classification difficult.

Fungi formerly considered non-pathogenic or limited to only one organ system, under proper circumstances and in a compromised host, can cause disease. The clinician must be aware that the recovery of certain fungal species from the skin, mucous membranes, or other sites may not represent localized disease but a manifestation of disseminated involvement. Further studies, including culture of several secretions, especially sputum and urine, are required to determine the extent of involvement. The mucocutaneous presentation of *Histoplasma capsulatum, Blastomyces dermatitidis,* and *Cryptococcus neoformans* in particular most commonly indicates disseminated disease. Therefore, except in cases of classic superficial cutaneous dermatophyte infections which are known to remain localized, it is probably wise to assume that virtually any fungus species recovered in a symptomatic host potentially can represent disseminated disease, and a complete evaluation of the patient is indicated.

GENERAL SYMPTOMS OF MYCOTIC DISEASE

Deep-seated or disseminated fungal diseases may clinically mimic a number of other generalized diseases, such as tuberculosis, brucellosis, syphilis, sarcoidosis, and disseminated carcinomatosis, to name a few. It is necessary to recover the etiologic agent in culture or demonstrate it in biopsy specimens before a final diagnosis can be made.

Such non-specific complaints as fever, night sweats, weight loss, lassitude, easy fatigability, cough, chest pain, and so forth may be common to all of these conditions. Abnormal laboratory test results, such as leukocytosis (neutrophilia, lymphocytosis, and monocytosis), elevation in the erythrocyte sedimentation rate or elevation in serum enzymes or protein fractions only indicate that some type of an inflammatory response is present, but are of little aid in making a differential diagnosis. Positive x-ray findings, such as pulmonary infiltrates or evidence of inflammatory processes in other organs, are rarely specific. In some patients with severely compromised host resistance, these general symptoms may be minimal, if present at all.

Therefore, the initial clue to the presence of possible fungal disease in a given patient often must come from the recognition of more specific signs and/or symptoms or from information derived from the clinical history. Since fungal diseases are rarely if ever transmitted from man to man, but rather are contracted from the environment, it is important that the physician elicit important historical information from the patient, such as past or recent travel into geographic areas known to be endemic for certain fungi, or exposure to soil, dust, or other materials having a high probability of contamination.

SPECIFIC SIGNS AND SYMPTOMS OF FUNGAL DISEASE

Tables 50-1 to 50-4 outline the clinical types of fungal diseases, specific symptomatology, modes of infection, and some of the differential diagnoses to be considered for the fungi most commonly causing human infections. The mycotic diseases included in Tables 50-1 to 50-4 are listed in Table 50-5. Table 50-1 includes those fungi that routinely cause deep-seated mycoses and can be generally considered pathogenic whenever isolated from a human host. Table 50-2 lists those fungi that are opportunistic pathogens, causing localized organ disease or, rarely, disseminated mycoses in hosts with compromised immune resistance. Table 50-3 includes those fungi that are most commonly incriminated in various types of subcutaneous diseases, although reported cases of deep visceral or disseminated diseases can be found in the literature. Table 50-4 lists those fungi that cause only superficial cutaneous disease limited to the keratinized integument and are not known to cause invasive or disseminated mycotic disease.

These tables have been constructed to provide the physician with a quick review of the fungal diseases most commonly encountered in clinical practice. These tables are in no way complete, and other references are recommended for more detailed coverage. It is hoped, however, that this manner of presentation will provide those symptoms and epidemiologic factors necessary to formulate inductively a working diagnosis when confronted by a patient with certain leading signs and symptoms, as outlined in these tables.

The morphologic characteristics by which the laboratory diagnosis for each of the fungi discussed can be made will be presented in later sections of this chapter.

Approach to the deep-seated mycoses

The various clinical parameters of the deep-seated mycoses are summarized in Table 50-1. One of these mycotic diseases must be considered in the differential diagnosis of any patient who presents with signs and symptoms of chronic inflammatory or debilitating disease. Symptoms such as low grade fever, weight loss, malaise or persistence of single organ symptoms should draw one's attention to the potential for mycotic disease, although tuberculosis, systemic bacterial infections, and neoplasm must be ruled out.

If one of the deep-seated mycoses is suspected, it is important that the physician carefully examine the skin and mucous membranes. Histoplasmosis, for example, may first manifest itself with non-healing ulcerating lesions of the buccal mucosa, tongue, or posterior pharynx. Purulent material must be obtained from any suspicious lesion, direct mounts or stained smears for microscopic examination prepared, and a portion submitted for culture. Direct microscopic examination of purulent or serous material may provide an immediate diagnosis if "sulfur granules," budding yeasts, hyphal forms, or other fungal structures are identified.

If exudative material cannot be obtained from the lesion, a biopsy may be necessary. It is important that the physician alert the tissue laboratory if he suspects mycotic disease so that the biopsy specimen can be handled properly and small portions of tissue submitted for culture. Tissue biopsy specimens should be submitted to the laboratory in a sterile 4 by 4 inch gauze. Larger specimens should be submitted in sterile containers, and formalin fixative or "saline for injection," to which anti-bacterial substances have been added, should be avoided.

More than one specimen should be obtained from any patient in whom a deep-seated mycotic disease is suspected. For example, if spinal fluid is obtained from a patient with suspected fungal meningitis, sputum, urine, and possibly blood should also be submitted for culture. It is not uncommon for *Cryptococcus neoformans* to be recovered from the blood or urine when spinal fluid cultures fail to yield organisms.

Patients should be carefully questioned concerning travel to known endemic areas or about exposure to materials that may be potentially contaminated with fungal spores. History of a recent traumatic injury involving breaks in the skin or mucous membrane may be an extremely important point of information. The epidemiology of the fungal species causing deep-seated mycoses is outlined in Table 50-1.

Approach to the opportunistic mycoses

Table 50-2 outlines the clinical parameters of the more commonly encountered fungi that may be incriminated in the mycoses caused by certain species of opportunistic fungi. The various species of *Aspergillus, Candida, Geotrichum,* and Zygomycetes, as well as the bacteria *Actinomyces* and *Nocardia,* are widely distributed in nature and often are found as commensal inhabitants of the skin, respiratory passages, or gastrointestinal tract. Therefore, whenever one of these species is recovered from a patient with suspected infectious disease, it is necessary that the organism be isolated on repeated cultures directly from the site of infection before any given isolate can be considered pathogenic.

Physicians should be on the alert for opportunistic fungal infection in any patient whose immunologic response is compromised. The prolonged administration of broad-spectrum antibiotics or treatment with anticancer drugs inhibits both cellular and immune responses so that the usual symptoms and signs of infection may be obscure. Therefore, culture of secretions may be indicated even in the absence of clinical signs of infection. However, the recovery of an opportunistic fungal species from an immunosuppressed host should not preclude a thorough examination of the patient in search for a second microorganism of potentially greater significance that may be

(*Text continued on p. 1679*)

Table 50-1.   CLINICAL PARAMETERS OF THE DEEP-SEATED MYCOSES

FUNGAL DISEASE	ETIOLOGIC AGENTS	CLINICAL DISEASE MANIFESTATIONS: SIGNS AND SYMPTOMS	EPIDEMIOLOGY AND MODES OF INFECTION	DIFFERENTIAL CONSIDERATIONS

Blastomycosis	*Blastomyces dermatitidis*	*Primary Pulmonary Blastomycosis*
		Self-Limited Disease: Symptoms of non-specific respiratory disease—non-productive cough, intermittent chest pain, low grade fever, joint and muscle aches.
		Progressive Disease: Onset may be insidious, acting as a persistent "chest cold." Weight loss and progressive disability may be first signs. Cough productive of purulent or blood-tinged sputum, dyspnea, chest pain may increase in severity. Lung consolidation, pneumonia, and hilar adenopathy become evident on x-ray.
		Primary Cutaneous Blastomycosis
		Gilchrist's Disease: Rare. Lesions first appear on unclothed areas of skin, hands, face, and forearms. Firm, coalescing skin nodules first appear, with suppuration of their centers. Lesions become wartlike, spreading over the surface with verrucous borders.
		   Cutaneous involvement usually means disseminated disease, which must always be ruled out.
		Disseminated Blastomycosis
		Patient experiences increase in fever, night chills, sweating, and progressive weakness. Skin is involved in large proportion of cases. Bone lesions occur in $\frac{2}{3}$ of patients, usually in ribs or vertebrae. Spinal cord compression may result from vertebral collapse. Liver, spleen, kidneys, and prostate are the viscera most commonly involved; central nervous system lesions occur in $\frac{1}{3}$ of patients.
			No known animal to man or man to man transmission.
			Soil is thought to be the most probable source, although *B. dermatitidis* has only rarely been cultured from that source.
			Endemic disease in patients living in the Mississippi and Ohio river valleys, particularly those in close contact with the soil.
			Pulmonary disease is most common manifestation, presumably from inhalation of spores.
			Primary cutaneous disease results from inoculation of traumatic breaks in the skin with contaminated soil, dung, or other material.
				Pulmonary
				-Tuberculosis
				-Aspiration pneumonia
				-Carcinoma of the lung
				-Other mycoses:
				   Histoplasmosis
				   Coccidioidomycosis
				   Nocardiosis
				Cutaneous
				-Basal cell carcinoma
				-Leishmania: tropical sore
				-Other mycoses
				Disseminated
				-Tuberculosis
				-Metastatic carcinomatosis
				-Kala azar
				-Other mycoses

Coccidioidomycosis	*Coccidioides immitis*	*Primary Pulmonary Coccidioidomycosis* 60% of infected individuals are asymptomatic. Remainder have "grippe" or influenza-like symptoms: fever, chills, headache, arthralgia, and dyspnea ("valley fever"). Chest pain aggravated by breathing, or sharp pleuritic pains simulating traumatic rib fracture or myocardial infarction. Cough usually nonproductive and hemoptysis is rare. 2% of infected individuals ultimately present with residual cavitary or solid "coin lesions."	*C. immitis* is endemic in the dry desert regions of the southwestern United States and in Mexico. Man acquires the disease from exogenous sources, after contact with infected soil or inhalation of dust-laden spores. One reported incidence of man to man transmission occurred in six medical staff members attending a patient with osteolytic coccidioi-	Clinical manifestations are protean, and primary disease can simulate many other bacterial, mycotic, or disseminated neoplastic diseases. Cavitary lesions may simulate tuberculosis, particularly when the lesions involve the upper lobes of the lungs.

(*Table continued on following page*)

FUNGAL DISEASE	ETIOLOGIC AGENTS	CLINICAL DISEASE MANIFESTATIONS: SIGNS AND SYMPTOMS	EPIDEMIOLOGY AND MODES OF INFECTION	DIFFERENTIAL CONSIDERATIONS
		Cavities are thin-walled, peripheral in location, and can closely simulate tuberculosis *Primary Cutaneous Coccidioidomycosis* Primary skin lesions are rare, usually self-limited, and heal without sequelae. Erythema multiforme and erythema nodosum are common complications and are thought to portend a good prognosis. Erythematous rash is a frequent manifestation, secondary to a hypersensitivity reaction. *Disseminated Coccidioidomycosis* Fever, rapidly progressing weight loss, and weakness are usual manifestations. Headache may be severe with CNS involvement, secondary to hydrocephalus. Cutaneous lesions are usually due to disseminated disease; destructive lymphadenopathy, osteomyelitis, meningitis, and visceral involvement often seen in fatal cases.	domycosis where the infective mycelial form developed in the plaster cast. Spores disseminated in air currents were inhaled by the attendees (Emmons, 1977).	"Coin" lesions are often surgically removed, since they cannot be distinguished radiologically from solitary bronchiolar carcinoma or metastatic neoplasm.
Cryptococcosis	*Cryptococcus neoformans*	*Central Nervous System Cryptococcosis* Insidious or abrupt onset of neurologic symptoms usually bring patient to physician: headache, increasing in frequency and severity; ataxia and vertigo; vomiting; memory lapses; and, less commonly, seizures of the Jacksonian type. *Pulmonary Cryptococcosis* Symptoms often less than extent of disease: fever is usually mild or absent; cough is usually minimal, with production of scanty mucoid, blood-tinged sputum. Pleural pain occasionally present; pleural effusion rare. Rales and rhonchi are minimal because there is little exudation into the bronchial tree. *Disseminated Cryptococcosis* All viscera and organ systems may be involved. Cutaneous manifestations in 5% of cases: papules and vesicles of the face. Widely disseminated osseous lesions occur in 10% of cases. Weight loss, malaise, and persistence of fever often seen. Headache, vomiting, dizziness, restlessness, hallucinations, and personality changes simulating psychosis may be initial manifestations.	Cryptococci have a natural habitat in the soil. *C. neoformans* may be particularly found in the dust of pigeon droppings due to the alkaline medium rich in nitrogen which promotes growth. Man is particularly susceptible to infection when cleaning up dung-infested areas. Pigeons act as carriers of the organism but do not develop primary disease, presumably because of their high body temperature. The possibility of endogenous infection is still debated. Development of virulence in latent yeast cells inhaled at some previous time is a possibility.	*CNS* -Tubercular meningitis -Meningeal carcinomatosis *Pulmonary* -Tuberculosis -Other mycoses. The cavitary lesions of cryptococcosis can be distinguished from tuberculosis and histoplasmosis in that the thick wall or areas of calcification do not develop. *Disseminated* -Tuberculosis -Other mycoses -Mucin secreting carcinoma. It may be particularly difficult to differentiate gelatinous cysts of cryptococcus from mucin-secreting carcinoma.

Table 50-1.   CLINICAL PARAMETERS OF THE DEEP-SEATED MYCOSES (*Continued*)

FUNGAL DISEASE	ETIOLOGIC AGENTS	CLINICAL DISEASE MANIFESTATIONS: SIGNS AND SYMPTOMS	EPIDEMIOLOGY AND MODES OF INFECTION	DIFFERENTIAL CONSIDERATIONS
Histoplasmosis	*Histoplasma capsulatum*	*Pulmonary Histoplasmosis* *Acute Form:* Disease usually mild or may be asymptomatic. Process usually self limited. Non-productive cough, shortness of breath, chest pain, hoarseness, hemoptysis, and cyanosis may be present. *Chronic Form:* Chronic cavitary lesions may develop in adults. Symptoms may include chronic cough, low-grade fever, and occasional hemoptysis. X-rays may be diagnostic if a radiodense, thick, laminated and calcified "histoplasmoma" is present. *Disseminated Histoplasmosis* Pulmonary symptoms may be minimal. Hepatosplenomegaly and diffuse lymphadenopathy are usually present in varying degrees of severity due to propensity of fungus to invade the cells of the reticuloendothelial system. Fever, anemia, leukopenia, weight loss, and lassitude often portend disseminated disease. Solitary or multiple ulcerations of the skin, mucous membranes, or intestinal lining may be initial indication of disseminated disease. Any of the viscera may be involved; adrenal gland disease leading to Addison's disease may lead to fatal outcome.	Infections in the United States are most prevalent in the Mississippi River valley and its tributaries. Source of human infection is probably the soil. Soil laden with excreta of chickens, turkeys, birds, and bats ("cave fever") may have a high concentration of *H. capsulatum* organisms. Human infections most commonly result from inhalation of spore-laden dust. Serious acute infections have been reported following clean-up of chicken houses or turkey pens or removal of the dung from city squares under trees inhabited by starlings or other birds.	*Pulmonary* -Tuberculosis -Viral pneumonia -Lipoidal pneumonia -Hamman-Rich syndrome -Interstitial fibrosis -Sarcoidosis *Disseminated* -Hodgkin's disease -Lymphosarcoma -Kala azar
Paracoccidioidomycosis	*Paracoccidioides brasiliensis*	*Mucous Membrane Paracoccidioidomycosis* Ulcerating lesions present in the nasal or oral mucosa, gingivae; less commonly in the conjunctiva or anorectal mucosa. The ulcerations spread slowly and have a mulberry-like reddened appearance with yellow speckles. Extension to the tonsils is common. Lymphadenitis of the face and neck is severe. *Cutaneous Paracoccidioidomycosis* Lesions occur most commonly on the face, particularly in a perioral distribution, in association with oral mucous membrane disease. The lesions characteristically are ulcerative, have a crusted surface and a serpiginous border. Cervical lymph nodes are involved early in the disease.	Paracoccidioidomycosis is limited to the South American continent. Prevalence is highest in Brazil, Venezuela, and Colombia; the disease has not been reported in Chile, Guyana, and Surinam in South America, or in El Salvador, Nicaragua, or Panama in Central America. Most common portal of entry is still debated; however, current theory implicates the lungs. Infections through traumatic areas in the nasal mucosa, gums, oral mucosa, or pharynx have not been totally discounted. Primary inoculation may result from eating of raw vegetables.	*Mucocutaneous* -Cutaneous tuberculosis -Syphilis -Yaws -Cutaneous leishmaniasis (tropical sore) -Sporotrichosis -Basal cell carcinoma *Pulmonary* -Tuberculosis -Other mycoses *Disseminated* -Tuberculosis -Tuberculous adenitis -Tertiary syphilis

FUNGAL DISEASE	ETIOLOGIC AGENTS	CLINICAL DISEASE MANIFESTATIONS: SIGNS AND SYMPTOMS	EPIDEMIOLOGY AND MODES OF INFECTION	DIFFERENTIAL CONSIDERATIONS
		Pulmonary Paracoccidioidomycosis Pulmonary disease occurs in a high percentage of cases and the lungs may represent the portal of entry. Signs and symptoms often indicate less than degree of involvement would indicate. Productive cough, hemoptysis, dyspnea, fever, malaise, weight loss, and easy fatigability are experienced in varying degrees. *Disseminated Paracoccidioidomycosis* The lymphatic system, spleen, intestines, and liver are most commonly involved. Extensive pulmonary disease, central nervous system disease, adrenal insufficiency, or perforation of intestinal ulcers is a more common cause of death.	Inhalation of spores results in primary lung infections.	

5

Table 50–2. CLINICAL PARAMETERS OF THE OPPORTUNISTIC MYCOSES

FUNGAL DISEASE	ETIOLOGIC AGENT	CLINICAL DISEASE MANIFESTATIONS: SIGNS AND SYMPTOMS	EPIDEMIOLOGY AND MODES OF INFECTION	DIFFERENTIAL CONSIDERATIONS
Aspergillosis	*Aspergillus fumigatus* *Aspergillus flavus* *Aspergillus niger* Other *Aspergillus* species	*Pulmonary Aspergillosis* *Invasive:* Chief symptom is hemoptysis, resulting from necrotizing bronchopneumonia and pulmonary infarction (thromboses occur because of the propensity of the fungal hyphae to invade blood vessels). Dyspnea, fever, and tachypnea occur in progressive disease. *Allergic:* Most commonly develops in asthmatics who develop hypersensitivity to aspergilli antigens. Wheezing, cough, fever, and pleuritic pain are common symptoms. The presence of mucous plugs containing eosinophils and Charcot-Leyden crystals in expectorated sputum samples is highly suggestive of this form of the disease. *Fungus Ball:* Congenital bronchial cysts or cavitary lesions caused by tuberculosis, bronchiectasis, or carcinoma may become colonized with one of the aspergilli, notably *A. fumigatus.* The fungus colony tends to remain localized to the cyst cavity, only rarely invades into the adjacent pulmonary tissue, and is most commonly asymptomatic. *Otomycotic Aspergillosis* An aspergillus, notably *A. niger,* becomes colonized within a cerumen plug in the external auditory canal. Irritation of the canal mucosa occurs, resulting in itching, superficial erosion of the tympanic membrane, and impaired hearing. The exudate is usually foul smelling.	The spores of aspergilli are ubiquitous in nature, produced from mycelial forms that grow as saprobic fungi on decaying vegetation. Since aspergillus spores are commonly inhaled, aspergilli of various strains may be recovered from the upper respiratory passages of asymptomatic individuals. In the presence of suspicious symptoms, the same strain of *Aspergillus* must be recovered from multiple samples of respiratory secretions before the diagnosis can be accepted. *Aspergillus fumigatus* most commonly causes invasive pulmonary aspergillosis; *A. flavus* is usually incriminated in allergic bronchopulmonary disease; *A. fumigatus* and *A. niger* most commonly are recovered from cavitary fungus ball infections, and *A. niger* is most commonly implicated in otomycosis.	*Zygomycosis (Phycomycosis)* Hyphal fragments may be detected in direct mounts of sputum or other material. Those of aspergilli are slender, tend to have parallel walls, are septate, and branch dichotomously at 45 degree angles. Those of the Zygomycetes are irregularly broad, ribbon-like, aseptate, and branch at irregular angles. *Candidosis* Pneumonitis in compromised hosts caused by *Candida* species or other yeasts can closely simulate aspergillosis. Budding blastoconidia and focally constricted pseudohyphae are characteristic of *Candida.*
Candidosis	*Candida albicans* *Candida* species	*Cutaneous Candidosis* Generalized cutaneous, intertriginous, paronychia, onychia: redness, edema, scaling. *Mucous Membrane Candidosis* Vulvovaginal and oropharyngeal thrush: redness, edema, soft white patches on tonsils, gums, tongue, and vaginal mucosa. *Pulmonary Candidosis* Bronchial and bronchopulmonary varieties: cough, sputum production at times tinged with blood, pleuritis, and pleural effusion. *Endocarditis and Septicemia* Fever, splenomegaly, heart murmur, congestive heart failure, and anemia may be seen in varying combinations.	Infections with *Candida* are endogenous. Various species of *Candida* colonize the skin and mucous membranes. Clinical disease may arise in conditions in which there is an alteration in host defenses or suppression of the normal bacterial flora. Conditions predisposing to candidosis are: -Pregnancy -Diabetes mellitus -Indwelling venous catheters -Chronic debilitating diseases -Prolonged therapy with broad-spectrum antibiotics	*Cutaneous and Mucous Membrane* -Bacterial infections -Avitaminosis -Contact dermatitis -Trichomonas (vaginal) -Vaginal gonorrhea *Pulmonary* -Aspergillosis -Geotrichosis -Other yeast infections *Septicemia* -Bacterial endocarditis

FUNGAL DISEASE	ETIOLOGIC AGENT	CLINICAL DISEASE MANIFESTATIONS: SIGNS AND SYMPTOMS	EPIDEMIOLOGY AND MODES OF INFECTION	DIFFERENTIAL CONSIDERATIONS
Geotrichosis	*Geotrichum candidum*	*Respiratory Geotrichosis* Acute bronchitis and tracheitis: Cough productive of mucoid or purulent sputum. Pulmonary: Cough, low grade fever, pleuritis. Allergic variant causing wheezing and asthma-like attacks. Thin-walled cavities form rarely. Oral: Simulates candidal thrush. *Gastrointestinal Geotrichosis* Colitis	Common environmental saprobe on tomatoes and other fruit, in soil, and in dairy products. Infections probably endogenous, since *Geotrichum* may colonize skin, mucous membranes, and gastrointestinal tract. Disease most commonly occurs in debilitated patients with primary diseases, such as diabetes mellitus, leukemia, lymphoma, and other neoplasms.	Geotrichosis cannot be clinically differentiated from other yeast infections, notably those caused by *Candida*. Allergic bronchopulmonary disease closely simulates a similar disease caused by aspergilli.
Zygomycosis (Phycomycosis) (Mucormycosis)	*Rhizopus* sp. *Absidia* sp. *Mucor* sp.	*Orbitocerebral Zygomycosis* Nasal: A thick, dark, blood-tinged nasal discharge may be found. The nasal turbinate appears black, malar anesthesia may be present, and a necrotic palatal ulcer may be observed. Signs of sinusitis. Ocular: Edema of the eyelids and retina, proptosis and signs of retinal artery thrombosis. Complete internal and external ophthalmoplegia may occur in severe cases. Cerebral: Cerebral zygomycosis usually occurs as a direct extension of nasal, sinus, or orbital disease. Headache, drowsiness, or semistupor portend possible cerebral involvement. Nuchal rigidity indicates meningeal involvement. This form can be rapidly fatal, with symptoms suggesting cerebrovascular accident due to propensity for hyphae to invade and cause thrombosis of cerebral vessels. *Pulmonary Zygomycosis* Onset may be insidious or sudden. Chest pain, hemoptysis, sputum production, and cough are seen in varying degrees of severity. Sudden development of chest pain and development of a pleural friction rub are found when the pleura is invaded. *Disseminated Zygomycosis* Rare occurence, almost always in immunodepressed hosts. Virtually all organs may be involved, and the gastrointestinal tract in particular may be invaded, particularly the gastroesophageal region. Fever, weight loss, lassitude, and somnolence are common manifestations. Disease is rapidly fatal.	*Orbitocerebral* Diabetes mellitus is the most common predisposing condition. Uremic acidosis is less commonly a predisposing cause. *Pulmonary and Disseminated* Usually contracted as a nosocomial, hospital-acquired infection in patients being treated for leukemia or other disseminated neoplastic disease; or in those receiving corticosteroids for chronic renal disease or other immune related diseases. The *Zygomycetes* (*Phycomycetes*) comprise a group of fungi that are widely distributed in nature in soil and dung, and on vegetable matter. Spores are readily disseminated in the air. Portal of entry in man is by inhalation, either into the nasal passages or into the lungs. Gastrointestinal disease may occur from ingestion of contaminated foodstuffs. In disease, the fungus tends to invade blood vessels, causing extensive thrombosis and necrosis.	The triad of diabetic acidosis, ophthalmoplegia, and signs of diffuse cerebral vascular disease is virtually diagnostic of zygomycosis (phycomycosis). The nasal or external ocular exudation may become secondarily infected and simulate bacterial disease. It is important that the disease not be mistaken for bacterial infection. Since the fungus often does not exfoliate into the secretions, a tissue biopsy may be required to confirm the diagnosis. Pulmonary disease must be differentiated from other mycoses, particularly candidosis and aspergillosis.

(Table continued on following page)

5

Table 50–2.   CLINICAL PARAMETERS OF THE OPPORTUNISTIC MYCOSES (*Continued*)

FUNGAL DISEASE	ETIOLOGIC AGENT	CLINICAL DISEASE MANIFESTATIONS: SIGNS AND SYMPTOMS	EPIDEMIOLOGY AND MODES OF INFECTION	DIFFERENTIAL CONSIDERATIONS

Actinomycosis*	*Actinomyces israelii*	*Facial Actinomycosis*
		  "Lumpy jaw" is the classic disease. There is painful induration and swelling of the subcutaneous tissue of the jaw and upper neck. As the disease progresses, deeply penetrating fistulae that break out on the skin surface develop, and exuding purulent material within which "sulfur granules" may be seen.
		Thoracic Actinomycosis
		  Disease develops as a pneumonitis in the hilar or basal regions of the lung. The disease spreads by direct extension into the pleura, and adhesions are prominent. There may be direct extension through the thoracic wall with formation of suppurative cutaneous fistulae. Cough, spiking fever, pleural pain, and production of a mucopurulent blood sputum may be observed.
		Abdominal Actinomycosis
		  Disease commonly occurs in the right lower abdomen, simulating appendicitis. The appendix and adjacent organs may be involved in a dense, suppurative fibrosing lesion. Right lower abdominal pain and presence of a cecal tumor mass are common symptoms. Penetration of the abdominal wall with development of suppurative cutaneous fistulae may occur. Rarely, disease may result from perforation of a gastric ulcer, with involvement of the liver and extrahepatic biliary system. Jaundice may occur.
		  Salpingitis, cystitis, pyelonephritis, psoas muscle abscess, and direct extension into the spine are other complications of abdominal actinomycosis.
			Various species of *Actinomyces* are harbored in the oral cavity, within carious teeth, or in tonsilar crypts. This accounts for the source of most infections.
			Facial disease often follows tooth extraction, oral surgery, or breaks in the oral mucosa either from stabbing the lining with bits of straw or other vegetative matter or from compound fractures of the mandible.
			Pulmonary disease also is thought to be endogenous, following aspiration of infected materials from the tonsils or other areas in the oral cavity.
			Abdominal disease most commonly occurs secondary to a perforation of the gastrointestinal tract, either from ulceration or rupture of the appendix.
				Actinomycosis may resemble many other suppurative inflammatory diseases.
				Cervical, pulmonary, and intestinal tuberculosis must be ruled out.
				Syphilitic gumma may closely resemble actinomycotic lesions.
				Appendicitis, carcinoma of the cecum, and ameblasis are all abdominal diseases which may simulate actinomycosis.

Nocardiosis†	*Nocardia asteroides*	*Pulmonary Nocardiosis* Cough is the most common symptom, usually productive of a thick, at times bloody sputum. As the disease progresses chest pain, dyspnea, malaise, weight loss, low grade fever, and night sweats may be seen in varying degrees of severity. Cavitary disease, closely simulating tuberculosis, may lead to massive hemop-	*Nocardia asteroides* has a natural habitat in the soil. The portal of entry is through the respiratory tract through inhalation of dust-borne spores. Susceptibility to infection increases in certain debilitating diseases such as Cushing's syndrome, in alveolar	Pulmonary nocardiosis mimics tuberculosis and can be clinically difficult to differentiate. The organism does withstand the digestion and decontamination procedure and if viable, can grow on Lowenstein-Jensen cul-

FUNGAL DISEASE	ETIOLOGIC AGENT	CLINICAL DISEASE MANIFESTATIONS: SIGNS AND SYMPTOMS	EPIDEMIOLOGY AND MODES OF INFECTION	DIFFERENTIAL CONSIDERATIONS
		tysis. Sinus tracts, simulating actinomycosis, may penetrate the chest wall. Suppurative pneumonia with consolidation of one or more lobes of the lungs is common in some patients, complicated by pleuritis. *Cerebral Nocardiosis* Nearly one third of patients with progressive pulmonary disease develop metastatic brain abscesses. Brain lesions often are multiple. Severe headache and localizing sensory or motor disturbances often have an acute onset. *Disseminated Nocardiosis* The kidney is the next most frequently involved organ in disseminated disease. Involvement of the spleen, liver, and adrenal glands occurs; bone disease is rare. Endocarditis, myocarditis, and pericarditis also may occur. The disseminated form is usually fatal within months to a few years. *Subcutaneous Nocardiosis* See Table 50–3: Mycetoma	proteinosis, and in subjects with leukemia or lymphoma who are under chemotherapy. The recovery of *Nocardia asteroides* from pulmonary secretions usually indicates disease, although the organism has been recovered as a saprophyte from asymptomatic subjects. Nocardiosis occurs in all parts of the world, has no racial or occupational predelection, and has its highest age incidence at 30 to 50 years.	ture medium. Nocardia filaments may be missed in Ziehl-Neelsen stained smears because they are only partially acid fast. Pleural or chest wall involvement must be differentiated from actinomycosis. Disseminated disease is most commonly mistaken for carcinomatosis, particularly in the presence of brain lesions.

*Actinomycosis is currently classified as a bacterial and not a fungal disease.
†Nocardiosis is currently classified as a bacterial and not a fungal disease.

Table 50-3. CLINICAL PARAMETERS OF THE SUBCUTANEOUS MYCOSES

FUNGAL DISEASE	ETIOLOGIC AGENT	CLINICAL DISEASE MANIFESTATIONS: SIGNS AND SYMPTOMS	EPIDEMIOLOGY AND MODES OF INFECTION	DIFFERENTIAL CONSIDERATIONS
Chromomycosis	*Fonsecaea pedrosoi* *Fonsecaea compactum* *Phialophora verrucosa* *Cladosporium carrionii*	*Subcutaneous Chromomycosis* With few exceptions, chromomycosis is limited to the skin and subcutaneous tissue, most commonly involving the feet and legs. The initial lesion is a small papular or pustular ulcer, probably representing the site of inoculation, that exudes a serous exudate and forms a crust on the surface. As the disease becomes more chronic, the ulcer is replaced by a dry, crusted, warty, violaceous lesion that spreads locally but tends to remain restricted to the area of infection for months or years. In time the lesions become raised to form a cauliflower-like tumor having a dark brown or violaceous appearance, and in time the entire extremity may be covered. There is little pain. Secondary infections with bacteria may lead to lymphatic stasis and varying degrees of elephantiasis. *Cerebral Chromomycosis* A few cases of cerebral chromomycosis have been reported, probably representing hematogenous spread from primary subcutaneous sites of infection. Cerebral chromomycosis is indistinguishable clinically from other types of brain abscess.	The organisms causing chromomycosis have their natural habitat in the soil, and human infections occur secondary to skin penetration by infected thorns, splinters, or traumatic wounds contaminated with soil. Agricultural workers, field and jungle laborers, and mine workers make up a high percentage of reported cases, particularly individuals who work without protection of shoes. *F. pedrosoi* is the most common agent, and since this species prefers warm, moist conditions, most infections occur in the tropics. *F. pedrosoi* has been isolated from tree branches, bark, and trunks, rotten vegetative matter, and soil. *C. carrionii* and *P. verrucosa*, on the other hand, survive well in drier, colder conditions and can cause chromomycosis in more temperate climates.	*Cutaneous blastomycosis:* The early lateral spread with a tendency to heal centrally with a flat, thin scar that is commonly seen in cutaneous blastomycosis is not seen in the lesions of chromomycosis. *Cutaneous tuberculosis:* Recovery of the etiologic agent may be needed to make an early diagnosis. Tuberculosis usually does not form the advanced cauliflower tumors. *Leishmaniasis:* Lymphadenopathy is usually far more prominent. *Tertiary syphilis* *Yaws*
Mycetoma	Eumycotic *Petriellidium (Allescheria) boydii* (Imperfect form: *Monosporium apiospermum).* *Exophiala (Phialophora) jeanselmei* *Madurella grisea* Actinomycotic *Nocardia asteroides* *Nocardia brasiliensis* *Nocardia caviae* *Actinomyces israelii*	Lesions most commonly occur on the foot. The neck or back (pack carriers), the hand, the scalp, or rarely other body sites may also be infected where traumatic breaks in the skin may occur. The initial lesion is a small area of swelling, usually on the sole or the dorsum of the foot, presumably at the primary site of inoculation. Swelling, suppuration, and healing occur in a cyclic pattern, but with slow progression until in severe cases the entire foot may be involved. Swelling can become so pronounced that the sole of the foot assumes a convex curvature. Multiple sinus tracts develop, exuding purulent material from cutaneous ostia onto the surface of the skin. Often a variety of "grains" or "granules" composed of aggregates of microorganisms mixed with purulent and necrotic debris may be observed within the exudate, at times helpful in making a genus identification.	The organisms causing mycetomas have their natural habitat in the soil and enter the body through traumatic breaks in the skin. The disease is not contagious. Mycetomas are more common in males, generally rural farmers. Most cases have been reported from Mexico, Africa, and South America, although cases have been reported from the southern United States. There are geographic differences in species distribution. Actinomycotic mycetomas tend to be more universal in distribution; eumycotic mycetomas predominate in tropical countries. *Petriellidium (Allescheria) boydii* is the most common cause of my-	-*Bacterial cellulitis:* Subcutaneous staphylococcal abscesses (so called botryomycosis) may cause confusion; however, they rarely reach the severity of involvement as with the mycetomatous agents. -Elephantiasis secondary to filariasis. -Chromomycosis where mycetomas take on a more verrucous appearance.

FUNGAL DISEASE	ETIOLOGIC AGENT	CLINICAL DISEASE MANIFESTATIONS: SIGNS AND SYMPTOMS	EPIDEMIOLOGY AND MODES OF INFECTION	DIFFERENTIAL CONSIDERATIONS
	Actinomyces bovis *Actinomadura* species *Streptomyces* species	Hematogenous spread to other parts of the body does not occur; however, secondary bacterial infections may lead to bacterial septicemia. Although eumycotic mycetomas caused by a number of fungal species are separated from actinomycotic mycetomas caused by the Actinomycetes (Schizomycetes), they cannot be distinguished clinically. Experienced mycologists can separate the two by microscopically examining the grains and granules that form in the exudates. Actinomycosis is excluded from the actinomycotic mycetomas because the granules are more minute and the microaerophilic actinomycetes are endogenous in habitat and the mode of infection is different (Emmons, 1977).	cetomas in the United States.	
Sporotrichosis	*Sporothrix schenckii*	*Cutaneous Lymphatic Sporotrichosis* Following a penetrating wound of the skin with a splinter or thorn infected with spores, a small ulcerated lesion develops within one or two weeks, gradually enlarging into a sporotrichotic chancre which is slow to heal. Fever is uncommon. The lymphatics commonly become secondarily involved. As the fungus spreads up the lymphatic channels, a series of secondary subcutaneous nodules form. These become fixed to the skin, undergo necrosis, and ultimately surface to form secondary chancroid ulcers. Lesions often become infected with bacteria. *Cutaneous Non-lymphatic Sporotrichosis* Rarely, the primary lesion remains localized without lymphatic spread. The lesions may appear ulcerative, papular, or acneform. The neck, trunk, and arm are other sites beside the fingers and hand that may be involved. *Disseminated Sporotrichosis* Despite the propensity for primary lesions to spread via lymphatics, disseminated disease is rare. Constitutional symptoms are marked and the disease may be rapidly fatal. Widespread nodular and papular skin lesions, involvement of oral and nasal mucous membranes, and dissemination to the viscera have been seen. The central nervous system is not involved; pulmonary disease, lesions of bone (periostitis and osteomyelitis), joints, (synovitis) and muscle are the most common extracutaneous sites of infection.	The classic method of infection is through traumatic puncture of the skin by a prick from a thorn, piece of shrub, or hay. The fungus may also be present on wood, bark, straw, soil, and even on insects. Insect bites may cause infections. The rose gardener is particularly vulnerable, or nursery workers who handle sphagnum moss. Alcoholic gardeners are also highly susceptible because of a diminution in peripheral pain sensation. The fungus also lives under old brick or masonry stone and can infect masonry workers by entering through cracks or fissures in the hands. In the United States most infections occur in the midwest particularly in the states adjoining the Missouri and Mississippi River valleys.	The classic clinical presentation of a slow-to-heal ulcer on a finger or the hand, with a string of secondary lesions associated with a chain of enlarged lymph nodes extending up the arm is virtually diagnostic of sporotrichosis. Tularemia is a far more acute disease, with acute necrosis of the lymphatics and lymph nodes. Fever commonly accompanies tularemia infections. Disseminated sporotrichosis must be differentiated from other systemic mycoses, from miliary tuberculosis, glanders, anthrax, or chronic disseminated bacterial diseases of other types.

5

Table 50-4. CLINICAL PARAMETERS OF THE SUPERFICIAL MYCOSES

FUNGAL DISEASE	ETIOLOGIC AGENT	CLINICAL DISEASE TYPES: SIGNS AND SYMPTOMS	EPIDEMIOLOGY AND MODES OF INFECTION	DIFFERENTIAL CONSIDERATIONS
Dermatophytosis	*Microsporum audouinii* *Microsporum canis* *Microsporum gypseum* *Epidermophyton floccosum* *Trichophyton mentagrophytes* *Trichophyton rubrum* *Trichophyton tonsurans* *Trichophyton verrucosum* *Trichophyton schoenleinii* *Trichophyton violaceum*	The dermatophytes are a group of fungi that infect the superficial keratinized portion of the integument—skin, hair, and nails—without spread into the deeper skin, viscera, or dissemination. Various clinical types have only a rough correlation with specific dermatophyte species with considerable overlapping between types. *Tinea Pedis* (dermatophytosis of the foot) Ringworm of the foot or athlete's foot, the most common type of dermatophytosis, begins as a weeping, peeling lesion between the web of the 4th and 5th toes. Lesions extend to involve other toe webs and the subdigital and interdigital surfaces of the toes. In chronic cases, spread as a dry scaling condition over the sole, arch, heel, and even dorsum of the foot may occur. Acute lesions are pruritic; chronic disease may be asymptomatic. *T. rubrum*, *T. mentagrophytes*, and *E. floccosum* are most common species. *Tinea Corporis* (dermatophytosis of the body) Most common in children, involving the glabrous portions of the face, shoulders, arms, or other exposed surfaces. The lesions vary in size, are circular, and exhibit a raised, red, serpiginous margin, accounting for the anachronistic term "ringworm." *M. canis*, *M. gypseum*, *T. mentagrophytes*, and *T. rubrum* most common. *Tinea Barbae* (dermatophytosis of the beard) A severe pustular folliculitis involving the beard or other hairy areas of the face and neck. *T. verrucosum* and *T. mentagrophytes* are the most common species. *Tinea Cruris* (dermatophytosis of the groin) Chronic, severely pruritic involvement of the groin and perineal and perianal areas. May be in epidemic form on shipboard or in locker rooms where community towels may transmit the disease. Lesions may remain localized (*E. floccosum*) or may spread widely over the buttocks or waist (*T. rubrum*).	Dermatophytic infections may be contracted in a variety of ways. Dermatophytes have been recovered from floors of shower stalls and locker rooms. It is probable that tinea pedis infections are incurred exogenously by walking barefoot over these contaminated areas. *M. audouinii*, the most frequent cause of inflammatory tinea capitis, can be transmitted from man to man by direct contact, or through contaminated fomites such as hair brushes, combs, or caps. *T. tonsurans* may be similarly transmitted. *E. floccosum*, *T. violaceum*, and *T. schoenleinii* may be directly transmitted from man to man through contaminated towels or clothes. Zoophilic sources are numerous. Tinea corporis is commonly secondary to *M. canis* transmitted from an infected cat or dog which is fondled by the patient. *T. verrucosum*, a cause of tinea barbae, is most commonly contracted from cattle. Farmers who hand milk cows have the habit of resting the bearded surface of their face against the side of the cow. Dogs, chinchillas, guinea pigs, mice, horses, and other animals have been incriminated as sources for human ringworm infections.	Allergic dermatitis of the hands and feet can simulate dermatophytosis. These usually lack the reddened serpiginous margin of a classic ringworm lesion. Dermatophytid ("id") reactions are vesicular eruptions of the fingers caused by circulating antigens from a focus of mycotic infection elsewhere. These are allergic lesions and are not primary sites of fungal infection. Onychomycosis must be differentiated from *Candida* spp. infections, which can appear quite similar. It is essential that direct mounts be made to establish the correct etiology before dermatophyte therapy is instituted. Skin and nail lesions must also be differentiated from psoriasis, which can produce similar appearing alterations. Seborrhea of the scalp can also be mistaken for tinea capitis.

FUNGAL DISEASE	ETIOLOGIC AGENT	CLINICAL DISEASE TYPES: SIGNS AND SYMPTOMS	EPIDEMIOLOGY AND MODES OF INFECTION	DIFFERENTIAL CONSIDERATIONS
		Lesions are sharply demarcated, marginated, centrally red, and usually dry. *Tinea Capitis* (dermatophytosis of the scalp) Classic type: *M. audouinii* Primary involvement of the hairs of the scalp in which the fungus invades the hair follicle, forming a sheath of spores around the hair shaft (ectothrix invasion). Hairs often break 1 to 2 mm above the surface and produce a bright green-yellow fluorescence under an ultraviolet Wood's lamp. Varying degrees of inflammation of the skin are noted, particularly severe with *M. canis*. Black dot type: *T. tonsurans* and *T. violaceum* Dry, diffuse, scaly lesions of the scalp in which the hair shaft is invaded internally (endothrix invasion) with destruction of the keratin. The hair becomes fragile and breaks off beneath the surface of the skin, producing a "black dot." Boggy lesions known as kerions may develop in this type. *T. tonsurans* and *T. violaceum* are most common causes of black dot hair infection. *T. verrucosum* and *T. mentagrophytes* cause kerions. Onychomycosis (*Tinea Unguium*) Ringworm of the nails may involve either the feet or the hands, or both. The infected nails have a chalky, crumbling consistency or "moth-eaten" appearance or may become hypertrophic and project above a thickened nail bed of keratinized cells and debris. *T. rubrum* and *T. mentagrophytes* are the most common causes.	*M. gypseum* is the most important geophilic fungus that causes ringworm in man. The soil is its natural habitat, where the fungus grows on keratinous debris. Children may become infected by direct contact during play (mudpies, etc.)	

(*Table continued on following page*)

5

Table 50–4. CLINICAL PARAMETERS OF THE SUPERFICIAL MYCOSES (*Continued*)

FUNGAL DISEASE	ETIOLOGIC AGENT	CLINICAL DISEASE TYPES: SIGNS AND SYMPTOMS	EPIDEMIOLOGY AND MODES OF INFECTION	DIFFERENTIAL CONSIDERATIONS
Tinea Nigra Palmaris	*Exophiala* (*Cladosporium*) *werneckii*	Superficial fungus infection of the skin, most commonly involving the palms of the hands but rarely other sites, with asymptomatic brown or black macules which may be discrete or become confluent. The dark pigmentation has been likened to skin stained with silver nitrate. Pigmentation is often most intense at the periphery of the macule, simulating a ringworm. Inflammation is not a feature, and pruritus is mild if present at all.	The disease is prevalent in South and Central America, but has been reported in the coastal southeastern United States. The fungus resides as a saprophyte in nature, and man presumably contracts the disease by direct contact with infected materials. Familial spread of the disease is a possibility.	Tinea nigra differs from tinea versicolor by its distinct dark pigmentation. The pigmented lesions of pinta can cause confusion, as can pigmented lesions of Addison's disease and syphilis. Laboratory examinations are required.
Pityrosporum (Tinea) Versicolor	*Malassezia* (*Pityrosporum*) *furfur*	The disease is recognized as an asymptomatic cream-tan discoloration of the superficial skin, most commonly of the chest or trunk, but may also involve groin, thighs, arms, face, and scalp. The lesions are non-inflammatory and covered by thin scales and generally are sharply marginated. The fungus interferes with sun tanning and may appear as light blotches in exposed areas.	The fungus exists as a free-living saprophyte and probably spreads from person to person by exposure to desquamated scales. Lack of personal hygiene facilitates development of skin lesions.	Tinea corporis can usually be distinguished by its distinct border and presence of inflammatory reaction. Seborrhea, secondary syphilis, and pinta must be considered and ruled out by laboratory examination.
Piedra Black Piedra White Piedra	*Piedraia hortae* *Trichosporon beigelii*	Infection of hairs, characterized by the presence of firmly adherent black, hard, gritty nodules (black piedra) or soft, mucilaginous nodules (white piedra). Scalp, beard, mustache, and genital hairs may be involved. The patient suffers no discomfort, since the lesion is limited to the hairs.	Prevalent in South America and tropical Africa. Reservoir may be in primates. White piedra is also found in Central Europe, England, and Japan.	The only major differential problem is in the recognition of nits of pediculosis capitis and bacterial trichomycoses that are not true "mycoses."

Table 50-5. MYCOTIC DISEASES INCLUDED IN
TABLES 50-1 to 50-4

TABLE 50-1 DEEP-SEATED MYCOSES	TABLE 50-2 OPPORTUNISTIC MYCOSES	TABLE 50-3 SUBCUTANEOUS MYCOSES	TABLE 50-4 CUTANEOUS MYCOSES
Blastomycosis	Actinomycosis*	Actinomycosis*	Dermatomycoses
Coccidioidomycosis	Aspergillosis	Chromomycosis	Piedra
Cryptococcosis	Candidosis	Maduromycosis	Tinea versicolor
Histoplasmosis	Geotrichosis	Nocardiosis*	Tinea nigra
Paracoccidiodomycosis	Nocardiosis*	Sporotrichosis	palmaris
	Zygomycosis (Phycomycosis)		

*The actinomycetes, including *Actinomyces* sp. and *Nocardia* sp., are not
fungi, but rather are bacteria belonging to the *Schizomycetes*.

masked by the more rapidly growing oppor-
tunist.

Approach to the subcutaneous mycoses

Table 50-3 outlines the clinical parameters
of several fungi that are known to cause subcutaneous mycoses. In the United States,
*Sporothrix schenckii, Petriellidium (Alles-
cheria) boydii,* and members of the Actinomycetes (*Nocardia* and *Actinomyces*) will be the
organisms most commonly recovered from
cases of subcutaneous mycosis. A few cases of
Exophiala (Phialophora) jeanselmei infections
have been reported from the southeastern
United States. The agents of chromomycosis
are endemic only in the tropical regions of the
world.

In suspected mycetomatous disease, serous
or purulent material from the draining sinuses
should be directly examined for the presence
of granules or grains, and a presumptive diagnosis can often be made. The morphology of
these grains is discussed later in this chapter.
Specimens should be cultured both aerobically
and anaerobically, in that *Actinomyces* grows
only anaerobically.

The clinical parameters of sporotrichosis, as
outlined in Table 50-3 are virtually diagnostic.
This disease should be suspected when any
non-healing ulcers of the fingers, hand, or
forearm are clinically encountered, particularly if there is concomitant involvement of
the lymphatics draining the arm. Direct examination of any exudate that may be present
or review of tissue sections of biopsy specimens will usually not reveal the characteristic
yeast-like organisms. Therefore, the diagnosis
can be confirmed only by recovering the causative organism in culture.

Approach to the superficial mycoses

Table 50-4 outlines the clinical parameters
of the superficial mycoses. Ringworm infections caused by several species of dermatophytes are the most common mycoses encountered in clinical practice.

A variety of tinea infections may be encountered, as outlined in Table 50-4. The advent of griseofulvin has to some degree precluded the necessity to make a species identification, and fewer cutaneous cultures are
referred to laboratories. However, physicians
must confirm their clinical impression of dermatophyte infection by performing a direct
potassium hydroxide mount of skin scales,
hairs, or nail scrapings, because other microorganisms, notably species of *Candida*, can
closely simulate tinea infections.

In collecting specimens for culture, the
growing outer serpiginous border of typical
ringworm lesions should be scraped with a
blade, and the scales collected in a sterile Petri
dish. Before cultures are taken, the skin should
be cleansed with 70 per cent alcohol or other
suitable disinfectant to remove contaminating
surface bacteria. In collecting specimens from
infected nails, some of the softened material
from beneath the nail surface should be selected. The use of a Wood's lamp is useful in
selecting infected hairs when *M. audouinii* or
M. canis are the agents involved, since they
produce a bright yellow-green fluorescence.

Dermatophyte infections remain confined to
the keratinized portion of the integument and
subcutaneous or visceral invasion does not
occur.

The other superficial mycoses listed in Table
50-4 have little clinical significance. Pityriasis
versicolor is relatively frequent, and is most

commonly diagnosed by direct examination of KOH mounts of superficial skin scales. The other conditions are only rarely encountered in the United States.

Miscellaneous mycotic diseases

A number of other fungal species, many commonly recovered as saprobic contaminants in the laboratory, can occasionally cause mycotic disease. Species of *Aspergillus, Fusarium, Candida,* and *Acremonium (Cephalosporium)* can cause mycotic keratitis, following corneal trauma or postoperatively. Keratitis begins as a small corneal ulcer which develops into a slightly raised, gray-white nodule with an opaque halo around the center. The cornea may become inflamed. Scarring may develop and the disease can progress to invade the anterior chamber if not treated. Corneal scrapings should be taken and microscopically examined for fungal mycelial elements.

Otomycosis was discussed above and is commonly caused by *A. fumigatus* and *A. niger.* Species of *Scopulariopsis, Rhizopus, Candida,* and some of the dermatophytes have also been recovered. The tympanic membrane is rarely perforated.

A condition known as cerebral chromomycosis can be caused by generally non-pathogenic species of *Cladosporium,* notably *C. trichoides.* This fungus species has been recovered from brain abscesses and focal parenchymal lesions.

Rhinosporidiosis is a chronic granulomatous infection of the nasal passages resulting in the production of polyps or a hyperplastic mucous membrane. The etiologic agent is *Rhinosporidium seeberi.* The eyes, ears, larynx, and occasionally the mucous membranes of the vagina or penis may be involved, where the disease must be differentiated from warts or condylomata.

Aflatoxins, toxic products of a number of fungal species that may cause gastrointestinal, neurologic, or allergic manifestations in man and animals, may be encountered more frequently than suspected. Many foodstuffs or commercial products made from vegetative by-products (sugar cane refuse, for example) may become infected with aflatoxin-producing species of fungi during storage. The toxic products accumulate in these foodstuffs and may be either ingested or inhaled. Gastrointestinal upset, transient neurologic symptoms such as headache, dizziness or neuromuscular manifestations, or allergic interstitial pulmonary disease simulating Hamman-Rich syndrome (bagassosis, byssinosis) may be encountered. A careful history of exposure to any of these materials must be elicited when encountering these clinical syndromes.

HISTOPATHOLOGY OF FUNGAL INFECTIONS

Surgical pathologists often play an important role in the diagnosis of mycotic disease. The referring physician should always inform the pathologist when he suspects one of the fungal diseases so that the biopsy or surgical specimen can be properly prepared for study and a portion can be submitted for culture.

Unfortunately, the specimen request slip does not routinely have this information, and the presence of fungal disease may be suspected only when suspicious fungal forms are detected in routine hematoxylin and eosin (H & E) sections of surgical or autopsy tissue. Often cultures have not been obtained, and it may be difficult to make a definitive identification based on tissue section morphology alone. The use of special stains that have a specific avidity for the carbohydrate-rich cell walls, capsules, or hyphal forms of fungi, such as the periodic acid–Schiff (PAS), Gomori methenamine silver (GMS), or mucicarmine stains, can be helpful. However, it should be pointed out that fungal forms can often be well visualized in routine H & E sections, and in many instances the use of special stains merely confirms an initial impression.

The discussion in this section will include a practical approach that surgical pathologists may find helpful in making a presumptive diagnosis when fungal elements are observed in tissue sections. Unfortunately, fungal forms are often distorted beyond recognition by the host's inflammatory response, making a diagnosis other than "fungal disease" difficult. Nevertheless, the approach outlined here will prove helpful in many instances in which fungal elements are present in tissue sections, and occasionally a definitive diagnosis may be possible.

ASSESSMENT OF INFLAMMATORY TISSUE REACTIONS

The invasion of organs or tissues by fungi produces a variety of inflammatory reactions. Although these reactions are often non-specific, fungal disease should be suspected when certain inflammatory patterns are recognized. The presence of granulomatous inflammation,

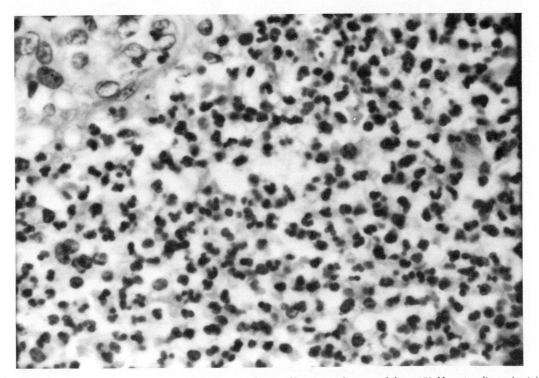

Figure 50-3. Suppurative inflammatory reaction showing dense infiltration with neutrophils. $\times$ 450. Hematoxylin-eosin stain.

caseous necrosis, or infiltration with multinucleated giant cells is highly suggestive of fungal disease.

In the following paragraphs are reviewed commonly encountered tissue inflammatory reactions and a brief discussion of some of the specific fungi that may be associated with each.

Suppurative Inflammation. The term *suppurative* refers to an inflammatory reaction in which polymorphonuclear leukocytes predominate (Fig. 50-3). Suppurative inflammation indicates the presence of pus, which may be loculated within walled-off abscesses, may cover the surface of mucous membranes, or may exude from the stomas of fistulae or sinus tracts.

Actinomycosis or nocardiosis should always be suspected when a dense suppurative inflammatory response is seen in tissue sections from patients in whom fungal disease is suspected. Direct mounts of the purulent exudate or the stained tissue sections should be carefully examined for the presence of sulfur granules (Fig. 50-4). A Gram stain or silver stain may be necessary to make the final diagnosis by demonstrating the characteristic del-

icate, branching filamentous forms within the sulfur granule (Fig. 50-5).

Blastomyces dermatitidis also frequently produces suppurative inflammation, particularly within the characteristic intraepithelial microabscesses that are found in primary or secondary cutaneous disease (Fig. 50-6). The additional detection of yeast forms 8 to 15 μ in diameter, with some having the single bud attached by a broad base, is virtually diagnostic (Fig. 50-7).

Chronic "Round Cell" Inflammation. If an acute suppurative inflammatory reaction does not resolve with healing in a relatively short time, the exudate begins to take on a different appearance, and a predominance of lymphocytes, monocytes, or other mononuclear inflammatory cells will be noted (Fig. 50-8). Polymorphonuclear leukocytes are either few in number or totally absent. This "round cell" response is referred to as chronic inflammation. This reaction is non-specific and may be seen in many different fungal infections and other chronic inflammatory responses as well.

An admixture of eosinophils in an inflammatory reaction often suggests an allergic or hypersensitivity response; a preponderance of

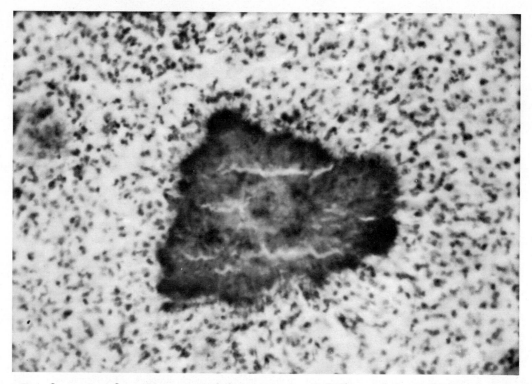

Figure 50–4. Suppurative inflammatory reaction including an actinomycotic "sulfur granule." ×250. Hematoxylin-eosin stain.

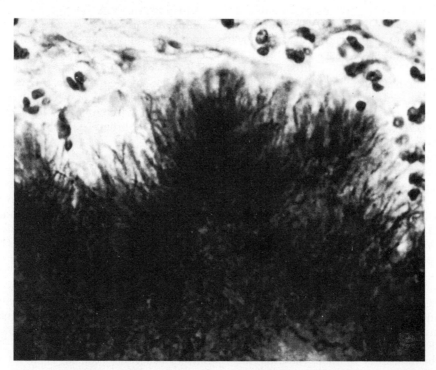

Figure 50–5. Margin of "sulfur granule" showing delicate branching filaments. ×950. Hematoxylin-eosin stain.

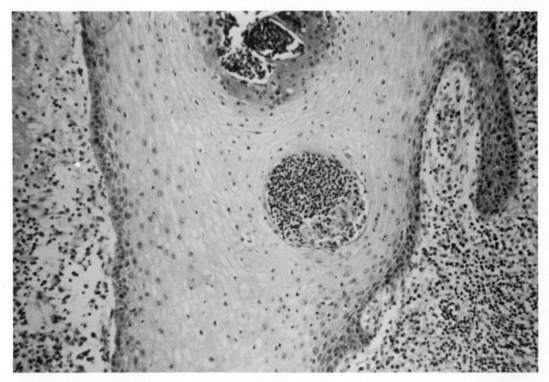

Figure 50–6. Section of skin showing hyperplastic squamous epithelium including epithelial microabscess. ×100. Hematoxylin-eosin stain. (From Dolan, C. T., Funkhouser, J. W., Koneman, E. W., Miller, N. G., and Roberts, G. D.: Atlas of Clinical Mycology II. Chicago, Ill., American Society of Clinical Pathologists, 1975.

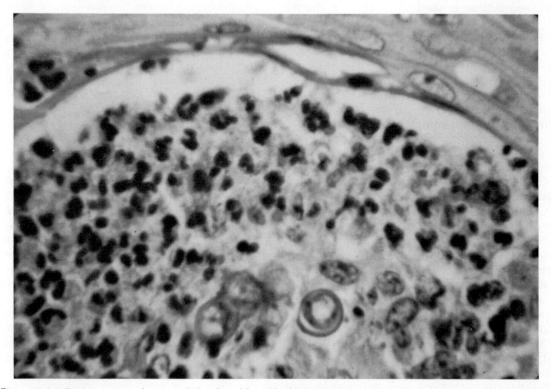

Figure 50–7. Cutaneous microabscess including broad-based budding yeast forms of *Blastomyces dermatitidis.* ×450. Hematoxylin-eosin stain. (From Dolan, C. T., Funkhouser, J. W., Koneman, E. W., Miller, N. G., and Roberts, G. D.: Atlas of Clinical Mycology II. Chicago, Ill., American Society of Clinical Pathologists, 1975.)

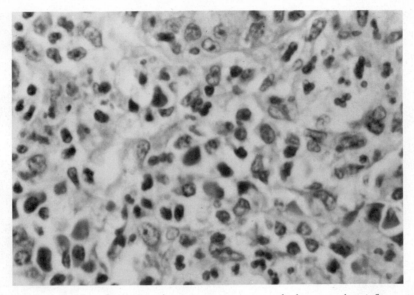

Figure 50-8. Chronic "round cell" inflammation showing reaction composed of mononuclear inflammatory cells. ×450. Hematoxylin-eosin stain.

plasma cells usually indicates an adequate immunologic response with production of type-specific proteins.

Granulomatous Inflammation. The term *granulomatous* is used to describe a specific type of chronic inflammation in which the cellular response is almost entirely composed of large macrophages or histiocytes, which often aggregate to form multinucleated giant cells.

The prototype of granulomatous inflammation is the tubercle, a focal collection of large mononuclear inflammatory cells surrounded by a cuff of lymphocytes, with varying degrees of caseous necrosis and infiltration with varying numbers of giant cells (see Fig. 50-11). Although most commonly produced by various species of mycobacteria, notably *M. tuberculosis*, tubercle-like reactions may also be seen with many fungal diseases.

The characteristic multinucleated giant cell in tuberculosis is the Langhan's giant cell, characterized by the arrangement of the cell nuclei around the periphery of the cytoplasm, simulating a spoke wheel (Fig. 50-9). These are to be distinguished from foreign body or tumor giant cells, in which the nuclei are arranged irregularly throughout the cytoplasm (Fig. 50-10). Although tuberculosis is suspected when Langhan's giant cells are seen in inflammatory reactions, they may also be seen in a number of mycotic infections as well.

Caseation necrosis is another feature that often accompanies granulomatous inflammation. *Caseation* is a term that is used to designate a degenerative tissue response in which there develops a cheese-like consistency. When examined microscopically, areas of caseation necrosis are devoid of viable cells, but rather consist entirely of a homogeneously staining, finely granular material, within which Langhan's giant cells are often scattered (Fig. 50-11). Caseation necrosis is also one of the hallmarks of tuberculosis, thought to represent a hypersensitivity reaction to antigenic substances produced by the tubercle bacilli. However, caseation necrosis is not infrequently seen in mycotic infections, notably *Histoplasma capsulatum* and *Coccidioides immitis*, and Langhan's giant cells may be seen as well.

Necrotizing Inflammation, With or Without Infarction. *Infarction* is a term used to describe that process by which a portion of an organ or segment of tissue undergoes cellular death due to sudden loss of blood supply. Infarctions are commonly observed in mycotic infections caused by *Aspergillus fumigatus* or one of the *Zygomyces (Phycomyces)* species of fungi because of their peculiar predilection for directly invading blood vessels (Fig. 50-12), causing vascular occlusion (thrombosis).

Necrosis is a term used to describe the "mopping up" cellular reaction in response to

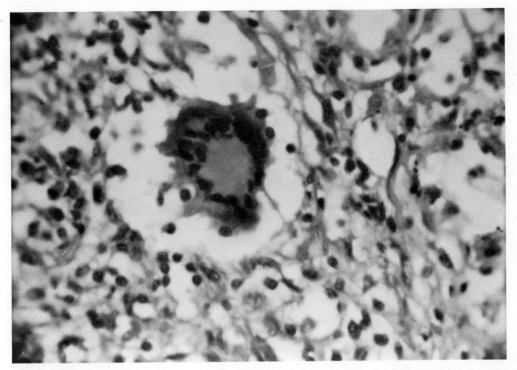

Figure 50-9. Inflammatory reaction including a Langhan's giant cell with characteristic peripheral arrangement of nuclei. ×250. Hematoxylin-eosin stain.

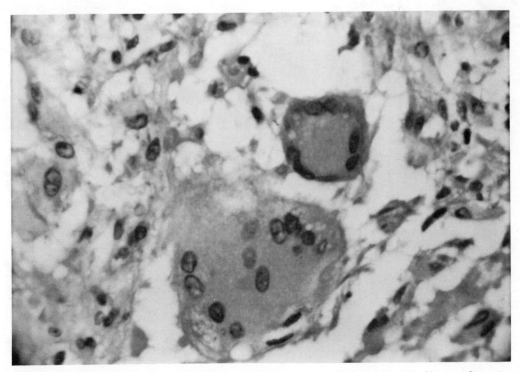

Figure 50-10. Comparison of Langhan's giant cell (top) with tumor giant cell (bottom). ×250. Hematoxylin-eosin stain.

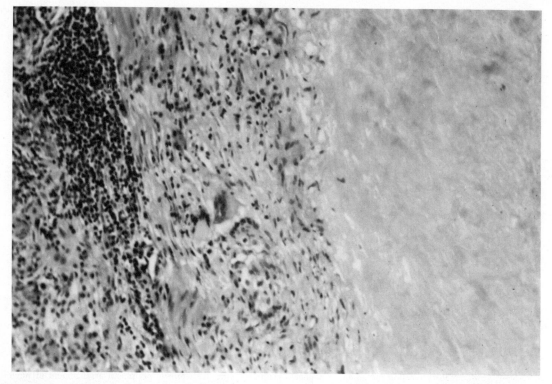

Figure 50–11. Portion of a "tuberculoma." Caseation necrosis is present on the left, adjacent to a band of fibrosis including giant cells and a collection of lymphocytes on the right. ×100. Hematoxylin-eosin stain.

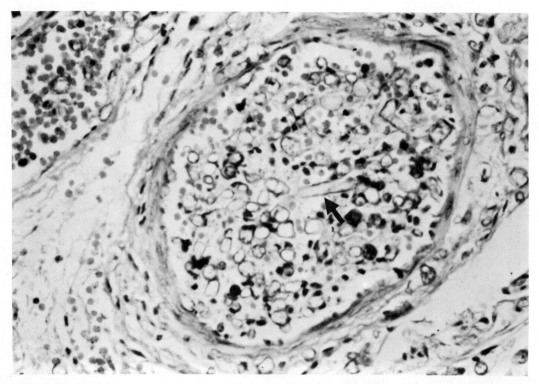

Figure 50–12. Arteriole showing a lumen occluded by aseptate hyphae (zygomycosis). ×250. Hematoxylin-eosin stain.

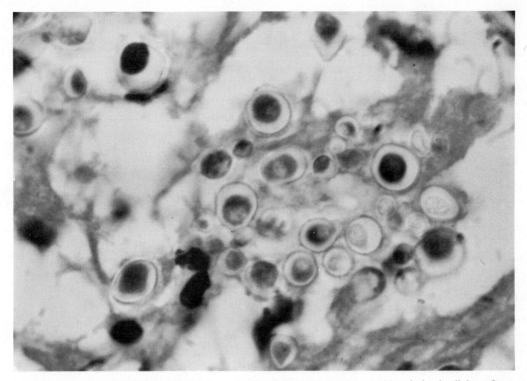

Figure 50–13. Tissue invasion with encapsulated yeast cells of *Cryptococcus neoformans*. Note lack of cellular inflammatory response. ×250. Hematoxylin-eosin stain.

focal infarction. Virtually every type of inflammatory cell may be present in necrotizing inflammation, and a large amount of degenerate cellular debris is present. A large number of vacuolated, lipid-containing histiocytes are often present. Varying degrees of hemorrhage with the deposition of hemosiderin pigment in the areas of necrosis are seen. It is this type of reaction that produces the burned eschar appearance of tissue specimens that have been obtained from areas of necrosis secondary to *Zygomyces* infections.

Inert Response. Patients with immune deficiency disease or individuals under immunosuppressive therapy often do not produce a cellular inflammatory response to invading fungi or other microorganisms. So-called agranulocytic pneumonia is a prime example. For reasons not totally understood, *Cryptococcus neoformans* characteristically does not elicit a cellular inflammatory response, even in patients who are immunologically competent (Fig. 50-13). The lack of cellular response, together with the production of abundant polysaccharide capsular substance by *C. neoformans*, may lead to a misdiagnosis of mucin-secreting carcinoma.

In summary, fungal infections should be considered in the differential diagnosis of any of the tissue reactions described above, and special stains may be necessary to make an identification if either the yeast or hyphal forms cannot be recognized in routine H & E sections.

PRESUMPTIVE IDENTIFICATION OF FUNGI IN TISSUE SECTIONS

Fungi may assume one of two basic forms in tissues:

1. A mycelial form, characterized by the presence of filamentous structures called hyphae.
2. A yeast or "tissue" form in which only yeast cells are present.

Tissue forms of commonly encountered fungi are listed in Table 50-6.

Some fungi produce only a yeast form in tissues, others only a mycelial form. Rarely do the two occur together in the same organ or tissue. The dimorphic fungi, which include most of the species causing deep-seated mycotic disease in man, are called "dimorphic"

Table 50-6. TISSUE FORMS OF FUNGI OF MEDICAL IMPORTANCE TO MAN

ETIOLOGIC AGENT	DIAGNOSTIC TISSUE FORM	SIZE	COMMENTS
I. Deep-seated Mycoses			
Blastomyces dermatitidis	Thick-walled, double-contoured yeast cells, producing single bud attached by a broad base.	8–20 μ	
Coccidioides immitis	Thick-walled spherules enclosing numerous non-budding endospores.	10–60 μ	Rudimentary mycelium may rarely develop in open cavitary lesions.
Cryptococcus neoformans	Irregularly sized yeast cells, budding singly and attached by a hair-like neck, surrounded by a thick mucoid capsule.	4–15 μ	*Cryptococcus neoformans* never forms a true mycelium.
Histoplasma capsulatum	Small yeast cells located within reticuloendothelial cells. Pseudocapsules account for the species name.	2–4 μ	True capsules do not form.
Paracoccidioides brasiliensis	Large yeast cells producing multiple buds arranged in the form of a mariner's wheel.	8–20 μ	
II. Opportunistic Mycoses			
Aspergillus species	Hyaline, septate hyphae, dichotomously branching and regular in diameter with parallel opposing walls.	5–10 μ	Rarely, conidial-bearing fruiting bodies may develop in fungus ball cavities.
Candida species	Pseudohyphae composed of elongated blastospores, showing regular points of constriction simulating link sausages. Budding oval or spherical blastospores also present.	5–10 μ (Pseudohyphae) 3–4 μ (Blastospores)	
Geotrichum candidum	Hyphae producing arthrospores.		
Zygomycetes *Mucor* sp. *Rhizopus* sp. *Absidia* sp.	Broad, aseptate, irregularly branching, ribbon-like hyphae with non-parallel opposing walls.	10–30 μ	Rarely, sporangial fruiting bodies may form in fungus ball cavities.
Actinomyces israelii	Delicate, branching, minute filaments often within "sulfur granules."	Less than 1 μ	*A. israelii* is an anaerobic bacterium.
Nocardia asteroides	Delicate, branching, minute filaments often within "sulfur granules."		Branching filamentous, "partially" acid-fast bacterium.
III. Subcutaneous Mycoses			
Chromomycosis group: *Fonsecaea pedrosoi* *Fonsecaea compactum* *Phialophora verrucosa* *Cladosporium carrionii*	Dark yellow or brown, septate, hyphal segments. Also, rounded or crescent-shaped, thick-walled deep yellow or brown sclerotic bodies.	5–8 μ (Hyphae) 8–15 μ (Sclerotic bodies)	
Petriellidium (Allescheria) boydii	Production of yellow-gray granules containing wide mycelial forms often clubbed at the periphery of the granule.	6–8 μ	10–12 μ oval to round conidia may be produced in fungus ball cavities.
Actinomycetes	Delicate, branching filaments within "sulfur granules."	Less than 1 μ	*Nocardia* sp. filaments are partially acid-fast
Sporothrix schenckii	Tiny, irregular, elongated cigar-shaped yeast forms.	3–5 μ	Yeast forms are extremely difficult to demonstrate in human tissues.

Table 50–6.   TISSUE FORMS OF FUNGI OF MEDICAL IMPORTANCE TO MAN (*Continued*)

ETIOLOGIC AGENT	DIAGNOSTIC TISSUE FORM	SIZE	COMMENTS
IV. Superficial Mycoses Dermatophyte group: *Microsporum* sp. *Epidermophyton* sp. *Trichophyton* sp.	Slender hyphal forms, often breaking into arthrospore-like segments in the stratum corneum of the skin. Endothrix and ectothrix minute spores in hair infections.	3–5 μ (Hyphae) 1–2 μ (Spores)	Fungal forms best demonstrated in direct KOH mounts of infected skin scales, nail scrapings, or plucked hairs
Exophiala (*Cladosporium*) *werneckii*	Delicate, twisting, tortuous hyphal segments confined to the stratum lucidum.	1–2 μ	Fungal elements best demonstrated in direct KOH mounts.
Malassezia (*Pityrosporum*) *furfur*	Many short, stubby hyphal segments, admixed with budding spheroidal cells, limited to the stratum corneum.	3–5 μ (Hyphae) 4–6 μ (Cells)	Fungal elements best demonstrated in direct KOH mounts

because they can assume either a mycelial or a yeast form depending upon environmental temperature.

The mycelial form is produced at temperatures less than 37°C. This is the natural form of filamentous fungi in the environment, is the form most commonly used for culture identification in the laboratory, and is the form that is most commonly infective for man.

The yeast form of the dimorphic fungi is assumed at 37°C. incubation, the normal body temperature of man. Only in rare instances will a dimorphic fungus assume the mycelial form in tissues. One example is shown in Fig-

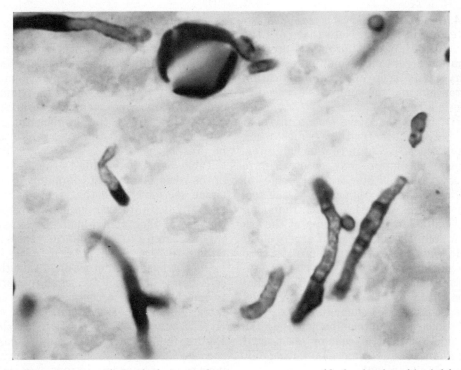

Figure 50–14.   Tissue invasion with *Coccidioides immitis* showing rare occurrence of both spherule and hyphal forms. ×450. Gomori methenamine silver stain.

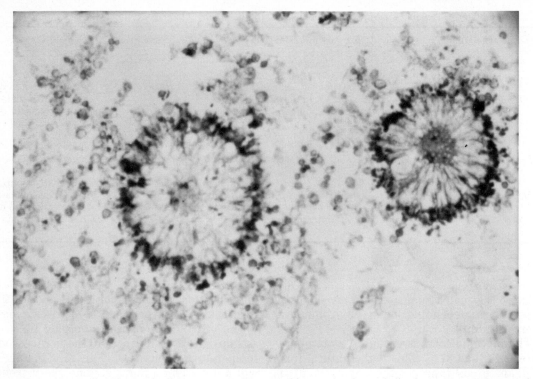

Figure 50–15. Aspergillus "fruiting heads" seen in tissue section of lung with a fungus ball infection. ×450. Hematoxylin-eosin stain.

ure 50-14, a case of cavitary *Coccidioides im-mitis* infection in a lung. Note that both the spherule and the mycelial forms are present. This situation occurs most commonly when a pulmonary cavity is in open communication with a bronchus and the fungus is exposed to atmospheric air.

Similarly, fungi that have only a mycelial form do not produce fruiting bodies when present in tissues, except in fungus ball infections when sporulation may occur. Figure 50-15 is an example of how fruiting bodies of *Aspergillus* species may appear in tissue sections. Shown are two vesicles with radiating phialides and a few brown conidia at the periphery. A definitive diagnosis of aspergillosis is possible when these structures are observed in tissue sections.

Therefore, the initial observations that should be made by the surgical pathologist when suspected fungal elements are seen in tissue sections is to determine whether the form being observed is mycelia or yeast, or, if possible, if one of the dimorphic pathogenic species might be present.

IDENTIFICATION OF YEAST FORMS IN TISSUES

Fungi that do not produce hyphae in tissue, rather remaining in the yeast form only, can be presumptively identified by evaluating the following: (1) The size of the individual yeast cells; (2) the arrangement and location of the yeast cells; and (3) the number and mode of attachment of buds (blastoconidia) that may be present.

Table 50-7A is a guide to the identification of the yeast forms most commonly observed in tissue sections. Note that these yeasts have been divided into two major groups based on the size of their individual cells: small yeasts ranging from 1 to 7 μ and large yeasts ranging from 8 to 20 μ.

Once it has been determined that the yeast cells being observed are small, generally between 1 and 4 μ, ascertain if any cells are intracellular. This assessment can be made on H & E stained tissue section, as shown in Figure 50-16. Intracytoplasmic yeast cells, such as those seen in Figure 50-16, that appear to be encapsulated are highly suggestive

Table 50-7A. IDENTIFICATION OF TISSUE YEAST FORMS

YEAST SPECIES	SIZE OF YEAST CELLS	IDENTIFYING CHARACTERISTICS
I. Yeast cells of small size (1-4 μ)		
Coccidioides immitis (endospores)	Regular: 2-4 μ	Spherical, easy to identify when contained within characteristic spherule
Cryptococcus neoformans (non-encapsulated)	Irregular size: range from 1-7 μ	Easy to identify when surrounded by thick mucinous capsule. Budding forms may be present, with daughter cell attached by narrow thread.
Histoplasma capsulatum	Regular: 2-4 μ	Have a characteristic pseudocapsule when observed within reticuloendothelial cells. May be extremely difficult to differentiate from coccidioides endospores or non-encapsulated cryptococcal cells when lying free in tissues.
Torulopsis glabrata	Tiny: Less than 1-2 μ	Cells usually lie in compact clusters within tissue spaces. Identification may be suspected on basis of extremely small size.
II. Yeast cells of large size: (8-20 μ)		
Blastomyces dermatiditis	Irregular: 8-20 μ	Characteristic thick, doubly refractile wall, forming single bud attached with a broad base.
Coccidioides immitis (spherules)	Irregular: Immature spherules 5-20 μ; mature 50 μ and greater	Immature spherules may simulate yeast cells of *B. dermatitidis* due to thick refractile wall. Identification is made when endospores are identified within the spherule space.
Cryptococcus neoformans (encapsulated)	Irregular: 5-20 μ if capsule is measured	Thick mucinous capsule is virtually diagnostic. Look for small buds attached by hair-like threads.
Paracoccidioides brasiliensis	Irregular: 8-20 μ or more	Mature yeast cells have thick capsule, with multiple daughter buds around the periphery, simulating a mariner's wheel.

Table 50-7B. IDENTIFICATION OF TISSUE HYPHAL FORMS

HYPHAL MORPHOLOGY OBSERVED	ETIOLOGIC AGENT SUSPECTED	COMMENTS
Hyphae aseptate, irregularly broad, and ribbon-like, 10-30 μ in diameter, irregularly branching, opposing hyphal walls not parallel.	*Zygomycetes (Phycomycetes)* *Mucor* species *Rhizopus* species *Absidia* species	In fungus ball cavities also look for diagnostic sporangial fruiting heads.
Hyphae appear septate, with points of constriction at septations, simulating link sausages. Oval 3-5 μ budding yeast cells may also be seen.	*Candida* species *Candida albicans*	Diagnostic chlamydospores do not form in tissues
Hyphae clearly septate, regular in diameter, breaking into distinct arthrospores.	*Geotrichum candidum* Dermatophyte species: keratin skin only.	*Coccidioides immitis* only rarely forms rudimentary mycelial structures in tissues. Spherules usually can be found.
Hyphae distinctly septate, hyaline, branch regularly and dichotomously at 45 degree angles, regular in diameter (5-10 μ) with opposite walls parallel	*Aspergillus* species *Aspergillus fumigatus* *Aspergillus flavus* *Aspergillus niger*	In fungus ball cavities also look for diagnostic vesicular, conidia-bearing fruiting heads.
Hyphae distinctly septate, dark yellow or brown in color (dematiacious), in short segments without branching	Chromomycosis group: *Fonsecaea pedrosi* *Fonsecaea compactum* *Phialophora verrucosa* *Cladosporium carrionii*	Also search the inflammatory areas for the presence of spherical, multi-celled, dark yellow or brown sclerotic bodies.
Hyphae in form of delicate, gram-positive, branching filaments, either free in the inflammatory infiltrate or confined within "sulfur granules" ("Ray fungus").	Actinomycetes: *Actinomyces* species *Nocardia* species *Streptomyces* species	If *Actinomyces* species is suspected, tissue must be submitted for anaerobic culture. *Nocardia* sp. filaments are "partially" acid-fast.

5

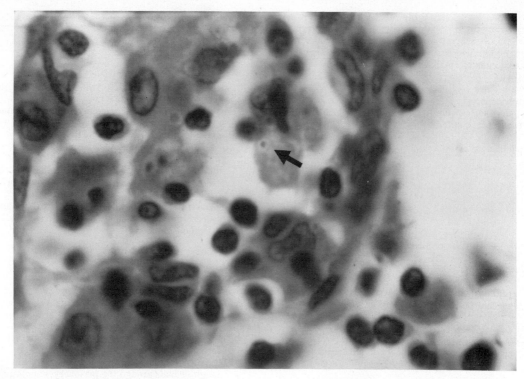

Figure 50–16. Section of an inflammatory reaction showing aggregates of large reticuloendothelial histiocytic cells within the cytoplasm of which are contained small pseudoencapsulated yeast forms of *Histoplasma capsulatum.* ×950. Hematoxylin-eosin stain.

of *Histoplasma capsulatum*. *H. capsulatum*, despite its species name, does not possess a true capsule; rather, the pseudoencapsulated effect is produced in stained preparations from the shrinkage of the yeast cell from the outer membrane during the fixation process. Figure 50-17 is a photomicrograph of a silver-stained section showing clusters of the tiny (2 to 4 μ) yeast forms of *H. capsulatum*.

The yeast forms of *Cryptococcus neoformans* can generally be readily identified by the presence of a thick, mucinous capsule (Fig. 50-13). The small central yeast cells vary from 2 to 7 μ in diameter; however, the presence of the capsule makes them appear as much as 20 μ in diameter. Variation in cell size is one helpful characteristic by which *C. neoformans* can be distinguished from other yeast cells of similar size. This feature is best demonstrated in silver-stained preparations. Figure 50-18 shows marked differences in size of the individual yeast cells.

The endospores of *Coccidioides immitis* are not difficult to identify when they are enclosed within the characteristic spherules to be described below. However, when 2 to 4 μ individual yeast cells are seen lying free in tissues

(Fig. 50-22), it may be extremely difficult to differentiate extracellular forms of *H. capsulatum*, non-encapsulated forms of *C. neoformans* (irregularity in size may be one aid), and endospores of *C. immitis* that have been released from their spherules. In such instances, an extensive search throughout the tissue sections may be necessary to locate a few yeast forms that may still be intracellular, a few forms that have retained a mucinous capsule, or remnants of a spherule before a presumptive identification can be made. In the absence of any of these, the final diagnosis may be possible only by recovering the causative agent in culture.

Torulopsis glabrata is another yeast that is encountered in human infections with increasing frequency. *T. glabrata* may be suspected in tissue sections because of the extremely small size of the yeast cells (1 to 2 μ) and their tendency to cluster together (Fig. 50-19). However, *T. glabrata* may on occasion be intracellular within non-nuclear inflammatory cells, and because of tissue shrinkage, may also appear pseudoencapsulated, closely simulating *H. capsulatum*. In these instances, recovery of the etiologic yeast in culture may

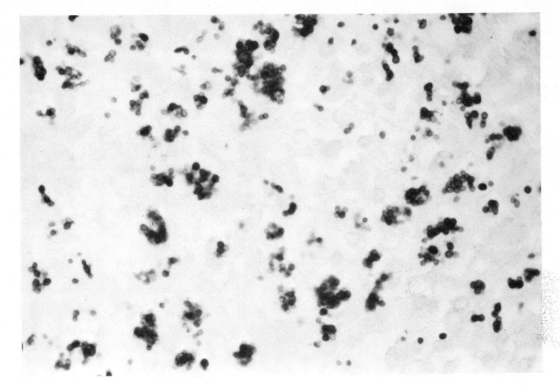

Figure 50-17. Section of lung showing intracellular clusters of tiny (2-3 μ) yeast forms of *Histoplasma capsulatum.* ×450. Gomori methenamine silver stain.

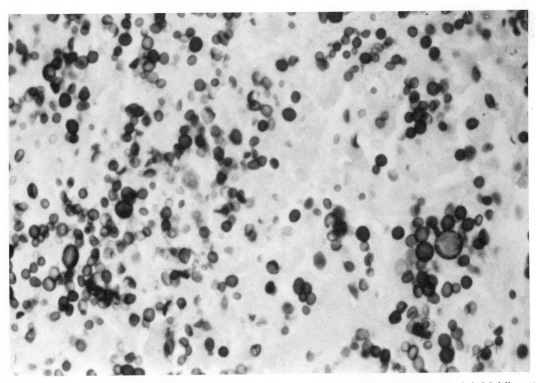

Figure 50-18. Section of lung illustrating the marked variation in size of cells of *Cryptococcus neoformans*, a helpful differential clue in the identification of this yeast. ×450. Gomori methenamine silver stain.

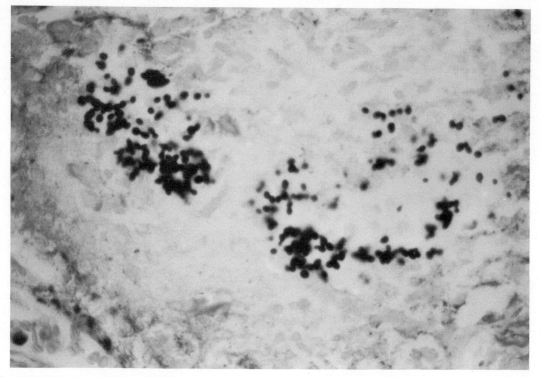

Figure 50–19. Inflammatory reaction showing clusters of minute yeast forms of *Torulopsis glabrata*. ×450. Gomori methenamine silver stain.

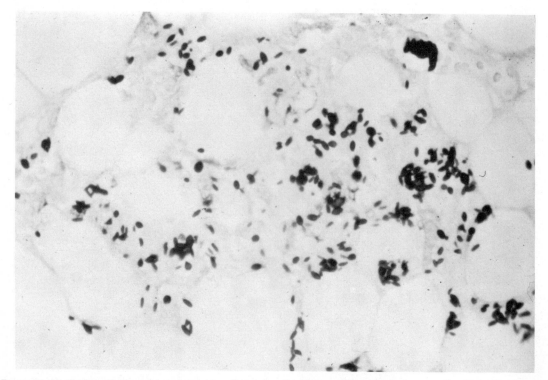

Figure 50–20. Section of animal tissue showing small (2-5 μ) oval to elongated (cigar bodies) yeast cells of *Sporothrix schenckii*. ×450. Gomori methenamine silver stain.

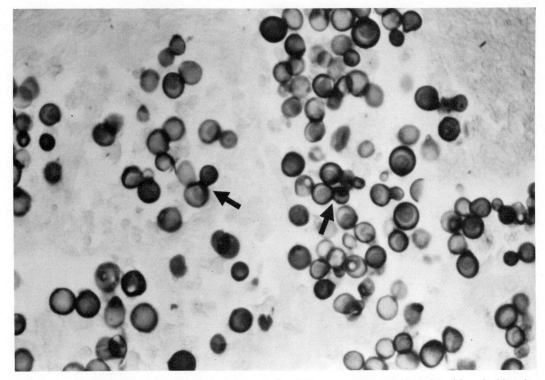

Figure 50-21. Section of lung showing large (8-15 μ) yeast cells of *Blastomyces dermatitidis*. Note broad-base budding forms. ×450. Gomori methenamine silver stain.

be the only means for making a definitive identification.

The yeast forms of *Sporothrix schenckii* are also small but are rarely seen in human tissue. They can be demonstrated in animal tissue as illustrated in Figure 50-20. Characteristic cells are 2 to 5 μ, oval to "cigar-shaped," and produce one or more buds at either or both poles.

The group of yeasts producing larger cells are generally identified in tissue sections with less difficulty than the smaller forms.

Blastomyces dermatitidis produces yeast cells that vary from 8 to 20 μ in diameter and have thick, doubly contoured walls that appear refractile. A definitive identification can be made if yeast cells having a single bud attached by a broad base are identified (Fig. 50-21). If budding forms cannot be found, there may be difficulty in distinguishing *B. dermatitidis* from immature spherules of *Coccidioides immitis* which are devoid of endospores. In these instances, additional tissue sections should be screened for mature spherules containing endospores or for broad-based budding forms. If not found, the final diagnosis may have to await positive culture results.

A typical spherule of *C. immitis* containing mature endospores is shown in Figure 50-22. Spherules are generally greater than 20 μ in diameter, reaching as much as 60 μ. Figure 50-22 is virtually diagnostic when observed in tissue sections.

Although the encapsulated yeast forms of *C. neoformans* may approach the size of *B. dermatitidis* in tissue sections, identification is usually not difficult. The mucicarmine stain is virtually specific for the capsular material of *C. neoformans* and can be useful if confusion should arise. The presence of the thick capsule, together with the narrow attachment of the budding cell, is usually sufficient to make a presumptive identification of *C. neoformans* in tissues. Because of the frequent lack of a cellular response and the dense infiltration of tissues with encapsulated *C. neoformans*, the differential diagnosis of mucin-secreting carcinoma may at times be difficult. However, the small central yeast cells and the lack of large pleomorphic nuclei are generally sufficient to suspect *C. neoformans*.

The large yeast forms of *Paracoccidioides brasiliensis* are not difficult to identify in tissue sections when the multiple peripheral

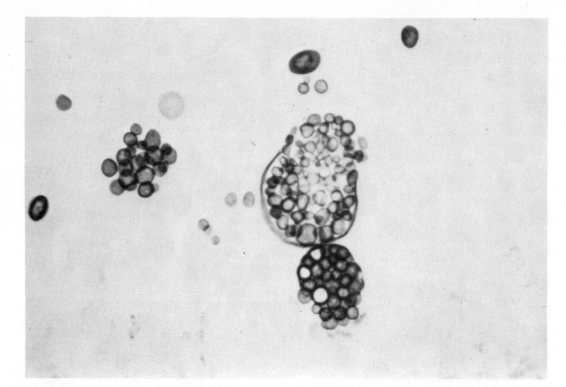

Figure 50-22. Section of lung showing a classic spherule of *Coccidioides immitis* containing numerous endospores. ×450. Gomori methenamine silver stain.

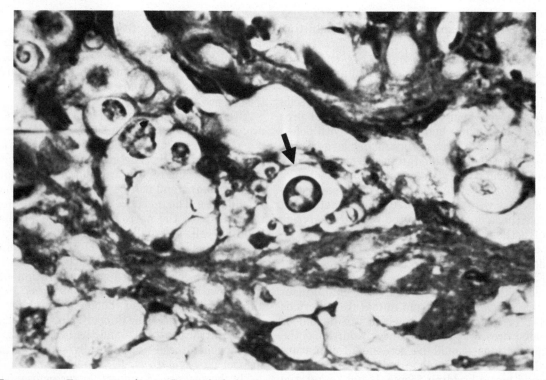

Figure 50-23. Tissue section showing *Paracoccidioides brasiliensis*. Note the characteristic large yeast cell (arrow) with multiple buds simulating a "mariner's wheel." ×450. Hematoxylin-eosin stain. (From Dolan, C. T., Funkhouser, J. W., Koneman, E. W., Miller, N. G., and Roberts, G. D.: Atlas of Clinical Mycology II. Chicago, Ill., American Society of Clinical Pathologists, 1975.)

budding cells simulating a mariner's wheel are seen (Fig. 50-23). However, in the absence of multiple buds, the large mother yeast cells may be impossible to distinguish from *B. dermatitidis* in tissue sections, and cultures may be required to make the final identification. The clinical history and geographic location of the patient would also be helpful in making the differentiation.

IDENTIFICATION OF MYCELIAL FORMS IN TISSUES

The detection of delicate filaments or hyphal strands in tissue sections suggests one of the etiologic agents outlined in Table 50-7B.

If the hyphal forms appear irregular in diameter, ranging between 10 and 60 μ, are ribbon-like, branch irregularly, and are devoid of septa, one of the fungal species belonging to the Zygomycetes (Phycomycetes) should be suspected (Fig. 50-24). In older lesions, the tissue reaction may distort the hyphae to the point that recognition becomes difficult (Fig. 50-25). Silver-stained preparations may not be useful, since the stain may not penetrate the hyphae (Fig. 50-26).

All other filamentous fungi produce septate hyphae in tissue sections. The mycelium of *Candida* species is actually composed of pseudohyphae, recognized by regular points of constriction along the strands, closely resembling link sausages (Fig. 50-27). Pseudohyphae are elongated blastoconidia, and the points of constriction represent the residual points of attachment of the primitive buds. The ability to recognize pseudohyphae is helpful in differentiating *Candida* from *Aspergillus*. *Candida* also commonly produce budding yeast cells along with the pseudohyphae, structures never formed by *Aspergillus* (Fig. 50-27).

When observing septate hyphae in tissue sections, an initial determination should be made whether or not arthroaleuriospores are being formed. *Coccidioides immitis* is the most common pathogenic fungus that forms arthroaleuriospores; however, as discussed above, these rarely form at 37°C. Therefore, the presence of arthroaleuriospores in tissue sections is virtually diagnostic of geotrichosis. Geotrichosis, caused by *Geotrichum candidum*, is a relatively rare disease, and arthroaleuri-

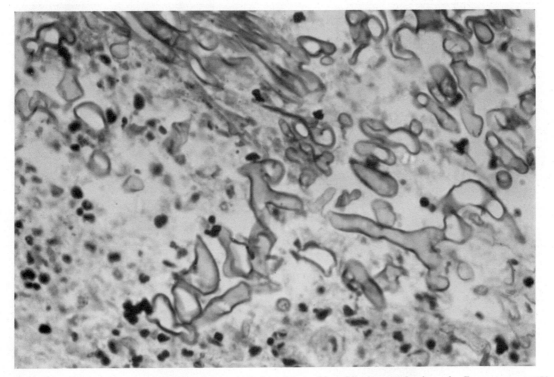

Figure 50-24. Tissue section showing broad, irregularly branching, ribbon-like aseptate hyphae of a Zygomycete. ✕450. Hematoxylin-eosin stain.

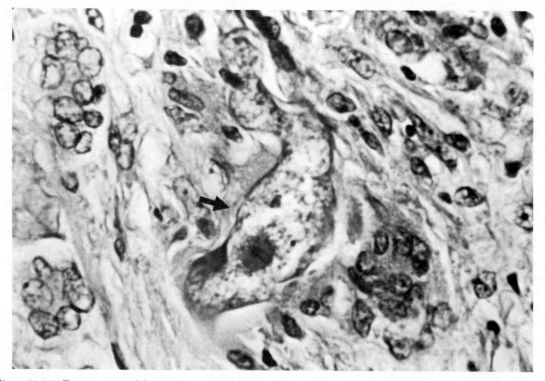

Figure 50-25. Tissue section exhibiting Zygomycete infection. Illustrated is a giant cell granulomatous reaction and a distorted ribbon-like hyphal fragment with severe cystic degeneration that makes identification difficult. ×450. Hematoxylin-eosin stain.

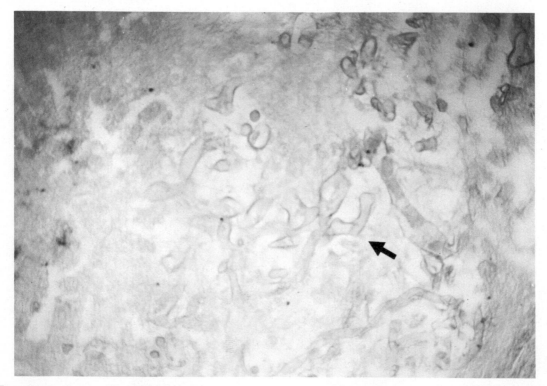

Figure 50-26. Section of lung tissue showing poor penetration of the hyphal forms of a Zygomycete by the silver stain. ×450. Gomori methenamine silver stain.

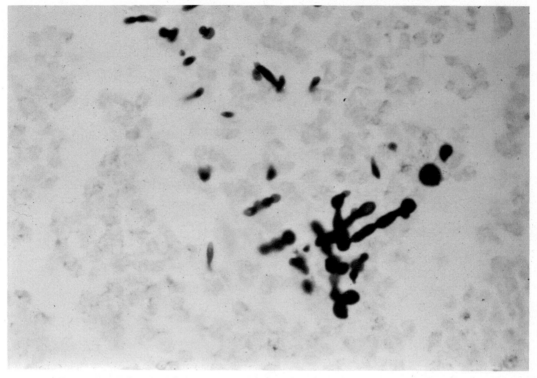

Figure 50–27.   Tissue section showing infection with *Candida albicans*. Pseudohyphae with sausage-like points of constriction and a few budding cells are illustrated. ✕450. Gomori methenamine silver stain.

ospores do not always form in tissues. The dermatophytic fungi also may produce arthroaleuriospores; however, they are limited to the superficial corneum of the skin, and tissue biopsies are rarely procured to diagnose dermatophytoses.

Aspergillus is the most common fungal agent that will be observed in tissue sections. Unless there is considerable tissue distortion, the hyphae of *Aspergillus* species can be readily identified. They are distinctly septate (the septa appear more prominent in special fungal stained preparations), are uniform in diameter, range from 5 to 10 μ wide, have parallel walls, and branch dichotomously at 45 degree angles (Fig. 50–28). Sporulation does not occur except in cavitary fungus ball infections, and the detection of the vesicular fruiting heads with radiating phialides and chains of spores can lead to a definitive diagnosis. A species identification may also be possible if the vesicle is club-shaped and sporulation is seen to take place only from the top half of the vesicle (Fig. 50–29). These features are characteristic of *A. fumigatus*, the species most commonly causing aspergillosis in man. Globose vesicles

covered with densely packed, black conidia are highly suggestive of *A. niger* infection.

Septate hyphae that have a distinctly dark yellow or brown appearance in H & E stained tissue sections suggest infection with one of the dematiacious fungal agents responsible for chromomycosis (Fig. 50–30). Hyphae are generally short and fragmented and may appear distorted by the inflammatory reaction. The presumptive diagnosis of chromomycosis in tissue sections of suspected lesions can be strengthened by detecting the characteristic spherical, multicelled brown-staining sclerotic bodies (Fig. 50–31).

The presence of thin, delicate filaments that average no more than 1 μ in diameter and are freely branching is highly suspicious for infection with *Actinomyces* species, *Nocardia* species or *Streptomyces* species (Fig. 50–32). These forms are actually bacterial in nature and may lie free within a purulent exudate or be confined within "sulfur granules."

Nocardia species can be presumptively identified by demonstrating that the branching filaments are partially acid-fast. By "partially acid-fast" is meant that a dilute mineral

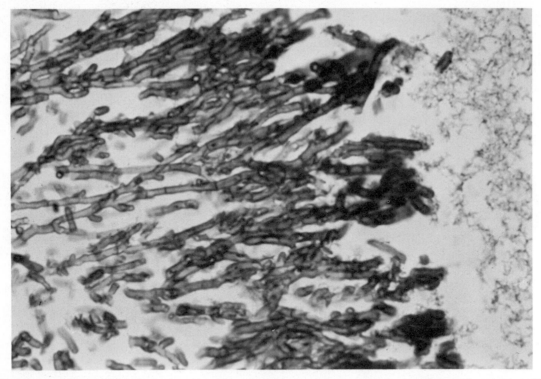

Figure 50-28. Tissue section showing invasion with septate, dichotomously branching hyphae of *Aspergillus* species. ×450. Gomori methenamine silver stain.

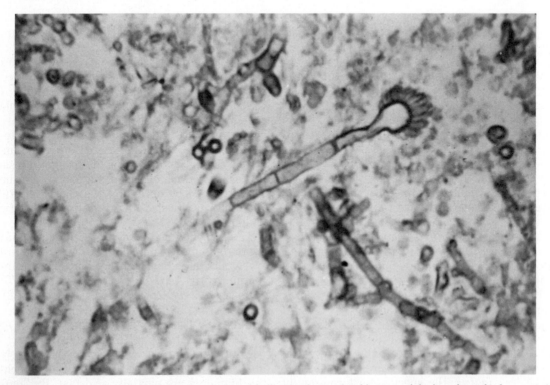

Figure 50-29. Tissue section showing portion of a fungus ball with a fruiting head having a club-shaped vesicle characteristic of *Aspergillus fumigatus.* ×100. Periodic acid–Schiff stain. (From Dolan, C. T., Funkhouser, J. W., Koneman, E. W., Miller, N. G., and Roberts, G. D.: Atlas of Clinical Mycology III. Chicago, Ill., American Society of Clinical Pathologists, 1975.)

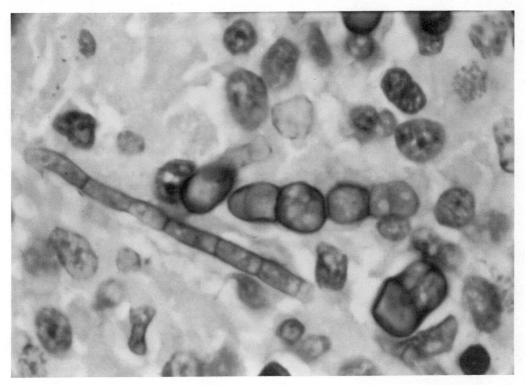

Figure 50–30. Inflammatory tissue reaction including short brown hyphal fragments suggestive of chromomycosis infection. ×950. Hematoxylin-eosin stain.

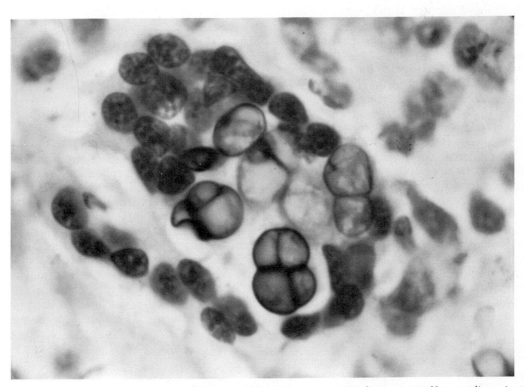

Figure 50–31. Multicelled brown sclerotic bodies characteristic of chromomycosis infection. ×950. Hematoxylin-eosin stain.

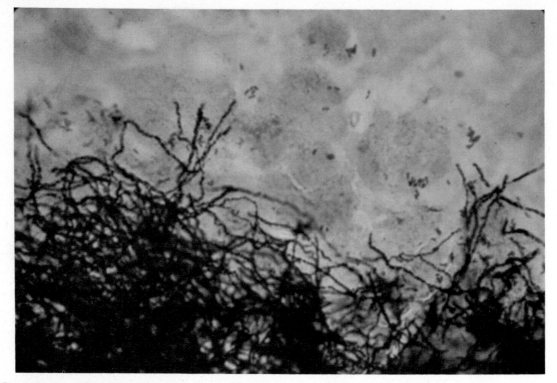

Figure 50–32. Tissue section showing infection with one of the aerobic actinomycetes. Note presence of delicate (1 μ) branching filaments. ×950. Gram stain.

acid, such as 1 per cent H_2SO_4, was used as the decolorizer, rather than the more potent acid alcohol solutions used in the routine Ziehl-Neelsen acid-fast stain. These filamentous forms can be confused with the rapidly growing species of mycobacteria. However, mycobacteria rarely if ever branch, an important feature in distinguishing them from the *Actinomycetes*. In some instances, however, culture may be necessary before a definitive diagnosis can be rendered.

When examining tissue sections from suspected cases of subcutaneous mycetoma infection, careful examination of the grains and granules is important in rendering a presumptive diagnosis. The sulfur granules characteristic of the *Actinomycetes* have been described above. A gray-white granule in which club-shaped, true hyphae are present is highly suggestive of infection with *Petriellidium* (*Allescheria*) *boydii* (*Monosporium apiospermum*), the most common cause of eumycotic mycetomatous infections in the United States (Fig. 50–33).

Pathologists are urged to collect as many tissue sections containing fungal structures as possible. These serve not only as a means for self study and instruction of others, but as a valuable reference resource for comparing new cases of presumptive fungal infections. These reference slides are particularly useful for comparing new slides from those fungal infections that are only rarely encountered.

LABORATORY DIAGNOSIS OF FUNGAL INFECTIONS

The recovery of fungi from clinical specimens depends on the collection of an appropriate specimen and its rapid transport to the laboratory. If rapid transportation to the laboratory is impossible, the specimens should be refrigerated at 4°C. to prevent overgrowth by contaminating bacteria and yeasts which may be present. Once received by the laboratory, the specimen should be examined and inoculated onto appropriate culture media. The following section will be devoted to the processing and culturing of clinical specimens for mycologic examination.

CEREBROSPINAL FLUID

One to three ml of freshly collected cerebrospinal fluid should be filtered through a 0.45 μ

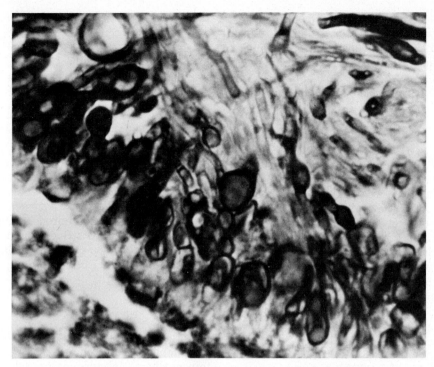

Figure 50-33. Section through a subcutaneous granule of *Petriellidium boydii* showing swollen cells at periphery. ×450. Gomori methenamine silver stain.

Swinnex filter (Millipore Corporation) attached to a sterile syringe. The filter is removed and placed on an appropriate culture medium so that the side containing the concentrate touches the agar surface. Cultures should be examined daily and the filter pad moved to another location on the medium surface. If more than 3 ml of specimen is collected, equal amounts of 2 ml or more should be separately filtered and cultured onto the appropriate media. If less than 2 ml of sample is collected, the cerebrospinal fluid should be centrifuged for 10 minutes and one-drop aliquots of the sediment should be placed onto several areas on the agar surface. This method is preferable to streaking the sample onto the agar surface with a loop, since it allows the organism to acclimate more easily to environmental conditions. Cultures should be examined daily for visible evidence of growth.

Media which are suitable for culturing cerebrospinal fluid specimens include brain-heart infusion agar, chocolate agar, Sabouraud's dextrose agar, Sabhi agar, and inhibitory mold agar. Cerebrospinal fluid specimens should not be cultured onto media which contain cycloheximide, since some important pathogens are known to be inhibited by this antifungal agent.

BLOOD

Blood culture bottles containing soybean-casein digest (e.g., Trypticase or Tryptic soy) broth or Columbia broth are satisfactory for the recovery of fungi from blood. It is recommended that these be vented with a sterile cotton-plugged needle throughout the duration of incubation. However, it is recommended that a biphasic brain-heart infusion agar-brain-heart infusion broth bottle be used, since the recovery rate of fungi is somewhat quickened using this system. Blood culture bottles should be examined daily for visible evidence of growth. If the biphasic brain-heart infusion agar-broth bottle is used, the surface of the agar should be flooded with the blood and cultures should be examined daily. All blood culture bottles should be incubated at 30°C. for a minimum of 30 days. Growth may appear either on the agar slant or in the broth. If either Columbia broth or soybean-casein digest broth is used, subcultures after 24 and 48 hours should be made onto brain-heart infusion agar or Sabouraud's dextrose agar. Small laboratories may prefer to inoculate 5 to 10 ml of blood onto the surface of Sabouraud's dextrose agar or brain heart infusion agar. Although not as efficient as those previously described, this method is adequate.

URINE

Currently there is debate concerning the value of quantitating urine cultures, and it is not recommended. All urine samples should be centrifuged and the sediment inoculated onto an appropriate medium. Specimens should be streaked with a loop to ensure adequate isolation of colonies. Contamination by gram-negative bacteria is often observed, making it necessary to use media containing antibacterial antibiotics.

RESPIRATORY SECRETIONS

Properly collected, respiratory secretions (sputum, bronchial washings, and transtracheal aspirations) are among the most important of all clinical specimens received for fungal cultures. Many mycotic infections have pulmonary manifestations, and respiratory secretions often provide the only microbiologic evidence of infection.

Respiratory secretions are commonly contaminated with bacteria and rapidly growing molds which may suppress or overgrow the slower growing true mycotic pathogens. It is necessary that culture media containing antibacterial antibiotics be included in the battery of media to be used. Cycloheximide, an antifungal antibiotic which prevents the rapid overgrowth of cultures by rapidly growing molds, should also be incorporated into one of the culture media used. As much specimen as possible (up to 0.5 ml) should be inoculated onto the surface of appropriate media. Cultures should be incubated at 30°C. and examined every other day for visual evidence of growth.

TISSUE, BONE MARROW, AND BODY FLUIDS

All biopsy tissues should be minced or ground before being cultured. As much specimen as possible should be inoculated onto the surface of appropriate culture media. If a zygomycete infection is suspected, the tissue

should be minced and not ground, as the former reduces the destruction of hyphal elements. Five-tenths ml of tissue homogenate should be placed onto the surface of appropriate media, and cultures should be examined daily for visual evidence of growth.

CORNEAL SCRAPINGS AND EAR CULTURES

Mycotic keratitis and external otomycosis are most often caused by the rapidly growing saprobic molds. For the recovery of these organisms, it is necessary that media be used which contain no antifungal antibiotics. As much specimen as possible should be inoculated onto the surface of appropriate media. Cultures should be examined daily for visual evidence of growth.

ORAL MUCOSA

Material from lesions in the mouth or pharynx should be cultured onto media which contain antibacterial and antifungal antibiotics. Cultures should be incubated for a minimum of 30 days before being reported out as negative, since slower growing pathogens (e.g., *H. capsulatum*) are commonly recovered from oropharyngeal lesions.

SKIN SCRAPINGS, NAILS, AND HAIR

Most specimens submitted for dermatophyte culture are contaminated with bacteria and rapidly growing molds. It is necessary that a medium be used which contains antibacterial and antifungal antibiotics. The specimen should be inoculated onto the surface of the appropriate culture medium and incubated for a minimum of 30 days. Cultures should be examined periodically for visual evidence of growth.

MEDIA REQUIREMENTS AND INCUBATION CONDITIONS

Table 50-8 provides a description of specimen types and culture requirements for the recovery of fungal etiologic agents. The selection of appropriate culture media may be based upon the information presented in this table.

The culture media used for the recovery of

fungi need not be elaborate or complex. Obviously one can enhance the recovery rate by using a number of media; however, the problem of economics arises. The combinations of penicillin (20 units/ml) and streptomycin (40 units/ml) or gentamicin (5 μg/ml) and chloramphenicol (16 μg/ml) have proved satisfactory to prevent most bacterial overgrowth. Cycloheximide (Actidione) in a concentration of 0.5 mg/ml is satisfactory for the prevention of overgrowth by rapidly growing molds; however, some pathogens, including *Cryptococcus neoformans* and *Aspergillus fumigatus*, may be totally or partially inhibited, and it is necessary to include a medium lacking cycloheximide in the battery of media used.

A number of commercially prepared culture media are available for the cultivation of fungi from clinical specimens. Included are Sabouraud's dextrose, Sabouraud's dextrose (Emmon's modification) containing 2 per cent dextrose, Sabhi, inhibitory mold, brain-heart infusion, and mycobiotic and mycosel agars. It is recommended that at least one culture medium be supplemented with 5 to 10 per cent sheep blood. This enhances the chances of recovery of some fastidious pathogens. It should be kept in mind that media containing blood, e.g., brain-heart infusion containing 5 to 10 per cent sheep blood, are excellent isolation media; however, they are not adequate as identification media. It is necessary to subculture the organisms that are recovered on media containing blood onto other media that will allow characteristic sporulation to occur. Media suitable for subculture include cornmeal agar, Sabouraud's dextrose agar, inhibitory mold agar, brain-heart infusion agar, or any of the previously mentioned media.

Cultures should be incubated only at 25 to 30°C.; incubation of duplicate cultures at 37°C. is unnecessary and costly. The recovery rate of the dimorphic pathogens is not significantly enhanced by incubating cultures at 37°C. All cultures should be incubated at 30°C. (optimal) for a minimum of 30 days before being discarded. Six weeks of incubation is optimal; however, limitation of space often prevents this.

Petri dishes or culture tubes are satisfactory for the recovery of fungi. For those laboratories not thoroughly acquainted with the handling of fungi, it is suggested that large, screw-capped tubes be used. The slants should be thick and, after inoculation, the caps should be screwed on but left slightly loose. The dis-

advantages of this method include relatively poor aeration of cultures and a reduced surface area, which results in poorly isolated colonies. Culture tubes are more easily stored, require less space, are obviously safer for small laboratories, and have a lower dehydration rate. Although somewhat more hazardous, culture dishes may be used by those laboratories which are familiar with the handling of fungal cultures; however, they are not recommended for the inexperienced laboratory. The advantages include better aeration of cultures, a large surface area which provides better isolation of colonies, and greater ease of examination and subculture of fungal colonies. The disadvantages include an increased dehydration rate and an increased chance of laboratory contamination. Dehydration may be reduced by preparing the culture dishes to contain at least 40 ml of medium; lids should be taped down in two locations to prevent inadvertent opening, and dishes should be incubated in an atmosphere containing 30 to 40 per cent relative humidity.

DIRECT EXAMINATION OF CLINICAL SPECIMENS

In many instances the direct microscopic examination of a clinical specimen allows one to make a rapid tentative diagnosis. All laboratories will find the direct examination of a clinical specimen practical, since most already examine skin and nail scrapings microscopically for the presence of dermatophytes. The use of the direct examination may be extended to include all clinical specimens except blood.

The procedure is simple and consists of mixing a small amount of the specimen with a drop of 10 per cent potassium hydroxide on a microscope slide. A coverslip is positioned and the slide may be gently flamed and examined microscopically. Brightfield microscopy is satisfactory if the light is reduced; however, phase contrast microscopy is optimal because it provides more detail. Figures 50-34 to 50-41 present organisms commonly seen on direct microscopic examination with a detailed description of their characteristic features.

The India ink preparation is commonly used for the detection of *Cryptococcus neoformans* in cerebrospinal fluid. Although only positive in less than 50 per cent of the cases of cryptococcal meningitis, this examination is diag-

(*Text continued on p. 1712*)

Table 50–8. SPECIMEN AND MEDIA REQUIREMENTS FOR THE RECOVERY OF FUNGI FROM SPECIFIC MYCOTIC INFECTIONS

INFECTION	SPECIMEN TYPE	COMMON CULTURE MEDIA
Histoplasmosis	Respiratory secretions; blood; bone marrow; urine; cerebrospinal fluid; mucocutaneous ulcers	Sabouraud's dextrose agar[a]; brain-heart infusion agar; inhibitory mold agar; Sabhi agar; brain-heart infusion blood agar with antibiotics[b]; brain-heart infusion blood agar with antibiotics and cycloheximide[c]. Biphasic brain-heart infusion agar/broth recommended for blood cultures.[d]
Blastomycosis	Respiratory secretions; skin; bone; urine; mucocutaneous ulcers	Sabouraud's dextrose agar[a]; brain-heart infusion agar; inhibitory mold agar; Sabhi agar; brain-heart infusion blood agar with antibiotics[b]; brain-heart infusion blood agar with antibiotics and cycloheximide.[c]
Coccidioidomycosis	Respiratory secretions; skin; cerebrospinal fluid; urine; mucocutaneous ulcers	Sabouraud's dextrose agar[a]; brain-heart infusion agar; inhibitory mold agar; Sabhi agar; brain-heart infusion blood agar with antibiotics[b]; brain-heart infusion blood agar with antibiotics and cycloheximide.[c]
Paracoccidioidomycosis	Respiratory secretions; mucocutaneous ulcers; skin; intestine	Sabouraud's dextrose agar[a]; brain-heart infusion agar; inhibitory mold agar; Sabhi agar; brain-heart infusion blood agar with antibiotics[b]; brain-heart infusion blood agar with antibiotics and cycloheximide.[c]
Cryptococcosis	Respiratory secretions; cerebrospinal fluid; bone; urine; skin; pleural fluid; bone marrow; blood	Sabouraud's dextrose agar[a]; inhibitory mold agar; brain-heart infusion agar; Sabhi agar; brain-heart infusion blood agar with antibiotics.[b] Media containing cycloheximide inhibit the growth of *Cryptococcus neoformans*. Biphasic brain-heart infusion agar/broth recommended for blood cultures.
Candidosis	Respiratory secretions; urine; mucocutaneous lesions; blood; stool; vagina; nails	Most common fungal and bacterial culture media are satisfactory; however, those containing cycloheximide inhibit some species. Biphasic brain-heart infusion agar/broth recommended for blood cultures.[d]
Aspergillosis	Respiratory secretions; mucous plugs; external ear	Sabouraud's dextrose agar[a]; brain-heart infusion agar; inhibitory mold agar; Sabhi agar; brain-heart infusion blood agar containing antibiotics.[b] Media containing cycloheximide are unsatisfactory and inhibit the growth of aspergilli.
Nocardiosis[e]	Respiratory secretions; blood; cutaneous abscesses	Sabouraud's dextrose agar[a]; brain-heart infusion agar; Sabhi agar; biphasic brain-heart infusion agar/broth recommended for blood cultures.[d] Media containing antibiotics inhibit the growth of nocardiae.
Zygomycosis (Phycomycosis)	Respiratory secretions; rhino-orbital lesions; skin	Sabouraud's dextrose agar[a]; brain-heart infusion agar; inhibitory mold agar; Sabhi agar; brain-heart infusion blood agar with antibiotics.[b] Media containing cycloheximide inhibit the growth of zygomycetes.
Geotrichosis	Respiratory secretions; oropharynx; stool	Sabouraud's dextrose agar[a]; brain-heart infusion agar; inhibitory mold agar; Sabhi agar; brain-heart infusion blood agar with antibiotics[b]; brain-heart infusion blood agar with antibiotics and cycloheximide.[c]
Sporotrichosis	Respiratory secretions; lymphocutaneous abscesses; synovial fluid; nasal sinuses	Sabouraud's dextrose agar[a]; brain-heart infusion agar; inhibitory mold agar; Sabhi agar; brain-heart infusion blood agar with antibiotics[b]; brain-heart infusion blood agar with antibiotics and cycloheximide.[c]

Table 50-8. SPECIMEN AND MEDIA REQUIREMENTS FOR THE RECOVERY OF FUNGI FROM SPECIFIC MYCOTIC INFECTIONS (*Continued*)

INFECTION	SPECIMEN TYPE	COMMON CULTURE MEDIA
Mycetoma	Draining cutaneous sinuses; bone	*Eumycotic mycetoma:* Sabouraud's dextrose agar[a]; brain-heart infusion agar; inhibitory mold agar; Sabhi agar; all media should contain antibiotics and cycloheximide.[c] *Actinomycotic mycetoma:* Sabouraud's dextrose agar[a]; brain-heart infusion agar; Sabhi agar. Media containing antibiotics inhibit the growth of aerobic actinomycetes.
Chromomycosis	Skin; brain	Sabouraud's dextrose agar[a]; brain-heart infusion agar; inhibitory mold agar; Sabhi agar; All media should contain antibiotics and cycloheximide.[c]
Dermatomycosis	Hair; skin; nails	Mycosel agar or mycobiotic agar.[f]
Mycotic keratitis	Corneal scraping	Sabouraud's dextrose agar[a]; brain-heart infusion agar; Sabhi agar. Media containing antibiotics or cycloheximide are unsatisfactory.
Otomycosis	External ear	Sabouraud's dextrose agar[a]; brain-heart infusion agar; inhibitory mold agar; Sabhi agar; brain-heart infusion blood agar containing antibiotics.[b] Media containing cycloheximide are unsatisfactory and inhibit the growth of several etiologic agents.

[a]Contains 2% dextrose, pH 7.0.

[b]Contains gentamicin, 5 μg/ml, and chloramphenicol, 16 μg/ml, or penicillin, 20 units/ml, and streptomycin, 40 units/ml.

[c]Contains gentamicin, 5 μg/ml, and chloramphenicol, 16 μg/ml, or penicillin, 20 units/ml, and streptomycin, 40 units/ml, and cycloheximide, 0.5 mg/ml.

[d]See Roberts, 1975.

[e]Not a mycotic infection; however, organisms are often recovered on fungal culture media.

[f]Contains chloramphenicol, 50 μg/ml, and cycloheximide, 0.5 mg/ml.

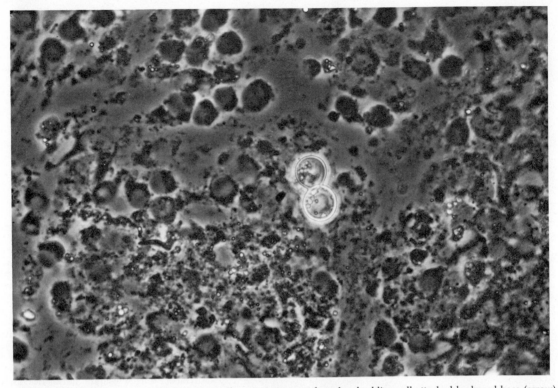

Figure 50–34. *Blastomyces dermatitidis* in sputum. Characteristic yeast form has budding cell attached by broad base (arrow). Also note "double contoured" appearance of cell wall and large size of cell. ×450. (From Roberts, G. D.: J. Clin. Microbiol., 2:261, 1975.)

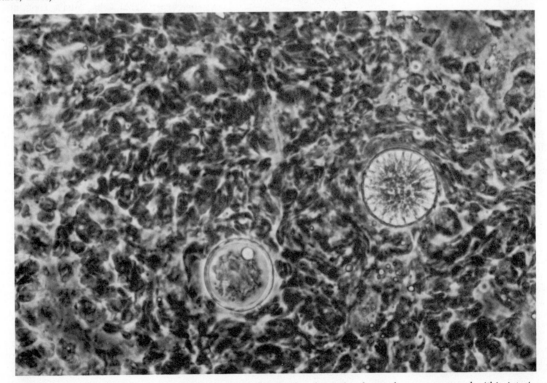

Figure 50–35. *Coccidioides immitis* in sputum. Large thick-walled spherules with a few endospores scattered within interior of spherule or cleavage furrows developing along periphery to form endospores. ×450. (From Roberts, G. D.: J. Clin Microbiol., 2:261, 1975.)

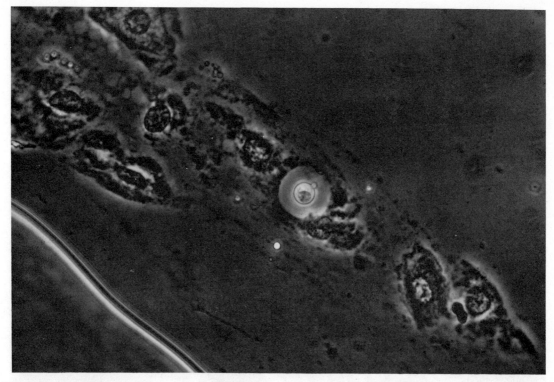

Figure 50–36. *Cryptococcus neoformans* in sputum. Spherical yeast cell is surrounded by large capsule with small bud arising from parent cell. ×450. (From Roberts, G. D.: J. Clin. Microbiol., 2:261, 1975.)

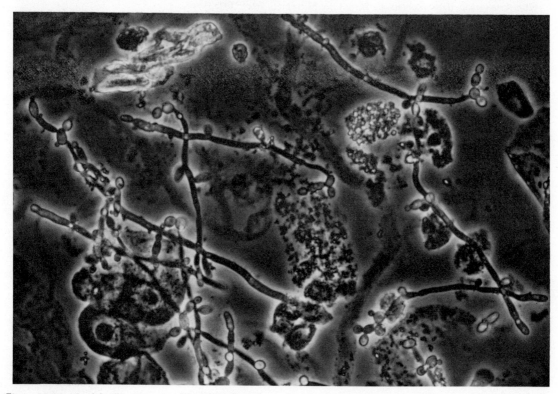

Figure 50–37. *Candida albicans* in urine. Hyphae and budding yeasts appear among epithelial cells. ×450. (From Roberts, G. D.: J. Clin. Microbiol., 2:261, 1975.)

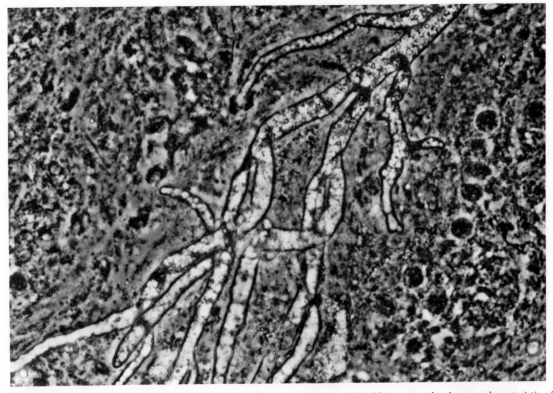

Figure 50–38. *Mucor* species in pus from skin lesion. The large, branching, ribbon-like aseptate hyphae are characteristic of a phycomycete. ×450. (From Roberts, G. D.: J. Clin. Microbiol., 2:261, 1975.)

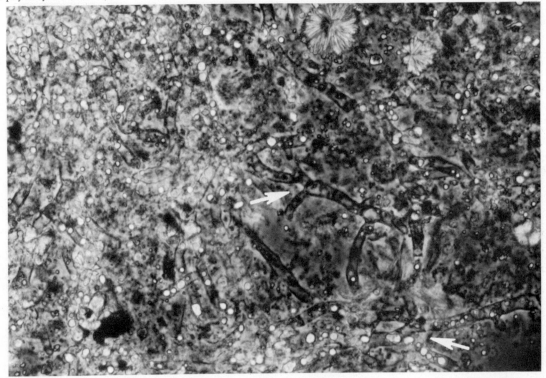

Figure 50–39. *Aspergillus fumigatus* in sputum. The septate hyphae show dichotomous branching (arrows). ×450. (From Roberts, G. D.: J. Clin. Microbiol., 2:261, 1975.)

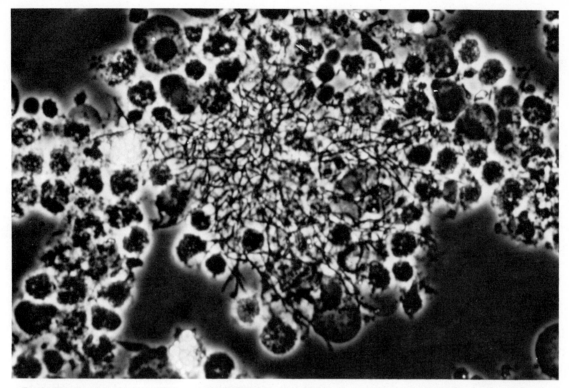

Figure 50-40. *Nocardia asteroides* in sputum. Small branching filaments are interpositioned among leukocytes. ×450.

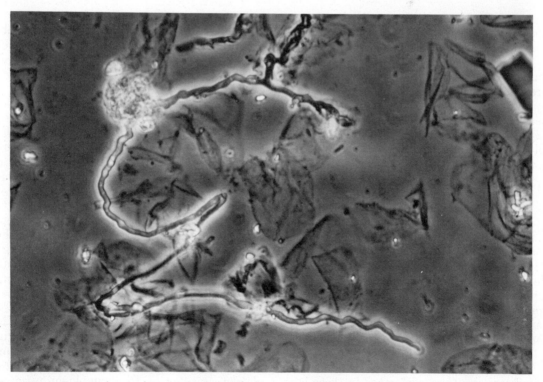

Figure 50-41. Dermatophyte in skin scraping. Septate hyphae intertwine among squamous cells. ×450. (From Roberts, G. D.: J. Clin. Microbiol., 2:261, 1975.)

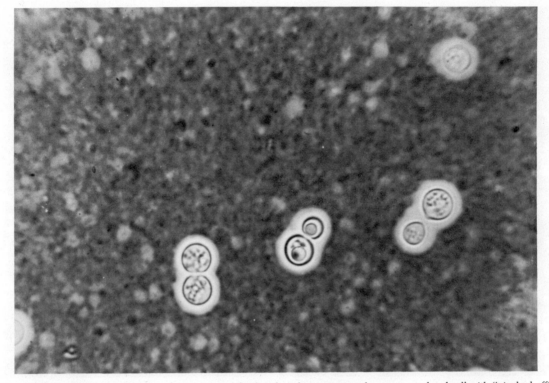

Figure 50-42. *Cryptococcus neoformans* in cerebrospinal fluid. India ink preparation shows encapsulated cell with "pinched off" buds. Also note that cells are spherical and vary in size. ×450. (From Dolan, C. T., Funkhouser, J. W., Koneman, E. W., Miller, N. G., and Roberts, G. D.: Atlas of Clinical Mycology I. Chicago, Ill., American Society of Clinical Pathologists, 1975.)

nostic when encapsulated organisms are present. A drop of India ink is mixed with a drop of sediment from centrifuged cerebrospinal fluid and is observed microscopically for the presence of encapsulated yeast cells. Cells of *C. neoformans* are usually encapsulated, may be budding, and are variable in size (Fig. 50-42). In most instances only a few cells are seen on direct examination.

THE IDENTIFICATION OF FILAMENTOUS FUNGI

Until recently, the filamentous fungi were considered to be either pathogens or saprobes. Saprobes previously thought to be non-pathogenic have been implicated as the etiologic agents of severe, often fatal, infections in compromised patients. Currently, it is necessary to consider all filamentous fungi as potential pathogens, and they should be handled with extreme caution in the laboratory.

The laboratory identification of the filamentous fungi should be performed in those laboratories equipped with biologic safety cabinets

to prevent laboratory-acquired infection. Laboratories which do not have adequate facilities for handling filamentous fungal cultures should send suspected pathogens to a reference laboratory for proper identification.

Generally, the growth rate for the strict pathogens, including *Blastomyces dermatitidis*, *Histoplasma capsulatum*, and *Coccidioides immitis*, is slow, and one to six weeks are required before colonies become apparent; however, most appear within three to four weeks. *Coccidioides immitis* in some instances may produce visible growth within three to five days. When specimens contain an exceptionally high number of organisms, the growth rate may be somewhat shortened, e.g., *Blastomyces dermatitidis* may be seen within six days of incubation. It is recommended that all fungal cultures be kept for a minimum of 30 days before being discarded.

The colonial morphology is of little value in identifying the filamentous fungi due to natural variation among isolates and variation which is culture medium-dependent. *Histoplasma capsulatum*, for example, on primary isolation often appears yeast-like on a blood-enriched medium, but on Sabouraud's dextrose agar or a similar medium it grows as a white tan fluffy colony. The growth rate usually provides more helpful information than colonial morphology. The definitive identification of the filamentous fungi is based on the characteristic microscopic morphology (type and arrangement of spores) and demonstration of both the saprobic and parasitic form of the dimorphic fungi. The ability to identify visually the filamentous fungi is based on experience and exposure to a wide variety of fungi which occur in nature.

The fungi may be prepared for microscopic observation by several methods. The procedure most familiar to clinical microbiology laboratories is the wet mount, which is prepared by adding a small portion of the culture and supporting agar to a drop of lactophenol aniline blue on a microscope slide. A coverslip is positioned on the slide and gentle pressure is applied to disperse the sample so that microscopic features are easily observed. This method is helpful if characteristic spores are found; however, it is unsuitable for the detection of characteristic spore arrangements. The most helpful procedure to use is the adhesive transparent plastic tape (Scotch tape) method of preparing cultures for microscopic examination. The adhesive side of the tape is gently touched to the surface of a colony and then is adhered to a slide on which a drop of lactophenol aniline blue has been placed. (The mounting medium consists of 15 grams of polyvinyl alcohol, 100 ml of distilled water, 39 ml of lactic acid, 39 ml of phenol [melted], and 0.1 g of aniline blue. The polyvinyl alcohol is added to the water and is heated at 80°C. until clearing occurs. The lactic acid is added, followed by the phenol and aniline blue.) This technique allows one to observe the spores and supporting structures arranged somewhat as they were when part of the original colony. This method is inexpensive, rapid, and simple for observing the filamentous fungi and is preferred by most laboratories.

The most important feature required for the identification of filamentous fungi is the characteristic arrangement of spores. As has been previously mentioned, the wet mount is unsuitable for this purpose. The Scotch tape method, in most instances, allows one to visualize the characteristic arrangement of spores. However, in some instances no characteristic arrangements can be seen, and it is necessary to prepare a microslide culture as follows: a small agar block is placed on a sterile microscope slide; the four corners are lightly inoculated, and a coverslip is placed on top. The culture is incubated in a moist chamber and after adequate growth occurs, the coverslip is removed and placed on a slide to which a drop of lactophenol aniline blue has been added. This allows the undisturbed spores to be observed as they were arranged during growth under the coverslip. It is recommended that two microslide cultures be made concurrently, since it is often difficult to determine when the culture is mature enough for examination. If necessary, the agar block may be removed and a drop of lactophenol aniline blue and a coverslip are added to the microscope slide. Often, the characteristic arrangement of spores may be observed in this manner. This provides another opportunity to observe an organism using a single microculture.

All these techniques allow one to observe the microscopic features of the filamentous fungi. Initially, the hyphae should be examined to determine if they are septate. If no septae are present, the organism may be classified as a Zygomycete, e.g., *Rhizopus, Mucor*, or *Absidia*. The size of the hyphae is important also; Zygomycetes have large, ribbon-like, twisted hyphae which are quite distinct. The strict pathogens exhibit hyphae which are septate but quite small in diameter. Many of the other fungi, including *Aspergillus* and *Penicillium*, etc., have hyphae of intermediate size between those of the Zygomycetes and the strict pathogens. In many instances when a characteristic arrangement of spores is absent, a tentative identification of a potential pathogen may be made based strictly on the growth rate and the size of the hyphae present as seen by microscopic examination. Usually, it is necessary to subculture the organism to another medium to induce sporulation.

The definitive identification of the dimorphic fungi, including *Blastomyces dermatitidis, Sporothrix schenckii, Histoplasma capsulatum*, and *Coccidioides immitis*, requires that both the parasitic and saprobic forms be observed in the laboratory. Conversion to the parasitic form may be accomplished by placing a large inoculum of the filamentous form onto the surface of a fresh, moist slant of an enriched medium containing blood. Brain-heart infusion agar containing 5 to 10 per cent sheep blood is preferred as the best conversion medium. Cultures are incubated at 37°C., and transfers are made to fresh media as soon as growth is apparent. Rarely, conversion may be completed overnight or within two to three days; however, usually several transfers are necessary for complete conversion, and this may require 7 to 21 days. This *in vitro* conversion procedure is satisfactory for demonstrating the yeast forms of the dimorphic fungi with the exception of *Coccidioides immitis*, which has only spherules and endospores.

The *in vitro* conversion of *Coccidioides immitis* to the spherule form may be accomplished; however, it is often done so only with difficulty. As an alternative, animal inoculation appears to be the best method to employ. A small amount of a suspension of the filamentous form of *Coccidioides immitis* is injected intraperitoneally into white mice. Animals are autopsied within one to two weeks after injection, the liver, spleen, and omental lesions are removed, and direct microscopic examinations are made. Methenamine silver-stained histologic sections are preferable, since they more readily reveal the tissue forms of the organism and provide for a permanent record of the culture conversion. Animal inoculation is a satisfactory method for converting all the dimorphic fungi from the saprobic form to the parasitic form. However, most laboratories find it impractical, and use is limited to reference laboratories.

Recognition of the characteristic microscopic features is determined by the experience. It requires a careful comparison of the microscopic features of fungi with photographs and descriptions available in current texts and laboratory manuals. Figure 50-43 presents the microscopic features of filamentous organisms commonly encountered in the clinical microbiology laboratory; it is not within the scope of this chapter to present a detailed description of each organism (see general references).

The clinical significance of the presence of most filamentous fungi in clinical specimens is undetermined. The laboratory has an obligation to identify and to report all organisms that are present in clinical specimens, and the clinician then must determine the significance of the organisms to the patient. In many instances the presence of the filamentous fungi is unimportant; however, the same fungi recovered from a compromised patient may play an important role in causing infection. Table 50-9 presents filamentous fungi commonly recovered in clinical specimens, time required for their identification, probable recovery sites, and infections with which they have been associated.

IDENTIFICATION OF YEASTS AND YEAST-LIKE ORGANISMS

During recent years there has been a definite increase in the number of yeast infections caused by *Candida albicans* and *Cryptococcus neoformans;* moreover, other species previously thought to be non-pathogenic have also been implicated. This has resulted from the clinical alteration of host defense mechanisms by underlying disease processes and chemotherapeutic agents, including steroids, antibiotics, and immunosuppressive agents. Many infections are the result of long-term intravenous therapy combined with inadequate catheter care. It is well documented that infections produced by yeasts and yeast-like organisms occur primarily in the compromised patient.

The identification of yeasts and yeast-like organisms from clinical specimens is currently of interest to most laboratories; however, the significance of these organisms is questionable. Since yeasts are considered to be normal flora in the oropharynx and gastrointestinal tract, their recovery might be expected from most clinical specimens, including respiratory secretions, gastric washings, vaginal secretions, stool specimens, and throat cultures. Other sites where yeasts are commonly recovered include urine, skin, and nail scrapings. Yeasts and yeast-like organisms are not usually recovered from normally sterile body fluids, including blood, cerebrospinal fluid, and synovial fluid, where their presence should be considered an abnormal finding. Table 50-10 lists the most common yeast-like organisms that are encountered in the clinical microbiology laboratory and infections with which they have been associated.

Since many yeasts and yeast-like organisms are considered normal flora and others under appropriate circumstances are pathogens, the question of whether all laboratories should identify them is a valid one. Their repeated recovery from multiple specimens from the same patient indicates either colonization or infection with the organism. When this occurs, the clinical microbiology laboratory should speciate the organisms, since this information is often important in making a decision concerning which therapeutic agent is to be used for treatment. Other situations which warrant

(*Text continued on p. 1723*)

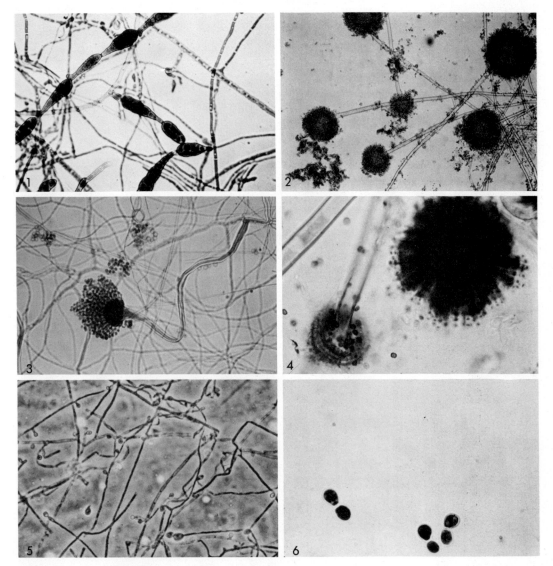

Figure 50–43. Common filamentous fungi which may be recovered from clinical specimens, microscopic features, lactophenol cotton blue preparation. ×450. (From Dolan, C. T., Funkhouser, J. W., Koneman, E. W., Miller, N. G., and Roberts, G. D.: Atlas of Clinical Mycology V and VI. Chicago, Ill., American Society of Clinical Pathologists, 1976.)

1. *Alternaria* species, conidia
2. *Aspergillus flavus*, conidial heads
3. *Aspergillus fumigatus*, conidial head
4. *Aspergillus niger*, conidial head
5. *Blastomyces dermatitidis*, filamentous form, conidia
6. *Blastomyces dermatitidis*, yeast form

(Illustration continued on following page)

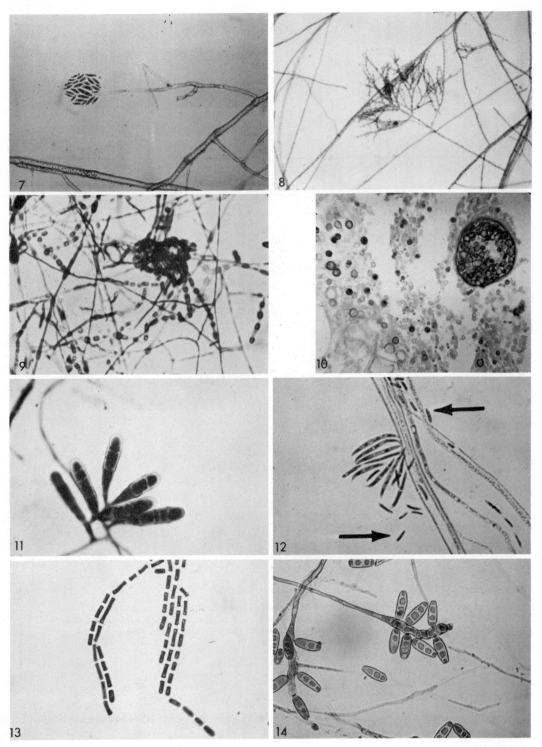

Figure 50–43 *continued.*   *(See opposite page for legend.)*

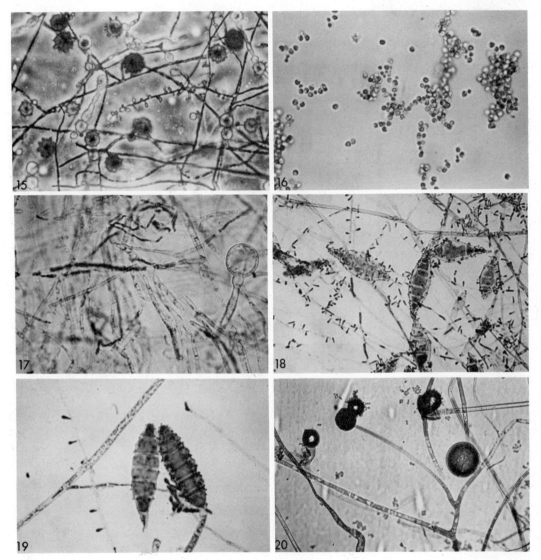

Figure 50–43 *continued.*

7. *Cephalosporium* species, conidia
8. *Cladosporium* species, conidia
9. *Coccidioides immitis,* filamentous form, arthrospores
10. *Coccidioides immitis,* spherule form
11. *Epidermophyton floccosum,* macroaleuriospores
12. *Fusarium* species, macroconidia
13. *Geotrichum* species, arthrospores
14. *Helminthosporium* species, conidia
15. *Histoplasma capsulatum,* filamentous form, macroaleuriospores and microaleuriospores
16. *Histoplasma capsulatum,* yeast form
17. *Microsporum audouinii,* terminal chlamydospore
18. *Microsporum canis,* macroaleuriospores and microaleuriospores
19. *Microsporum gypseum,* macroaleuriospores and microaleuriospores
20. *Mucor* species, sporangia

(*Illustration continued on following page*)

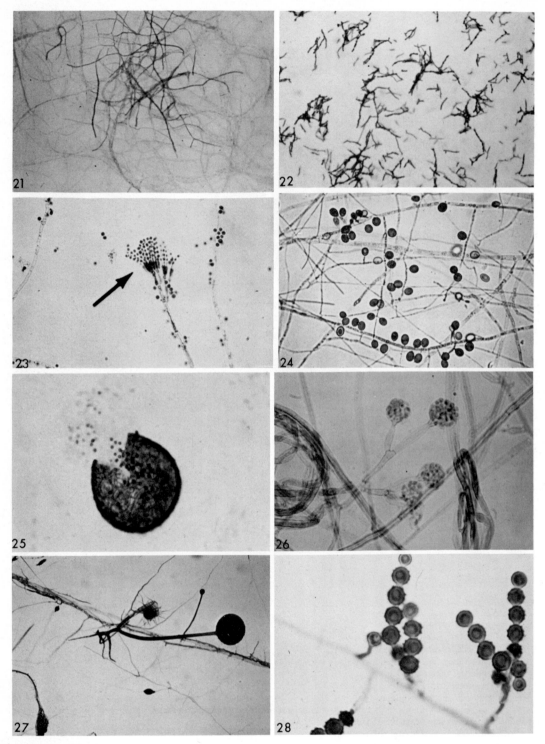

Figure 50–43 *continued.*
21. *Nocardia asteroides,* branching filaments
22. *Nocardia asteroides,* coccobacillary form
23. *Penicillium* species, conidial head
24. *Petriellidium boydii,* conidial stage
25. *Petriellidium boydii,* cleistothecia
26. *Phialophora verrucosa,* flask-shaped phialide
27. *Rhizopus* species, sporangia and rhizoids
28. *Scopulariopsis* species, conidia

(Illustration continued on opposite page)

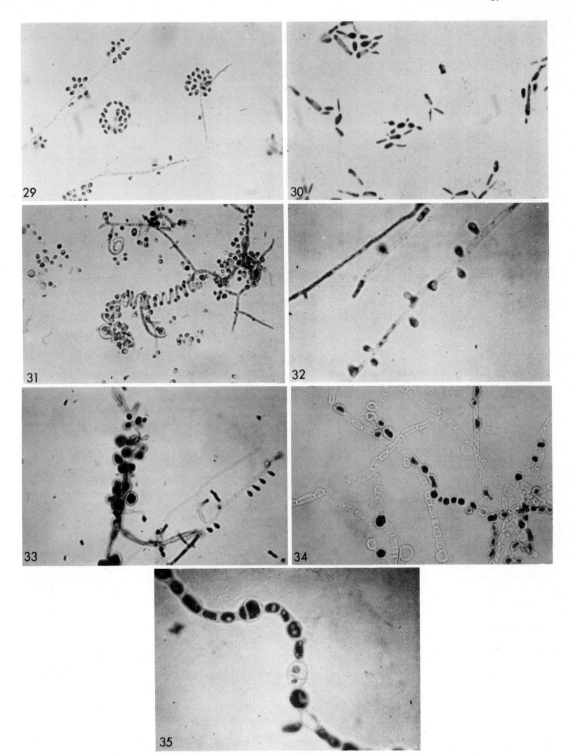

Figure 50–43 *continued.*

29. *Sporothrix schenckii,* filamentous form, flowerette and sleeve arrangements of conidia
30. *Sporothrix schenckii,* yeast form, cigar bodies
31. *Trichophyton mentagrophytes,* microaleuriospores and spiral hyphae
32. *Trichophyton rubrum,* tear-shaped microaleuriospores
33. *Trichophyton tonsurans,* swollen (balloon forms) microaleuriospores
34. *Trichophyton verrucosum,* chains of chlamydospores at 37°C.
35. *Trichophyton violaceum,* swollen hyphae containing cytoplasmic granules

Table 50-9. COMMON FILAMENTOUS FUNGI IMPLICATED IN HUMAN MYCOTIC INFECTIONS

ETIOLOGIC AGENT	TIME REQUIRED FOR IDENTIFICATION	PROBABLE RECOVERY SITES	CLINICAL IMPLICATION(S)
Alternaria species	2-6 days	Skin, nails, conjunctiva, and respiratory secretions	Skin and nail infections, conjunctivitis, hypersensitivity pneumonitis
Aspergillus flavus	1-4 days	Skin, respiratory secretions, gastric washings, nasal sinuses	Skin infections, allergic bronchopulmonary infection, sinusitis, myocarditis, disseminated infection, renal infection, subcutaneous mycetoma
Aspergillus fumigatus	2-6 days	Respiratory secretions, skin, ear, cornea, gastric washings, stool, nasal sinuses	Allergic bronchopulmonary infection, fungus ball, invasive pulmonary infection, skin and nail infections, external otomycosis, mycotic keratitis, sinusitis, myocarditis, renal infection
Aspergillus niger	1-4 days	Respiratory secretions, gastric washings, ear, skin	Fungus ball, pulmonary infection, external otomycosis, mycotic keratitis
Blastomyces dermatitidis	6-21 days (recovery time) [additional 3-14 days required for confirmatory identification]	Respiratory secretions, skin, oropharyngeal ulcers, bone, prostate	Pulmonary infection, skin infection, oropharyngeal ulceration, osteomyelitis, prostatitis, arthritis, CNS infection
Cephalosporium (Acremonium) species	2-6 days	Skin, nails, respiratory secretions, cornea, vagina, gastric washings	Skin and nail infections, mycotic keratitis
Cladosporium species	6-10 days	Respiratory secretions, skin, nails, nose, cornea	Skin and nail infections, mycotic keratitis. Chromoblastomycosis, brain abscess and tinea nigra palmaris caused by *Cladosporium carrionii*, *C. trichoides*, and *E. werneckii*, respectively.
Coccidioides immitis	3-21 days	Respiratory secretions, skin, bone, cerebrospinal fluid, synovial fluid, urine, gastric washings	Pulmonary infection, skin infection, osteomyelitis, meningitis, arthritis, disseminated infection
Epidermophyton floccosum	7-10 days	Skin, nails	Tinea cruris, tinea pedis, tinea corporis, onychomycosis
Fusarium species	2-6 days	Skin, respiratory secretions, cornea	Mycotic keratitis, skin infection (in burn patients)
Geotrichum species	2-6 days	Respiratory secretions, urine, skin, stool, vagina, conjunctiva, gastric washings, throat	Bronchitis, skin infection, colitis, conjunctivitis, thrush
Helminthosporium species	2-6 days	Respiratory secretions, skin	Pulmonary infection (rare)
Histoplasma capsulatum	10-45 days (recovery time) [additional 7-21 days required for confirmatory identification]	Respiratory secretions, bone marrow, blood, urine, adrenals, skin, cerebrospinal fluid, eye, pleural fluid, liver, spleen, oropharyngeal lesions, vagina, gastric washings, larynx	Pulmonary infection, oropharyngeal lesions, CNS infection, skin infection (rare), uveitis, peritonitis
Microsporum audouinii	10-14 days (recovery time) [additional 14-21 days required for confirmatory identification]	Hair	Tinea capitis
Microsporum canis	5-7 days	Hair, skin	Tinea corporis, tinea capitis, tinea barbae, tinea manuum
Microsporum gypseum	3-6 days	Hair, skin	Tinea capitis, tinea corporis

Table 50–9. COMMON FILAMENTOUS FUNGI IMPLICATED IN HUMAN MYCOTIC INFECTIONS (*Continued*)

ETIOLOGIC AGENT	TIME REQUIRED FOR IDENTIFICATION	PROBABLE RECOVERY SITES	CLINICAL IMPLICATION(S)
Mucor species	1-5 days	Respiratory secretions, skin, nose, brain, stool, orbit, cornea, vitreous humor, gastric washings, wounds, ear	Rhinocerebral infection, pulmonary infection, gastrointestinal infection, mycotic keratitis, intraocular infection, external otomycosis, orbital cellulitis
*Nocardia asteroides**	4-25 days	Respiratory secretions, skin, urine, blood, brain, conjunctiva, bone, cornea, gastric washings	Pulmonary infection, mycetoma, brain abscess, conjunctivitis, osteomyelitis, mycotic keratitis
Penicillium species	2-6 days	Respiratory secretions, gastric washings, skin, urine, ear, cornea	Pulmonary infection, skin infection, external otomycosis, mycotic keratitis, endocarditis
Petriellidium (Allescheria) boydii	2-6 days	Respiratory secretions, gastric washings, skin, cornea	Pulmonary fungus ball, mycetoma, mycotic keratitis
Phialophora species	6-21 days	Respiratory secretions, gastric washings, skin, cornea, conjunctiva	Some species produce chromoblastomycosis or mycetoma; mycotic keratitis, conjunctivitis, intraocular infection
Rhizopus species	1-5 days	Respiratory secretions, skin, nose, brain, stool, orbit, cornea, vitreous humor, gastric washings, wounds, ear	Rhinocerebral infection, pulmonary infection, mycotic keratitis, intraocular infection, orbital cellulitis, external otomycosis
Scopulariopsis species	2-6 days	Respiratory secretions, gastric washings, nails, skin, vitreous humor, ear	Pulmonary infection, nail infection, skin infection, intraocular infection, external otomycosis
Sporothrix schenckii	3-12 days (recovery time) [additional 2-10 days required for confirmatory identification]	Respiratory secretions, skin, subcutaneous tissue, maxillary sinuses, synovial fluid, bone marrow, bone, cerebrospinal fluid, ear, conjunctiva	Pulmonary infection, lymphocutaneous infection, sinusitis, arthritis, osteomyelitis, meningitis, external otomycosis, conjunctivitis, disseminated infection
Trichophyton mentagrophytes	7-10 days	Hair, skin, nails	Tinea barbae, tinea capitis, tinea corporis, tinea cruris, tinea pedis, onychomycosis
Trichophyton rubrum	10-14 days	Hair, skin, nails	Tinea pedis, onychomycosis, tinea corporis, tinea cruris
Trichophyton tonsurans	10-14 days	Hair, skin, nails	Tinea capitis, tinea corporis, onychomycosis, tinea pedis
Trichophyton verrucosum	10-18 days	Hair, skin, nails	Tinea capitis, tinea corporis, tinea barbae
Trichophyton violaceum	14-18 days	Hair, skin, nails	Tinea capitis, tinea corporis, onychomycosis

*Although *N. asteroides* is a bacterium, it is commonly recovered on fungal culture media due to its slow growth rate.

5

Table 50-10. COMMON YEAST-LIKE ORGANISMS IMPLICATED IN HUMAN INFECTION*

ETIOLOGIC AGENT	PROBABLE RECOVERY SITES	CLINICAL IMPLICATION(S)
Candida albicans	Respiratory secretions, vagina, urine, skin, oropharynx, gastric washings, blood, stool, transtracheal aspiration, cornea, nails, cerebrospinal fluid, bone, peritoneal fluid	Pulmonary infection, vaginitis, urinary tract infection, dermatitis, fungemia, mycotic keratitis, onychomycosis, meningitis, osteomyelitis, peritonitis, myocarditis, endocarditis, endophthalmitis, disseminated infection, thrush, arthritis
Torulopsis glabrata	Respiratory secretions, urine, vagina, gastric washings, blood, skin, oropharynx, transtracheal aspiration, stool, bone marrow, skin (rare)	Pulmonary infection, urinary tract infection, vaginitis, fungemia, disseminated infection, endocarditis
Candida tropicalis	Respiratory secretions, urine, gastric washings, vagina, blood, skin, oropharynx, transtracheal aspiration, stool, pleural fluid, peritoneal fluid, cornea	Pulmonary infection, vaginitis, thrush, endophthalmitis, endocarditis, arthritis, peritonitis, mycotic keratitis, fungemia
Candida parapsilosis	Respiratory secretions, urine, gastric washings, blood, vagina, oropharynx, skin, transtracheal aspiration, stool, pleural fluid, ear, nails	Endophthalmitis, endocarditis, vaginitis, mycotic keratitis, external otomycosis, paronychia, fungemia
Saccharomyces species	Respiratory secretions, urine, gastric washings, vagina, skin, oropharynx, transtracheal aspiration, stool	Pulmonary infection (rare), endocarditis
Candida krusei	Respiratory secretions, urine, gastric washings, vagina, skin, oropharynx, blood, transtracheal aspiration, stool, cornea	Endocarditis, vaginitis, urinary tract infection, mycotic keratitis
Candida guilliermondii	Respiratory secretions, gastric washings, vagina, skin, nails, oropharynx, blood, cornea, bone, urine	Endocarditis, fungemia, dermatitis, onychomycosis, mycotic keratitis, osteomyelitis, urinary tract infection
Rhodotorula species	Respiratory secretions, urine, gastric washings, blood, vagina, skin, oropharynx, stool, cerebrospinal fluid, cornea	Fungemia, endocarditis, mycotic keratitis
Trichosporon species	Respiratory secretions, skin, oropharynx, stool	Pulmonary infection, brain abscess, disseminated infection, piedra
Cryptococcus neoformans	Respiratory secretions, cerebrospinal fluid, bone, blood, bone marrow, urine, skin, pleural fluid, gastric washings, transtracheal aspirations, cornea, orbit, vitreous humor	Pulmonary infection, meningitis, osteomyelitis, fungemia, disseminated infection, endocarditis, skin infection, mycotic keratitis, orbital cellulitis, endophthalmic infection
Candida pseudotropicalis	Respiratory secretions, vagina, urine gastric washings, oropharynx	Vaginitis, urinary tract infection
Cryptococcus albidus/albidus	Respiratory secretions, skin, gastric washings, urine, cornea	Meningitis, pulmonary infection
Cryptococcus luteolus	Respiratory secretions, skin, nose	Not commonly implicated in human infection
Cryptococcus laurentii	Respiratory secretions, cerebrospinal fluid, skin, oropharynx, stool	Not commonly implicated in human infection
Cryptococcus albidus/diffluens	Respiratory secretions, urine, cerebrospinal fluid, gastric washings, skin	Not commonly implicated in human infection
Cryptococcus terreus	Respiratory secretions, skin, nose	Not commonly implicated in human infection

*Arranged in order of occurrence in the clinical laboratory.

the speciation of yeasts and yeast-like organisms include their recovery from patients who are compromised from an underlying disease process or by chemotherapy. The laboratory should always speciate an organism from any site which the clinician feels is important.

Many different procedures are available for the identification of yeasts and yeast-like organisms, and the decision concerning which method should be used must be made by each individual laboratory. Obviously, some methods are better suited for large laboratories that have extensive experience and other methods are suitable for smaller laboratories. Representative methods which may be utilized by laboratories of all sizes will be presented in the following paragraphs.

GERM TUBE TEST

The germ tube test is the most widely used test for the identification of *Candida albicans*. A very small inoculum from an isolated colony is suspended in a tube containing 0.5 ml of sterile normal human serum or another suitable substrate. The suspension is incubated for three hours at 37°C. and is observed microscopically for the presence of germ tubes. A germ tube is characterized by the production of an appendage one half the width of and three to four times the length of the cell from which it extends (Fig. 50-44). The presence of a germ tube provides a definitive identification of *Candida albicans* if the test is performed as described above. Some laboratories prefer to make the distinction between *Candida albicans* and *Candida stellatoidea*, although most laboratories consider *C. stellatoidea* to be a variant of *Candida albicans*. *Candida stellatoidea* may be differentiated from *Candida albicans* by its inability to assimilate sucrose. When performing the germ tube test, *Candida albicans* should be included as a positive control and *Candida tropicalis* as a negative control. If the germ tube test is incubated longer than three hours, *Candida tropicalis* may produce pseudogerm tubes which appear much wider and more hypha-like than true germ tubes.

Many other substrates, including sheep

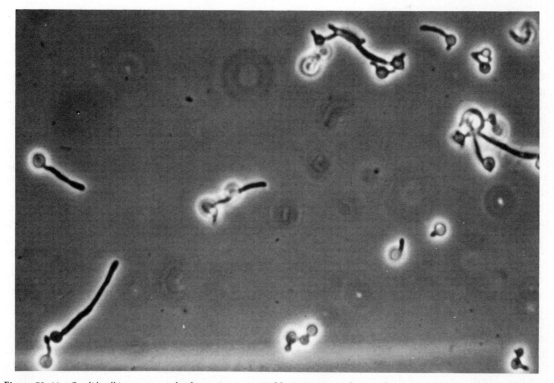

Figure 50-44. *Candida albicans,* germ tube formation in normal human serum after incubation at 37°C. for three hours. ×450. (From Dolan, C. T., Funkhouser, J. W., Koneman, E. W., Miller, N. G., and Roberts, G. D.: Atlas of Clinical Mycology I. Chicago, Ill., American Society of Clinical Pathologists, 1975.)

serum, fetal calf serum, Trypticase soy broth, Sabouraud's dextrose broth, and others, have been utilized for the germ tube test. Most of these substrates are satisfactory; however, extensive quality control testing should be performed to ensure reliable results.

UREASE TEST

Urease production is most helpful for the detection of cryptococci. All common species of cryptococci produce urease; however, *Candida krusei*, members of the genus *Rhodotorula, Sporobolomyces,* and *Trichosporon* also exhibit this characteristic.

Rapid urease production may be detected by placing a large inoculum from a single colony onto the surface of the upper portion of the slant in a tube of Christensen's urea agar. The tube is incubated at 37°C. for at least 72 hours. Most members of the genus *Cryptococcus* will produce urease within several hours, and this is indicated by the production of a pink to red color. The urease test is best utilized as a screening tool for the detection of *Cryptococcus neoformans* when characteristic colonies are observed.

CARBOHYDRATE UTILIZATION (ASSIMILATION)

Carbohydrate utilization tests are the most widely used methods for the definitive identification of clinically important yeasts and yeast-like organisms. Most laboratories are prepared to perform these tests; however, little standardization of methods exists. Generally, all methods utilize a basal medium (yeast nitrogen base) which supports the growth of yeasts when an appropriate carbohydrate substrate is added. The medium is observed for the presence of growth, which indicates utilization of a particular carbohydrate substrate by the organism.

Many methods have been developed for detecting carbohydrate utilization patterns: auxanographic plate methods utilizing carbohydrate-impregnated disks (Roberts, 1976) or carbohydrate nutrient-impregnated disks (Huppert, 1975); agar slant utilization methods involving individual carbohydrate sources contained within yeast nitrogen base agar slants (Adams, 1974); broth tube methods containing individual carbohydrate sources within yeast nitrogen base broth (Wickerham, 1948); and numerous commercially available

systems which contain carbohydrate utilization tests (Bowman, 1976). Carbohydrate utilization patterns for yeasts commonly encountered in the clinical laboratory are presented in Table 50-11.

CARBOHYDRATE FERMENTATION

Carbohydrate fermentation tests are useful to supplement carbohydrate assimilation test results when there is difficulty in making the definitive identification of an organism. Fermentation tests are less reliable when used alone and are most commonly used as supplementary tests.

Fermentation media contain peptone, beef or yeast extract, an indicator (bromcresol purple), and individual carbohydrate sources. Fermentation is detected by the production of gas only. Acid production (carbohydrate utilization), as indicated by a change in color of the indicator, is not an indication of fermentation. Most fermentation tests require an extended incubation period of 6 to 10 days before final results can be reported. Characteristic fermentation reactions are also presented in Table 50-11.

NITRATE UTILIZATION

Nitrate utilization tests are most helpful for the speciation of cryptococci. Basically most methods consist of placing an organism in an environment which contains potassium nitrate as the only inorganic nitrate source. This substrate can be reduced to nitrite and be detected using sulfanilic acid and α-naphthylamine reagents (Rhodes, 1975). The rapid nitrate reduction test (swab method) (Hopkins, 1977) is currently the method of choice for most clinical laboratories. The test is simple to perform, reagents are easy to prepare, and results are available within 10 minutes. This test is particularly helpful in making a rapid, tentative identification of *Cryptococcus neoformans* which does not reduce nitrate.

PIGMENT PRODUCTION MEDIA FOR THE IDENTIFICATION OF CRYPTOCOCCUS NEOFORMANS

Cryptococcus neoformans is known to possess an enzyme, phenoloxidase, which reacts with caffeic acid to produce a brown to black pigment. The thistle seed or niger seed agar developed by Staib and Senka (1973) is com-

Table 50-11. CHARACTERISTIC BIOCHEMICAL FEATURES OF YEASTS COMMONLY RECOVERED FROM CLINICAL SPECIMENS

ORGANISM	UTILIZATION (ASSIMILATION)							FERMENTATION[a]					UREASE PRODUCTION	NITRATE UTILIZATION
	Dextrose	Maltose	Sucrose	Lactose	Raffinose	Trehalose	Inositol	Dextrose	Maltose	Sucrose	Lactose	Galactose		
Cryptococcus neoformans	+	+	+	–	±	+	+	–	–	–	–	–	+	–
C. albidus var albidus	+	+	+	+[b]	+	+[b]	+	–	–	–	–	–	+	+
C. albidus var. diffluens	+	+	+	–	+	+	+	–	–	–	–	–	+	+
C. luteolus	+	+	+	–	–[b]	+	+	–	–	–	–	–	+	–
C. laurentii	+	+	+	+[b]	+[b]	+	+	–	–	–	–	–	+	–
Candida albicans[c]	+	+[c]	+[c]	–	–	+	–	G	G	–[b]	–	G	–	–
C. tropicalis	+	+	+[b]	–	–	+	–	G	G	G	–	G	–	–
C. parapsilosis	+	+	+	–	–	+	–	G	–	–	–	G[b]	–	–
C. krusei	+	–	–	–	–	–[b]	–	G	–	–	–	–	+[b]	–
C. guilliermondii	+	+	+	–	+	+[b]	–	G	G	G	–	G	–	–
C. pseudotropicalis	+	–	+	+	+	–	–	G	G	G	G	G	–	–
Rhodotorula rubra	+	+	+	–	+[b]	+	–	–	–	–	–	–	+	–
Torulopsis glabrata	+	+	–	–	–	+	–	G	–	–	–	–	–	–
Geotrichum candidum	–	–	–	–	–	–	–	–	–	–	–	–	–	–
Trichosporon cutaneum	+	+[b]	+[b]	+	+[b]	+[b]	+[b]	–	–	–	–	–	+	–

[a] G = Fermentation detected by gas production.
[b] Strain variation.
[c] *Candida stellatoidea* is included with *C. albicans* here; the only difference is in sucrose assimilation.

5

Table 50–12. COMMONLY AVAILABLE FUNGAL SEROLOGIC TESTS

INFECTION	ANTIGEN(S)	TEST(S)	INTERPRETATION
Aspergillosis	*Aspergillus fumigatus* *Aspergillus niger* *Aspergillus flavus*	Immunodiffusion	One or more precipitin bands suggestive of active infection. Precipitin bands shown to correlate with complement-fixation titers—the greater the number of bands, the higher the titer. When cultural proof is presented in the presence of a positive test, it is diagnostic of active infection. Precipitins can be found in 95% of the fungus ball cases and 50% of the allergic bronchopulmonary cases. Sometimes positive in invasive infection, depending on the immunologic status of the patient.
Blastomycosis	*Blastomyces dermatit-idis*		
	Yeast form	Complement-fixation	Titers of 1:8 to 1:16 are highly suggestive of active infection; titers of 1:32 or greater are indicative. Cross-reactions occur in patients having coccidioidomycosis or histoplasmosis; however, titers are usually lower. A decreasing titer is indicative of regression. Most patients (75%) having blastomycosis have negative tests.
	Yeast culture filtrate	Immunodiffusion	Preliminary results show that it is more sensitive than complement-fixation—80% detection rate.
Candidosis	*Candida albicans* (Hollister-Stier Laboratories)	Immunodiffusion, Counterimmunoelectrophoresis	Test difficult to interpret because precipitins are found in 20–30% of the normal population, and reports in the literature are conflicting. Clinical correlation must exist for the test to be useful.
Coccidioidomycosis	Coccidioidin	Complement-fixation	Titers of 1:2 to 1:4 have been seen in active infection. Low titers should be followed by repeat testing at 2–3 week intervals. Titers of greater than 1:16 are usually indicative of active infection. Cross-reactions occur in patients having histoplasmosis, and false-negative results occur in patients with solitary pulmonary lesions. Titer parallels severity of infection.
	Coccidioidin	Immunodiffusion	Results correlate with complement-fixation test and can be used as a screening test—should be confirmed by performing complement-fixation test.
	Coccidioidin	Latex agglutination	Precipitins occur during first three weeks of infection and are diagnostic, but not prognostic. Useful as a screening test for precipitins in early infection. False-positive tests frequent when diluted serum or cerebrospinal fluid specimens are used.
Cryptococcosis	No antigen—latex particles coated with hyperimmune anticryptococcal globulin (IBL Laboratories)	Latex agglutination for cryptococcal antigen	Presence of cryptococcal polysaccharide in body fluids is indicative of cryptococcosis. Rheumatoid factor presents false-positive reactions and RA test must be performed as a control. Decrease in antigen titer indicates regression. Positive tests (in CSF) have been seen in 95% of cryptococcal meningitis cases and 30% of non-meningitis cases. Serum is less frequently positive than CSF. Disseminated infections usually present positive results in serum. Test may be performed using serum, CSF, and urine. Test more sensitive than India ink preparation.

Table 50–12. COMMONLY AVAILABLE FUNGAL SEROLOGIC TESTS (*Continued*)

INFECTION	ANTIGEN(S)	TEST(S)	INTERPRETATION
Histoplasmosis	Histoplasmin and yeast form of *Histoplasma capsulatum*	Complement-fixation	Titers of 1:8 to 1:16 are highly suspicious of infection; however, titers of 1:32 or greater are usually indicative of active infection. Cross-reactions occur in patients having aspergillosis, blastomycosis, and coccidioidomycosis, but titers are usually lower. Several follow-up serum samples should be tested—drawn at 2-3 week intervals. Rising titers indicate progressive infection and decreasing titers indicate regression. Some disseminated infections are nonreactive to the complement-fixation test. Recent skin tests in persons who have had prior exposure to *H. capsulatum* will cause an elevation in the complement-fixation titer. This occurs in 17-20% of persons tested. The yeast antigen gives positive reactions in 75-80% of cases, and the histoplasmin gives positive reactions in 10-15% of cases. In 10% of cases both are positive simultaneously.
	Histoplasmin	Immunodiffusion	H and M bands appearing simultaneously are indicative of active infection. M band may appear alone and can indicate early infection or chronic infection. Also the M band may appear after a recent skin test. The H band appears later than the M band and disappears earlier, and its disappearance may indicate regression of the infection.
	Histoplasmin	Latex agglutination	Test is unreliable. Many false-positive and negative tests may be observed. Any positive test should be confirmed by the complement-fixation test.
Sporotrichosis	Yeast of *Sporothrix schenckii*	Agglutination	Titers of 1:80 or greater usually indicative of active infection. Some cutaneous infections present negative tests; however, extracutaneous infections present positive tests.

5

monly used for the detection and identification of *Cryptococcus neoformans*. Most isolates of *Cryptococcus neoformans* produce the characteristic brown pigment within one to three days of incubation.

A medium containing Tween-80-Oxgall caffeic acid has been developed which allows pigment production by *Cryptococcus neoformans* within six hours (Fleming, 1977) and may prove useful for the definitive identification of *Cryptococcus neoformans*. Another method which utilizes caffeic acid that has been impregnated into paper disks has been developed and also provides a rapid identification of *Cryptococcus neoformans* within six hours (Hopfer, 1975). However, a number of false positive and false negative tests have been observed with the latter method, and its usefulness is limited as a screening tool for the tentative identification of *Cryptococcus neoformans* (Wang, 1977). The latter two tests offer the advantage of being rapid and when combined with results of the rapid nitrate utilization test and urease test can provide a tentative identification of *Cryptococcus neoformans* within a few hours.

CORNMEAL AGAR MORPHOLOGY

Cornmeal agar has been successfully used for the detection of chlamydospores produced by *Candida albicans* and *Candida stellatoidea*. This method is currently satisfactory for the definitive identification of *Candida albicans* and *Candida stellatoidea* if sucrose assimilation testing is incorporated. However, it has been shown that distinct characteristic microscopic morphologic features of several common species of the genus *Candida* may be observed on cornmeal agar (Dolan, 1971). The morphology is distinct enough to provide a definitive identification of the following members of the genus Candida: *Candida albicans, Candida krusei, Candida parapsilosis, Candida tropicalis,* and *Candida pseudotropicalis*. Microscopic features are also helpful in distinguishing between members of the genera *Cryptococcus, Torulopsis,* and *Saccharomyces*, although their definitive identification cannot be made on the basis of microscopic morphology on this medium. It is necessary to use biochemical tests to provide confirmation for the latter organisms. Cornmeal agar morphology is often difficult to determine, and perhaps its use should be limited to those laboratories with large volumes of yeasts submitted for identification.

It is not within the scope of this chapter to provide detailed descriptions of all methods useful for the identification of yeasts. Appropriate general references are provided which will allow a laboratory to select and perform those methods appropriate for each laboratory setting. Kits are commercially available for the identification of yeasts and most appear to be satisfactory. However, such factors as cost, stability of reagents, and adaptability to the laboratory setting should be considered before they are purchased. In many instances commercially available yeast identification kits are preferable to individually selected tests.

FUNGAL SEROLOGIC TESTS

The definitive diagnosis of mycotic infections is based on the successful recovery and identification of the etiologic agent from a clinical specimen. However, there are instances in which cultural proof cannot be obtained and other laboratory information must be utilized. Fungal serologic tests play an important role in the diagnosis of mycotic infections, although they often provide only tentative evidence of infection. These tests are helpful to supplement cultural or histopathologic evidence of etiology. Many of the tests used in fungal serology require difficult reagent preparation and precise technical expertise and are useful only in reference laboratories. Recently, commercially available sources for reagents have become available, making fungal serologic testing feasible for laboratories other than reference laboratories. Demand, costs, expiration rates of reagents, and technical expertise requirements should be considered by individual laboratories before making a decision to institute such a testing program.

As with other serologic tests, false-negative results may occur when blood is drawn at an inappropriate time or if blood is drawn from a patient who is immunosuppressed by chemotherapy or underlying disease and whose antibody production is therefore diminished. Many of the antigens used for testing are crude extracts of the fungi and contain many common components that cross-react with other fungi to give false-positive results. For example, the antigens of *Histoplasma capsulatum* are similar to those of *Blastomyces dermatitidis* and *Coccidioides immitis*. Occasionally, a patient with histoplasmosis will have serologic tests that are positive to all the antigens. In most instances, however, the antibody titer is greater to the antigen from the organism which is the actual cause of infection, *H. capsulatum* in this instance. In addition, it is preferable to repeat serologic tests at two to three week intervals to detect a rise in titer to the antigen of the responsible etiologic agent.

Since most laboratories find it necessary to refer serum samples submitted for serologic testing to reference laboratories, it is necessary to discuss the collection and transport of those samples. Serum aseptically collected from at least 10 ml of blood is adequate for most serologic testing. Samples should be as fresh as possible; however, if short-term storage is required, 4°C. is satisfactory. If longer term storage within the laboratory is necessary, then temperatures of −20°C. to −60°C. are recommended.

When serum or cerebrospinal fluid samples are sent by mail, they should be packed in dry or wet ice to prevent bacterial contamination. Another suitable alternative is to add a preservative, e.g., merthiolate, so that the specimen contains a final concentration of 1:5000. Samples containing the preservative may be mailed without refrigeration.

All samples should be properly packaged and labeled according to governmental regulations before shipping. Air mail or air express routes of shipping are recommended to reduce the transit time.

Table 50-12 presents commonly utilized serologic tests and an interpretation of each. Used properly, these serologic tests can provide very helpful diagnostic information to the clinician in a much shorter time than is required for fungal cultures to become positive. In most instances fungal serologic tests provide enough information when combined with the clinical presentation and can provide a presumptive diagnosis of mycotic infection; their use is highly recommended.

REFERENCES

Specific References

Adams, E. D., Jr., and Cooper, B. H.: Evaluation of a modified Wickerham medium for identifying medically important yeasts. Am. J. Med. Technol., *40*:377, 1974.
Bowman, P. I., and Ahearn, D. G.: Evaluation of commercial systems for the identification of clinical yeast isolates. J. Clin. Microbiol., *4*:49, 1976.
Dolan, C. T.: A practical approach to identification of yeast-like organisms. Am. J. Clin. Pathol., *55*:580, 1971.
Fleming, W. H., Hopkins, J. M., and Land, G. A.: New culture medium for the presumptive identification of *Candida albicans* and *Cryptococcus neoformans.* J. Clin. Microbiol., *5*:236, 1977.
Hopfer, R. L., and Gröschel, D.: Six hour pigmentation test for the identification of *Cryptococcus neoformans.* J. Clin. Microbiol., *2*:96, 1975.
Hopkins, J. M., and Land, G. A.: Rapid method for determining nitrate utilization by yeasts. J. Clin. Microbiol., *5*:497, 1977.
Huppert, M., Harper, G., Sun, S. H., and Delanerolle, V.: Rapid methods for identification of yeasts. J. Clin. Microbiol., *2*:21, 1975.
Rhodes, J. C., and Roberts, G. D.: Comparison of four methods for determining nitrate utilization by cryptococci. J. Clin. Microbiol., *1*:9, 1975.
Roberts, G. D.: Laboratory diagnosis of fungal infections. Human Pathol., *7*:161, 1976.
Roberts, G. D., and Washington, J. A., II: Detection of fungi in blood cultures. J. Clin. Microbiol., *1*:309, 1975.
Staib, F., and Senska, M.: Der Braunfarbeffekt (BFE) bei *Cryptococcus neoformans* auf Guizzotia abyssinica-kreatinin-agar in Abhängigkeit vom Ausgangs-pH-wert. Zentralbl. Bakteriol. [Orig. A], *225*:113, 1973.
Wang, H. S., Zeimis, R. T., and Roberts, G. D.: Evaluation of a caffeic acid-ferric citrate test for rapid identification of *Cryptococcus neoformans.* J. Clin. Microbiol., *6*:445, 1977.
Wickerham, L. J., and Burton, K. A.: Carbon assimilation tests for the classification of yeasts. J. Bacteriol., *56*:363, 1948.

General References

Ajello, L.: Epidemiology of human fungous infections. *In* Dalldorf, G. (ed.): Fungi and Fungous Diseases. Springfield, Ill., Charles C Thomas, Publisher, 1962, p. 69.
Baker, R. D.: Human Infection With Fungi, Actinomycetes and Algae. New York, Springer-Verlag, 1971.
Braude, A. I.: Diseases caused by fungi. *In* Thorn, G. W., Adams, R. D., Braunwald, E., Isselbacher, K. S., and Petersdorf, R. G. (eds.): Harrison's Principles of Internal Medicine, 8th ed. New York, McGraw-Hill Book Co., 1977, p. 937.
Conant, N. F., Smith, D. T., Baker, R. D., and Callaway, J. L.: Manual of Clinical Mycology, 3rd ed. Philadelphia, W. B. Saunders Company, 1971.
Emmons, C. W., Binford, C. H., Utz, J. P., and Kwon-Chung, K. J.: Medical Mycology, 3rd ed. Philadelphia, Lea and Febiger, 1977.
Kaufman, L.: Serodiagnosis of fungal diseases. *In* Rose, N. R., and Friedman, H. (eds.) Manual of Clinical Immunology. Washington, D.C., American Society for Microbiology, 1976, p. 363.
Kersting, D. W.: The pathology of deep fungous infections. *In* Robinson, H. M. (ed.): The Diagnosis and Treatment of Fungal Infections. Springfield, Ill., Charles C Thomas, Publisher, 1974, p. 277.
Koneman, E. W., Roberts, G. D., and Wright, S. F.: Practical Laboratory Mycology, 2nd ed. Baltimore, Williams and Wilkins Company, 1978.
Rippon, J. W.: Medical Mycology: The Pathogenic Fungi

and the Pathogenic Actinomycetes. Philadelphia, W. B. Saunders Company, 1974.

Schwartz, J.: The pathogenesis of histoplasmosis, *In* Ajello, L., Chick, E. W., and Furcolow, M. F. (eds.): Histoplasmosis. Springfield, Ill., Charles C Thomas, Publisher, 1971, p. 244.

Silva-Hutner, M., and Cooper, B. H.: Medically important yeasts. *In* Lennette, E. H., Spaulding, E. H. and Truant, J. P. (eds.): Manual of Clinical Microbiology, 2nd ed. Washington, D.C., American Society for Microbiology, 1974, p. 491.

Wilson, J. W., and Plunkett, O. A.: The Fungous Diseases of Man. Berkeley, University of California Press, 1965.

51

MEDICAL PARASITOLOGY

James W. Smith, M.D.,
and Yezid Gutierrez, M.D., Ph.D.

5

Parasitic diseases are of great importance to the world and contribute significantly to economic, social, and medical problems. As a result of improved sanitation and better control of insect hosts, the incidence of parasitic diseases has decreased, particularly in "developed" countries such as the United States. With increasing world travel, however, the possibility of seeing various parasitic infections in visitors or returning citizens has increased.

Diagnosis of parasitic diseases is generally established by morphologic demonstration of parasites or by immune response to parasites. Occasionally, culture or animal inoculation may be used. Proper diagnosis requires that (1) the physician consider that a parasite might be a cause of the disease, (2) appropriate specimens be obtained and properly transported to the laboratory, (3) the laboratory competently examine the specimens, (4) the laboratory results

be effectively communicated to the physician, and (5) these results be correctly interpreted and applied to the care of the patient. A basic knowledge of the natural cycle of the disease is important in determining the diagnostic approach. Parasites may cause clinical disease at a time when diagnostic forms are not yet present in the usual site; for example, Ascaris larval migration may cause symptomatology weeks before eggs are present in feces. The overall expansion of medical knowledge has led to a decrease in the time devoted to parasitology during physician training, and thus clinicians may not be knowledgeable about parasitic diseases. In addition, most laboratories in the United States see few positive parasitology specimens from patients, often seeing a wider variety of parasites in material from proficiency testing programs than from patients. To use the laboratory optimally, the clinician must have an understanding of the adequacy of the methods and personnel in the laboratory examining specimens from his patients.

Figures on parasite prevalence are difficult to obtain. Laboratory methods used, population studied, and criteria for diagnosis vary. A recent review of the incidence of various intestinal parasites in fecal specimens examined by State Health Department Laboratories (CDC, Aug. 1977) (Table 51-1) gives some indication of the relative importance of various infections. However, in interpreting those figures, the following facts should be considered. These are results of specimens submitted for parasite examinations and thus do not represent prevalence figures. There is variation in methods used and in proficiency of various laboratories. Patterns of physician use

of these laboratories vary in different states. Examination of fecal specimens does not reflect accurately the incidence of enterobiasis, as fecal examination is not the best way to diagnose this infection. The incidence of specific parasites varies in different parts of the country. It is interesting to note that, nationwide, 15.5 per cent of specimens were positive for fecal parasites, with the frequency of positive specimens, in individual states, varying from 1 to 35 per cent.

Another recent review of helminth infections in the United States (Warren, 1974) estimates a similar incidence of *Trichuris trichiura*, *Strongyloides stercoralis*, hookworm, and *Hymenolepis nana*, a higher (4 per cent) incidence of *Ascaris lumbricoides*, and a much higher (42 per cent) incidence of *Enterobius*

Table 51-1. INCIDENCE OF INTESTINAL PARASITES IN 388,745 FECAL SPECIMENS EXAMINED BY STATE HEALTH DEPARTMENT LABORATORIES, 1976*

PARASITE	NUMBER	PER CENT OF SPECIMENS	PER CENT OF POSITIVE SPECIMENS	PER CENT OF ALL IDENTIFICATIONS
Protozoa	48,353			61.1
Giardia lamblia	14,773	3.8	24.5	18.7
Entamoeba histolytica	2,486	0.6	4.1	3.1
Dientamoeba fragilis	1,588	0.4	2.6	2.0
Balantidium coli	21	†		
Isospora belli	3			
Non-pathogenic	29,482	7.6		37.3
Nematodes	29,107			36.8
Ascaris lumbricoides	9,207	2.4	15.2	11.6
Trichuris trichiura	8,796	2.3	14.6	11.1
Enterobius vermicularis	7,088	1.8	11.7	9.0
Hookworm	3,216	0.8	5.3	4.1
Strongyloides stercoralis	757	0.2	1.3	1.0
Trichostrongylus sp.	22			
Heterodera sp.	21			
Trematodes	396			0.5
Clonorchis/opisthorchis	210	0.05	0.3	0.3
Schistosoma mansoni	143	0.04	0.2	0.2
Fasciolopsis buski	5			
Heterophyes heterophyes	3			
Fasciola hepatica	1			
Metagonimus yokogawai	1			
Paragonimus westermani	1			
Cestodes	1,205			1.5
Hymenolepis nana	946	0.2	1.6	1.2
Taenia sp.	209	0.05	0.3	0.3
T. solium	6			
T. saginata	45			
Taenia sp. unknown	158	0.04	0.2	0.2
Hymenolepis diminuta	23			
Diphyllobothrium latum	25			
Dipylidium caninum	2			

*Adapted from Center for Disease Control: Intestinal Parasite Surveillance. Annual Summary, 1976. Issued August, 1977. Does not include laboratories in Guam, Puerto Rico, or Virgin Islands.

†Percentages are not calculated for parasites identified less than 100 times.

vermicularis infections. It also estimates a greater incidence of taenia (0.2 per cent) and schistosome (0.2 per cent) infections.

Parasitic life cycles may be simple, as in amebae and pinworms, or complex, as in malaria and schistosomiasis. If there are multiple hosts, the definitive host harbors the sexual stage of the life cycle and the intermediate host(s) the asexual stage(s). A reservoir host is a host other than man that may also be parasitized by the same stage(s) of the parasite as man and thus serve as a source of infection. Man is an incidental host of some animal parasites.

The transmission of parasitic diseases is often influenced by sanitation, housing, diet, cooking, and social customs. In addition, geographic factors, such as rivers, climate, and altitude may play a significant role. Control efforts are aimed at breaking the life cycle in one or several places; for instance, eliminating a host, removing the reservoir of infection, assuring a safe water supply, or developing sanitary means of disposal of feces.

In this section, emphasis is on laboratory diagnosis. Sufficient information is given about parasitology, epidemiology, clinical disease, and pathology to allow the reader to have a basic understanding of the disease. For more detailed information, the reader is referred to some of the many excellent books on parasitology and tropical medicine (Adams, 1976; Belding, 1965; Brown, 1975; Faust, 1970; 1975; Hunter, 1976; Manson-Bahr, 1966; Markell, 1976) and pathology (Edington, 1969; Marcial-Rojas, 1971; Spencer, 1973).

In parasitology, as in other areas of biologic science, there are disagreements about taxonomy, pathogenesis, and methodology. We have not attempted to resolve these but have attempted to take a middle ground. Laboratory results that are not of direct diagnostic value will not be discussed. The amount of discussion given to each parasitic infection is in part based on the frequency and importance of the infection.

LABORATORY METHODS

Numerous methods for diagnosis of parasitic diseases have been described; some are useful in detecting a wide variety of parasites, and others are particularly useful for one or a few parasites. It is better for the laboratory to offer a limited number of procedures compe-

tently performed than to offer a wide variety of infrequently and poorly performed tests. The methods described are widely used and should provide good results in the hands of proficient laboratory personnel. Some methods useful in special situations are briefly described or referenced in the text under appropriate organisms. Descriptions of a variety of procedures of general and limited usefulness may be found in various parasitology and tropical medicine books and in books emphasizing methodology (Garcia, 1975; Lennette, 1974; U.S. Naval Medical School, 1965; Melvin, 1974).

The type of specimen collected will depend upon the species and form of parasite suspected. Knowledge of the life cycle of the parasite aids in determining the type, number, and frequency of specimens for diagnosis.

CALIBRATION OF AN OCULAR MICROMETER

Measurement of size of parasites is important for accurately identifying both protozoa and helminths and should be done using an ocular micrometer that has been properly calibrated for each objective of each microscope with which it is to be used (Fig. 51-1).

CALIBRATION OF OCULAR MICROMETER

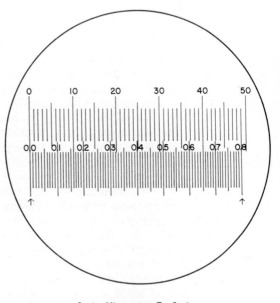

Ocular Micrometer–Top Scale
Stage Micrometer–Bottom Scale

Figure 51-1. Example of calibrated ocular micrometer. From Melvin, D. M. and Brooke, M. M.: Laboratory Procedures for the Diagnosis of Intestinal Parasites. U. S. Department of Health, Education, and Welfare, Public Health Service, 1974.

1. An ocular micrometer is inserted into the ocular element so that the scale is in focus when the microscope is in focus.
2. A ruled stage micrometer is placed on the microscope stage, the iris diaphragm is partially shut to reduce light, and the ruled scale is brought into focus.
3. The ocular micrometer scale and the stage micrometer scale are moved until the 0's align. Then the ocular micrometer is examined until a division is found which also aligns with a division on the stage micrometer. Each large division of the stage micrometer equals 0.1 mm (100 microns) and each small division equals 0.01 mm (10 microns).
4. Distance between small ocular units is calculated by determining the distance in microns between two aligned divisions on the stage micrometer and dividing by the number of small ocular units between the same aligned divisions. The result is the distance between ocular units in microns. In the example in Figure 51-1, 10 ocular units = 0.16 mm (160 μ); therefore, one ocular unit = 0.016 mm or 16 μ.
5. Record the unit value of an ocular micrometer division (in microns) using each objective of the microscope. Each microscope must be calibrated separately.
6. To determine the size of an object, count the number of ocular units that represent the dimension to be measured and multiply this number by the value calculated in Step 4 for the magnification used.

BLOOD EXAMINATION

Two types of blood films are prepared for diagnosis of blood parasite infections: thin films and thick films. In the thin film, the blood is spread over the slide in a thin layer and the red blood cells are intact after staining. In the thick film, the blood is concentrated in a small area and is many cell layers deep. During staining, the red cells are lysed, and only white blood cells, platelets, and parasites (if present) will be visible. The thick film is preferred for diagnosis, since it contains 16 to 30 times as much blood per microscopic field as does the thin film, thus increasing the chances of detecting minimal ("light") infections and decreasing the time needed for a reliable examination. In well-prepared films, approximately the same amount of blood can be examined with the oil immersion lens in a thick film in five minutes as can be examined in a thin film in 30 minutes.

Parasite species can usually be determined from thick films by an experienced examiner. However, since morphologic characteristics, particularly those of the malarial parasites, are more definitive in thin films, these preparations may sometimes be needed for definite species identification. For routine examination both thick and thin films should be prepared. They may be prepared on separate slides, but a combination slide, with the thin film on one end and the thick film on the other, is often used.

Preparation of slides

Blood for examination may be obtained by finger stick, ear lobe puncture, or venipuncture. If obtained by venipuncture, the first drop of blood (anticoagulant-free) from the needle is used to prepare the films. Films, especially for diagnosis of malaria, should *not* be prepared from anticoagulated or clotted blood. Anticoagulants may cause distortion of the organisms and interfere with staining, particularly of the older malarial stages that may stain palely and appear degenerate. Anticoagulants do not interfere with the staining of microfilariae. If 70 per cent alcohol is used to disinfect the site of the stick, it must be wiped off or allowed to dry to assure that it does not fix blood cells and prevent dehemoglobinization. Slides (even if new and "precleaned") should be cleaned with alcohol or acetone and polished dry with a lint-free cloth to assure that thick film will adhere and thin film will spread evenly.

A thin film is prepared in the manner described in the hematology section. Thick films may be prepared by touching the undersurface to a drop of blood on a stuck finger and rotating the slide to cover an area the size of a dime (1.5 cm). An alternate method is to puddle several small drops of blood with the corner of a slide. A proper thick film should be thin enough that newspaper print may be read through it. If too thick, the film may peel from the slide.

Slides may be prepared with a thin film on one end and thick film on the other. In such instances, only the thin film should be fixed with methyl alcohol (30 seconds) and contact of the thick film with alcohol fumes must be avoided. Thick films should be allowed to dry flat at room temperature, usually overnight. Excess heat may fix erythrocytes and prevent dehemoglobinization.

Staining

Blood begins to lose its affinity for stain in about three days and older thick films do not dehemoglobinize well. Staining is best performed with Giemsa stain. Wright's stain may be used for thin films, but is unsatisfactory for thick films because it fixes the erythrocytes. Fresh working Giemsa stain solution must be made each day by diluting stock Giemsa stain (commercially available) with M/150 phosphate buffered water, pH 7.0 to 7.2.* One part stock is added to 50 parts water in a Coplin jar and slides are stained for 50 minutes. (Thin films may alternatively be stained for 20 minutes with a stain of one part Giemsa stock added to 20 parts buffered water.)

After staining, thin films are rinsed by briefly dipping the slide in buffered water. Thick film should be rinsed an additional 3 to 5 minutes in buffered water. Slides are allowed to air dry and are then examined with low power for microfilariae and with high power and oil immersion for blood and tissue protozoa.

FECAL SPECIMENS

Infection with intestinal helminths can in most instances be diagnosed by demonstration of eggs or larvae in feces. Intestinal protozoan infections are diagnosed by finding trophozoites or cysts in feces. For many parasites, the number of diagnostic forms in feces varies little from day to day; however, there may be marked variations of some such as *Strongyloides* and *Giardia*. Some helminths produce many eggs per day and others produce few. It is advisable to select methods for routine examination that will allow identification of both helminth and protozoan parasites with use of other methods only when special situations require. As a minimum, laboratories performing fecal examinations for parasites should be capable of performing direct examination, a concentration procedure, and a permanent stain method.

Specimen collection and handling

Detection and identification of parasites depends upon properly collected and handled specimens. Old, poorly preserved, or contaminated specimens are of little value. Specimens should not be collected for one week after the patient has been taking materials which leave

*Buffered water for Giemsa stain—pH 7.0-7.2
Acid buffer M/15 NaH$_2$PO$_4$—39 ml
Alkaline buffer M/15 Na$_2$PO$_4$—61 ml
Distilled water—900 ml
Check pH

crystalline residue, such as anti-diarrheal compounds, antacids, bismuth, and barium. In addition, oily laxatives, such as mineral oil, may interfere with examination. Antibiotics and contrast media may decrease the numbers of organisms, particularly protozoa, in the stool for two to three weeks. Specimens should be free of urine and should not be contaminated with toilet water or soil, as these may contain free living protozoa and helminths or may destroy trophozoites. Water stored in the laboratory may also become contaminated with these organisms. Specimens may be collected directly into clean, dry paper cartons, or may be collected in bed pans or, if not diarrheic, by squatting over wax paper. They should be submitted to the laboratory in containers with tight-fitting lids.

Because the number of diagnostic forms of some parasites may vary, it is advisable to examine specimens obtained every second or third day with a total of three specimens being a minimum to assure freedom from infection.

When a series of normally passed stools has been examined without identification of parasites, purged specimens may be desirable, particularly when protozoan infections are suspected. Saline purgatives, such as sodium sulfate or buffered phosphosoda, should be used rather than mineral oil or magnesia compounds, which may interfere with examination because of oil globules or crystalline debris. If a purged series is being collected, each specimen should be collected separately and submitted to the laboratory as soon as possible after collection. It is wise to alert the laboratory prior to submitting a purged series.

Each specimen must be appropriately labeled with proper identification information and must include the date and time of collection. Specimens should be submitted to the laboratory as soon as possible and should be handled expeditiously on arrival in the laboratory. Time is particularly important for loose and watery specimens because protozoan trophozoites may degenerate rapidly. Ideally, liquid specimens should be examined or placed in fixatives within one hour after passage. Specimens that cannot be processed immediately should be left at room temperature or refrigerated and should not be placed in an incubator, as this only speeds disintegration of parasites.

If specimens must be collected at home or must be mailed to the laboratory, it is advisable to use a two-vial preservation technique with one portion of the specimen being fixed in three parts of 5 to 10 per cent buffered formalin and another portion of the specimen being fixed in three parts of polyvinyl alcohol (PVA) fixative. The specimen must be thoroughly mixed when placed in these fixatives. Specimens that arrive in the laboratory late in the day or during evening hours or that cannot be examined promptly may also be preserved by this two-vial technique. Other systems of preservation have been described (see Melvin, 1974), but most do not provide material with which to make permanently stained slides.

Gross examination

Fecal specimens should be examined grossly. The consistency of the specimen should be noted and recorded as formed, soft, loose, or watery. Protozoan trophozoites are most likely to be found in watery, loose, or soft specimens and cysts in formed, soft, or loose specimens. Proglottids or adult worms may be detected by gross examination and, in addition, flecks of blood or mucus may be specifically selected for examination.

Many parasites are uniformly distributed in the stool as a result of the mixing action of the cecum (Martin, 1965); however, eggs that enter the fecal stream in the lower colon and rectum (such as schistosomes) may be unevenly distributed, as may taenia eggs and pinworm eggs that are released by rupture of parasites.

Microscopic examinations

Specimens may be examined microscopically by direct wet mounts of fresh or preserved material, concentrated wet mounts, or permanent stains. Each procedure has specific advantages. Direct saline wet mounts of fresh feces allow detection and observation of motile protozoan trophozoites and helminth larvae. Direct mounts of preserved feces may allow detection of parasites that do not concentrate well. Concentration procedures increase the ability to detect protozoan cysts and helminth eggs and larvae, but generally are unsatisfactory for detecting protozoan trophozoites. Permanent stains are useful for detection and morphologic examination of protozoan trophozoites and cysts.

At a minimum, formed stool specimens should be examined by direct wet mounts and concentration; watery stools should be examined by permanent stains and direct wet mounts; and soft and liquid stools should be examined by direct wet mounts, concentration, and permanent stain procedures.

Wet Mounts. Direct wet mounts or wet mounts of concentrated material are best made using 3 by 2 inch slides (rather than 3 by 1 inch) and 22 mm No. 1 coverslips. This prevents leaking of specimen onto the microscope and allows room to seal the coverslip with vaspar if desired (see below). Fecal preparations should be thick enough that newspaper print can just be read through them. Large particles should be avoided, as they prevent a proper fit of the coverslip. Air bubbles should also be avoided. Generally a double mount will be made, one unstained and one stained with a drop of iodine solution. The iodine should be that of Dobell and O'Connor (Lennette, 1974)* or a 1:5 dilution of Lugol's iodine. An overly strong iodine solution, such as straight Lugol's or Gram's iodine, will cause clumping of material and will obscure organisms. Iodine makes nuclear structure of protozoan cysts more evident and stains glycogen masses; however, chromatoid bodies are less visible than in saline mounts and cysts are less refractile and thus may be more difficult to find. The unstained mount of fresh feces should be made in physiologic saline (0.85 per cent). For preserved feces, diluent is needed only if the preparation is too dense. Wet mounts may be used to examine a variety of body fluids in addition to feces.

Sealing of the wet mount with vaspar allows use of the oil immersion objective to examine the slide and prevents drying of the preparation. Vaspar is a 50/50 mixture of Vaseline and paraffin, which is heated on a hotplate till melted. A camel's-hair brush or cotton tipped applicator is dipped in the melted vaspar and touched to opposite corners of the coverslip to attach it to the 3 by 2 inch slide, then with even strokes, vaspar is applied to the edges of the coverslip until it is completely sealed. This may require several dips.

Microscopically examine the mount in a sys-

---

*Dobell and O'Connor's Iodine Solution
    Iodine (powdered crystals)   1 g
    Potassium iodide   2 g
    Distilled water   100 ml
Dissolve potassium iodide in water. Add iodine crystals and shake thoroughly. Filter or decant into dark bottle. Store away from light. Solution should be color of medium strong tea. Shelf life is at least two weeks.

tematic fashion so that the entire coverslip is scanned. A good method is to begin in one corner and, using the stage, move up and down so that each field can be methodically scanned with the 10× objective. It may be worthwhile also to scan across the coverslip several times with the high dry or oil immersion objective to ensure that small protozoa are not missed. Identification of protozoa should be with the 40× or 100× oil immersion objective. 20× dry and 50× oil immersion objectives, in addition to the usual 10× and 40× dry and 100× oil, may be useful in parasitology.

Concentration Procedures.   Concentration procedures increase the ability to detect protozoan cysts and helminth eggs and larvae by decreasing the amount of background material in the preparations and by an actual concentration of organisms. Concentration procedures may be performed on fresh or preserved specimens. A wide variety of methods and modifications have been described; some of which are useful only for specific parasites. For routine use, a method should be selected that will allow reliable detection of both protozoan cysts and helminth eggs. Concentration methods generally employ sedimentation, in which the heavier parasites settle to the bottom owing to gravity or centrifugation, or flotation, in which the parasites rise to the surface of a solution of high specific gravity.

The two most widely used procedures in the United States are the zinc sulfate centrifugal flotation technique of Faust and the formalin-ether sedimentation technique of Ritchie or modifications of them. Methods are described below for performing each technique on fresh specimens or formalin-preserved feces. The formalin-ether sedimentation technique has somewhat greater sensitivity in detecting most parasites but requires the use of ether, which may present storage, handling, and disposal problems. The formalin-zinc sulfate method described is recommended for laboratories that cannot use ether. Formalin fixation prevents distortion of eggs, cysts, and larvae and prevents popping of opercula. Centrifugation in both concentration procedures should be done in a free-swinging rather than an angle centrifuge.

FORMALIN-ETHER PROCEDURE. This concentration procedure is efficient in recovering most protozoan cysts and helminth eggs and larvae, including operculate eggs, and is moderately effective for schistosome eggs. Less distortion of cysts occurs with this technique than with the zinc sulfate method. *Hymenolepis nana* eggs may be missed, however, and concentration of *Giardia lamblia* and *Iodamoeba bütschlii* cysts may not be very good.

Technique for Fresh Specimens
Adapted from Melvin, 1974)

1. Comminute a portion of stool about 2 cm diameter in sufficient saline so that 10 ml of suspension will yield about 1 ml of sediment upon centrifugation. The suspension can be prepared in the carton in which it is submitted (if portions for permanent staining are removed first) or in a beaker or a flat-bottom paper cup. Water may be used in place of saline.

2. Strain about 10 ml of the suspension through a small funnel containing wet gauze or cheesecloth into a 15 ml conical centrifuge tube. (To conserve glassware, a cone-shaped paper cup [about a 4-ounce size] with the point cut off can be substituted for a funnel.)

3. Centrifuge at 650 g for 1 to 2 minutes. Decant supernatant. About 1 to 1.5 ml of sediment should be present. If the amount is much larger or smaller, adjust to the proper quantity in the following manner.

   a. Amount too large

      Resuspend the sediment in saline (or water) and pour out a portion. For example, if the amount is twice the desired quantity, pour out about half of the suspension and then add saline (or water) to bring the fluid level to about 10 ml and centrifuge again.

   b. Amount too small

      Pour off the supernatant and strain a second portion of the original fecal suspension into the tube. The amount to be strained can be determined from the amount of sediment; that is, if about half of the quantity necessary is obtained with the first centrifugation, strain another 10 ml into the tube. Centrifuge again. It is not necessary to have an exact quantity of sediment in the tube, but the quantity should approximate the amount indicated above.

4. Resuspend the sediment in fresh saline (or water), centrifuge, and decant as before.

5. Add about 9 ml of 10 per cent formalin to the sediment, mix thoroughly, and allow to stand for 5 minutes or longer. At this point, the formalin-feces mixture may be stoppered and saved until a later time.

   Note: Plastic squeeze bottles for saline and formalin will facilitate dispensing these solutions into the tubes.

6. Add 3 ml of ether, stopper the tube, and shake vigorously in an inverted position for at least 30 seconds. Remove the stopper with care.

7. Centrifuge at 450 to 500 g for 1 minute. Four layers should result as follows: (1) layer of

ether, (2) plug of debris, (3) layer of formalin, and (4) sediment.

8. Free the plug of debris from the sides of the tube by ringing with an applicator stick and carefully decant and discard the top three layers. Use a cotton swab to clean debris from the walls of the tube.

9. With a pipette, mix the remaining sediment with the small amount of fluid that drains back from the sides of the tube and prepare iodine and unstained mounts for microscopic examination. If not enough fluid is left in the tube, a drop of saline or 10 per cent formalin can be added to the sediment.

10. If examination of the specimen is delayed, add 1 or 2 ml of 10 per cent formalin to the sediment and stopper the tube. Formalinized sediments may be kept for some time if they do not dry. Remove the excess formalin before making mounts.

Technique for Formalin-preserved Specimens

1. Thoroughly stir the formalinized specimen.

2. Depending on the size and density of the specimen, strain a sufficient quantity through wet gauze into a conical 15 ml centrifuge tube to give 0.5 to 0.75 ml of sediment. Usually 4 to 5 ml is sufficient unless the fecal suspension is thin. In formalin-preserved specimens, the formalin has clarified the feces to some extent, and further clarification is caused primarily by the ether. Therefore, the sediment volume during concentration is not as great as with fresh feces, and the initial quantity must be less.

3. Add tap water to make 10 ml of suspension, mix thoroughly, and centrifuge at 500 to 650 g for 1 to 2 minutes.

4. Decant supernatant and, if desired, wash again with tap water. The amount of sediment should be about 0.5 to 0.75 ml. If too much or too little is present, adjust the quantity by the method described for fresh material.

5. Add 9 ml of 10 per cent formalin (preferably buffered) to the sediment and mix thoroughly.

6. Add 4 ml of ether, stopper the tube, and shake ;orously in an inverted position for at least 30 .onds. Remove the stopper with care.

7. ɪ .oceed as with fresh specimen.

FORMALIN-ZINC SULFATE FLOTATION PROCEDURE. The original zinc sulfate flotation procedure was developed by Faust in 1938 for the recovery of both helminth eggs and larvae and protozoan cysts. Since that time various modifications have been described. The modification described here is performed on formalin-fixed fecal suspensions. This helps to clear the specimen and prevents popping of opercula and distortion of parasites. The method is unsatisfactory for detecting schistosome eggs.

Procedure

1. Strain a well-mixed fecal suspension through one layer of gauze into a round-bottomed 100 by 16 mm tube to within 2 cm of the rim (the specimen must have been fixed in formalin for at least 30 minutes).

2. Centrifuge at approximately 750 g for $3\frac{1}{2}$ minutes. A free-swinging centrifuge must be used. Allow the centrifuge to come to a full stop without braking before lifting the lid.

3. Decant the supernatant from each tube, draining the last drop against a clean section of paper towel, and place upright in a test tube rack.

Steps 4 through 10 must be done without interruption.

4. Add zinc sulfate to within 2.5 cm of the rim of each tube. To prepare the zinc sulfate solution, dissolve about 400 g of $ZnSO_4$ in one liter of water. Check the specific gravity with a good hydrometer and adjust as necessary to between 1.195 and 1.200, preferably closer to 1.200. Store in tightly stoppered container. Specific gravity should be checked at least once a week.

5. Mix the packed sediment thoroughly with two applicator sticks until no coarse particles remain.

6. Immediately centrifuge at 500 g for one and one half minutes in a free-swinging centrifuge.

7. As soon as the centrifuge comes to a full stop (without braking), very carefully transfer the tubes to a rack. Avoid disturbing the surface films, which now contain the floating parasites.

8. Allow the tubes to stand undisturbed for one full minute; then with a wire loop in which the loop is at a right angle to the stem, carefully transfer two loops of the surface film to the corresponding drops of saline or Dobell and O'Connor's iodine on a 3 by 2 inch glass slide. Touch the loop carefully to the surface film without dipping below the surface and deposit the drop in the loop beside a drop of saline or iodine. Then, using the heel of the loop, mix the fecal drops first in the saline then in the iodine.

9. Place a clean 22 by 30 mm, No. 1 coverslip on the fluid mount, avoiding trapped air bubbles.

10. Flame the wire loop, then proceed with steps 8 and 9 on the next tube.

11. Place each prepared slide mount in a Petri dish containing a moist paper towel to retard evaporation.

12. Examine the mounts immediately or at least within the hour. A longer holding period may make the identification of some stages more difficult.

Permanent Stain Technique. A variety of different permanent stains have been described and have advantages and disadvantages. The most widely used technique in the United States is the Wheatley trichrome method, and it is the only stain which will be described. Iron hematoxylin and phosphotungstic acid hematoxylin stains are other widely used stains for fixed fecal smears. Chlorazol black E is also a satisfactory stain but must be used on fresh fecal material; thus, it cannot be used on material fixed with polyvinyl alcohol fixative.

Films for permanent staining may be prepared on clean 1 by 3 inch glass slides. Fresh films are made by smearing the fecal sample on a slide with applicator sticks in an even uniform smear, then fixing immediately in Schaudinn's fixative (slides must not be allowed to dry). After fixation of one hour or longer at room temperature, staining may be performed. PVA-fixed material should be well mixed and then smeared on the slide as described above, being sure the smear extends to the edges of the slide to prevent peeling. Leave smears at room temperature or in an incubator overnight to ensure they are dry before staining.

WHEATLEY TRICHROME STAIN (Melvin, 1974). Trichrome stain is relatively simple and rapid and uses reagents that are stable. It may be used with either fresh or PVA-fixed material, the only difference being in the timing of some staining steps. The method is simple in that overstaining and differentiation are not necessary to bring out the morphologic details of the parasites, nor is it necessary to treat with a mordant before staining. However, destaining the smears gives better differentiation of the organisms, and this step should be included. The stain solution is stable and may be used repeatedly, the lost volume being replaced by adding stock solution. Staining over 15 smears daily (in 50 ml of stain), however, tends to weaken the stain. If stain is allowed to evaporate, strength will return. This can be accomplished by leaving the cover off the staining dish for several hours or overnight. The staining of fresh and PVA-fixed material differs chiefly in the increased time required for the latter and in the omission of the fixative step, since the material in the PVA solution is already fixed. Both procedures are given below. Each numbered step indicates a different Coplin jar. Control slides of known staining quality should be run with each batch of slides stained. Positive material is preferred, but negative material is satisfactory.

Staining Technique with Fresh Specimens
1. Schaudinn's fixative
   (Solution No. 1) ......5 min at 50°C. or 1 hr at room temperature. Do not allow smear to dry before placing it in Schaudinn's
2. 70% alcohol plus iodine
   (Solution No. 3) ......1 min (to remove mercuric chloride)

3. 70% alcohol ....1 min
4. 70% alcohol ....1 min
5. Stain (trichrome)
   (Solution No. 4) ......2-8 min
6. 90% alcohol, acidified
   (Solution No. 5) ......5-10 sec, total; usually a brief dip (in and out) is sufficient.

Since the acid alcohol continues to destain as long as it is in contact with the material, the time allowed *should include the few seconds between the time the slide is removed from the destain and rinsed in 95 per cent alcohol* (step 7). For more effective removal of the acid destain, two 95 per cent alcohol washes are suggested instead of one. These should be changed frequently to prevent them from becoming so acid that the destaining process will continue. Prolonged destaining in acid alcohol (over 20 seconds) may cause the organisms to be poorly differentiated, although larger trophozoites, particularly those of *Entamoeba coli*, may require slightly longer periods of decolorization.

Note: If several slides are being stained simultaneously, they should be destained separately. Remove only one slide at a time from the stain, destain it, rinse in the 95 per cent alcohols, and place it in the carbol-xylene (step 9).

7. 95% alcohol..............................Rinse briefly
8. 95% alcohol..............................Rinse twice
9. 100% alcohol or carbol-xylene......1 min
10. Xylene.....................................1-3 min
11. Mount with coverslip using Permount or other mounting medium.

Staining Technique with PVA Films
1. 70% alcohol plus iodine
   (Solution No. 3) .....10-20 min
2. 70% alcohol.................3-5 min
3. 70% alcohol.................3-5 min
4. Trichrome stain
   (Solution No. 4).........8 min
5. 90% alcohol, acidified
   (Solution No. 5).........10-20 sec, total (See previous paragraph on destaining.)
6. 95% alcohol.................Rinse to remove acid destain
7. 95% alcohol.................5 min
8. Carbol-xylene...............5-10 min
9. Xylene........................10 min
10. Mount with coverslip using Permount or other mounting medium.

TRICHROME STAIN REACTIONS. The cytoplasm of thoroughly fixed and well-stained cysts and trophozoites is blue-green tinged with purple. Occasionally, *Entamoeba coli* cysts may stain slightly more purplish than cysts of other species. The nuclear chromatin, chromatoid bodies, and ingested red cells and bacteria stain red or purplish red. Other ingested particles, such as yeasts or molds, generally stain green, but variations frequently occur in the color reaction of ingested particles. Background material usually stains green, thus contrasting with the protozoa.

Non-staining cysts and those staining predominantly red are most frequently associated with incomplete fixation. Unsatisfactorily stained organisms obtained from specimens submitted in PVA-fixative usually indicate incomplete fixation associated with poor mixing of feces with fixative. Thorough mixing will yield critically stained cysts and trophozoites. Organisms, especially trophozoites, in soft or liquid specimens often stain better than those from formed specimens. Degenerate forms stain pale green, although understained or overstained organisms may also appear green.

Eggs and larvae stain red and contrast strongly with the green background. Thin-shelled eggs often collapse when placed in mounting medium, although some diagnostic features may be retained, especially if the smear is examined immediately.

Mononuclear and polymorphonuclear leukocytes and *Blastocystis* must be differentiated from protozoa. The nuclei of pus cells and tissue cells stain red and the cytoplasm green. However, the cytoplasm of these cells does stain more greenish than that of the protozoa.

Preparation of Solutions

Solution No. 1—Schaudinn's fixative

    Ethyl alcohol, 95%..............................1 part
    Saturated aqueous mercuric chloride......2 parts

Prepare saturated aqueous mercuric chloride by adding 90 g of mercuric chloride crystals to one liter of distilled water. Dissolve by heating and then let cool (excess mercuric chloride will crystallize out). Filter the clear solution and store in a glass-stoppered bottle. Before use, add 5 ml of glacial acetic acid per 100 ml of solution.

Solution No. 2—PVA fixative

1. Stirring constantly, slowly add 5 g polyvinyl alcohol (PVA) powder to 100 ml modified Schaudinn's fixative at room temperature. (Modified Schaudinn's fixative contains 1.5 ml glycerol per 100 ml in addition to the other ingredients described above.)
2. Heat (to approximately 75°C.) while stirring until powder dissolves and solution clears (do not boil).
3. Cool to room temperature. Material should not be cloudy and should not gel. It is stable for months if visual examination is satisfactory. Prepared PVA fixative, or PVA powder, may be obtained from commercial sources (Delkote Inc., 76 So. Virginia Ave., Penns Grove, N.J. 08069). When ordering powder; specify pretested powder for use in making PVA fixative.

Solution No. 3—Iodine alcohol

Prepare a stock solution by adding enough iodine crystals to 70 per cent alcohol to make a dark, concentrated solution. Either ethyl or isopropyl alcohol may be used. For use, dilute some of the stock with 70 per cent alcohol until a strong tea-colored solution is obtained. The exact concentration is not important, but the solution should not be too dark, since the iodine may stain the protozoa and interfere with subsequent hematoxylin or trichrome staining. If it is too light, the mercuric chloride in the fixative will not be removed and mercuric chloride crystals in the finished preparation will interfere with examination.

Solution No. 4—Trichrome stain

    Chromotrope 2R ....0.6 g
    Light green SF..................0.15 g
    Fast green FCF..................0.15 g
    Phosphotungstic acid ....0.7 g
    Acetic acid (glacial) ....1.0 ml
    Distilled water....................100.0 ml

Put the dry stains into a clean, dry flask. Add the glacial acetic acid, stir to mix, and dampen all of the stain powder. Allow the mixture to stand ("ripen") for 30 minutes. Add the distilled water. Shake to mix thoroughly. The stain is stable and is used without diluting. Good stain is deep purple, almost black.

Solution No. 5—Acidified alcohol

    Acetic acid..........................0.45 ml
    90% ethyl alcohol.................99.55 ml

Cellulose tape technique for pinworms

Follow the directions in Figure 51-2 as described below:

1. Apply a strip of transparent cellulose tape 2½ to 3 inches in length to a glass slide so that the tape is wrapped around one end of the slide. (Frosted or opaque tape is not satisfactory.) A small portion of the end should be folded on itself to provide a non-sticky surface for handling the tape.
2. To obtain a sample, pull the folded tab so that the sticky side of the tape is freed, still leaving some of it stuck to the back of the slide.
3. Carry the freed tape over the end of a tongue blade so that the sticky side is out.
4. Hold the tape and slide against the tongue depressor.
5. Press the sticky surface onto the right and left perianal folds but do not insert the blade into the rectum.
6. Replace the tape onto the slide (these slides can be carried or sent by mail to the laboratory).
7. Pull tape back from the slide, leaving a small portion attached.
8. Add a drop of toluene and replace the tape on the slide. (The toluene clears everything except the eggs and adults, if present.)
9. Smooth out the tape with a piece of gauze, which should be disinfected and discarded. Examine for the eggs and female adults under the low power objective. In old or mailed-in specimens sometimes only empty egg shells are seen. (Other helminth eggs, especially *Taenia*, may occasionally be seen on the cellulose tapes.)

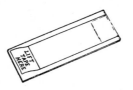
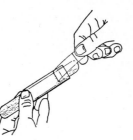

a. Cellulose-tape slide preparation

b. Hold slide against tongue depressor one inch from end and lift long portion of tape from slide

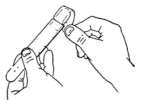
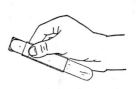

c. Loop tape over end of depressor to expose gummed surface

d. Hold tape and slide against tongue depressor

Figure 51-2. Use of cellulose tape slide preparation for diagnosis of pinworm infections. (Adapted from Brook, 1949.)

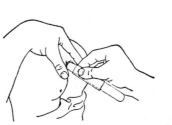

e. Press gummed surfaces against several areas of perianal region

f. Replace tape on slide

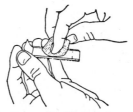

g. Smooth tape with cotton or gauze

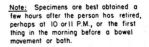

Note: Specimens are best obtained a few hours after the person has retired, perhaps at 10 or 11 P.M., or the first thing in the morning before a bowel movement or bath.

10. Remember that pinworm eggs are infectious, and specimens must be handled carefully to prevent infection.

Culture methods

Culture methods have been developed for a wide variety of protozoan parasites of man and for development of larvae of *Strongyloides stercoralis* and hookworm. Some, such as those for amebae (Melvin, 1974) may be of diagnostic aid, although they are not widely used. Cultures may also be used for research and teaching and for preparing antigens for various immunodiagnostic methods. For example, procedures have been developed for culturing malaria, leishmania, and pneumocystis. Infection of experimental animals has also proved helpful in similar ways but is not widely applied for diagnostic studies.

Immunodiagnostic methods

A variety of immunodiagnostic methods for parasitic diseases have been described (Kagan, 1976). Some are of proven value, and the reagents that are commercially available are those for amebiasis, toxoplasmosis, and trichinosis. Most others are available only from reference laboratories, such as the Center for Disease Control (via State Health Department Laboratories), are in development stages, or are research procedures. Various antigens and various serologic techniques are used, and interpretation is dependent on the specific method being used. These methods are constantly being modified and improved; therefore, specific interpretation criteria will not be given except for well-defined tests.

Various types of tests are described. Agglutination tests use whole organisms or, more commonly, antigen-coated particles. These include tests such as bentonite flocculation, indirect hemagglutination, latex agglutination, and cholesterol-lecithin flocculation. Complement fixation tests have been developed using various antigens from various organisms. Precipitin tests described include capillary precipitin, double gel diffusion, counterimmunoelectrophoresis, and circumlarval precipitin tests. Indirect immunofluorescence has been applied to a wide variety of protozoal and helminthic infections; however, problems exist with both sensitivity and specificity, and interpretation of results may be difficult. Serologic tests are most helpful when diagnostic forms cannot be readily demonstrated, as in tissue parasite infections such as amebic abscess of liver, trichinosis, and toxoplasmosis.

Quality control and safety

Quality control in parasitology is similar to quality control in other areas of the laboratory in that reagents and equipment must be monitored to assure that they will perform properly. In addition, performance of personnel should be monitored periodically with internal and/or external unknown specimens. Ready availability and use of reference material such as positive slides and fecal specimens, printed atlases (Spencer, 1961; Peters, 1977) or colored slide atlases (Smith, 1976 a, b, and c) containing diagnostic stages will aid in maintaining proficiency.

Unpreserved specimens submitted for parasitic examination should be considered potentially infectious, and in fact some preserved specimens may be infectious, as *Ascaris* eggs may survive and embryonate in 5 per cent formalin. Cysts of fecal protozoa, eggs of *Taenia solium, Enterobius vermicularis*, and *Hymenolepis nana*, and larvae of *Strongyloides stercoralis* may be infective in fresh specimens. *Trichuris trichiura, Ascaris lumbricoides*, and hookworm may be infective in older specimens. Malaria and hemoflagellates in blood or tissues may be infective. Parasites are not the only potentially infective forms in specimens. For example, feces submitted for parasitic examination may contain *Salmonella, Shigella, Vibrio cholerae*, enterotoxigenic *Escherichia coli*, or viruses. Strict observance of proper technique and proper disposal of contaminated material is essential. Personnel should not eat, drink, or smoke in the laboratory and should wash hands before doing any of these. Ether must not be used near a flame and should be purchased in small containers. Small quantities may be stored on an open shelf but larger amounts must be stored in approved storage cabinets for flammable solvent. Ether, which has a very low flash point ($-49°$F.), should not be stored in a refrigerator, not even an "explosion proof" refrigerator. Fumes may accumulate in the refrigerator and be released when the door is opened. If an ignition source is present in the room, an explosion may result.

PROTOZOA

MALARIA

Malaria is an acute and chronic protozoal infection which is characterized by fever, anemia, and splenomegaly. It generally occurs between 45° North and 40° South latitude (Coatney, 1971). The sporozoan parasites of the genus *Plasmodium* are spread by female anopheline mosquitoes. Four species of plasmodia cause human malaria: *P. vivax, P. falciparum, P. malariae*, and *P. ovale. P. falciparum* infection occurs principally in tropical areas, whereas *P. vivax* infections occur in a wider area, including temperate zones. *P. ovale* is the least frequent of the malarias, with most cases being acquired on the west coast of Africa.

Because of increasing world travel, malaria must be considered as a cause of fever even in malaria-free countries, and history of travel in endemic geographic areas should be sought. Diagnosis is established by demonstrating parasites in blood films.

Life cycle

Malaria parasites have a sexual phase termed sporogony in *Anopheles* mosquitoes and an asexual stage termed schizogony in man (Fig. 51-3). The female anopheline mosquito, when feeding on an infected individual, obtains microgametocyte (male) and macrogametocyte (female) sex cells of the malaria parasites. In the mosquito, these gametocytes mature and fertilization occurs. An oocyst is then formed on the stomach of the mosquito, and within this oocyst numerous spindle-shaped sporozoites are formed. The mature oocyst ruptures into the body cavity, releasing the sporozoites, which then migrate through the tissues to the salivary glands from which they are injected into the vertebrate host as the mosquito feeds. The time required for development in the mosquito ranges from 8 to 21 days.

The sporozoites injected into the vertebrate host reach the hepatic parenchymal cells, in which they undergo extensive proliferation. This stage is known as the pre-erythrocytic

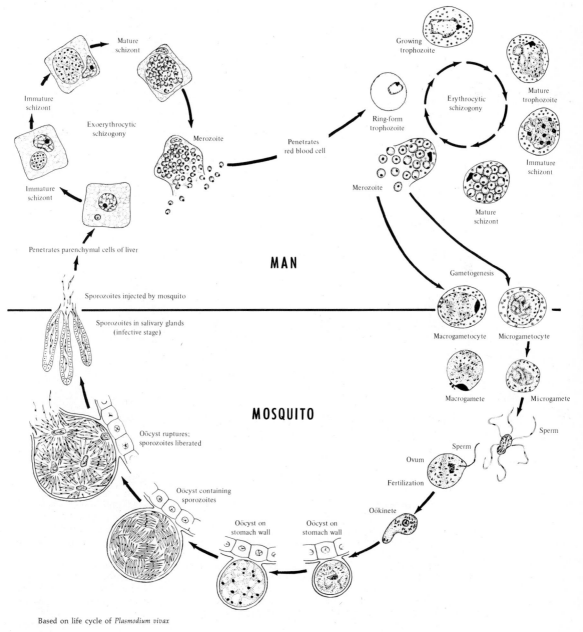

Based on life cycle of *Plasmodium vivax*

Figure 51-3. Life cycle of malaria. (Courtesy of the Center for Disease Control, Parasitology Training Branch, Atlanta, Ga.)

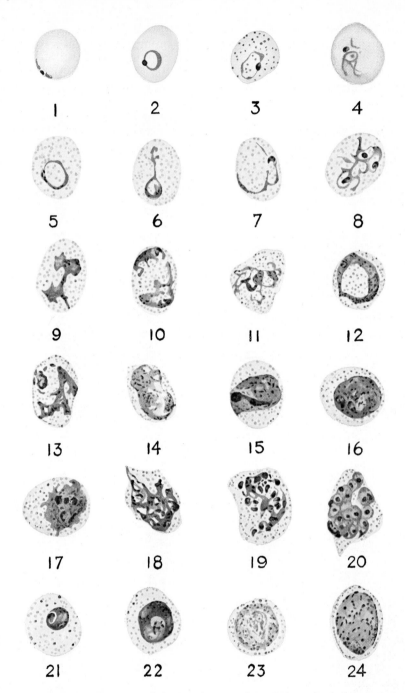

Figure 51–4. *Plasmodium vivax. 1.* Normal-size erythrocyte with marginal ring form trophozoite. *2.* Young signet-ring form of trophozoite in macrocyte. *3.* Slightly older ring form trophozoite in erythrocyte showing basophilic stippling. *4.* Polychromatophilic erythrocyte containing young tertian parasite with pseudopodia. *5.* Ring form of trophozoite showing pigment in cytoplasm of an enlarged cell containing Schüffner's stippling. This stippling does not appear in all cells containing the growing and older forms of *Plasmodium vivax,* but it can be found with any stage from the fairly young ring form onward. *6* and *7.* Very tenuous medium trophozoite forms. *8.* Three ameboid trophozoites with fused cytoplasm. *9, 11, 12,* and *13.* Older ameboid trophozoites in process of development. *10.* Two ameboid trophozoites in one cell. *14.* Mature trophozoite. *15.* Mature trophozoite with chromatin apparently in process of division. *16, 17, 18,* and *19.* Schizonts showing progressive steps in division (presegmenting schizonts). *20.* Mature schizont. *21* and *22.* Developing gametocytes. *23.* Mature microgametocyte. *24.* Mature macrogametocyte. (From Wilcox, A.: Manual for the Microscopical Diagnosis of Malaria in Man. Bulletin No. 180, National Institute of Health, 1942.)

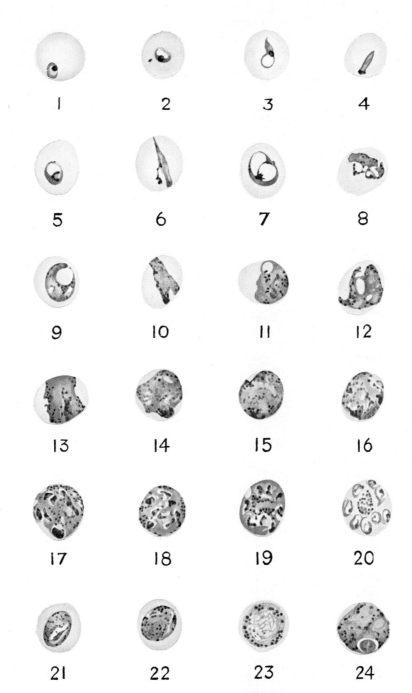

Figure 51–5. *Plasmodium malariae.* *1.* Young ring form trophozoite of quartan malaria. *2, 3,* and *4.* Young trophozoite forms of the parasite showing gradual increase of chromatin and cytoplasm. *5.* Developing ring form of trophozoite showing pigment granule. *6.* Early band form of trophozoite—elongated chromatin, some pigment apparent. *7, 8, 9, 10, 11,* and *12.* Some forms which the developing trophozoite of quartan may take. *13* and *14.* Mature trophozoites—one a band form. *15, 16, 17, 18,* and *19.* Phases in the development of the schizont (presegmenting schizonts). *20.* Mature schizont. *21.* Immature microgametocyte. *22.* Immature macrogametocyte. *23.* Mature microgametocyte. *24.* Mature macrogametocyte. (From Wilcox, A.: Manual for the Microscopical Diagnosis of Malaria in Man. Bulletin No. 180, National Institute of Health, 1942.)

phase of the disease. The parasites of *P. falciparum* and *P. malariae* do not persist within the hepatic cells, whereas those of *P. vivax* and *P. ovale* may persist in liver cells. This is important, for *P. vivax* and *P. ovale* may cause relapses arising from liver forms, whereas *P. falciparum* and *P. malariae* do not. Any recurrences of the latter are termed recrudescences and are felt to arise from persisting blood forms. The infected liver cells rupture, releasing numerous merozoites which then infect erythrocytes. *P. vivax* primarily infects young erythrocytes (Fig. 51-4), *P. malariae* primarily infects old erythrocytes (Fig. 51-5), and *P. falciparum* infects erythrocytes of all ages (Fig. 51-6).

The stages seen in the erythrocytes are trophozoites (growing forms), schizonts (dividing forms), and gametocytes (sexual forms). The youngest trophozoites have a globose shape with a central vacuole, a red chromatin mass, and a blue cytoplasm. In slides they appear to be rings and are generally referred to as rings or ring forms. Growing trophozoites beyond the ring stage have more abundant cytoplasm but still a single chromatin mass and may be irregular (ameboid) or compact. Mature trophozoites are usually compact but still have only one chromatin mass. Hemozoin (hematin) pigment from metabolized hemoglobin is not usually evident in ring forms but becomes evident in growing trophozoites. Schizonts are divided into immature schizonts, which are those that have two or more chromatin masses and an undivided cytoplasm, and mature schizonts, which have both cytoplasm and chromatin completely divided so that individual merozoites are evident. The mature schizont ruptures and the merozoites infect additional red cells. This erythrocytic cycle takes 48 hours in *P. falciparum*, *P. ovale*, and *P. vivax* infections and 72 hours in *P. malariae* infections (Figs. 51-5 to 51-7). Gametocytes (sex cells) develop directly from some merozoites. Those of *P. vivax*, *P. malariae*, and *P. ovale* are rounded, whereas those of *P. falciparum* are elongated (sausage-shaped). Macrogametocytes (female) are characterized by a compact chromatin mass, whereas microgametocytes (male) have chromatin that is more dispersed. Developing gametocytes are more compact than growing trophozoites.

Epidemiology

Endemic spread of malaria requires a reservoir of infection, an appropriate mosquito host, and a susceptible host. Control of malaria is directed at elimination of appropriate mosquitoes, removal of the reservoir of active cases, and prophylaxis of susceptible persons. However, emergence of mosquitoes resistant to insecticides (DDT) and lack of adequate funding have made control difficult in many areas. Blacks with sickle cell trait are less susceptible to *P. falciparum* malaria, and persons who lack certain Duffy blood group determinants show protection against *P. vivax* infections. Most patients who develop *P. falciparum* infection become symptomatic within one month, whereas there may be a delay of six months or more with other species of malaria. In 1976 only 35 per cent of *P. vivax* infections in the United States were manifest within one month, whereas 76 per cent of *P. falciparum* infections had onset within one month. Transfusion-induced malaria may occur when blood donors have subclinical malaria and, if not recognized, may be fatal. The number of civilian cases of malaria reported in the United States has gradually increased from 38 in 1959 to 401 in 1976 (CDC, 1977: Fig. 51-8); 171 of the cases of imported malaria in 1976 occurred in United States citizens, particularly tourists, businessmen, and college students or teachers. Approximately two thirds were males, and the peak age group was 20 to 29 years old. Of the four cases indigenous to the United States, one was transfusion-induced, two were congenital, and one was unexplained. The other 225 cases occurred in foreign visitors, especially college students or teachers. Table 51-2 shows the area where malaria infection was acquired. Table 51-3 shows the distribution of species causing malaria.

Clinical disease

The common presenting symptoms of malaria are chills and fever which are often associated with splenomegaly. In the early stages of the disease, the temperature spikes may occur in irregular fashion but become more periodic, with repeated spikes assuming a tertian (48 hour) pattern in *P. vivax*, *P. falciparum*, and *P. ovale*, and a quartan (72 hour) pattern in *P. malariae* infections. Patients with malaria may develop anemia, and may have variable manifestations, such as diarrhea, abdominal pain, headache, and muscle aches and pains. *P. falciparum* malaria can have high density parasitemias with as many as 50 per cent of the red cells being parasitized which can lead to severe hemolysis with hemo-

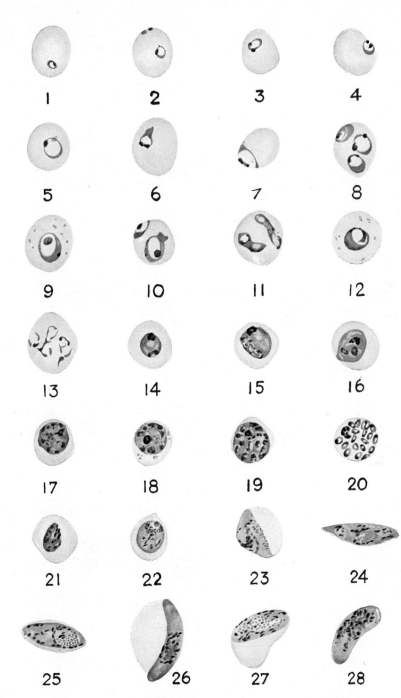

Figure 51-6. *Plasmodium falciparum. 1*, Very young ring form trophozoite. *2*, Double infection of single cell with young trophozoites, one a "marginal form," the other "signet ring" form. *3, 4*, Young trophozoites showing double chromatin dots. *5, 6, 7*, Developing trophozoite forms. *8*, Three medium trophozoites in one cell. *9*, Trophozoite showing pigment, in a cell containing Maurer's dots. *10, 11*, Two trophozoites in each of two cells, showing variation of forms which parasites may assume. *12*, Almost mature trophozoite showing haze of pigment throughout cytoplasm. Maurer's dots in the cell. *13*, Estivo-autumnal "slender forms." *14*, Mature trophozoite, showing clumped pigment. *15*, Parasite in the process of initial chromatin division. *16, 17, 18, 19*, Various phases of the development of the schizont (presegmenting schizonts). *20*, Mature schizont. *21, 22, 23, 24*, Successive forms in the development of the gametocyte—usually not found in the peripheral circulation. *25*, Immature macrogametocyte. *26*, Mature macrogametocyte. *27*, Immature microgametocyte. *28*, Mature microgametocyte. (Courtesy National Institutes of Health, U.S.P.H.S.)

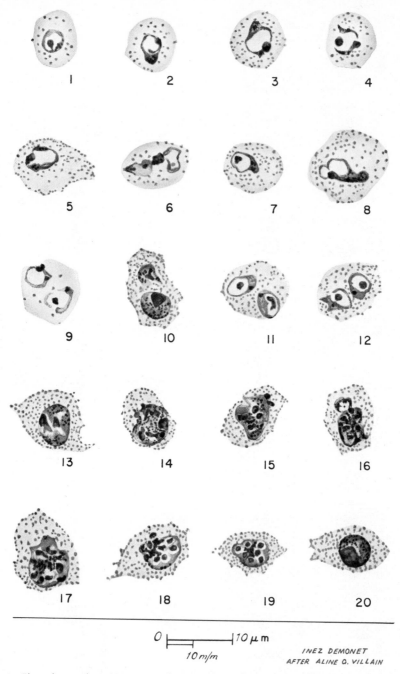

Figure 51-7. *Plasmodium ovale. 1,* Young ring-shape trophozoite. *2, 3, 4, 5,* Older ring-shaped trophozoites. *6, 7, 8,* Older ameboid trophozoites. *9, 11, 12,* Doubly infected cells, trophozoites. *10,* Doubly infected cell, young gametocytes. *13,* First stage of the schizont. *14, 15, 16, 17, 18, 19,* Schizonts, progressive stages. *20,* Mature gametocyte.

Free translation of legend accompanying original plate in "Guide pratique d'examen microscopique du sang appliqué au diagnostic du paludisme" by Georges Villain. Reproduced with permission from "Biologie Medicale" supplement, 1935.

(Courtesy of Aimee Wilcox, National Institutes of Health Bulletin No. 180, U.S.P.H.S.)

globinuria and severe anemia. Erythrocytes infected with growing trophozoites and schizonts of *P. falciparum* become sequestered in small vessels of the body and may lead to occlusion of these vessels, causing symptoms related to capillary obstruction. If there is obstruction of small vessels in the brain, there may be "cerebral malaria," in which the patient becomes disoriented and progresses to delirium and often death.

MILITARY AND CIVILIAN CASES OF MALARIA, UNITED STATES, 1959-1976

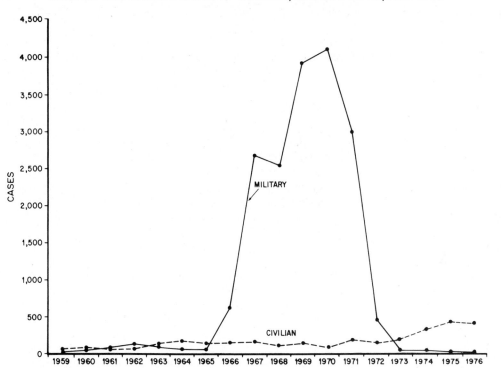

Figure 51-8. Military and civilian cases of malaria in the United States from 1959 to 1976. (From Center for Disease Control: Malaria Surveillance Summary 1976, issued September 1977.)

Patients with malaria may have biologically false positive serologic tests for syphilis and peripheral smears may show leukocytes that contain malaria pigment. Increased reticulocyte counts may be associated with the rapid erythrocyte turnover.

Therapy and prophylaxis of malaria may be directed against proliferative forms in the blood stream (trophozoites and schizonts), gametocytes, and exoerythrocytic forms. Except for resistant falciparum infections, the usual drug used for the blood forms is chloroquine. Primaquine is used in *P. vivax* and *P. ovale* infections to eradicate exoerythrocytic forms. Use of primaquine may be dangerous in patients who have glucose 6-phosphate dehydro-

Table 51-2. GEOGRAPHIC ORIGIN OF IMPORTED MALARIA CASES SEEN IN THE UNITED STATES IN 1976

	NUMBER	PER CENT
Asia*	196	48.1
Africa†	119	29.1
Central America‡	59	14.6‡
North America	17	4.4
South America	11	2.7
Oceana	3	0.7
Europe	1	0.2

Adapted from Center for Disease Control: Malaria Surveillance. Annual Summary, 1976. Issued September 1977.

*130 (66 per cent) were from India.

†29 (24 per cent) were from Nigeria.

‡26 (44 per cent) were from Nicaragua and 19 (32 per cent) were from El Salvador.

Table 51-3. MALARIA CASES BY PLASMODIUM SPECIES, UNITED STATES, 1976*

SPECIES	NUMBER	PER CENT
P. vivax	269	66.5
P. falciparum	83	20.2
P. malariae	21	5.2
P. ovale	5	1.2
Mixed infections	2	0.5
Undetermined	26	6.4
Total	406	100.0

*Adapted from Center for Disease Control: Malaria Surveillance. Annual Summary, 1976. Issued September 1977.

genase (G6PD) deficiency and in whom the drug may cause hemolysis of older erythrocytes.

The course of untreated malaria depends on the species. Most fatal cases of malaria are due to *P. falciparum*. With time, in non-fatal cases, the febrile paroxysms become less severe and the disease gradually subsides. Patients with *P. vivax* or *P. ovale* infection may have relapses arising from the latent exoerythrocytic stages after months or even years. Persons with *P. malariae* infection often have a low-grade parasitemia and may be asymptomatic with recrudescences occuring sporadically. Relapses and recrudescences may be associated with changes in the host's defense mechanisms or possibly with antigenic changes in the infecting organisms.

Diagnosis

In patients with fever, malaria should be included in the differential diagnosis, and a history of travel, drug addiction, and blood transfusion should be sought. Diagnosis is generally established by demonstrating parasites in blood films. Both thin and thick blood films should be made. Thick films allow detection of parasites, whereas thin films are better for study of the morphology of parasites and infected erythrocytes. Blood films several hours apart may sometimes be required to demonstrate infection, as the number and morphologic stages of parasites can vary in different parts of the cycle. Parasites can be seen in blood of almost all patients with clinical malaria by examining thick films.

Identification of malaria parasites in thin blood films requires a systematic approach to the examination of infected erythrocytes. There are three major factors to be considered: appearance of erythrocytes, appearance of parasites, and stages found (Table 51-4). The erythrocytes in *P. vivax* and *P. ovale* infection become enlarged. Those infected with early ring forms may be of normal size but, as growing trophozoites and schizonts develop, the *P. vivax* infected erythrocytes will be 1.5 to 2 times the diameter of normal erythrocytes. The erythrocytes in *P. ovale* infections are generally enlarged but to a lesser extent than those of *P. vivax*. Erythrocytes in *P. malariae* and *P. falciparum* infection are of normal size. The erythrocytes infected with parasites of *P. ovale* are often oval, as the name implies, or they may be fimbriated (have irregular projections of the cell margins). Erythrocytes infected with *P. vivax* may occasionally (less than 6 per cent of infected cells) be oval, whereas in *P. ovale* infection over 20 per cent of the parasitized erythrocytes are oval or fimbriated. Schüffner's stippling, numerous small uniform pink granules in the erythrocyte, is usually present in erythrocytes infected with *P. vivax* and *P. ovale*, although it may not be evident in cells infected with ring forms or in improperly stained slides. This type of stippling is not seen in *P. malariae* or *P. falciparum* infection, although Maurer's dots (irregular red dots) may be seen in *P. falciparum* infection and Ziemann's dots (scattered small pink granules) may be seen in *P. malariae* infections. The latter two are not seen in properly stained Giemsa films. As the trophozoites grow in the infected cells, the amount of hemoglobin in the erythrocyte will decrease and is reflected by less intense staining of the erythrocyte and accumulation of hemozoin pigment. The amount and appearance of the pigment varies among the species. Ring forms of all parasites may have a similar appearance and if only occasional ring forms are found, the species may not be identifiable. Marginal forms (spindle-shaped parasites with a central red chromatin mass that appear to be lying on the surface of the erythrocyte) are often seen in *P. falciparum* infection but are rarely seen in other types of infection. Young rings of *P. falciparum* are smaller than those of the other species (one sixth the diameter of the red blood cell, as opposed to one third the diameter of the red blood cell for the other species). Rings of *P. falciparum* that have grown will be similar in size to those of the other species. Infections of erythrocytes by multiple organisms may occur with any of the species but are most common in *P. falciparum*. Double chromatin dots in the rings are more common in *P. falciparum* infections but can occur with the other species.

Growing trophozoites of *P. vivax* have irregular shapes and are termed ameboid. Those of *P. malariae* and *P. ovale* are compact and, although they may have some vacuoles, do not show the ameboid appearance of those of *P. vivax*. Growing trophozoites of *P. falciparum* are not seen in the peripheral blood except in very severe infections. The number of merozoites in the mature schizont stage is helpful in identifying the various species.

The gametocytes of *P. falciparum* are quite distinctive because of their sausage shape; however, the gametocytes of *P. vivax*, *P. malariae*, and *P. ovale* are difficult to differ-

Table 51-4. COMPARISON OF PLASMODIUM SPECIES AFFECTING MAN*

| SPECIES | APPEARANCE OF ERYTHROCYTE | | APPEARANCE OF PARASITE | | | |
	Size	Schüffner's Stippling	Cytoplasm	Pigment	Number of Merozoites	STAGES FOUND IN CIRCULATING BLOOD
Plasmodium vivax	Enlarged. Maximum size (attained with mature trophozoites and schizonts) may be 1½-2 times normal erythrocyte diameter.	+ With all stages except early ring forms.	Irregular, ameboid in trophozoites. Has "spread-out" appearance.	Golden-brown inconspicuous.	12-24 Average is 16.	All stages. Wide range of stages may be seen on given film.
Plasmodium malariae	Normal.	− (Ziemann's dots rarely seen.)	Rounded, compact trophozoites with dense cytoplasm. Band-form trophozoites occasionally seen.	Dark-brown, coarse, conspicuous.	6-12 Average is 8. "Rosette" schizonts occasionally seen.	All stages. Wide variety of stages usually not seen. Relatively few rings or gametocytes generally present.
Plasmodium ovale	Enlarged. Maximum size may be 1¼-1½ times normal red blood cell diameter. Approximately 20% or more of infected red blood cells are oval and/or fimbriated (border has irregular projections).	+ With all stages except early ring forms.	Rounded, compact trophozoites. Occasionally slightly ameboid. Growing trophozoites have large chromatin mass.	Dark-brown conspicuous.	6-14 Average is 8.	All stages.
Plasmodium falciparum	Normal. Multiply-infected red blood cells are common.	− (Maurer's dots occasionally seen.)	Young rings are small, delicate, often with double chromatin dots. Gametocytes are crescent or elongate.	Black. Coarse and conspicuous in gametocytes.	6-32 Average is 20-24.	Rings and/or gametocytes. Other stages develop in blood vessels or internal organs but are not seen in peripheral blood except in severe infections.

*From Smith, J. W., Melvin, D. M., Orihel, T. C., et al.: Diagnostic Parasitology—Blood and Tissue Parasites. Chicago, American Society of Clinical Pathologists, 1976.

entiate based on parasite morphology, although characteristics of infected red cells can aid in identifying *P. malariae*. The varieties of developmental stages found in the peripheral blood may aid in diagnosis. In *P. falciparum* there will usually be only ring forms, and finding numerous ring forms without more mature stages is good evidence of *P. falciparum* infection. In *P. vivax*, *P. malariae*, and *P. ovale* infections, various stages of parasites will be found with some predominance of one stage depending on the part of the cycle. There are usually relatively few rings in *P. malariae* infections.

Thick films are preferred for detecting malaria infections, as approximately 16 to 30 times the volume of blood may be examined in the same amount of time. In these preparations, the erythrocytes will be lysed so that the background will consist of white cell nuclei and platelet debris (Fig. 51-9). The ring forms will often have the appearance of punctuation marks rather than complete rings, and the presence of red chromatin and blue cytoplasm should be required to identify them as parasites. Schüffner's stippling may still be a helpful identifying characteristic, and it may be recognized around growing trophozoites as a pink halo rather than the distinct granules seen in thin films. The ameboid character of *P. vivax* trophozoites is not as evident in thick films and thus is not as helpful a characteristic. In thick films, the number of merozoites in the mature schizonts is helpful. Macro- and microgametocytes usually cannot be differentiated in thick films. The distinctive sausage shape of *P. falciparum* gametocytes is still evident, although they may be more stubby than in thin films.

Mixed infections occur occasionally, but caution should be used in making such diagnoses unless there is definite evidence of two species. The most common mixed infections are *P. falciparum* and *P. vivax*. Finding gametocytes of *P. falciparum* in a person obviously infected with *P. vivax* is diagnostic. Sometimes only occasional rings will be found and the species cannot be identified.

There are multiple artifacts that may be confused with malaria parasites in thick and thin films. Malaria parasites should have deep red chromatin mass, blue cytoplasm, and (except for rings) some pigment. Probably the most commonly confused artifacts in thin films are blood platelets that are superimposed on red cells. These should be readily differentiated because they do not have a true ring form and do not show the differentiation of the chromatin and cytoplasm. Clumps of bacteria or platelets may be confused with schizonts. At times, masses of fused platelets may resemble gametocytes of *P. falciparum*

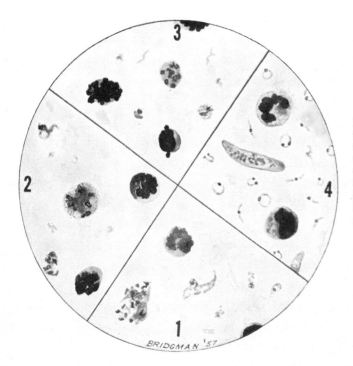

Figure 51-9. The human plasmodia as seen in thick film: *1, Plasmodium vivax:* young and older trophozoites and schizont; *2, P. ovale:* developing trophozoite and schizonts, one within a "ghost cell"; *3, P. malariae:* trophozoites and schizont; *4, P. falciparum:* young trophozoites and gametocyte. (From Markell, E. K., and Voge, M.: Medical Parasitology. Philadelphia, W. B. Saunders Company, 1976.)

but once again do not show the differential staining or the pigment. Precipitated stain and contaminating bacteria, fungi, or spores may also be confused with parasites.

A variety of serologic tests have been developed for malaria but are not usually used to diagnose clinical infections. They are particularly useful for epidemiologic surveys and detection of infected blood donors. Those most commonly used are the indirect fluorescent antibody (IFA) and the indirect hemaglutination (IHA) tests. IFA titers equal to or greater than 1:16 are suggestive of recent infection with malaria. These serologic tests show a false positive rate of 1 per cent or less and have a sensitivity of over 95 per cent. In the United States, they may be obtained from the Center for Disease Control via State Health Department Laboratories.

BABESIA

These sporozoan blood parasites of animals are spread by the bite of tick vectors. Man may occasionally be infected, and fatal infections have occured, especially in splenectomized individuals. Patients develop fever, malaise, and anemia. An outbreak that recently occurred on Nantucket Island off the coast of New England was caused by *Babesia microti*, which normally infects field and deer mice (Rubush, 1977). Investigation showed that some patients harbored the parasite for months and that some individuals showed serologic evidence of infection without a history of clinical disease. Thus, as with many other infections, the first cases recognized were severe, but with investigation, mild and subclinical cases were recognized.

This parasite divides by binary fission, both in erythrocytes and in the tick. The trophozoites of many species are pear-shaped, but those of *B. microti* usually look like rings and may be confused with malaria, especially *P. falciparum* (Fig. 51-10). As a result of divi-

sion of the organisms, erythrocytes may have multiple rings, often tetrads with the rings touching in the center. *Babesia* can be differentiated from malaria by the lack of blood pigment, large growing trophozoites, and gametocytes. History of travel to Nantucket or of a recent tick bite might suggest this infection. Malaria serology is negative. A serologic test for babesiosis is available from the Center for Disease Control via the State Health Department Laboratory.

PNEUMOCYSTIS CARINII

Pneumocystis carinii is a parasite of uncertain taxonomy, probably a sporozoan. It causes serious pulmonary infections in malnourished and premature infants; however, most infections in the United States occur in severely immunosuppressed patients, such as leukemic patients on chemotherapy and transplant recipients (Hughes, 1975). It has become more frequent as immunosuppressive therapy has become more effective and more widely used. Rapid diagnosis and early institution of therapy are important in improving survival.

The epidemiology is not understood because techniques to culture the organisms have only recently been developed and serologic tests do not have good sensitivity and specificity. It appears, however, that the disease is often a latent infection that becomes activated when the patient is immunosuppressed. The organism is spread by the respiratory route, possibly from normal patients with asymptomatic infection or from carriers (Walzer, 1977).

The organisms grow as free trophozoites and as cysts. Proliferation apparently occurs both in trophozoites by binary fission and in cysts, with up to eight organisms present in mature cysts.

The infection may produce an interstitial pneumonia with alveoli filled with foamy exudate containing numerous extracellular and sometimes intracellular *Pneumocystis* orga-

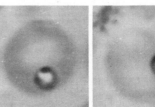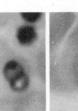

Figure 51–10. *Babesia microti.* The cell on the left contains one ring, that in the center has two rings, and the cell on the right has four small pyriform organisms.

nisms. The amount of cellular reaction varies depending on the underlying disease and the duration and severity of infection. Malnourished infants have extensive interstitial plasma cell infiltration. Immunosuppressed patients often show little cellular infiltration. Patients present with fever and an interstitial pneumonia; Po_2 is low, often out of proportion to the degree of radiologic change. Although organisms have been described in other organs, the disease process involves primarily the lung.

The principal means of diagnosis is demonstration of the organisms in pulmonary material (see Chap. 22, p. 734). Examination is tedious and time consuming and must be done by a competent examiner. The examination of sputum is less productive, as the yield is extremely small. Other types of specimens that have been examined include bronchial washings and transbronchial lung biopsies, transthoracic needle biopsies, transthoracic needle aspirates, and open lung biopsies. Bronchial washings and transbronchial biopsies are often negative in patients proven to have the disease. Open lung biopsies provide the most accurate means of establishing the diagnosis by demonstrating typical organisms in sections or imprints. Open biopsies have the additional advantage that if the pulmonary infiltrate is of a different etiology than *Pneumocystis*, the etiology can usually be established. Imprints should be made in addition to sections because results may be available faster (2 to 3 hours) and internal cyst morphology is discerned more readily than in tissue sections. In Giemsa stains, trophozoites and individual organisms within cysts have red nuclei and pale blue cytoplasm; cyst walls do not stain (Fig. 51-11). Cysts are generally 5 to 7 μ in diameter and trophozoites are 1.5 to 4 μ. Methenamine silver stains the cyst wall and does not stain trophozoites. If organisms are numerous, methenamine silver stains show non-budding cysts that are often cup-shaped and have a darker staining central area. However, if only occasional organisms are seen, cysts and yeasts may be confused and it may not be possible to establish a diagnosis. The Gram-Weigert stain may be used on imprints, frozen sections, or permanent sections to detect the presence of cysts (or fungi). It stains the cyst wall and takes only 20 minutes. A cresyl violet stain for cysts has been described (Bowling, 1973) which is relatively simple to perform. Another rapid stain for

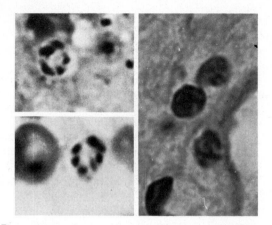

Figure 51-11. *Pneumocystis carinii.* Two Giemsa stained mature cysts are present on the left and are slightly smaller than an erythrocyte. Methenamine silver stain on the right stains only cyst walls.

P. carinii in impression smears is toluidine blue 0 (Chalvardjian, 1963).

An indirect fluorescent antibody serologic test is available from the Center for Disease Control, but the sensitivity and reproducibility of the test are not ideal at this time. Culture procedures have recently been developed (Latorre, 1977) and show promise for allowing development of better antigens and thus better serologic tests.

TOXOPLASMA GONDII

This sporozoan of the coccidian group has a worldwide distribution in man and in domestic and wild animals, especially those that are carnivorous. It generally produces an asymptomatic or mild infection but may cause serious congenital and ocular infections and acute, severe infections in immunosuppressed patients (Remington, 1976).

The life cycle has a sexual phase in the intestinal epithelium of cats and other feline definitive hosts. This phase is similar to *Isospora* intestinal infections. In the intestinal epithelium, asexual schizogony or sexual gametogony may occur. The latter leads to the development of immature oocysts that are passed in the feces and mature to the infective stage in 1 to 5 days. Ingestion of these sporocysts by a wide variety of susceptible intermediate hosts may cause infection in which the trophozoites (tachyzoites) may infect any nucleated cells. Proliferation of these trophozoites may lead to cell death or, if immunity has devel-

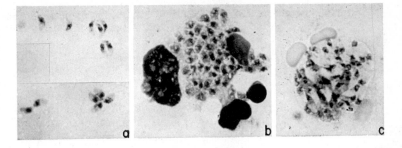

Figure 51-12. Toxoplasmata as seen (*a*) free in stained films of peritoneal exudate or tissue, (*b*) intracellularly, and (*c*) as pseudocyst in film of brain. Wright's stain (×800) reduced from a photomicrograph with a magnification of 1000 diameters. (Courtesy of Dr. A. B. Sabin and J.A.M.A.)

oped, to the formation of tissue cysts containing up to 3000 organisms. This cyst stage is seen in chronic infections. All stages of the life cycle occur in felines, but only the trophozoite and cyst stages occur in man and other intermediate hosts. Man may acquire infection by ingestion of inadequately cooked tissues of other infected intermediate hosts or ingestion of infective oocysts from material contaminated by cat feces. Congenital infection may occur if the mother develops an acute infection during pregnancy. Such transplacental infection is more likely to occur in the latter part of pregnancy.

Most infections are asymptomatic, but there may be fever and lymphadenopathy with an illness resembling infectious mononucleosis. The most significant infections in man are chorioretinitis, which may lead to blindness, and congenital infections, which may cause intrauterine death. Microcephaly or hydrocephaly with intracranial calcifications may develop if infection is acquired in the first half of pregnancy. Infections in the second half of pregnancy are usually asymptomatic at birth, with chorioretinitis or central nervous system manifestations developing months or years later, although there may be fever, hepatosplenomegaly, and jaundice at the time of birth. Congenital toxoplasmosis is a significant cause of blindness, psychomotor retardation, and convulsive disorders.

Severe toxoplasmosis may develop in immunosuppressed hosts, either as a result of acquiring acute infection or by reactivation of latent infection. The disease usually presents with central nervous system manifestations, myocarditis, or pneumonitis.

Diagnosis of toxoplasmosis may be established by morphologic demonstration of organisms, growth of the organisms in tissue culture or mice, or serology. Trophozoites are oval and measure approximately $3 \times 7\ \mu$. They are usually difficult to find in tissue sections and

smears of body fluids with routine stains (Fig. 51-12). Cysts may be seen in sections of infected tissues. The infection may be suspected on the basis of the histologic appearance of lymph nodes, although organisms are rarely seen.

Serology is the most common way to establish the diagnosis. The Sabin-Feldman dye test and indirect fluorescent antibody (IFA) test are the most accurate, although the former is rarely used now. IFA reagents are commercially available. Antibodies appear in 1 to 2 weeks and titers peak at 6 to 8 weeks. An IFA test for IgM may be helpful in diagnosing congenital and acute infection. An indirect hemagglutination (IHA) test is also available but measures different antigens and may be negative in patients with congenital infections. Thus, the IHA cannot replace the IFA test. Because of the large number of persons who have had asymptomatic infections, low titers are of little significance. Titers of $\geq 1{:}128$ with IFA and $\geq 1{:}256$ with IHA are suspicious, but it is best to demonstrate a rise in titer. Titers in patients with chronic ocular infections may be lower.

HEMOFLAGELLATES

Man can be infected by hemoflagellates of the genera *Trypanosoma* and *Leishmania*. The exact taxonomy of the members of these genera is not agreed upon, as there are geographic differences in the clinical disease, the pathogenicity of the organisms, the reservoir hosts infected, the vectors, and the responses to therapy. All of these organisms have stages in insects and stages in man, and many have non-human reservoir mammalian hosts.

The organisms may occur in a variety of stages in man and insect vectors (Fig. 51-13). The currently acceptable terminology of Hoare (1966) will be used, with the older ter-

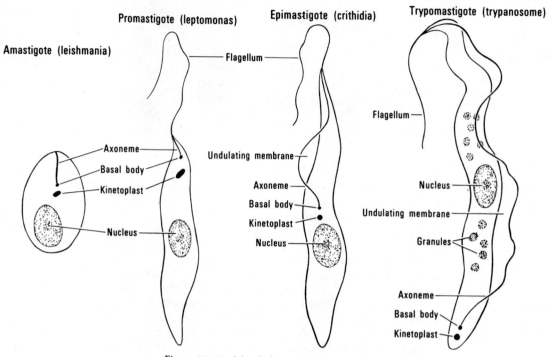

Figure 51-13. Morphology of hemoflagellates.

minology given parenthetically. The amastigote (leishmania) is an intracellular parasite that is round or oval and measures 2 to 5 μ in greatest dimension. The nucleus is generally toward one end of the organism. Near it is a kinetoplast, basal body, and axoneme that usually cannot be separately distinguished and appear as one elongated structure. The amastigote does not have a free flagellum. The promastigote (leptomonas) is elongate and slender with the basal body and kinetoplast at the anterior end and a free flagellum. The epimastigote (crithidia) is an extracellular form that is long and slender with a slightly posterior nucleus. Just anterior to the nucleus are the kinetoplast and basal body with an undulating membrane bordered by the axoneme extending to the anterior end where it projects as a free flagellum. The trypomastigote is an extracellular form that may be found in both arthropod vectors and human or other mammalian hosts. It is long and slender, with the nucleus generally located centrally. The kinetoplast and basal body are posterior, with the axoneme forming the outer margin of the undulating membrane that extends to the anterior end of the organism from which a free flagellum projects.

The number of stages present in the life

cycle varies with the genus and species. The genus *Leishmania* has only two stages, amastigote in man and promastigote in the arthropod vector. The African trypanosome (*T. brucei* group) has a trypomastigote in man and epimastigote in the arthropod vector, although recent evidence suggests that there may be an amastigote stage in the choroid plexus of the mammalian host. *T. cruzi* may have all four stages: the amastigote and trypomastigote are the principal forms in man, but promastigote and epimastigote occur as transitional forms during the change from amastigote to trypomastigote. Promastigote and epimastigote predominate in the insect host, but amastigote and trypomastigote also occur. In *T. rangeli* infection, only the trypomastigote is present in man.

TRYPANOSOMES

There are three trypanosome infections of man: African trypanosomiasis (sleeping sickness) caused by the *T. brucei* group, South American trypanosomiasis (Chagas' disease) caused by *T. cruzi*, and trypanosomiasis caused by *T. rangeli*. A main form found in *T. brucei* and *T. rangeli* infections is the trypomastigote that divides in the peripheral blood and tissues of the infected individual. In *T. cruzi* infection, the intracellular amastigote form and the peripheral blood trypomastigote form are present, but division occurs only in the amastigote stage.

African trypanosomiasis, caused by trypanosomes of the *T. brucei* group, is spread by the bite of certain *Glossina* spp. (tsetse flies). Two different clinical forms of the disease are recognized (Mahmoud, 1976a). The gambiense form occurs in western African areas, with man being the only host of the disease, and the rhodesiense form occurs in east Africa and has animal reservoir hosts. The disease is characterized by an acute febrile stage with lymphadenopathy and subsequent development of central nervous system involvement. The rhodesiense form causes a more severe and rapidly progressive infection, and patients often die before central nervous system involvement is prominent, whereas the gambiense form has prominent central nervous system involvement with somnolence, confusion, and fatigue, progressing to stupor and coma with eventual death. Not all infections progress; some appear to resolve spontaneously.

Trypanosomiasis can be suspected based on geographic history and increased levels of immunoglobulin, particularly IgM, in blood and cerebrospinal fluid. There may be false-positive reaginic tests for syphilis. Cerebrospinal fluid will also have increased cell counts (predominantly mononuclear) of 50 to 500 cells per cu mm. Diagnosis is best established by demonstrating parasites in blood. This can be done by examining a direct mount of blood in which the motile parasites may be detected or by examining stained thin or thick films. Parasites are readily demonstrated in the acute stages of the disease. If there is central nervous system involvement, trypomastigotes may be demonstrated in the spinal fluid after centrifugation at 1000 g by staining and examining the sediment. Concentration procedures for blood have been described and may be attempted. The rhodesiense type of *T. brucei* may be diagnosed by experimentally infecting animals such as hamsters, but this is not effective for the gambiense type of *T. brucei*. Trypomastigotes are somewhat variable in size and shape, with some short, blunt forms. The typical trypomastigote is long and thin with graceful curves. It measures up to 30 microns long. The kinetoplast is near the posterior end. Serologic tests of various types have been described, and some are available from reference laboratories such as the Center for Disease Control.

T. rangeli is transmitted by the bite of triatomid bugs and causes asymptomatic trypanosomiasis in parts of South and Central America. It is important that *T. rangeli* infections be differentiated from the more serious infections caused by *T. cruzi* in the same geographic area. The trypomastigotes of *T. rangeli* are long and thin, and the kinetoplast is a moderate distance from the tapered posterior end.

South American trypanosomiasis (Chagas' disease), caused by *T. cruzi*, occurs in South and Central America and Mexico. The organism and appropriate arthropod hosts are present in the southern United States, but infections are rarely described. This disease is spread by reduviid bugs, and, in contrast to the other trypanosomiases, it is the feces of the bug that are infective. The particular strains of reduviid bugs that are the principal vectors of this disease are those that defecate at the time of obtaining their blood meal. Man becomes infected when infective trypomastigotes in the bug feces are rubbed into the bite, other wounds, or mucous membranes as the victim scratches.

The trypomastigotes are ingested by macrophages, become amastigotes, and begin to proliferate by binary fission in the cells of the reticuloendothelial system. A primary lesion (chagoma) often develops at the site of the bite and regional lymph nodes will be involved. The organisms proliferate intracellularly as amastigotes, then transform into trypomastigotes and invade the blood stream, carrying the infection to all parts of the body. Amastigote forms then multiply within various types of cells in organs and tissues of the body and cause fever and lymphadenopathy. Trypomastigotes can often be demonstrated in the peripheral blood during the febrile phase of the disease; however, the number of parasites is usually small. The reticuloendothelial system; cardiac, skeletal, and smooth muscle; and neuroglia cells are preferentially invaded.

The acute stage of the disease is most prominent in infants and is characterized by malaise, chills, fever, and aches and pains with acute hepatosplenomegaly (Mahmoud, 1975). In older individuals, the acute stage is not as prominent and may be asymptomatic or may present as a febrile illness with lymphadenop-

5

athy and hepatosplenomegaly. During the acute stage, trypomastigotes may be demonstrable in the peripheral blood, although they are more commonly found in the blood of infected children than in that of infected adults. Trypomastigotes of *T. cruzi* do not divide. In infants, the infection may involve the nervous system, causing meningoencephalitis and leading to death in a short time. Nervous system involvement is usually not manifest in adults and older children. In patients with asymptomatic initial infections, the first clinical signs of the disease can be related to cardiac involvement or dilatation of the digestive tract in the chronic stages of the disease. The heart shows myocarditis and fibrosis and the digestive tract and heart show damage to the autonomic nervous system, which in the intestine leads to dilatation, causing megaesophagus or megacolon.

Diagnosis of trypanosomiasis in the acute stage is usually made by demonstration of the trypomastigotes in Giemsa-stained thick or thin blood films, or by direct examination of blood (Fig. 51-14). In addition, procedures have been described utilizing larger volumes of blood in which the erythrocytes are lysed to further concentrate the trypanosomes. Trypomastigotes of *T. cruzi* vary somewhat in appearance but are usually 15 to 20 μ long and have a larger kinetoplast than the *T. brucei* group or *T. rangeli*. "C" or "S" shaped trypomastigotes are common in stained smears. In tissue, the amastigotes resemble those of the *Leishmania* spp., although *T. cruzi* amastigotes are slightly larger. Other means of diagnosis are culture, animal inoculation, and xenodiagnosis. The latter is performed by allowing disease-free reduviid bugs to feed on the patient and examining their rectal content in 10 days and one to two months later to see if parasites are present. This method is not available in the United States.

Complement fixation, indirect hemagglutination, and agglutination tests are usually positive in patients with Chagas' disease. The disease may sometimes be spread by blood transfusion, and quiescent infections may sometimes be exacerbated by immunosuppression.

LEISHMANIA

There are three general forms of leishmaniasis: cutaneous, mucocutaneous, and visceral (Mahmoud, 1977). Cutaneous leishmaniasis is caused by *Leishmania tropica* and occurs from the bite of sand flies belonging to the genus *Phlebotomus*. The infections occur in tropical areas and in countries bordering the Mediterranean, with different clinical syndromes occurring in different areas. In the eastern hemisphere, *L. tropica* causes oriental sore, which begins as a localized lesion at the site of the bite with formation of a papule that enlarges and finally ulcerates. It may take from two weeks to six months after a bite for such lesions to first appear. The lesions, if left untreated, will generally heal unless there is secondary bacterial infection. Lesions seen in the western hemisphere differ from those seen in the rest of the world. The organism causing infection in Central America and southern Mexico is sometimes referred to as *L. tropica mexicana* or *L. mexicana* and causes a lesion known as a chiclero ulcer. This has a predilection for the ear where slowly healing lesions of the pinna develop.

Mucocutaneous leishmaniasis caused by *Leishmania braziliensis* often begins as a cutaneous disease similar to that described but with involvement extending to the mucous membranes. Lesions of the mucous membranes do not heal as readily as cutaneous lesions and continue to extend, leading to destruction of mucous membranes, eventually

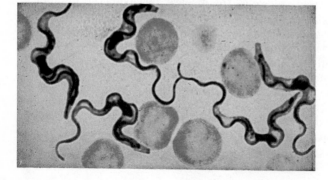

Figure 51-14. *Trypanosoma brucei* in stained blood film; ×about 2000. (Krall.)

including all of the soft parts of the nose, lips, and palate. The disease is very slowly progressive and, if untreated, death may occur from secondary infection.

Diagnosis of cutaneous and mucocutaneous leishmaniasis is usually by demonstration of amastigotes in reticuloendothelial cells in the lesion. Material is best obtained by avoiding the contaminated ulcerated area by biopsying, aspirating, or curetting the margin of the lesion and preparing imprints or smears. The organisms can be recognized in Giemsa stains by their characteristic kinetoplast, which allows differentiation from fungal diseases such as histoplasmosis. Culture of promastigotes on artificial media may also allow diagnosis. A skin test, the Montenegro test, is usually positive in cutaneous and mucocutaneous leishmaniasis, although it is not usually positive in visceral leishmaniasis. A variety of serologic tests have been described, including indirect hemagglutination, indirect fluorescence, complement fixation, and agglutination.

Visceral leishmaniasis or kala-azar is caused by *Leishmania donovani* and is endemic in some parts of South America, Africa, China, India, and the Mediterranean area. It is maintained in various mammalian reservoir hosts. The disease may begin with a skin lesion but primarily is a disease involving the reticuloendothelial system of the visceral organs with massive hepatosplenomegaly. The patient will often present with a febrile disease that may be confused with typhoid fever or malaria and may complain of abdominal swelling. Serum globulin level is increased. Without treatment the disease is progressive, with death rates of up to 75 per cent.

Diagnosis is usually established by demonstration of organisms in reticuloendothelial cells (Fig. 51-15). Bone marrow aspiration is most frequently done and will allow diagnosis of approximately 80 per cent of the cases. The most sensitive method is splenic aspiration, which will allow diagnosis of 90 per cent of the cases but is dangerous and is not recommended. Serologic tests, such as complement fixation and fluorescent antibody, may be helpful in establishing the diagnosis.

SOIL AMEBAE

Meningoencephalitis may be caused by ameboflagellates of the genus *Naegleria* (especially *N. fowleri*) and occasionally by ameba of the *Acanthamoeba/Hartmannella* (A-H) group. Infection is usually acquired by swimming in fresh or brackish stagnant water containing the amebae. It appears that the amebae invade from the nasopharynx through or around the olfactory bulb to reach the subarachnoid space. The infection is usually rapidly progressive and fatal, although some cases of A-H infection are more slowly progressive.

Diagnosis is established by demonstrating the organisms in cerebrospinal fluid by light or phase microscopy, by culture in tissue culture or on cell-free media, or by animal inoculation (Culbertson, 1974). *Naegleria* measure 8 to 15 μ and have blunt pseudopodia, whereas A-H are large (10 to 15 μ) and have spinelike pseudopodia. Differentiation is important, as it affects therapy.

INTESTINAL AND ATRIAL PROTOZOA

Protozoa may frequently inhabit the intestinal tract or atrial cavities of man (Table 51-5), most being amebae and flagellates with occasional instances of ciliate and coccidian infection. In a review of fecal specimens submitted to State Health Department Laboratories (see Table 51-1), non-pathogenic protozoa were found in 7.6 per cent of specimens with the potential pathogens *Giardia lamblia* in 3.8

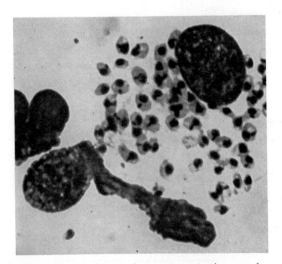

Figure 51-15. *Leishmania donovani* in stained smear from spleen puncture. (From Hunter, G. W., Swartzwelder, J. C., and Clyde, D. F.: A Manual of Tropical Medicine. Philadelphia, W. B. Saunders Company, 1976.)

Table 51-5. INTESTINAL AND ATRIAL PROTOZOA

	INTESTINAL	ATRIAL
Amebae	*Entamoeba histolytica** *Entamoeba coli* *Entamoeba hartmanni* *Entamoeba polecki* *Endolimax nana* *Dientamoeba fragilis** *Iodamoeba bütschlii*	*Entamoeba gingivalis*
Flagellates	*Giardia lamblia** *Chilomastix mesnili* *Trichomonas hominis* *Enteromonas hominis* *Retortamonas intestinalis*	*Trichomonas tenax* *Trichomonas vaginalis**
Ciliate	*Balantidium coli**	
Coccidia	*Isospora belli** *Sarcocystis sp.*	

* Potential pathogens.

per cent, *Entamoeba histolytica* in 0.6 per cent, and *Dientamoeba fragilis* in 0.4 per cent. Most of the intestinal infections (except some coccidia) are acquired by fecal/oral contamination, either directly, as by flies and food handlers, or indirectly via contaminated water.

For most laboratories, identification of intestinal protozoa is the most difficult aspect of parasitology. The parasites are small and the pathogenic organisms must be differentiated from the non-pathogenic organisms, as well as from inflammatory cells, epithelial cells, and other confusing objects. There are a number of characteristics that may be helpful in identifying intestinal protozoa. Size is a helpful characteristic (Fig. 51-16), and a properly calibrated ocular micrometer must be available. Amebae must be differentiated from flagellates. This is relatively easy in wet mounts of fresh material where the amebae

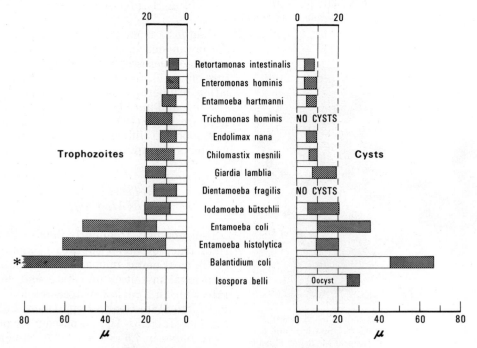

Figure 51-16. Size ranges of intestinal protozoa.

can be seen to move in the typical ameboid fashion, whereas flagellates move more rapidly and in a "falling leaf," darting, or tumbling fashion. It is important to differentiate macrophages from amebae, and this may be difficult for inexperienced examiners; however, permanently stained slides of the material make differentiation easier.

Number and size of nuclei and pattern of chromatin distribution are helpful. These are best seen in permanently stained preparation but may be evident in iodine-stained wet mounts.

Helpful cytoplasmic characteristics include fibrils and special structures in flagellates, ingested materials in trophozoites, and glycogen masses and chromatoid bodies in amebic cysts.

Flagellates will generally have a long axis with a nucleus or nuclei at one end and tapering at the opposite end. Finding this configuration in multiple organisms should make one suspect flagellates.

Organisms may degenerate before or after feces are passed, and some organisms may be too degenerated to be identified. Multiple organisms may need to be examined in order to assess accurately the characteristics present and thus arrive at an identification. It may not be possible to identify definitively each individual parasite. In addition, before identifying two species of protozoa, there should be two distinct populations of organisms, not just an occasional organism with an atypical appearance.

Direct wet mounts of fresh material are helpful for identification of trophozoites or cysts, whereas formalin-fixed material is helpful primarily for detection of cysts. Permanently stained preparations are used to detect and examine in detail both trophozoites and cysts.

AMEBAE

There are four genera of amebae that may inhabit the intestinal tract of man: *Entamoeba*, *Endolimax*, *Iodamoeba*, and *Dientamoeba*. The life cycle of the amebae (except for *Dientamoeba fragilis* and *Entamoeba gingivalis*) is similar, with the cyst form being the infective stage. The cysts are ingested and excyst in the small intestine. The resulting trophozoites proliferate in the lumen of the colon. Cysts and trophozoites may be passed in feces. Mature cysts are the infective stage. The genus *Entamoeba*, characterized by

having chromatin on the nuclear membrane, is the most important and includes *E. histolytica*, the etiologic agent of amebiasis, *E. hartmanni* and *E. coli*, which are commonly found, and *E. polecki*, which is occasionally found in people who have contact with pigs (Figs. 51-17 to 51-19). *Entamoeba gingivalis* may inhabit the oral cavity of people, particularly those with poor oral hygiene. *Endolimax nana* and *Iodamoeba bütschlii* are non-pathogenic. *Dientamoeba fragilis* probably causes diarrhea on some occasions (Yang, 1977).

Entamoeba histolytica

In most instances, the *E. histolytica* organisms lead a commensal existence in the intestinal lumen without clinical disease, and it is debated whether these commensal organisms cause lesions. *E. histolytica* may cause various clinical diseases, most commonly amebic dysentery, non-dysenteric amebic colitis, and liver abscesses (Adams, 1977; Mahmoud, 1976b). General host defense mechanisms, previous contact with parasite, diet, and the strain of *E. histolytica* may influence the manifestations of infection in the individual. Amebic dysentery is a severe acute disease characterized by severe bloody diarrhea with abdominal cramping. There is extensive invasion of the mucosa with ulceration that may lead to perforation and peritonitis, severe hemorrhage, or secondary bacterial infection. This form of the disease is infrequently seen in the United States. The more common form in the United States is amebic colitis, which has various symptoms such as diarrhea, constipation, abdominal cramping, and weight loss but without the severe dysentery with blood and mucus seen in amebic dysentery. There are small, pinpoint mucosal ulcerations that may expand in the submucosa to form flask-shaped ulcers. The cecal area is most frequently involved, with the rectosigmoid area and the ascending colon also being involved often.

The most common form of extraintestinal amebiasis is amebic abscess of the liver, which occurs in approximately 5 per cent of symptomatic patients. Symptoms are fever and right upper quadrant pain. These liver abscesses are usually diagnosed by radioisotope scans, ultrasound, demonstration of amebae in stool, aspiration of the abscess, and serologic tests. Often, amebae are not present in the stool, so their absence is not helpful. Another condition

5

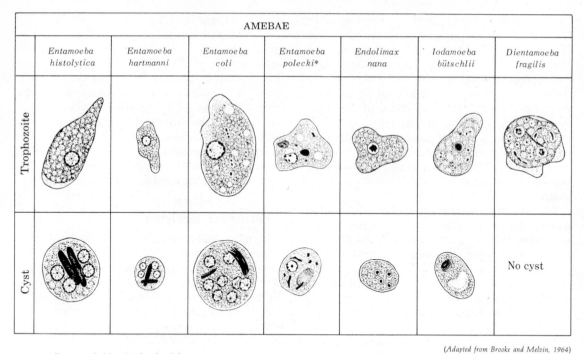

*Rare, probably of animal origin

(Adapted from Brooke and Melvin, 1964)

Figure 51-17.   Amebae found in stool specimens of man.

known as amebic hepatitis may occur in some cases and is characterized by an enlarged, tender liver in someone with intestinal amebiasis. It is debatable whether this state is a result of bacterial, toxic, or direct amebic involvement of the liver. Rarely, amebic abscesses may appear in other organs, such as the lung and brain, either by direct spread from the intestinal disease or by secondary spread from a liver abscess.

Rarely there may be granulation tissue masses, known as amebomas, formed in response to amebae. In the intestine, they may cause "napkin ring" lesions and be confused with carcinomas. Very rarely amebic ulcerations may occur in perianal or other areas of skin. Diagnosis is by morphologic or cultural demonstration of the organisms, although serology is usually positive in these patients.

Diagnosis.   Examination of stool speci-

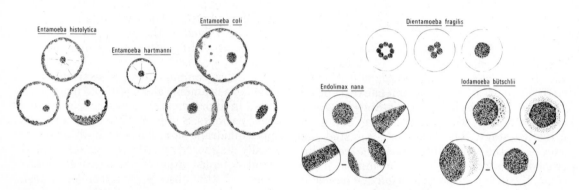

Figure 51-18.   Nuclei of amebae. This drawing shows some of the various appearances of amebic nuclei in stained preparations.

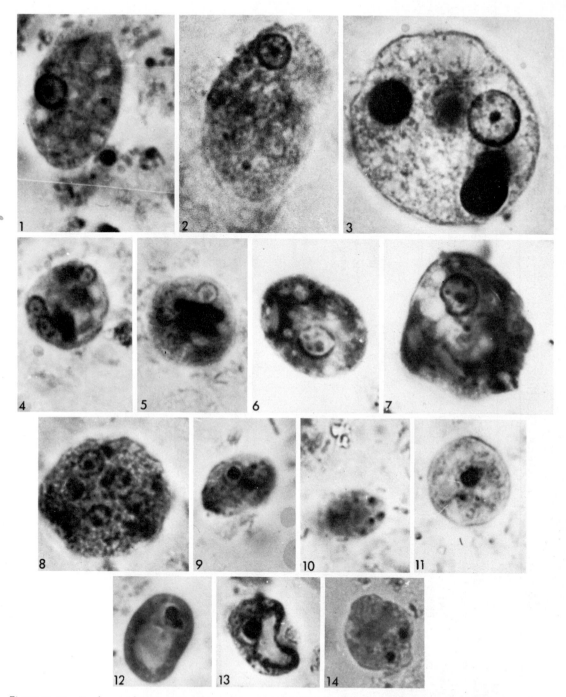

Figure 51–19.   Amebae, trichrome stain, oil immersion. *1* and *2. Entamoeba histolytica* trophozoites. *3. E. histolytica* trophozoite with ingested erythrocytes. *4. E. histolytica* cyst with three nuclei visible, chromatoid bodies, and glycogen vacuoles. *5. E. histolytica* cyst with chromatoid bodies. *6* and *7. E. coli* trophozoites. *8. E. coli* cyst. *9. Endolimax nana* trophozoite. *10. E. nana* cyst with four nuclei. *11. Iodamoeba bütschlii* trophozoite with achromatic granules above karyosome. *12. I. bütschlii* cyst with achromatic granules below karyosome and glycogen vacuole. *13. I. bütschlii* cyst without evident achromatic granules and with glycogen vacuole and irregular shape. *14. Dientamoeba fragilis* trophozoite.

Table 51-6. MORPHOLOGY OF TROPHOZOITES OF INTESTINAL AMEBAE*

SPECIES	SIZE (IN DIAMETER OR LENGTH)	MOTILITY	NUCLEUS			CYTOPLASM	
			Number§	Peripheral Chromatin	Karyosomal Chromatin	Appearance	Inclusions
Entamoeba histolytica	10-60 μ. Usual range, 15-20 μ—commensal form. ‡Over 20 μ—invasive form.	Progressive, with hyaline, finger-like pseudopods.	1 Not visible in unstained preparations.	Fine granules. Usually evenly distributed and uniform in size.	Small, discrete. Usually central but occasionally eccentric.	Finely granular.	Erythrocytes occasionally. Non-invasive contain bacteria.
Entamoeba hartmanni	5-12 μ. Usual range, 8-10 μ.	Usually non-progressive, but may be progressive occasionally.	1 Not visible in unstained preparations.	Similar to *E. histolytica.*	Small, discrete, often eccentric.	Finely granular.	Bacteria.
Entamoeba coli	15-50 μ. Usual range, 20-25 μ.	Sluggish, non-progressive, with blunt pseudopods.	1 Often visible in unstained preparations.	Coarse granules, irregular in size and distribution.	Large, discrete, usually eccentric.	Coarse, often vacuolated.	Bacteria, yeasts, other materials.
Endolimax nana	6-12 μ. Usual range, 8-10 μ.	Sluggish, usually non-progressive, with blunt pseudopods.	1 Visible occasionally in unstained preparations.	None.	Large, irregularly shaped.	Granular, vacuolated.	Bacteria.
Iodamoeba bütschlii	8-20 μ. Usual range, 12-15 μ.	Sluggish, usually non-progressive.	1 Not usually visible in unstained preparations.	None.	Large, usually central. Surrounded by refractile, achromatic granules. These granules are often not distinct even in stained slides.	Coarsely granular, vacuolated.	Bacteria, yeasts, or other material.
Dientamoeba fragilis	5-15 μ. Usual range, 9-12 μ.	Pseudopodia are angular, serrated, or broad lobed and hyaline, almost transparent.	2 (In approximately 20% of organisms only 1 nucleus is present.) Nuclei invisible in unstained preparations.	None.	Large cluster of 4-8 granules.	Finely granular, vacuolated.	Bacteria.

* Adapted with permission from Brooke, M. M., and Melvin, D. M.: Morphology of Diagnostic Stages of Intestinal Parasites of Man, USDHEW PHS Publication No. 1966, 1969.
† Usually found in asymptomatic or chronic cases; may contain bacteria.
‡ Usually found in acute cases; often contain red blood cells.
§ Visibility is for unfixed material. Nuclei may sometimes be visible in fixed material.

mens will allow diagnosis of the intestinal infection in most cases. If the patient has been given antibiotics or gallbladder dyes, the amebic infection may be suppressed for a period of time. If there is a strong suspicion of amebiasis and stool examinations are negative, collection of a purged series is recommended. Some laboratories use culture procedures to grow the amebae.

Aspirated material from liver abscesses can be examined microscopically to detect trophozoites. Usually the last material aspirated is most likely to contain trophozoites and may be examined by direct microscopic examination or permanently stained slides. If tissue is available, tissue sections may show organisms. Culture procedures may be attempted but since bacteria are not present in the liver abscesses, they (e.g., *Clostridium perfringens*) will need to be added to the culture medium. The trophozoites of *Entamoeba histolytica* vary from 10 to 60 μ, with the commensal forms usually 15 to 20 μ and the invasive forms over 20 μ in greatest dimension (Table 51-6, Figs. 51-17 to 51-19). In direct wet mounts, the trophozoites show progressive motility with hyaline pseudopodia that are rapidly formed by sharp demarcation between endoplasm and ectoplasm, but unstained nuclei are not visible. In severe disease, some trophozoites may contain ingested erythrocytes, a feature diagnostic of *E. histolytica* infection. The peripheral chromatin is present in moderate amounts and is typically distributed evenly as fine granules around the nucleus, although it may appear to be a smooth layer of chromatin material rather than granules. The karyosome is small and centrally located, with fine fibrils attaching it to the nuclear membrane; however, these fibrils are not generally visible. Nuclei vary, and eccentric karyosomes and irregularly distributed peripheral chromatin may be seen. It should be emphasized that the appearance of amebae may vary, and there is no single characteristic that is pathognomonic except the phagocytosis of erythrocytes, which very rarely occurs with other species. The cytoplasm is finely granular and in the invasive organisms, there are either no inclusions or only erythrocyte inclusions. Non-invasive organisms may occasionally contain ingested bacteria. In degenerating organisms, the cytoplasm may become vacuolated and nuclei may show abnormal chromatin clumping. Cysts of *E. histolytica* are spherical and 10 to 20 μ in diameter, with the usual range being

12 to 15 μ (Table 51-7, Figs. 51-17 to 51-19). The precyst stage has a single nucleus and is rounded but does not have a refractile cyst wall. The cyst as it matures develops four nuclei, each of which is approximately one sixth the diameter of the cyst. The nuclei show characteristics similar to those of trophozoite nuclei, but it should be emphasized that nuclear characteristics are not as helpful in differentiation of *Entamoeba* cysts as they are in differentiation of trophozoites. The cytoplasm of the cyst may contain glycogen vacuoles and chromatoid bodies with blunted or rounded ends. The number and size of nuclei and the appearance of chromatoid bodies are good diagnostic criteria for cysts.

Serologic tests are very helpful in establishing the diagnosis. Both latex agglutination and counterimmunoelectrophoresis tests for detecting amebic antibodies are commercially available, and others are available from the Center for Disease Control. They are positive in over 95 per cent of patients with amebic liver abscesses. Serology may be positive in 70 per cent or more of patients who have invasive intestinal amebiasis and in approximately 5 per cent of those who carry the organism but do not have clinical disease.

Entamoeba hartmanni

E. hartmanni was formerly called small race *E. histolytica*, and its taxonomic position and relationship to *E. histolytica* small race are still not entirely settled. These organisms have morphologic characteristics similar to those of *E. histolytica* except that the trophozoites have a maximum diameter of 12 μ and the cysts have a maximum diameter of 10 μ. The cytoplasm of *E. hartmanni* trophozoites is fine and delicate and may contain bacteria. Differentiation between *E. histolytica* and *E. hartmanni* is primarily on the basis of measurement with a properly calibrated ocular micrometer.

Entamoeba coli

E. coli is a frequent lumen-dwelling ameba and may be difficult to differentiate from *E. histolytica* (Tables 51-6 and Figs. 51-17 to 51-19). The trophozoites are 15 to 50 μ in diameter but usually measure 20 to 25 μ. These organisms have sluggish non-progressive motility in direct wet mount preparations and the nucleus may be visible, in contrast to *E. histolytica*, in which nuclei are generally

5

Table 51-7. MORPHOLOGY OF CYSTS OF INTESTINAL AMEBAE*

SPECIES	SIZE	SHAPE	NUCLEUS			CYTOPLASM	
			Number	Peripheral Chromatin	Karyosomal Chromatin	Chromatoid Bodies	Glycogen
Entamoeba histolytica	10–20 μ. Usual range, 12–15 μ.	Usually spherical.	4 in mature cyst. Immature cysts with 1 or 2 occasionally seen.	Peripheral chromatin present. Fine, uniform granules, evenly distributed.	Small, discrete, usually central.	Present. Elongated bars with bluntly rounded ends.	Usually diffuse. Concentrated mass often present in young cysts. Stains reddish brown with iodine.
Entamoeba hartmanni	5–10 μ. Usual range, 6–8 μ.	Usually spherical.	4 in mature cyst. Immature cysts with 1 or 2 often seen.	Similar to *E. histolytica*.	Similar to *E. histolytica*.	Present. Elongated bars with bluntly rounded ends.	Similar to *E. histolytica*.
Entamoeba coli	10–35 μ. Usual range, 15–25 μ.	Usually spherical. Occasionally oval, triangular, or of another shape.	8 in mature cyst. Occasionally, supernucleate cysts with 16 or more are seen. Immature cysts with 2 or more occasionally seen.	Peripheral chromatin present. Coarse granules irregular in size and distribution, but often appear more uniform than in trophozoites.	Large, discrete, usually eccentric, but occasionally central.	Present. Usually splinter-like with pointed ends.	Usually diffuse, but occasionally well-defined mass in immature cysts. Stains reddish brown with iodine.
Endolimax nana	5–10 μ. Usual range, 6–8 μ.	Spherical, ovoid, or ellipsoidal.	4 in mature cysts. Immature cysts with less than 4 rarely seen.	None.	Large, usually centrally located.	Occasionally, granules or small oval masses seen, but bodies as seen in *Entamoeba* species are not present.	Usually diffuse. Concentrated mass seen occasionally in young cysts. Stains reddish brown with iodine.
Iodamoeba bütschlii	5–20 μ. Usual range, 10–12 μ.	Ovoid, ellipsoidal, triangular, or of another shape.	1 in mature cyst.	None.	Large, usually eccentric. Refractile, achromatic granules on one side of karyosome.	Granules occasionally present, but bodies as seen in *Entamoeba* species are not present.	Compact, well-defined mass. Stains dark brown with iodine.

*Adapted with permission from Brooke, M. M., and Melvin, D. M.: Morphology of Diagnostic Stages of Intestinal Parasites of Man, USDHEW PHS Publication No. 1966, 1969.

not visible. *E. coli* has more abundant peripheral chromatin than *E. histolytica,* and it is distributed more irregularly and in coarse granules. The karyosome is large and usually eccentric and there may be additional fragments of karyosome material in the karyolymph space. The cytoplasm stains somewhat more darkly than the cytoplasm of *E. histolytica* and is more vacuolated, containing numerous ingested bacteria, yeasts, and other materials. *E. coli* trophozoites do not ingest erythrocytes. It should be emphasized that occasional *E. coli* nuclei may have evenly distributed chromatin and/or may have central karyosomes.

Cysts of *E. coli* measure from 10 to 35 μ in diameter, with most in the 15 to 25 μ range. These spherical cysts, when mature, contain eight nuclei, with occasional supernucleate cysts containing sixteen or more nuclei. Immature cysts with four nuclei are not common and, when present, the individual nuclei are larger (one-fourth the diameter of the cyst) than those of *E. histolytica* (one sixth the diameter of the cyst). The nuclei will have peripheral chromatin and the karyosomes may be either central or eccentric, emphasizing that distribution of peripheral chromatin and karyosomes should not be given great emphasis in identification of *Entamoeba* cysts.

Chromatoid bodies, when present, are irregular in shape with fibrillar, splintered, or pointed ends rather than the rounded ends seen in *E. histolytica.* Glycogen may be present in immature cysts.

E. polecki is an infrequently seen parasite and is not further described (Figure 51-17).

Endolimax nana

E. nana (Tables 51-6 and 51-7; Figs. 51-17 and 51-18) is a small ameba (6 to 12 μ in diameter) that shows sluggish movement in direct wet mounts of fresh material. Its nucleus does not have peripheral chromatin and has a large, irregular karyosome. The trophozoites may have atypical nuclei that contain a triangular chromatin mass, a band of chromatin across the nucleus, or two discrete masses of chromatin on opposite sides of the nuclear membrane. Finding these atypical forms may be quite helpful in the identification of this species and its differentiation from *Iodamoeba bütschlii.* The karyolymph space of *E. nana* is usually quite clear and halo-like, another feature that differs from *I. bütschlii.* The cytoplasm of *E. nana* is granular and vacuolated, sometimes containing numerous ingested bacteria. Cysts of *E. nana* are 5 to 10 μ in diameter and spherical or oval with four nuclei in mature cysts. Cysts with less than four nuclei are infrequently seen. The nuclei are smaller than those of trophozoites but similar in appearance. Chromatoid bodies as such are rarely seen, but there may be small, irregular portions of chromatoid material. Glycogen, when present, is usually diffuse rather than a discrete mass. Cysts are usually not hard to differentiate from those of other amebae but may be confused with *Blastocystis hominis* organisms, which show granules but do not have the distinct karyolymph space around these granules as seen in *E. nana* nuclei and have variable sizes and numbers of granules (Table 51-7).

Iodamoeba bütschlii

I. bütschlii trophozoites (Table 51-6; Figs. 51-17 and 51-18) measure 8 to 20 μ in diameter and in direct wet mount material usually show sluggish, non-progressive motility. In stained mounts, the nucleus has a large, centrally located karyosome that is frequently surrounded by achromatic granules. These achromatic granules may not be distinct but appear only as a muddy karyolymph space. In some nuclei, the karyolymph space will be clear without evident achromatic granules and thus be indistinguishable from *E. nana* nuclei. The cytoplasm of *I. bütschlii* is coarsely granular and vacuolated, containing numerous bacteria and yeasts. Differentiation between *I. bütschlii* and *E. nana* is primarily on the basis of nuclear characteristics of the trophozoites and size, but often numerous organisms must be examined to make this differentiation. The cytoplasm of *I. bütschlii* is more coarse with more ingested material than that of *E. nana.* Differentiation is not clinically important, as neither is pathogenic.

Cysts of *Iodamoeba bütschlii* (Table 51-7, Figs. 51-17 to 51-19) measure from 5 to 20 μ in diameter but usually are 10 to 12 μ in diameter. They are usually oval but may be of various shapes. The cyst usually contains only one nucleus in which the karyosome is often eccentric with a nearby crescent of achromatic granules. The cyst is characterized by a prominent vacuole of glycogen that stains reddish brown in iodine-stained wet mounts, thus the name of the organism. Glycogen is dissolved by aqueous fixatives and thus may not be demonstrable in material that has been stored.

Table 51-8. MORPHOLOGY OF INTESTINAL FLAGELLATES*

TROPHOZOITES

SPECIES	SIZE (LENGTH)	SHAPE	MOTILITY	NUMBER OF NUCLEI	NUMBER OF FLAGELLA†	OTHER FEATURES
Trichomonas‡ *hominis*	8-20 μ. Usual range, 11-12 μ.	Pear-shaped.	Rapid, jerking.	1 Not visible in unstained mounts.	3-5 anterior. 1 posterior.	Undulating membrane extending length of body.
Chilomastix mesnili	6-24 μ. Usual range, 10-15 μ.	Pear-shaped.	Stiff, rotary.	1 Not visible in unstained mounts.	3 anterior. 1 in cytostome.	Prominent cytostome extending 1/3-1/2 length of body. Spiral groove across ventral surface.
Giardia lamblia	10-20 μ. Usual range, 12-15 μ.	Pear-shaped.	"Falling leaf."	2 Not visible in unstained mounts.	4 lateral. 2 ventral. 2 caudal.	Sucking disk occupying 1/2-3/4 of ventral surface.
Enteromonas hominis	4-10 μ. Usual range, 8-9 μ.	Oval.	Jerking.	1 Not visible in unstained mounts.	3 anterior. 1 posterior.	One side of body flattened. Posterior flagellum extending free, posteriorly or laterally.
Retortamonas intestinalis	4-9 μ. Usual range, 6-7 μ.	Pear-shaped or oval.	Jerking.	1 Not visible in unstained mounts.	1 anterior. 1 posterior.	Prominent cytostome extending approximately 1/2 length of body.

CYSTS

SPECIES	SIZE	SHAPE	NUMBER OF NUCLEI	OTHER FEATURES
Chilomastix mesnili	6-10 μ. Usual range, 8-9 μ.	Lemon-shaped, with anterior hyaline knob or "nipple."	1 Not visible in unstained preparations.	Cytostome with supporting fibrils. Usually visible in stained preparation.
Giardia lamblia	8-9 μ. Usual range, 11-12 μ.	Oval or ellipsoidal.	Usually 4. Not distinct in unstained preparations. Usually located at one end.	Fibrils or flagella longitudinally in cyst. Cytoplasm often retracts from a portion of cell wall.
Enteromonas hominis	4-10 μ. Usual range, 6-8 μ.	Elongated or oval.	1-4, usually 2 lying at opposite ends of cyst. Not visible in unstained mounts.	Resembles *E. nana* cyst. Fibrils or flagella are usually not seen.
Retortamonas intestinalis	4-9 μ. Usual range, 4-7 μ.	Pear-shaped or slightly lemon-shaped.	1 Not visible in unstained mounts.	Resembles *Chilomastix* cyst. Shadow outline of cytostome with supporting fibrils extends above nucleus.

*Adapted with permission from Brooke, M. M., and Melvin, D. M.: Morphology of Diagnostic Stages of Intestinal Parasites of Man, USDHEW PHS Publication No. 1966, 1969.

†Not a practical feature for identification of species in routine fecal examinations.

‡*Trichomonas hominis* does not have a cyst form.

Dientamoeba fragilis

D. fragilis (Table 51-6, Fig. 51-17 and 51-18) is an ameboid pathogen without a cyst stage which infects the colon and has been associated with diarrhea (Yang, 1977). Its taxonomic position is uncertain, but it appears to be more closely related to some flagellates than to the amebae. Symptoms include diarrhea and abdominal pain. Pathogenesis is not well defined, but some feel that there is mucosal damage and that erythrophagocytosis may be seen. Recent evidence suggests that dientamebiasis is a more frequent cause of diarrhea than previously thought, with 4.2 per cent of patients in a recent study harboring this organism. Approximately 25 per cent of persons infected with this parasite have symptomatic disease. In contrast to amebiasis, this infection is not usually associated with other fecal protozoa, but it shows a 10 to 20 times greater than expected association with enterobiasis (pinworms). This association and some experimental evidence suggest that *D. fragilis* infection may be spread by ingestion of pinworm eggs infected with *D. fragilis* (Burrows, 1956). The infection may easily be overlooked unless permanently stained slides are examined. The number of parasites in feces may vary from day to day and the number of parasites is greater in the last than in the first portion of a bowel movement.

The trophozoites measure 5 to 15 μ in diameter and in direct wet mounts of fresh material show angular pseudopodia. Two-thirds to four-fifths of the organisms will contain two nuclei. These nuclei do not have peripheral chromatin but do have a cluster of four to eight karyosomal granules. These may appear to be one large irregular karyosome in some instances; thus, a uninucleate *D. fragilis* may be confused with an *E. nana* or *I. bütschlii* trophozoite. The cytoplasm of *D. fragilis* is delicate; therefore, trophozoites may be easily overlooked. The finely granular cytoplasm often contains ingested bacteria.

FLAGELLATES (Table 51-8)

Giardia lamblia

G. lamblia is a pathogenic intestinal protozoan that causes both endemic and epidemic disease with recent outbreaks described in Aspen, Colorado; Leningrad, Russia; and Rome, New York (Shaw, 1977). This organism may also cause infections in children, particularly those attending newborn nurseries (Black, 1977). It was the most frequent pathogenic parasite identified in fecal specimens by State Health Laboratories during 1976 (3.8 per cent of specimens). It appears that some of the large outbreaks have been related to problems in the water supply. Pathogenic protozoa are not killed by the usual concentrations of chlorine in municipal water supplies and thus, unless the water supply is filtered, it may serve as a source of infection as it did in the Rome, New York, outbreak.

G. lamblia is shaped like half a pear (Figs. 51-20 and 51-21). When viewed in its broad dimension, it is pear-shaped with a tapered posterior end and measures 10 to 20 μ long. When viewed from the side, the anterior end of the organism is thicker and tapers posteriorly, with the anterior half to three-fourths consisting of a sucking disc. This organism has eight flagella: four lateral, two ventral, and two caudal. Down the center of the organism are two blepharoplasts that divide the organism into symmetrical halves, and in the middle of this are two darkly stained structures, the median bodies. The nuclei are round with prominent, usually central karyosomes, and there is no peripheral chromatin. When viewed from the broad aspect, the organism has the appearance of a smiling face with prominent eyes. The flagella are not usually evident in wet mounts or in stained preparations. In direct wet mount, the organism is motile, with the motion being described as a "falling leaf."

Cysts of *G. lamblia* are oval and measure 8 to 19 μ long. Mature cysts contain four nuclei. Fibrils are evident within the cyst, and the cytoplasm is often retracted from the wall in some areas. *G. lamblia* is readily differentiated from other protozoa of man by the binucleate trophozoite with its distinctive structures and the quadrinucleate cyst with fibrils. Generally when organisms are not identified in specimens that contain them, it is because they are overlooked rather than because they are misidentified.

G. lamblia causes an infection of the small intestine. There are often asymptomatic individuals, and the disease may vary from mild diarrhea with vague abdominal complaints to a full malabsorption syndrome with diarrhea and steatorrhea, similar to sprue. The organisms appear to cause disease both by the mechanical blockage of the absorptive surface and by damage to the mucosal epithelium. *G.*

5

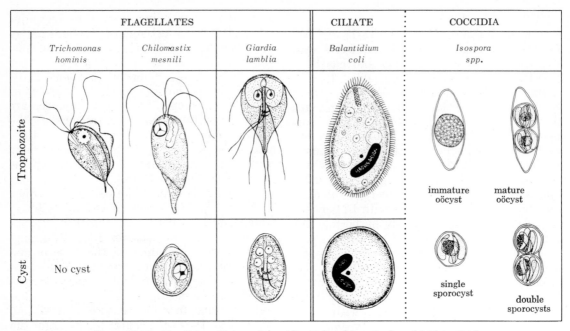

FLAGELLATES			CILIATE	COCCIDIA
Trichomonas hominis	*Chilomastix mesnili*	*Giardia lamblia*	*Balantidium coli*	*Isospora* spp.
Trophozoite				immature oöcyst mature oöcyst
No cyst (Cyst)				single sporocyst double sporocysts

Figure 51–20. Flagellates, ciliate, and coccidia. (*Adapted from Brooke and Melvin, 1964*)

lamblia does not infect other organs of the body. The disease occurs worldwide and is increasingly recognized in the "developed" areas of the world. Giardiasis should be considered in any patient presenting with diarrhea of over 10 days' duration.

Diagnosis is established by demonstration of *Giardia* trophozoites and/or cysts in fecal specimens. The passage of organisms may vary from day to day; therefore, multiple specimens, collected over a period of time, need to be examined. Direct wet mounts are particularly helpful for demonstrating the motile trophozoites, although they may also be used to show cysts. Cysts can be demonstrated

by concentration techniques and both trophozoites and cysts may be demonstrated and carefully studied in permanently stained slides. In some cases, the organisms cannot be demonstrated in fecal specimens, and aspirates of small bowel material may be required to demonstrate them. In such instances, the laboratory should be advised ahead of time so that it will be able to perform a direct wet mount when the specimen is received.

Chilomastix mesnili

C. mesnili (Table 51-8, Figs. 51-20 and 51-22) is a non-pathogenic lumen-dwelling flagel-

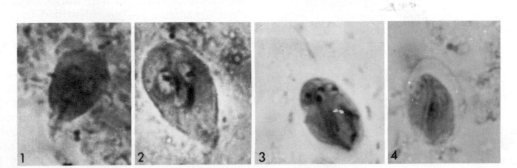

Figure 51–21. *Giardia lamblia,* trichrome stain, oil immersion. *1* and *2*. Trophozoites with prominent nuclei, median bodies, and tapered posterior ends. *3* and *4*. Cysts with nuclei and fibrils. The cyst on the right has retracted from the cyst wall.

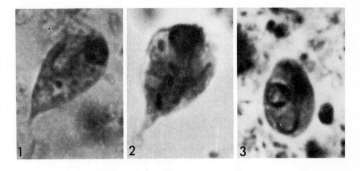

Figure 51–22. *Chilomastix mesnili,* trichrome stain, oil immersion. *1* and *2.* Trophozoites with anterior nuclei and tapered posterior ends. The cytostome is to the left of the nucleus in *1* and to the right of the nucleus in *2. 3* is a cyst with the typical lemon shape. Nucleus is on the left. Curved fibrils are prominent at the bottom of the cyst.

late of man and may occasionally be seen in stool specimens. The organisms are oval with a tapered posterior end and usually measure 10 to 15 μ long. In direct wet mounts, the organism moves in a stiff rotary fashion. The organism has a cytostome extending one third to one half the length of the body adjacent to the nucleus, but it is not always visible. In addition, there is a spiral groove across the ventral surface of the organism, and the indentations of the margin of the organism are a reflection of this. The nucleus is anterior, and the chromatin may be distributed in various patterns, including a large chromatin mass on the nuclear membrane, or a more diffuse distribution of chromatin and fragmented chromatin, or a large central karyosome. Within the organism is a cytostomal fibril that curves posteriorly around the cytostome. In addition, there are three anterior flagella and a short flagellum that arises from the cytostome and curves posteriorly. These organisms must be differentiated from trophozoites of amebae in stained smears. The consistent location of the *C. mesnili* nucleus at one end of the organism and the tapering of the end opposite the nucleus are helpful. If multiple organisms are examined, the cytostome will be visible in some. The flagella are usually not visible in stained or formalin-fixed preparations. The cysts of *Chilomastix* are generally 3 to 9 μ long and lemon-shaped, with an anterior hyaline knob or nipple. The single nucleus has an appearance similar to that of the trophozoite, and the cytoplasm contains various curved cytostomal fibers that sometimes have a "safety-pin" appearance.

Trichomonas hominis

T. hominis (Table 51-8, Fig. 51-20) is a less frequent non-pathogenic flagellate, which does not have a cyst form. The organism measures 11 to 12 μ long and also tapers at the posterior end. It has an anteriorly situated nucleus with an axostyle that runs the length of the organism and protrudes posteriorly. An undulating membrane arises at the anterior end and runs the length of the body, where the axoneme protrudes as a free flagellum. The base of this undulating membrane is a fibril known as the costa. There are three to five anterior flagella. In wet mounts of fresh material, *T. hominis* has rapid jerking movements. The organisms do not stain particularly well but in stained material have a nucleus with a small karyosome and unevenly distributed chromatin. They may be confused with *Entameoba hartmani* or small *E. histolytica* trophozoites. The axostyle may be visible and aids in identification. Several organisms may need to be examined in order to demonstrate the undulating membrane, flagella, axostyle, or costa, which are important diagnostic characteristics.

Trichomonas vaginalis

T. vaginalis causes a common vaginal infection characterized by inflammation with itching and vaginal discharge. Occasionally the urinary tract may be involved, with dysuria being associated with vaginal involvement. The infection may be spread by sexual intercourse. Males may have asymptomatic infections or occasionally symptomatic prostatitis. *T. vaginalis* infections are usually diagnosed by the physician in his office using the simple procedure of direct wet mount to look for the typical jerky motile organisms. Media have also been developed for culture of these organisms but are not widely used, although they are useful for demonstration and teaching purposes.

Morphologically, *T. vaginalis* resembles *T. hominis* but is larger (30 μ), and the undulating membrane extends only half the length of the body. Because of the differences in habitat,

5

Table 51-9. MORPHOLOGY OF INTESTINAL CILIATE AND COCCIDIA*

SPECIES	SIZE (LENGTH)	SHAPE	MOTILITY	NUMBER OF NUCLEI	OTHER FEATURES
Balantidium coli					
Trophozoite	50-70 μ or more. Usual range, 40-50 μ.	Ovoid with tapering anterior end.	Rotary, boring.	1 large, kidney-shaped macronucleus. 1 small, micronucleus immediately adjacent to macronucleus. Macronucleus occasionally visible in unstained preparations.	Body surface covered by spiral, longitudinal rows of cilia. Contractile vacuoles are present.
Cyst	45-65 μ. Usual range, 50-55 μ.	Spherical or oval.	- - - - -	1 large macronucleus visible in unstained preparations.	Macronucleus and contractile vacuole are visible in young cysts. In older cysts, internal structure appears granular.
Coccidia (*Isospora belli* and *Sarcocystis* sp.)	Oocyst: 25-30 μ. Usual range, 28-30 μ. Immature oocyst not usually seen in *Sarcocystis* sp. Sporocyst: *I. belli*—12-14 μ. *Sarcocystis* sp.—14-16 μ.	Ellipsoidal. Round or oval.	Non-motile.		Mature oocyst contains 2 sporocysts with 4 sporozoites each. *I. belli:* Usual diagnostic stage is immature oocyst with single granular mass (zygote) within. *Sarcocystis* sp.: Mature sporocysts, singly or in pairs, are usually passed in feces. Oocyst wall not apparent.

* Adapted with permission from Brooke, M. M., and Melvin, D. M.: Morphology of Diagnostic Stages of Intestinal Parasites of Man, USDHEW PHS Publication No. 1966, 1969.

it is generally not necessary to differentiate these trichomonads morphologically.

Two small infrequently found intestinal flagellates, *Enteromonas hominis* and *Retortamonas intestinalis*, will not be described other than in Table 51-8. *Trichomonas tenax* is a trichomonad that occasionally infects the oral cavity but does not cause disease.

CILIATES

Balantidium coli

The ciliate *B. coli* (Table 51-9, Fig. 51-20) may cause a severe intestinal infection similar to the intestinal phase of amebiasis with colonic ulcerations, but it does not cause liver abscesses and other systemic lesions. It appears that man acquires the infection from association with hogs, which are commonly infected. The trophozoites vary greatly in size, from 40 to over 200 μ in greatest dimension, with most measuring 40 to 70 μ. The body is uniformly covered with cilia that are slightly longer at the anterior end adjacent to the cytostome. There is a larger macronucleus, which is readily seen, and a smaller micronucleus, which is infrequently visible. There are numerous food vacuoles and contractile vacuoles in the cytoplasm. The encysted organism is rounded and when young, will still show cilia that disappear as the cyst ages. This organism does not present diagnostic problems other than sometimes being overlooked because of its large size. Specimens contaminated with stagnant water may contain other ciliates, which can usually be distinguished from *B. coli* by differences in their ciliary pattern.

SPOROZOA

There are two intestinal sporozoan infections of man that are infrequently diagnosed and that are in some ways similar to the feline stage of toxoplasmosis. Isosporiasis is caused by the coccidian *Isospora belli*, which infects the epithelium of the small intestinal mucosa and sometimes gives rise to diarrheal disease. The disease is acquired by fecal-oral contamination and occasionally may cause a malabsorption syndrome similar to that seen in giardiasis. Infection is maintained in the intestinal tract by asexual schizogony. The diagnostic sexual stage in the feces is the oocyst (Table 51-9, Fig. 51-20). Immature oocysts, 30 by 12 μ, are passed in the stool. The immature oocyst contains a zygote that divides to form two sporoblasts. These then develop heavy cyst walls and become sporocysts. Within each sporocyst, four curved sausage-shaped sporozoites develop. *Isospora* oocysts in these various stages of development may be seen by direct examination or by concentration procedures.

Sarcocystis sp., which infect pigs and cattle, may infect man with the sexual stage in the epithelium of the intestinal tract. Such infection is acquired by eating undercooked infected meat and is asymptomatic. These *Sarcocystis* sp. organisms were formerly called *Isospora hominis*. In contrast to *I. belli*, in which the oocyst is usually intact and is immature, *Sarcocystis* usually is found in the form of mature sporocysts, singly or in pairs, that have ruptured out of the oocyst (Fig. 51-20).

Non-parasitic Objects. There are various inflammatory and tissue cells, yeasts, and other substances that may be seen in feces. Table 51-10 lists characteristics that may aid in their differentiation from protozoa.

INTESTINAL HELMINTHS

Helminths occur both as free-living and as parasitic forms. They are classified into nematodes (roundworms) and platyhelminths (flat worms). Platyhelminths in turn are divided into trematodes (flukes) and cestodes (tapeworms). The adult worms vary in size from barely visible to the naked eye to 10 meters in length.

The life cycles of helminths are variable and include both direct and indirect cycles. The direct type of development requires only one host, who is infected by the embryonated egg or larva. In some instances the egg is infective when passed, and in others it requires a soil maturation period to reach the infective stage. Indirect cycles are more complex and include intermediate hosts, in which the larval stages develop, and definitive hosts, which harbor the adults. The adult and larval stages, depending upon specific requirements of each, occur in the intestinal lumen or in host tissues. Most living organisms, including man, serve as habitat for larval and/or adult parasitic helminth stages.

Signs and symptoms of helminth infections

Table 51-10. NON-PARASITIC OBJECTS THAT MAY BE CONFUSED WITH INTESTINAL PROTOZOA*

ARTIFACT	RESEMBLANCE	SALINE MOUNT	DIFFERENTIAL CHARACTERISTICS OF ARTIFACT PERMANENT STAIN	
			CYTOPLASM	NUCLEUS
Polymorphonuclear leukocytes (Seen in dysentery and other inflammatory bowel diseases.)	E. histolytica cyst	Usually not a problem. Granules in cytoplasm. Cell border irregular.	Less dense, often frothy. Border less clearly demarcated than that of ameba.	More coarse. Larger, relative to size of organism. Irregular shape and size. Chromatin unevenly distributed. Chromatin strands may link nuclei.
Macrophages (Seen in dysentery and other inflammatory bowel diseases. May be present in purged specimens.)	Amebic trophozoite, especially E. histolytica	Nuclei larger and of irregular shape, with irregular chromatin distribution. Cytoplasm granular; may contain ingested debris. Cell border irregular and indistinct. Movement irregular and pseudopodia indistinct.	Coarse. May contain inclusions.	Large and often irregular in shape. Chromatin irregularly distributed.
Squamous epithelial cells (from anal mucosa)	Amebic trophozoite	Nucleus refractile and large. Cytoplasm smooth. Cell border distinct.	Stains poorly.	Large and single. Large chromatin mass may resemble karyosome.
Columnar epithelial cells (from intestinal mucosa)	Amebic trophozoite	Nucleus refractile and large. Cytoplasm smooth. Cell border distinct.	Stains poorly.	Large with heavy chromatin on nuclear membrane. Often large central chromatin mass resembling karyosome.
Blastocystis hominis (Yeastlike organism that frequently grows in feces. Ruptures in water.)	Protozoan cyst	Spherical to oval. 6-15 μ in length. Central clear area. Peripheral refractile granules (3-7) may resemble nuclei.	Central mass may stain light or dark. Prominent wall.	Peripheral granules may resemble nuclei. Granules vary in size and appearance. True nuclear structure not present.
Yeasts (Normal constituent of feces.)	Protozoan cyst	Oval. Thick wall. No internal structure. Budding forms may be seen.	Oval. Little internal structure. Refractile cell wall. Budding forms may be seen.	None.
Starch granules	Protozoan cyst	Rounded or angular. Very refractile. No internal structure. Stain pink to purple in iodine mounts.	Not a problem in permanently stained slides.	

Note: Other artifacts, such as contaminating plant cells and pollen grains, are occasionally seen. These should not be difficult to differentiate.
*From Smith, 1976.

may be variously caused by adults, larvae, or eggs. Eosinophilia is common, especially in early stages of infection in which parasites are in tissue.

A clear understanding of the life cycles of the parasites, the tissues likely to be compromised, and the geographic distribution are necessary if parasitic infection is to be suspected and diagnosed. Final diagnosis usually depends upon the morphologic identification of a stage of the parasite (egg, larva, embryo, or adult). However, in some infections only a clinical diagnosis is possible, or diagnosis is established indirectly by serologic methods. There are some infections in which the diagnosis must be established by the surgical pathologist.

Identification of helminth eggs in feces is particularly important and should be approached systematically. A variety of factors must be considered. Size of eggs is particularly important and requires use of a properly calibrated ocular micrometer (Fig. 51-23 and 51-24). Shape and thickness of the shell should be noted. Special structures, such as a mammillated covering, operculum, shoulders adjacent

to the operculum, abopercular knob, polar plugs, or spines should be sought. The egg should be examined to determine if it contains an undeveloped ovum, a developing ovum, or a larva, and hooklets should be sought in larvae. If these various characteristics are considered and used and the examiner is familiar with the background material in feces, there should be no difficulty identifying eggs in fecal specimens.

NEMATODES

Nematodes are the most common helminths parasitizing man. The intestinal nematodes are usually diagnosed by finding eggs, larvae, or adult worms in the feces.

Enterobius vermicularis. Enterobiasis, sometimes called oxyuriasis, is the most common helminthic infection in children of all social strata in the United States. The infection rate is not known, but there have been estimates of 30 per cent of children and 16 per cent of adults. Rates are often higher in institutions (Warren, 1974).

The normal habitat is the lumen of the cecum and adjacent areas where both males

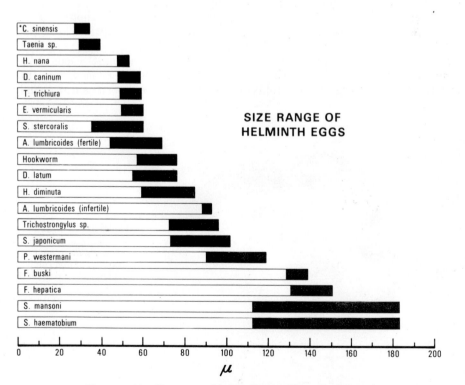

Figure 51-23.   Size range of helminth eggs. (From Smith, 1976.)

RELATIVE SIZES OF HELMINTH EGGS

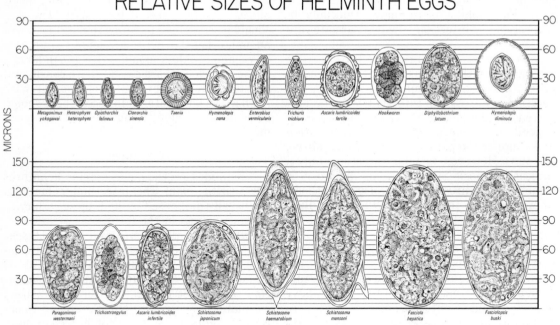

Figure 51-24. Relative sizes of helminth eggs. (From Parasitology Training Branch, Center for Disease Control, Atlanta, Ga.)

and females live. The female worm measures up to 13 mm in length and has a pointed posterior end which gives the common name of pinworm. A characteristic of both adult worms is a cephalic knob which is seen as alae (Fig. 51-25).

The gravid female migrates from the cecum to the perineal area, usually during the evening or night, and deposits eggs in the folds of the perineal skin. The eggs (Fig. 51-26) are ovoid with one side flattened, measure 50 to 60 by 20 to 30 μ, are embryonated when laid, and are infective within hours. If eggs are ingested by the appropriate host, the life cycle is completed.

Clinically, in most cases enterobiasis is asymptomatic or causes very mild disease. There may be *pruritus ani*, usually at night,

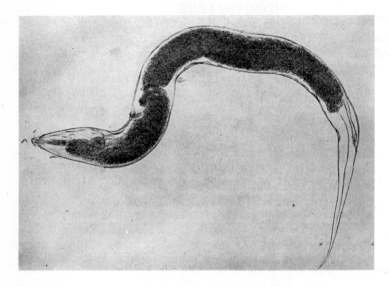

Figure 51-25. Adult female *E. vermicularis* showing bulb behind esophagus, vulva, egg mass, anus, and pointed posterior end. (From Hunter, C. W., Swartzwelder, J. C., and Clyde, D. F.: A Manual of Tropical Medicine. Philadelphia, W. B. Saunders Company, 1976.)

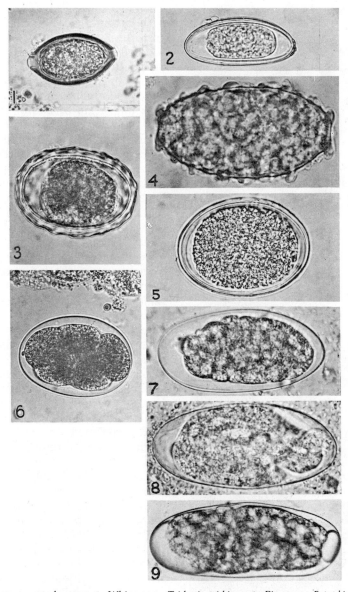

Figure 51–26. Common nematode eggs. *1.* Whipworm, *Trichuris trichiura. 2.* Pinworm, *Enterobius vermicularis. 3.* Large roundworm, *Ascaris lumbricoides*, fertilized egg. *4. Ascaris*, unfertilized egg. *5. Ascaris*, decorticated egg. *6.* Hookworm egg. *7.* Immature egg of *Trichostrongylus orientalis. 8.* Embryonated egg of *T. orientalis. 9.* Egg of *Heterodera marioni*, a plant nematode which sometimes is found in stools. All figures ×500. (*5, 6* courtesy of Photographic Laboratory, AMSGS; photos by Mild Cheskis. *7, 8,* and *9* courtesy of Dr. T. B. Magath, Mayo Clinic. All others courtesy of Dr. R. L. Roudabush, Ward's Natural Science Establishment, Rochester, N.Y.; photos by T. Romaniak.)

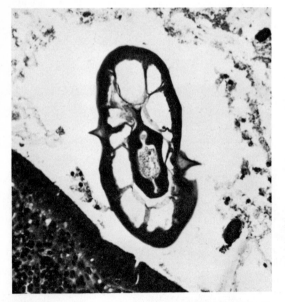

Figure 51-27. *Enterobius vermicularis* in appendix. Note the characteristic lateral alae. ×200.

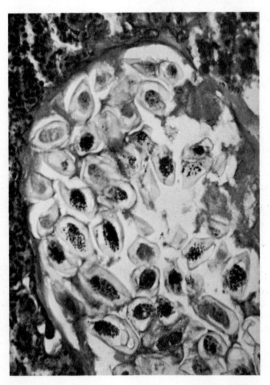

Figure 51-28. *Enterobius vermicularis* in omentum. Note the mass of typical eggs surrounded by remnants of the uterine wall, and the inflammatory reaction. ×300.

which is related to the migration of the parasites to the perineal area, and there may be irritability. Pinworms may be found in surgical specimens of the appendix, either in the lumen or buried in the mucosa. They are identified by their size and typical morphology with lateral alae (Fig. 51-27). A role for the parasite in development of some cases of appendicitis has been questioned but not resolved. It appears that in most cases the worm is just an incidental bystander.

Ectopic localizations are produced by aberrant migration of adult females, which may find their way into the vagina where the eggs can be visualized in Papanicolaou smears. Further, they can migrate to the uterus and peritoneal cavity via the fallopian tubes. In the uterus endometrial granulomatous lesions can be produced by the parasite eggs. In the peritoneum a single granuloma 1 to 2 cm in diameter is usually formed. Microscopically, it shows the remnants of the adult parasite or a mass of eggs (Fig. 51-28) (Symmers, 1950).

Diagnosis of the infection is usually made by recovery of typical eggs from the perianal folds. This is best accomplished with the cellulose tape technique (see p. 1740) because only 5 to 10 per cent of the cases are detected with routine stool examination for ova and parasites. The sample should always be taken at night after the child has gone to sleep or in the morning before a bath. Visual examination of the anal area may allow detection of adult worms. Both eggs and adult worms are easily identified.

Diagnosis may require examination of several samples taken on different days before the eggs can be found; in fact, one method of determining severity of infection is to determine the number of days out of six when cellulose tape preparations are positive.

Trichuris trichiura. A common nematode worldwide, especially in tropical and subtropical areas, *Trichuris* is the causative agent of trichuriasis (whipworm infection) in man.

Trichuris adults are located in the large intestine, especially the cecum, but in more severe infections the parasites can be found in the entire colon and rectum. The worms are easily identified because the anterior portion of their bodies is long and slender with a thicker posterior end, thus the name whipworm (Fig. 51-29). Adult worms measure up to 50 mm in length and live attached to the intestinal mucosa by their slender anterior portions. Like most nematodes, the posterior end

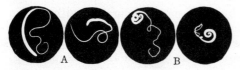

Figure 51-29. Whipworms (*Trichuris trichiura*). *A,* Females; *B,* males. The posterior portion of the male is usually coiled as is shown at the right. Photographs of mounted specimens. Natural size.

of the male is curved ventrally. *Trichuris* is one of the soil-transmitted helminths with a rather simple life cycle. The unembryonated eggs (Figs. 51-23, 51-26, 51-30) passed with the stools find their way into the appropriate soil, following which there is a period of maturation of several weeks before they contain infective larvae. When swallowed by the appropriate host, larvae are released and mature into adults. Attachment to the mucosa occurs early, and the worms apparently remain attached during their lifetime (estimated to be four to five years).

The clinical manifestations of trichuriasis in man depend upon the number of worms present (Jung, 1951). In light to moderate infections (most cases) there are no symptoms. However, with larger numbers (150 worm pairs) there may be diarrhea, and in the most severe cases there is dysentery, clinically indistinguishable from that caused by amebae, with mucus and blood in the stools. A common complication in children is rectal prolapse which is not caused by the worm itself but rather is a consequence of the patient's repeated efforts to void when there is diarrhea.

Histopathologically, the intestine shows only mild non-specific polymorphonuclear cell infiltrate with some eosinophils.

The diagnosis is made by finding the typical eggs measuring 52 to 57 by 22 to 23 μ (Figs. 51-26, 51-30) in either the saline or iodine fecal smears or with the concentration techniques. The eggs are barrel-shaped with refractile polar plugs at both ends. If eggs are found in the direct mount, they may be quantitated in various ways. A simple method is to determine the number of eggs in a standard smear (which is equivalent to 2 mg of stool). When counts are used, light infections will be represented by less than 5 eggs per slide and heavy infections by over 25 eggs. Watery stools or those containing large amounts of mucus or undigested food are not suitable for egg counts. The egg size varies under normal conditions. Oversized eggs or eggs with atypical shape may result from previous treatment with anthelmintics.

Ascaris lumbricoides. This is the largest nematode of the human intestinal tract. The infection (ascariasis) is common in many parts of the world, and it is estimated that there are over half a billion people infected with *Ascaris*. It is a soil-transmitted helminth that occurs mainly in areas where sanitation is poor, such as the tropics (W.H.O., 1964). Like *Trichuris*, it is especially common in children, who are also more likely to have heavy infections.

The female measures up to 35 cm in length by 6 mm in diameter. The male is smaller and has the posterior end curved ventrally. The adult parasites generally live in the small intestine, especially the duodenum and proximal jejunum. Each female will lay approximately 200,000 non-embryonated eggs per day. They measure 45 to 70 by 35 to 50 μ. When the eggs are deposited in a satisfactory environment, they become embryonated (infective) in two to four weeks. If the infective eggs are swallowed by the susceptible host, they will hatch in the intestine and release larvae. These then penetrate the intestinal mucosa and enter the blood stream, which carries them to the lungs where they develop for several days in the alveolar capillary bed. When the larvae have

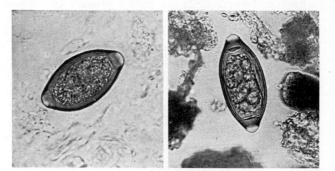

Figure 51-30. Eggs of *Trichuris trichiura* in feces ($\times$500).

developed to the proper stage, they break into the alveoli, migrate upward in the respiratory tree to the epiglottis where they are swallowed, reach the small intestine, and grow to adulthood. The entire development from embryonated egg to adult takes approximately two months.

Ascariasis varies from asymptomatic infection to severe disease. In the intestine a few worms will not usually cause noticeable symptoms, but heavy infections may produce pain, abdominal discomfort, and diarrhea, all of which are non-specific. A mass of worms may cause intestinal obstruction, especially in young children. Migration of the worms with invasion of the common bile duct may cause biliary colic and biliary obstruction and can lead to cholangitis and intrahepatic abscesses if the worms reach the liver. Worms in the appendix may cause appendicitis. Worms may migrate to the stomach and be vomited. Fever or drug therapy (especially anesthetics) may stimulate this migration.

Migration of the young larvae through the lungs may cause Loeffler syndrome, which is characterized by diffuse mottled infiltrates of both lungs in radiographs and peripheral eosinophilia and mild bronchitis. Severity of clinical manifestations varies with the number of larvae migrating through the lungs and the severity of the host response. The syndrome is rarely diagnosed even in endemic areas, and only seldom have patients come to the autopsy table with it (Spillmann, 1975).

Diagnosis of the infection is made by demonstrating the eggs in feces or occasionally by examining an adult which has been passed or vomited. The direct smear will almost always reveal infection even if there is only one female worm. The 200,000 eggs that one female produces every 24 hours will give at least 5 eggs per slide of 2 mg of feces. If counts are done, less than 20 eggs per slide indicates light infections and over 100, heavy infections.

Fertile *Ascaris* eggs are round to slightly oval with a yellow-brown, irregular external mamillated layer and a thick shell. The ovum is round and, in fresh specimens, undivided with a clear space between the ovum and shell at each end. Sometimes the egg is decorticate (the mamillated layer is missing) and the thick shelled egg may be confused with other helminth eggs (see Fig. 51-26). However, the *Ascaris* egg has a much thicker shell, and the *Ascaris* ovum is not developed (in a fresh specimen). Unfertilized eggs are larger, up to 94 by 44 μ, more elongated with a thinner, more irregular external layer, and have irregular globules of yolk material filling the egg without clear areas at the ends (see Fig. 51-26).

Various non-parasitic objects in the stools such as vegetable fragments may be mistaken for *Ascaris* eggs, especially infertile ones.

Hookworms. These nematodes commonly infect the small intestine of man. The two principal species causing disease in man are *Ancylostoma duodenale*, the old world hookworm, and *Necator americanus*, the new world hookworm. The infection is most frequent in the tropics but also occurs in subtropical areas. In Europe, hookworms were once very prevalent, and in the United States there are still some endemic areas in the southeastern part of the country.

The hookworm female measures up to 12 mm in length and the male slightly less. The males are easily distinguished by the fan-shaped copulatory bursa at the posterior end. Male and female parasites attach to the small intestinal mucosa but often change attachment site (in contrast to *Trichuris*, which do not change sites).

The females lay the characteristic eggs which are passed in feces (see Fig. 51-26). When the eggs are deposited on the soil, they develop and (depending on conditions) produce in one day or more rhabditiform larvae that hatch and develop to the infective filariform stage in about seven days. If they contact the skin of an appropriate host, they will actively penetrate it, gain access to the host's circulation, travel to the lungs where they penetrate into the alveoli, following a route similar to that of *Ascaris*, and mature to adults in the small intestine. Ingested *A. duodenale* larvae can develop into adults in the intestine without tissue migration.

Hookworms may produce various clinical manifestations in man. In the skin, if the host has been previously sensitized to the parasite, there may be marked inflammation, redness, and blister formation with intense itching, a condition known as "ground itch." In the lungs, if the number of larvae migrating at one time is large, there may be Loeffler syndrome. In the intestine, also depending on the worm burden, the infection can result in gastrointestinal symptoms, such as diarrhea, abdominal pain, and nausea. However, the main clinical manifestations of hookworm infections are caused by chronic blood loss with secondary iron deficiency anemia due to laceration of the small intestinal mucosa by the parasites. It has been estimated that there is between 0.15 and 0.25 ml of blood lost per day for each adult *A. duodenale* and 0.03 ml for each adult *N. americanus*. The blood loss and number of worms in hookworm infections have been shown to correlate with the number of eggs per gram of stool, so that egg counts may aid in determining need to treat (Layrisse, 1964a and b).

The diagnosis is made by finding the characteristic eggs in the stools. The oval eggs measure 58 to 76 μ long by 36 to 40 μ wide and have a thin shell. The egg is usually in the four to eight cell segmented stage when passed but may vary from unsegmented to embryonated, the latter in specimens from constipated patients. Embryonated eggs or free larvae may be found in unpreserved specimens that are not examined promptly. Hookworm larvae must be differentiated from larvae of *Strongyloides stercoralis*. Hookworm rhabditiform larvae have a longer buccal chamber and an inconspicuous genital primordium. Filariform hookworm larvae have a pointed posterior end and an esophagus approximately one fourth the length of the larva (Fig. 51-31).

If specimens are contaminated with soil, the larvae must also be differentiated from larvae of free-living nematodes. Hookworm eggs must be differentiated from eggs of *Trichostrongylus* species (which are longer and more pointed) and of *Meloidogyne* (*Heterodera*) sp., which are longer and narrower, have blunt ends, and are often asymmetrical. *Meloidogyne* spp. are plant parasitic nematodes, the eggs of which are accidentally ingested when eating root vegetables such as potatoes, carrots, and onions.

In direct wet mounts, egg counts of less than 5 eggs per slide denote light infections, which are unlikely to cause symptoms or anemia, whereas more than 25 denote heavy infections. Eggs from different human hookworm species cannot be differentiated; therefore, "hookworm eggs" should be reported.

Adults of human hookworms can be differentiated on the basis of the types of mouth parts. *Ancylostoma* have teeth, whereas *N. americanus* adults have a pair of cutting plates. Configuration of the male copulatory bursa and other characteristics are used to identify species.

Trichostrongylus spp. These small nematodes live with their anterior ends embedded

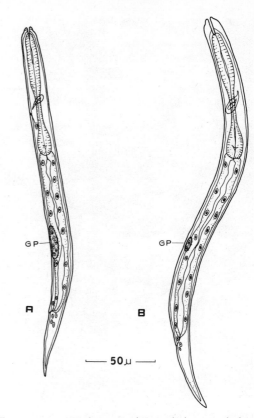

Figure 51-31. Hookworm and *Strongyloides stercoralis* larvae. *A, S. stercoralis* rhabditoid larva in human stools. Note the short size of the buccal cavity and the large genital primordium (GP). *B,* Hookworm rhabditoid larva as seen in a few instances in stools left for at least 24 hours at room temperature. The buccal cavity is longer and the genital primordium is smaller.

in the small intestinal epithelium of man and animals. Several species may infect man, including *T. colubriformis, T. axei, T. orientalis,* and *T. brevis. Trichostrongylus* infections in man have been described mainly in the Far East, India, and Russia, with sporadic cases in Latin America and the United States (Faust, 1975).

The females lay eggs that are passed with the stools. After a short period of maturation in the soil, larvae emerge and then develop to the infective stage. Infective larvae crawl on soil and vegetation and infect a new host when ingested with contaminated food or water. They develop to adults in the intestine without migration through the lungs. The disease is usually asymptomatic, but heavy infections may produce abdominal pain and diarrhea, usually with a mild eosinophilia. The diagnosis is made by finding the typical eggs

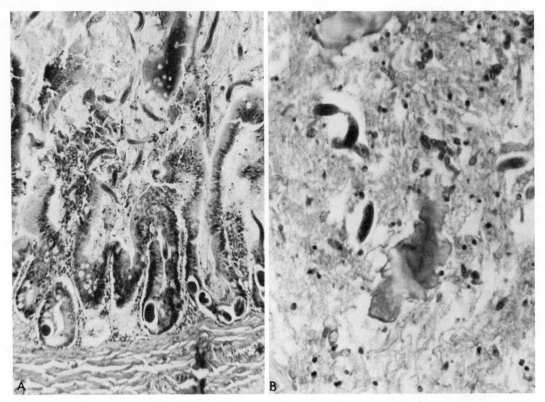

Figure 51-32. *Strongyloides stercoralis.* Autopsy specimens from patient with massive strongyloidiosis. *A,* Larvae and eggs in duodenal mucosa. ×120. *B,* Larvae in sputum (cell block) ×300.

in the patient's stools. Eggs resemble those of hookworm but are narrower and longer (see Fig. 51-26), measuring 78 to 98 μ by 40 to 50 μ, and have somewhat pointed ends. Eggs from different species of *Trichostrongylus* cannot be differentiated; therefore, only a generic identification is made.

Strongyloides stercoralis. *Strongyloides* is a small nematode which lives buried in the mucosa of the duodenum and jejunum (Fig. 51-32). The infection is more common in warm climates, but there are also cases in temperate zones.

The small parasitic female is 2 mm long and reproduces parthenogenetically. There is probably no parasitic male in the vertebrate phase of the cycle. The female lays eggs deep in the mucosa. These develop rhabditiform larvae, which hatch and find their way into the intestinal lumen to be passed with the patient's stools (Fig. 51-33). Therefore, eggs are

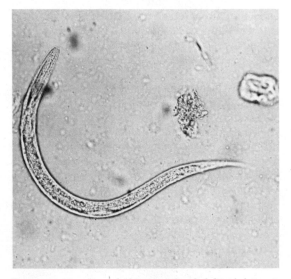

Figure 51-33. *Strongyloides stercoralis* rhabditoid larva in human stool (×300).

almost never found in the stools. Larvae, if deposited in appropriate areas, will mature to infective filariform larvae in a short time. Infective larvae, after contact with the skin of susceptible hosts, will penetrate and migrate via the circulatory system to the lungs, then migrate to the small intestine and grow to adult females. Under certain circumstances, larvae in soil may develop a free-living generation in which there are male and female adults, eggs, and larvae.

Rhabditiform larvae traveling with the intestinal contents may sometimes develop into infective filariform larvae that are capable of penetrating the mucosa and traveling via the circulation to the lungs, thereby completing the life cycle. The factor or factors that allow for this development of internal autoinfection are not known. However, it is known that this rhabditiform to filariform transformation usually occurs in patients who have compromised defenses due to conditions such as malnutrition or immunosuppression.

The clinical manifestations that strongyloidiasis produces in man are variable. As with hookworm, parasites in the skin may produce irritation with pruritus and redness at the site of entry, and migration of large numbers of larvae through the lungs may produce a Loeffler syndrome with peripheral eosinophilia (Purtillo, 1974).

The intestinal phase of the infection produces no symptoms in the great majority of cases. However, some patients may have gastrointestinal symptoms varying from a mild to severe diarrhea and some may develop a malabsorption syndrome.

The major importance of *Strongyloides* infections, however, lies in the cases of internal autoinfection (superinfection) in which massive strongyloidiasis develops. These patients have a high peripheral eosinophilia. Massive numbers of infective larvae migrating through the lungs for a prolonged period of time result in marked pulmonary disease with radiographic infiltrates and consolidation. In the intestine, because of the massive number of parasitic females, there may be marked diarrhea and enteritis. Larvae may invade a wide variety of tissues. Unfortunately, diagnosis is usually made at the autopsy table (see Fig. 51-32).

Strongyloidiasis is generally diagnosed by the recovery and identification of the typical rhabditiform larvae in the stools (Fig. 51-33). Morphology of larvae must be carefully stud-

ied to be certain that they are *Strongyloides* larvae. *Strongyloides* rhabditiform larvae have a short buccal cavity and a prominent genital primordium, whereas hookworm rhabditiform larvae have a long buccal cavity and an indistinct genital primordium. *Strongyloides* filariform larvae have a notched tail and an esophagus approximately half the length of the body, whereas hookworm filariform larvae have a pointed tail and an esophagus approximately one fourth the length of the body (see Fig. 51-31). In fresh saline mounts the moving parasites may be easily detected under low power. If large numbers of infective larvae are found in a recently passed stool sample, then the diagnosis of superinfection is warranted (Eveland, 1975).

Finally, there are cases in which the infection is suspected clinically and the laboratory cannot demonstrate the parasite in repeated fecal examinations. In these cases, examination of duodenal aspirates may be helpful, or the Baerman concentration technique for stools may be used (Melvin, 1974).

TREMATODES

Trematodes or flukes are platyhelminths (flattened dorsoventrally). They are hermaphroditic except for the schistosomes, which have two separate sexes. Sizes of mature worms vary greatly. Those infecting man range in length from 1 mm (*Metagonimus*) to 70 mm (*Fasciolopsis*). There are two suckers: one oral, through which the digestive tract opens, and one ventral for attachment. There are male and female reproductive organs and the cuticle may be smooth or rough depending on species.

The adult hermaphroditic flukes infecting man live in various areas such as intestine, lungs, and biliary tree. The eggs are operculate and may be unembryonated or contain larvae when laid depending on the species. After being laid, eggs reach the exterior environment in the stool, urine, or sputum. Trematodes infecting man complete their life cycle in fresh water and require two intermediate hosts. The first of these intermediate hosts is usually a specific molluscan and the second are plants, crabs, fish, ants, etc. The manner of disposal of feces so that trematode larval stages reach water, as well as availability of appropriate intermediate hosts, is an important factor in perpetuating the infection. Dietary customs must allow the infective stage to

5

be ingested by man for the life cycle to be completed in most cases.

Epidemiologically, the distribution of human trematode infections is in the tropical and subtropical areas of the world, with different areas having different types of trematodes. There is not a single place where all of these infections co-exist in man. In spite of control campaigns, some of these infections are spreading each year because of man-made environmental changes, such as dams and irrigation systems. The symptomatology in man varies depending upon the number of worms parasitizing the host at a given time and the tissues and organs involved. Many infections are asymptomatic.

Diagnosis is established by demonstrating eggs in fecal specimens. Direct mounts and formalin-ether concentration are useful for all trematodes. Zinc sulfate flotation methods are not satisfactory for hermaphroditic fluke eggs unless specimens are first fixed in formalin.

Human trematodes are located in the intestine, liver, lungs, and blood vessels. Since most are diagnosed by stool examination, they will all be included in this section (Faust, 1970, 1975).

Fasciolopsis buski. This trematode occurs naturally in pigs, other animals, and man in China and some other countries of Southeast Asia (Faust, 1975). The parasite is a fleshy worm measuring up to 70 mm long by 20 mm wide and 3 mm thick (Fig. 51-34).

The worms lived attached to the mucosa of the duodenum and jejunum by means of a ventral sucker. The characteristic eggs are found in the stools (Fig. 51-35). The eggs re-

quire a long maturation period in fresh water, after which they release an embryo that seeks a particular species of snail for its further development. In the snail, after a complicated life cycle, the parasite gives rise to numerous larval forms that leave the molluscan and encyst on some water plants. When these plants are ingested by appropriate hosts, the parasites grow to adulthood in the intestine in approximately three months.

The symptomatology is related to the number of worms. Ulceration of the superficial mucosa and obstruction can occur if there are enough worms, but apparently most of the symptomatology is due to "toxic" effects. Diarrhea and epigastric pain are the main presenting symptoms, but anorexia, nausea, and vomiting can occur accompanied by eosinophilia. The infection may be asymptomatic.

The diagnosis is made by finding eggs in the stools. The oval, operculate eggs measure 130 to 140 μ by 80 to 85 μ and are unembryonated. The shell is of moderate thickness and does not have other distinctive structures. Differentiation from *Fasciola* eggs (see below) is generally not possible, and they can be differentiated from *Echinostoma* sp. eggs only because the latter are smaller.

***Heterophyes* spp. and *Metagonimus* spp.** These two genera of trematodes comprise a large number of species represented by minute worms measuring 1 to 3 mm long. Both groups have several species that may infect man. They usually live attached to the mucosa of the small intestine by means of the ventral sucker. The operculate eggs are passed with the stools. The life cycle requires a molluscan

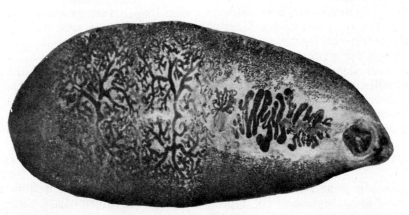

Figure 51-34. *Fasciolopsis buski.* (From Markell, E. K., and Voge, M.: Medical Parasitology. Philadelphia, W. B. Saunders Company, 1976.)

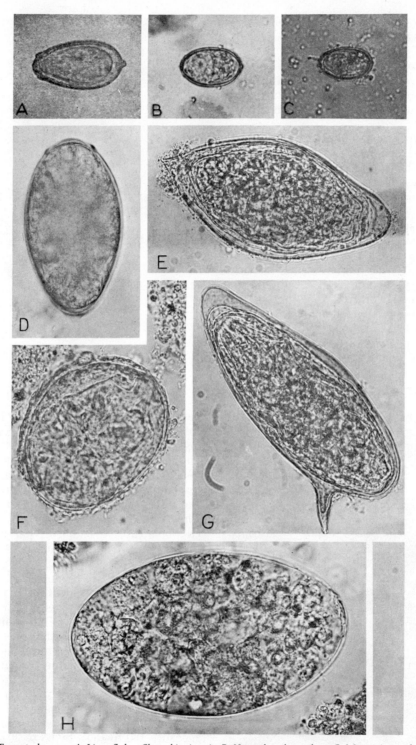

Figure 51-35. Trematode eggs. *A,* Liver fluke, *Clonorchis sinensis. B, Heterophyes heterophyes. C, Metagonimus yokogawai. D,* Lung fluke, *Paragonimus westermani. E,* Blood fluke, *Schistosoma haematobium. F,* Oriental blood fluke, *Schistosoma japonicum. G,* Manson blood fluke, *Schistosoma mansoni. H,* Large intestinal fluke, *Fasciolopsis buski.* All figures ×500 except *A,* which is ×830. (*A* courtesy of Dr. E. C. Faust, in Brenemann: Practice of Pediatrics, W. F. Prior Co.; *B* and *C* courtesy of Lt. L. W. Shatterly, MSC, School of Aviation Medicine, Gunter AFB, Alabama. All others courtesy of Dr. R. L. Roudabush, Ward's Natural Science Establishment, Rochester, New York; photos by T. Romaniak.)

as the first intermediate host and a fresh water fish as the second. Infection occurs after ingestion of uncooked fish.

The clinical manifestations vary with the number of worms present. There are minute areas of inflammation at the attachment sites, and diarrhea and abdominal pain may be present.

The diagnosis is established by finding the embryonated, operculate eggs which measure less than 30 by 17 μ. These eggs may be difficult or impossible to differentiate from those of *Clonorchis* and *Opisthorchis* sp. (Fig. 51-35).

Fasciola spp. There are at least two species of *Fasciola* that parasitize man: *F. hepatica* and *F. gigantica*. Both are parasites of domestic and wild animals, such as cattle, sheep and goats, and accidentally of man. *F. hepatica* has a worldwide distribution, while *F. gigantica* is restricted to Africa and the Orient (Faust, 1970).

The adult parasites live in the biliary tree (Fig. 51-36) where they lay eggs that are

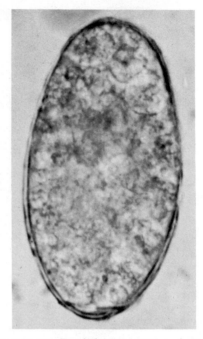

Figure 51-37. *Fasciola hepatica* egg in stools (×500).

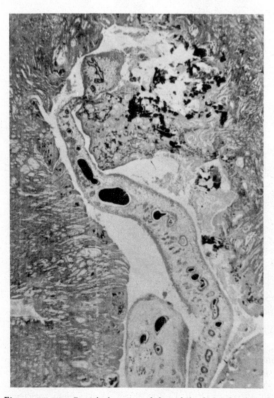

Figure 51-36. *Fasciola hypatica* adult in bile duct of infected cow. There is marked hyperplasia of biliary duct epithelium (×11).

passed in feces. After developing in water and following a life cycle similar to that of *Fasciolopsis* (see above), the infective larvae encyst on aquatic plants such as water chestnuts. When ingested, the infective larvae are released from their cysts and penetrate through the intestinal wall into the peritoneal cavity. They migrate to the liver, bore through the Glisson's capsule and liver parenchyma, and finally reach the bile ducts, where they mature and live.

The young larvae produce little or no symptomatology during migration. In the liver they elicit an inflammatory response in the biliary ducts with hyperplasia of the epithelium and eventually fibrosis of the ducts. The bile drainage may be slowed and bile salt precipitation may result in stone formation. Eosinophilia is present in the early stages, especially during larval migration.

The diagnosis is established by finding eggs in stools. The unembryonated, operculate eggs measure 130 to 150 μ by 63 to 90 μ and cannot be distinguished from those of *Fasciolopsis* (Fig. 51-37). Care must be taken to differentiate between a real parasitism and a spurious presence of eggs resulting from ingestion of infected liver. These can be differentiated by advising the patient to abstain from ingesting liver for three days or more and then repeating the stool examination. If eggs are still found, infection is present.

***Clonorchis sinensis* and *Opisthorchis* spp.** These closely related trematodes are inhabitants of the biliary system of man and other carnivorous mammals, such as cats and dogs. Many authors consider *Clonorchis* to be synonomous with *Opisthorchis* and call all *Opistorchis*. *Clonorchis sinensis* occurs mainly in Japan, Korea, China, Taiwan, and Vietnam. *Opisthorchis* spp. are found mainly in central and eastern Europe, as well as in Turkey and Siberia, but there are also foci in Vietnam, and they have been recorded sporadically in India and Japan. The parasites are delicate trematodes measuring up to 25 mm in length and produce small eggs that enter the duodenum with the bile and are passed in stools. After a cycle in the molluscan first intermediate host, the parasite enters muscles of one of several species of fresh water fish, where infective larvae develop. Infection is acquired by the ingestion of uncooked fish. After excystation in the duodenum, the infective larvae migrate via the ampulla of Vater and common bile ducts into bile ducts of the liver where they mature and live.

The infection in man is generally asymptomatic or very mild (Strauss, 1962), however, large numbers of parasites produce a variety of gastrointestinal disturbances.

The diagnosis is made by recovering the eggs from stools (Fig. 51-35). Eggs measure 23 to 35 μ by 12 to 20 μ, and the eggs of *Opisthorchis* cannot be differentiated from those of *Clonorchis*. These eggs are difficult to differentiate from those of the *Heterophyes/Metagonimus* group. Eggs of *Clonorchis/Opisthorchis* often have a hook on the abopercular end and are narrower at the end with the flattened operculum. *Heterophyes/Metagonimus* do not have the hook and are wider and more rounded at the opercular end. Specific differentiation of the eggs is not possible, and a generic diagnosis of *Clonorchis/Opisthorchis* spp. may be reported.

***Paragonimus* spp.** There are several *Paragonimus* spp. that may parasitize the lungs of man and other carnivores. The first species to be described was *P. westermani*, which is found in Japan, Korea, Formosa, China, Manchuria, Phillipines, and Southeastern Asia. Isolated cases of *Paragonimus* infection have been reported in other places such as Africa and South, Central, and North America. Some

of these cases have been caused by *Paragonimus* spp. other than *P. westermani*.

The adult parasites measure up to 12 mm by 6 mm and live in the lungs, where they are encapsulated by the host's fibrous reaction (Fig. 51-38). Usually each "capsule" measures less than 20 mm in diameter and contains two or three adult worms bathed by fluid. There is usually a communication between the capsule and the bronchi through which the eggs find their way into the respiratory tree. The eggs are generally passed in the stools, but may reach the environment in expectorated sputum. The parasite needs a molluscan as first intermediate host and crabs or crayfish as the second. Infective larvae encyst in the muscles of these second intermediate hosts and, if uncooked, infection follows their ingestion. Larvae are released in the stomach and migrate through the intestinal wall into the peritoneal cavity, reaching the lungs from there after boring through the diaphragm.

Symptoms may be caused by larvae migrating through the tissues or by adults estab-

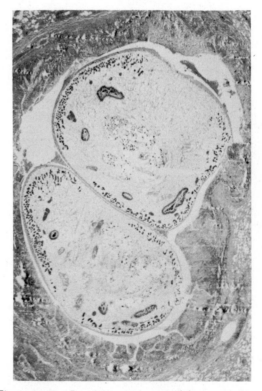

Figure 51-38. *Paragonimus westermani* adults in experimentally infected dog. Note the fibrous capsule surrounding the parasites (×9.5). (Material courtesy of Dr. M. D. Little, Tulane University Medical School.)

lished in the lungs. Light infections are generally asymptomatic. The onset of the disease is usually associated with slight chills, fever, and high eosinophilia. Once the worms are well established in the lungs, the main symptoms are those of chronic cough with abundant mucus production and episodes of hemoptysis. Radiographs vary considerably but may show nodular shadows, calcifications, or patchy infiltrations. If the eggs are not passed via the bronchial tree, they are deposited in the pulmonary parenchyma where they may cause an extensive granulomatous reaction. The parasites do not always successfully reach the lungs and have been found in many other locations, including peritoneum, subcutaneous tissues, and brain (Fig. 51-39). In these cases, there is a marked granulomatous inflammatory reaction to the eggs. The symptomatology varies with the organ involved, and the

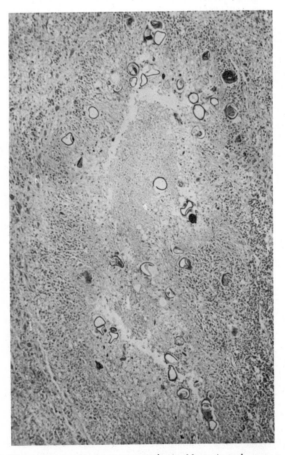

Figure 51-39. *Paragonimus* sp. in brain. Necrosis and granulomatous inflammation to eggs deposited by aberrantly localized adult (×48).

histopathologic diagnosis is usually based on the morphology of the eggs in the granulomas.

Diagnosis is accomplished by finding the typical eggs in either the stools or the sputum (Fig. 51-35). The operculate, unembryonated eggs measure 80 to 120 μ by 48 to 60 μ and have a moderately thick shell. The operculum is flattened and is usually set off from the rest of the shell by prominent shoulders. The abopercular end is sometimes thickened but does not have a knob. Size allows ready distinction from the eggs of *D. latum* and *Fasciola* or *Fasciolopsis* with which they may be confused.

Schistosomes. These trematodes inhabit blood vessels of many animals including man. There are separate male and female worms and in that respect they resemble the nematodes. Man is infected by at least three species or species complexes (i.e., *S. mansoni, S. japonicum,* and *S. haematobium*). Each species complex is composed of several related subspecies or strains, which are usually difficult to differentiate morphologically.

Schistosomes are the most important trematodes in man in terms of incidence and severity of infection. The incidence of *Schistosoma* infection is increasing in most areas of the world in spite of aggressive control campaigns in many endemic areas.

The adult female parasites are slender, measuring up to 26 mm by 0.5 mm (Fig. 51-40). The males are slightly shorter and have a longitudinal canal resulting from the infolding of the lateral aspects of the body toward the center. The female takes up residence in this canal early in development, and the worms stay together in this fashion for the rest of their lives. The adult parasites live in the smaller venules of the mesenteric and vesicle plexuses (Fig. 51-41) where they elicit little or no inflammatory reaction. The female deposits eggs in the smallest venules of the intestine or the bladder wall near the superficial layers of the mucosa. The eggs elicit a marked inflammatory reaction with both mononuclear and polymorphonuclear cellular infiltrates and formation of microabscesses. These usually rupture into the lumen of the viscus, allowing the eggs to enter feces or urine. In addition, the larvae in the eggs may produce enzymes that aid in their penetration through the tissues.

The eggs develop as they move through the tissues and are fully embryonated when they are passed into the environment. The swimming larvae must find an appropriate fresh

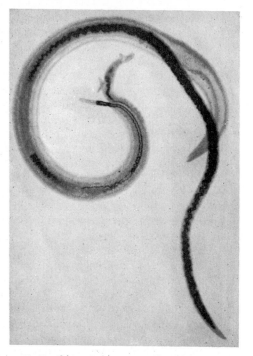

Figure 51–40. *Schistosoma mansoni,* male and female *in copula.* (From Markell, K., and Voge, M.: Medical Parasitology. Philadelphia, W. B. Saunders Company, 1976.)

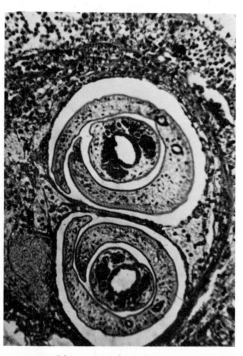

Figure 51–41. *Schistosoma mansoni* cross section of adults in mesenteric vein ($\times$140).

water snail as intermediate host. In the snail, a complicated proliferative life cycle occurs, ending with the liberation from the snail of many thousands of small larvae known as cercariae. Cercariae swim freely in the water for only a few hours. If they contact susceptible hosts, they actively penetrate exposed skin.

After penetration, the parasites enter the circulation and pass through the lungs to establish themselves in the liver for a short period of maturation, then migrate via the portal system to the mesenteric or vesicle venules where sexual maturity occurs and oviposition starts.

The infection is similar in all three species of human schistosomes in that disease results from the eggs rather than from the adult worms. The parasite attempts to shed as many eggs as possible into the external environment; however, some eggs are trapped in the tissues, and the host's reaction to the egg antigens results in microabscesses that can progress to granulomas and eventual fibrosis. The granuloma formation has been related to hypersensitivity reaction in the host (Warren, 1972, 1973). Moreover, some eggs, especially in *S. japonicum* and *S. mansoni* infections, may be carried by the portal vein into the liver (Fig. 51-42), where they lead to the development of granulomas that can coalesce, resulting in so-called "pipe stem" fibrosis of the liver and eventually in portal hypertension with its associated manifestations.

Diagnosis is usually established by demonstrating eggs in fecal or urine specimens by direct mount or formalin-ether concentration. Zinc sulfate concentration is not satisfactory for the heavy schistosome eggs. Eggs may sometimes be demonstrated in biopsies of rectal or bladder tissue either by crush preparation or by section, and they may sometimes be found in liver biopsies. Eggs may be difficult to speciate in sections because of folds and shrinkage. If eggs are not found by routine fecal or urine examination, hatching may be attempted. This method may be especially helpful in light infections or in chronic infections in which many eggs are trapped in fibrous tissue and few reach the lumen. Feces mixed with distilled water are placed in a flask that is painted black or wrapped with foil to keep out light, with only the neck or a side arm exposed to a bright light. In the presence of water, the eggs hatch and the swimming larvae seek light in the neck or side arm. With a hand lens they can be detected swimming

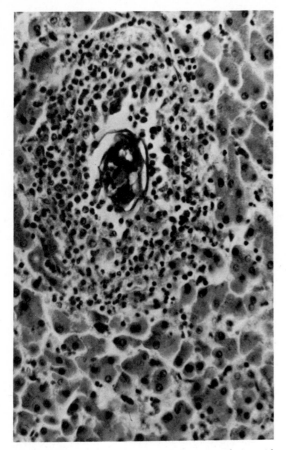

Figure 51–42. *Schistosoma mansoni.* Recent granuloma with egg in liver. Note the miracidium inside the egg and distortion of shell due to fixation. There is a polymorphonuclear cell infiltrate, mostly eosinophiles (×250).

near the surface and removed with a capillary pipette for more detailed examination. Species cannot be identified with this technique.

Many serologic techniques for schistosomiasis have been investigated. Some currently used are the cholesterol-lecithin (CL) flocculation, bentonite flocculation (BF), complement fixation (CF), and indirect immunofluorescent (IF). Results are sometimes difficult to interpret, since there is cross-reactivity between schistosomiasis and other parasitic diseases.

The CL flocculation technique uses a cercarial extract as antigen and has a sensitivity varying from 77 to 90 per cent in confirmed cases. The BF technique uses an antigen similar to that for CL technique and has a similar sensitivity, but it gives approximately 15 per cent false positives. The IF test is the newest and uses a section of adult worm as antigen. It is probably the most sensitive and most spe-

cific. The CF technique uses a delipidized adult worm antigen and is usually employed in conjunction with one of the above (Kagan, 1970, 1976).

Schistosoma mansoni. *S. mansoni* occurs in Africa, especially in the tropical areas and the Nile delta. In the Western Hemisphere it occurs in Brazil, Venezuela, Surinam, and the West Indies. Puerto Rico has several foci, and there are many infected Puerto Ricans who have moved to the United States, particularly to urban areas.

S. mansoni adults live in the mesenteric venous plexuses of the large intestine, and the symptomatology they produce depends on the stage of the infection. During the prepatent period, there may be urticarial skin rash, fever, eosinophilia, or diarrhea, and the liver may be enlarged and tender. After the parasites lodge in the mesenteric veins, there may be abdominal pain and dysentery with abundant blood and mucus in the stools. During this period, the characteristic eggs are usually found in stools. These symptoms eventually subside and the chronic phase of the disease with granuloma formation and fibrosis ensues. The chronic phase can last for many years depending on the number of worms present, occasionally resulting in liver fibrosis and the portal hypertension syndrome. This disease is generally less severe than that caused by *S. japonicum*. Eggs measure 116 to 180 μ by 45 to 58 μ and are oval, with a large distinctive lateral spine that protrudes from the side of the egg near one end. If it is not visible, the egg may be rotated by tapping the coverslip. Movement of the larva within the egg may be evident in unfixed material if the larva is viable (Fig. 51–35).

Schistosoma japonicum. This species is limited mainly to China, Korea, and the Phillipines. It causes disease that is clinically similar in most aspects to *S. mansoni* but causes more severe disease in all stages of the infection. Eggs readily reach the liver, and fibrosis with portal hypertension is a common complication of chronic *S. japonicum* infection.

The eggs are broadly oval, measuring 70 to 105 μ by 50 to 65 μ (Fig. 51–35) and often have a characteristic rudimentary lateral spine, though it may sometimes be difficult to demonstrate.

Schistosoma haematobium. This trematode occurs in the African continent, where its distribution includes both the tropical and subtropical areas. The Nile river banks and delta have a particularly high incidence. There are also foci in the Middle East and Madagascar.

The parasites migrate via the hemorrhoidal veins to the venous plexuses of the urinary bladder, prostate, uterus, and vagina. One of the earliest and most common symptoms of the infection is hematuria, especially at the end of micturition. In the chronic stages there may be pelvic pain and bladder colic with increased desire to urinate. Accumulation of eggs in the bladder wall results in hypertrophy of the epithelium, squamous metaplasia, and marked fibrosis, which are responsible for the above symptoms and may lead to urinary obstruction. An association between urinary schistosomiasis and squamous cell carcinoma of the urinary bladder has been repeatedly noted, but there is not as yet conclusive proof that it is a cause-and-effect relationship.

The eggs are elongated, measuring 112 to 180 μ by 40 to 70 μ, and have a terminal spine (Fig. 51-35). Examining urine sediment may allow detection of eggs. Late morning specimens are usually best.

SWIMMERS ITCH. This entity, also known as schistosome cercarial dermatitis, is produced by the cutaneous penetration of cercariae of non-human schistosomes. Generally, they are cercariae of blood flukes of birds and mammals and may affect persons exposing skin to fresh or salt water. In all these cases, man is a non-compatible host and the life cycle cannot be completed. Probably some degree of prior sensitization to the cercariae is required. The cercariae apparently cannot penetrate beyond the superficial layers of the skin. The disease is a dermatitis with erythema and urticaria which can progress to the formation of papules. The reaction is most intense within 48 to 72 hours after exposure to contaminated waters and eventually subsides spontaneously. The disease has a worldwide distribution, and it is well known in the United States, especially in the western and northern parts of the country. The diagnosis is established on clinical grounds.

CESTODES

Cestodes (tapeworms) are platyhelminth parasites characterized by a body or strobila that is composed of a chain of segments called proglottids and an anterior portion known as a scolex. Tapeworm scoleces have various structures for attachment to the intestinal mucosa depending on species. These include suckers, grooves or bothria, and a rostellum with hooks. Behind the scolex is the neck from which new proglottids develop. Each proglottid has one or two complete sets of male and female organs. Proglottids develop from immature to mature to egg-producing, with those furthest from the neck being most developed. In some species there is active oviposition, but in most species eggs are stored in the uterus, which thus becomes gravid. A prominent structure usually visible with the naked eye is the genital pore where the male and female organs meet. The adults parasitize the small intestine of vertebrates. Size varies considerably from species in which adults are barely visible with the naked eye to species 20 to 25 feet long. Adult and larval stages of cestodes contain basophilic laminated bodies known as calcareous corpuscles, which aid in recognition of cestode tissue (Wardle, 1952).

Eggs are passed with the stools and usually require one, two, or more intermediate hosts for the asexual larval stages to develop. Intermediate hosts include both invertebrates and vertebrates.

Cestode larval stages of various types develop to the infective stage in the tissues of the intermediate host. The life cycle is completed when infective larvae are ingested by the appropriate definitive host. The types of cestode larval stages that may infect man are cysticerous, hydatid, coenurus, and sparganum, and the infections in man are known as cysticercosis hydatid disease, coenurosis, and sparganosis.

***Taenia saginata* and *Taenia solium*.** Man is the sole definitive host for *T. saginata*, the beef tapeworm, and *T. solium*, the pork tapeworm. *T. solium* is common in Eastern Europe, Latin America, China, Pakistan, and India, and cases found in the United States are imported. *T. saginata* has a wider distribution with a greater incidence in the Middle East, Africa, Europe, and Latin America, and it occurs occasionally in the United States.

Both human *Taenia* live in the small intestine and produce large numbers of eggs that are stored in the uterus. Eggs reach the stools and the outside when gravid proglottids drop from the strobila. Proglottids either rupture in the intestine, freeing the eggs (usual in *T. solium*), or are passed with the stools intact and still active (usual in *T. saginata*). When the appropriate intermediate hosts, such as cattle in *T. saginata* and pigs in *T. solium*,

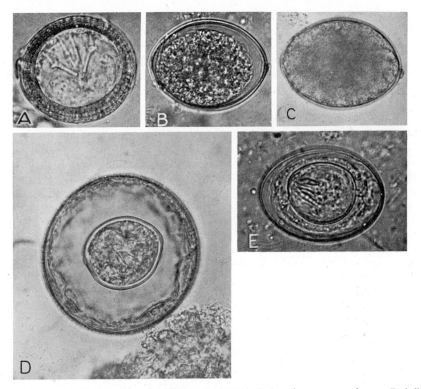

Figure 51–43.   Cestode eggs. *A,* Human tapeworm, *Taenia* sp. (×750). *B,* Broad tapeworm of man, *Diphyllobothrium latum* (×500). *C,* Broad tapeworm of man, *Diphyllobothrium latum* (×500). *D,* Rat tapeworm, *Hymenolepis diminuta* (×650). *E,* Dwarf tapeworm, *Hymenolepis nana* (×750). (*B* courtesy of Lt. L. W. Shetterly, School of Aviation Medicine, Gunter AFB, Alabama; all others courtesy of Dr. R. L. Roudabush, Ward's Natural Science Establishment, Rochester, New York; photos by T. Romaniak.)

swallow the eggs, the larvae (cysticerci) develop in the tissues. After ingestion of poorly cooked contaminated meat, the cysticercus develops into an adult in the small intestine of the definitive host (usually only one adult in each infection).

The symptomatology produced by both of these parasites in man is minimal, but gastrointestinal disturbances have been described. A striking biologic difference of practical importance is that *T. solium* eggs, if ingested by man, can develop into cysticerci (see below).

The diagnosis of the infection is made by finding eggs in the stools using direct or concentration techniques, or in the perianal folds with the scotch tape technique. The eggs are spherical and measure 31 to 43 μ in diameter (Fig. 51–43). The shell is thick, radially striated, and contains a six-hooked embryo. Unfortunately, the eggs of the two *Taenia* species cannot be differentiated morphologically and are reported as "*Taenia* spp. eggs."

Grossly, both parasites have a similar strobila up to 7 meters in length. However, on close examination the uterus of *T. saginata* is seen to have 15 to 20 branches, and the genital pores sometimes alternate regularly from side to side, while *T. solium* has 7 to 13 uterine branches and the genital pores alternate with great irregularity (Fig. 51–44). Microscopically, the scolex of *T. solium* has a rostellum composed of two rows of hooks, while that of *T. saginata* has no rostellum and no hooks.

In many instances passed proglottids are brought to the laboratory for identification. Careful handling and clearing of these specimens overnight in glycerol should be done so that the branches of the uterus can be counted and a specific identification can be made. If a larger segment of the strobila with scolex is available, more conclusive identification can be done.

Dipylidium caninum. This tapeworm is worldwide in distribution and dogs are usually the definitive hosts.

The life cycle involves an arthropod intermediate host, usually a flea, which ingests the egg and in which the infective larvae develop.

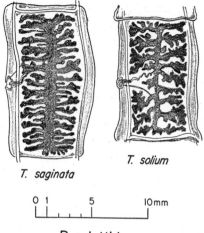

Proglottids

Figure 51-44. Gravid proglottids of *Taenia saginata* and *T. solium.* Notice the number of uterine branches. (From Mackie, T. T., Hunter, G. W., and Worth, C. B.: Manual of Tropical Medicine, 2nd ed.)

The definitive host acquires the infection by ingesting a flea infected with the larval stage. Larvae attach to the small intestinal mucosa and mature to adult parasites, which measure approximately 70 cm in length. The proglottids are barrel-shaped with a genital pore and sex organs on each side. The uterus of the gravid proglottid consists of numerous small capsules each containing 8 to 20 eggs (Fig. 51–45.

The parasitism results in little or no symptomatology. The diagnosis is made by finding the spherical eggs, measuring 24 to 40 μ, singly or in packets, and containing a six-hooked embryo (Fig. 51-46). Sometimes a segment of the strobila is passed, and it can be identified by the double genital pores and the egg packets.

Hymenolepis nana. *H. nana,* known as the dwarf tapeworm of man, has worldwide distribution. This is the most frequently found tapeworm in the United States. The parasite has a delicate strobila measuring up to 40 mm in length, genital pores are located on one side, and the scolex has a rostellum with hooks. The life cycle has a dual pathway, which is of practical importance. The first is a direct type of development occurring when the host ingests freshly passed eggs. After the embryos are released from the eggs in the intestine, they penetrate the mucosal villi, where development to infective larvae occurs. The larvae drop into the lumen and develop to adults in a

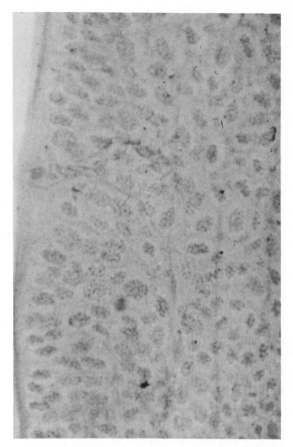

Figure 51-45. *Dipylidium caninum,* detail of gravid proglottid showing uterus with egg capsules and genital pore ($\times 30$).

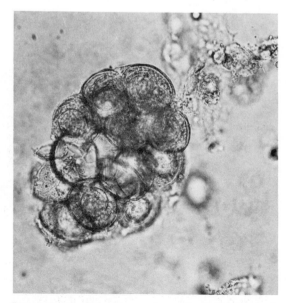

Figure 51-46. *Dipylidium caninum* egg packet in stools ($\times 300$).

5

number that correlates with the number of eggs ingested. The tissue phase, though only of a few days duration, is apparently sufficient to confer a strong immunity to the host (Heyneman, 1963).

The second type of development is infrequent and is similar to that of *H. diminuta* in that infection is acquired by ingesting an infected arthropod (see below). Therefore, the host does not develop immunity to the larval parasite and when adults start oviposition, the eggs may hatch in the intestine, invade the mucosa, and undergo a development similar to that described above, with infection by many thousands of worms. This mechanism has been demonstrated in experimental animals and has been proposed as an explanation for the massive infections sometimes seen in man.

Symptomatic infection develops in patients with large numbers of worms attached to the small intestinal mucosa as a result of the irritation they produce. Non-specific general and gastrointestinal symptoms have been described in patients with this tapeworm. The diagnosis is made by the recovery of the characteristic eggs in the stool. The oval colorless eggs measure 30 to 43 μ in diameter (Fig. 51-43) and have a medium-thick shell. They contain a developed six-hooked embryo when passed and have polar thickenings at each end of the inner membrane from which polar filaments arise external to the outer membrane. Portions of the strobila or complete worms may occasionally be passed (Fig. 51-47).

Hymenolepis diminuta. This cestode in-fects rats, mice, and other rodents, and is found throughout the world. Sporadic cases have been reported in man in almost every country.

Embryonated eggs passed in stools are ingested by flea larvae or other arthropods in which the infective larvae develop. Accidental ingestion of infected arthropods results in infection. Adults develop in the small intestine and measure up to 60 cm in length. The strobila is delicate, and all genital pores are located on one side (Fig. 51-47). The scolex has no hooks and the eggs are released when the gravid proglottids detach from the body of the adult worm. Infections are usually asymptomatic, although occasional cases with intestinal symptoms have been reported. The diagnosis is made by finding the characteristic eggs in the feces, 60 to 82 μ by 72 to 86 μ (Fig. 51-43D). They are almost spherical with an inner membrane with two rudimentary polar thickenings, but there are no polar filaments. They contain a six-hooked embryo.

***Diphyllobothrium* spp.** This group is composed of large cestodes that infect many wild and domestic carnivores in addition to man (Vik, 1964). They are widely distributed in the temperate zones, especially in central and northern Europe, northern USSR, and central Siberia. In Asia they occur in Manchuria and Japan. In North America the main endemic areas are in the vicinity of the lakes in the northern United States and Canada. There are isolated foci in Chile, Uganda, and Palestine.

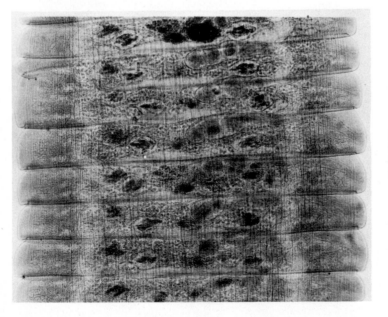

Figure 51-47. *Hymenolepis diminuta* portion of strobila with internal anatomy and genital pores on one side (right) (×47).

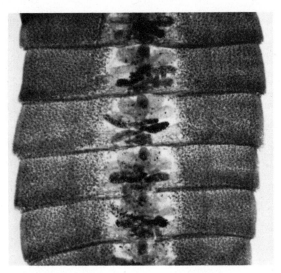

Figure 51-48. *Diphyllobothrium latum.* Proglottids showing uterus with medial genital pore (×15).

The parasite inhabits the small intestine and can reach a length of up to 10 meters. The scolex is elongated with a pair of deep longitudinal grooves (bothria) that are distinctive for this group of tapeworms. There is a genital pore located medially and ventrally, and next to it is an opening for oviposition from which the eggs are passed (Fig. 51-48). The eggs are unembryonated when passed. They are elongate, measuring 58 to 76 μ by 40 to 51 μ and have an operculum (in contrast to other cestodes). They often have a small, round, knoblike protrusion of the shell on the abopercular (posterior) pole (Fig. 51-43). There are no shoulders adjacent to the operculum.

Eggs are passed in stools and must reach a fresh water stream or lake to continue the life cycle. A first intermediate host may be one of many species of small aquatic arthropods. The second intermediate host is a small fish that ingests the arthropods, and the third intermediate host is a larger fish that ingests the smaller fish. In the muscles of the large fish the larva (sparganum) develops to the infective stage. The life cycle is completed when the larva is ingested by any of the definitive hosts in raw or inadequately cooked fish.

There are several species of *Diphyllobothrium* that may parasitize man, but the most common is *D. latum.* These parasites are closely related and differentiation cannot be based on morphology of eggs.

The symptomatology produced by *Diphyllobothrium* infections in man is variable. Usually the worms are harbored for many years without appreciable symptomatology. Passage of a portion of the strobila may be what brings the patient to the physician. In northern Europe where the parasite is endemic a small percentage of patients develop findings of vitamin B_{12} deficiency, including megaloblastic anemia. The parasite selectively competes with the host for vitamin B_{12}, which thus accumulates in the worm tissues in large amounts. This syndrome is rarely seen in North America or in endemic foci other than northern Europe.

The diagnosis is made by finding eggs in the stools by either direct or concentration methods.

TISSUE HELMINTHS

NEMATODES

Filariae. These nematodes are widely distributed in nature, with representatives occurring in almost every vertebrate species. The adults are long and slender, measuring many centimeters in length, and may inhabit almost any tissue (i.e., subcutaneous tissues, lymphatics, blood vessels, peritoneal and pleural cavities, heart, brain, etc.). Some species wander about in tissues, whereas others remain stationary and become encased in a nodular fibrous tissue reaction. Usually, both male and female worms are found together in these tissues. The progeny are microfilariae which are slender, motile embryos found either in the circulating blood or wandering in the subcutaneous tissues, depending upon the species. Microfilariae are not infective to vertebrates but must be ingested by a biting arthropod, usually a mosquito or fly, in which they mature to the infective stage. These infective larvae are passed into the new hosts when the arthropod takes another meal. After skin penetration, the larvae will migrate to the appropriate location and develop into adults. Maturation requires from several months to a year.

DIAGNOSIS OF FILARIASIS. Geographic location, type of disease, and time of obtaining a specimen may aid in diagnosis, but the actual diagnosis is usually based on identification of microfilariae in blood or material obtained from the skin. Species identification of blood microfilariae is particularly important, as some may cause serious disease while others rarely do. Diagnostic laboratory identification usually uses Giemsa- or hematoxylin-stained thick films, although special, more sensitive procedures, such as Knott's concentration or saponin lysis, may be useful in some cases. Microfilariae may sometimes be seen moving in direct mounts of blood or tissue fluid.

There are numerous special anatomic landmarks in microfilariae, some of which may be demonstrated with special stains, but all of these are not needed for routine diagnosis.

The principal characteristics that are used in diagnostic laboratories are the presence of a sheath and its staining characteristics, the shape and nuclear distribution in the tail, the size of the cephalic space, and the appearance of the nuclear column. The length is helpful, but it is difficult to measure and is rarely needed in the routine clinical laboratory. *Wuchereria* and *Brugia* microfilariae usually have a nocturnal periodicity, so the blood sample should be drawn between 10 P.M. and 2 A.M. *Loa loa* has a diurnal periodicity, and microfilariae are best found in blood at around noon. *Dipetalonema* and *Mansonella* are characteristically non-periodic. Serologic tests using extracts of *Dirofilaria immitis* as antigen include indirect hemagglutination and flocculation tests, but they allow only a diagnosis of the filarial group rather than the species. Moreover, there is frequent cross-reactivity with other parasites (false positives), as well as many false negatives (Kagan, 1970, 1976).

Wuchereria bancrofti. This filarial worm lives in the lymphatic channels (Fig. 51-49) and usually those draining the lower extremities (Sasa, 1976). It occurs mainly in central and north Africa, Southeast Asia, India, northern South America, the West Indies, and some South Pacific Islands.

The female worms produce microfilariae that enter the blood stream of the patient and circulate mainly during the hours of 10 P.M. to 2 A.M. This phenomenon is known as nocturnal periodicity. The time of microfilaremia corresponds to the peak activity of the mosquitoes that serve as vectors, usually species of *Culex*, *Aedes*, *Anopheles*, or *Mansonia*. In some Pacific Islands *W. bancrofti* microfilaremia is continuous, although it is higher in the afternoon and is called subperiodic. The clinical manifestations of *Wuchereria* infection vary. People who are in endemic areas for only a short time and get infected usually suffer a few acute bouts of transient lymphangitis and lymphadenopathy, which resolve in a short time without microfilaremia (Beaver, 1970). People who live in endemic areas are continu-

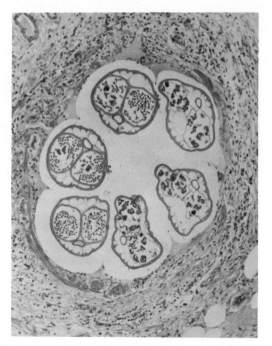

Figure 51-49. *Wuchereria bancrofti.* Cross-section of adult in human lymph node. Note fibrosis surrounding the worm. (×120).

ously re-exposed to the parasite over many years and develop heavy infection. The infection can become a chronic condition with protracted lymphadenopathy and lymphangitis, which may progress to lymphedema and fibrosis with resultant elephantiasis, usually most severe in the lower extremities and male or female genital organs.

Specimens for diagnosis must be obtained at the time when microfilaremia would be expected to occur. The microfilaria of *W. bancrofti* has a sheath that does not stain well with Giemsa stain. The tail is pointed, and there are no nuclei in the tip. The cephalic space is not as long as it is wide and the nuclei in the nuclear column are distinct (Fig. 51-50).

Brugia malayi. This is similar in most respects to *W. bancrofti* but has a more restricted geographical distribution, occurring mainly in India, Southeast Asia, Korea, and Japan. The disease in man is usually milder and more frequently involves the lymphatics of the upper extremities (Sasa, 1976).

The microfilaria of *B. malayi* has a sheath that stains well with Giemsa stain. The tail has a swelling at the tip and has two solitary nuclei in the tail, beyond the end of the nuclear column, which may be called terminal and subterminal nulei. They may be smaller

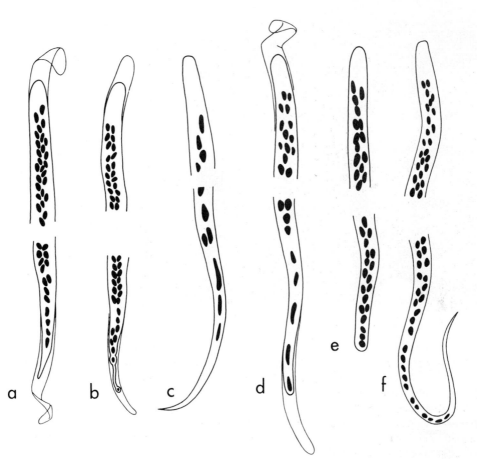

Figure 51–50. Anterior and posterior ends of microfilariae found in man. *a, Wuchereria bancrofti. b, Brugia malayi. c, Onchocerca volvulus. d, Loa loa. e, Dipetalonema perstans. f, Mansonella ozzardi.* (Adapted from Smith, 1976c, with permission.)

5

than other nuclei and are not always seen. The cephalic space may be much longer than it is wide, and the nuclear column may be blurred in Giemsa stains (Fig. 51-50).

Loa loa. The agent of "loaisis" or "fugitive swellings" is found primarily in the rain forests of Africa, where horse flies of the genus *Chrysops* are the vectors (Sasa, 1976).

The adult worms live in the subcutaneous tissues, where they seem to move freely and produce repeated swellings less than 30 mm in diameter that last two to three days. The parasite elicits high eosinophilia, and the infection has been seen in the United States in people with a history of travel to Africa. The microfilaria of *Loa loa* has a sheath that does not stain with Giemsa stain. The tail has nuclei to the rounded tip. The nuclear column is distinct, and the cephalic space is short (Fig. 51-50).

Dipetalonema perstans and Mansonella ozzardi. Infections by both of these filarial worms are usually asymptomatic in man. *Dipetalonema* infections are found in Africa and the northern part of South America, whereas *Mansonella* is restricted to Central and South America, as well as the West Indies. The vectors of both of these nematodes are "gnats" belonging to the genus *Culicoides*. The adult parasites live in the peritoneal, pleural, or pericardial cavities, and the microfilariae (Fig. 51-50) appear in the peripheral blood at all hours of the day and night. Microfilariae of both species are unsheathed. *M. ozzardi* microfilariae have a thin, pointed tail without nuclei, whereas the tail of *D. perstans* is broad and blunt with nuclei extending to the tip.

Onchocerca volvulus. The filaria causing onchocerciasis lives in the subcutaneous tissues of man, and the microfilariae inhabit the

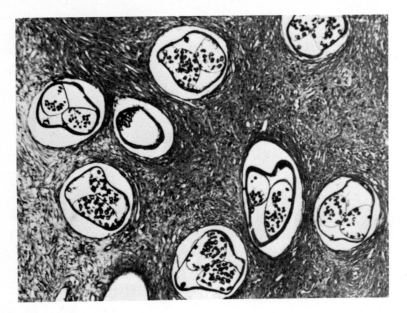

Figure 51-51. *Onchocerca volvulus* nodule. Section showing fibrous tissue with several cross-sections of adult parasite (×48).

skin. *Onchocerca* occurs mainly in Africa, but there are some endemic foci in Central America (Mexico and Guatemala), Columbia, Venezuela, and Brazil (Sasa, 1976).

There are various clinical manifestations of the disease. The adult parasites in the subcutaneous tissues are tightly coiled upon themselves and elicit a host response of fibrosis and inflammation that results in the formation of a hard subcutaneous nodule measuring up to 40 mm in diameter (Fig. 51-51). In general, these nodules are on the upper half of the body in patients in Central America and in the lower half of those in Africa. The main complications arise from the microfilariae that migrate throughout the skin, with greatest numbers near the nodules. There is itching, which can be accompanied by changes in the skin varying from atrophy to edema and hypertrophy. The microfilariae may cause keratitis, corneal opacity, and damage to the anterior chamber and iris, thus leading to blindness in a significant percentage of the infected population.

In *Onchocerca* (Figs. 51-50 and 51-51) infections the microfilariae are detected in teased skin snips coverslipped in saline or stained sections. Cases with skin microfilariae in the Western Hemisphere (Central and South America) are usually *Onchocerca*. Those from Africa present more problems, as there are other filaria with skin microfilariae that may infect man but usually do not cause disease.

Dirofilaria spp. Zoonotic filariases have become important in this country because they can result in potentially expensive hospitalization and surgery in some patients. Although several species of such zoonotic infections have been described, only the two most likely to be found are discussed here (Beaver, 1965: Orihel, 1965).

Dirofilaria immitis is commonly known as the dog heart worm. It has a life cycle similar to that of the other filarial worms and is widely distributed in the tropics and subtropics. In the United States it is endemic, especially in the Southeast, although it is also present in other parts of the country.

In the dog, the adult worm usually lives in the right ventricle and the major branches of the pulmonary artery and may cause chronic heart failure. In man, accidental infections are probably acquired by the bite of the intermediate host and results in one worm, seldom more, usually lodged in the right heart or pulmonary artery. Microfilariae are not produced. When the worm dies, it is embolized to a smaller branch of the pulmonary artery, resulting in an area of infarction that heals and may appear as a coin lesion in a chest radiograph (Fig. 51-52). The patient may undergo resection of the lesion because of suspicion of a malignancy. Microscopic examination reveals the typical cross-sections of the parasite, and if enough morphologic characteristics are evident in the dead parasite, the specific diag-

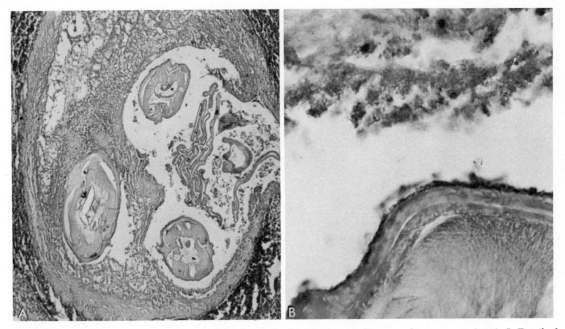

Figure 51–52. *Dirofilaria immitis. A,* Cross-section of embolized adult worm in human pulmonary vein (×48). *B,* Detail of cuticle showing the smooth outer surface (×480).

nosis can be made (Fig. 51–52). The cuticle has been described as thick and smooth in the sense that the outer surface has no longitudinal ridges (see below for comparison). The diameter of the worm varies considerably but it is generally less than 0.4 mm (Fig. 51-52) (Beaver, 1965).

Dirofilaria tenuis is usually found in the subcutaneous tissues of the racoon in the southeastern part of the United States. Accidental infections occur in man and are manifest as small subcutaneous inflammatory nodules. These may be removed surgically. On section the parasite is encased in a marked inflammatory reaction with granulation tissue. The worm usually is dead before its removal. The cuticle measures 5 to 8 μ thick, is delicate, and has characteristic longitudinal ridges that are spaced at about 10 μ intervals. The transverse diameter is usually less than 0.3 mm (Fig. 51-53) (Orihel, 1965).

Trichinella spiralis. Trichinosis in man occurs mainly in temperate zones of the Northern and Southern Hemispheres. In the United States the incidence of trichinosis has been in steady decline, and currently around 100 cases are reported per year.

The adult *Trichinella* lives in the mucosa of the small intestine of man and other carnivo-

rous animals. The female measures 3 to 4 mm long and deposits larvae measuring 80 to 120 μ, which enter the lymphatics and venules, reach the general circulation, and are distributed throughout the body. In striated muscles, the larvae invade muscle fibers and mature to the infective stage. The larvae will be curled and measure up to 1.0 mm long. They produce muscle damage, and the host's inflammatory response leads to the formation of a fibrous capsule around each larva. Such larvae are often referred to as encysted, though the "cyst" is of host origin. Larvae may remain viable for extended periods of time (years), and "cysts" may eventually become calcified. Ingestion by the appropriate host of muscle containing infective larvae will complete the life cycle. Larvae mature to adults rapidly, and larviposition begins in about one week. Pork and pork products, especially various cured sausages, are the main source of human infection, although bear meat or beef that has been adulterated with pork may be sources. Adequate cooking or extended freezing will destroy larvae.

Symptoms principally relate to intestinal tract, skeletal muscle, or allergic manifestations. The intestinal phase of the infection begins following ingestion of infected meat

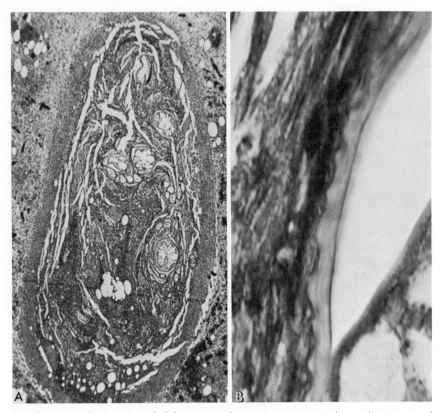

Figure 51–53. *Dirofilaria tenuis.* Cross-section of adult worm in subcutaneous tissues. *A,* Abscess showing several cross-sections of worm (×300). *B,* Cuticle with characteristic longitudinal ridges (×400). (Case of Dr. Jose Suarez-Hoyos, Tampa, Florida.)

and may cause nausea, vomiting, diarrhea, and pain depending upon the patient's susceptibility and the number of worms present and may last for several days. Migration of larvae into muscles begins in 10 to 14 days and results in high eosinophilia, fever, muscle pain, and in some cases, difficulty in breathing, swallowing, and speech. Periorbital edema is frequent and may be associated with photophobia. After the parasites are encysted, there is little symptomatology. Adult worms are usually eliminated from the intestine after two to three weeks by the host's immune response, although corticosteroid therapy may delay this elimination and thus prolong larviposition.

The diagnosis is usually made clinically in the acute stage. Larvae or adults are rarely recovered from stools during the diarrheic phase. During the migration stage, larvae have been occasionally recovered from blood by using a technique such as Knott's concentration.

Clinically, the best clues are a history of exposure, clinical findings of intestinal symptoms, muscle pain, periorbital edema, and eosinophilia. Creatine phosphokinase and other serum enzymes may be elevated. There are often "clusters" of cases with a common infection source. After larval migration to the muscles, the diagnosis may be established by a muscle biopsy, but in light infections larvae may not be detected in multiple sections (Fig. 51-54).

Diagnosis is often established indirectly by serologic tests. Several serologic tests are described and some are commercially available. The most commonly used are bentonite flocculation (BF), fluorescent antibody (FA), and complement fixation (CF). The bentonite flocculation test is very sensitive and usually becomes negative two to three years after an infection; thus, a positive test usually indicates active infection. The test becomes positive after the third week of infection and is most helpful when a fourfold rise in paired serum specimens can be demonstrated. The

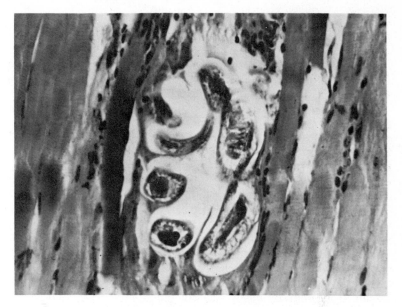

Figure 51-54. *Trichinella spiralis* cross-section of larva in deltoid muscle (×300).

CF test detects antibodies slightly earlier than the BF test, and the FA is considered to be as good as the BF (Kagan, 1970, 1976).

Larva migrans. Larva migrans is produced by the prolonged wandering through the tissues of nematode larvae. If this migration occurs within the layers of the skin where tracks may be seen, then the entity is called cutaneous larva migrans. The syndrome is produced by several human and non-human species of hookworm and *Strongyloides.* It is manifested by tortuous, markedly pruritic red tracks on the skin.

Visceral larva migrans is produced by larvae from non-human nematodes, especially the dog ascarid, *Toxocara canis,* but also occasionally *T. cati.* When man accidentally ingests infective eggs, the larvae hatch and penetrate into the circulation. In man, an abnormal host, the larvae are unable to complete their cycle, and there is prolonged migration of the larvae through various tissues and organs, producing the visceral form of this disease (Beaver, 1952, 1969).

The patient is usually a child between $1\frac{1}{2}$ and 4 years of age who presents with a clinical picture of failure to thrive, low-grade fever, hepatomegaly, and sometimes pulmonary infiltrates. Laboratory studies reveal hypergammaglobulinemia and high eosinophilia (up to 80 per cent in half of the cases) with absolute eosinophil counts greater than 20,000/cu mm.

The diagnosis is difficult to confirm because the parasite usually cannot be recovered. Open liver biopsy may show larvae of 18 μ diameter surrounded by an inflammatory granuloma (Fig. 51-55) but this procedure is seldom done because of the risk. Serologic tests may aid in establishing the diagnosis. Different methods vary in sensitivity and specificity. Both the indirect hemagglutination (HA) and the bentonite flocculation (BF) tests may employ antigens extracted from *Ascaris* or *Toxocara canis.* Positive or negative results must be evaluated with the clinical picture because there may be a high percentage of false reactions. Positive titers, therefore, do not neces-

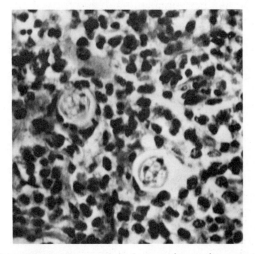

Figure 51-55. *Toxocara canis.* Larva in human liver granuloma. Note the polymorphonuclear cell infiltrate. Larval diameter is 18 μ (×450).

sarily mean infection. A titer of 1:400 or greater in the HA or of 1:5 or greater in BF can be of diagnostic significance, but serologic results are of greatest significance when a fourfold rise in titer is demonstrated (Kagan, 1970, 1976).

Angiostrongylus cantonensis. The agent of angiostrongyloidiasis or eosinophilic meningoencephalitis in man is a nematode up to 25 mm in length that usually lives in the pulmonary artery of rodents. Man is an incidental host. The parasite occurs mainly in Southeast Asia and the Pacific Islands, including Hawaii.

The female worm lays eggs in the pulmonary parenchyma of rodents, where they hatch, and the larvae migrate up the trachea and then to the gastrointestinal tract, from which they are passed with the stools. The larvae develop to the infective stage in molluscan intermediate hosts, usually slugs or land snails. Ingestion of the molluscan by the rodent results in the infection. Larvae enter the circulation, then migrate to the brain, where they mature. They then migrate to the lungs.

In man, who acquires the infection by eating the uncooked molluscan, the entire life cycle is usually not completed, but central nervous system invasion occurs. Infection produced by the larvae may present as meningitis with a high spinal fluid eosinophilia. It is seldom fatal. The few cases that have been autopsied have shown typical immature *Angiostrongylus* worms in the brain and spinal cord. The diagnosis is made clinically and the spinal fluid eosinophilia is highly suggestive. The infection may occur in epidemic form if there has been a common exposure.

CESTODES

Several diseases in man result from the development of cestode larval stages in tissues of man. In some patients the location of the parasite can result in serious disease (Abuladze, 1964).

Cysticercus. This is a cyst with a single inverted scolex representing the larval stage of a large number of tapeworms, including *Taenia* spp. The cysticerci of the two human species of *Taenia* develop in cattle (*T. saginata*) and in pigs. (*T. solium*) and are known as *Cysticercus bovis* and *C. cellulosae*, respectively. They may be differentiated because *T. solium* has a characteristic rostellum with hooks, similar to that of the adult, and *T. sagi-*

nata does not. Most cysticerci in man are morphologically indistinguishable from those of *T. solium* (i.e., they have a rostellum) so that all have been ascribed to this species. However, it is possible that related species of animal tapeworms with similar cysticerci could exist in man. This would explain some of the epidemiologic inconsistencies between the distribution of *T. solium* (adult) and *C. cellulosae* (larva) in man.

The infection in man results from the accidental ingestion of the eggs with food or water following the oral-fecal route. The larvae hatch from the eggs, penetrate the intestinal mucosa, and reach other organs of the body via blood. Infections range from a single cysticercus to thousands of them. The usual location is in the skeletal muscles, but they can be found in almost any organ, including heart, brain, eye, etc. (Fig. 51-56). Symptomatology is related to the number of cysticerci, their location, and the amount of host reaction. In the brain, the infection can cause seizures or symptoms of a space-occupying lesion.

In endemic areas, diagnosis is usually made

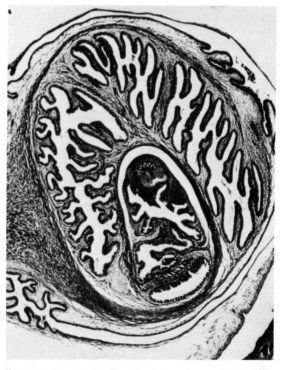

Figure 51-56. *Taenia solium.* Cysticercus in muscle. The larva has scolex tightly invaginated in the bladder. There is a crown of hooks tangentially cut (×30).

clinically. In non-endemic areas, diagnosis may be difficult. Serologic tests, such as indirect hemagglutination, are available, but they are overly sensitive and cross-react with other diseases. Radiographs have been used to demonstrate calcified cysticerci but are not effective in diagnosing recent infections. Definitive diagnosis may be established by identification of larvae removed by surgery.

Hydatid.   Hydatidosis or hydatid cysts in man are caused by the larval stages of cestodes belonging to the genus *Echinococcus.*

There are several species of *Echinococcus* that have as definitive hosts various wild and domestic carnivores including dogs. The adults live attached to the mucosa of the small intestine, measure up to 6 mm in length, and are usually composed of a scolex with a rostellum plus three segments. Eggs are passed in the stools and are ingested by the intermediate hosts, which include sheep, cattle, pigs, rodents, etc. (considered to be the main reservoirs in nature). Man is occasionally an accidental intermediate host.

In the intermediate host the eggs hatch in the intestine, and the young embryos penetrate the intestinal wall and then migrate to different organs where growth of the hydatid cyst begins. Development is slow, taking many years for the formation of a cyst 10 to 15 cm in diameter. The cyst is lined by a germinal membrane consisting of a single cell layer from which numerous infective larvae grow. The cyst lumen is filled with clear fluid. The larvae number in the thousands and may be attached to the germinal membrane but can also be found free in the cyst fluid. Next to the germinal membrane there is an acellular friable membrane called the laminated layer. On the outside of this layer is the host's fibrous reaction surrounded by normal tissue. Sometimes, there is a focal mononuclear cell infiltrate around the fibrous capsule.

Symptoms in man correspond to those of a space-occupying lesion growing very slowly, usually in the liver, lungs, or brain, but other organs can be involved.

There are several species of *Echinococcus* that may cause hydatid cyst in man. The most common is *E. granulosus,* which is found mainly in countries with large sheep and cattle industries, such as Australia, the southern part of South America, northern and eastern Europe, northern China, the Middle East, and southern and northern Africa. In the United States occasional cases, usually imported but occasionally autochthonous, are reported. A variety of domesticated and wild animals are the usual intermediate hosts.

The next most frequent species is *E. multilocularis,* which produces the multiloculated or alveolar hydatid disease. It is found principally in southern Germany, Switzerland, USSR, France, Italy, Argentina, Uruguay, New Zealand, Australia, and Alaska. The usual intermediate hosts are small rodents such as mice.

The diagnosis of the infection is usually made serologically. The serologic tests used include the indirect hemagglutination (HA), bentonite flocculation (BF), and latex agglutination (L). Low titers with any of these tests do not necessarily mean infection, since sera from patients with other conditions, such as liver cirrhosis and collagen diseases, cross-react. Cross-reactions with other cestode larvae such as cysticercus are also common. In addition, patients with hydatid cyst of the lung frequently have negative serology.

The tests employ hydatid fluid as antigen. The HA is considered positive in titers of 1:400 and the BF in titers of 1:5. The specificity of the three tests is similar and is between 82 and 88 per cent. Healthy people are consistently negative, but patients suffering from diseases other than hydatid cyst give up to 10 per cent positivity, which makes interpretation of the tests somewhat difficult.

In surgical and autopsy material there are morphologic differences among the *Echinococcus* cysts mentioned above. *E. granulosus* is unilocular (Fig. 51-57), while *E. multilocularis* is composed of many different compartments. Both have a thick acellular membrane.

Coenurus.   This is the agent of coenurosis, a sporadic, accidental infection of man following ingestion of eggs of a tapeworm belonging to the genus *Multiceps.* The adult parasites live in the intestine of dogs. Goats, cattle, and occasionally man are the intermediate hosts (Templeton, 1971).

The larval coenurus stage usually develops in the brain or spinal cord of the intermediate hosts, but other organs can also be involved. It is composed of a transparent large cyst up to 10 cm in diameter filled with clear fluid and containing up to several hundred larvae growing on the inner side of the cyst membrane. Cases of coenurosis have been reported in Africa, France, England, and Brazil, as well as in

5

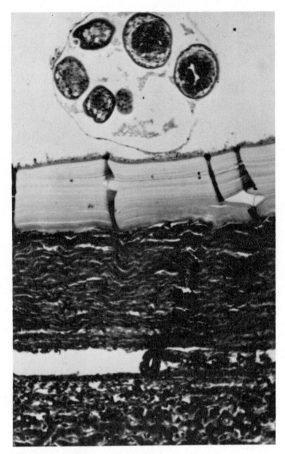

Figure 51–57. *Echinococcus granulosus.* Hydatid cyst in human liver. There is a brood capsule with at least 6 scolices, a thin germinal membrane, thick laminated membrane, and a fibrous host reaction (×150).

the United States. The diagnosis is made clinically and by study of cyst morphology after its removal. Species identification is not possible based on examination of the cyst alone.

Sparganum. Sparganosis in man is caused by larval stages of various *Spirometra* species, which are tapeworms closely related to *Diphyllobothrium* (Schwartzwelder, 1964). *Spirometra* are widely distributed in many domestic and wild animals, including both cats and dogs, which are the definitive hosts. Although the life cycle is not completely known, it has been assumed to be similar to that of *Diphyllobothrium* with vertebrates other than fish serving as second intermediate hosts.

The infection in man is thought to occur by ingestion of water contaminated with the arthropod first intermediate host harboring the larvae. The *Sparganum* larva develops in man, who therefore acts as the second intermediate host.

Symptoms of the infection are related to the localization of the larva, which is usually subcutaneous. An area of inflammation with redness, edema, and pain is usually the main presentation. Removal of the parasite reveals a delicate, slender, white worm measuring 60 to 80 mm long by 1 to 2 mm wide. The morphology in cross-sections is typical of that of a larval cestode with thick layered cuticle and a basement membrane (Fig. 51–58). There is not a cavity as seen in the nematodes, and it contains numerous calcareous corpuscles.

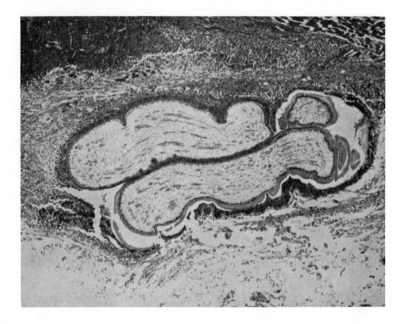

Figure 51–58. Sparganosis. Larva of *Spirometra* sp. in tissues with surrounding inflammation. (From Hunter, G. W., Swartzwelder, J. C., and Clyde, D. F.: Tropical Medicine. Philadelphia, W. B. Saunders Company, 1976.)

MEDICAL ENTOMOLOGY

Arthropods are of great medical importance because they transmit a wide variety of infectious agents, some of which are listed in Table 51-11. In addition, arthropods such as flies may mechanically transmit microorganisms from contaminated material to food, skin, or mucous membranes. Arthropods are very widespread in the environment, and excrement and fragments (frass) of various arthropods are present in soil and dust of various types. Persons may become hypersensitive to these arthropod materials and develop allergic manifestations, such as asthma and "hay fever." Chemical substances in the bodies of some arthropods may be irritating to persons who come in contact with them, as by crushing the arthropod.

The arthropods that will be discussed in this section are some of those that bite, sting, or live on man. There is no attempt to describe all such arthropods, but rather those which the laboratory is most likely to be asked to identify.

Many of the biting arthropods are attempting to obtain a blood meal, which is essential for their development. In contrast, stinging arthropods use their caudal stingers as a defense mechanism. Reaction to the arthropods may result from mechanical damage, toxic substances produced by the arthropod, or hypersensitivity to various arthropod antigens. In addition, there may be secondary mechanical damage from scratching or secondary infection from microorganisms borne by the arthropod or arising from the host's environment.

The arthropods may have egg, larval, nymph, and adult stages, and their effect on man may be caused by one or more of these. Identification of these parasites is dependent on morphologic recognition of the arthropod in one of its stages. Identification is based on various structural characteristics described in many books and manuals (CDC, 1969; Horsfall, 1962; James, 1969; U.S. Naval Medical School, 1967; Smith, 1973). If the laboratory is not proficient, the specimens may be referred to a competent entomologist.

Small arthropods, such as mosquitoes, flies, lice, and fleas, may be submitted live or dead without preservative, but the morphology of larval stages and larger arthropods will be better preserved in 10 per cent formalin or 70 per cent alcohol. Examination with a hand

Table 51-11. DISEASES TRANSMITTED BY ARTHROPODS

VECTOR	DISEASE TRANSMITTED
CRUSTACEA	
Copepod—*Cyclops* and *Diaptomus*	*D. latum* infection
Crayfish and crabs	*P. westermani* infection
ARACHNIDA	
Mites	Tsutsugamushi fever (scrub typhus); rickettsial pox
Ticks	Tularemia; Russian spring-summer encephalitis; Q fever; Colorado tick fever; Rocky Mountain spotted fever, relapsing fever, babesiosis
INSECTA	
Lice	Epidemic typhus; relapsing fever; trench fever
Fleas	Plague; murine typhus; *Dipylidium caninum* infection
Bugs	Chagas' disease (American trypanosomiasis)
Beetles (some species)	*Hymenolepis diminuta* infection
Bloodsucking flies	
Phlebotomus (sand fly)	Leishmaniasis; bartonellosis
Glossina (tsetse fly)	African trypanosomiasis
Simulium (black fly)	Onchocerciasis
Culicoides (midge, gnat)	*Dipetalonema perstans* and *Mansonella ozzardi* infections
Chrysops (deer fly)	Loaiasis; tularemia
Culex mosquito	Filariasis; viral encephalitides
Anopheles mosquito	Malaria; Bancroftian filariasis; Malayan filariasis
Aedes mosquito	Yellow fever; dengue; viral encephalitides; Bancroftian filariasis
Mansonia mosquito	Malayan filariasis

5

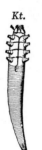

Kt.

Figure 51-59. The "face insect," *Demodex folliculorum* (× 100); *Kt.*, biting jaws. (After R. Blanchard in Brumpt.)

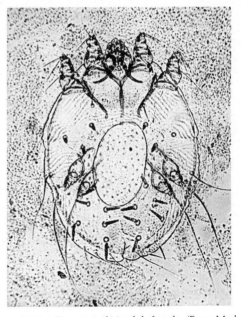

Figure 51-60. *Sarcoptes scabiei*, adult female. (From Markell, E. K., and Voge, M.: Medical Parasitology. Philadelphia, W. B. Saunders Company, 1976.)

lens, dissecting microscope, or light microscope will allow study of the characteristics of the parasite.

CLASS ARACHNIDA

This class includes mites, scorpions, spiders, and ticks and represents those arthropods with adults having a cephalothorax, abdomen, and eight legs.

Mites. Mites are of microscopic size, most measuring less than 1 mm in length. They are widely distributed in the environment. Allergens from mites in the environment may be responsible for allergy to "dust" in some individuals. Various species of mites parasitize the skin of animals, including man, and cause a disease called mange. Man is commonly infested by three mites, *Domodex folliculorum*, the follicle mite; *Sarcoptes scabiei*, the itch mite, which causes a disease known as scabies; and larval trombiculid mites, called red bugs, chiggers, or harvest mites. Man may occasionally be an accidental host for various animal mites in the environment.

D. folliculorum (Fig. 51-59) parasitizes hair follicles or sebaceous glands, particularly of the face, and is widespread in man, probably infesting over half of middle-aged adults.

The infestation is usually asymptomatic but may be associated with skin problems such as blackheads and acne in some cases. These parasites may often be seen as an incidental finding in histologic sections of facial skin. They are recognized by their elongated shape and stubby legs.

S. scabiei females (Fig. 51-60) tunnel in the superficial layers of skin, particularly in the interdigital areas and the flexor surfaces of the wrists and forearms, but they may also infest other areas. The female lays eggs (Fig. 51-61) in the tunnels which embryonate and larvae hatch (Fig. 51-62). The disease is spread by person-to-person contact, as in sleeping in the same bed or holding hands, or contact with contaminated clothing or other articles. The itching results from a sensitization reaction to the parasites and their products and varies in severity from patient to patient (Mellanby, 1972). There may be itching in areas in which there are no mites. Lesions often become secondarily infected (Orkin, 1975). The diagnosis is established by dissecting organisms or eggs from the tunnels, placing them in 20 per cent potassium hydroxide or mineral oil for clearing, and examining them under the microscope.

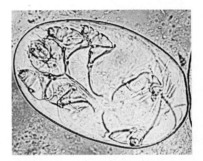

Figure 51-61. *Sarcoptes scabiei* egg containing fully developed larva. (From Markell, E. K., and Voge, M.: Medical Parasitology. Philadelphia, W. B. Saunders Company, 1976.)

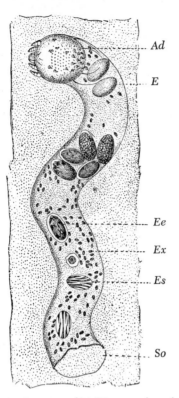

Figure 51-62. *Sarcoptes scabiei.* Diagram of a subcutaneous burrow; *Ad,* adult female; *E,* eggs; *Ee,* embryo egg; *Ex,* excrement; *Es,* egg shell; *So,* skin orifice. (After Railliet in Brumpt.)

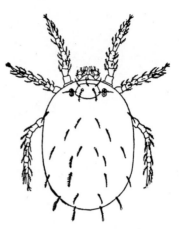

Figure 51-63. The North American chigger, *Trombicula irritans* (larva, ×100). (Ewing: A Manual of External Parasites. Springfield, Ill., Charles C Thomas, Publisher.)

Eggs, six-legged larvae, eight-legged nymphs, or adults may be detected and are diagnostic. Unfortunately, these cannot be readily demonstrated in all patients.

When scabies has been detected in a place, such as a school, there are often numerous individuals who develop itching without evidence of disease, probably of psychological origin. Care must be taken to properly diagnose the disease to prevent such pseudoepidemics. A particularly severe form of the disease may occur, especially in institutionalized patients, and is called "Norwegian scabies."

Trombiculid mites infest grasses and bushes, and their six-legged larvae, chiggers (red bugs, harvest mites) (Fig. 51-63), may attack man. The larvae attach to the skin, usually in areas of tight clothing such as elastic bands or belts. In sensitive individuals there is reaction to the secretions of the larvae with swollen itching areas at the sites of attachment which persist for days. Excoriations may become secondarily infected. Diagnosis is established on clinical grounds. Other trom-

biculid mites may be vectors of scrub typhus caused by *Rickettsia tsutsugamushi.*

Scorpions. Scorpions are found in the southern United States and other warm areas of the world. They have a stinger at the tip of the caudal end (Fig. 51-64) which injects a neurotoxin. Stings may produce local weakness and numbness, as well as systemic paralysis and abdominal pain. Fatalities may occasionally occur in children, usually as a result of respiratory paralysis.

Spiders. Spiders of a wide variety may bite man, but most produce minor lesions. The black widow spider, *Latrodectus mactans* (Fig. 51-65), bites in self defense. There is instant pain at the site of the bite, which becomes swollen and more painful. Of major significance are the systemic manifestations, including abdominal cramps and pain with muscle pains in the legs, chest, and back. There may be fever, vomiting, headache, and occasionally hypertension. Symptoms last 12 to 48 hours. Fatalities are rare, usually occurring in young children. The adult female spider is identified by the bright red hourglass on the midventral surface of its otherwise dark black body.

The bite of the brown recluse spider, *Loxosceles reclusus* in the United States and *L. laeta* in South America, produce severe necrotic skin lesions that may require grafting. Occasional fatalities have been described. *L. reclusa* is identified by a dark brown violin-shaped area on the dorsal cephalothorax.

Ticks. Ticks belong to the superfamily *Ixodoidea* and are important as vectors of infectious diseases (Table 51-11), but in addition

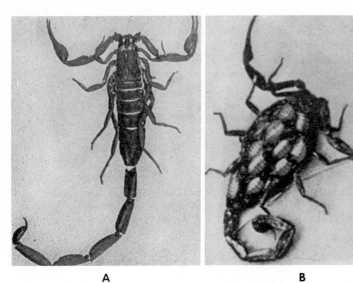

A   B

Figure 51–64. *A*, Male specimen of scorpion (*Centruroides*). ×1. (After C. C. Hoffmann, Anat. del Inst. de Biol., Mexico, from Faust, in Brennemann's Practice of Pediatrics; courtesy of W. F. Prior Company.) *B*, *Centruroides sculpturatus*, female with newly born young. ×1. (After Stahnke, Turtox News; courtesy of General Biological Supply House.)

Figure 51–65. Black widow spiders, *Latrodectus mactans*.

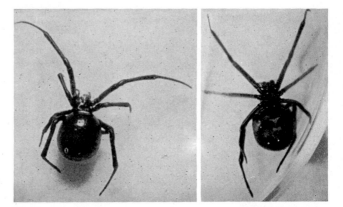

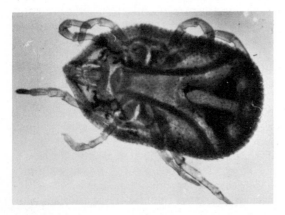

Figure 51–66. *Ornithodoros kellyi*, a soft tick, photographed with transmitted light.

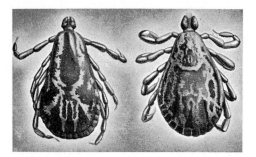

Figure 51-67. *Dermacentor andersoni* and *Dermacentor variabilis;* vectors of Rocky Mountain spotted fever rickettsiae. (Courtesy of Merck, Sharp & Dohme, Inc.)

may cause local damage from bites and may cause tick paralysis. There are two groups of ticks. Soft ticks belonging to the family *Argasidae* (Fig. 51-66) have a soft leathery body, and mouthparts are not visible from above. Hard ticks belonging to the family *Ixodidae* have a hard dorsal plate, and mouth parts are visible from above (Fig. 51-67). The dorsal plate covers the entire dorsum of the male, but only the anterior portion of the female, allowing the body to swell when engorged. Unengorged ticks are generally 3 to 4 mm long, but engorged ticks may be up to 1.5 cm long. The stages in development are egg, larva, nymph, and adult. Blood meals are essential for the development of ticks. Infestation is acquired in grassy or bushy

areas where the ticks reside between blood meals on various mammals.

Tick paralysis is an ascending paralysis that develops in occasional patients, especially children, bitten by various ticks and is due to a toxic substance introduced by the tick. This disease may be confused with Guillain-Barré syndrome, poliomyelitis, botulism, and other paralytic diseases. Removal of ticks results in recovery.

CLASS INSECTA

Members of the class Insecta are characterized by a body divided into head, thorax, and abdomen and having three pair of legs. There are usually two pairs of wings. Insects of medical importance include lice, fleas, bugs, mosquitoes, and flies. Bees and wasps may cause severe reactions, particularly in sensitive individuals, but will not be further described.

Lice. Lice are flattened dorsoventrally and are wingless. There are three lice that infest man and obtain nourishment by biting and sucking on the human host. They are named according to the region of the body that they usually (but not exclusively) inhabit. *Pediculus humanus capitis* is the head louse and is 1 to 2 mm long. *P. humanus corporis* is the body louse and is 2 to 4 mm long, and *Phthirus*

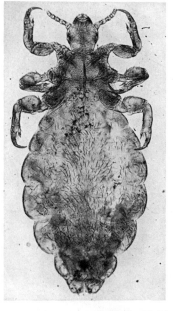

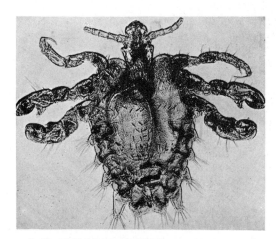

Figure 51-68. *Pediculus humanus* (left) and *Phthirus pubis* (right).

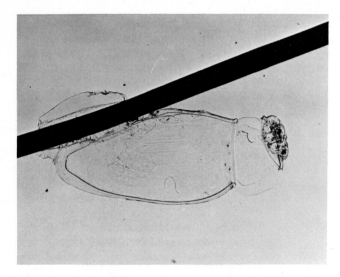

Figure 51–69. *Pediculus capitis.* Empty egg case ("nit") attached to hair (×60). (From Raphael, S. S.: Lynch's Medical Laboratory Technology. Philadelphia, W. B. Saunders Company, 1976.)

pubis is the pubic or crab louse and is approximately 1 mm long (Fig. 51-68). The body louse is particularly important as the vector of epidemic typhus. Infections with lice usually occur when people live in crowded conditions with little opportunity for bathing and laundering. Infestation may be spread by intimate contact, as in bed partners, or by contaminated hats, clothing, blankets, or furniture. Eggs of *P. humanus capitis* and *P. pubis* are attached to hairs and are known as "nits" (Fig. 51-69). Eggs of *P. humanus corporis* are laid in clothing. Diagnosis is suspected from finding bites but established by finding adults, usually in hairy areas, such as the head, eyebrows, armpits, and genital areas, or by detecting "nits" attached to hairs (*P. humanus capitis* and *P. pubis*) or eggs in clothing (*P. humanus corporis*). "Nits" should be examined microscopically to be certain they are truly eggs and not globs of hair spray or some other material.

Fleas. Fleas are bloodsucking wingless insects that are laterally compressed and have large hind legs for jumping. They average 2 to 4 mm long and have bloodsucking mouthparts. The oriental rat flea (*Xenopsylla cheopis*) is the vector of plague, and fleas may be associated with other infections (Table 51-11). Flea bites cause little trouble to some persons but are quite irritating to others, probably as a result of sensitization of the host. Man may be infected by the human flea (*Pulex irritans*) (Fig. 51-70) or may be an incidental host for fleas of other animals, particularly the dog flea (*Ctenocephalides canis*) and the cat flea (*C. felis*). Eggs develop in dog and cat bedding and in carpets and furniture. They usually cause little difficulty for man unless the pet is no longer present, for then they will bite man. This usually occurs after moving, boarding, or death of pets.

Bugs. Reduviid bugs are bloodsucking bugs that are vectors of South American trypanosomiasis and will not be discussed further.

The bed bug, *Cimex lectularius* (Fig. 51-71) is reddish brown and about 5 mm long and has short wing pads but cannot fly. Bites of these bloodsucking insects vary in severity depending on the degree of sensitivity that the host has developed. In some individuals they may cause wheals up to 3 mm in diameter with intense itching; in others they cause almost no reaction. During the day the bugs live in mattresses, bedsteads, cracks in walls, furniture, etc., and at night come out to bite the sleeping victim. Diagnosis is established by identifying the adult bugs or on clinical grounds.

Flies. Mosquitoes are flies with two pairs of wings with scales and a proboscis for sucking. They are important in transmission of a number of serious infectious diseases (Table 51-11). In addition, they are a nuisance, since their bites make living in some environments quite uncomfortable. The severity of reaction to their bite is related to the degree of sensitivity in the host.

Bloodsucking flies of various types may be important as vectors of infectious diseases (Table 51-11) or may be important only as

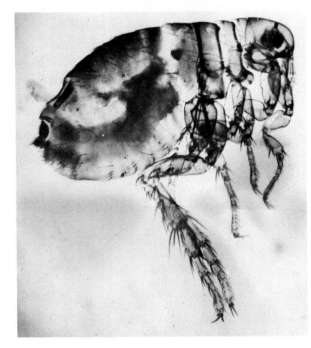

Figure 51-70. *Pulex irritans* female flea. Note the powerful hind legs.

pests that inflict painful wounds. Other flies (filth flies) may spread a variety of infectious diseases, such as salmonellosis, typhoid fever, shigellosis, and poliomyelitis, by mechanical means.

Larvae of various flies (maggots) may be seen in a variety of conditions and are often brought to the laboratory as "worms." There are characteristics that allow their identification by experienced entomologists, although sometimes they must be allowed to develop to adult flies for specific identification.

Specific myiases are caused by flies that deposit eggs on the tissues of specific hosts. The larvae invade the host and are thus truly parasitic. These are usually infestations of other animal species. For example, the primary screw-worm, *Cochliomyia hominivorax*, is a serious economic problem to the cattle industry in the southern United States. When man is infected, the disease may be particularly severe if the larvae invade the eye, nose, or mouth.

Semispecific myiases are caused by flies which usually lay their eggs on dead animals or rotting vegetation but which may lay eggs on open wounds or around the nose or other mucous membranes. The larvae usually live a saprophytic existence on necrotic material or secretions and on occasion have been proposed as agents for debridement of wounds. The larvae may be irritating, especially in the nasal area, where they cause increased mucus flow.

Accidental myiasis involving the gastrointestinal tract occurs when eggs or larvae are accidentally ingested and survive the digestive juices. They may be asymptomatic or may be associated with nausea, abdominal pain, and diarrhea. The maggots are usually found in vomitus or feces and submitted to the laboratory as "worms." Care should be taken to assure that the larvae were present in the specimen when passed and did not develop later. The latter is particularly common in larvae detected when the mother is washing diapers.

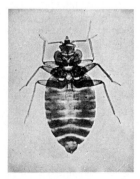

Figure 51-71. The common bedbug, *Cimex lectularius,* male (×5). In the female the posterior end of the abdomen is more rounded. (Cleared with sodium hydroxide to bring out the structure more clearly.)

REFERENCES

Abuladze, K. I.: Taeniata of animals and man and diseases caused by them. In Skrjabin, K. I. (ed.): Essentials of Cestodology, vol. 4 (Translated from Russian). Washington, D.C., United States Department of Agriculture, 1964.

Adams, A. R. D., and Maegraith, B. G.: Clinical Tropical Diseases, 6th ed. Oxford, Blackwell Scientific Publications, 1976.

Adams, E. B., and MacLeod, I. N.: Invasive amebiasis. I. Amebic dysentery and its complications. Medicine, 56:315, 1977a.

Adams, E. B., and MacLeod, I. N.: Invasive amebiasis. II. Amebic liver abscess and its complications. Medicine, 56:325, 1977b.

Beaver, P. C.: The nature of visceral larva migrans. J. Parasitol., 55:3, 1969.

Beaver, P. C.: Filariasis without microfilaremia. Am. J. Trop. Med. Hyg., 19:181, 1970.

Beaver, P. C., and Orihel, T. C.: Human infection with filariae of animals in the United States. Am. J. Trop. Med. Hyg., 14:1010, 1965.

Beaver, P. C., Snyder, C. H., Carrera, G. M., Dent, J. H., and Lafferty, J. W.: Chronic eosinophilia due to visceral larva migrans: Report of three cases. Pediatrics, 9:7, 1952.

Belding, D. L.: Textbook of Parasitology, 3rd ed. New York, Appleton-Century-Crofts, 1965.

Black, R. E., Dykes, A. C., Sinclair, S. P., and Wells, J. G.: Giardiasis in day-care centers: Evidence of person-to-person transmission. Pediatrics, 60:486, 1977.

Bowling, M. C., Smith, I. M., and Wescott, S. L.: A rapid staining procedure for Pneumocystis carinii. Am. J. Med. Technol., 39:267, 1973.

Brooke, M. M., and Melvin, D. M.: Morphology of Diagnostic Stages of Intestinal Parasites of Man (Publication No. [CDC] 74-8116). Washington, D.C., United States Department of Health, Education, and Welfare, 1969.

Brown, H. W.: Basic Clinical Parasitology, 4th ed. New York, Appleton-Century-Crofts, 1975.

Burrows, R. B., and Swerdlow, M. A.: Enterobius vermicularis as a probable vector of Dientamoeba fragilis. Am. J. Trop. Med. Hyg., 5:258, 1956.

Center for Disease Control: Intestinal Parasite Surveillance. Annual Summary, 1976. Issued August, 1977.

Center for Disease Control: Malaria Surveillance. Annual Summary, 1976. Issued September, 1977.

Chalvardjian, A. M., and Grawe, L. A.: A new procedure for the identification of Pneumocystis carinii cyst in tissue sections and smears. J. Clin. Pathol., 16:383, 1963.

Coatney, G. R., Collins, W. E., Warren, M., and Contacos, P. G.: The Primate Malarias. Washington, D.C., U.S. Government Printing Office, 1971.

Culbertson, C. G.: Soil amoeba infection. In Lennette, E. H., Spaulding, E. H., and Truant, J. P.: Manual of Clinical Microbiology, 2nd ed. Washington, D.C., American Society for Microbiology, 1974, p. 602.

Edington, G. M., and Gilles, H. M.: Pathology in the Tropics. London, Edward Arnold (Publishers), 1969.

Eveland, L. K., Kenney, M., and Yermakov, V.: Laboratory diagnosis of autoinfection in strongyloidiasis. Am. J. Clin. Pathol. 63:421, 1975.

Faust, E. C., Beaver, P. C., and Jung, R. C.: Animal Agents and Vectors of Human Disease, 4th ed. Philadelphia, Lea & Febiger, 1975.

Faust, E. C., Russell, P. F., and Jung, R. C.: Craig and Faust's Clinical Parasitology, 8th ed. Philadelphia, Lea & Febiger, 1970.

Garcia, L. S., and Ash, L. R.: Diagnostic Parasitology: Clinical Laboratory Manual. St. Louis, The C. V. Mosby Company, 1975.

Heyneman, D.: Host-parasite resistance patterns—some implications from experimental studies with helminths. Ann. N.Y. Acad. Sci., 113:114, 1963.

Hoare, C. A., and Wallace, F. G.: Developmental stages of trypanosomatid flagellates: A new terminology. Nature, 212:1385, 1966.

Horsfall, W. R.: Medical Entomology: Arthropods and Human Disease. New York, Ronald Press Company, 1962.

Hughes, W. T.: Current status of laboratory diagnosis of Pneumocystis carinii pneumonitis. CRC Crit. Rev. Clin. Lab. Sci., 6:145, 1975.

Hunter, G. W., III, Swartzwelder, J. C., and Clyde, D. F.: Tropical Medicine, 5th ed. Philadelphia, W. B. Saunders Company, 1976.

James, M. T., and Harwood, R. F.: Herms's Medical Entomology, 6th ed. New York, Macmillan Company, 1969.

Jung, R. C., and Beaver, P. C.: Clinical observations on Trichocephalus trichiurus (whipworm) infestation in children. Pediatrics, 8:548, 1951.

Kagan, I. G., and Norman L.: Serodiagnosis of parasitic diseases. In Blair, J. E., Lennette, E. H., and Truant, J. P.: Manual of Clinical Microbiology. Bethesda, Md., American Society for Microbiology, 1970, p. 453.

Kagan, I. G., and Norman, L.: Serodiagnosis of parasitic diseases. In Rose, N. R., and Friedman, H.: Manual of Clinical Immunology. Washington, D.C., American Society for Microbiology, 1976, p. 382.

Latorre, C. R., Sulzer, A. J., and Norman, L. G.: Serial propagation of Pneumocystis carinii in cell line cultures. Appl. Environ. Microbiol., 33:1204, 1977.

Layrisse, M., Blumenfeld, N., Carbonell, L., Desenne, J., and Roche, M.: Intestinal absorption tests and biopsy of the jejunum in subjects with heavy hookworm infection. Am. J. Trop. Med. Hyg., 13:297, 1964a.

Layrisse, M., and Roche, M.: The relationship between anemia and hookworm infection: Results of surveys of rural Venezuelan population. Am. J. Hyg., 79:279, 1964b.

Lennette, E. H., Spaulding, E. H., and Truant, J. P.: Manual of Clinical Microbiology, 2nd ed. Washington, D.C., American Society for Microbiology, 1974.

Mahmoud, A. A. F., and Warren, K. S.: Algorithms in the diagnosis and management of exotic diseases. IV. American trypanosomiasis. J. Infect. Dis., 132:121, 1975.

Mahmoud, A. A. F., and Warren, K. S.: Algorithms in the diagnosis and management of exotic diseases. XI. African trypanosomiases. J. Infect. Dis., 133:487, 1976a.

Mahmoud, A. A. F., and Warren, K. S.: Algorithms in the diagnosis and management of exotic diseases. XVII. Amebiasis. J. Infect. Dis., 134:639, 1976b.

Mahmoud, A. A. F., and Warren, K. S.: Algorithms in the diagnosis and management of exotic diseases. XXIV. Leishmaniases. J. Infect. Dis., 136:160, 1977.

Manson-Bahr, P. H.: Manson's Tropical Diseases: A Manual of the Diseases of Warm Climates, 16th ed. London, Baillière, Tindall & Cassell, 1966.

Marcial-Rojas, R. A.: Pathology of Protozoal and Helminthic Diseases with Clinical Correlation. Baltimore, Williams & Wilkins Company, 1971.

Markell, E. K., and Voge, M.: Medical Parasitology, 4th ed. Philadelphia, W. B. Saunders Company, 1976.

Martin, L. K.: Randomness of particle distribution in human feces and the resulting influence on helminth egg counting. Am. J. Trop. Med. Hyg., *14*:747, 1965.

Mellanby, K.: Scabies. Middlesex, England, E. W. Classey, 1943 (Reprinted, 1972).

Melvin, D. M., and Brooke, M. M.: Laboratory Procedures for the Diagnosis of Intestinal Parasites (DHEW Publication [CDC] 75-8282). Atlanta, Ga., Bureau of Laboratories, Laboratory Training and Consultation Division, 1974.

National Communicable Disease Center: Pictorial Keys to Arthropods, Reptiles, Birds and Mammals of Public Health Significance, 2nd ed. (Publication No. 1955). Washington, D.C., U.S. Government Printing Office, 1969.

Orihel, T. C., and Beaver, P. C.: Morphology and relationship of *Dirofilaria tenuis* and *Dirofilaria conjunctivae*. Am. J. Trop. Med. Hyg., *14*:1030, 1965.

Orkin, M.: Today's scabies (editorial). Arch. Dermatol., *111*:1431, 1975.

Peters, W., and Gilles, H. M.: A Colour Atlas of Tropical Medicine and Parasitology. London, Wolfe Medical Publications, 1977.

Purtilo, D. T., Meyers, W. M., and Connor, D. H.: Fatal strongyloidiasis in immunosuppressed patients. Am. J. Med., *56*:488, 1974.

Remington, J. S., and Desmonts, G.: Toxoplasmosis. *In* Remington, J. S., and Klein, J. O.: Infectious Diseases of the Fetus and Newborn Infant. Philadelphia, W. B. Saunders Company, 1976, p. 191.

Ruebush, T. K., II, Cassaday, P. B., Marsh, H. J., Lisker, S. A., Voorhees, D. B., Mahoney, E. B., and Healy, G. R.: Human babesiosis on Nantucket Island: Clinical features. Ann. Intern. Med., *86*:6, 1977.

Ruebush, T. K., II, Juranek, D. D., Chisholm, E. S., Snow, P. C., Healy, G. R., and Sulzer, A. J.: Human babesiosis on Nantucket Island: Evidence for self-limited and subclinical infections. N. Engl. J. Med., *297*:825, 1977.

Sasa, M.: Human Filariasis: A Global Survey of Epidemiology and Control. Baltimore, University Park Press, 1976.

Shaw, P. K., Brodsky, R. E., Lyman, D. O., Wood, B. T., Hibler, C. P., Healy, G. R., MacLeod, K. I. E., Stahl, W., and Schultz, M. G.: A communitywide outbreak of giardiasis with evidence of transmission by a municipal water supply. Ann. Intern. Med., *87*:426, 1977.

Smith, J. W., Ash, L. R., Thompson, J. H., McQuay, R. M., Melvin, D. M., and Orihel, T. C.: Diagnostic parasitology—intestinal helminths. Chicago, American Society of Clinical Pathologists, 1976a.

Smith, J. W., McQuay, R. M., Ash, L. R., Melvin, D. M., Orihel, T. C., and Thompson, J. H.: Diagnostic parasitology—intestinal protozoa. Chicago, American Society of Clinical Pathologists, 1976b.

Smith, J. W., Melvin, D. M., Orihel, T. C., Ash, L. R., McQuay, R. M., and Thompson, J. H.: Diagnostic parasitology—blood and tissue parasites. Chicago, American Society of Clinical Pathologists, 1976c.

Smith, K. G. V.: Insects and Other Arthropods of Medical Importance. London, British Museum of Natural History, 1973.

Spencer, F. M., and Monroe, L. S.: The Color Atlas of Intestinal Parasites, Springfield, Ill., Charles C Thomas, Publisher, 1975.

Spencer, H., Dayan, A. D., Gibson, J. B., Huntsman, R. G., Hutt, M. S. R., Jenkins, G. C., Koberle, F., Maegraith, B. G., and Salfelder, K.: Tropical Pathology. Berlin, Springer-Verlag, 1973.

Spillman, R. K.: Pulmonary ascariasis in tropical communities. Am. J. Trop. Med. Hyg., *24*:791, 1975.

Strauss, W. G.: Clinical manifestations of clonorchiasis: A controlled study of 105 cases. Am. J. Trop. Med. Hyg., *11*:625, 1962.

Swartzwelder, J. C., Beaver, P. C., and Hood, M. W.: Sparganosis in southern United States. Am. J. Trop. Med. Hyg., *13*:43, 1964.

Symmers, W. St. C.: Pathology of oxyuriasis with special reference to granulomas due to the presence of oxyuris vermicularis (Enterobius vermicularis) and its ova in the tissues. Arch. Pathol., *50*:475, 1950.

Templeton, A. C.: Anatomical and geographical location of human coenurus infection. Trop. Geogr. Med., *23*:105, 1971.

United States Naval Medical School: Medical Protozoology and Helminthology. Bethesda, Md., National Naval Medical Center, 1965.

United States Naval Medical School: Medical Entomology. Bethesda, Md., National Naval Medical Center, 1967.

Vik, R.: The genus *Diphyllobothrium:* An example of the interdependence of systematics and experimental biology. Exp. Parasitol., *15*:361, 1964.

Walzer, P. D., Schnelle, V., Armstrong, D., and Rosen, P. P.: Nude mouse: A new experimental model for *Pneumocystis carinii* infection. Science, *197*:177, 1977.

Wardle, R. A., and McLeod, J. A.: The Zoology of Tapeworms. Minneapolis, University of Minnesota Press, 1952.

Warren, K. S.: Helminthic diseases endemic in the United States. Am. J. Trop. Med. Hyg., *23*:723, 1974.

WHO Expert Committee on Helminthiases: Soil-transmitted helminths. WHO Tech. Rep. Ser. No. 277, 1964, p. 1-70.

Yang, J., and Scholten, T.: *Dientamoeba fragilis:* A review with notes on its epidemiology, pathogenicity, mode of transmission, and diagnosis. Am. J. Trop. Med. Hyg., *26*:16, 1977.

5

52

LABORATORY DIAGNOSIS OF VIRUSES, RICKETTSIA, AND CHLAMYDIA

C. George Ray, M.D., and
Mary Jane Hicks, M.D.

VIRAL INFECTIONS

Virology (Latin: *virus* = poison) is a relatively new discipline when compared with bacteriology. The beginning of the modern era of virology can best be credited to Walter Reed, who demonstrated in 1901 that yellow fever was caused by a viral agent. Since 1949, when John Enders and his collaborators reported the growth of viruses in tissue culture with resultant cytopathic effects, both our knowledge of viral infections in humans and the ability to identify them have increased in logarithmic fashion.

It is now generally accepted that viruses as a group are the single most common cause of human disease. Their capabilities for infection and disease production follow a number of different options, including subclinical infection, acute illness, latency with the potential for reactivation (e.g., varicella-zoster virus), chronic, productive infection (e.g., hepatitis B and chronic active hepatitis; "slow" virus infections of the central nervous system), and chronic, non-productive infection, wherein part of the viral genome has been integrated into the host genome, altering cell function (e.g., possibly some or all forms of human cancer, although not yet proven).

Traditionally, diagnostic virology has usually been left to the public health laboratories, which have relied heavily on serologic diagnosis. While much valuable information has been gained from these laboratories, and the public health has benefited considerably, these services do have admitted deficiencies. First of all, when diagnosis is based primarily upon serology, the number of agents for which the laboratory can reliably and economically test is limited. Secondly, with rare exceptions, serologic diagnosis requires paired serum samples collected 10 days to 6 weeks apart in order to reliably interpret the data. This results in a relatively long delay in etiologic diagnosis, and less benefit to the individual patient.

It is now reasonable, and indeed, important to consider wider application of diagnostic virology for direct patient management in the community-based hospital. In addition to public health and epidemiologic benefits, more rapid diagnosis can aid the clinician greatly in considering further diagnostic and therapeutic maneuvers—the result of a rapid viral diagnosis can be consideration for fewer other tests and therapies, and even shortening of hospitalization times in many cases. Furthermore, the results can aid the physician in prognostication and in understanding the clinical behavior of such infections. Specific antiviral therapy is available for a few infections, but an armamentarium comparable to that presently available for bacterial diseases will probably not be realized for several years. Nevertheless, the prospects are clear: in each future year there will be a greater demand on the diagnostic laboratory to make rapid etiologic diagnoses of viral infections with the

possibility of specific therapy in mind. This has already been shown to be true for herpes simplex encephalitis, and perhaps influenza A infections.

Our present experience has been in a community-based diagnostic laboratory, where we have found that it is not unreasonable to expect a 30 to 40 per cent diagnostic yield for viral infections among all patients studied. Such a laboratory, of course, includes specimens accompanied by a specific request to rule out certain viral possibilities and others from patients with illnesses of obscure nature for which viral cultures are included as part of the screening process; therefore, in a competent laboratory, negative results can also be of value.

We have also found, as have others, that rapid diagnosis is often a possibility. With standard cell culture methods alone, 25 per cent of infections can be detected within 48 hours, and over 70 per cent are found within 5 days or less. In addition, special rapid diagnostic procedures, including cytology, immunofluorescence, immunoperoxidase and electron microscopy can sometimes yield definitive positive answers within a few hours, and many of these are not beyond the scope of a well-equipped hospital laboratory.

We would point out, however, that diagnostic virology does require a reasonable degree of technical expertise and an adequate volume of specimens to sustain a quality operation and yet be economical. Therefore, we recommend that such diagnostic services not be considered a necessity in every laboratory in a given community. It is preferable to consider the potential volume involved, and designate one laboratory in a given population sector to serve as the regional virology diagnostic laboratory.

The specific approaches to viral diagnosis include (1) serologic studies, in most cases requiring acute and convalescent sera; (2) cytologic studies, with particular attention to intracellular inclusions, and possible giant-cell formation; (3) direct examination by electron microscopy; (4) isolation of viruses from tissue or body fluids in appropriate tissue culture, animal, or avian host systems; and (5) demonstration of viral antigen in clinical samples or host cell systems by immunologic methods. Any or all of these approaches may be considered in the workup of a patient, and require knowledge of the possible agents that might be associated with the illness in question, as well as their behavior in the laboratory. At the

5

present time, greatest emphasis is placed upon direct isolation and demonstration of the agent in host cell systems, but this should not discount the other approaches, which may complement or even speed diagnosis. Chlamydia and rickettsia, which are more like bacteria in their biology, do share a property common with viruses in that they require living cells in order to replicate. This property, and the fact that the principles of diagnosis are similar for these agents and for viruses, make it logical to include them in this chapter.

SELECTION AND COLLECTION OF SPECIMENS

C. R. Madeley, in his excellent discussion of collection and transport of specimens (Madeley, 1977), has appropriately emphasized the need for careful communication between the physician caring for the patient and the laboratory prior to collection of specimens. The decision regarding which types of specimens are to be obtained and how they should be transported and processed requires clinical and epidemiologic considerations, as well as an understanding of the biology of the agents which are to be sought. For these reasons, we would urge that such studies not be undertaken until after there has been a discussion with the virologist in charge.

The agents most commonly sought in the major syndrome categories encountered in a diagnostic laboratory, and the yield of the agents from various specimens (on a relative scale of − to + + + +) are listed in Table 52–1. In addition, it is usually advisable to request 5 to 10 ml of clotted blood in the acute phase of illness, separate the serum, and store it frozen (at least −20°C.) for possible reference in

Table 52–1. APPROPRIATE SPECIMENS FOR VIRUS ISOLATION*

DISEASE CATEGORY AND AGENTS GENERALLY SOUGHT	SPECIMENS					
	Throat	Stool	CSF	Urine	Vesicle Fluid	Other
Meningitis-Encephalitis						
Mumps	+ + + +	− −	+ +	+	− −	
Enteroviruses	+ + +	+ + + +	+ +	− −	− −	
Herpes simplex	±	− −	±	− −	+	Brain Biopsy + + + +
Arboviruses†	− −	− −	+	− −	− −	Brain + + Blood +
Respiratory Disease						
Myxoviruses						
Paramyxoviruses	+ + + +	− −	− −	− −	− −	
Rhinoviruses						
Adenoviruses	+ + + +	+ + + +	− −	− −	− −	
Exanthems and Enanthems						
Rubella† (Measles)	+ + + +	− −	− −	+	− −	
Variola	+ +	− −	±	±	+ + + +	
Vaccinia	− −	− −	− −	− −	+ + + +	
Varicella-Zoster	− −	− −	− −	− −	+ + + +	
Herpes simplex	+ + +	− −	− −	− −	+ + + +	
Enteroviruses	+ + +	+ + + +	− −	− −	+	
Myocarditis-Pericarditis						
Enteroviruses†	+ +	+ + +	− −	− −	− −	Pericardial Fluid + +
Myxoviruses†	+ + +	− −	− −	− −	− −	
Paramyxoviruses†	+ + +	− −	− −	− −	− −	
Other						
Cytomegalovirus	+ +	− −	− −	+ + +	− −	Leukocytes + Lung, Liver Biopsy +

*In general, it is important to remember that virus shedding often diminishes rapidly after the onset of illness; therefore, it is important to attempt to collect specimens as early as possible, including an acute serum sample for future testing.

†Because it is frequently very difficult to isolate and/or associate these agents with the disease in question, it is emphasized that serologic tests are particularly important in order to insure a diagnosis.

− − − = no yield; ± to + + + + = relative yield on culture.

Table 52–2. APPROPRIATE SEROLOGIC TESTS

MENINGOENCEPHALITIS		RESPIRATORY SYNDROMES		MISCELLANEOUS	
Agent	Serologic Test	Agent	Serologic Test	Agent	Serologic Test
ECHO	Neutralization	Influenza	CF or HI*	Varicella	CF
Coxsackie	Neutralization	Respiratory syncytial	CF or neutralization	Rubella	HI or CF
Polio	Neutralization, CF	Parainfluenza	CF or HI	Measles	CF or HI
Herpes	Neutralization, CF	Adenovirus	CF or neutralization	Cytomegalovirus	CF
Mumps	CF, HI, or neutralization	Psittacosis	CF		
Arboviruses	HI, CF	Mycoplasma	CF		

*CF = complement fixation; HI = Hemagglutination-inhibition.

serologic testing, if it later becomes apparent this will be useful. Table 52–2 lists the serologic tests which are most commonly used.

The relationship of stage of illness to the expected laboratory diagnostic yield is shown in Table 52–3. It is apparent that the best chances for viral detection will exist when specimens are taken and processed as early in the acute phase of illness as is possible.

There are some simple guidelines concerning specimen collection. For swabs and other samples which may dry out during transport

Table 52–3. RELATION OF STAGE OF ILLNESS TO PRESENCE OF VIRUS IN TEST MATERIAL AND TO APPEARANCE OF ANTIBODY*

STAGE OF ILLNESS	VIRUS DEMONSTRABLE IN APPROPRIATE TEST MATERIAL	SPECIFIC ANTIBODY PRESENT IN SERUM
Incubation period	Rarely	–
Prodromal period	Rarely	–
Onset	Frequently	–
Acute phase	Frequently	Frequently or generally†
Recovery phase	Rarely	Generally
Convalescence	Very rarely	Usually

*From Lennette, E. H., and Schmidt, N. J., (eds.): Diagnostic Procedures for Viral and Rickettsial Infections, 4th ed. New York, American Public Health Association, 1969, p. 31.

†In certain widespread endemic diseases, antibody representing prior experience with the agent is generally encountered in acute-phase blood (e.g., influenza, herpes simplex). In other instances (Western equine encephalomyelitis, poliomyelitis), antibody is frequently present in acute-phase serum; antibody formation apparently is well under way by the time the acute-phase specimen is taken.

Whether antibody is encountered will also depend upon the type of antibody (neutralizing, CF, or HI), because of temporal differences in persistence after infection.

to the laboratory, a virus transport medium (VTM) is necessary. Buffered saline with protein as a stabilizer and added antibiotics, such as penicillin, gentamicin, and amphotericin B, to suppress bacterial and fungal overgrowth, is commonly used. Veal infusion broth, 1 per cent bovine serum albumin, or even skimmed cow's milk are all usable alternatives; most bacteriologic media, particularly reducing media and semisolid vehicles, should be avoided. It should be remembered that antibiotic-containing media should not be used to moisten swabs applied to denuded skin or mucosal surfaces if the patient has a history of allergy to any of the components. The VTM can be dispensed in 2 ml aliquots into screw-capped tubes or vials with non-toxic cap liners, and kept frozen at −20°C. until used.

The following comments are useful to remember when collecting samples for different viral agents:

Respiratory Syndromes. The primary sampling site is the respiratory tract. Cotton-tipped throat swabs, well saturated with pharyngeal secretions, and nasopharyngeal swabs are preferred, both immersed into a single vial of VTM. The ends may be broken off for transport to the laboratory, or, if wooden throat swabs are used which may contain toxic preservatives, the swabs may be vigorously agitated in the VTM, the excess fluid expressed on the side of the vial, then discarded. Alternative methods which have produced high yields of respiratory viruses are nasopharyngeal washings, using buffered saline, or, in patients able to cooperate, pharyngeal washings after gargling with antibiotic-free VTM. Some investigators have reported excellent results when nasopharyngeal washings are immediately inoculated into cell cultures without further processing.

5

Central Nervous System Syndromes.
Feces, throat swabs, and cerebrospinal fluid should be obtained from patients with aseptic meningitis or encephalitis. If mumps is suspected, urine may also be of value. Feces, 5 to 10 g collected in screw-capped bottles, are preferred for enterovirus isolation, but this may delay workup while one waits for the patient to defecate. A useful alternative is a rectal swab, immersed in VTM; however, it must be emphasized that rectal swabs are greatly inferior to feces unless the swab is well soiled with fecal material.

Cerebrospinal fluid, 1 to 3 ml, is collected in a sterile tube and held without further processing until inoculation.

Exanthems and Enanthems. Throat and rectal swabs or feces should be obtained; in addition, any ulcerated lesions should be directly swabbed and the swabs placed in VTM. If vesicular or bullous lesions are present, these can be aspirated into a tuberculin syringe or capillary tube, the contents discharged into VTM, followed by rinsing of the tube or syringe with VTM. Smaller lesions can be gently unroofed, and the fluid obtained by thorough soaking of a swab. It is often useful to sample several lesions and pool the sample into one vial of VTM in order to increase the virus yield. In addition, the fluid may be collected for direct electron microscopic examination, and it may be desirable to scrape the base of the lesion for cytologic study.

Ophthalmologic Syndromes. Conjunctivitis is best approached by obtaining a swab of conjunctival exudate and immersing it in VTM. Conjunctival scrapings for cytologic examination can also be of value, particularly when evidence of chlamydial infection is sought. Occasionally, corneal scrapings or aqueous humor may be submitted for study by the ophthalmologist. It is usually best to inoculate these samples directly into tissue culture, without transport in VTM.

Congenital Infections. Viral agents most commonly involved in congenital or perinatal infections include cytomegalovirus, rubella, herpes simplex, and enteroviruses. Cultures to be considered include throat, stool or rectal swab, cerebrospinal fluid, urine, and vesicle fluid.

Other Specimens. Urine is often a useful culture source for acquired or congenital cytomegalovirus infection, acute hemorrhagic cystitis associated with adenoviruses, and possibly other agents. Occasionally mumps virus may also be detected in the urine for up to two weeks after onset of illness. Clean-voided specimens, 5 to 10 ml, are preferred, with transport to the laboratory as quickly as possible. Some laboratories prefer, if there is to be a delay of several hours before processing, to alkalinize the urine to a pH of 7.0; however, the evidence that this is crucial is not convincing. Other body fluids, such as pleural fluid, tracheobronchial washings, joint fluid, etc., are collected in sterile containers without further processing before transport.

Blood is usually not cultured for viruses; however, it is worthwhile to consider doing so in some situations, such as suspected viral hemorrhagic fevers, certain arboviral infections, and in situations of special interest to both the clinician and the virologist. While not wishing to completely discourage blood culture for viremia, we would point out that the yield of such cultures is usually quite low in contrast to the expense and effort of performing the studies. This is most likely due to the fact that the detectable viremic phase in many acute viral infections is often gone by the time the illness is manifest and cultures are considered. Isolation attempts can be made on serum or on buffy coat material from heparinized or citrated blood samples.

Biopsy materials can also be handled with relative ease by simply placing the tissue in a sterile screw-capped bottle or vial for transport. In general, 1 to 3 g of tissue are preferred. If only very small pieces of tissue are available, these should be placed in a vial of VTM to keep them from drying out.

Postmortem specimens, 2 to 3 g of each tissue, are obtained with separate, sterile instruments in order to prevent cross-contamination, and handled in the same way as biopsy tissues. The selection of sites for sampling depends on the individual case and the viral agents suspected. Table 52–4 serves as a general guide in this selection.

Transport of Specimens.   In general, prompt transport to the laboratory gives the best assurance of viral detection. If there is a delay of more than a few minutes, it is best to keep the specimens cooled to approximately 4°C., *but not frozen.* Freezing can destroy the infectivity of some viruses quickly, and should be done only if there is to be a prolonged delay of a day or more between collection and processing of specimens. Table 52–5 summarizes the relative stability of various viral agents in clinical samples.

Table 52-4. POSTMORTEM SPECIMENS
OF CHOICE

SYNDROME	SPECIMENS
Respiratory	Lung, tracheal swab
Central nervous system	Brain, spinal cord, cerebrospinal fluid, feces
Undiagnosed febrile illnesses	Brain, liver, lung, spleen, kidney, blood, feces, skin lesions, pharyngeal swab
Cardiovascular	Myocardium, pericardium, and pericardial fluid, feces
Hepatitis	Liver, blood, feces

Transport to the laboratory in the cool, unfrozen state can be accomplished in several ways, including the use of sealed, frozen ice packs in insulated or styrofoam containers, wet ice in bags, or, if short distances are involved over a brief time, placement of the sealed vials into a carton of crushed ice. When freezing is unavoidable, such as for shipment that may take many hours, the best alternative is to "snap-freeze" the sample in Dry Ice, Dry Ice and alcohol, or liquid nitrogen and transport the specimens in either Dry Ice or liquid nitrogen. It must be remembered that specimens that are being shipped by air or by mail must be appropriately labeled as infectious material and properly packaged according to federal guidelines.

Table 52-5. STABILITY OF VIRUSES IN
CLINICAL SPECIMENS

Relatively stable*	Variola, Adenoviruses, Enteroviruses
Variably stable†	Influenza, Parainfluenza, Arboviruses, Herpes simplex, Measles, Mumps, Rubella, Rhinoviruses
Highly unstable‡	Respiratory syncytial, Varicella-Zoster, Cytomegaloviruses

*Stable at room temperature for several hours or more; Variola can survive drying and room temperature for weeks. All can be frozen at −70°C. without significant loss of infectivity.

†Stable at room temperature for at least 1 to 3 hours; freezing at −70°C. can result in variable loss of infectivity.

‡Very unstable at room temperature; specimens should be kept cool and inoculated as soon as possible; infectivity can be totally lost on freezing.

TISSUE CULTURE TECHNIQUES

The cornerstone of diagnostic virology is the establishment and maintenance of tissue cultures. There are several cell culture techniques, including organ cultures and co-cultivation methods, that are applicable to special situations in medical virology. However, monolayer cell cultures are most commonly used in the clinical laboratory, and this discussion will focus on these. Excellent, detailed instructions and discussion of the monolayer methods can be found in the texts by Lennette (1969) and Grist (1974). Kruse (1973) also has edited a thorough text dealing with both simple and complex cell and organ culture methods, which serves as a useful laboratory reference.

Monolayer cultures are prepared by dispersing tissue cells, usually with a proteolytic enzyme such as trypsin, suspending in a nutrient growth medium, and aliquoting into stationary tubes or bottles. The cells settle to the most dependent surface, adhere, and proliferate until a confluent monolayer one cell in thickness develops. When this has occurred, the growth medium is replaced with maintenance medium (a liquid with only enough nutrients to keep the cells viable and containing no viral inhibitors). These cells are then ready for virus isolation and can remain viable for up to several weeks.

TYPES OF CELL CULTURES

There are three basic types of monolayer cell cultures. *Primary cultures* are derived directly from the parent tissue, such as human embryonic kidney, rhesus monkey kidney, human amnion, etc. These epithelial cells may be subcultured once, by trypsinizing and dispersing a primary monolayer, giving *secondary cultures*, which usually have similar appearance and virus sensitivity. Often, when one has an organ which has been minced and treated with trypsin to disperse the cells, many more cells are obtained than may be needed immediately. The excess cells in suspension can be placed in a freezing medium and kept frozen in liquid nitrogen until needed, then thawed and dispensed into bottles or tubes for use.

Diploid cell lines are usually derived from human embryonic lung or tonsil tissues. They are prepared in a manner similar to primary cultures, or by explantation of small (1 sq mm)

5

fragments of tissue in bottles with growth medium to allow outgrowth of fibroblastic cells. The resultant fibroblast monolayers retain a diploid chromosome number, and can be subcultured 20 to 50 times before they lose viability.

Heteroploid cell lines are, for practical purposes, "immortalized" cells which can be subcultured indefinitely. Most are derived from human epithelial carcinomas or otherwise transformed cells. The most popular are HeLa from a cervical carcinoma, KB from a carcinoma of the nasopharynx, Hep-2, and HL cells. These cells grow rapidly, and have a heteroploid chromosome count.

SELECTION OF
CULTURE SYSTEMS

Each of these cell types has distinctive uses in the virus laboratory, much as special and selective media do in bacteriology. They differ significantly in their susceptibility to various viruses, and these differences will be mentioned in the sections to follow. In general, it is preferable to have representatives of all three types available for use, and, when a

variety of possible agents are being sought in an individual patient, all three are often inoculated simultaneously.

Primary (or secondary) rhesus monkey kidney (RMK) cells are currently the single best available cell culture source because of their broad sensitivity to human viruses, especially influenza, parainfluenza, mumps, many of the enteroviruses, and some adenoviruses. Recently, it has been suggested that cynomolgus monkey kidney is a useful alternative to RMK, with the possible exception that it may be less sensitive for parainfluenza viruses.

Human diploid fibroblasts complement primary RMK, extending the viral spectrum to particularly include herpes simplex, varicella-zoster, cytomegaloviruses, rhinoviruses, and some enteroviruses and adenoviruses.

Heteroploid cell lines have been particularly useful in the detection of respiratory syncytial virus, many adenoviruses, and some herpes simplex and enterovirus isolates.

There are many other cell cultures to choose from that have excellent broad-spectrum viral sensitivity (e.g., primary human embryonic kidney), or special sensitivity (e.g., primary African green monkey kidney for rubella virus isolation). However, the problems of cost and

Table 52-6. VIRUS CULTURE SYSTEMS AND THEIR SENSITIVITY TO DIFFERENT VIRUSES *

VIRUS	PRMK	HDF	HET	MICE	EGGS
Adenoviruses	+(var)	+(var)	++(var)	−	−
Herpes simplex	0	++	+(var)	+	+
Cytomegalovirus	−	++	−	−	−
Varicella-Zoster	−	++	−	−	−
Variola	+	0	+	−	++
Vaccinia	+	0	+	−	++
Echoviruses	++	++(var)	0	−	−
Polioviruses	++	++	++	−	−
Coxsackie A	0(var)	0(var)	0	++†	−
Coxsackie B	++	−	+	++†	−
Arboviruses	−	−	−	++†	−
Influenza	++	−	−	−	++
Parainfluenza	++	−	−	−	0
Respiratory syncytial	+	+	++	−	−
Rhinoviruses	0	++	0	−	−
Mumps	++	0	0	0	+
Measles	++	0	0	−	−
Rubella‡	−	−	−	−	−
Rabies	−	−	−	++†	−

*PRMK = Primary rhesus monkey kidney; HDF = human diploid fibroblast cell strains; HET = heteroploid cell lines; var = variable. A + + means maximum sensitivity for a virus; + means that the system is usually satisfactory for routine use; 0 means that the system is not reliable by itself for routine use; − means that the system is completely insensitive to the virus.

†Newborn mice required.

‡Special culture systems usually required (see text).

availability must be weighed against the relative usefulness of the culture systems in a clinical laboratory; for example, acute rubella infection can often be diagnosed serologically with paired sera obtained 10 to 14 days apart, while rubella virus isolation and identification, which is somewhat less sensitive, may take 8 to 20 days.

Other culture systems that should be available to the clinical laboratory include mice and embryonated hen's eggs. Suckling mice less than 24 hours of age are sensitive indicators of Coxsackievirus A or B infection; in fact, many Coxsackie A viruses will be missed if newborn mice are not inoculated. This is not to imply that mice should be used frequently in the diagnostic laboratory, but when clinical and epidemiologic findings suggest such infections, and other culture systems do not yield an answer, mice can be valuable. Newborn mice are also susceptible to rabies, herpes simplex, and most arboviruses.

Embryonated hen's eggs are very sensitive to most strains of influenza A and B viruses, sometimes allowing isolation of these agents when cell culture attempts have failed. They are also useful in the isolation and identification of variola and vaccinia viruses, and are susceptible to herpes simplex viruses, but not to other agents of the herpesvirus group.

Table 52-6 summarizes the relative virus sensitivity of the different major culture systems in current use; however, this serves only as a rough guideline. Different strains of viruses, even within a given serotype, sometimes behave variably in different systems, or even in different laboratories. Some infections, including several not listed in Table 52-6, are better diagnosed by serologic or other methods that will be discussed in their specific sections. In general, it is best to select at least two systems, and sometimes more, when seeking a specific agent.

MEDIA

While a variety of culture media can be used, only a few are required in the clinical laboratory. These can be purchased ready for use as a concentrated (10 ×) solution, or as a powder that is mixed with deionized distilled water and then sterilized by pressure filtration through a Millipore or nucleopore filter. The powder can be stored in the refrigerator in a dessicator for many months, and the liquid media are usually quite stable for several months when stored frozen at $-20°C$. All media should be checked for sterility before use.

Hanks' and Earle's balanced salt solutions serve as the base for most media and are excellent general diluents in the virology laboratory. They differ in buffering capacity, with Earle's solution being a stronger buffer for use in maintenance media where established cells produce large amounts of acid. Hanks' solution is useful in growth media where minimal acid is produced by the growing cultures. The composition of each is shown in Table 52-7.

Phenol red, a non-toxic pH indicator, is also a useful component of media. It is purple at a pH of 8.4 or greater, which is above that tolerated by most cell cultures, yellow at a pH of 6.8 or below, and orange to red in the physiologic range of 7.0 to 7.4.

Serum is required for growth and often is also necessary in maintenance media. It should have the properties of preservation of cell viability, and relative absence of antibodies or non-specific inhibitors of viruses. Fetal or agamma calf serum is generally useful in this regard, and is used at a 5 or 10 per cent concentration in growth media, depending upon the needs of the cell type. For maintenance or viral isolation, the serum concen-

Table 52-7. COMPOSITION OF HANKS' AND EARLE'S BALANCED SALT SOLUTIONS*

	CONCENTRATION (GRAMS PER LITER) IN 1X SOLUTION	
COMPONENT	Hanks' BSS	Earle's BSS
NaCl	8.00	6.80
KCl	0.40	0.40
CaCl$_2$	0.14	0.20
MgSO$_4$·7H$_2$O	0.20	0.20
Na$_2$HPO$_4$·12H$_2$O	0.12	—
NaH$_2$PO$_4$	—	0.125
KH$_2$PO$_4$	0.06	—
NaHCO$_3$	0.35†	2.20‡
Glucose	1.00	1.00
Phenol red, 1% solution	1.60 ml§	1.60 ml

*From Lennette, E. H., and Schmidt, N. J. (eds.): Diagnostic Procedures for Viral and Rickettsial Infections, 4th ed. New York, American Public Health Association, 1969, p. 93.

†Prepared as a 2.8 per cent stock solution and added at the time of use.

‡Prepared as an 8.8 per cent stock solution and added at the time of use.

§If a somewhat deeper red color is preferred, 2.0 ml may be used.

tration should be reduced as much as possible to a point which allows cell viability and minimizes the risk of serum inhibition of viruses. For respiratory agents, particularly influenza or parainfluenza virus, the less serum the better. In general, a 2 per cent serum concentration in maintenance media works well for routine use.

Bicarbonate ion is necessary for cell growth, and almost all media use a carbonic acid–sodium bicarbonate buffer system. Since the carbonic acid is volatile, cell cultures must be tightly sealed to avoid an excessive rise in pH. For tissue work in microtiter plates or other semi-open systems, a CO_2 incubator can be used to compensate the buffer system, or non-volatile buffers such as tricine can be added. We have found, even in closed culture systems, that adding approximately 10 ml of 1 M tricine buffer and 10 ml of 8.8 per cent $NaHCO_3$ to 500 ml of media serves to maintain an optimum pH and is not deleterious to the cells or viruses. Leibovitz Medium No. 15 contains galactose instead of glucose and is useful when a low bicarbonate concentration is required, such as for isolation of some rhinoviruses.

Of the various chemically defined media available, Eagle's minimum essential medium (MEM) and Medium 199 are the most popular in the virology laboratory. We prefer MEM because of its lesser cost and its proven performance. In summary, we currently suggest that MEM with Hanks' BSS base, added tricine and sodium bicarbonate, and 5 to 10 per cent fetal calf serum be used for growth purposes, and MEM with Earle's base, tricine, sodium bicarbonate, and 1 to 2 per cent fetal calf serum be used for maintenance and virus isolation.

REAGENTS

The selection of water for use in tissue culture work is important. We prefer sterile distilled water which has been deionized to a resistance of greater than 1 million ohms. In some areas, double distilling or the use of simple deionizing units can achieve this level of purity.

There are a number of satisfactory antibiotic combinations for use in treating bacterial, fungal, and mycoplasmal contaminants in inoculated tissue cultures and clinical samples. Our preference is Hanks' BSS containing aqueous penicillin G at a concentration of 1000 units per ml, gentamicin at 0.5 mg per ml, and amphotericin B at a concentration of 10 μg per ml. This solution is stable for months when frozen.

Sodium bicarbonate, 8.8 per cent, is prepared in water, filter sterilized or autoclaved, and stored at room temperature.

Other essential reagents include trypsin, 0.25 per cent solution with EDTA, and GKN (glucose, KCl, NaCl) solution for rinsing cell monolayers prior to trypsinization; phosphate buffered saline (PBS) at a pH of 7.0 is a useful general diluent, and 2 per cent phosphotungstic acid at pH 7.0 for electron microscopy preparations.

Our virus transport medium consists of veal or heart infusion broth with antibiotics added to a final concentration of 2000 units/ml penicillin G, 0.2 mg/ml gentamicin, and 5 μg/ml amphotericin B. The pH is adjusted to 7.2 to 7.4 and the solution dispensed in 2-ml aliquots and frozen until used.

PREPARATION OF SPECIMENS

Swabs. Swabs of throat, rectum, and other sites are vigorously agitated in 2 ml of transport media, wrung out on the side of the tube, and discarded. If it is expected that bacterial or fungal contamination of the specimen will be a problem, the solution can be left at room temperature for 30 minutes to allow the added antibiotics to be effective. In some situations, such as use of rectal swabs, 0.5 to 1.0 ml of Hanks' BSS with antibiotics can be added, followed by centrifugation at 3000 rpm for 10 minutes to clarify the medium. Aliquots of 0.2 ml are placed into tissue culture tubes.

Feces. Approximately 2 g of feces are thoroughly mixed with 12 ml of Hanks' BSS with antibiotics in a centrifuge tube and held at room temperature for 30 minutes. The suspension is then centrifuged at 3500 rpm in a refrigerated centrifuge for 15 minutes, and 0.2 ml of the supernatant inoculated into each tissue culture tube.

Urine. While some authorities recommend adjustment of urine pH to 7.0 to 7.2 with sodium bicarbonate, we have not found this to be particularly advantageous unless there is going to be an unavoidable delay of several hours before inoculation. It is preferable to obtain a fresh, clean-voided morning urine, add 0.5 ml of Hanks' BSS with antibiotics to

2 ml of the sample, and inoculate 0.2 ml into the tissue culture tubes as quickly as possible. The pH of the tubes may then be adjusted if the color change is too acid. It is advisable to change the media 16 to 24 hours after inoculation.

Cerebrospinal Fluid. Aliquots of 0.2 ml of CSF are placed directly into tissue culture tubes without prior treatment. Virus isolation may occasionally be enhanced by first draining the culture tubes, adding the CSF inoculum, incubating in a stationary rack for 30 to 60 minutes, then adding fresh media. This method has also been employed for other inocula when scanty amounts of infectious particles are expected.

Tissues. When biopsy tissue or autopsy materials are received, 1 to 2 g are ground in a mortar and pestle wth sterile sand, and a 10 per cent suspension (w/v) prepared in Hanks' BSS with antibiotics. Alternatively, a Pyrex glass tissue grinder may be used.

In either case, special care must be taken to avoid aerosol contamination of the work area; such preparation must be done in a biologic safety cabinet. The suspension is centrifuged at 3500 rpm for 15 minutes, and 0.2 ml of supernatant is inoculated into each tissue culture tube. The media should be changed after 16 to 24 hours of incubation, since many such inocula are toxic to tissue cultures.

In special situations, such as herpes simplex encephalitis, the virus yield is often enhanced by careful trypsinization of the biopsy tissue and co-cultivation of the resultant cell suspension by inoculation directly on the tissue culture monolayer. This requires care in allowing the viable cells to attach to the monolayer, then later changing the media to remove unattached, non-viable material and toxic products. Methods such as this, as well as explant cultures, are also particularly useful when seeking fastidious, highly cell-associated viruses or attempting to detect latent virus infection; however, their use in the routine clinical laboratory is limited.

Blood. While attempts to culture blood or bone marrow are not often made, there are occasions when this may be desirable. Serum, buffy coat, or anticoagulated whole blood (0.05 to 0.2 ml.) can be inoculated directly into tissue culture tubes or mice. The tubes should be kept stationary for 2 to 4 hours to allow adsorption of free virus or leukocytes; then the medium is changed, followed by a second change the following day.

INOCULATION INTO OTHER HOST SYSTEMS

It may be desirable to inoculate the prepared specimens directly into mice or embryonated eggs, in addition to tissue culture tubes. Newborn mice, less than 48 hours of age, are preferable for most virus work, because of their greater susceptibility to infection. When seeking arboviruses, rabies, or herpes simplex virus, 0.015 ml of suspension is inoculated intracerebrally with a tuberculin syringe and the mice are observed for 21 to 28 days for mortality or encephalitic signs. If coxsackie A or B viruses are suspected, we prefer several routes of inoculation: 0.015 ml intracerebrally, 0.05 ml intraperitoneally, and 0.03 ml subcutaneously. They are observed for 14 days for mortality, encephalitic signs with spastic paralysis (coxsackie B), or flaccid paralysis and cyanosis (coxsackie A). Deaths in the first postinoculation day are considered as nonspecific or post-traumatic and can be disregarded.

Inoculation into embryonated hen's eggs can be into the amnionic, allantoic, or yolk sacs, or onto the chorioallantoic membrane. Of these sites, the amnionic sac is most commonly used for influenza virus isolation. The chorioallantoic membrane is particularly useful in isolation and identification of variola and vaccinia viruses.

RECOGNITION OF VIRUSES IN CELL CULTURES

There are several ways in which viruses affect cell cultures. The most common is induction of morphologic changes in the cell cultures, called cytopathic effect (CPE), as the viruses replicate. The type of CPE induced varies with the viral agent involved and the cells affected. These changes can usually be easily seen on low-power ($30 \times$) microscopic inspection, and the different appearances are often distinctive enough to permit a tentative virus group identification. These will be illustrated in the appropriate sections in this chapter.

Some agents, such as influenza and parainfluenza viruses, may or may not induce CPE; however, they induce hemagglutination antigens on the tissue culture cell surface which will adsorb red blood cells from various animal and avian species. As infection progresses, these hemagglutinins are released into the media, as part of the envelope of intact virions. Virus infection of the cell culture can be detected after a few days of incubation by adding guinea pig red blood cells to the cell cultures, incubating at 4°C. for 30 minutes, then reading the tubes microscopically to determine if the red cells have become adherent to the cell culture surfaces (*hemadsorption*) or have agglutinated in the medium (*hemagglutination*). Incubation in the cold enhances this phenomenon, except for parainfluenza type 4 virus, where incubation at room temperature is preferred for detection of hemadsorption.

Another method, called the *interference* test, is more tedious, but has been found useful for rubella virus detection. Rubella virus infects and replicates well in primary African green monkey kidney; however, no CPE or hemadsorption occurs. The presence of rubella virus is demonstrated by incubating the infected cell cultures for seven days or more, then adding another "challenge" virus (usually an enterovirus) which is known to infect the cell culture and produce CPE. If the challenge fails to cause CPE, it is likely that rubella virus is present and has interfered with the replication of the second virus, probably by stimulating interferon production.

Sometimes, despite careful precautions and media changes, specimens will be toxic to tissue culture cells, producing what appears to be CPE. This is particularly a problem with feces, urine, and tissue homogenates. The changes usually occur within 24 hours, and toxicity can be recognized by transferring a small amount of material to new cell cultures. Toxic products are usually diluted by this method so that no change occurs; if a virus is responsible for the effect, it will again produce CPE on transfer.

Occasions frequently arise when cell infection is either equivocal, definite but so minimal that it appears it will be difficult to further identify the virus, or undetectable after prolonged incubation of a specimen which was felt to have a high probability of being positive. In any of these situations, the culture can be "passed" by subculturing 0.2 ml of the contents into fresh tissue culture tubes. This can be done by transfer of media, media and scraped or trypsinized cells, or media and cells disrupted by sonication or freeze-thawing, depending upon the viral agent suspected. Passing cultures enhances the propagation of viruses with the development of greater and

often more rapid and recognizeable CPE or hemadsorption. It also serves to "adapt" the viruses to the cell culture, making it easier to identify them by serologic methods.

IDENTIFICATION OF AN ISOLATE

Preliminary virus group identification of an isolate can often be made quickly, on the basis of differential growth in certain cell cultures, mice or eggs, type of CPE produced, or ability to induce hemagglutination or hemadsorption. In many situations, the site from which the isolate was obtained and the clinical syndrome further aid in definitive early identification. For example, an isolate from the respiratory tract of an infant with bronchiolitis, which produces syncytia in heteroploid cell cultures and does not hemadsorb, is most likely to be respiratory syncytial virus. An isolate from the urine of a newborn infant with suspected congenital infection, growing only in human diploid fibroblasts and producing multiple foci of groups of rounded cells, is most likely to be a cytomegalovirus.

Utilizing these principles mentioned above, the laboratory can then proceed to specific confirmation and serotyping, as needed. The most common method employed is *neutralization* of the effect of the virus in the culture system in which it was detected. Briefly stated, this involves mixing a standard amount of the unknown virus with type-specific antisera, incubating the serum-virus and positive control (virus-PBS) mixtures at 35°C. for 30 to 60 minutes, and inoculating into the appropriate cultures. Identity of the isolate is confirmed when the specific antiserum inhibits the effect of the virus as compared with the positive control. This principle can be applied to inhibition of CPE, hemadsorption, hemagglutination, or illness in animals.

Other, less commonly employed methods include identification by complement fixation, immunodiffusion, or immune electron microscopy. In some instances, immunofluorescence or immunoperoxidase methods may be directly applied to the infected cells for rapid identification (Gardner, 1974; Kawamura, 1977).

In the sections that follow, identification of specific viruses is discussed in more detail.

OTHER SYSTEMS OF VIRUS DETECTION

Besides cell cultures, suckling mice, and embryonated eggs, there are several other methods which are useful for viral diagnosis. Of these, one of the oldest, and still occasionally useful, is histologic or cytologic examination. While not nearly so sensitive as virus isolation, such findings can guide the laboratory and sometimes be of immediate help to the clinician. For example, cytologic examination of the base of a vesicle may reveal intranuclear inclusions and multinucleated giant cells, indicating a herpes simplex or varicella-zoster infection. There are numerous examples, which will be considered in sections dealing with specific viruses.

Immunofluorescence or immunoperoxidase methods have also become increasingly popular in the virology laboratory and have the advantages of speed and flexibility. These methods can be employed for rapid detection of viral antigens in cells obtained directly from the patient, such as exfoliated nasopharyngeal cells, CSF or urine sediment, vesicle scrapings, or biopsy tissues, and have been particularly successful in the rapid diagnosis of infections due to mumps, measles, herpes simplex, and some of the respiratory viruses. As mentioned before, the same methodology can also be applied to identification of an isolate in cell cultures.

Radioimmunoassay for the detection of viral antigen in body fluids and secretions is rapid and sensitive. It is the method of choice for the detection of hepatitis B viral infections, and may eventually be useful in several other infections.

Direct electron microscopy has further extended the capability of viral diagnosis. For years, it has been an excellent method for discerning between pox virus and herpes virus infections in vesicular eruptions. More recently, it has become particularly helpful in diagnosing infections due to viral agents which grow poorly, or not at all, in present culture systems. For example, rotaviruses and several other agents responsible for acute diarrhea in infants and young children have been detected by direct examination of the diarrheal stool. A positive result can often be found in 2 hours by this method, and it can also be used to group viral isolates from tissue cultures where CPE is unusual. A further refinement, immune electron microscopy, has been used to identify viral serotypes and to detect antibodies in human sera. This method allows visualization of virus-antibody aggregates when specific reactions have occurred.

SERODIAGNOSIS

While the emphasis on viral diagnosis has shifted somewhat away from serology and emphasized direct demonstration of viruses or their antigens, serodiagnosis continues to have significant value. In general, it is wise to obtain a sample of serum from most patients being cultured, and make plans to collect a convalescent serum, usually after two to three weeks. There are two important reasons to do this:

1. The viral agent may be missed on culture for a variety of reasons, and serodiagnosis may be the only method of detecting it. In some diseases, such as coxsackie B virus myopericarditis, virus shedding may have ceased by the time clinical disease is apparent, and serology is particularly valuable. Other infections, such as rubella, infectious mononucleosis, and arbovirus encephalitis represent situations where routine culture is difficult or particularly slow, and serology is the preferred method of diagnosis.

2. In some instances, a viral isolate may be obtained, but it is unclear whether that agent is temporally or causally related to the illness in question. For example, an enterovirus isolated only from the feces of a patient with encephalitis may be involved in the illness or may represent a transient "carrier" state of several weeks' duration, related to asymptomatic infection, but not to the current illness. If a significant rise in antibodies to that agent is demonstrated, it becomes likely that the virus was causative. However, one must be careful of over-interpretation of such data; dual viral infections can occur, and, if the epidemiologic and clinical data are suggestive, one may even wish to do serologies for other viral agents on the same sera to rule out other possible infections.

The interpretation of serologic data is easiest when paired, acute and convalescent sera are tested simultaneously. A *fourfold or greater rise* in antibody titer strongly supports a current infection. A fourfold or greater fall in titer, when the first serum is collected late in the course of an acute illness, assumes some significance, but must be interpreted with caution; similarly, single, late acute or convalescent sera with high titers may be occasionally useful, but one must be careful about over-interpretation. In some diseases, e.g., arbovirus infections, a "presumptive" diagnosis based on a single high titer may be made. This is based on a knowledge of the duration and level of specific antibodies in these infections, and the fact that persons with infections months to years in the past do not have antibody titers approaching those found in the patient. Another special instance is mumps virus infection, wherein antibodies to the "S" (soluble) antigen and a modest titer to the "V" antigen would be considered as presumptive evidence of recent mumps infection. Finally, antibody responses to primary viral infections usually follow classic patterns in that much of the early antibody is of the IgM class, which will later be replaced almost totally by IgG antibodies. In critical situations where only a single serum is available, it may be possible to determine whether the specific antiviral antibody is primarily IgM or IgG. If it is determined to be mostly IgM, this suggests a close temporal association to the disease in question. However, we do not recommend this as a routine test for the clinical virology laboratory. While the methodology for removal or quantitation of specific IgM or IgG antibodies appears to be simple, there are potential pitfalls, and strict quality control is mandatory.

The most common serologic test employed in a routine laboratory is the complement fixation (CF) test. Others include hemagglutination-inhibition (HI), neutralization, and indirect immunofluorescent antibody tests. These and other tests are discussed further in the sections dealing with specific viruses.

A particularly vexing problem encountered in both public health and clinical laboratories is the receipt of paired sera (or, worse yet, a single serum) with an order marked "viral serology." It is very important to emphasize to the ordering physcian the need to provide vital data, including the age of the patient, type of illness and date of onset, and the dates the sera were drawn. If no viral isolates were obtained from the patient, a decision can still be made regarding the choice of tests, based on these data. Most laboratories design serologic "batteries" to test these sera accordingly. For example, if a respiratory illness is involved, the "battery" might include influenza A and B, adenoviruses, and *Mycoplasma pneumoniae;* if the diagnosis is encephalitis,

mumps and herpes simplex would be tested for; and, if the illness occurred in the summer or autumn, arbovirus serologies might be added, including those agents known to exist in the area.

CAPITAL AND EXPENDABLE EQUIPMENT

CAPITAL EQUIPMENT

The laboratory facility need not be elaborate, unless one is working with agents such as some arboviruses, rickettsia, rabies, arenaviruses, variola virus, or Marburg-like agents. These should be sought and propagated only in specially equipped isolation facilities and are not part of the usual clinical virology laboratory workload. If any of these is suspected, state or federal public health authorities should be notified immediately, and special arrangements made for transport and processing of specimens.

We suggest at least a three-component laboratory: a separate, small room for sterile tissue culture preparation and storage, another room for specimen processing and inoculation, and a third, larger area for specimen receipt, paperwork, tube reading, and serology.

The tissue culture room is ventilated by filtered air under positive pressure, to prevent or minimize airborne contamination of cultures. All cell cultures should be handled as if potentially virus-contaminated. Accidental laboratory infections have occurred as a result of contact with unsuspected agents in "normal" cell cultures. The most common has been *Herpesvirus simiae*, an occasional contaminant of tissue cultures from old world monkeys, which can cause serious or even lethal disease in humans. This room should be equipped with a 35°C. incubator for cell culture stocks, an inverted microscope, and, if contamination is a serious concern, a biologic safety cabinet.

The specimen processing and inoculation room should have a negative pressure ventilation system, preferably with exhaust through HEPA filters or to the outside, to minimize the risk of accidental spread of infection to other areas of the laboratory. A well-exhausted and filtered biologic safety cabinet is mandatory for this room, particularly when grinding or homogenization of tissues is being done.

The general laboratory area capital equipment inventory includes refrigerators for storage of reagents, sera, etc., at 4°C. or −20°C., and an ultra-low temperature (−70°C.) freezer for storage of specimens and virus stocks; a liquid nitrogen freezer (−196°C.) is also desirable for optimal long-term storage of cell culture suspensions and reference virus stocks to be used in quality control or teaching. While most mammalian cells and viruses will tolerate freezing at −70°C., they cannot be preserved for long periods without loss of viability or infectivity. Furthermore, the risk of a mechanical breakdown, with inadvertent thawing and loss of valuable stocks, is minimized with liquid nitrogen freezers.

Separate incubators for clinical specimens and uninoculated cell culture tubes are usually maintained at 35 to 36°C. The incubator for clinical specimens should be large enough to handle several tissue culture roller drums, and internal electrical outlets are also necessary for these.

While inoculated tissue culture tubes may be incubated in stationary racks after inoculation, there is evidence that the development of CPE may be enhanced for some viruses by slow rotation (12 to 15 revolutions per hour) in roller drums. Such roller drums are also much more convenient for use by technical personnel, particularly when tube reading, because they allow rapid screening of cultures without concern that the tubes be placed in a stationary position which assures that the cells are completely covered by media.

Tube reading microscopes are of the standard type, and should be equipped with a low-power objective to allow screening at 30 × or 40 × magnification, as well as metal "tracks" which may be clamped to the stage to cradle the tube under the objective. We prefer that at least one microscope be a two-headed, teaching type.

Other necessary equipment includes a centrifuge, preferably refrigerated, with a capability of at least 3500 rpm, a water bath, a torsion or open-beam balance, a magnetic stirrer, and a vortex mixer. There are, of course, other equipment items which are useful, but the needs and desires for these vary from place to place.

SMALL AND DISPOSABLE ITEMS

Measuring pipettes, either glass or disposable, in sizes ranging from 1 ml to 10 ml, as well as Cornwall syringes and pasteur pipettes, are essential. Disposable tissue culture tubes (16 by 125 mm) are preferred over reusable tubes, and may be sealed with non-toxic silicone rubber stoppers or plastic screw caps with non-toxic silicone liners. Tissue culture bottles can be disposable or reusable. We prefer milk dilution bottles and 32-ounce prescription bottles with screw caps and non-toxic cap liners. There are several types of tissue culture racks available, and the choice varies with the needs of the individual laboratory.

Other small items include pipette jars, autoclavable discard pans, and pipette fillers. These are extremely important for laboratory safety. Any spills of potentially infectious material must be cleaned up immediately and the area disinfected, preferably with a 2 per cent phenolic compound or 70 per cent alcohol, the cleaning materials (paper towels, etc.) discarded into a solution containing at least 100 ppm available chlorine, and autoclaved. For obvious reasons, mouth pipetting of *any* materials in the laboratory is strictly prohibited.

Many other small items may be useful, depending upon the scope of serologic and special studies planned for the individual laboratory.

SPECIFIC VIRAL AGENTS

VIRUS CLASSIFICATION

Virus classification has been an extremely confused issue and is constantly undergoing extensive revision. Classification has previously been attempted on the basis of means of transmission (Arboviruses), sites of isolation (Adenoviruses), disease produced (Pox viruses), and more recently on the basis of morphologic, chemical, and immunologic properties. There have been numerous important advances in viral taxonomy, including the comprehensive decisions made at the meetings of the International Committee on Taxonomy of Viruses (ICTV) held during the Third International Congress for Virology in September, 1975. The ICTV study groups continue to define and describe virus groups and report their decisions periodically in *Intervirology*. These reports form the basis for the viral classification and taxonomy presented here (Fig. 52–1 and 52–2 and Tables 52–8 and 52–9). The figures illustrate a comprehensive classification of DNA and RNA virus families

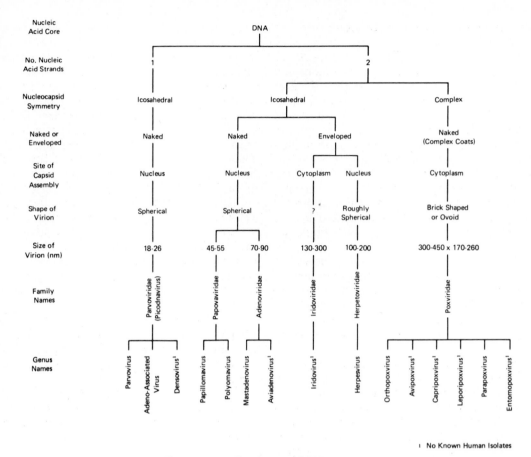

Figure 52-1. Classification of DNA viruses.

which infect primarily vertebrates, but including invertebrates and plants when the families contain genera which can infect more than one kind of host. For example, viruses of the Family Bunyaviridae, and five genera including Alphavirus, Flavivirus (Family Togaviridae), Orbivirus (Family Reoviridae), Vesiculovirus, and Lyssavirus (Family Rhabdoviridae) multiply both in arthropods and vertebrates. Such arthropods may act as vectors for producing disease in vertebrates. As one can see, classification based on means of transmission is antiquated. The present classification is based primarily on physical, morphologic, and chemical data to the family level, and immunologic criteria and natural host range are utilized primarily for division at the genus and species level. The remainder of this discussion will primarily involve viruses known to infect and cause disease in man.

The Mastadenovirus genus (Family Adenoviridae) contains the mammalian adenovirus species including human adenovirus types 1, 3 to 33. There is a common generic antigen shared by the Mastadenovirus species which is distinct from the corresponding Aviadenovirus antigen. "Mast" is derived from the Greek word *Mastos*, meaning breast, and is thus related to *mamma*, which is Latin for breast and from which is derived the word "mammalian."

Several viruses occur within the vertebrate Herpetoviridae family, but agreement on classification is difficult. Also, there is considerable serologic cross-reactivity (including neutralization antibodies) and genetic homology between mammalian herpetoviruses. Type species include human herpesvirus types 1 and 2. Other tentatively designated members which possibly represent different genera include human herpesvirus type 3 (varicella), human herpesvirus type 4 (Epstein-Barr virus), and human cytomegalovirus. Members of the Poxviridae family, which produce dis-

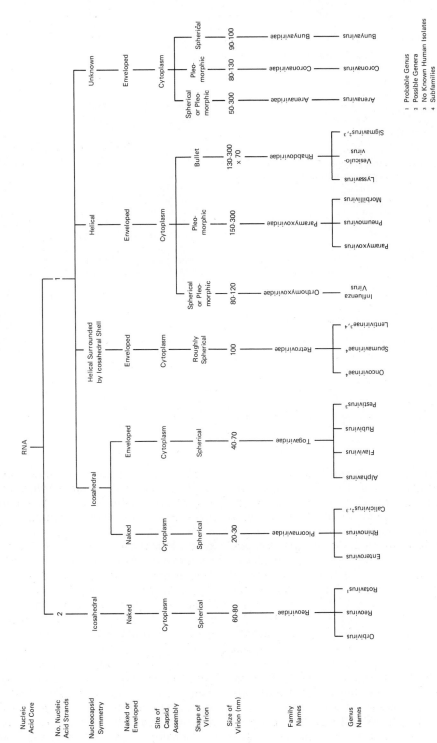

Figure 52-2. Classification of RNA viruses.

5

Table 52–8. DNA VIRUSES

FAMILY AND GENUS	REPRESENTATIVE SPECIES
Parvoviridae	
Parvovirus	Gastroenteritis virus of humans,[1] hepatitis virus[1]
Adeno-associated Group (vernacular name)	Human adeno-associated virus
Densovirus	
Papovaviridae	
Papillomavirus	Papillomavirus of man
Polyoma virus	BK virus and JC virus SV40 (monkey)
Adenoviridae	
Mastadenovirus	Human adenovirus
Aviadenovirus	
Iridoviridae (not known to infect man)	
Iriovirus	
Herpetoviridae	
Herpes virus	Human herpes virus types 1 and 2, Cercopithecid herpes virus 1 (B virus), human herpes virus type 3 (varicella),[2] human herpes virus type 4 (Epstein-Barr virus),[2] cytomegaloviruses[2]
Poxiviridae	
Orthopoxvirus (vaccinia subgroup)	Vaccinia, variola, cow pox virus
Avipoxvirus	
Capripox virus (sheep pox subgroup)	
Lepori pox virus (Myxoma subgroup)	
Parapox virus (Orf subgroup)	Orf virus, milker's nodule virus
Entomopox virus	

[1] Possible species.
[2] No general agreement on classification and may represent different genera.

ease sometimes clinically confused with those caused by members of the Herpetoviridae, include six genera, only two of which are associated with disease in man (Orthopoxvirus and Parapoxvirus). The familiar species which infect man include vaccinia, variola, and cowpox viruses, which are members of the Orthopoxvirus genus, and orf virus and milker's nodule virus, which are representatives of the Parapoxvirus genus. There are ten major family antigens, one of which cross-reacts with most poxvirus genera of vertebrates, and there is extensive serologic cross-reactivity between species within each genus of vertebrate poxviruses. The molluscum contagiosum virus of man is a member of the family Poxviridae, but has not yet been assigned to a genus.

Picornaviridae include two genera: Enterovirus and Rhinovirus. Enteroviruses are stable at pH 3 and are primarily viruses infecting the gastrointestinal tract. Species infecting humans include polio virus 1,2,3, coxsackie A1-24,

coxsackie B1-6, echo 1-34, and enteroviruses 68-71. In contrast, human rhinoviruses 1A, 1B-113 are unstable at pH 3 and infect the upper respiratory tract of man.

The Togaviridae family contains four genera (Alphavirus, Flavivirus, Rubivirus, and Pestivirus). Alphaviruses and Flaviviruses were previously designated Arbovirus Group A and Arbovirus Group B, respectively. From Table 52-9, it can be seen that these genera contain several species that infect man. All species of Alphavirus and probably all species of Flavivirus multiply in arthropod vectors. The Rubivirus genus contains only one species: rubella virus. All genera are physicochemically typical of the Togaviridae family, but serologically are distinct. All species within each genus, however, do show serologic relationships. The Bunyaviridae contain at least 84 antigenically related species within the single Bunyavirus genus. These agents are mostly transmitted by mosquito and tick vec-

Table 52-9. RNA VIRUSES

FAMILY AND GENUS	REPRESENTATIVE SPECIES
Reoviridae	
Orbivirus	Colorado tick fever
Reovirus	Human reovirus
Rotavirus[1]	Acute diarrhea virus of young children
Picornaviridae	
Enterovirus	Polio, coxsackie A, coxsackie B, echovirus, enterovirus 68-71
Rhinovirus	Human rhinovirus
Calicivirus[2]	
Togaviridae	
Alphavirus (arbovirus group A)	WEE, EEE, Venezuelan encephalitis
Flavivirus (arbovirus group B)	Yellow fever virus, dengue, St. Louis encephalitis, Japanese B encephalitis
Rubivirus	Rubella virus
Pestivirus	
Retroviridae	
Oncovirinae[3] (leukovirus)	
Type C oncovirus group[4]	
Mammalian type C oncovirus group[5]	Murine sarcoma and leukemia virus, feline sarcoma and leukemia viruses
Avian type C oncovirus group[5]	
Reptilian type C oncovirus group[5]	
Type B oncovirus group[4]	Mouse mammary tumor viruses
Spumavirinae[3] (genera not defined)	Human foamy virus group
Lentivirinae[3] (genera not defined)	
Visnavirus	
Maedivirus	
Orthomyxoviridae	
Influenza virus	Influenza A, B; Influenza C[1]
Paramyxoviridae	
Paramyxovirus	Parainfluenza virus, mumps virus, Newcastle disease virus
Pneumovirus	Respiratory syncytial virus
Morbillivirus	Measles virus
Rhabdoviridae	
Lyssavirus	Rabies virus
Vesiculovirus	Chandipura virus
Sigmavirus[2]	
Arenaviridae	
Arenavirus	Lymphocytic choriomeningitis virus, Lassa virus, Argentinian and Bolivian hemorrhagic fever viruses
Coronaviridae	
Coronavirus	Human coronaviruses, avian infectious bronchitis virus
Bunyaviridae (previously designated Togaviridae)	
Bunyavirus	Bunyamwera virus, California encephalitis virus

[1] Probable genus.
[2] Possible genus.
[3] Subfamilies.
[4] Genera.
[5] Subgenera.

tors, and previously had been loosely grouped with the Togaviridae family. The species are named primarily by geographic site of original isolation, which results in many unusual and colorful species names. The bunyamwera virus and California encephalitis virus are two species in this genus.

The influenza viruses belong to the Orthomyxoviridae family. Influenza A and influenza B are the two accepted genera, with influenza C being a probable third. The genera contain specific nucleoprotein antigens. Hemagglutinin (HA) and neuraminidase (NA) antigens, two protein peplomers which project from the surface of the virion envelope, antigenically distinguish species and variants within types. Fifteen HA (H) and nine NA (N) types have been recognized. Only HO-H3, HSW, and N1 and N2 have been identified on influenza isolates from man. Genetic recombination occurs frequently within species, but not between species or other genera. Influenza C differs from influenza A and B in HA receptor characteristics and NA functions. The Paramyxoviridae family contains three genera: Paramyxovirus, Pneumovirus, and Morbillivirus. The Paramyxoviruses contain a hemagglutinin and a neuraminidase and include the following human species: parainfluenza viruses 1-4 and mumps virus. The Morbillivirus genus contains a hemagglutinin but no neuraminidase, and all species possess a common generic antigen. Measles virus is the type species and only one known to infect man. The type species for the Pneumovirus genus is the respiratory syncytial virus. This genus contains neither an hemagglutinin nor a neuraminidase. The single Coronavirus genus (Family Coronaviridae) contains human coronavirus species of several serotypes which cross-react with other vertebrate coronavirus species. These also have been associated with respiratory disease. Projecting from the envelope are club shaped peplomers giving the virus the appearance of a "crown," which is derived from the Latin word *corona*, hence, coronavirus.

The bullet or rod shaped virus family, Rhabdoviridae (derived from the Greek word *rhabdos*, meaning "rod") contains three genera: Lyssavirus, Vesiculovirus, and Sigmavirus. The type species of the Lyssavirus genus (derived from *lyssa*, the Greek word for "rage"), is the rabies virus. There is serologic cross-reactivity between species, but this genus is serologically distinct from the other genera which it morphologically resembles.

Members of the Vesiculovirus genus multiply in insects as well as vertebrates, and several species are serologically related. The chandipura virus species has been isolated from man.

The Parvoviridae family contains two genera, Parvovirus and Densovirus, plus the adeno-associated virus group, which requires an adenovirus as a helper virus for replication. This family is composed of the only known single-stranded DNA viruses. The type of single strand of DNA (positive strand only versus positive or negative strands) and the requirement for a helper virus are the main criteria for classification of these genera. Possible species of the Parvovirus genus include some human gastroenteritis viruses (e.g., Norwalk agent). Human adeno-associated virus types 1-4 of unknown significance have also been identified. The Parvoviridae are the smallest of the DNA viruses and their name derives from the Latin word *parvus*, meaning "small."

The Reoviridae family contains two genera, Reovirus and Orbivirus, and a probable genus, Rotavirus. This group of viruses is also unique in that it contains the only double-stranded RNA viruses. Reovirus species multiply only in vertebrates and include human agents. In contrast, all Orbivirus species multiply in insects and several, in addition, multiply in vertebrates. The Orbivirus genus includes Colorado tick fever virus, which infects man. The proposed new genus, Rotavirus (Melnick, 1976), closely resembles the orbiviruses physicochemically and has previously been called "duovirus" and "reovirus-like agent." Isolates from this probable genus are associated with a rather severe gastroenteritis syndrome of infants and young children.

The Retroviridae family is unique in that the characteristic biochemical feature is a reverse transcriptase (RNA-dependent DNA polymerase). Classification within this family is complicated by the diversity of agents included within the three subfamilies: Oncovirinae, Lentivirinae, and Spumavirinae. The Oncovirinae (previously known as leukovirus) are a large complex group in which many members cause neoplastic diseases, especially leukemias and sarcomas, in many species of animals. Genera are divided into subgenera on the basis of type of animal host (see Table 52-9). The significance of this subfamily in human oncogenesis is currently unknown. The Spumavirinae subfamily does not have a defined genus, but one of the species, human foamy virus, has been isolated from man. It is of unknown significance. The Lentivirinae subfamily also does not have a defined genus and is primarily a pathogen of sheep. Although chemically and morphologically similar to Oncovirinae, the latter two subfamilies do not have known oncogenic potential in host animals.

The Papovaviridae family contains the Papillomavirus and Polyomavirus genera. Various Papillomavirus species cause papillomas in a variety of specific hosts, including man. Papillomaviruses have never been isolated in tissue culture systems, and there is evidence that this virus group may be mechanically transmitted by arthropods. The various polyomavirus species infect multiple hosts and have oncogenic potential in immunosuppressed hosts different from the natural animal host. There is no serologic cross-reactivity between polyomavirus species. Human polyomaviruses include BK virus and JC virus. JC virus has been isolated from the brains of lymphoma patients with progressive multifocal leukoencephalopathy, and BK virus has been isolated from the urine of renal transplant patients. The simian virus SV40 is also a species of the Polyomavirus genus.

The single Arenavirus genus (Family Arenaviridae) includes the type species lymphocytic choriomeningitis virus. This and other members of the genus have a single restricted rodent host in which persistent infection with viremia and/or viruria characteristically occurs. Natural spread to man and other mammals has occurred. The virus particles of this family have a sandy appearance in electron microscope sections and the name Arenavirus derives from *arenosus*, which means "sandy" in Latin.

We have attempted to describe briefly all the current virus families and genera with emphasis on human viruses, and to comment on special chemical, physical, and serologic properties and host range when indicated. Not included in this classification are the unconventional viruses, such as scrapie, Creutzfeldt-Jacob, and Kuru agents, since little is currently known of their physical and chemical nature.

ADENOVIRUSES

Initially isolated from adenoid tissue by Rowe in 1953, adenoviruses have since become recognized as important causes of disease in humans. There are at least 33 different antigenic types which can be cultivated in the laboratory, of which types 1, 2, 3, 5, 6, and 7 comprise the bulk of isolates.

It has been estimated that adenoviruses are responsible for up to 10 per cent of all febrile illnesses occurring in the first 2 years of life, and 5 per cent of febrile episodes in the 2-to-4-year age group. In older schoolchildren and young adults, sharp outbreaks are not unusual. Table 52-10 lists the recognized adenovirus-associated syndromes and the serotypes that have been usually associated with these. The most common illnesses include undifferentiated febrile illnesses in younger children, and upper or lower respiratory syndromes, often associated with tonsillitis and occasionally also with conjunctivitis (pharyn-

Table 52–10. CLINICAL SYNDROMES SHOWN TO BE ASSOCIATED WITH ADENOVIRUS INFECTIONS

SYNDROMES	SEROTYPES ASSOCIATED*
Childhood febrile illness; pharyngoconjunctival fever	1, 2, <u>3</u>, 5, 6, <u>7</u>, <u>7a</u>, (14, 21)
Pneumonia in infants; acute respiratory illness and pneumonia in adults	1, 2, <u>3</u>, 5, <u>7</u>, <u>7a</u>, (21)
Pertussis-like illness	1, <u>2</u>, <u>3</u>, 5, 19, 21.
Conjunctivitis	2, 5, <u>7</u>, <u>8</u>, <u>19</u>, (1,4,6,9,10,11,15, 16,17,20,22)
Keratoconjunctivitis	<u>3</u>, <u>8</u>, <u>9</u>, <u>19</u>, (2,7a)
Acute hemorrhagic cystitis	11, (21)

*Underlined serotypes are those which have more commonly been associated with outbreaks; serotypes in parentheses are only occasionally associated with the syndrome.

goconjunctival fever). The upper respiratory illnesses sometimes mimic acute streptococcal pharyngitis and tonsillitis with exudates and cervical lymphadenopathy. Pneumonia can be severe and occasionally fatal. It sometimes resembles an acute bacterial process that is unresponsive to antibiotics and may persist for several weeks. In some instances, chronic pulmonary disease has resulted. Pertussis-like illnesses have also been well described, with episodes of severe paroxysmal cough associated with lymphocytosis.

Aside from the febrile respiratory syndromes, eye infections are also commonly associated with adenoviruses, particularly acute follicular conjunctivitis and the more severe keratoconjunctivitis, which may produce symptoms lasting for 3 weeks or more. Some of these infections occur in sharp outbreaks related to inadequately chlorinated swimming pools ("swimming-pool conjunctivitis"), and other outbreaks have been attributed to such items as contaminated eye droppers or tonometers in ophthalmology clinics and sharing of cloth towels.

In addition, adenoviruses have occasionally been associated with maculopapular or petechial exanthems and disseminated illnesses which may include encephalitis, myocarditis, hepatitis, and diarrhea. However, the association between the recognized serotypes and primary viral diarrhea per se is debatable and largely unproven. There is evidence, mostly circumstantial, that adenoviruses may also be important in the pathogenesis of childhood intussusception, acute appendicitis, and mesenteric adenitis. One syndrome of interest is acute hemorrhagic cystitis. This has been associated with adenovirus type 11 in particular, usually lasts 2 weeks or less, and most commonly affects children aged 5 to 15 years.

Aside from direct or indirect contact with infected secretions, most adenovirus infections are spread via respiratory droplets. Fecal-oral spread is also possible.

LABORATORY DIAGNOSIS

The viruses can be isolated from throat swabs and rectal swabs, as well as other clinically affected sites (conjunctiva, lung, urine). While primary embryonic human kidney cell cultures are considered very sensitive for isolation, most types will also grow more or less readily in human heteroploid or diploid fibroblast cell cultures, and some also produce CPE in RMK cultures. The CPE is characteristic (Fig. 52-3) with rounded, often uniformly swollen cells that tend to form grapelike clusters. As CPE progresses, the cell sheet often appears lacy and later detaches from the tube wall. The speed with which CPE develops varies from strain to strain and may take from two days to four weeks.

The viruses contain both group-specific and type-specific antigens. The former is sometimes used in either a complement-fixation or gel-diffusion procedure for serologic confirmation of the isolate as an adenovirus; however, specific serotyping requires neutralization by type-specific antiserum. Our usual approach is to select specific antisera for typing of the unknown isolate, based upon the clinical syndrome and known epidemiology. Table 52-10 serves as a useful guideline in this regard. For

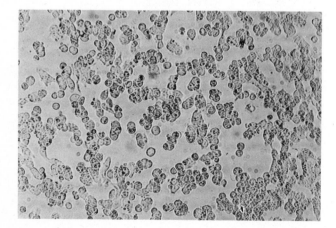

Figure 52-3. Adenovirus CPE in HeLa cells. (×125.) (Courtesy of T. F. Smith, Ph.D., Section of Clinical Microbiology, Mayo Clinic.)

isolates which are not readily identified by a limited battery of antisera to common types, it is possible to classify them into one of three groups, depending on their ability to agglutinate rat or monkey erythrocytes, then proceed to neutralization tests, or hemagglutination-inhibition tests, depending upon their behavior. However, before expending a great deal of time and effort on specific serotyping of all adenovirus isolates, it should be determined whether such identification could have significant relevance to the patient, the illness, or the epidemiologic situation.

Serologic diagnosis, using paired sera, is useful in situations where the virus was not detected, or as further confirmation that the virus isolated was temporally associated with the illness in question. The usual test utilizes the group antigen in a CF test, which is convenient and sometimes helpful. However, the CF serology is not as sensitive as a neutralization test. Portnoy (1967) showed that in patients with adenovirus isolates the neutralizing antibody titer to the homologous virus rose significantly at least twice as often as did the CF antibody titer to the group antigen.

INTERPRETATION OF LABORATORY FINDINGS

There is little difficulty in associating an adenovirus with a disease if it has been directly isolated from a biopsy of clinically affected tissue, e.g., lung. The association is even more firm if "smudgy" intranuclear inclusions typical of adenoviruses are also seen on histologic examination.

In other situations, epidemiologic evidence has been sufficiently convincing to allow rather firm conclusions about the association of some adenovirus isolates with specific clinical syndromes. For example, the isolation of adenovirus type 11 from the urine of a child with acute hemorrhagic cystitis would be considered significant; similarly, any adenovirus isolate from a conjunctival swab from a patient with acute conjunctivitis, in the absence of evidence for bacterial, chlamydial, or other concomitant viral infection, would strongly suggest an etiologic association.

The difficulties in interpretation which commonly arise are related to several facts. Adenoviruses are extremely ubiquitous, particularly in patients between the ages of four months and four years, and subclinical infections with seroconversions are common. Furthermore, these agents can lead to persistent,

asymptomatic infections of the adenoid and tonsillar tissues as well as the lymphoid tissues of the small bowel. As a result, intermittent virus shedding into the respiratory secretions or the feces may last for as long as 6 to 18 months after primary infection, and such shedding may be enhanced by stress, such as other viral or bacterial infections. For these reasons, adenovirus isolates from throat or fecal samples must be interpreted with caution, even when supported by antibody seroconversions. This dilemma is particularly difficult in the younger age groups (under four years).

Extensive epidemiologic studies (Brandt, 1969; Fox, 1977) have helped our understanding of these problems, but the interpretive difficulties remain. Based upon the epidemiologic findings relevant to the recognized adenoviral febrile and respiratory syndromes, we have developed the following rough guidelines for interpretation: simultaneous isolation from both throat and feces has approximately a 70 to 85 per cent probability of etiologic association with the illness, based upon the ability also to demonstrate a significant seroconversion. Isolation from the throat, and not the feces, has approximately a 50 to 60 per cent probability of such an association, and isolation only from the feces drops this figure to between 20 and 35 per cent. The interpretation of the significance of the isolates or serologies can be further aided if the laboratory has made an attempt to exclude other common viral agents, such as enteroviruses, parainfluenza and influenza viruses, and if bacterial pathogens have also been reasonably excluded. Also, the finding of such isolates in older children and adults with compatible illnesses assumes somewhat greater significance, since chronic carriage appears to diminish with advancing age.

HERPES VIRUSES

HERPES SIMPLEX VIRUS (HSV, OR HERPESVIRUS HOMINIS)

The comon cold sore, or fever blister (herpes labialis), the most usual manifestation of HSV infection, has been described since antiquity. The virus was first isolated in 1919 by inoculation of herpes labialis vesicle fluid into a rabbit cornea, and transmissibility was demonstrated by reinoculation from the infected rabbit cornea to the cornea of a blind man.

Following the successful growth of HSV in tissue culture the virus was shown to be etiologically related to a wide variety of clinical syndromes, as well as subclinical infection, occurring with either primary or recurrent disease. Immunologic investigation in the early 1960's established two broadly cross-reacting antigenic types of HSV: herpes simplex virus type 1 (HSV-1) and herpes simplex virus type 2 (HSV-2). In general HSV-1 is found primarily in and around the oral cavity and in skin lesions above the waist, while HSV-2 is isolated primarily from the genital tract and skin lesions below the waist. Neonatal disease usually results from HSV-2 infection, and HSV encephalitis in adults is usually caused by HSV-1 infection. The vast majority (approximately 99 per cent) of all primary HSV infections are asymptomatic, and the host-parasite relationship can be seen in Figure 52-4. Recurrent HSV disease usually occurs at the site of primary infection, but other distant sites may be involved. Recurrence with cell-to-cell spread of virus occurs in the presence of serum-neutralizing antibodies. Fever, sunlight, environmental temperature extremes, infection, physical trauma, emotional stress, neoplasia, and pregnancy are some of the factors noted to trigger recurrent HSV disease. Recurrent infection is usually the result of reactivation of latent virus residing in paraspinal or cranial nerve ganglia innervating the site of primary infection. The activated virus presumably travels down the axon to the skin (or other site) and induces disease. However, in some instances exogenous reinfection cannot be ruled out.

Epidemiology

The HSV are widespread, and man is the only natural host or known reservoir of infection for the human herpesviruses (herpesviruses of other vertebrates occur). The incubation period usually lasts 2 to 12 days, and there is no apparent sexual or seasonal predilection for infection. Based on serologic evidence, by age 25 years approximately 70 to 80 per cent have experienced contact with virus, and by 45 years this rises to nearly 100 per cent in some populations. However, the range of antibody prevalence in adults varies greatly with socio-economic class. Approximately 30 to 50 per cent of upper socioeconomic class adults compared to 80 to 100 per cent of adults in lower socio-economic groups have detectable antibody to HSV. HSV can be cultured from the oropharynx in about 1 per cent of healthy adults and from the genital tract of slightly less than 1 per cent of non-pregnant, asymptomatic adult women.

Malnutrition, concurrent debilitating disease, a variety of acute childhood illnesses, and prematurity all predispose to disseminated primary infections in infants and young children.

The transmission of HSV-1 is usually non-venereal but probably requires close contact, i.e., hand-to-mouth and kissing. HSV-2 is venereally transmitted and is most often acquired by newborns passing through an infected birth canal (perinatal transmission). Mechanisms of antenatal transmission are less well understood. Beyond the neonatal period, young children and preadolescents are infected almost exclusively with HSV-1, while

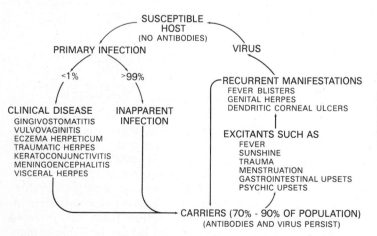

Figure 52-4. The host-parasite relationship of herpes simplex virus in man. (From Krugman, S., and Ward, R.: Infectious Diseases of Children. St. Louis, The C. V. Mosby Co., 1968.)

HSV-2 is isolated most commonly from the 15-to-30-year age group, usually from genital lesions.

Clinical aspects

Acute gingivostomatitis is the commonest manifestation of primary HSV-1 infection and is most frequent in the 1-to-4-year age group. The differential diagnosis includes aphthous stomatitis and herpangina. Other manifestations of primary HSV infections include rhinitis, keratoconjunctivitis, meningoencephalitis, eczema herpeticum (Kaposi's varicelliform eruption), traumatic herpes, e.g., herpetic whitlow, and generalized infection. Primarily acquired HSV-1 infection in young adults may frequently produce an acute upper respiratory illness with pharyngitis and tonsillitis (Glezen, 1975). Primary HSV-1 infection may also cause follicular conjunctivitis with chemosis, edema, and corneal ulcers. The ulcers may progress from small dendritic ulcers to large "geographic" ulcers. Secondary bacterial infection may then lead to opacification of the lens. Herpes labialis and dendritic corneal ulcers are the commonest manifestations of symptomatic, recurrent HSV-1 infection.

Immunosuppressed patients with primary or recurrent disease show a predilection for esophageal ulceration and interstitial pneumonitis as well as disseminated disease.

Occasionally, HSV-1 will also cause a severe necrotizing encephalitis usually affecting the temporal or frontal lobes. This is the commonest cause of sporadic encephalitis in the United States. It is often fatal (average mortality of about 50 per cent), and more than half of the survivors are left with significant neurologic sequelae. However, a specific antiviral agent, adenine arabinoside, has provided a good therapeutic index. There appears to be no age, sex, or socio-economic predilection for HSV encephalitis. About 15 per cent have a history of recurrent herpes labialis, which is similar to the frequency observed in the general population, and about one third of patients with encephalitis will manifest herpes labialis during the course of encephalitis.

The commonest form of HSV-2 primary and recurrent disease has been recognized for approximately 200 years, but reawakened interest is related to the discovery of widespread venereal transmission, neonatal infection, and a possible, but unproved, association with carcinoma of the cervix. HSV-2 is the commonest cause of genital vesicular lesions in women and is second only to syphilis in men.

Occasionally during primary HSV-2 genital infection in adults, a concurrent, usually benign aseptic meningitis develops, either from neuronal ascent or via hematogenous spread. Transient myelitis or myeloradiculitis can also occur.

Neonatal HSV infections may be acquired in the antenatal (intrauterine) or perinatal period. The majority, however, are acquired perinatally as the result of exposure to an infected birth canal during delivery. The greatest risk (approximately 40 per cent) to the fetus occurs as a result of primary acquired HSV infection in the mother's genital tract late in pregnancy, with active lesions present at the time of birth. If primary genital infection occurs at 32 weeks gestation or later, without active lesions at birth, the neonatal risk of infection is about 10 per cent. The risk of neonatal infection in a pregnant woman with recurrent genital herpes, active or not, at the time of delivery is unknown. When virus is present in the vagina or cervix and if membranes have been ruptured for four hours or greater prior to delivery, there is an increased chance that ascending virus may have infected the infant. Approximately half of clinically infected infants are born to asymptomatic mothers. Figure 52-5 outlines a method for managing a pregnancy complicated by herpes genitalis.

The mode of transmission of intrauterine

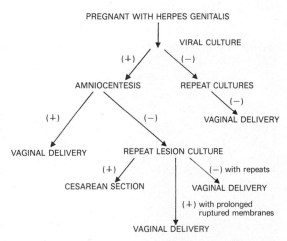

Figure 52-5. Summary of the management of patients with genital herpes infection in pregnancy based on positive (+) and negative (−) viral cultures. (From Amstey, M. S.: Obstet. Gynecol., *37*:519, 1971.)

infection is less well defined and probably involves hematogenous, transplacental spread, as well as ascending infection with associated chorioamnionitis. The best indicators of intrauterine acquisition of infection are manifestations of disease at birth or sooner than the usual incubation period after birth, or delivery of an affected child with histologic evidence or clinical signs suggesting a process that would necessarily have begun prior to perinatal exposure to virus, i.e., cerebral calcifications, microcephaly, or skin lesions at birth. The spectrum of disease in an infected neonate varies from subclinical to severe, with symptoms and signs reflecting the organs of involvement, i.e., lungs, liver, adrenals, brain, retina, and skin. In overwhelming generalized infection encephalitis, respiratory and/or hepatic failure with increasing jaundice and adrenal insufficiency may occur. Infants that survive infection are often, but not always, left with some degree of neurologic damage and may manifest recurrent vesicular skin lesions for years.

Although HSV-1 and HSV-2 generally have different modes of transmission and associated clinical disease, there is overlap. HSV-2 infection may occur in the oral cavity and HSV-1 may infect the genital tract. When HSV-1 genital disease occurs in pregnant women, it may cause neonatal disease as well. Both types of virus may cause cutaneous vesicular eruptions indistinguishable from varicella-zoster; also, erythema multiforme, probably the result of an immune reaction to HSV, has been associated with both HSV-1 and HSV-2.

Laboratory diagnosis

Viral isolation is the best means of documenting HSV infection. The virus has been isolated from vesicular fluid, ulcer scrapings, throat swabs, saliva, cervical secretions, CSF, paraspinal and cranial nerve ganglia, and clinically infected tissues. Other sites from which virus is isolated less frequently include buffy coat, urine, and rectal cultures. The virus grows rapidly *in vitro*, with cytopathogenic effects (CPE) often apparent by 24 hours. The human diploid fibroblast is the tissue culture system of choice, and HSV produces a rather specific pattern of CPE with large, round, "balloon" cells (Fig. 52-6). Less commonly there is formation of multinucleated syncytial giant cells.

A HSV isolate from a typical lesion is diagnostic with regard to the etiology of the lesion. Isolates from normally sterile, clinically infected tissues from patients with compatible syndromes, such as brain, lung, or liver, are also highly significant, especially in the absence of other etiologic possibilities. However, isolation of HSV from throat cultures or vesicular lesions of patients with undifferentiated febrile illness could result from reactivation of HSV without being causally related to the acute disease process. In fact, the potential reactivation of a HSV at any site during another febrile illness must be considered in interpreting a HSV isolate.

Differentiating a HSV isolate into type 1 or 2 is rarely indicated, and the available HSV typing sera show extensive cross-reactivity, as would be expected. Antiserum prepared from HSV-1 antigen usually has a higher titer to

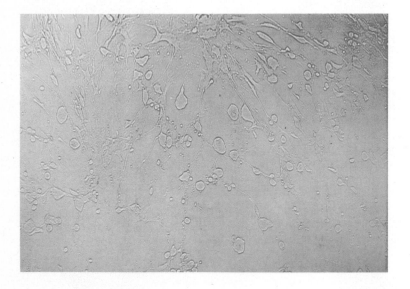

Figure 52-6. Typical CPE of H. hominis in WI-38 cells. (Courtesy of R. Martins, M.D., and W. Walker, Ph.D.)

HSV-1 than to HSV-2, but antiserum prepared from HSV-2 antigen usually has about equal titers to HSV-1 and 2. Therefore, if HSV-1 antisera is diluted, it will show increased specificity for HSV-1, but HSV-2 antisera usually shows similar reactivity to both HSV-1 and 2. With these facts in mind, immunofluorescent, immunoperoxidase, and indirect hemagglutination inhibition methods have been used to type HSV isolates (Stewart, 1976).

Serology is a useful epidemiologic tool for determining prevalence of exposure to HSV and for diagnosing primary infection when a fourfold or greater rise in antibody titer is demonstrated. However, in the adult population the prevalence of previous virus exposure is so great that detection of antibody gives no information as to when disease was first acquired, and since most primary infections are asymptomatic, there is little opportunity to demonstrate the initial titer rise. Early recurrent infections may significantly boost antibody titers, but following multiple recurrences, titers usually become stabilized at moderately high levels, as measured by com-

plement fixation (CF) or neutralization (NA) techniques.

CF antibodies are sensitive, stable, and long lasting, but they are reactive against broadly held antigens in both HSV-1 and HSV-2, making it impossible to distinguish type 1 from type 2 primary or recurrent infection. This difficulty in serodifferentiation of type 1 versus type 2 infections extends to other serologic techniques, including NA and indirect hemagglutination (IHA). All three methods are more sensitive for HSV-1 than for HSV-2 infections, but CF and NA tests are more sensitive than IHA for HSV-1 infections. However, IHA appears slightly more sensitive than the other methods in early HSV-2 infections, but titers are often already high by the time acute serum is drawn, making demonstration of a significant titer rise difficult (Back, 1974).

To further complicate matters, primary or recurrent infection by either HSV-1 or 2 usually causes elevation of antibody titer to both strains of HSV, and the greatest titer rise may be heterotypic. Therefore, serologic determination of which virus induced a recent infec-

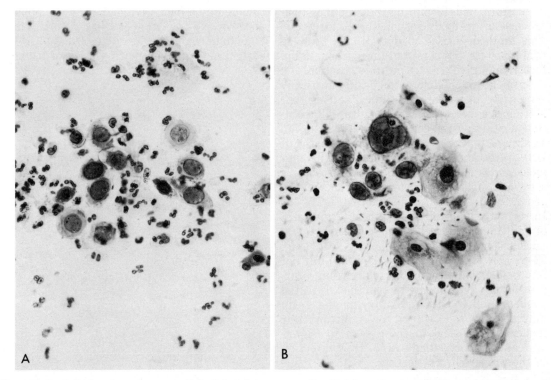

Figure 52-7. *A,* Early primary herpes genitalis. Infected squamous cells with intranuclear vacuolization and "ground glass" nuclear appearance ($\times 500$). *B,* Multinucleated viral infected cells with a predominantly "ground glass" nuclear appearance. Intranuclear inclusions are identified in some of the cells ($\times 500$). (From Ng, A. B. P., Regan, J. W., and Lindner, E.: Acta Cytol., *14:*125, 1970.)

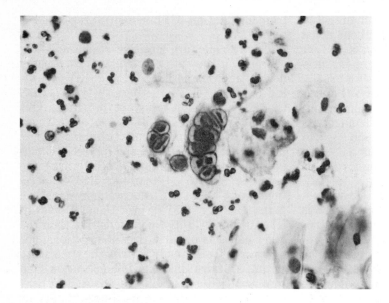

Figure 52-8. Recurrent herpes genitalis. Tight aggregates of infected cells with intranuclear acidophilic inclusions (× 500). (From Ng, A. B. P., Regan, J. W., and Lindner, E.: Acta Cytol., *14*:126, 1970.)

tion is extremely difficult. Neutralization (NA) kinetics and plaque reduction techniques have been employed (Plummer, 1973). The indirect immunofluorescence method using HSV infected cells and appropriate antihuman globulin is useful in determining the immunoglobulin class of antibody responding to infection. This method is used in detecting a primary IgM response, but sera containing rheumatoid factor may give a false positive reaction.

Cytology and histology can be diagnostically supportive in the proper clinical setting, but neither is as sensitive as viral culture. Papanicolaou staining of cervical or vesicle lesion scrapings may reveal cells characteristic of HSV infection. In primary disease the uninucleated or multinucleated viral infected cells show occasional intranuclear inclusions with a ground glass nuclear appearance (Fig. 52-7). In recurrent genital herpes, tight aggregates of multinucleated cells demonstrating intranuclear inclusions are frequently seen (Fig. 52-8). However, it is extremely difficult, if not impossible, to distinguish primary from recurrent herpes genitalis by this method. Infected tissues stained with hematoxylin and eosin may also reveal Cowdry type A intranuclear inclusions identical to those seen in Figure 52-8 and support a diagnosis of HSV infection in the proper clinical setting.

croscopy from its close relatives, herpes simplex and varicella. CMV infection results in distinctive histologic changes characterized by striking epithelial cell cytomegaly with a single, large, red intranuclear inclusion surrounded by a halo, giving the cell the appearance of an owl's eye (Fig. 52-9). These histologic changes were first observed in the early nineteenth century in tissues of stillborn

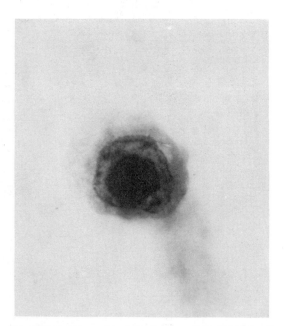

Figure 52-9. Intranuclear inclusion in a renal epithelial cell. Urinary sediment from a child with congenital cytomegalovirus disease. (From Blanc, W. A., and Goetz, R.: Pediatrics, *29*:61, 1962.)

CYTOMEGALOVIRUS

Human cytomegalovirus (CMV) is indistinguishable by negative staining electron mi-

infants and in salivary glands of infants apparently dying of other causes. Because of their large size, the intranuclear inclusions were initially thought to be protozoan-like structures, and associated disease was called "protozoan cell disease." Subsequently, the terms "syndrome of unknown etiology," "salivary gland disease," and finally "cytomegalic inclusion disease" were used to describe what was regarded as a severe, disseminated, congenital disease. A viral etiology was first suspected in 1920, but not confirmed until 1956, when the virus was first isolated in tissue culture. However, with the advent of viral isolation and development of serologic techniques, it became obvious that congenital infections were often asymptomatic, and infection, which was usually asymptomatic, could be acquired in the perinatal or postnatal periods. In addition, CMV infections have been associated with a growing number of different syndromes in previously healthy adults, patients with lymphoreticular or hematopoietic disorders, chronic disease, and those receiving immunosuppressive therapy or massive blood transfusions.

CMV infections have a long incubation period (weeks to months) which parallels the slow replicative cycle in tissue culture. Infections may be local or systemic and can be either active or latent.

Epidemiology

CMV infection is endemic world wide with the highest prevalence rates among very young children, particularly those living under crowded, intimate conditions. The infection may be congenital, but it is most often acquired in the perinatal or postnatal periods. The prevalence of viral excretion in the urine, reflecting active infection, varies from 0.5 to 2.0 per cent at birth to 10 to 56 per cent at six months of age, depending upon the population studied. By one year of age the prevalence of viral excretion usually stabilizes or declines, and less than 1 per cent of normal, healthy adults excrete virus in the urine. The rate of viruria, however, increases during pregnancy to 4 to 13 per cent in the third trimester, and the incidence of positive cervical cultures has been reported to be as high as 28 per cent in late pregnancy. On the other hand, the rate of serologic positivity, also reflecting experience with CMV, increases slowly through childhood. During adolescence the infection rate rises significantly, until 35 to 100 per cent of adults by age 35 have detectable complement fixation (CF) antibodies. The incidence of seropositivity varies greatly depending on the socio-economic status and living conditions of the population surveyed. Serologic evidence also indicates that adult women have higher rates of CF positivity than men of the same age.

Congenital infection

CMV is probably the commonest cause of congenital infection in humans. The mode of natural transmission of virus from mother to fetus is ill-defined because of the usual lack of either maternal or fetal signs or symptoms. Maternal CMV infections, like herpes simplex virus infections, are subject to recurrence, especially in the genital tract, and the role of recurrent infection in intrauterine transmission is poorly understood. More often, a congenitally infected infant is a first child of a younger mother, suggesting a relationship to a primarily acquired maternal infection, but sequentially infected children born to the same mother have been occasionally reported. The frequency of congenital CMV infection varies with socio-economic class (greater frequency in lower classes) and is more prevalent in low birth weight infants.

The vast majority of congenital CMV infections are asymptomatic or characterized by mild hepatomegaly with moderately abnormal liver functions and jaundice. However, symptoms vary from these minor manifestations to severe, disseminated disease with growth retardation, chorioretinitis, pneumonitis, thrombocytopenic purpura, maculopapular or hemorrhagic skin rash, and hemolytic anemia. Congenitally infected infants sometimes excrete extremely high titers of infectious CMV in the urine for periods as long as a year or more after birth, and, therefore, could function as a source of acquired infection for others. It is estimated that 10 per cent of newborn virus excretors are neurologically damaged, but this is probably a conservative figure.

Acquired infections and reactivated latent infections

By adulthood most persons have experienced asymptomatic contact with CMV virus as evidenced by the presence of CF antibodies. Persons experiencing acquired infection, reinfection with the same or different CMV strains, or reactivation of a latent infection

5

can excrete virus in titers as high as 10^6 infective units/ml in the urine and/or saliva for weeks or months. Dissemination of infection to others is known to occur and can be via oral, respiratory, or venereal routes, or parentally by organ transplantation or blood transfusion.

Clinical manifestations reflect the organ(s) of involvement with preferential targets being liver, spleen, hematopoietic system, kidney, and lungs. A heterophile negative mononucleosis-like syndrome with fever, splenomegaly, and atypical lymphocytosis following open-heart surgery utilizing extracorporeal circulation and multiple blood transfusions, and a similar syndrome unrelated to transfusion and seen mostly in adults (rarely under 20 and usually over 30 years) are both caused by CMV infection. Studies of the acquisition rate of CMV infection following blood transfusion suggest a 5 to 12 per cent blood donor CMV carrier rate, although the possibility exists that transfusions may simply reactivate latent virus in the recipient. The severe exudative tonsillopharyngitis and marked lymphadenopathy seen with heterophile-positive infectious mononucleosis are usually absent in CMV mononucleosis.

Cases of anicteric and icteric hepatitis have also been related to acquired CMV infection. Despite the frequent histologic evidence of renal involvement, symptomatic renal disease is not seen. Reactivation or primary CMV infections are known to complicate a wide variety of chronic debilitating diseases, in particular hematopoietic and lymphoreticular malignancies, post-allograft transplantation patients, and others undergoing immunosuppressive therapy. In immunosuppressed patients, the lungs appear to be the primary target organ, accompanied by frequent liver involvement. Asymptomatic involvement is common and often diagnosed only by the distinctive histologic changes. The non-specific symptoms and chest x-ray findings, when they occur, are those of an interstitial pneumonitis of variable severity.

Prospective studies of renal transplant patients receiving immunosuppressive therapy have shown that the majority developed active CMV infection, and reactivation of latent infection appeared to be the most probable pathogenetic mechanism. However, recent data indicate the highest mortality risk for such patients occurs when tissue from a seropositive donor is transplanted into a seronegative recipient. This suggests that primary CMV infection is more severe than reactivation in this group. Symptoms may include fever, arthralgia, pneumonitis, leukopenia, and hepatitis. Other diseases in the post-transplant patients included retinitis and glial-nodule encephalitis. The majority of immunosuppressed patients with CMV infection have a normal serum antibody response to the virus. Therefore, it seems more likely that the CMV infection (primary or reactivated) may be related to defective cell-mediated immunity.

Laboratory diagnosis and interpretation

Viral culture is the method of choice for confirming CMV infection. Virus is most often recovered from the urine during active infection, but may also be isolated from blood leukocytes, saliva, semen, cervix, and other infected tissues (lung, liver, kidney). CMV exhibits strict species-specific growth requirements, and viral replication occurs best in human diploid fibroblasts. The virus exhibits somewhat unpredictable thermal and chemical instability. Some workers report that the virus is more stable at 22°C. or 37°C. than at 4°C. and that freezing causes complete loss of virus infectivity. However, if stored at −80°C. or lower, the virus is relatively stable. For best results, a fresh specimen from any source should be inoculated into tissue culture as soon as possible. The virus is highly cell-associated and sometimes slow growing, occasionally requiring four to six weeks for primary isolation. Human CMV are identified by distinctive cytopathogenic effects in tissue culture (Fig. 52-10). Small nests of enlarged, rounded, refractile cells surrounded by normal fibroblasts are scattered throughout the cell sheet.

Isolation of CMV from clinically infected tissues is etiologically significant. However, one must remember that other opportunistic organisms, especially *Pnemocystis carinii*, may simultaneously infect a compromised host and may be contributing significantly to the symptomatology. In view of the high prevalence of CMV viruria during infancy and in institutionalized children, caution is necessary in these populations in equating viral isolation from the urine with acute disease. In older, immunologically normal children and adults viruria assumes greater diagnostic importance. Isolation of CMV from the blood leukocytes also requires some interpretive caution, since asymptomatic carriage of virus

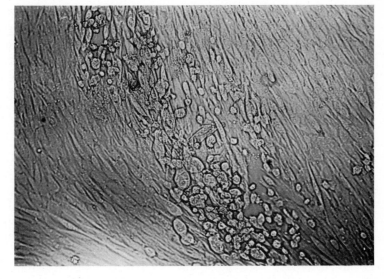

Figure 52-10. Cytopathic effect of CMV in human embryonic lung fibroblasts; focal lesion, strain C87. Unstained preparation (×140). (From Lennette, E. H., and Schmidt, N. J. (eds.): Diagnostic Procedures for Viral and Rickettsial Infections. 4th ed ed. New York, American Public Health Association, 1969.)

has been demonstrated. However, when associated with a compatible clinical syndrome for which no other cause can be demonstrated, the significance of the isolation increases.

Serology plays a supportive role in diagnosing CMV infection. There is a qualitative and quantitative antigenic heterogeneity within human CMV with several different strains being recognized. This becomes important when interpreting serologic data based on the use of a single antigenic strain of CMV.

A microtiter CF test is the easiest and most commonly used method for determining the presence of CMV antibodies. Although a broadly reactive CMV antigen (strain AD169) is used, some degree of strain specificity is still demonstrated. The CF test measures IgG antibody, and a titer of 1:8 or greater is considered evidence of prior exposure to CMV. In association with compatible clinical and virologic isolation data, a fourfold or greater rise in CF titer is good evidence for acquired or reactivated CMV infection. Following acquired infection and seroconversion, CF titers have declined to undetectable levels and, to further complicate interpretation, wide, spontaneous fluctuations in CF titers have been observed prospectively in apparently normal, healthy adults (Waner, 1973). Therefore, both the absence of a CF titer and a fourfold change in the titer must be interpreted with caution. The indirect fluorescent antibody test is also relatively easy to perform and allows measurement of antibodies of specific immunoglobulin classes. The detection of IgM anti-

bodies correlates well with active disease in the newborn and has been suggested for detection of primary acquired infection. The CMV IgM antibody test has shown cross-reactivity with Epstein-Barr (heterophile-positive infectious mononucleosis), varicella, and herpes simplex viruses. Therefore, the IgM antibody appears to detect broadly held antigens of the human herpes virus group. Also, sera containing rheumatoid factor may give a false positive IgM reaction. Neutralizing antibodies show greater strain specificity and are detected by cumbersome plaque reduction techniques. Since this method is not often used or available, it will not be discussed further.

Examination of a stained (hematoxylin-eosin, Giemsa, or Papanicolaou) urinary sediment of a fresh, filtered (membrane filter with $0.5~\mu$ pore size) urine specimen for typical inclusion bearing cells (Fig. 52–9) is rarely helpful, being 60 to 80 per cent less sensitive than urine culture and not entirely specific. Infected cells are shed only intermittently. Tissue biopsy for histologic examination is also less sensitive than culture of the infected tissue. Typical histologic changes are rarely seen in absence of a positive culture. However, positive cultures (for example, postmortem lung) can occur in the absence of any typical histologic changes, i.e., epithelial cytomegaly and intranuclear inclusions. In the latter instance it may be difficult to interpret the significance of the CMV isolate, especially when it occurs unassociated with recognizable symptomatology.

VARICELLA-ZOSTER VIRUS

Man is the only known natural host of varicella-zoster (V-Z) virus. The name reflects the two diseases associated with the virus, i.e., varicella (chicken pox) and zoster (shingles). Primary infection with V-Z virus results in the clinical manifestations of chicken pox. Following this the virus enters a latent phase, presumably within nuclei of neurons in dorsal root ganglia. Reactivation of virus results in the clinical manifestations characteristic of zoster.

Zoster infection has been recognized since antiquity and was called *zona*, meaning "girdle," by the Greeks. Varicella was considered a mild form of smallpox until the mid-eighteenth century, when the relationship between zoster and varicella was suggested by the observation that susceptible children exposed to a patient with zoster developed typical varicella.

Following isolation in tissue culture in 1953 the common etiology for both diseases was confirmed. In tissue culture the virus is strongly cell associated, and it is best passed *in vitro* using intact, infected cells.

Epidemiology

Varicella is endemic with superimposed winter or spring epidemics every 2 to 5 years. The 2-to-8-year age group is primarily affected, but susceptible individuals of any age may become infected. The disease is highly contagious, with an 80 to 90 per cent clinical attack rate. Immunity to varicella is lifelong. The presumed mode of transmission is via the respiratory tract, but virus is only rarely isolated from this site.

Zoster is a sporadic disease of older persons, the majority being over 45 years of age, and there is no sex, racial, geographic, or seasonal predilection for infection.

Zoster is less communicable than varicella, probably because it is usually a more localized disease, but infected persons can transmit typical varicella infection to exposed susceptible persons. Humoral immunity to varicella does not protect against reactivation and clinical zoster. Depressed host immune response is associated with reactivation of V-Z virus, and the following specific factors have been associated with triggering the onset of zoster: manipulation of the spinal cord, local radiation therapy, and underlying diseases or therapy which suppress cellular immunity.

Clinical aspects

The incubation period of varicella is usually 14 to 17 days. There may be a 1 to 3 day prodromal period of fever, headache, and malaise prior to eruption of the red macular rash which progresses to papules, vesicules, and pustules which crust over and are shed without scarring. The vesicle is described as a "dew drop on a rose petal". The eruption is centripetal, involving the trunk more heavily than the extremities, palms and soles, in contrast to the eruption in smallpox. Successive crops of lesions continue to appear in the same area for 2 to 6 days, leading to lesions in different stages of development at one time.

Complications of varicella include an interstitial, nodular pneumonitis, especially in adults. This occurs concomitantly with the typical skin rash and follows a course of variable severity depending on the host's immune competence. There are several rare hemorrhagic varicella syndromes which may complicate primary infection. Febrile purpura occurs in both children and adults, usually within a few days of the onset of eruption, and is characterized by thrombocytopenia with hemorrhage into the vesicles. Postinfectious purpura is another complication also characterized by thrombocytopenia with gastrointestinal, genitourinary, cutaneous, and mucous membrane hemorrhage, beginning one to two weeks after appearance of the rash. More severe hemorrhagic manifestations include malignant varicella with purpura, and purpura fulminans.

Encephalitic complications of varicella most commonly include acute cerebellar ataxia, which has an excellent prognosis, and cerebral involvement. Other complications include Reye's syndrome, nephritis, nephrosis, arthritis, and myocarditis. Immune-suppressed susceptible individuals have an increased risk of complications following exposure to V-Z virus.

Zoster infection is heralded by neuralgia for a few days to weeks, followed by the characteristic eruption typically confined to one or two adjacent dermatomes. Occasionally the distribution involves multiple dermatomes or may cross the midline. Severity of the infection increases with advancing age. Older patients have a greater tendency to develop persistent neuralgia, which is often severe and may last several months to a year. Children and younger adults characteristically develop brief, mild zoster infections. Zoster usually involves the thoracic dermatomes, followed in frequency by lumbar, cervical, and trigeminal nerve distributions. When cranial nerve roots are involved, encephalomyelitis may develop; pleural inflammation may accompany a thoracic eruption.

Cell-mediated immunity (CMI) correlates best with immunity to zoster. Patients with Hodgkin's disease have a greatly increased risk (25 per cent) of zoster, especially those with advanced, recurrent disease or those recently finishing radiation therapy, and up to 70 per cent with zoster may develop disseminated disease. Between 5 and 10 per cent of non-Hodgkin's lymphoma and leukemia patients may also develop zoster.

Neonatal varicella occurs and may be acquired in utero or in the perinatal period. A few reports have associated primary V-Z virus infection in pregnant women with congenital anomalies in their infants. The greatest risk to the infant appears to be when the onset of maternal illness occurs within four days or less prior to delivery (Meyers, 1974).

Approximately 9 per cent of parturient women in one study (Gershon, 1976a) lacked antibodies to varicella, thus making their newborn infants likewise susceptible to varicella infection.

Laboratory diagnosis

Clinical diagnosis of typical varicella infection in children and zoster infection in adults can be made with great accuracy. However, herpes simplex virus infection can cause a vesicular eruption identical to V-Z virus infection, and should be strongly suspected in patients with "recurrent" zoster. The best way to confirm infection is to recover the virus in human diploid fibroblast cell cultures. Vesicle fluid is the most reliable source of virus for isolation attempts.

Serologic methods have been employed for epidemiologic surveys for determining prevalence of past exposure to infection as well as documenting recent infection. The CF test is most often used for determining V-Z virus antibody. The major disadvantage is its relative insensitivity, especially after a year or more following infection. Therefore, CF is most useful for confirming recent infection. Heterologous antibody response following infection with another herpes virus can also interfere with the CF test. An indirect immunofluorescent technique for detecting antibodies directed against specific membrane antigens (FAMA) acquired by infected tissue culture

cells is a more sensitive and specific serologic technique which is useful in determining susceptibility to infection in epidemiologic studies (Williams, 1974). This method is also rapid and hence particularly useful in determining susceptibility to infection in immunosuppressed patients exposed to varicella. The FAMA method can usually detect antibody within two days after onset of rash, unless the patient is immunosuppressed. Other serologic methods which have been developed but not widely used for diagnosis include agar gel diffusion (Uduman, 1972) and immune adherence hemagglutination (Gershon, 1976b). The latter test appears particularly promising.

Other methods for presumptively diagnosing V-Z virus infection include scraping the base of a vesicular lesion and histologically observing multinucleated giant cells containing intranuclear inclusions or observing herpes virus particles by electron microscopy; however, these techniques will not differentiate between V-Z and herpes simplex virus infections.

EPSTEIN-BARR VIRUS

Epstein-Barr virus (EBV) was first discovered in 1964 when Dr. M. A. Epstein and associates demonstrated a herpes-like virus by EM in cell cultures from a Burkitt's lymphoma. Subsequently, EBV antibody was later demonstrated in the sera of nearly all patients with African Burkitt's lymphoma and nasopharyngeal carcinoma. However, unexpectedly, EBV antibody was shown to be highly prevalent within the general population as well.

EBV was serendipitously linked to infectious mononucleosis (IM) in 1967, when a laboratory technician working with EBV developed classic heterophile-antibody positive IM. During the course of the disease, antibodies to EBV appeared and rose to high titer. The virus can be demonstrated *in vitro* by its ability to transform lymphocytes into indefinitely propagating lymphoblastoid cell lines, and the transformed cells contain EBV antigen demonstrable by immunofluorescent staining.

Epidemiology

EBV is present world wide, and, based upon seroepidemiologic survey data, it is apparent that EBV infection during childhood is quite frequent, especially in lower socio-economic groups. In socio-economically deprived areas

80 per cent of 5-year-old children are seropositive, while 40 to 50 per cent of 5-year-old children from higher socio-economic groups are seropositive (Andiman, 1976). By 40 years of age most persons have acquired EBV infection. In young children EBV infection is usually asymptomatic or associated only with an undifferentiated febrile illness or mild upper respiratory symptoms. If EBV infection is acquired by an adolescent or adult, which happens in 40 to 50 per cent of persons who missed childhood exposure, the IM syndrome develops. Infectious mononucleosis shows no seasonal trends in the general population, but early fall and spring are periods of high frequency among college students.

The evidence linking IM to EBV etiology is as follows: (1) IM occurs only in persons lacking prior EBV antibody; (2) all patients with classical heterophile-positive IM have high antibody titers to EBV; (3) IM does not occur in persons with pre-existing EBV antibody; (4) EBV antigen can be detected in lymphocytes; (5) throat washings from IM patients contain a lymphocyte-transforming agent which induces lymphocyte proliferation and the appearance of EBV-like antigens in susceptible cells; and (6) no other infectious agent has been consistently linked to heterophile-positive IM.

The evidence linking EBV to both African Burkitt's lymphoma and nasopharyngeal carcinoma includes demonstration of EBV-associated antigens in cultured lymphoblasts from both tumors. Proof of etiologic involvement in these tumors is difficult, but some species of animals inoculated with EBV or EBV-containing lymphoid cells develop malignant lymphomas. Supportive evidence includes the fact that EBV can transform lymphoid cells into permanent cell lines.

Clinical aspects

Infectious mononucleosis is characterized by a 3- to 5-day prodromal period of non-specific symptoms including fever, asthenia, fatigue, and anorexia. This is followed most commonly by severe pharyngitis, lymphadenitis, and splenomegaly. Other less common manifestations include mild hepatitis, conjunctivitis, and a fleeting maculopapular rash. This stage of illness usually lasts 10 to 20 days. Fatigue and asthenia persist thoughout the illness into the convalescent stage which may extend for months.

Infectious mononucleosis is usually a self-limited benign disease, but occasionally severe complications and rarely death have occurred. Complications include severe hepatic involvement, neurologic manifestations with encephalitis, pneumonitis, thrombocytopenia, splenic rupture, hemolytic anemia, airway obstruction, and transient cutaneous hypersensitivity to ampicillin.

IM appears to be transmitted primarily by close contact with infective oropharyngeal secretions. Other reported routes of transmission include blood transfusion and transplacental spread.

As occurs with the other herpes viruses, there is a persistent viral carrier state after primary infection, which may be followed by asymptomatic reactivation of endogenous EBV. Immunosuppressed patients have a higher prevalence (35 to 47 per cent) of oropharyngeal excretion of EBV as compared to healthy controls (17 per cent) (Strauch, 1974).

Laboratory diagnosis

Since there is no convenient *in vitro* system for isolation and identification of the EBV, diagnosis of IM is based primarily on clinical, hematologic, and serologic data. In the adolescent and young adult the clinical signs and symptoms can strongly suggest the diagnosis of IM. The peripheral blood picture usually shows an absolute lymphocytosis with 10 to 20 per cent or more atypical lymphocytes. Early, the lymphocytosis results from increased B- and T-lymphocytes, but later there is a predominance of T-lymphocytes. The EBV appears to infect only B-lymphocytes, while the atypical lymphocytes are uninfected T-lymphocytes.

Heterophile antibody usually, but not always, appears in patients with IM. There are multiple types of heterophile antibodies, all of which agglutinate sheep red blood cells (RBC) and are IgM immunoglobulins. The heterophile antibody produced during IM can be differentiated from the Forssman type by differential absorption techniques. Forssman antigen (found in guinea pig or horse kidney cells) will not absorb IM-induced heterophile antibody from serum, but the non-specific antisheep RBC agglutinins found in normal persons and in serum sickness patients are absorbed by Forssman antigen. Beef RBC will absorb IM-induced heterophile antibody and serum sickness antibody. Therefore, a pa-

Table 52–11. HETEROPHILE
ANTIBODY RESPONSES

		AFTER ABSORPTION WITH	
	Heterophile	Guinea pig kidney	Beef RBC
Infectious mononucleosis	+ +	+, + +	–
Serum sickness	+ +	–	–
Normal serum (Forssman)	+	–	+

tient's serum with IM heterophile antibodies differentially absorbed with both antigens will show little or no reduction in sheep RBC agglutination activity following absorption with Forssman antigen, but will show loss of agglutinating activity following absorption with beef RBC's. A patient with serum sickness will show loss of activity following absorption with both cell types (Table 52–11). During the first two weeks of EBV infection, approximately 60 per cent of patients develop a positive classic heterophile test with titers of 1:56 or greater. This increases to 80 to 90 per cent by one month, then declines to undetectable levels in most cases by three to six months.

Formaldehyde-treated horse RBC, ox RBC, and enzyme treated and untreated sheep cells are also acceptably sensitive and specific for detection of IM heterophile antibodies and can be used in rapid, qualitative "spot" screening tests. The horse RBC agglutination test is almost as sensitive as the EBV-IgM test (96 per cent vs 97 per cent), and it stays positive at a titer of 1:40 or greater for 12 months or more in 75 per cent of cases. Sheep and beef cell hemolysin tests are each 81 to 85 per cent sensitive for the diagnosis of IM.

The classic heterophile antibody test will be negative in about 10 per cent of IM cases subsequently shown to have acute EBV infection by specific EBV serology. The false negative rate is even higher in young children. In comparison with the classic heterophile test, the Monospot test has a 2 per cent false negative rate and a 6 to 13 percent false positive rate. A positive Monospot correlates with a heterophile titer of 1:28 or greater. False positives have been associated with hepatitis A, hepatitis B, leukemia, lymphomas, and pancreatic carcinoma. It is estimated that of all IM-like illnesses, as many as one fourth will be heterophile negative. Of these, 20 to 45 per cent will

demonstrate EBV antibodies suggestive of infection. Cytomegalovirus and *Toxoplasma gondii* infections probably account for most of the remainder.

During primary infection with EBV, antibodies develop to a wide variety of antigens including the viral capsid antigen (VCA), early antigens (EA), membrane antigens (MA), and nuclear antigens (NA). Antibodies to early antigens have been subdivided into diffuse (D) and restricted (R) types based upon the location in infected cells. More broadly reactive antibodies to crude extracts of lymphoblastoid cell lines can also be detected by complement fixation, immunoprecipitation, and neutralization techniques. Indirect immunofluorescence, using EBV-infected lymphoblastoid cells and fluorescein-conjugated immunoglobulin, is employed for detecting antibodies to the VCA and EA, and complement fixation is used to detect antibodies to the NA (Andiman, 1976).

During primary EBV infection, early acute phase sera often already contain VCA antibodies in high titers, and paired sera will demonstrate a significant titer rise in only about 20 per cent. Anti-VCA titers then slowly decline to low levels, but persist for life. Sera from about 80 per cent of acutely infected persons also contain antibody to the D form of EA. These antibodies usually decline to undetectable levels following the acute illness. The R form of anti-EA appears much less commonly, and its continuing presence has been correlated with a persistent IM-like syndrome (Horwitz, 1975). Anti-EBNA begins to appear in a minority of patients in the convalescent stage of illness (three to four weeks), but by six months nearly all infected persons demonstrate this antibody, which then persists for life. The persistent anti-EBNA suggests continued stimulation by viral genomes in lymphoid cells (Henle, 1974).

In summary, serologic diagnostic criteria for primary EBV infection include (1) *early, acute serum* with anti-VCA titer of 1:320 or greater, presence of anti-D or IgM specific anti-VCA, and absence of anti-EBNA; and (2) *later serum* with rising anti-VCA or anti-D titers, or declining anti-VCA titers, or loss of anti-D, and appearance of anti-EBNA. Elevated anti-VCA and detectable anti-D in the presence of anti-EBNA suggest reactivation of infection (Sumaya, 1977).

It should also be mentioned that high anti-VCA titers as well as antibodies to EA are

5

often found in patients with African Burkitt's lymphoma and nasopharyngeal carcinoma. However, diagnosis of these tumors is
based upon biopsy and demonstration of typical histologic patterns.

POXVIRUSES

Historically, the most important poxvirus
affecting humans has been variola, the cause
of smallpox. There are two variants of this
agent—variola major, which is a severe disease with mortality rates ranging as high as
35 per cent, and variola minor (also called
alastrim), a milder disease with mortality
rates of only 1 to 2 per cent. The two strains
are not distinguishable from one another in
the laboratory. At the present time, smallpox
has been almost totally eradicated throughout
the world, but must still be considered in patients with fever and papular eruptions who
have traveled to potentially endemic areas. In
future years, it is expected that the risk of
smallpox, even in a few remaining endemic
areas in Africa, will become nil.

Vaccinia virus is closely related antigenically to variola and cowpox viruses. Its exact
origin is obscure; some believe it is an attenuated variola strain, others believe it is a variant of cowpox, and still others have proposed
that it is a hybrid of both. Regardless of its
origin, it has been used for many years for
effective immunization against smallpox. Unfortunately, vaccinia virus can sometimes produce severe, disseminated disease or progressive local necrosis, particularly in patients
with atopic dermatitis or immunodeficiency.
Use of vaccinia virus for immunization is no
longer routine in the United States.

Both variola and vaccinia viruses can be
isolated in routine cell cultures, such as the
heteroploid cell lines, and they also grow well
and can be distinguished from one another on
the basis of pock development on chorioallantoic membranes in embryonated eggs. However, *if smallpox is suspected, laboratory assistance should be immediately requested from
the nearest public health laboratory!*

Other methods used to distinguish these
viruses from other causes of vesicular, vesicu-
lopustular, or papular eruptions (e.g., herpes
simplex, varicella-zoster viruses) include direct
examination of the vesicular fluid or crusts by
electron microscopy and cytologic examination of scrapings taken from the base of the
lesion. In the latter method, air-dried and
fixed smears are stained with methyl violet
(Gutstein's method), or Giemsa stain. The
presence of intranuclear inclusions and/or
multinucleated giant cells suggests the diagnosis of a herpes group infection and tends to
rule out poxvirus. Poxvirus infections are
characterized by swollen epithelial cells containing intracytoplasmic inclusions surrounded by a halo (Guarnieri bodies). Poxvirus
antigens may also be detected in skin lesions
by agar gel precipitation or complement fixation methods.

Cowpox and paravaccinia (milker's nodules)
are bovine poxviruses which are occasionally
transmitted to humans in direct contact with
infected cows or calves. Cowpox is characterized in humans by low grade fever and multiple papular lesions on the fingers and hands
which later become vesicular and pustular,
resolving after several weeks. Paravaccinia is
somewhat similar, except that the lesion is
usually solitary, progressing to a firm nodule 1
to 2 cm in diameter in 10 days, then crusting
and healing in another two to three weeks. A
clinical picture nearly identical to paravaccinia
is also seen with orf, a poxvirus of sheep (ec-
thyma contagiosum), and is an occupational
hazard among sheep farmers (Fig. 52-11).

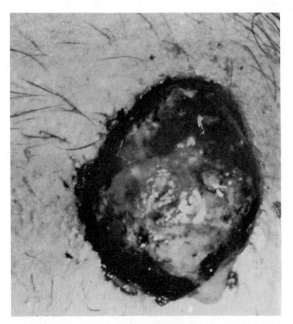

Figure 52-11. The acute stage of orf showing a nodule with a
weeping, ulcerated surface. (From Leavell, U. E., et al.:
J.A.M.A., *204*:660, 1968.)

The diagnosis of these diseases is usually made on clinical and epidemiologic grounds; confirmation of orf infection can be made by determining specific CF antibody responses, a special procedure not generally available except in some public health laboratories.

Molluscum contagiosum, a poxvirus disease affecting humans only, produces smooth, "pearly" skin papules, averaging about 4 mm in diameter. This agent cannot be cultured in the laboratory. Diagnosis is by clinical and histologic examination.

ENTEROVIRUSES

Enteroviruses include polio, coxsackie, and echo virus species, for which man is the only known natural host. Poliovirus was the first virus to be described and propagated in tissue culture in1949 by Enders, Weller, and Robbins. During the peak incidence of poliomyelitis in the United States in the mid-twentieth century, about 1500 deaths and 7000 cases of residual paralysis occurred annually. This, plus the successful growth of virus in tissue cul-

ture, provided a great stimulus for vaccine research which resulted in the Salk and Sabin vaccines. The use of these vaccines has nearly eradicated poliomyelitis from developed countries. There are three distinct poliovirus serotypes recognized and all grow well in tissue culture.

The other two enterovirus species were discovered during intense epidemiologic studies of poliomyelitis. Coxsackie viruses were first recovered in 1949 in suckling mice inoculated with the fecal extracts from two children with a paralytic poliomyelitis-like syndrome. They derive their name from the fact that both isolates were discovered in Coxsackie, New York. Two groups of coxsackie viruses were later defined on the basis of unique clinical and pathologic effects on suckling mice: group A coxsackie viruses cause flaccid paralysis, myositis, and death within a week, whereas group B viruses produce encephalitis with a spastic paralysis, myocarditis, and other visceral inflammatory changes. All the coxsackie B, but only a few coxsackie A viruses, grow in tissue culture; therefore, inoculation into suckling mice is necessary for isolation of

Table 52–12. CLINICAL SYNDROMES ASSOCIATED WITH ENTEROVIRUS INFECTIONS: RELATIVE FREQUENCIES AND COMMON SEROTYPES INVOLVED

| | ENTEROVIRUS SEROTYPES | | |
| | Coxsackie | | |
SYNDROME	Group A	Group B	Echo
Aseptic meningitis	+ 2,4,7,9,10	+ + 1,2,3,4,5,6	+ + + + most serotypes
Muscle paralysis and weakness	+ 7*,9	+ 2,3,4,5	+ + 2,4,6,9,11,30
Encephalitis and radiculitis	+ 2,5,6	+ + + + 1,2,3,4,5	+ 2,6,9,10
Pleurodynia (epidemic myalgia)	−	+ + + + 1,2,3,4,5	+ 1,6,9
Pericarditis, myocarditis	+ 4,16	+ + + + 1,2,3,4,5	+ 1,6,8,9,19
Rashes	+ + + 4,5,6,9,16	+ + 2,3,5	+ + + 2,4,6,9,11,16,18
Respiratory illness	+ + 9,16,21,24	+ + 1,3,4,5	+ + + 4,9,11,20,25
Hand-foot-and-mouth disease	+ + + + 16,5,10	+ 2,5	−
Herpangina	+ + + + 1,2,3,4,5,6,8,10,22	+ 1,2,3,4,5	+ 9,16,17
Generalized disease (infants)	+ 9	+ + + 1,2,3,4,5	+ 5,11,16,19

Code: − = not reported
+ = uncommon
+ + to + + + + = relative frequencies of isolation
*Coxsackie A 7 is second to poliovirus as a cause of neuromuscular disease.

5

most of the latter. No single antigen is common to all coxsackie viruses, although there may be some heterotypic cross-reactivity between coxsackie A viruses. There is a common coxsackie B antigen, however, which is also shared with one coxsackie A virus. Currently, 24 coxsackie A and 6 coxsackie B virus serotypes are recognized.

Beginning in 1950, many new non-polio, non-coxsackie human enteric viral isolates were discovered. These viruses were initially called "orphans" because they were often not associated with recognized disease. All the isolates grew well in tissue culture, producing cytopathogenic changes. Subsequently in 1955 the name was changed to ECHO, an abbreviation for "enteric cytopathogenic human orphans." There is no common echovirus group antigen, and 34 different echovirus serotypes were originally recognized. Echovirus 10, however, has been reclassified as a reovirus, and echovirus 28 is now classified as a rhinovirus. Echovirus 9 is now reclassified as coxsackie A23, because of its behavior in suckling mice.

Enteroviruses are ubiquitous agents that are spread primarily by fecal-oral contamination, but respiratory transmission also occurs. The viruses initially colonize the alimentary tract, growing in the lymphoid tissues of the nasopharynx and intestinal tract. Viremia subsequently occurs, allowing secondary localization in other viscera and lymphoid tissues. Infection is often asymptomatic (30 to 90 per cent), but a wide variety of notable syndromes may also occur, including paralytic disease, aseptic meningitis, encephalitis, pleurodynia, pericarditis, herpangina, and lymphonodular pharyngitis. However, the most common clinical picture is that of an undifferentiated febrile illness with malaise, headache, myalgia, and sore throat. Enteroviruses may also cause a generalized disease of variable severity in newborn infants. Table 52-12 shows which non-polio enteroviruses are most commonly associated with the various syndromes.

POLIOVIRUS

Polioviruses are found in a world wide distribution. In many underdeveloped countries poliomyelitis is still endemic and nearly all infections are subclinical. When symptomatic disease occurs it primarily involves infants and children. With improved sanitation the age distribution changes to include older children and adults. In temperate climates, the wild viruses are most commonly isolated during the summer and autumn months.

Clinical disease usually occurs in one of three forms: (1) non-specific febrile illness, (2) aseptic meningitis, or (3) poliomyelitis, which is classically an asymmetrical, flaccid paralysis of variable extent. Maximum involvement is evident within a few days after onset of paralysis, and is followed by gradual recovery of temporarily damaged motor neurons which may continue for up to six months.

Laboratory diagnosis is based on viral isolation in tissue culture followed by identification by neutralization techniques using type-specific antisera. The virus is readily isolated from throat swabs early in the infection and from feces after onset of symptoms. It is rarely isolated from the CSF. Following oral polio vaccination with the live attenuated virus, fecal excretion may be observed for up to 18 weeks. In countries where there is widespread vaccination with live attenuated vaccine, a polio isolate from a patient with a compatible clinical syndrome and recent vaccine exposure should be forwarded to a reference laboratory to determine if it is a wild virus strain or a vaccine strain. A fourfold or greater rise in complement fixation antibody titer is indicative of recent infection or polio vaccination. However, CF titers may decline to undetectable levels, and neutralization techniques may be required to determine immune status.

COXSACKIE AND ECHOVIRUS

These viruses have the same pathogenesis, mode of spread, and seasonal occurrence that poliovirus infections demonstrate. In contrast, however, these viruses produce a wider variety of clinical syndromes (Table 52-12) and have a greater tendency to infect the meninges and cerebrum with only rare involvement of motor neurons of the spinal cord. Also, these infections can pursue a relapsing course for several weeks, manifesting a variety of different clinical syndromes. Recurrent infection by some coxsackie B serotypes and rarely by echovirus serotypes may occur.

Additional diseases that have been etiologically linked to enteroviruses include hepatitis, transverse myelitis, cranial nerve palsies, and acute hemorrhagic conjunctivitis (AHC). AHC was epidemic in Africa, Asia, India, and parts of Europe from 1969 to 1974. It is now endemic in these areas, and the viral isolate from af-

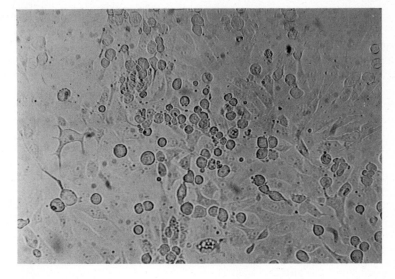

Figure 52–12. Typical CPE of enteroviruses in primary monkey kidney culture (coxsackievirus B) (×125), (From Herrmann, E.C., Jr., et al.: Mayo Clin. Proc. 47:577, 1972.)

fected persons has been called enterovirus 70. Coxsackie viruses have been implicated in a wide variety of other syndromes, including acute cerebellar ataxia, hemolytic-uremic syndrome, hepatitis, nephritis, and chronic myopathies.

Both coxsackie and echoviruses have been implicated in occasionally fatal, generalized infections of newborns manifested by fever, meningitis, rash, diarrhea, or shock. This occurs primarily in the summer and fall and is often associated with recent maternal infection with the same virus. Sometimes the infected infant exhibits only signs of sepsis and shock with a negative bacteriologic workup, thus emphasizing the need to include these agents in the differential diagnosis of neonatal sepsis.

Laboratory diagnosis

These viruses can be grown best in primary monkey kidney cell cultures in which they produce distinctive cytopathic effects (Fig. 52-12) or in suckling mice (Coxsackie A). Most enteroviruses will become apparent in tissue culture within a few days, allowing a rapid presumptive identification, which is followed by confirmation techniques using type-specific antisera.

The pattern of growth in multiple tissue culture systems often suggests the species of enterovirus being isolated (Table 52-13). Since there are so many serotypic possibilities within species, pools of several different antisera are used, often in an intersecting pattern

(Fig. 52-13) for viral neutralization studies. For confirmation of these results, a neutralization test using a single specific antiserum is then performed to identify the isolate.

During the course of an enteroviral infection, the virus is present in the oropharynx and often in the feces at the onset of disease. After one or two weeks the virus disappears from the throat, but will continue to be excreted in the feces for as long as 16 to 18 weeks. Virus may also be isolated from specimens taken from clinically infected, sites, i.e., CSF, blood, or tissues. Recovery of virus from these ordinarily sterile sites is diagnostic. Isolation of virus from the throat only or from both the throat and feces early in the course of a compatible illness also supports an etiologic relationship. Viral recovery from the feces alone, with or without seroconversion (discussed below), however, must be interpreted

Table 52–13. PATTERN OF ENTEROVIRUS GROWTH IN SELECTED CULTURE SYSTEMS

	RMK[1]	HDF[2]	HET[3]	MICE
Polio virus	+*	+	+	−
Echo virus	+	+	−	−
Coxsackie A virus	±	±	−	+
Coxsackie B virus	+	−	+	+

[1] Primary Rhesus monkey kidney.
[2] Human diploid fibroblasts.
[3] Human heteroploid cells.
* + = growth
  ± = growth in some strains
  − = no growth

5

Composition of serum pools

Identification of isolates

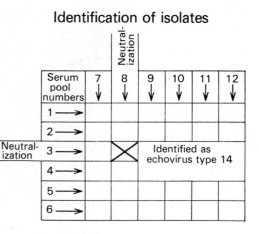

Serum pool numbers	7	8	9	10	11	12
1 →	E1*	E2	E3	E4	E5	E6
2 →	E7	E8	E9	Reo 1**	E11	E12
3 →	E13	E14	E15	E16	E17	E18
4 →	E19	E20	E21	E22	E23	E24
5 →	E25	E26	E27	E28+	E29	E30
6 →	E31	E32	E33	E11 prime	Cox A9	‡

Neutralization

Neutralization

Serum pool numbers	7	8	9	10	11	12
1 →						
2 →						
3 →		✕	Identified as echovirus type 14			
4 →						
5 →						
6 →						

*Echovirus immune serum type

**Serum also neutralizes reovirus types 2 and 3

+Now classified as rhinovirus type la

‡Immune serum to enterovirus candidate strains

Figure 52–13. Twelve-pool intersecting serum schema for identification of echoviruses by neutralization tests. (From Lennette, E. H., and Schmidt, N. J. (eds.): Diagnostic Procedures for Viral and Rickettsial Infections, 4th ed. New York, American Public Health Association, 1969.)

with caution, since viral excretion and gradual decline of antibody titers may continue for several weeks beyond initial infection. This is particularly a diagnostic problem with young children in whom the prevalence of asymptomatic fecal excretion may range from 3 to 4 per cent in the northern United States to 30 per cent in the Gulf States during the summer and early fall. Therefore, a fecal isolate may not necessarily be etiologically related to the acute disease being investigated. This becomes less of a diagnostic problem with adults because of the somewhat lower incidence of asymptomatic fecal excretion.

Serum-neutralizing antibodies develop rapidly, often reaching high titers shortly after the onset of symptoms, and may persist at high titers for years, sometimes making demonstration of a fourfold or greater change in titer difficult. Neutralizing antibodies are the most serotypically specific, but because of the large numbers of viral serotypes, performing neutralizing antibody titers on paired sera becomes a laborious and time-consuming technique. Use of information contained in Table 52–12, as well as local epidemiologic data, aids in determining which viruses one should select for use in neutralization serology.

Complement fixation antibodies develop more slowly and decline to low levels, rarely being detectable after three years. Also, CF serologies are insensitive and rather non-specific owing to heterotypic cross-reactivity. They are of little practical value except in poliovirus serodiagnosis. Only a few enteroviral serotypes produce hemagglutination inhibition antibodies, thus limiting the usefulness of this serologic technique. To further complicate the situation, there may be considerable variability in antibody response; therefore, a lack of seroconversion does not exclude the possibility of a coxsackie or echovirus infection. Despite these disadvantages, a fourfold or greater rise or fall in antibody titer is considered significant when interpreted in the context of the clinical syndrome and epidemiologic data.

In some enterovirus infections, such as myocarditis or pericarditis due to coxsackie B viruses, virus isolation rates are usually less than 10 per cent, even when affected tissue or pericardial fluid is cultured. The clinical and experimental data would suggest that the syndrome is immunologically mediated, particularly by T-lymphocytes (Woodruff, 1974), and virus excretion may have ceased or considerably diminished by the time symptoms are manifest. In these situations, diagnosis by neutralization antibody testing of paired sera is usually much more sensitive than culture.

ARBOVIRUSES

The term *arbovirus* indicates those agents which share in common a similar mode of transmission by hemophagous insects, especially ticks and mosquitoes. There are over 250 viruses in this category, including representatives from the Togaviridae, Bunyaviridae, Reoviridae (Orbivirus), and Rhabdoviridae families, as well as some unclassified agents. The arboviruses which have been found associated with disease in the United States are summarized in Table 52-14.

The major syndromes are loosely categorized as:
1. fever, malaise (any of these viruses);
2. fever, encephalitis, or aseptic meningitis (the encephalitis agents, California, Powassan, and occasionally Colorado tick fever);
3. fever, myalgia, and headache (Colorado tick fever);
4. fever, myalgia, headache, rash, lymphadenopathy (dengue);
5. fever, hemorrhagic diathesis (yellow fever, sometimes dengue).

The most important of these agents in the United States are: St. Louis encephalitis,

Table 52-14. IMPORTANT ARBOVIRUSES IN THE UNITED STATES

TOGAVIRIDAE FAMILY
   Alphavirus group
      Eastern equine encephalitis
      Western equine encephalitis
      Venezuelan equine encephalitis*
   Flavivirus group
      St. Louis encephalitis
      Yellow fever*
      Powassan
      Dengue types 1, 2, 3, 4*
BUNYAVIRIDAE FAMILY
   California group
      California (La Crosse)
REOVIRIDAE FAMILY (ORBIVIRUS)
   Colorado tick fever

*Venezuelan equine encephalitis, yellow fever, and dengue are not now indigenous to the continental United States; however, imported cases from adjacent tropical and subtropical areas are occasionally diagnosed, and the potential vectors for these agents do exist in North America.

western equine encephalitis, and California (La Crosse) virus. Eastern equine encephalitis and Colorado tick fever infections are identified only occasionally; Powassan infections of humans appear to be rare.

Virus isolation attempts are only occasionally successful in these infections. The most common method used is inoculation of serum (whole blood is preferable for Colorado tick fever), CSF, or brain homogenates into suckling mice. Confirmation and identification of isolates usually require the aid of a public health laboratory. However, serologic diagnosis has been shown to be a much more practical approach and is preferable. A knowledge of the epidemiologic behavior of these viruses, coupled with the clinical history, helps one to select the appropriate serologies to be done.

The seasonal distribution parallels the activity of the insect vector—the encephalitides are common from mid-summer through early autumn (usually July through September), then disappear; Colorado tick fever is more common during late spring and early summer, the period of greatest tick activity.

Eastern equine encephalitis is confined primarily to wooded, swampy areas along the eastern seaboard, from New England to Florida. Young children are most commonly affected. Serologic diagnosis is by CF or HI antibody titer rises between acute and convalescent sera.

St. Louis and western equine encephalitis viruses have been responsible for outbreaks of central nervous disease in many areas of the United States and are not at all as geographically restricted as the names suggest. Interestingly, the highest attack and sequelae rates are among individuals over 40 years of age with St. Louis encephalitis, while infants and young children are more severely affected during western equine encephalitis outbreaks.

In both of these infections, HI and CF antibodies are usually significantly elevated within two to three weeks after onset, and serologic confirmation is based upon a fourfold or greater antibody titer rise between acute and convalescent sera. If the first serum sample has been obtained later than seven days after onset, a diagnosis is considered likely if the HI titer is ≥ 1:80 or the CF titer is ≥ 1:16 for either antigen ("presumptive" case). Single HI titers of 1:40 are suggestive of recent infection but are usually regarded as "equivocal" or inconclusive cases.

California virus is a major cause of encepha-

5

litis during the summer season in Minnesota, Ohio, Indiana, and Wisconsin, but is actually very rare in the western states. It most commonly affects children between the ages of five and nine years and is associated with suburban or rural environments (Balfour, 1973). Serologic diagnosis can be made on paired sera utilizing either a CF or HI test. However, the CF titer tends to rise more slowly in this infection, reaching a peak usually by three to five weeks after onset. Precipitating antibody to the La Crosse strain of California virus has also been shown to appear during the infection and to disappear within one year. Balfour (1974) has shown that counterimmunoelectrophoresis of the patient's serum, using the La Crosse strain as the antigen, will detect precipitating antibody in 41 per cent of acute phase sera and 100 per cent of convalescent sera in proved cases. This method appears sensitive and can be completed in 1.5 hours.

Colorado tick fever (mountain fever, tick fever) is found in brushy, wooded mountain areas in the western United States, corresponding to the habitat of the vector *Dermacentor andersoni*. It is usually an acute febrile illness with headache and myalgia beginning three to five days after the tick bite. Occasionally, encephalitis and hemorrhagic complications may also develop. The diagnosis is usually made serologically by CF testing, but antibody develops slowly and a significant rise may not be detected until four to six weeks after the onset of illness.

INFLUENZA VIRUSES

Influenza viruses exist as three distinct types, A, B, and C, based on immunologically different soluble nucleoprotein antigens. These viruses are characterized by hemagglutinin (HA) and neuraminidase (NA) protein spikes projecting from the surface of the lipid-containing envelope. The HA attaches to specific glycoprotein receptors on a variety of cell surfaces including erythrocytes. The neuraminidase destroys these receptor sites, releasing the absorbed virus from the surface of cells. This activity may facilitate the spread of virus within the infected host. There are antigenically variable HA ($H_{0,1,2,3}$) and neuraminidase ($N_{1,2}$) antigens which are used for subtyping and determining specific immunity to influenza A subtypes. Within each subtype there are strains which show minor serologic

differences and are designated in the following example: A/Hong Kong/68 (H_3N_2), i.e., virus type/site of original isolation/year of initial isolation, followed by H, N notation. The HA and NA of influenza B viruses are less well characterized and therefore not used in the nomenclature (Table 52-15).

The outstanding characteristic of influenza viruses (primarily type A) is the tendency to cause periodic local epidemics and major pandemics owing to their ability to undergo minor and major antigenic changes. Probable influenza epidemics have been described for several centuries; at least four major pandemics have occurred within the past century.

Epidemiology

Influenza A infections occur most frequently during the winter in temperate climates and cause major epidemics every two to four years. Influenza B occurs more sporadically or in localized outbreaks. Influenza C usually causes mild or undetected disease, but serologic evidence reveals a high prevalence of infection.

The periodicity of influenza A infection results from the antigenic drifts and shifts which occur, leaving the population susceptible to reinfection by different strains or different subtypes when they occur. Antigenic drifts involve no major change in HA or NA antigens, but antisera prepared in animals against specific strains vary in ability to inhibit hemagglutination of similar strains isolated from differing geographic locations or time periods. Major antigenic shifts occur when there is a major change in HA and/or NA types. This occurs approximately every 10 to 15 years and is responsible for severe pandemics (Table 52-15).

Influenza A epidemics develop rapidly over three to six weeks, with the peak prevalence of infection occurring within two to three months, and then subside rapidly. From 10 to 50 per cent of an urban population may be affected, and serologic testing suggests that up to 25 per cent may experience subclinical infection. The highest attack rates often occur in children, and serologic evidence indicates that by school age most persons have been infected at least once. Influenza B spreads more slowly but otherwise behaves similarly to type A. Influenza C probably never causes significant epidemics.

The doctrine of "original antigenic sin" is

Table 52–15.   CLASSIFICATION AND EPIDEMIOLOGY OF INFLUENZA VIRUSES

NUCLEOPROTEIN TYPE	HEMAGGLUTININ SUBTYPE	NEURAMINIDASE SUBTYPE	REPRESENTATIVE STRAIN	EPIDEMIC YEAR
A	H_{sw}	N_1	Swine-like agent	1918*
A	H_o	N_1	A/PR/34 (H0N1) (formerly A_o)	1933
A	H_1	N_1	A/FM/47 (H1N1)	1947
A	H_2	N_2	A/Singapore/57 (H2N2) (formerly A_2; Asian)	1957*
A	H_3	N_2	A/Hong Kong/68	1968*
			A/England/72	1972
B			B/Mass/66	
			B/Vic/70	
			B/Hong Kong/72	
C			C/Taylor/47	

* Pandemics occurred at these times.

an interesting immunologic phenomenon which has been observed with influenza A infections. The first influenza A strain to infect a person produces a specific immunologic response to the hemagglutinin which remains the predominant antibody response following all subsequent influenza A infections with any subtype or strain. For example, each different influenza A infection produces its own specific antibody response, but usually in lower titer than the anamnestic antibody response to the original infecting strain. This phenomenon can be used to determine not only the original infecting strain, but, considering the age of the person and the epidemiology of infection, can establish approximately when a given strain was causing disease in a susceptible population. These types of serologic studies have led to the hypothesis that antigenic types recycle after many years. For example, during the Hong Kong influenza A epidemic in 1968, the attack rate among persons born before 1890 was one third the rate of those born after 1890 (Schoenbaum, 1976). This implies a high antibody prevalence to the Hong Kong influenza A virus and suggests it may have been the cause of the 1889-90 pandemic. Other studies have also supported this "recycling" hypothesis. Similar work suggests that the agent responsible for the 1918 pandemic may have been similar to the swine-like influenza virus. If there is an orderly cyclic pattern to the reemergence of influenza strains (Schoenbaum, 1976), a swine type of influenza virus could be predicted to cause a major epidemic between 1975 and 1985. It has been suggested that animals (swine, horses, and fowl) may function as reservoirs for different antigenic strains of influenza A, allowing reemergence and infection of man after many years.

Clinical aspects

During outbreaks of influenza A or B, the disease manifests the typical pattern of rapid onset, following an incubation period of one to three days, with headache, myalgia, fever, chills, and marked prostration accompanied by rhinitis, sore throat and often a cough with chest pain. The acute disease usually lasts three days to a week, but convalescence with fatigue, malaise, and cough may last an additional two to three weeks. The disease in infants can be very severe, associated with febrile convulsions and/or severe croup, occasionally requiring tracheostomy.

A more serious form of influenza infection is primary viral pneumonia which occurs within the first one to three days after onset of initial symptoms. During the pandemic of 1918 there was a high mortality in young adults due to influenza pneumonia. Other respiratory complications include a mixed bacterial and viral pneumonia also occurring within one to three days of onset, or a superimposed bacterial pneumonia developing later in the illness or during the convalescent period.

Another problem complicating influenza infection is congestive heart failure and pulmonary edema in persons with marginal cardiovascular or respiratory status. Some additional described complications include disseminated intravascular coagulation with hemolytic-uremic syndrome, severe myositis with elevated muscle enzymes, Reye's syndrome, acute renal failure, encephalopathy, and pericarditis.

5

Laboratory diagnosis

Influenza A and B viruses are readily isolated from throat swabs taken during the first three days of acute illness and inoculated into primary monkey kidney cell cultures or amnionic sacs of embryonated hen's eggs. The presence of virus is indicated by hemadsorption of guinea pig erythrocytes to infected tissue culture cells (see section on parainfluenza viruses) or detection of hemagglutinating activity in the amnionic or allantoic fluid. Both systems are often used simultaneously to increase the sensitivity of detection. Further identification is based on neutralization of this activity by specific antisera *in vitro*. Influenza C is isolated best by inoculation of the amnionic sac of embryonated eggs.

Serologic diagnosis is useful when a fourfold or greater rise in antibody titer to a specific, currently infecting strain of influenza is demonstrated. However, a single elevated titer to a totally new antigenic strain in convalescent sera during an outbreak caused by the same virus offers supportive evidence of infection.

There may be variable antibody responses to any of the four major influenza antigens: matrix (M) protein, nucleoprotein (NP), neuraminidase (NA), and hemagglutinin (HA). The M and NP antigens are stable in contrast to NA and HA antigens. Antibodies to M antigen usually occur only following severe illness and hence are rarely sought, but antibody rises to NP antigens are more predictable, and tests for NP antibody are quite sensitive.

Complement fixation (CF) techniques may be utilized for serodiagnosis in laboratories already equipped for CF procedures. Either the NP antigen or whole virion (HA and NA) may be used as the antigen in the system, thereby affording the degree of specificity desired. Results using the whole virion compare with those obtained by hemagglutination inhibition (HI). However, the HI test system is simpler and less technically demanding than CF and hence is the commonest serologic technique employed for both serodiagnosis and epidemiologic studies. The choice of antigen in the HI test should be a strain most closely related antigenically to the suspected current epidemic strain. Another serologic method less commonly employed is single radial immunodiffusion (Mostow, 1975).

PARAINFLUENZA (PI) VIRUSES

First discovered in 1953, the PI viruses are now recognized as four distinct serologic types, designated as types 1, 2, 3, and 4. They share some common antigens among themselves, as well as with some other human and animal viruses. Most notable is the antigenic sharing between PI type 2 and mumps, as well as simian virus-5 (SV-5). The latter agent is a common contaminant of monkey kidney cell cultures; it causes hemadsorption and occasionally is misidentified as a parainfluenza virus in clinical samples. This mistake can be prevented by including appropriate cell culture controls when identifying suspected human hemadsorbing agents, and, when SV-5 is specifically suspected as a contaminant, neutralization by specific antiserum to SV-5 should also be checked when typing an isolate.

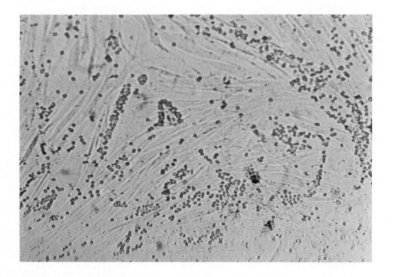

Figure 52–14. Hemadsorption with guinea pig erythrocytes in monkey kidney cells infected with parainfluenza 3. (From Herrmann, E. C., Jr., and Hable, K. A.: Mayo Clin. Proc., 45:185, 1970.)

All four serotypes are primarily respiratory tract pathogens. Of these, type 4 is the least frequent, and generally associated with only mild upper respiratory symptoms. Types 1, 2, and 3 are extremely important and common agents, particularly among infants and young children, producing croup, tracheobronchitis, bronchiolitis, pneumonia, or a combination of these syndromes. In older children and adults, the symptoms are more often those of a "common cold," pharyngitis, or laryngitis. Infections may occur in any season, but are generally more common in the autumn and winter.

Virus shedding from the respiratory tract can be detected for up to a week after onset, then disappears rapidly. Pooled nasopharyngeal and throat swabs or nasopharyngeal washings are the best sources for isolation attempts.

Primary or secondary rhesus monkey kidney cell cultures are preferred for isolation. The PI viruses are recognized by the fact that infected cultures will produce hemagglutinin on the cell surfaces, and eventually release this into the media. After three days of incubation, and at two- to three-day intervals thereafter, the cell cultures are tested for the presence of hemadsorption by the addition of 0.1 ml of a 0.5 per cent suspension of guinea pig red blood cells in either PBS or Hank's BSS. A fresh suspension of guinea pig cells is usually stable for up to seven days at 4°C. The tubes are incubated horizontally at 4°C. with the cell culture down for 30 minutes, then examined microscopically for hemadsorption (Fig. 52-14). The tubes should also be inspected to determine if hemagglutination has occurred in the media as a result of excess free hemagglutinin release. This may block the hemadsorption phenomenon, but nevertheless indicates virus presence. Types 1, 2, and 3 hemadsorb at 4°C., with reversal above 25°C. for types 1 and 3; type 4 hemadsorbs only at 25 to 37°C. If cultures are negative at 4°C., reincubation at 25°C. for 30 minutes will detect type 4. If the cultures are hemadsorption- or hemagglutinin-positive, they can be passed into fresh culture tubes for further identification, or the infected cells may be directly examined by immunofluorescent or immunoperoxidase methods for rapid typing (Benjamin, 1974). If the cultures are read as negative, the medium is removed and fresh maintenance medium added, followed by reincubation. Virus detection in cell cultures is usually made in 3 to 14 days. Cytopathic effect is often non-descript or absent, with the exception of PI type 2, which will often produce syncytia (Fig. 52-15).

The classic methods of PI virus indentification are hemadsorption-inhibition (HadI) or neutralization. Antisera for either test must first be treated with receptor-destroying enzyme and heat inactivated to remove non-specific inhibitors. In the HadI test, infected cell cultures are washed three times with Hank's BSS, then 0.8 ml of diluted antiserum is added. After 30 minutes incubation at room temperature, 0.2 ml of 0.4 per cent guinea pig red blood cells is added, and the cultures are reincubated at 4°C. for 30 minutes. The serum which inhibits hemadsorption as compared with controls identifies the isolate. The neutralization test differs only in that the fluid harvest from infected cell cultures is first in-

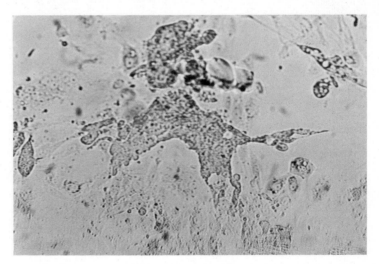

Figure 52-15. Typical syncytial pattern of cytopathic effect produced in monkey kidney cells by parainfluenza virus. (From Herrmann, E. C., Jr., and Hable, K. A.: Mayo Clin. Proc., 45:184, 1970.)

cubated with treated antisera, then inoculated into fresh cell cultures and tested periodically for hemadsorption.

Interpretation of the significance of clinical isolates is usually not difficult, since asymptomatic carriers of PI viruses are rare. However, if the diagnosis of PI infection is suspected, but cannot be confirmed by isolation, serologic testing may be desired. Either the HI or neutralization tests are preferred.

RESPIRATORY SYNCYTIAL VIRUS (RSV)

RSV is considered the single most important respiratory virus affecting infants and young children. Infection with severe illness can occur as early as the first month of life and is manifested primarily in infants as bronchiolitis, pneumonia, or both. Older children and adults are also susceptible, and reinfection is common. This latter group usually develops mild coryza and cough in response to infection, but croup and tracheobronchitis can also occur. RSV has also been associated with acute flare-ups of asthmatic bronchitis or chronic bronchitis in older individuals.

Infections are most commonly seen during the winter and early spring. Outbreaks among infants in a community usually last 8 to 12 weeks, and are often associated with a high degree of morbidity. Mortality in hospitalized infants is estimated to be as high as 2 per cent, and epidemic spread in a hospital setting is recognized as a serious problem. The virus is extremely labile and does not tolerate freezing well at all. The usual method of diagnosis is to obtain pooled nasopharyngeal and throat swab specimens (some workers prefer nasopharyngeal washings), and inoculate these as quickly as possible into cell cultures. As with parainfluenza viruses, shedding of virus is most prominent in the first week of illness.

RSV will grow in the three basic types of cell cultures, but is most reliably isolated in human heteroploid cell cultures. The CPE is characteristically fusion of cells to form multinucleated syncytial or "giant" cells (Fig. 52-16) and may appear anytime from 2 to 12 days after inoculation. RSV does not possess or produce a hemagglutinin. The characteristic CPE, the lack of hemadsorption with guinea pig red blood cells, and the usual syndromes associated with RSV often allow the laboratory to make a presumptive etiologic diagnosis and distinguish this virus from other agents which produce syncytia, such as parainfluenza type 2, mumps, and measles viruses. Definitive identification, if necessary, can be done by immunofluorescent or immunoperoxidase, neutralization, or complement fixation tests.

Rapid identification of RSV infections has also been made by immunofluorescent examination of infected epithelial cells shed from the respiratory tract (Gardner, 1974).

As with parainfluenza viruses, interpretation of the significance of a clinical isolate of RSV is usually not difficult, since asymptomatic carriage is exceedingly rare. Serologic diagnosis, if deemed necessary, is usually by CF or neutralization; however, there are diffi-

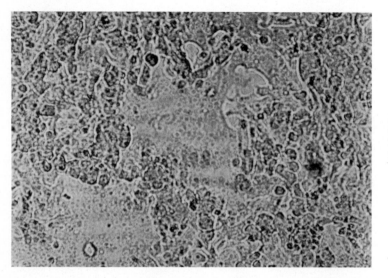

Figure 52-16. Typical RSV syncytial CPE in HeLa cells (× 110). (From Smith, T. F., et al.: Mayo Clinic Proc., 46:610, 1971.)

culties. Young infants do not always respond serologically to such infections; therefore, absence of a significant antibody response does not rule out infection. There is also a disparity between CF and neutralizing antibody responses, in that as many as 50 per cent of sera containing CF antibody may have no detectable neutralizing antibody (Fulginiti, 1974).

RHINOVIRUSES

There are over 89 serotypes of rhinoviruses which are currently recognized. They are acknowledged as important causes of the common cold, but are very rarely and questionably associated with more severe disease, such as lower respiratory illnesses. Rhinovirus infections have also been blamed for some acute exacerbations of illness in asthmatics and patients with chronic bronchitis.

While they are important causes of morbidity in the general population, the nature of the illness produced is usually such that a diagnostic virology laboratory is only occasionally requested to specifically seek them by culture. The highest yield of virus isolation from nasopharyngeal and throat specimens is in the first three to five days of illness.

The rhinoviruses have been isolated in monkey kidney, human embryonic kidney, human diploid fibroblasts, and occasionally in heteroploid cell lines. Of these, the human diploid fibroblasts, particularly WI-38 cells, have been the most sensitive. Most rhinoviruses grow best at 33°C. incubation, a factor which is also likely to explain their growth and pathology as limited primarily to the cooler environment of the upper respiratory tract in humans. In addition, continuous rotation of cultures in roller drums is usually required for primary isolation. These special incubation requirements are usually not all met in a diagnostic laboratory unless there is a special interest in rhinovirus infections. The CPE produced consists of irregular-sized, rounded cells which often glisten like dewdrops when fine focusing adjustment is made microscopically. As CPE progress, cell disintegration and granularity become more apparent (Fig. 52-17). The CPE bears a close resemblance to that seen with some enterovirus isolates.

Because of the multiplicity of serotypes, neither specific serotyping nor serologic diagnosis are feasible in other than a research laboratory. If an isolate is suspected of being a

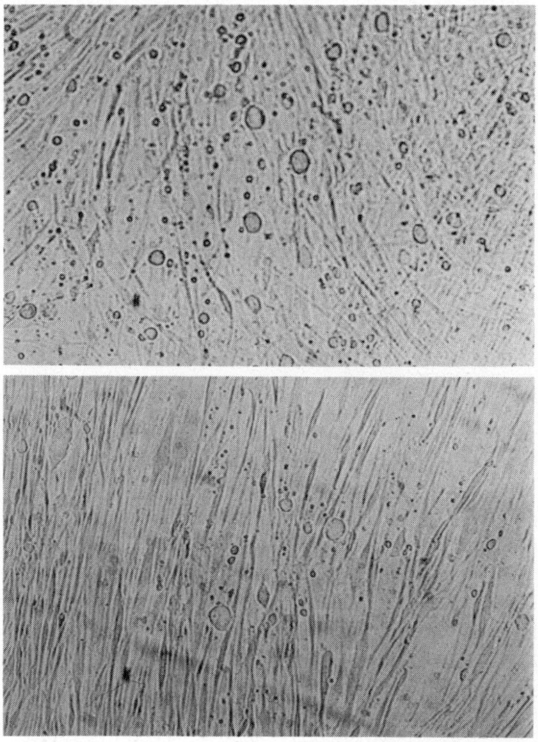

Figure 52-17. Rhinovirus CPE in WI-38 cell culture (×125). (From Person, D. A., and Herrmann, E. C., Jr.: Mayo Clin. Proc., 45:521, 1970.)

rhinovirus, it can be confirmed by demonstrating resistance to chloroform or ether inactivation (ruling out herpesviruses) and by acid lability. In the latter test, rhinovirus infectivity is lost when the harvest is diluted at 1:10 in a solution at a pH of 2.0 to 2.2 and held at room temperature for two hours. Enteroviruses, which can be confused with rhinoviruses, are not inactivated by this procedure.

CORONAVIRUSES

Like the rhinoviruses, coronaviruses are considered to be important causes of mild upper respiratory illnesses, particularly among adults. Also, based on serologic surveys, they may be associated with some cases of lower respiratory disease in young children (McIntosh, 1974).

The number of serotypes is unknown; two strains (229E and OC43) have been studied to some extent epidemiologically, and their overall contribution to human disease is presently not known. Coronaviruses are rarely, if ever, specifically sought in a hospital or public health laboratory. They have been isolated with some difficulty on human diploid lung fibroblasts, human embryonic trachea organ cultures, and in human embryonic intestinal fibroblasts. Some strains have been adapted to grow in human cell lines with plaque production. Most coronavirus isolates have been identified by electron microscopy or immune electron microscopy of culture supernatant fluids (Kapikian, 1973).

Most infections have been identified serologically, using either CF or HI tests, but these have not yet been routinely employed for clinical diagnosis.

MUMPS VIRUS

There is only one serotype of mumps virus, although minor antigens are shared with other paramyxoviruses. Man is the only known host and reservoir of infection. The typical parotitis syndrome was accurately described by Hippocrates in the fifth century. The name *mumps* was derived from the mumbling speech of patients whose jaws were too painful to move.

The virus contains a hemagglutinin (HA), neuraminidase (NA), and hemolysin associated with the viral envelope. Two antigens elicit immunologic responses in an infected host. These are the soluble S antigen derived from the nucleocapsid and the V antigen derived from the surface hemagglutinin.

Epidemiology

The infection is endemic worldwide and primarily affects the 6-to10-year age group. Infections occur predominately in the spring, with mumps virus infection being the commonest cause of aseptic meningitis during this time period. Approximately 85 per cent of exposed susceptible contacts become infected, but 25 to 40 per cent of infections are asymptomatic. Seroepidemiologic surveys indicate that 80 to 90 per cent of adults have evidence of prior mumps virus infection. Virus is transmitted by infective salivary secretions and possibly by urine. Oral secretions contain virus for about six days before onset of parotitis until as long as two weeks afterwards. Viruria may persist for two to three weeks. The incubation period ranges from two to four weeks. Symptomatology coincides with onset of viremia, and multiple organ systems may be subclinically seeded with virus. Direct spread from the respiratory tract to the parotid gland is also a possibility.

Clinical aspects

Onset of parotitis is typically sudden and may or may not be preceded by non-specific prodromal symptoms. Often there are few systemic manifestations of disease. The parotid swelling usually resolves within a week. Twenty to thirty-five per cent of postpubertal men who acquire mumps develop epididymo-orchitis within one to two weeks following parotitis. Only 1 to 12 per cent of cases are bilateral; hence sterility is an uncommon late sequela. Pancreatitis complicating mumps may be difficult to diagnose, since both conditions may cause hyperamylasemia. A lipase determination in this instance may be helpful.

Mumps virus is a very common cause of benign aseptic meningitis. Approximately half of patients with mumps show CSF pleocytosis, but meningeal symptoms are less common. Conversely, 30 to 40 per cent of proven cases of mumps meningitis are unassociated with parotitis. Encephalitis is an unusual complication, but may lead to a variety of neurologic sequelae. Other rare CNS complications include a mild poliomyelitis-like syndrome, transverse myelitis, cerebellar ataxia, and Guillain-Barré syndrome. Additional complications include oophoritis, myocarditis, hepatitis, thrombocytopenic purpura, lower respiratory tract disease, polyarthritis, and thyroiditis.

Laboratory diagnosis

The typical parotitis syndrome can be diagnosed clinically with great accuracy by physicians and laymen alike. Diagnosis by viral isolation or serologic techniques is most useful when the patient presents with a non-parotitis syndrome in which mumps virus infection is part of the differential diagnosis. Viral isolation from blood, CSF, oropharyngeal secretions, and urine confirms the diagnosis of current mumps virus infection. Best isolation results are obtained by using primary monkey kidney cell cultures. Characteristic CPE with large syncytial giant cells (Fig. 52-18) may or may not be produced; therefore, hemadsorption, employing guinea pig erythrocytes, should be performed periodically as described for the parainfluenza viruses. Specific identification is based on hemadsorption inhibition using mumps virus antiserum.

Complement fixation (CF), neutralization, hemagglutination inhibition (HI), and radioimmunoassay (Daugharty, 1973) methods have

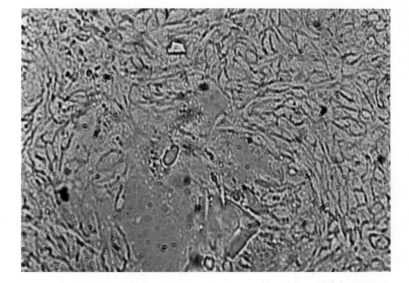

Figure 52–18. Typical syncytial CPE produced by mumps virus in RMK cells. (From Person, D. A., Smith, T. F., and Herrmann, E. C., Jr.: Mayo Clin. Proc., 46:544–548, 1971.)

all been employed for serologic diagnosis. The HI method is simple, but too non-specific, because of cross-reactions with other paramyxoviruses, to be generally useful. The CF method is most widely used. The S and V antigens elicit characteristic specific CF antibody responses. The S antibody develops early, rises rapidly, and often peaks within the first week of symptoms. Afterward the S antibody declines to undetectable levels within 6 to 12 months. The V antibody rises more slowly, peaking in 2 to 3 weeks, and then usually persists for a lifetime. Therefore, an acute serum demonstrating an elevated S antibody titer suggests acute or very recent disease. For definitive diagnosis of acute disease, a fourfold or greater change in antibody (usually V antibody) is required. Serum demonstrating only a V antibody titer indicates past infection and immunity. The V antigen elicits a delayed hypersensitivity reaction when used as an intradermal skin test in persons previously infected with mumps virus. However, the skin test has not been shown to be sufficiently specific to be used as a sole criterion for immunity or susceptibility.

MEASLES VIRUS

Measles virus or morbillivirus (previously called rubeola) has man as the only known natural host, but serologically related viruses infect animals, e.g., canine distemper and rinderpest viruses. Infection is characterized by the formation of large syncytial giant cells in tissues both *in vivo* and *in vitro*. Clinical measles has been known since antiquity but was not distinguished from other exanthems until the seventeenth century. Transmissibility of disease to man and non-human primates, by blood and oropharyngeal secretions, from measles patients was demonstrated in the early 1900's, but tissue culture isolation was not achieved until 1954.

Epidemiology

Prior to widespread vaccination practices, measles epidemics occurred approximately every two years, usually in the late winter and spring, and primarily affected children. The disease is highly contagious, with secondary infections occurring in approximately 90 per cent of susceptible contacts, and the clinical attack rate of infected persons is greater than 95 per cent. By age 20 years about 95 per cent of persons in populous areas have been infected. The disease is communicable for five days before to five days after onset of the rash, and the infection is transmitted by oropharyngeal secretions introduced into the respiratory tract. The incubation period ranges from 7 to 18 days.

In 1963 both an attenuated live and a killed measles vaccine were licensed. The killed vaccine proved less effective, and children who received this vaccine were at risk of developing an atypical, severe form of disease with severe hypersensitivity manifestations following subsequent exposure to live wild measles virus. However, following widespread use of the live attenuated vaccine there has been approximately a 90 per cent reduction in reported cases of measles. There is now, however, a large group of susceptible older children and young adults who are experiencing outbreaks of measles. The live attenuated vaccine is recommended for all children 12 months of age or older, as well as potentially susceptible older children. Revaccination is also recommended for children previously immunized with killed vaccine or those who received immune serum globulin simultaneously with a previous vaccination.

Clinical manifestations

There is an initial three- to four-day prodromal period characterized by malaise, high fever, rhinitis, cough, and conjunctivitis. The pathognomonic Koplik spots appear on the buccal mucosa one to two days before onset of the red maculopapular rash which begins on the forehead and extends downward over the face, trunk, and lower extremities. The rash resolves in the same sequence, lasting approximately six days.

Infections may extend into the lower respiratory tract, causing croup, bronchitis, bronchiolitis, and rarely a giant cell interstitial pneumonia, particularly in immunocompromised children. Other complications include myocarditis, thrombocytopenia, mesenteric lymphadenitis with abdominal pain, and superimposed bacterial pneumonia and otitis media. Encephalomyelitis occurs in about 0.1 per cent of cases. Subacute sclerosing panencephalitis (SSPE), also called Dawson's encephalitis or inclusion encephalitis, is a rare later CNS complication.

Transplacental infection results in an increased frequency of abortion and stillbirth, but a suggested increased incidence of congenital malformation lacks confirmation.

Laboratory diagnosis

Clinical diagnosis of a typical case of measles can be made with a high degree of accuracy, but demonstration of the virus or seroconversion is necessary to confirm the diagnosis. Best isolation results are achieved from specimens taken within the first few days of illness. Virus is present in the peripheral blood buffy coat during the first day of illness, in nasopharyngeal secretions during the first four to five days, and may be present in urinary sediment for as long as one week. Measles virus grows slowly in primary monkey or human kidney and human amnion cell cultures, producing characteristic multinucleate, syncytial giant cells after 7 to 10 days of incubation. The absence of hemadsorption with non-simian erythrocytes is useful to distinguish this virus from other paramyxoviruses, especially mumps. Identification is based on neutralization of cytopathic effects (CPE) with measles virus antiserum or by specific immunofluorescence of infected cell cultures. The presence of virus is diagnostic.

Hemagglutination inhibition (HI), neutralization (NA), and complement fixation (CF) methods have all been employed for the sero-

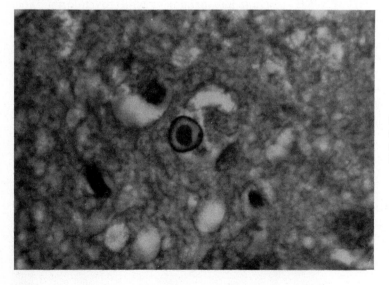

Figure 52–19. Cowdry type A intranuclear inclusion from a case of subacute sclerosing panencephalitis. (Courtesy of John Budinger, M.D.).

diagnosis of measles. The HI test is usually the most rapid and useful method, having sensitivity and specificity comparable to NA and greater than CF. Antibody detected by all three methods appears within one to two days after the onset of rash and titers peak ten days to two weeks later. Antibody titers decline very gradually, making serodiagnosis after the first week of illness often difficult. The presence of specific IgM antibody also documents recent infection. Serodiagnosis is based on a fourfold rise in antibody titer.

The diagnosis of suspected SSPE is supported by extremely high serum and CSF measles antibody titers. Titers in this disease are characteristically tenfold greater than titers in normal patients one year following typical measles. A serum HI titer of 1:1000 or greater in the proper clinical setting and without a history of recent measles is suggestive of SSPE; detectable CSF antibody further supports the diagnosis. Histologically, there are Cowdry type A intranuclear inclusions within neurons and glial cells of the brain (Fig. 52-19).

During measles, giant cells are characteristically formed at many sites of infection, including the skin, buccal mucosa, respiratory and occasionally urinary epithelium and within reticuloendothelial cells of lymph nodes or spleen (Warthin-Finkeldey cells). During active disease, histologic examination or indirect immunofluorescent staining of affected tissues, tissue scrapings, or urinary sediment may reveal the characteristic giant cells or antigen.

RUBELLA VIRUS

Clinical rubella (three-day measles or German measles) was first described in Germany about 200 years ago and was called *roetheln*. In the late 1930's the viral agent was transmitted to man and monkeys, but the virus was not isolated *in vitro* until 1962. In tissue culture systems used at that time the rubella virus produced no cytopathic effect, and hence was undetected until the interference or exclusion technique for identification was devised.

Rubella virus infection causes a benign, usually mild exanthematous illness when acquired postnatally; however, severe congenital anomalies can be produced in infants following maternal infection in the first trimester.

Epidemiology

Major epidemics of rubella have occurred in 6- to 10-year cycles, in the winter and spring, primarily involving school age children; however, this pattern has been altered by the widespread use of the live attenuated vaccine. The disease has now become more common in older children and adolescents.

Rubella is probably transmitted by inhalation of infective droplets into the oropharynx. It is highly communicable, but less so than measles infections. Approximately 15 to 20 per cent of adults have escaped infection. The overall clinical attack rate is about 30 per cent (range of estimate, 13 to 60 per cent). The incubation period varies from two to three weeks with an average of about 18 days, and the contagious period extends from a week before to a week after onset of the rash.

The incidence of congenital birth defects varies with time of maternal infection. Estimates of risk of fetal malformations following infection in the first month of gestation vary from 50 to 80 per cent, decreasing to approximately 25 per cent in the second month and 17 per cent in the third month. The overall risk following exposure in the first trimester is about 25 per cent. The incidence of viral excretion by congenitally infected infants declines with age, but some still excrete virus for up to three years, serving as reservoirs of infection.

Vaccination with live attenuated virus results in antibody production in approximately 95 per cent of recipients, but the degree and duration of immunity have not been completely evaluated. Virus can be detected in the oropharynx for as long as four weeks after vaccination; however, this vaccine strain is apparently not communicable and therefore may be administered to children who have contact with pregnant women. The vaccine strain is considered potentially teratogenic, and has been isolated from abortuses of women inadvertently vaccinated during the first trimester of pregnancy. For this reason, the vaccine should never be given to a pregnant woman or a woman who might become pregnant within two to three months following vaccination.

Clinical aspects

Infection acquired by children is a mild disease characterized by generalized lymphade-

5

Table 52-16. FREQUENCY OF MAJOR
FINDINGS IN SYMPTOMATIC
CONGENITAL RUBELLA INFECTIONS

FREQUENCY	MANIFESTATIONS
75%+	Congenital heart disease (patent ductus arteriosus, pulmonary stenosis, etc.)
50-75%	Eyes—cataracts, chorioretinitis, cloudy cornea, microphthalmia, glaucoma
75%+	Deafness
30-40%	Hepatosplenomegaly
40-60%	Thrombocytopenic purpura
40-60%	Intrauterine growth retardation

nopathy which is particularly prominent in the posterior cervical, suboccipital and posterior auricular locations. This is followed by a macular rash which varies in intensity, starting on the forehead and face and spreading downward over the trunk and extremities. It usually lasts for three days. An infected older individual may have prodromal symptoms of malaise, headache, and fever. Complications are few but include postinfectious encephalitis, thrombocytopenia, arthritis, and arthralgias. Since many other infectious agents can produce rubella-like illness, the proof of rubella infection can only be established with certainty by laboratory studies.

Congenital rubella traditionally was thought to be manifest by congenital heart disease (patent ductus arteriosus, ventricular septal defect, and pulmonary stenosis), corneal clouding, cataracts, chorioretinitis, microcephaly, mental retardation, and deafness. Following the 1964 epidemic, additional manifestations were described, leading to the term "expanded rubella syndrome." These include hepatosplenomegaly, thrombocytopenic purpura, intrauterine growth retardation, interstitial pneumonia, myocarditis, and metaphyseal bone lesions. Table 52-16 outlines the relative frequencies of the major findings in congenital infections. A delayed onset progressive panencephalitis has also been described as a result of congenital rubella (Townsend, 1975).

Laboratory diagnosis

The diagnosis of current or remote rubella infection is important in two circumstances: (1) diagnosis of congenital rubella, and (2) determination of immune status of women of reproductive age. Serodiagnosis of acute infection is indicated in a susceptible pregnant woman possibly exposed to rubella. Attempts to isolate the virus are most often indicated for the diagnosis of congenital infection, in which case viral excretion from the oropharynx and feces may continue for up to three years. Following postnatally acquired infection, virus can be isolated from the oropharynx for about seven days before to approximately two weeks after appearance of the rash and from the blood for a few days prior to onset of the rash. It may also be isolated occasionally from the feces, urine, and placental and fetal tissues of abortuses.

The virus can be grown in several continuous cell lines, including rabbit kidney (RK-13), rabbit cornea (SIRC), and green monkey kidney (VERO) in which microfoci of CPE have been described, but the usual way to demonstrate a rubella isolate is by the interference or exclusion method. By this technique primary African green monkey kidney cells are inoculated with a specimen, and after 7 to 10 days the cell culture and uninoculated control tubes are challenged by inoculation with another virus, usually an echovirus, and observed for the CPE characteristic of the superinfecting virus. Presence of CPE in control tubes, and absence of CPE in the inoculated tubes indicate the possible presence of rubella virus. Absolute identification requires specific neutralization of interference with rubella antiserum. The presence of virus is diagnostic for congenital infection; however, the vaccination history must be considered in interpreting isolates from older infants or children. A reliable way to differentiate wild from vaccine strains has not been developed.

Serologic techniques, usually quicker and simpler than viral isolation, are used primarily for the diagnosis of postnatally acquired infection and for determining immune status. Both hemagglutination inhibition (HI) and complement fixation methods may be employed. The virologic and serologic sequence of events following infection can be seen in Figure 52-20. HI antibodies usually become detectable about 14 to 17 days after primary exposure or about 2 to 3 days after onset of the rash. Peak titers are reached in about 2 weeks, slowly decline for a few years, and then persist for life. CF antibodies demonstrate a slower onset and peak, and then become undetectable after a few years. Neutralization and immunofluorescence tests are demanding and therefore not commonly performed.

The presence of any detectable HI titer in

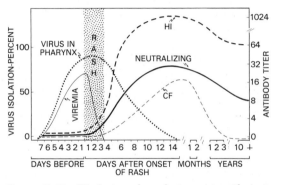

Figure 52-20. Virologic and serologic events with acute postnatal rubella infection. (From Krugman, S., and Ward, R. A.: Infectious Diseases of Children, 4th ed. St. Louis, The C. V. Mosby Co., 1968.)

the absence of disease indicates previous infection and hence immunity to reinfection. However, re-exposure to rubella virus has resulted in an asymptomatic anamnestic rise in antibody titers, but viremia has not been demonstrated to accompany this phenomenon. Therefore, a fetus would appear to be at little or no risk under these circumstances. A rubella HI titer is often routinely performed as part of a prenatal workup of pregnant women. If HI antibody is undetected, the woman is considered potentially susceptible and is followed accordingly. However, if a pregnant woman first comes to medical attention after a history of exposure to possible rubella, a HI titer done within the first two weeks after exposure will accurately reflect the woman's immune status prior to exposure. If HI antibodies are detected at any titer within this time frame, risk of damage to the fetus is assumed to be negligible. If no HI antibody is detected, a subsequent sample two weeks later should be obtained to determine whether a fourfold rise in HI antibody titer has occurred. If the woman has recently had a clinical syndrome compatible with rubella, it may be too late to demonstrate an antibody rise by HI methods, but CF antibodies, which develop more slowly, may still demonstrate a significant titer rise. The presence of specific IgM antibodies by indirect immunofluorescence or other methods may also be useful in diagnosing primary disease. It must be emphasized that paired sera should always be examined simultaneously in the same test run if reliable interpretations of quantitative antibody responses are to be made.

RABIES

Rabies is a worldwide zoonotic disease, affecting a wide variety of warm-blooded mammals and bats. Man is usually infected by contact with saliva or infected tissues through skin wounds (usually bites), and occasionally via the respiratory route by inhaling highly infectious aerosols. The incubation period in man and animals is usually 1 to 3 months, but can range from 10 days to 16 months or perhaps longer. There have been only three documented human survivors of clinical rabies to date—two infected with wild ("street") virus, and one laboratory worker presumably infected by an attenuated, live vaccine strain.

Because of the potential danger of lethal infection, and the obvious public health importance attached to this disease, it is recommended that *all rabies diagnostic work involving animals and humans be performed at a public health laboratory with special isolation facilities and trained, rabies-immunized personnel.*

In humans, the diagnosis is suggested by a history of possible or proved exposure (not always elicited), and a prodromal phase of non-specific complaints, hyperesthesia, and emotional changes progressing in two to four days to an "excitation" phase. This phase is characterized by increasing emotional lability, multiple cranial nerve weaknesses, spasmodic contractures of the muscles of swallowing and respiration, particularly when the patient attempts to swallow liquids (hydrophobia), and increased muscle tone. This is followed by progression to flaccid muscle paralysis, coma, and usually death.

The diagnosis of rabies in humans can be confirmed by culture, immunofluorescent, histologic, and serologic methods.

Culture of 20 per cent suspensions of brain biopsy or postmortem brain tissue is done by intracerebral inoculation of one- to two-day old mice, and observing for neurologic signs or death for 28 days. Virus has also been isolated from salivary secretions, myocardium, skeletal muscles, lung, liver, and kidney in fatal human cases.

Direct immunofluorescence to demonstrate the antigen is also a reliable diagnostic method and may be used on brain smears and corneal scrapings; it has also been reported that antigen may be detected by examination of skin biopsy material taken from the nape of the neck.

5

Intracytoplasmic inclusions in neurons, measuring 2 to 10 μm in diameter (Negri bodies), can be demonstrated in fixed brain sections or impression smears by staining with eosin and methylene blue, Giemsa, or Seller's stains.

Serologic diagnosis can be made by mouse-neutralization, indirect fluorescent antibody, fluorescent focus inhibition, or CF methods. Such testing is important, not only for rabies diagnosis, but to determine the adequacy of antibody responses in either pre- or postexposure courses of immunization. Rabies antibody testing and advice concerning immunization can be obtained from the Center for Disease Control through individual state health department laboratories.

HEPATITIS

The clinical diagnosis of viral hepatitis is usually not difficult, supported by elevations of SGOT or SGPT enzymes and bilirubin, a moderate increase in the serum alkaline phosphatase, and variable prolongation of the prothrombin time. While toxic, metabolic, obstructive, and bacterial causes need to be ruled out, the clinician is usually able to narrow the possibilities down to a viral etiology. The problem then is, which virus?

A number of different viral agents can cause acute hepatitis, either as an isolated infection or as part of a systemic illness. These include Epstein-Barr virus, cytomegalovirus, adenoviruses, enteroviruses, and yellow fever, as well as some others. However, the majority of cases of hepatitis are due to three different agents, which will be discussed in further detail. These are hepatitis A, hepatitis B, and a third candidate virus, called "non-A, non-B hepatitis" (also referred to by some authors as "hepatitis C").

While the clinical behavior of these three viruses is usually indistinguishable, they do have some differentiating characteristics, summarized in Table 52-17. There is no cross-immunity between these agents, and none have been grown in culture systems other than humans and other primates. It has been increasingly recognized that specific etiologic diagnosis in individual cases has important implications, both in terms of patient management and in epidemiologic control.

HEPATITIS A

Hepatitis A is ubiquitous, and is often associated with subclinical infection. Based on serosurveys, approximately 40 to 45 per cent of adults have evidence of prior infection. Outbreaks are not uncommon, often involving family members or groups exposed to a common source of food or water contamination. The illness tends to be milder and of shorter duration than hepatitis B, but fatalities have been recorded.

Hepatitis A probably rarely if ever spreads by parenteral mechanisms, even though transient viremia has been noted during infection. There is also no evidence that either a chronic viremic or intestinal carrier state exists. Cases are generally considered infectious from one to two weeks before the onset of abnormal enzyme levels to two weeks after the peak levels have been attained.

In the past, hepatitis A has been diagnosed after hepatitis B infection was excluded by appropriate laboratory tests; however, with the recognition that non-A, non-B hepatitis

Table 52-17. CHARACTERISTICS OF HEPATITIS VIRUSES

| | HEPATITIS AGENT | | |
CHARACTERISTIC	A	B	Non-A, Non-B
Agent type	Picornavirus (tentative)	Unclassified DNA virus	Unknown
Culture systems	Man, subhuman primates	Man, subhuman primates	Man, subhuman primates
Primary modes of transmission	Fecal-oral, urine, ?respiratory	Parenteral, sexual	Parenteral
Epidemiology	Sharp outbreaks common	Often sporadic	Sporadic
Incubation period	2-6 weeks	6 weeks-6 months	2-15 weeks
Chronic carriage	Not shown	Yes—chronic viremia	Yes—chronic viremia
Chronic hepatic disease	No	Yes	Probable
Gamma-globulin prophylaxis	Effective	Possibly effective	Not known

may be commoner than originally thought, this assumption becomes less tenable. Hepatitis A virus antigen has been identified in feces, and occasionally in serum, by somewhat laborious electron microscopic and radioimmunoassay methods, but these are not readily adapted to the clinical laboratory.

More recently, serologic tests utilizing antigen extracts from infected marmoset livers or infectious human feces have been devised. A CF test or a modification of the CF test, the immune adherence hemagglutination assay (IAHA), have both been used to demonstrate antibody titer responses to hepatitis A in paired sera obtained two or more weeks apart. The IAHA is based on the principle that human "O" erythrocytes are aggregated in the specific antigen-antibody-complement reaction (Miller, 1975). This test shows particular promise for clinical application.

HEPATITIS B

Initially thought to be the major cause of post-transfusion hepatitis (serum hepatitis), hepatitis B has now assumed major public health importance in a number of other situations. In the United States, 0.5 to 0.9 per cent of adults are potentially infectious carriers of the virus, and 8 to 12 per cent of adults are antibody-positive, indicating a relative ubiquity of the agent. These rates increase to significantly higher levels in some groups, such as individuals repeatedly exposed to blood or blood products (surgeons, dentists, immunosuppressed patients, and patients and staff in hemodialysis units), institutionalized groups, illicit drug users, and homosexual males. While parenteral infection is considered to be the most important mode of spread, infections can be acquired by rather casual contact with infective blood or serum, whereby inoculation may occur through often trivial or even unnoticed breaks in skin or mucous membranes. Sexual transmission is also strongly suggested, particularly by the studies of male homosexuals, and arthropod spread (mosquitos, bedbugs) is suspected in some tropical areas. All ages are susceptible; maternal transmission to the fetus or newborn is recognized, and frequently leads to chronic infection of the infant. While nearly all body secretions have been shown to contain the viral surface antigen (e.g., saliva, urine, semen, sweat, and colostrum), it still appears that the most dangerous source of infection is blood

and its byproducts. The infectivity titer of human serum which contains the surface antigen (HB_sAg) has been shown to be as high as $10^{7.5}$ ID_{50}/ml in primates, and very likely is similar in humans. The implications for the laboratory are clear: all bloods and serums must be handled with great care to avoid spillage or aerosolization, and disposal should be done so as not to endanger others who might come into contact with these samples.

Hepatitis B infection can be severe and prolonged, in contrast to the usual hepatitis A-associated illnesses. The usual course of infection is shown in Figure 52-21. After exposure, and approximately 1 to 7 weeks before illness or enzyme elevations appear, the viral surface antigen (HB_sAg) is detectable in the blood. The antigenemia persists for 1 to 12 weeks, then usually disappears after symptoms and laboratory evidence of hepatic dysfunction have resolved. CF antibody to the viral "core" antigen (anti-HB_c) usually appears at the time enzyme elevations are first seen, and disappears within one to two years after antigenemia is no longer detectable. Antibody to the surface antigen (anti-HB_s) usually appears later, sometimes being delayed by 6 to 12 months after the acute episode. It appears to be relatively protective against reinfection. Other findings include the frequent detection of complete infectious virions (HB virus, formerly called Dane particles) and HB virus-associated DNA polymerase during the active phase of disease (Robinson, 1976). Another antigen, HB_eAg, has also been described, which is sometimes detected in acute serum as well as in chronic carriers and seems associated with a higher degree of infectivity (Sher-

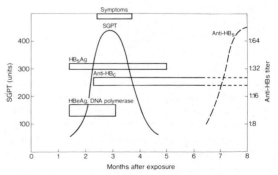

Figure 52-21. Typical course of acute hepatitis B infection.

lock, 1976; reviewed also by Robinson, 1976).

In some individuals, HB$_s$Ag is not eliminated, and antigenemia can persist indefinitely (chronic infection). In these patients, anti-HB$_c$, DNA polymerase activity, and sometimes HB$_e$Ag or antibody to HB$_e$ (anti-HB$_e$) will also persist, and anti-HB$_s$ is not detectable. These persons are not only potentially infectious to others, but can go on to develop either chronic persistent hepatitis (generally considered a benign, asymptomatic condition) or the more aggressive chronic active hepatitis, which may progress to cirrhosis. The various possible results of hepatitis B infection are illustrated in Figure 52–22. This demonstrates the importance of establishing whether or not a patient has hepatitis B, as well as to obtain appropriate follow-up to determine what the individual prognosis might be in proven cases. (See also Chaps. 11 and 38.)

Hepatitis B infection can also lead to extrahepatic manifestations. These can take the form of a serum sickness syndrome during the prodrome of an acute infection, or immune complex vasculitis, affecting a variety of organs and tissues, in chronic infections (Duffy, 1976).

The primary laboratory tests for diagnosis are those designed to detect HB$_s$Ag in the serum. These are used to detect active infections as well as to screen potential blood donors. Of these, immunodiffusion, counterimmunoelectrophoresis, complement fixation, and radioimmunoassay (RIA) have all been used. The relative sensitivities of these tests for detection of HB$_s$Ag are approximately 1, 10, 100, and 1000, respectively. Reversed passive hemagglutination, using antibody-sensitized sheep, turkey, or human red blood cells has also been used as a rapid screening test, with a sensitivity claimed to be near that of RIA (Vandervelde, 1974) but false positive results have been somewhat of a problem in many laboratories.

Our current preference is the so-called "third-generation" RIA test, which utilizes a "sandwich" principle. Plastic beads coated with guinea pig antibody are placed in tubes, and patient serum is added and incubated. If HB$_s$Ag is present, this is fixed to the antibody. After washing, antibody tagged with iodine-125 is added; it will bind to any HB$_s$Ag on the bead, creating an antibody-antigen-tagged antibody "sandwich" which can be detected by counting on a gamma scintillation detector.

This test will detect nearly all cases of acute hepatitis B and most chronic carriers. It has been suggested that adding a CF or RIA test to detect anti-HB$_c$ will enhance the sensitivity of detection, particularly for chronic carriers, but it is not clear that cost-benefit ratios justify adding this to a routine screening program.

Serologic testing for anti-HB$_s$ is usually not helpful for diagnosis, since the antibody often appears weeks to months after antigenemia has subsided. It can be detected rather simply by passive hemagglutination of antigen-sensitized red blood cells or by RIA. Such testing is primarily useful in determining past infection and possible immunity in individuals who may have been exposed to infection, or who are likely to work in situations where exposure risks are high, e.g., hemodialysis unit personnel.

HB$_e$Ag and anti-HB$_e$ can be detected by immunoprecipitation, such as the Ouchterlony method. While there may be prognostic implications of such detection, the sensitivity of such testing is not yet precisely determined, and it cannot yet be strongly recommended that these be sought in a routine setting.

There are also antigenic determinants of HB$_s$Ag that can be discerned with specific antisera. These include the "a" determinant, which is group-specific and found in all HB$_s$Ag samples, and subdeterminants, such as "d," "y," "w," and "r," which are type-specific. In all, there may be as many as 18 such subdeterminants. These are not clinically useful, but subtyping does occasionally play a very helpful role in epidemiologic investigations. Such testing is available in special situations by

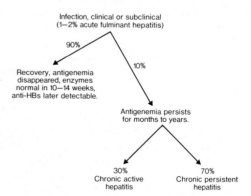

Figure 52–22. Outcome of hepatitis B infection.

consultation with the Center for Disease Control through state health laboratories.

NON-A, NON-B HEPATITIS

Until recently, most viral hepatitis that could not be proved to be associated with hepatitis B, cytomegalovirus, or Epstein-Barr virus infection has been presumed to be due to hepatitis A. With the advent of specific diagnostic methods for all these other agents, this has been shown to be an erroneous assumption. Non-A, non-B hepatitis (or "hepatitis C") has been shown to be quite common. It is estimated that as many as 90 per cent of the cases of post-transfusion hepatitis now seen in the United States may be related to this agent. Furthermore, chronic antigenemic carrier states may exist and may be associated with chronic active hepatitis. Sporadic cases have also been documented without known exposure to blood or blood products.

The diagnosis of non-A, non-B hepatitis is currently made only by excluding other known causes of hepatitis by appropriate laboratory tests. Nothing is currently known of the nature of the infectious agent, or even whether a heterogeneous group of viruses may be involved. Similarly, the epidemiology is as yet obscure, except for the known risk of transmission via transfusion. The disease produced is somewhat comparable to hepatitis A, usually being relatively mild, but the risks of chronic carriage and possible progressive liver disease are of great concern.

VIRAL GASTROENTERITIS AGENTS

Gastroenteritis accounts for approximately 12 per cent of all pediatric hospital admissions and is second only to the common cold as a cause of disease in infants and children. Overall, only approximately 30 per cent of cases in the United States and western Europe can be associated with bacterial pathogens. A viral etiology was first postulated in 1931, but studies in the 1940's attempting to demonstrate the communicability of the disease by using bacteria-free stool filtrates for oral ingestion by animals and human volunteers gave variable results.

Enteroviruses and adenoviruses have been suggested as possible etiologic agents of diarrhea, but subsequent studies have failed to show significantly different rates of isolation of these viruses from healthy controls versus patients with diarrhea.

With the use of immune-electron microscopy (IEM), Kapikian (1972) demonstrated 27 nm virus particles (later called the Norwalk agent) resembling parvoviruses in diarrheal stools and etiologically associated these with an acute non-bacterial gastroenteritis syndrome. Subsequently, several other parvovirus-like agents which were antigenically unrelated to the Norwalk agent have also been detected in diarrhea outbreaks. Later, 70 nm virus particles resembling reoviruses but antigenically different were demonstrated in duodenal mucosa by negative staining electron microscopy. This same virus was subsequently repeatedly demonstrated with high frequency in feces from patients with acute non-bacterial gastroenteritis, while it was consistently absent from healthy controls. This reovirus-like agent was subsequently called duovirus, orbivirus, and rotavirus. The most recent recommendation is to use the term rotavirus. It is possible that several antigenic types involve humans. Neither the parvovirus-like agents nor the rotaviruses can be reliably grown in tissue cultures. In addition to the above viruses, extensive electron microscopic studies of feces from children with non-bacterial gastroenteritis have revealed several additional candidate viruses: "minireovirus," morphologically similar to reoviruses but only about 30 nm in diameter; "adeno-like" viruses and "astroviruses," measuring about 28 to 30 nm in diameter and having a star-shaped periphery (Appleton, 1975; Middleton, 1977). The etiologic significance of these agents is still unclear. Coronavirus-like agents have also been suggested as possible etiologic agents (Caul, 1975). Of these agents, the rotavirus appears to be the most frequent cause of gastroenteritis. It is estimated that between 60 and 80 per cent of cases in infants and young children are due to this agent, and parvovirus-like agents are the next most common.

Epidemiology and clinical aspects

The rotavirus is associated with sporadic, moderate to severe diarrhea occurring most often in the 3-to-23-month age group, primarily during the winter. The incubation period is estimated to be 72 hours or greater. The diarrhea lasts 2 to 11 days and may be associated with mild to moderate vomiting for 1 to 5 days and fever for 2 to 4 days. Dehydration requiring hospitalization frequently occurs. When an

5

infant with this disease is hospitalized, strict isolation techniques are mandatory because of the high incidence of nosocomial infection in children on the same ward. One seroepidemiologic survey (Gomez-Barreto, 1976) revealed that about 60 per cent of the 6-month to 4-year age group, 30 per cent of those 4 to 10 years, 50 to 60 per cent of those 10 to 30 years, and 45 per cent of those over 30 years of age had complement fixing antibodies to the rotavirus. The significance of serum antibody is unknown because reinfection apparently can occur in the presence of antibodies.

The parvovirus-like agents cause an explosive, rapidly spreading epidemic disease manifested primarily by nausea, vomiting, abdominal cramps, malaise, and a mild to moderate diarrhea, with complete recovery usually with 24 to 48 hours. This disease can affect infants, children, and adults and is more prevalent from September to March. The incubation period is estimated to be 48 hours, and reinfection in the presence of humoral immunity may occur.

Laboratory diagnosis and interpretation

The clinical syndromes and epidemiology of these virus infections are quite helpful in suggesting the correct etiology, but definitive diagnosis requires demonstration of the virus. These viruses do not grow in tissue culture; therefore, direct electron microscopic examination of fluid extracts of diarrheal stools which have been negatively stained (Fig. 52–23) is the usual way to demonstrate their presence. However, an enzyme-linked immunosorbent assay (Yolken, 1977) and radioimmunoassay techniques have been developed for detection of the rotavirus. During convalescent stages virus is usually not detectable, further strengthening the diagnostic association of the agents with acute disease.

Complement fixation (CF) has been used to study antibody to the rotavirus. The antigen is prepared from stool filtrates of infected persons or calves infected with an antigenically similar virus. CF antibody titers have been shown to rise by fourfold or greater following acute rotavirus infections, but this is a variable observation. Furthermore, the significance of humoral immunity to this agent is unknown.

The usual method for demonstrating antibody to the parvovirus-like agents is by immune electron microscopy (Kapikian, 1972) which was used initially to demonstrate the virus in stools and to relate the agent serologically to acute disease. Reinfection frequently occurs in individuals with humoral antibodies, which questions their importance in disease prevention. There appear to be two kinds of immunity to the parvovirus-like agents: a short-term immunity which appears protective for one to two months and longer-term immunity lasting at least two to four years (Parrino, 1977). However, both forms of immunity appear to be imperfect and the mechanisms of each are unknown.

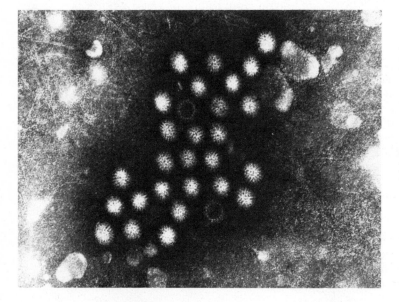

Figure 52–23. Rotavirus particles demonstrated by direct electron microscopy of diarrheal stool negatively stained with 2 per cent phosphotungstic acid. (Courtesy of Dr. Claire Payne.)

OTHER, LESS COMMONLY ENCOUNTERED VIRAL AGENTS

REOVIRUSES

Originally identified as ECHO virus type 10, reoviruses are now known to be double-stranded RNA viruses, totally unrelated to enteroviruses. They have been perhaps appropriately named, since they can be found in the respiratory and enteric tracts of humans and other mammals, and their association with disease in humans is still largely obscure. These features led to the term "respiratory-enteric orphans."

Reoviruses have been frequently isolated from healthy subjects, as well as from infants and children with fevers and exanthems or diarrhea. (These viruses should not be confused with the reovirus-like rotaviruses described in the section on gastroenteritis). There have also been isolated reports of encephalitis, hepatitis, and pneumonia associated with reovirus infections, and virus has been isolated from affected tissues in some of these cases. Nevertheless, their overall role and importance in human disease remains uncertain.

Three serotypes are known to infect humans (types 1, 2, and 3). They grow well in a variety of cell types, with rhesus monkey kidney cells being most commonly used. Cytopathic effects are often slow to develop, usually taking 10 to 21 days, and often appear only as a granular, non-specific degeneration. Serial passages of cultures are often necessary, and staining of the infected tissue culture cells is often helpful to distinguish the typical small cytoplasmic inclusions in a perinuclear array. Reoviruses will agglutinate human "O" erythrocytes, and identification of isolates as well as serologic determination of antibody response can be made by HI testing or by neutralization.

LYMPHOCYTIC CHORIOMENINGITIS VIRUS

Lymphocytic choriomeningitis virus is an arenavirus that is usually transmitted to humans from chronically infected rodents, either by aerosol, fomites, or contact with infected tissues. In the United States, most cases have been traced to contact with rodent breeding colonies in research or pet supply centers, and to pet hamsters in the home. The illness is usually febrile and flu-like with myalgia. Occasionally, meningitis or meningoencephalitis will also occur and has been associated with transient hydrocephalus, elevated CSF protein values to 290 mg/dl, and CSF lymphocyte counts to 8300/cu mm.

The diagnosis is suggested by a history of rodent contact. The virus can be isolated in the early stages of disease by intracerebral injection of CSF and whole blood into suckling or weanling mice or young guinea pigs. Serodiagnosis is most commonly employed, using either CF or indirect immunofluorescence testing.

ARENAVIRUSES ASSOCIATED WITH HEMORRHAGIC FEVERS

These viruses, like lymphocytic choriomeningitis, are thought to be transmitted primarily from infected rodents to humans, although person-to-person transmission has also been documented for most of them. They include the agents of the South American hemorrhagic fevers (Junin and Machupo viruses) and Lassa virus, the cause of Lassa fever in Africa. All are associated with severe, febrile illnesses usually accompanied by hemorrhagic manifestations, neurologic disturbances, bradycardia, and shock. Lassa fever also causes an exudative pharyngitis and frequently myocarditis and hepatitis. Mortality rates are estimated as 10 to 50 per cent for Lassa fever, and 5 to 30 per cent for the others. All are considered highly infectious and extremely dangerous. Imported cases to non-endemic areas have occurred with a significant risk of spread to medical and laboratory personnel. The virus can be isolated during illness from blood, respiratory secretions, urine, feces, and vomitus (Woodruff, 1973).

The diagnosis is suggested primarily by the clinical syndrome and the recent travel history of the patient. If one of these agents is suspected, *strict isolation precautions are mandatory, and public health officials should be immediately notified*. While virus isolation from blood and other sites can be made in suckling mice, hamsters, and some tissue cultures, and CF antibodies can be determined, *these attempts should not be made in a hospital diagnostic laboratory*. All specimens should be forwarded to a well-equipped isolation facility after consultation with public health authorities.

MARBURG AND EBOLA VIRUSES

In 1967, 26 cases of severe hemorrhagic fever occurred in Germany and Yugoslavia among persons caring for a group of African green monkeys imported from central Uganda. A smaller cluster of three cases was documented in South Africa in 1975. The agent in both instances was subsequently identified as Marburg virus.

In 1976, severe outbreaks of hemorrhagic fever appeared in northern Zaire and southern Sudan and were later found to be due to an agent now known as Ebola virus, named after a small river in Zaire.

While both agents produce a similar, highly fatal (30 to 80 per cent mortality) contagious disease and both have a similar physical appearance in cell cultures (filamentous particles averaging 100 nm in diameter and 300 to 1500 nm in length, with budding from cell membranes), each appears to be antigenically distinctive. The ecology and epidemiology of these agents is currently not well understood (Johnson, 1977).

Like the arenavirus-associated hemorrhagic fevers, the travel history of the patient and the hemorrhagic fever syndrome suggest the diagnostic possibilities, and precautions with regard to the patient and handling and processing of specimens are the same. The viruses have been grown in Vero cells (a continuous African green monkey kidney cell line), mice, and guinea pigs, but *this should never be attempted in a hospital diagnostic laboratory.*

RICKETTSIAL INFECTIONS

Rickettsia species are fastidious, obligate intracellular parasites with the exception of *R. quintana.* They are pleomorphic coccobacillary organisms possessing both RNA and DNA and both synthetic and energy-producing enzyme systems. These organisms are characterized by their natural proclivity to infect arthropods and other mammals (except for *R. prowazekii* and *R. quintana*), which serve as vectors and reservoirs of disease for incidental human infection.

Rickettsial disease, especially epidemic typhus, has historically been a major cause of worldwide morbidity and mortality and has been estimated as second only to malaria as a cause of human death from infectious disease. In the early twentieth century, Ricketts, for whom the microorganisms are named, successfully transmitted Rocky Mountain spotted fever, incriminated the wood tick as a vector, and observed the organisms in smears of tick tissue. Shortly thereafter, other rickettsial vectors were incriminated and further transmission studies performed. In 1926, rodents were recognized as natural reservoirs of infections. Brill recognized a mild form of epidemic typhus unassociated with the louse vector in 1910, and Zinsser in 1934 postulated that the disease was a recrudescent form of typhus occurring following stress or declining immunity. This was subsequently confirmed. In 1915 Weil and Felix recognized that agglutinins from typhus fever patients reacted with certain strains of *Proteus* sp., and this discovery lead to the widely used but non-specific Weil-Felix reaction.

The human pathogens can be divided into five antigenic groups: the typhus group, spotted fever group, scrub typhus, Q fever, and trench fever. The species within these groups as well as the epidemiology and natural cycles are outlined in Table 52-18. Rocky Mountain spotted fever (RMSF) and Q fever are the commonest rickettsial diseases in the continental United States, but Brill-Zinsser's disease, murine typhus, and rickettsialpox are also found occasionally.

Organisms enter through the skin or respiratory tract and probably replicate locally during the incubation period. This is followed by a rickettsemia, which coincides with initial symptoms and seeds organisms throughout the vascular system to infect endothelial cells, leading to the characteristic rash. Later, immunologic mechanisms may be important in enhancing vasculitis, and the toxic febrile state may be related to type-specific toxins. Rickettsial diseases in general are characterized by sudden onset of fever, chills, moderate to severe headache, malaise, and a variable degree of prostration and toxicity. In contrast to the other rickettsial infections, there is no rash in Q fever, and pneumonia is found in approximately half of the cases. A rash frequently develops a few days after onset of fever in all rickettsioses except Q fever, which is primarily a lower respiratory illness. An eschar or local skin lesion may be seen at the

Table 52–18. RICKETTSIAL DISEASES OF MAN*

DISEASE		NATURAL CYCLE			TRANSMISSION TO MAN	SEROLOGICAL DIAGNOSIS	
Group and Type	Agent	Geographical Distribution	Arthropod	Mammal		Weil-Felix Reaction	Complement Fixation
Typhus Epidemic	*R. prowazekii*	Worldwide	Body louse	Man	Infected louse feces into broken skin	Positive OX-19	Positive group- and type-specific
Brill's disease	*R. prowazekii*	N. America; Europe	Recurrence years after original attack of epidemic typhus			Usually negative	
Endemic	*R. mooseri*	Worldwide	Flea	Rodents	Infected flea feces into broken skin	Positive OX-19	
Spotted fever Rocky Mountain spotted fever	*R. rickettsii*	Western Hemisphere	Ticks	Wild rodents; dogs	Tick bite	Positive OX-19 OX-2	Positive group- and type-specific
Boutonneuse fever	*R. conori*	Africa; Europe; Middle East; India	Ticks	Wild rodents; dogs	Tick bite	Positive OX-19 OX-2	
Queensland tick typhus	*R. australis*	Australia	Ticks	Marsupials; wild rodents	Tick bite	Positive OX-19 OX-2	
North Asian tick-borne rickettsiosis	*R. sibiricus*	Siberia; Mongolia	Ticks	Wild rodents	Tick bite	Positive OX-19 OX-2	
Rickettsialpox	*R. akari*	North America; Europe	Bloodsucking mite	House mouse and other rodents	Mite bite	Negative	
Scrub typhus	*R. tsutsugamushi*	Asia; Australia; Pacific Islands	Trombiculid mites	Wild rodents	Mite bite	Positive OX-K	Positive in about 50% of patients
Q fever	*C. burnetii*	Worldwide	Ticks	Small mammals; cattle; sheep and goats	Inhalation of dried, infected material	Negative	Positive
Trench fever	*R. quintana*	Europe; Africa; North America	Body louse	Man	Infected louse feces into broken skin	Negative	None available

*From Lennette, E. H., and Schmidt, N. J. (eds.): Diagnostic Procedures for Viral and Rickettsial Infections, 3rd ed. American Public Health Association, New York, 1964, p. 744.

site of initial entry of the organism in rickettsialpox or scrub typhus infections. There is usually prominent lymphadenopathy in the region draining the area of the eschar of scrub typhus.

Epidemic typhus is caused by *R. prowazekii* and the vector is the body louse (*Pediculus humanis*). Man is the only vertebrate host and the disease is maintained in a man-to-louse-to-man cycle. Man is infected by rubbing infected feces deposited by the louse into broken skin. Epidemic typhus may be accompanied by circulatory disturbances, peripheral vascular collapse, and hepatic, renal, and CNS disturbances. Epidemic typhus has not occurred in the United States since the nineteenth century. Brill-Zinsser's disease, the recurrent form, is usually milder, but the disease is characterized by rickettsemia and is communicable to others if the proper vector is present.

Endemic (murine) typhus is caused by *R. mooseri* and the vector is primarily the rat flea (*Xenopsylla cheopis*). Again, disease is transmitted to man by rubbing infected feces from the vector into broken skin. Disease is maintained in nature by small rodents, and man is only an incidental host. This is one of the most benign of the rickettsiosis and occurs in the southeastern and Gulf Coast areas of the United States primarily in the summer and fall.

Scrub typhus is caused by *R. tsutsugamushi*, and a larval mite (usually *Leptotrobidium akamushi* or *L. deliense*) is the vector. Infection is transmitted when the chigger burrows beneath the skin to obtain a tissue fluid meal. Small rodents are the natural hosts, with only incidental human infection. Complications of disease are similar to those of epidemic typhus, but myocarditis more often occurs with scrub typhus. The disease occurs primarily in Asia, India, Australia, and the South Pacific Islands.

Rocky Mountain spotted fever is caused by *R. rickettsii*, and the wood tick (*Dermacentor andersoni*) or the dog tick (*D. variabilis*) are the vectors. Small mammals serve as natural hosts and reservoirs of infection, and man is incidentally infected by the bite of the tick. The disease may be quite severe, with delirium, shock, and renal failure complicating the usual clinical manifestations. The disease occurs throughout the United States and the Western hemisphere.

Rickettsialpox, caused by *R. akari* and transmitted by the bite of a mite vector (*Allodermanyssus sanguineus*) is maintained in nature in small rodents and mice and occasionally infects house mice. It produces a mild, non-fatal, febrile illness lasting about one week, and occurs sporadically in the United States.

Q fever, caused by *Coxiella burnetii*, has an extensive wild and domestic animal host range, and is transmitted in nature by ticks. However, man is infected by inhalation of droplets contaminated by salivary secretions or placental tissues of infected animals. Farm workers and slaughterhouse employees are at greatest hazard for infection, which is characterized by an interstitial pneumonitis. This organism also can cause a subacute bacterial endocarditis. There is no rash, and Weil-Felix agglutinins are not produced. The disease occurs worldwide, including the United States.

Trench fever is caused by *R. quintana*, which has been cultivated *in vitro* on blood agar. This characteristic makes one question the proper classification of this organism. The body louse (*P. humanis*) functions as the vector, and man is the only vertebrate host and reservoir of infection. Trench fever, primarily a disease of the military, is characterized by severe muscle, joint, and bone pains, primarily in the shins, and may puruse a relapsing course with persistent rickettsemia for several years. The disease has occurred in troops in Europe, Africa, and North America.

Prevention of rickettsial diseases has been based primarily on avoidance or elimination of the vector. Vaccines are available for RMSF, epidemic typhus, and Q fever and are recommended for persons in highly endemic areas or those most likely to be exposed, such as persons working in infectious disease laboratories. These preventive measures, coupled with the sensitivity of the rickettsial organisms to the broad spectrum antibiotics tetracycline or chloramphenicol, have reduced the mortality from rickettsioses in developed countries.

Laboratory diagnosis

Isolation of these organisms is extremely hazardous and should be attempted only by experienced, well-equipped reference laboratories. Aseptically collected tissues or whole blood that is flash frozen and maintained at −70°C. or lower during shipment maintain organism viability. Animal or embryonated egg inoculation methods are employed for isolation of *Rickettsia* sp., as well as tissue culture techniques for isolating *R. rickettsii* from blood or ticks (Wike, 1972). Smears of tissues infected *in vivo* or *in vitro* can be specially stained with Giménez, Macchiavello, or Giemsa stains. None of the above stains reliably differentiate these organisms from bacteria. *Rickettsia* sp. are usually seen in the cytoplasm of cells except for *R. rickettsii*, which may also be present within nuclei. Organisms in infected tissues, ticks, and tissue culture cells may also be demonstrated by direct immunofluorescence using specific antisera (Burgdorfer, 1970; Hanon, 1966).

The complement fixation (CF) test is useful for serodiagnosis of nearly all the rickettsioses except scrub typhus, in which mutually exclusive antigenic multiplicity of strains makes CF serodiagnosis too antigenically specific and hence impractical. For the other rickettsioses, CF tests detect partially group-reactive antibodies (see Table 52–18), and hence may not be entirely specific. Therefore, one must use caution in interpretation. Past immunizations and previous exposure in endemic areas may cause persistent low CF antibody titers that are uninterpretable. Nevertheless, the CF test on paired sera is usually the single most useful serodiagnostic tool. CF antibodies first appear one to two weeks after onset of symptoms, and a fourfold or greater titer rise can usually be detected during convalescence. Demonstrations of significant seroconversions in the proper clinical context is diagnostic for rickettsial group infection.

The Weil-Felix reaction depends on agglutination of OX-19, OX-2, of OX-K strains of *Proteus vulgaris* by antibody produced during typhus or spotted fever rickettsial infections. The usual pattern of reactions can be seen in Table 52–19. They vary in sensitivity and are frequently non-specific. False positive results are common, and may be the result of other infections, including urinary tract bacterial infections, leptospirosis, borreliosis, or severe hepatic disease.

Indirect immunofluorescence is an expensive, difficult technique for identifying rick-

Table 52-19   WEIL-FELIX REACTIONS*

RICKETTSIAL DISEASES	MAGNITUDE OF ANTIBODY RESPONSE Proteus Antigens		
	OX-19	OX-2	OX-K
Epidemic typhus (primary)	+ + + +	+	0
Murine typhus	+ + + +	+	0
Rocky Mountain spotted fever and other tick-borne spotted fever group infections	+ + + + +	+ + + +	0
Rickettsialpox	0	0	0
Scrub typhus	0	0	+ + + +
Q fever	0	0	0
Trench fever	0	0	0

*From Lennette, E. H., and Schmidt, N. J. (eds): Diagnostic Procedures for Viral and Rickettsial Infections, 3rd ed. American Public Health Association, New York, 1964, p. 761.

ettsial antibodies, but it shows promise for the diagnosis of scrub typhus infections because the antibody detected by this method is more group-reactive toward the multiple *R. tsutsugamushi* strains.

Rickettsial agglutinin titers may be useful in diagnosis of Q fever. In general, these antibodies appear and rise earlier to higher titer than CF titers, but both may persist for many years afterward. Since antibodies to *C. burneti* do not cross-react with other rickettsia, a significant rise in titer is considered diagnostic (except in recent vaccinees). This would make the test particularly useful for diagnosing subacute endocarditis caused by *C. burnetii*. In general, rickettsial agglutination tests (Fiset, 1969) appear to be more species-specific than the CF tests. This would be particularly useful in identifying murine typhus infection in individuals who have received epidemic typhus vaccine. The method is simple and reproducible, but the antigens used in the agglutination tests are not yet commercially available.

5

CHLAMYDIAL INFECTIONS

Formerly referred to as bedsonia, and originally thought to be viruses because of their obligate intracellular parasitism, the chlamydia are now recognized as a unique, bacte-

ria-like group of organisms. They possess a cell wall, divide by binary fission, contain both RNA and DNA, are unable to grow outside of an animal cell, and are susceptible to a variety

Table 52-20. CHLAMYDIAE AFFECTING HUMANS, AND DISEASES THEY PRODUCE.

GENUS	SPECIES	DISEASE	IMMUNOTYPES INVOLVED
Chlamydia			
	psittaci	Psittacosis (Ornithosis)	
	trachomatis	Trachoma ⎫	A, B, Ba, C
		Inclusion conjunctivitis ⎪	
		Non-gonococcal urethritis ⎪	
		Cervicitis ⎬	D, E, F, G
		Salpingitis ⎪	H, I, J, K
		?Pneumonia in infancy ⎭	
		Lymphogranuloma venereum	L₁, L₂, L₃

of antibiotics. While chlamydia affect a wide range of animal and avian hosts, this discussion will center on the agents known to affect humans. Table 52-20 represents a current classification of these and the syndromes with which they have been associated.

C. trachomatis has been distinguished from *C. psittaci* by the observation that the intracellular inclusions in the former are compact, contain glycogen, and are stained by iodine (Fig. 52-24), whereas *C. psittaci* inclusions are diffuse and are not stained by iodine.

All of the chlamydiae have a common CF antigen. In addition, there are several immunotypes of *C. trachomatis* which have some correlation with the diseases produced and their epidemiology (Table 52-20).

For isolation purposes, specimens may be collected as biopsy samples (e.g., lung), or as whole secretions or swabs from affected sites (e.g., eye, respiratory tract, cervix, urethra), and placed in a sucrose-phosphate buffer described by Gordon (1972), containing 50 μg of streptomycin per ml and 25 units of nystatin per ml, for transport to the laboratory. The organisms can withstand freezing at −70°C. or lower, but should not be kept frozen at higher temperatures. Tissue homogenates are prepared and inoculated as 20 per cent suspensions.

PSITTACOSIS (ORNITHOSIS)

Psittacosis, a disease of psittacine birds, such as parrots, parakeets, and cockatoos, is not as restricted in its host range as the name implies. The organisms can also infect pigeons, turkeys, chickens, and other avians, and the name ornithosis is currently preferred. Birds can infect humans via inhalation of contaminated aerosols or fomites, and person-to-

person transmission has also been documented. There is an incubation period of 7 to 14 days, and the syndrome is usually characterized by chills, fever, malaise, and pneumonia. Hepatosplenomegaly, jaundice, and myopericarditis may also occur.

The diagnosis is suggested by a history of bird contact and is a particular hazard for pet-shop workers, avian pet owners, and poul-

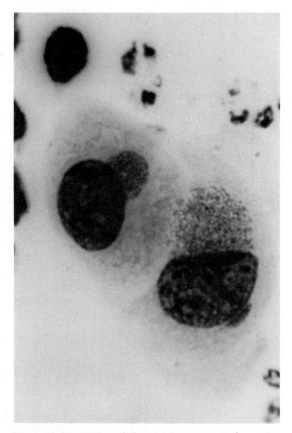

Figure 52-24. Chlamydial agent in conjunctival scraping (×1100). (Courtesy of Z. Naib, M.D.).

try workers. The agent can be cultivated in the yolk sac of embryonated eggs, by intraperitoneal inoculation of mice, or by inoculation into HeLa 229 or other cell cultures. The diagnosis is usually confirmed by demonstrating a significant rise in CF antibody titers in paired acute and convalescent sera.

LYMPHOGRANULOMA VENEREUM (LGV)

Lymphogranuloma venereum is venereally transmitted. The initial lesion is a small, painless 2- to 3-mm genital vesicle or ulcer, which often goes unnoticed and heals in a few days. This is followed by inguinal adenopathy which can be extensive, and may be associated with systemic signs of meningitis or meningoencephalitis, pneumonia, keratoconjunctivitis with eyelid edema and preauricular adenopathy, or polyarthritis. Erythema nodosum or erythema multiforme is also frequently associated with infection. Occasionally, severe proctitis or proctocolitis can develop, and rectal or urethral strictures may result from infection. The Frei test, a delayed hypersensitivity skin test using purified "Lygranum" chlamydial antigen, becomes positive as early as 10 days after infection and remains positive indefinitely. However, it does not necessarily distinguish recent LGV infection from past infection with this or other members of the chlamydia genus, and a negative test does not rule out such infection. CF or immunofluorescent testing is most commonly used for serodiagnosis. The antibody response has usually reached a peak titer before the diagnosis is considered, which often negates the opportunity to detect a rising titer during illness. A CF antibody titer of 1:16 or greater usually supports the clinical diagnosis. The agent has been isolated in cell cultures, in yolk sacs, and in mice after intracerebral or intraperitoneal inoculation.

TRACHOMA AND OTHER CHLAMYDIA TRACHOMATIS INFECTIONS

Endemic trachoma is present in many areas of the world, including some parts of the United States. It is usually spread by direct contact and begins as a conjunctivitis, which may persist for months to years. This can spread to the cornea, causing vascularization, scarring, and blindness. Immunotypes A, B, Ba, and C are most commonly involved.

The diagnosis can be made by examination by immunofluorescence, iodine, or Giemsa staining of methanol or acetone-fixed conjunctival scrapings, looking for intracytoplasmic inclusions in epithelial cells, as shown in Figure 52-24. Culture is a much more sensitive method, and is currently done more commonly in cell cultures than by other means. While several culture methods have been used, including irradiated McCoy cells (a strain of mouse heteroploid cells) and HeLa 229 cells pretreated with DEAE-dextran (Kuo, 1972), we prefer the 5-iodo-2-deoxyuridine (IUDR)-treated cell system described by Wentworth (1974).

In this procedure, McCoy cells are trypsinized and seeded into flat-bottomed 1 dram vials containing 12 mm circular cover slips. The cells are grown to confluence on the cover slips in the presence of 10 µg/ml of IUDR for 3 days. The medium is removed, and the cells are pretreated with 1 ml of 30 µg/ml DEAE-dextran in normal saline for 30 to 60 minutes. The DEAE-dextran is then aspirated, followed by inoculation of 0.1 ml of the specimen in sucrose-phosphate buffer, and centrifugation at 3200 rpm at room temperature for one hour. Maintenance medium is added, and the cultures incubated for three days. Following this, the contents are drained and the coverslips fixed, stained with iodine stain, and examined for the presence and quantity of chlamydial inclusions. This method can be employed for the isolation of all members of the genus, although HeLa 229 cells are preferred for *C. psittaci*. Antibody titers in serum, and even tears, can be measured by neutralization or microimmunofluorescent methods (Wang, 1975), but these are cumbersome tests not currently available in the diagnostic laboratory.

Other immunotypes of *C. trachomatis*, such as types D, E, F, G, H, I, J, and K, are being increasingly recognized as important disease-producing agents in humans. While these are thought to be spread primarily from a venereal reservoir, contact transmission by non-venereal routes is also possible. Inclusion conjunctivitis can occur at all ages. This is similar to trachoma, but is generally milder and usually self-limiting. In the United States, this is most often seen in infants, with onset at any time after 3 days of age. It can closely mimic acute neonatal gonococcal conjunctivitis. These strains have also been implicated as causes of non-gonococcal urethritis in adults and are thought to account for as many as 40 per cent of male cases.

In addition, some episodes of cervicitis, as well as salpingitis, have been associated with genital *C. trachomatis* infection in females. Recently, similar immunotypes have been isolated from respiratory tract secretions, associated with high type-specific antibody titers in serum, nasal, and lacrimal secretions, in infants from 3 weeks to 6 months of age with a protracted "pertussoid" pneumonia syndrome (Beem, 1977). Only about half of these infants had a history of preceding or concurrent conjunctivitis. The role of chlamydial infections in these syndromes is intriguing but requires further investigation before the significance of isolates can be fully interpreted. The diagnostic methods are the same as those described for trachoma.

GENERAL REFERENCES

Gardner, P. S., and McQuillin, J.: Rapid Virus Diagnosis. Application of Immunofluorescence. London, Butterworth and Company, Ltd., 1974.

Grist, N. R., Ross, C. A., and Bell, E. J.: Diagnostic Methods in Clinical Virology, 2nd ed. London, Blackwell Scientific Publications, 1974.

Hobson, D., and Holmes, K. K. (eds.): Nongonococcal Urethritis and Related Infections. Washington, D.C., American Society for Microbiology, 1977.

Kawamura, A. (ed.): Fluorescent Antibody Techniques and Their Applications, 2nd ed. Baltimore, University Park Press, 1977.

Kruse, P. F., and Patterson, M. K.: Tissue Culture. Methods and Applications. New York, Academic Press, 1973.

Lennette, E. H., and Schmidt, N. J.: Diagnostic Procedures for Viral and Rickettsial Infections, 4th ed. New York, American Public Health Association, Inc., 1969.

Lennette, E. H., Spaulding, E. H., and Truant, J. P. (eds.): Manual of Clinical Microbiology, 2nd ed. Washington, D.C., American Society for Microbiology, 1974.

Madeley, C. R.: Guide to the Collection and Transport of Virological Specimens. Geneva, World Health Organization, 1977.

Rose, N. R., and Friedman, H. (eds.): Manual Clinical Immunology. Washington, D. C., American Society for Microbiology, 1976.

REFERENCES

Andiman, W. A., et al.: Epstein-Barr virus. In Rose, N. R., and Friedman, H. (eds.): Manual of Clinical Immunology. Washington D.C., American Society of Microbiology, 1976.

Appleton, H., and Higgins, P. G.: Viruses and gastroenteritis in infants. Lancet, *1*:1297, 1975.

Back, A. F., et al.: Indirect hemagglutinating antibody response to *Herpesvirus* types 1 and 2 in immunized laboratory animals and natural infections in man. Appl. Microbiol., *28*:392, 1974.

Balfour, H. H., Jr., et al.: California arbovirus infections. Pediatrics, *52*:680, 1973.

Balfour, H. H., Jr., and Edelman, C. K.: Diagnosis of California (La Crosse) encephalitis by precipitin techniques: A prospective study. Appl. Microbiol., *28*:807, 1974.

Beem, M. O., and Saxon, E. M.: Respiratory-tract colonization and a distinctive pneumonic syndrome in infants infected with *Chlamydia trachomatis*. N. Engl. J. Med., *296*:306, 1977.

Benjamin, D. R., and Ray, C. G.: Use of immunoperoxidase for the rapid identification of human myxoviruses and paramyxoviruses in tissue culture. Appl. Microbiol., *28*:47, 1974.

Brandt, C. D., et al.: Infections in 18,000 infants and children in a controlled study of respiratory tract disease. 1. Adenovirus pathogenicity in relation to serologic type and illness syndrome. Am. J. Epidemiol., *90*:484, 1969.

Burgdorfer, W.: Hemolymph test. A technique for detection of rickettsia in ticks. Am. J. Trop. Med. Hyg., *19*:1010, 1970.

Caul, E. O., and Clarke, S. K. R.: Coronavirus propagated from a patient with nonbacterial gastroenteritis. Lancet, *2*:953, 1975.

Daugharty, H., Warfield, D. T., Hemingway, W. D., and Casey, H. C.: Mumps class-specific immunoglobulins in radioimmunoassay and conventional serology. Infect. Immunol., *7*:380, 1973.

Duffy, J., et al.: Polyarthritis, polyarteritis, and hepatitis B. Medicine, *55*:19, 1976.

Fiset, P., et al.: A microagglutination technique for the detection and measurement of rickettsial antibodies. Acta Virol. *13*:60, 1969.

Fox, J. P., et al.: The Seattle virus watch VII. Observations of adenovirus infections. Am. J. Epidemiol., *105*:362, 1977.

Fulginiti, V. A., and Stahl, M.: Parainfluenza and respiratory syncytial viruses. In Lennette, E. H., Spaulding, E. H., and Truant, J. P. (eds.): Manual of Clinical Microbiology, 2nd ed. Washington, D.C., American Society for Microbiology, 1974.

Gershon, A. A., et al.: Antibody to varicella-zoster virus in parturient women and their offspring in the first year of life. Pediatrics, *58*:692, 1976a.

Gershon, A. A., et al.: Detection of antibody to varicella zoster virus by immune adherence hemagglutination. Proc. Soc. Exp. Biol., Med., *151*:637, 1976b.

Glezen, W. P., et al.: Acute respiratory disease of university students with special reference to the etiologic role of *Herpesvirus hominis*. Am. J. Epidemiol., *101*:111, 1975.

Gomez-Barreto, J., et al.: Acute enteritis associated with reovirus-like agents. J.A.M.A., *235*:1857, 1976.

Gordon, F. B., et al.: Effect of ionizing radiation on susceptibility of McCoy cell cultures to *Chlamydia trachomatis*. Appl. Microbiol., *23*:123, 1972.

Hanon, N., et al.: Assay of *Coxiella burneti* by enumeration of immunofluorescent infected cells. J. Immunol., *97*:492, 1966.

Henle, G., et al.: Antibody to Epstein-Barr virus-associated nuclear antigen in infectious mononucleosis. J. Infect. Dis., *130*:321, 1974.

Horwitz, C. A., et al.: Clinical evaluation of patients with infectious mononucleosis and antibody to the R form of EB virus early antigen. Am. J. Med., *58*:330, 1975.

Johnson, K. M., et al.: Isolation and partial characterization of a new virus causing acute hemorrhagic fever in Zaire. Lancet, *1*:569, 1977.

Kapikian, A. Z., et al.: Detection of coronavirus strain 692 by immune electron microscopy. Infect. Immunol., *7*:111, 1973.

Kapikian, A. Z., et al.: Visualization by immune electron microscopy of a 27-nm particle associated with acute infectious nonbacterial gastroenteritis. J. Virol., *10*:1075, 1972.

Kuo, C. C., et al.: Primary isolation of TRIC organisms in HeLa 229 cells treated with DEAE-dextran. J. Infect. Dis., *125*:665, 1972.

McIntosh, K., et al.: Coronavirus infection in acute lower respiratory tract disease of infants. J. Infect. Dis., *130*:502, 1974.

Meyers, J. D.: Congenital varicella in term infants: Risk reconsidered. J. Infect. Dis., *129*:215, 1974.

Middleton, P. J., et al.: Viruses associated with acute gastroenteritis in young children. Am. J. Dis. Child., *131*:733, 1977.

Miller, W. J., et al.: Specific immune adherence assay for human hepatitis A antibody. Application to diagnostic and epidemiologic investigations. Proc. Soc. Exp. Biol. Med., *149*:254, 1975.

Mostow, S. R., et al.: Application of the single radial immunodiffusion test for assay of antibody to infleunza type A virus. J. Clin. Microbiol., *2*:351, 1975.

Parrino, T. A., et al.: Clinical immunity in acute gastroenteritis caused by the Norwalk agent. N. Engl. J. Med., *297*:86, 1977.

Plummer, G.: A review of the identification and titration of antibodies to herpes simplex viruses type 1 and 2 in human sera. Cancer Res., *33*:1469, 1973.

Portnoy, B., et al.: The sensitivity of the CF test for the detection of adenovirus infections in infants and children with lower respiratory disease. Am. J. Epidemiol., *86*:362, 1967.

Robinson, W. S., and Lutwick, L. I.: The virus of hepatitis, type B. N. Engl. J. Med., *295*:1168, 1232, 1976.

Schoenbaum, S. C., et al.: Epidemiology of influenza in the elderly: Evidence of virus recycling. Am. J. Epidemiol., *103*:166, 1976.

Sherlock, S.: Predicting progression of acute type-B hepatitis to chronicity. Lancet, *2*:354, 1976.

Stewart, J. A., et al.: Herpes simplex virus. *In* Rose, N. R., and Friedman, H. (eds.): Manual of Clinical Immunology. Washington, D.C., American Society for Microbiology, 1976.

Strauch, B., et al.: Oropharyngeal excretion of Epstein-Barr virus by renal transplant in immunosuppressed patients. Lancet, *1*:1234, 1974.

Sumaya, C. V.: Endogenous reactivation of Epstein-Barr virus infection. J. Infect. Dis., *135*:374, 1977.

Townsend, J. J., et al.: Progressive rubella panencephalitis-onset late after congenital rubella. N. Engl. J. Med., *292*:990, 1975.

Unduman, S. A., et al.: Rapid diagnosis of varicella zoster infection by agar gel diffusion. J. Infect. Dis., *126*:193, 1972.

Vanderwalde, E. M., et al.: User's guide to some new tests for hepatitis B antigen. Lancet, *2*:1066, 1974.

Waner, J. L., et al.: Patterns of cytomegalovirus complement-fixing antibody activity: A longitudinal study of blood donors. J. Infect. Dis., *127*:538, 1973.

Wang, S. P., et al.: Simplified microimmunofluorescence test with Trachoma-Lymphogranuloma venereum (*Chlamydia trachomatis*) antigens for use as a screening test for antibody. J. Clin. Microbiol., *1*:250, 1975.

Wentworth, B. B., and Alexander, E. R.: Isolation of *Chlamydia trachomatis* by use of 5-iodo-2-deoxyuridine-treated cells. Appl. Microbiol., *27*:912, 1974.

Wike, D. A., et al.: Plaque formation in tissue cultures by *Rickettsia rickettsi* isolated directly from whole blood and tick hemolymph. Infect. Immunol., *6*:736, 1972.

Williams, V., et al.: Serologic response to varicella-zoster membrane antigens measured by indirect immunofluorescence. J. Infect. Dis., *130*:669, 1974.

Woodruff, A. W., et al.: Lassa fever in Britain: An imported case. Br. Med. J., *3*:616, 1973.

Woodruff, J. F., et al.: Involvement of T lymphocytes in the pathogenesis of coxsackie virus B3 in heart disease. J. Immunol., *113*:1726, 1974.

Yolken, R. H., et al.: Enzyme-linked immunosorbent assay (ELISA) for detection of human reovirus-like agent of infantile gastroenteritis. Lancet, *2*:263, 1977.

5

53

MYCOPLASMAL INFECTION

Hjordis M. Foy, M.D., Ph.D. and
George E. Kenny, Ph.D.

BIOLOGY OF THE ORGANISMS

Mycoplasmata are the smallest (0.3 to 0.5 μm) free-living organisms known and differ from bacteria especially in their lack of a cell wall. They are unlike cell wall-defective bacteria (L-forms) in that the latter revert to their normal morphology when cultured on the appropriate media. Although the size and pliability of mycoplasmata allow them to pass filters that retain bacteria, they resemble bacteria more than viruses. Thus, they contain both RNA and DNA, grow on artificial media, and carry out their own replication processes. The biologic characteristics of human Mycoplasma are outlined in Table 53-1.

Mycoplasmata were originally designated as "PPLO," "*pleuropneumonia-like organisms*," because the agent first discovered in 1898 caused pleuropneumonia in cattle. The human species belong to two families, Mycoplasmataceae and Acholeplasmataceae, which are classified in the order Mycoplasmatales, class Mollicutes. *Mycoplasma* require sterols (cholesterol) for growth; *Acholeplasma* do not. The only *Acholeplasma* species found in humans, *Acholeplasma laidlawii*, is probably a saprophyte and is commonly found in sewage. The family Mycoplasmataceae is divided into two genera, *Mycoplasma* and *Ureaplasma;* the latter requires urea for growth. The nine species of mycoplasmata isolated from humans are described in Table 53-1. Mycoplasma species can be distinguished by their ability to ferment glucose and utilize arginine or by their requirements for urea. Serologically, they are heterogenous and can be divided into five quite dissimilar groups (Kenny, 1975). A large number of *Mycoplasma* species have also been isolated from animals, but these do not infect humans. However, they do pose problems as contaminants in tissue culture systems used for isolation of viruses (Barile, 1973).

NORMAL FLORA AND ROLE IN DISEASE

Four species, *Mycoplasma orale,* (formerly *Mycoplasma pharyngis* or *Mycoplasma orale type 1*), *Mycoplasma buccale* (formerly *Mycoplasma orale type 2*), *Mycoplasma faucium* (formerly *Mycoplasma orale type 3*), and *Mycoplasma salivarium*, inhabit the oral cavity and are considered normal flora (Table 53-1). *M. salivarium* is found in large quantities in periodontal crevices and is absent in edentulous persons; it may possibly play a role in periodontal disease.

Mycoplasma pneumoniae, formerly called Eaton agent after its discoverer, is a definite human pathogen, best known as a cause of pneumonitis (Grayston, 1969). The disease previously was called "atypical pneumonia" because it does not respond to penicillin. How-

Table 53-1. SPECIES OF MYCOPLASMATA FOUND IN HUMANS, THEIR LABORATORY CHARACTERISTICS, NORMAL SOURCES, AND ROLE IN DISEASE

SPECIES	SEROLOGIC GROUP*	GLUCOSE FERMENTATION	ARGININE UTILIZATION	UREA UTILIZATION	OPTIMUM pH	GROWTH† IN		NORMAL SOURCE	ROLE IN DISEASE
						AIR	95% N$_2$ 5% CO$_2$		
A. laidlawii	2	+	-	-	7.0-8.0	++++	++++	Skin, mouth, sewage	Unknown
M. orale (M. pharyngis)	7	-	+	-	6.0-7.0	+	+++	Mouth	None known
M. buccale (M. orale type 2)	7	-	+	-	6.0-7.0	+	+++	Mouth	None known
M. faucium (M. orale type 3)	7	-	+	-	6.0-7.0	+	+++	Mouth	None known
M. salivarium	7	-	+	-	6.0-7.0	+	+++	Periodontal crevices, mouth	Periodontal disease?
M. hominis	7	-	+	-	6.5-7.5	+++	+++	Genital tract, mouth	Opportunistic in pelvic inflammatory disease
M. pneumoniae	5	+	-	-	7.0-8.0	++++	+	Respiratory tract	Pneumonitis, bronchitis, pharyngitis
M. fermentans	6	+	+	-	7.0-8.0	++	+++	Genital tract	Rare, none known
U. urealyticum (T-strains)	?	-	-	+	5.5-7.0	+++	+++	Genital tract (rarely throat)	Urethritis? Dysfertility?

* According to Kenny, 1975.
† + = Marginal growth; ++++ = maximal growth

5

ever, it is but one of the atypical pneumonias. It is popularly known as "walking pneumonia" because the patient may appear only moderately ill, despite widespread pulmonary infiltrates. Indeed, mycoplasmal pneumonia may be associated with lobar infiltrates resembling those of pneumococcal pneumonia. Attack rates are highest among older children and young adults. The spectrum of manifestations comprises pharyngitis, bronchitis, tracheobronchitis, and bronchiolitis. Complications include hemolytic anemia, pleuritis, a variety of skin rashes, Stevens-Johnson syndrome, meningitis, encephalitis, and temporary arthritis. Death is a rare sequel but occasionally occurs in persons developing hemolytic anemia with thromboembolism or in those developing respiratory failure (Foy, 1976).

Mycoplasma hominis and *Ureaplasma urealyticum* normally inhabit the urogenital tract in sexually mature men and women; higher isolation rates are obtained from women than from men, possibly reflecting more favorable growth conditions in the vaginal tract. The degree of colonization with these species is related to sexual activity and to the number of sexual partners (McCormack, 1973). The isolation rate of *U. urealyticum* approaches 100 per cent for female prostitutes. The presence of *U. urealyticum* has been associated with abortions, dysfertility, and low birth weight of infants, but whether this association is etiologic or a reflection of a composite of other predisposing factors, including low socioeconomic status, smoking, and other concurrent infections, is not yet resolved. *M. hominis* may act as an opportunistic invader, and occasionally has been found as the sole isolate in salpingitis. Both *M. hominis* and *U. urealyticum* may be isolated in the blood stream post partum, not necessarily associated with postpartum fever. Colonization of newborn infants occurs temporarily without obvious ill effects. Although *Chlamydia trachomatis* is probably the most important cause of non-gonococcal urethritis, *U. urealyticum* may be the cause in a percentage of such infections, particularly among previously sexually inexperienced males (Bowie, 1977). A role for genital *Mycoplasma* in prostatitis and epididymitis is also suspected.

COLLECTION OF SPECIMENS

Since mycoplasmata are surface parasites, various secretions and body fluids, such as urine, vaginal discharge, saliva, and sputum are adequate for isolation attempts (Kenny, 1974). Sputum samples are frequently diluted 1:10 and 1:100 to avoid toxic effects. Similarly, washings of tissues are more useful for isolation than minced tissues. Pharyngeal swabs in respiratory infections and vaginal and urethral swabs in urogenital infections are also adequate. The tip of the swab is broken into the collection medium. Patients with *M. pneumoniae* pneumonia seldom have a productive cough at onset of illness; however, throat swabs are a good substitute for sputum, since the organisms colonize the pharynx, particularly in children. The organism is recovered even after treatment with tetracycline or erythromycin has been initiated, despite the fact that these drugs are known to shorten the duration of illness. The collection media commonly used contain 0.5 per cent bovine albumin with soybean-casein digest (e.g., Trypticase soy) broth (Grayston, 1969). Penicillin (100 U/ml) is usually added to control bacterial contamination. Specimens can be stored refrigerated at $-4°$C. for several days, and most mycoplasmata withstand transportation and freezing well. For long-term storage, $-70°$C. is recommended.

ISOLATION OF ORGANISMS

Mycoplasmata require special agar plates and broth cultures. The latter are especially advantageous for large inocula with small numbers of organisms (Kenny, 1974). Growth may cause faint turbidity or small spherules or colonies in fluid medium, but is better demonstrated by pH changes of indicators when appropriate substrates are used (Table 53-1). Subculture to agar plates is necessary for identification. *Mycoplasma* media are enriched with fresh yeast extracts, peptone, and animal serum. Penicillin is added to suppress bacterial growth; thallium acetate is also used for this purpose but is toxic for *U. urealyticum*. The organisms form small colonies that grow both on the agar surface and into the agar, with the resulting appearance of "fried eggs," or they may have a granular appearance (Fig. 53-1). For subculture, small blocks of agar have to be cut out and smeared face down on the surface of fresh plates. Most human *Mycoplasma* species can be seen with magnification within a couple of days, but it may take two to four weeks for *M. pneumoniae* colonies to become visible. Diphasic media, consisting of an agar

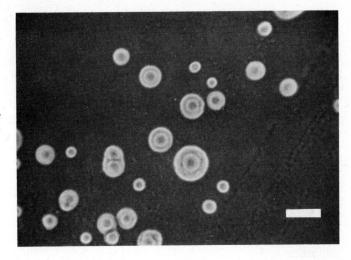

Figure 53-1. Colonies of *Mycoplasma pneumoniae* strain AP-164 on agar at 10 days of incubation. Bar = 100 μm.

base overlaid with a fluid medium with a pH indicator for glucose fermentation, are particularly useful for isolation of *M. pneumoniae* (Kenny, 1974). Although mycoplasmata can be separated by their ability to ferment glucose and utilize arginine, species identification is best carried out by inhibition with specific antisera, according to the method of Clyde (1964). *U. urealyticum*, discovered in the 1960's, forms minute colonies on agar media (Shepard, 1974). Thus they were first called T-strains for tiny. They are detected readily in well-buffered urea broth where their presence is recognized by alkaline changes (Kenny, 1974). Subculture must be done as soon as the pH increases, since the organisms die off rapidly. Lincomycin, 15 μg/ml, can be incorporated into the culture medium to suppress the growth of *M. hominis*, which otherwise may dominate over *Ureaplasma*.

SEROLOGY

SEROLOGY OF MYCOPLASMA PNEUMONIAE INFECTIONS

Detection of antibody in persons infected with *M. pneumoniae* is accomplished by three methods: (1) complement fixation with lipid or whole organism antigen, (2) fluorescent antibody, and (3) metabolic inhibition testing (Kenny, 1976). *M. pneumoniae* is unique among microorganisms in that glycolipids appear to be the major complement-fixing antigens: the role of other components, protein and polysaccharide, is less certain. Serodiagnosis by complement fixation using lipid ex-

tracts of the organism gives both greater titer rises and lower background antibody than the use of whole organism antigen. Antibody has also been measured by the indirect fluorescent technique. This method is more tedious but has the advantage of requiring less antigen than the complement-fixation test. The metabolic inhibition test measures the ability of antibody to stop growth of the organism as indicated by the prevention of the appearance of a metabolic product. Thus, in *M. pneumoniae* infections, acid from glucose (Taylor-Robinson, 1966) can be visualized by a pH indicator or by reduction of tetrazolium (Senterfit, 1966). Metabolic inhibition tests have the advantage of requiring only small numbers of organisms and are relatively easy to perform. The disadvantages consist of a dynamic endpoint (the endpoint changes from day to day) and the requirement of live organisms. The metabolic inhibition tests correlate well with the complement fixation test using lipid antigen. Complement fixation testing is the test most likely to be performed by Public Health and clinical laboratories because antigens are commercially available (Kenny, 1976). Serodiagnosis is best accomplished in retrospect by testing acute and convalescent sera for fourfold antibody increase. Because antibody is of long duration, the height of titer is only moderately useful in determining the occurrence of recent infections. A rise in *cold agglutinin* titer has traditionally been used for diagnosis of *M. pneumoniae;* however, although highly suggestive and convenient, this test is neither as specific nor as sensitive as the foregoing tests.

Routine methods for measuring immunologic response to *M. hominis* and *U. urealyticum* have not yet been established. Some of the difficulties are due to the heterogeneity of these organisms. *U. urealyticum* is divided into eight established serotypes, although as many as 11 different types have been recognized. Similarly, *M. hominis* appears to be serologically heterogenous. Additionally, the antibody response of infected humans appears poor, perhaps reflecting the superficial character of these infections. The methods used in research laboratories include the metabolic inhibition tests (the endpoint of the test is the prevention of production of the alkaline product ammonia from either arginine or urea) (Purcell, 1966a and b) and complement-mediated mycoplasmacidal tests (Lin, 1973). Although these tests are poor for serodiagnosis of infections, much of the knowledge we have obtained about the serologic heterogeneity of these organisms has been gained using these methods.

INTERPRETATION AND
CLINCIAL SIGNIFICANCE
OF LABORATORY RESULTS

Isolation of mycoplasmata requires experience among the laboratory personnel and cannot be carried out by most routine hospital laboratories. Because any constituents of the growth media, especially the serum, can have mycoplasmacidal components, new batches of media should be tested not only with known *Mycoplasma* stock strains but also with clinical materials (Kenny, 1974). Sometimes artifacts in the agar are mistaken for *Mycoplasma* colonies.

A throat culture is positive for *M. pneumoniae* in about two thirds of patients who by multiple diagnostic tests are shown to be infected with this organism. Since shedding ceases one to two months following onset of illness, a positive throat culture is practically diagnostic.

Genital mycoplasmata, *M. hominis* and *U. urealyticum*, isolated from urine, vagina, or cervix can be considered normal flora in sexually active persons. *M. hominis* and *U. urealyticum* have been isolated from infected salpinges and pelvic abscesses, as well as from postpartum blood, and the organisms may have a role in pelvic inflammatory disease and fever post partum (McCormack, 1973). However, since patients with these disease syndromes may also have a multitude of other organisms present, it is sometimes difficult to determine if the organisms are primary or secondary invaders. In males, ureaplasmata may play a role in non-gonococcal urethritis, although *Chlamydia trachomatis* is the major culprit in this syndrome. The role of *U. urealyticum* in fetal loss, low birthweight, and dysfertility is unresolved.

Serologic diagnosis of *M. pneumoniae* infections has been discussed above. Although results of serologic tests are usually not available until the patient has recovered, the proper diagnosis is helpful in epidemic situations. In family spread, the case-to-case interval averages three weeks. Most routine laboratories will carry out the cold agglutinin test, which is elevated (≤ 32) in about two thirds of *M. pneumoniae* patients, particularly those with the more severe symptoms. However, cold agglutinins may also appear in several other infectious diseases, so the test is not specific. Cold agglutinins and anti-MG (antibodies) are reviewed in Chapter 43 (p. 1444).

The presence of tetracyclines and macrolides in serum may interfere with the interpretation and reading of metabolic inhibition and tetrazolium reduction antibody titers by giving false positive reactions.

Serologic diagnosis for other human mycoplasmal infection has not advanced sufficiently to be of assistance in the routine management of patients.

REFERENCES

Barile, M. F.: Mycoplasmal contamination of cell cultures: Mycoplasma-virus-cell culture interactions. *In* Contamination in Tissue Culture. New York, Academic Press, Inc., 1973, p. 131.

Bowie, W. R., Wang, S. P., Alexander, E. R., Floyd, J., Forsyth, P. S., Pollock, H. M., Lin, J. S., and Holmes, K. K.: Etiology of nongonococcal urethritis. Evidence for *Chlamydia trachomatis* and *Ureaplasma urealyticum*. J. Clin. Invest., *59*:735, 1977.

Clyde, W. A., Jr.: Mycoplasma species identification based upon growth inhibition by specific antisera. J. Immunol., *92*:958, 1964.

Foy, H. M.: Pneumonia, *Mycoplasma pneumoniae. In* Top, F. H., and Wehrle, P. F. (eds.): Communicable and Infectious Diseases, 8th ed. St. Louis, The C. V. Mosby Company, 1976, p. 535.

Grayston, J. T., Foy, H. M., and Kenny, G. E.: The epidemiology of Mycoplasma infections of the human respiratory tract. *In* Hayflick, L. (ed.): The Mycoplasmatales and L-phase of Bacteria. New York, Appleton-Century-Crofts, 1969, p. 651.

Kenny, G. E.: Antigens of the Mycoplasmatales and Chlamydiae. *In* Sela, M. (ed.): The Antigens, vol. 3. New York, Academic Press, Inc., 1975, p. 449.

Kenny, G. E.: Mycoplasma. *In* Lennette, E. H., Spaulding, E. H., and Truant, J. P. (eds.): Manual of Clinical Microbiology. Washington, D.C., American Society for Microbiology, 1974, p. 333.

Kenny, G. E.: Serology of mycoplasmic infections. *In* Rose, N. R., and Friedman, H. (eds.): Manual of Clinical Immunology. Washington, D.C., American Society for Microbiology, 1976, p. 357.

Lin, J. S., and Kass, E. H.: Serotypic heterogeneity in isolates of human genital T-mycoplasmas. Infect. Immunol., *7*:499, 1973.

McCormack, W. M., Braun, P., Lee, Y.-H., Klein, J. O., and Kass, E. H.: The genital mycoplasmas. N. Engl. J. Med., *288*:78, 1973.

Purcell, R. H., Taylor-Robinson, D., Wong, D., and Chanock, R. M.: Color test for the measurement of antibody to T-strain mycoplasmas. J. Bacteriol., *92*:6, 1966a.

Purcell, R. H., Taylor-Robinson, D., Wong, D. C., and Chanock, R. M.: A color test for the measurement of antibody to the nonacid-forming human *Mycoplasma* species. Am. J. Epidemiol., *84*:51, 1966b.

Senterfit, L. B., and Jensen, K. E.: Antimetabolic antibodies to *Mycoplasma pneumoniae* measured by tetrazolium reduction inhibition. Proc. Soc. Exp. Biol. Med., *122*:786, 1966.

Shepard, M. C., Lunceford, C. D., Ford, D. K., Purcell, R. H., Taylor-Robinson, D., Razin, S., and Black, F. T.: *Ureaplasma urealyticum* gen. nov. sp. nov: proposed nomenclature for the human T (T-strain) mycoplasmas. Int. J. Syst. Bacteriol., *24*:160, 1974.

Taylor-Robinson, D., Purcell, R. H., Wong, D. C., and Chanock, R. M.: A color test for the measurement of antibody to certain Mycoplasma species based upon the inhibition of acid production. J. Hyg., *64*:91, 1966.

5

54

SERODIAGNOSTIC TESTS

Allen L. Pusch, M.D.

Serologic methods are used as an aid in the diagnosis of a wide variety of diseases. Many early studies involved the diagnosis of infectious diseases, especially bacterial. However, a serologic diagnosis is obtained after the fact in most acute infections and rather late for antimicrobial therapy to alter the disease process. In some instances the body sites involved by the organisms are not readily accessible, or the patient presents at a time when the organisms may not be viable for routine culture. Here a serologic diagnosis may be the only easily available method.

It is optimal to demonstrate a rise in antibody titer between two serum samples drawn at least 14 to 21 days apart (so-called acute and convalescent sera, also called paired serum samples). The "paired" serum samples must be tested together in the same test run with the same reagents to reduce spurious differences in titer resulting from day-to-day variation in the test. A two-tube (or fourfold) rise in titer, and preferably greater, is considered indicative of current infection. Attention must be paid to collection of the acute phase sample, ideally during the first week of symptoms, and proper labeling and storage of the serum (freezing at $-20°C.$ is considered adequate) until testing is accomplished.

In chronic or longstanding infections a single antibody titer may be used, but considerable care must be given to the interpretation of such titers. In geographic areas where certain infections are endemic, a low antibody titer may be considered "normal," while in other areas any titer suggests disease. It is important to know the mean titer response in various stages of the infection as generated by different test methods. Also, the patient's past history of infections and immunizations must be considered.

Cross-reactions occur between antigens of several organisms and a knowledge of these specific situations is important. Ideally, titers should be measured against all the antigens known to cross-react. The antigen giving the highest titer of antibody is considered to represent the organism evoking the antibody response.

In performing serologic determinations, it is important to follow the procedure rigidly. Any alterations to the method must be demonstrated to be fully comparable, in all titer ranges, to results obtained with the original method before being acceptable. When using commercial reagents, it is recommended that manufacturer's instructions be followed. Each new lot of reagents should be tested in parallel with the previous lot and used only if it gives results comparable to those obtained with the previous standardized lot. Every test run must include known negative and positive controls, and the results for these must be consistent with those of previous runs for the results to be acceptable.

Equipment must be kept clean and in good

working order. The temperatures of refrigerators and freezers must be monitored daily to insure proper specimen and reagent storage. Water bath temperatures must be checked at the start and finish of all incubation runs. Also, water baths must be checked for bacteria and molds growing within them which might contaminate tubes during incubation and create inaccurate results.

The speed of shaking and rotating machines must be checked by hand each time they are used. The precalibrated dial on the instrument should not be blindly accepted as the correct indicator of speed. Likewise, centrifuge speeds must be checked at regular intervals with a tachometer and automatic pipettes checked for accuracy of volume delivery. Glassware must be chemically clean. At times pipettes and other glassware become coated with protein or other organic material that is best removed by acid washing. Reagents must be handled properly, not cross-contaminated, and dating periods suggested by manufacturers properly observed. Date of purchase and the date the bottle is first opened should be noted on the bottle. Also, date of reconstitution of freeze-dried reagents should be recorded on the bottle.

Distilled water is used in making many reagents. Care must be taken to keep the still clean and functioning properly. Distilled water tends to absorb ions from gases present in the laboratory atmosphere and thus should be freshly distilled and kept in closed, hard glass containers. Chemicals used to prepare various reagents should be of reagent grade to obtain best results.

The host of methods developed in immunology are applied in the diagnostic serology laboratory. These are described in detail in Chapter 35. Hence, emphasis will be placed on the principles and interpretation of the more common serologic procedures available in many general hospital laboratories. Detailed procedures are available in the references and in the package inserts of commercial reagents. The *Manual of Clinical Immunology* edited by Rose and Friedman (1976) has detailed procedures for most diagnostic tests and can serve as a good general source.

SYPHILIS

Syphilis is seldom diagnosed by demonstrating the organisms in a primary or secondary lesion (see Chap. 49). Either the facilities for darkfield microscopic examinations are not readily available or the patient fails to present for medical care during these early stages of the disease. Serology thus becomes the most common laboratory tool used in diagnosis, and it is important that methods be standardized and well controlled. The United States Public Health Service (USPHS) through its Venereal Disease Research Laboratory of the Center for Disease Control (CDC) has done much to improve methods and reagents available to laboratories in the United States (USPHS, 1969). In addition, an active program of "check samples" is carried on through state laboratories to monitor the quality of syphilis serology throughout the United States.

Syphilis serology currently consists of two general groups of procedures: (1) the non-treponemal antigen tests, of which the VDRL is the prime example, and (2) the treponemal antigen tests, of which the fluorescent treponemal antibody-absorbed test (FTA-ABS) is currently the most important example.

NON-TREPONEMAL ANTIGEN TESTS

Wasserman in 1906 reported using an aqueous extract of syphilitic tissues from a human case as antigen to demonstrate antibodies in serum of syphilitic patients. He originally used a complement fixation procedure and presumed the reacting antigen to be treponemal antigen. Thereafter, it was demonstrated that alcoholic extracts of many normal animal tissues would give similar results and, indeed, alcoholic extracts of beef heart gave the best results. This obviously non-treponemal material, later called lipoidal, was rather crude and gave many non-specific reactions. The isolation and purification of two specific reactive substances in the beef heart muscle, cardiolipin and lecithin, led to a series of modifications and a more specific antigen used today in the VDRL (the letters VDRL refer to the Venereal Disease Research Laboratory, where the current procedure was developed). The antigen consists of a proper balance of cardiolipin, purified lecithin, cholesterol, and alcohol, which is standardized by adjustment of the lecithin content to give reproducible qualitative and quantitative results. The cholesterol provides adsorption centers so that agglutinated particles can be visualized. The 1 per cent sodium chloride solution with phosphate buffer (pH 6.0) is also important for proper agglutination of antigen in the presence of antibody, which in this system is called "reagin" (not to be confused with the term that was applied to allergic persons in the older literature).

The VDRL test was introduced in 1946 as a slide flocculation procedure. Heat-inactivated (56°C. for 30 minutes) serum is mixed with antigen diluted in buffer on a rotating glass slide. The endpoint is read microscopically ($100\times$ magnification). Very rigid procedures are outlined for mixing the antigen and buffer, the size of the drops of antigen mixed with the patient serum, and speed of the rotation of the slides. These must be followed strictly to obtain the greatest degree of comparable sensitivity and specificity among different laboratories. For laboratories preferring tube tests, a VDRL tube flocculation procedure in which the reaction is read macroscopically is available (USPHS, 1969).

The VDRL slide test results are graded as non-reactive (no flocculation), weakly reactive (slight flocculation), and reactive (definite flocculation). All reactive sera are then diluted—1:2, 1:4, and so forth—and each serum dilution giving a reaction is reported. Rarely, a patient with a high titer of reagin will have a negative VDRL with undiluted serum (prozone phenomenon). This phenomenon, when it occurs, is usually observed in secondary syphilis (Sparling, 1971).

Several authors have described modifications of the cardiolipin test, mostly involving alterations in the composition or preparation of antigen, concentrations of sodium chloride, or time of incubation. Many of these carry the name of the individual responsible for their development, such as Kline, Eagle, Manzzini, Hinton, and Kahn. These procedures are seldom used today and have largely been replaced by the VDRL or the RPR (Rapid Plasma Reagin) methods.

Complement fixation (CF) procedures became popular to confirm a reactive result in the flocculation procedures. The CF methods have gone through the same evolution of antigen use, i.e., aqueous extracts of syphilitic tissue, lipoidal, to cardiolipin, and more recently to a treponemal antigen, the Reiter protein (see below). The name Kolmer has figured prominently in CF syphilis serology. The first Kolmer modification of the Wasserman test was published in 1922 and became widely used.

It underwent many modifications, the most prominent being the "one fifth" Kolmer modification published in 1942, in which one fifth the volume of reagents is used. Generally, the results of the Kolmer CF procedures and the VDRL slide test are comparable, the Kolmer procedure, however, being somewhat less sensitive.

Several rapid test procedures employing the cardiolipin antigen have been developed, mostly as screening procedures in "field" situations where equipment may be limited (Wallace, 1970). These are known as "rapid reagin tests" and are commercially available in kit form. As a group, they are more sensitive and less specific than the VDRL, and any positive test must be followed by a VDRL or other more specific procedures. The Rapid Plasma Reagin (RPR) test was a prototype of this group, but has been developed into an acceptable alternative to the VDRL. The test is performed with unheated serum or plasma and a modified VDRL antigen containing choline chloride. Originally, the test was read microscopically, but addition of charcoal particles to the antigen permits macroscopic identification of the flocculation. The RPR (teardrop) card test uses plasma from a fingerstick blood specimen, and the reaction is carried out on a plastic-coated card that is rotated by hand. Another, known as the RPR (circle) card test, uses unheated serum and a plastic-coated card and requires a mechanical rotator. This latter procedure, which is comparable to the VDRL qualitatively but not always quantitatively, is now an accepted alternative to the VDRL as a general screening test for syphilis. The antigen from this procedure has been adapted to the AutoAnalyzer to provide an automated test known as the ART. This test is used today in some laboratories required to test large numbers of serum samples daily.

TREPONEMAL ANTIGEN TESTS

The first procedure using antigens of the treponemes themselves came in the form of the TPI (*Treponema pallidum* immobilization) test, which was introduced in 1949. The TPI uses as an antigen a strain of live *Treponema pallidum* cultured in rabbit testes and suspended in a survival medium. The antigen is mixed with the patient's serum and complement, incubated in an atmosphere of 5 per cent CO_2 and 95 per cent N_2, and then observed with a darkfield microscope to determine the proportion of treponemes immobilized relative to the controls. Sera causing immobilization are called TPI positive. This procedure has been recognized as the standard against which all other serologic tests for syphilis are measured. Unfortunately, the procedure is technically exacting, not well standardized, and few laboratories desire to maintain "cultures" of live *Treponema pallidum*. Only a few research laboratories still perform the test today.

In 1953 a method for preparing an antigen from the non-pathogenic Reiter treponemes, which are easily cultivated in the laboratory, was developed. This antigen was widely used as a treponemal antigen, although unfortunately not a *T. pallidum* antigen. The antigen was adapted to the one fifth volume Kolmer CF procedure and designated as the KRP (Kolmer Reiter Protein) test. This procedure, more widely available than the TPI, was not completely satisfactory because only 50 per cent of sera from late syphilis give a positive test.

Fluorescent antibody methodology was applied to syphilis in 1957 and led to the FTA-ABS procedure, which is highly specific and sensitive. With commercially available reagents and improvements in fluorescent microscopy, it is within the capability of most routine laboratories. The antigen consists of the Nichol's strain of *T. pallidum* (growth in rabbit testes) fixed to a slide. During the development of this method, a 1:5 dilution of patient serum was used, but this gave too many false positive reactions owing to non-specific antibodies in patient sera. Continued dilution of serum to 1:200 (the test known as FTA-200) removed the non-specific reactions, but many true positive reactions were also diluted out. Finally, the fluorescent treponemal antibody-absorbed (FTA-ABS) method was developed. In it the patient's serum is diluted 1:5 in "sorbent" (an extract of a culture of Reiter treponemes) to remove the non-specific antibodies before reacting the serum with the Nichol's strain of *T. pallidum*. Fluorescein-labeled anti-human globulin then demonstrates the presence of the patient's immunoglobulin on the surface of the treponemes. Such antibodies are considered specific for syphilis. The sensitivity of this procedure is at least equal to, and in several situations greater than, the TPI.

A recent addition to syphilis serology is the *Treponema pallidum* hemagglutination test (TPHA or, when microtechniques are used, the MHA-TP). Tanned sheep red cells are coated with antigen from the Nichol's strain of *T. pallidum*, and the serum is absorbed with sorbent similar to that in the FTA-ABS. A positive reaction is considered to be due to serum antibodies specific for syphilis. The reagents and equipment are less expensive than those for the FTA-ABS, and the procedure technically lends itself to automation. In this regard, it might be used as a highly specific screening test (see Chap. 35).

The enzyme-linked immunosorbent assay (ELISA) methodology is also being applied to syphilis serology. Tubes coated inside with *T. pallidum* antigen are incubated with dilute serum from patients. The tubes are washed, and then enzyme labeled anti-human immunoglobulin is added. The amount of enzyme (commonly, alkaline phosphatase) activity is measured by adding substrates to the tube and measuring the reaction product formed (see Chap. 35).

SEROLOGIC RESPONSE TO INFECTION

A comparison of positive serologic reactions in the various stages of untreated syphilis is presented in Figure 54-1. The RPR test is comparable to the VDRL in this regard. The FTA-ABS is the most sensitive in all stages, but it does not lend itself to screening large populations because of the more involved technical methodology and the incidence of weakly reactive results in certain groups (see below). The VDRL and RPR are, therefore, considered to be the best screening tests in the general population and in suspected primary and secondary syphilis. However, in patients with clinical findings suggesting late syphilis, the FTA-ABS is the procedure of choice, regardless of the VDRL result, since more than a third of such cases have negative VDRL's. The FTA-ABS gives a significantly greater number of positive results than the TPI in primary syphilis, while the two are comparable in the secondary stage; the TPI is only slightly less sensitive than the FTA-ABS in late syphilis (92 vs 98 per cent). The FTA-ABS is currently the best confirmatory test for a serum with a reactive VDRL. The hemagglutination procedure (see below) may prove to be an alternative to the FTA-ABS.

The quantitative titer with the VDRL is helpful both in diagnosis and in following the

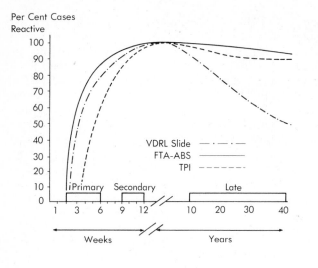

Per Cent Cases
Reactive

Figure 54-1. Serology of untreated syphilis.

course of treatment. Titers are usually low in primary syphilis—1:32 or less and only occasionally above this. In secondary syphilis the titers are virtually always above 1:32, and in late syphilis the titers are variable. Following successful treatment, the titer should fall significantly and often (two thirds of patients or more) the VDRL becomes negative, especially if treatment is rendered during the primary or secondary stages. Treatment during late syphilis seldom is associated with reversion of a reactive VDRL to negative. Documentation of this change in the VDRL over a 6-to 12-month period after completion of therapy is considered an indicator of success of treatment and permits one to suspect "re-infection" if the patient appears at a later time with an elevated titer. The TPI and FTA-ABS test results remain positive following therapy in most patients (Schroeter, 1972).

The newer procedures, the MHA-TP and ELISA, have most often been compared with the FTA-ABS in regard to their reactivity among patients. The MHA-TP has 90 to 95 per cent agreement with the FTA-ABS test. Most of the variance occurs in the primary stage, where the FTA-ABS appears more sensitive. In secondary and late syphilis the two are comparable. Thus, this procedure has potential both as a screening and as a confirmatory test; however, more experience is needed with the test and its automation. Also, a false-positive reaction in patients who have heterophile antibody must be ruled out in positive reactors (Ravel, 1976). The ELISA has not been extensively evaluated, but some have found it equal

in sensitivity to the FTA-ABS in all stages of the disease (Veldkamp, 1975).

The VDRL test is reactive in the serum of a significant number of patients who do not have syphilis. These are defined as sera with a reactive VDRL and a negative FTA-ABS and/or TPI from patients without a clinical history suggestive of syphilis. The VDRL in such cases is usually weakly reactive or has a reactive titer less than 1:8; such sera are designated biologic false positives (BFP). The incidence of these BFP's among reactive VDRL's varies from 10 to 50 per cent depending on the population being tested.

The BFP reactors are separated into two groups: the acute BFP in which the VDRL reverts to negative within six months, and the chronic BFP in which the serum reaction persists for a longer time. The acute BFP is usually associated with infectious disease, such as pneumonia, subacute bacterial endocarditis, chicken pox, infectious mononucleosis, scarlet fever, and atypical pneumonia; however, the incidence of BFP among patients with each of these conditions is rare. As many as 20 per cent of patients with lepromatous leprosy or those addicted to drugs exhibit chronic BFP reactions. Some laboratories report a significant incidence of BFP's or "rough" VDRL's in pregnant females, while others deny its existence during pregnancy. Any patient with a positive VDRL in pregnancy, even a weak reactor, must be studied thoroughly because of the untoward effects of untreated syphilis upon the fetus. The chronic BFP has had a well-recognized association with the immune complex diseases, especially systemic lupus erythematosus. A common trait in disorders causing chronic BFP reactions is hyperglobulinemia. A BFP may be attributed to aging alone, with as many as 10 per cent of persons in the eighth decade having such a reaction (Sparling, 1971).

The FTA-ABS may give borderline results and/or a "beaded" fluorescence along the treponemes (McKenna, 1973). These reactions are seen more commonly in the immune complex diseases and in the older age groups. When such is observed in an FTA-ABS, it is best to repeat the test on a second specimen. In the general population it has been estimated that as many as 2 per cent may have a false positive FTA-ABS. This low rate of false positivity forms the basis for the USPHS recommendation that the FTA-ABS not be used as a screening procedure, but should serve only as a confirmatory test in those with a positive VDRL or a clinical condition suspected of being syphilis. Wright(1975) reported 6 of 32 patients with acute genital herpes infections who had a positive FTA-ABS with negative RPR and MHA-TP tests. Patients with yaws or another treponemal infection also react positively with the FTA-ABS.

The serologic diagnosis of congenital syphilis may be a problem. Antibodies (IgG) from the mother with a positive VDRL and FTA-ABS can cross the placenta and transfer a positive reaction in these tests to serum obtained from the umbilical cord or from the newborn itself. A significantly higher titer in cord sera than in the mother would make one suspect infection involving the infant. Otherwise, serial VDRL titers of the infant's serum are needed. A progressive and significant fall in titer over a period of 6 to 12 weeks is expected when passively transferred IgG is metabolized; a steady or rising titer, on the other hand, suggests infection of the newborn. Quantitative IgM values on cord sera may serve as a general screen for intrauterine infection of the newborn. Unfortunately, in cases with subclinical or mild infection the cord IgM values are often borderline. A modification of the FTA-ABS test has been suggested in which IgM antibodies specifically against *T. pallidum* are sought in the cord or newborn serum. This requires the use of a specific fluorescein-labeled anti-human IgM antiserum in place of the polyvalent anti-human immunoglobulin antiserum used in the routine procedure. Kaufman (1974) has re-

viewed this procedure and finds that in newborns with symptomatic syphilis at birth or during the first month of life, 88 per cent react positively with the FTA-ABS (IgM procedure); those with delay of onset in symptoms beyond one month reacted only 65 per cent of the time at birth. In addition, it has been suggested that newborn IgM antibody directed against maternal IgG can give a falsely positive FTA-ABS (IgM) reaction. Thus, the best available procedure may still be serial VDRL titers.

Cerebrospinal fluid (CSF) examination is important in each case of syphilis, with increased leukocytes and/or protein being highly suggestive of central nervous system (CNS) involvement (see Chap. 18). However, this is not a sensitive indicator of CNS syphilis. In one series, the majority of patients with clinically apparent and serologically proven neurosyphilis had normal cerebrospinal fluid (CSF) protein levels and/or normal cell counts (Hooshmand, 1972). Unfortunately, CSF serology is not as sensitive and specific as is desirable.

Cerebrospinal fluid (CSF) specimens are traditionally tested by the VDRL and CF methods in attempts to diagnose neurosyphilis. The VDRL tube test requires 1 ml of CSF and is therefore unpopular. A modification of the VDRL on glass slides requires only 0.05 ml of CSF and gives results comparable to the tube test. However, in the patients studied by Hooshmand (1972), 40 per cent had non-reactive CSF-VDRL's in contrast to 100 per cent positive results with the FTA-CSF procedure (not the FTA-ABS on the CSF, as misprinted in Hooshmand's article [personal communication]).

The FTA-CSF is performed on CSF without the absorption step and is considered highly sensitive for neurosyphilis. It is lacking somewhat in specificity, however, with as many as 5 per cent of persons with negative serum FTA-ABS giving a positive CSF test. The false positive FTA-CSF results are thought to result from blood contaminating the CSF at the time of its collection or by alteration in the blood-brain barrier permitting serum proteins to enter the CSF. Unfortunately, no large group of "normal" CSF specimens has been studied with this procedure, so the lack of specificity may be even greater. This is the main rationale for the USPHS continuing to recommend the quantitative VDRL for testing CSF. Escobar (1970) recommended testing

5

fluids positive in the FTA-CSF test with a 1:3 dilution of CSF with sorbent (modification called by some FTA-ABS-CSF). In their experience this approach is highly specific but lacking in sensitivity (only 22 per cent of neurosyphilitic patients reacted positively). At this time, therefore, it appears that the serum FTA-ABS is the best starting place to document CNS syphilis by serologic methods. The quantitative VDRL on CSF will underdiagnose neurosyphilis, while the FTA-CSF will overdiagnose it and thus should not be used alone. The optimal procedure for establishing the diagnosis of neurosyphilis has yet to be developed.

ANTISTREPTOCOCCAL ANTIBODIES

Streptococcal infections of the pharynx and skin are rather common and easily documented by culture. However, such infection may not be clinically apparent, and the patient may not seek medical attention until after the onset of either acute rheumatic fever or poststreptococcal glomerulonephritis. In these situations, demonstration of a serologic response to streptococcal antigen provides evidence of antecedent streptococcal infection. Several extracellular products of the Group A streptococci, many of which have enzymatic as well as antigenic activity, are used as antigens. The antibodies produced block the enzymatic activity, and a reduction in activity of a standard enzyme preparation is used as an indicator of an antigen-antibody reaction. Antistreptolysin O (ASO), antihyaluronidase (AH), antistreptokinase, antidesoxyribonuclease B (anti-DNase-B) and antinicotinamide adenine dinucleotidase (anti-NADase) are the antibodies sought in clinical serology. The respective antigens are present in significant amounts in most strains of group A streptococci and in some members of other streptococcal groups. These antibodies offer no protection against streptococcal reinfection.

Titers to the extracellular antigens are demonstrated in most persons, especially school-age children, and attest to the frequency of streptococcal infections. The variation in titers has been defined with the ASO titer. The newborn has titers similar to those of the mother, but this falls significantly by the age of six months. Streptococcal infections under the age of two years are uncommon, and

persons in this age group usually have ASO titers less than 50 units. A child in the 5-to-12-year age group is repeatedly exposed to group A streptococci and often has titers up to 200 units without having experienced a recent clinically apparent infection. In adults the upper "normal" titer is in the range of 125 units. This same pattern is seen with all antistreptococcal antibodies. Paired serum samples are the best way to demonstrate a recent infection; however, streptococcal serology often is not measured until the patient is well into the convalescent stage and peak titers are present. Thus, interpretation of single titers or constant titers must be made with an understanding of the variations seen in "normals" of different ages. These stated "normal" values have been obtained by measuring titers in persons lacking evidence of recent group A streptococcal infections and by arbitrarily setting the upper normal limit to include 80 per cent of the group tested (Wannamaker, 1960).

Streptolysin O is an oxygen-labile hemolysin active against both human and rabbit erythrocytes. It is produced by most strains of Lancefield group A streptococci and a few strains of groups C and G. Measurement of antibodies against this antigen (the ASO titer) has been used for decades as an indicator of recent streptococcal infection. The antigen used in the procedure is obtained from the broth of an 18-hour culture of group A streptococci. It is mixed with dilutions of patient serum and buffer and incubated. Next, a 5 per cent suspension of human group O or rabbit erythrocytes is added to the tubes and reincubated. The endpoint is the highest serum dilution which gives no hemolysis (i.e., all the streptolysin is inactivated). In place of the usual serial twofold dilution, a more closely spaced dilution scheme using 0.1 log or a one and a quarter-fold increment in dilution of serum is used. The reciprocal of this endpoint is referred to as "Todd Units."

Patients with the non-suppurative complications of streptococcal infections (e.g., acute rheumatic fever and acute glomerulonephritis) have a higher incidence of elevated ASO titers and higher numerical titers than patients with uncomplicated streptococcal infection (Roy, 1956). ASO titers above 150 to 200 Todd Units are seen following streptococcal pharyngitis, while patients with non-suppurative complications more often have titers above 350 units. An interesting exception is lack of an ASO response in 75 per cent of the cases of streptococcal pyoderma, even if glomerulonephritis occurs (Kaplan, 1970).

Streptococcal desoxyribonuclease (also called streptodornase) has proved to be an especially helpful antigen in demonstrating a serologic response to streptococcal pyoderma. Some confusion may result from the fact that group A streptococci produce at least four antigenically distinct desoxyribonucleases. These are designated as A, B, C, and D. DNAse-B is the form most consistently antigenic and can be measured with commercially available reagents.

In measuring anti-DNAse titers, the patient's serum must first be heat-inactivated to remove its own DNAse. Appropriate dilutions of patients' sera are made, and antigen derived from cultures of appropriate streptococcal strains is added in standard amounts and incubated. Next, a standard solution of DNA substrate is added to each tube and incubated. Finally, an indicator of remaining intact DNA is added, which causes the polymerized DNA to form a mucin-like clot. Formation of a clot indicates inhibition of the enzyme, presumably due to the presence of antibody in the serum. The serial dilution scheme is similar to that used in the ASO test.

"Normal" subjects may have up to 250 units of anti-DNAse-B activity in their serum. The incidence of elevated titers in patients with acute rheumatic fever equals that of the ASO titer (80 per cent). Interestingly, fewer persons with post-streptococcal glomerulonephritis show anti-DNAse-B elevations (75 per cent) than ASO elevations (90 per cent) after streptococcal pharyngitis. This situation is reversed in glomerulonephritis following group A streptococcal pyoderma, in which 60 per cent show elevated anti-DNAse-B titers in contrast to 25 per cent with ASO titer elevations.

Hyaluronidase is another enzyme elaborated by the group A streptococci demonstrating antigenic activity. Titers of antihyaluronidase (AH) rise in the second week after infection and fall in three to five weeks. The antigen obtained from broth cultures is also available commercially. It is mixed with appropriate serum dilutions and incubated. Next, a standard amount of hyaluronate (substrate) is added to each tube and incubated, and uninhibited enzyme will accelerate its destruction. Finally, acetic acid is added to induce a mucin clot with any remaining intact hyaluronate. Tubes in which a clot forms are considered to contain significant antibody activity in that serum dilution.

The AH titer is elevated in approximately 60 per cent of documented streptococcal respiratory tract infections but is elevated in a much smaller percentage of streptococcal skin infections. It is less helpful than the ASO titer when used alone, but when the two are used in combination, 90 per cent of individuals with a recent streptococcal pharyngitis will have an elevated titer against at least one of the two antigens.

Streptococcal nicotinamide adenine dinucleotidase (NADase) also elicits an antibody response. The anti-NADase titers are determined by measuring enzyme activity remaining after appropriate serum dilutions are incubated with a standard enzyme preparation. The unbound NAD reacts with cyanide to form a complex absorbing light at 340 mm to demonstrate unbound antigen. The anti-NADase titer rises in the same proportion of situations as does the ASO titer. However, the difference between the upper "normal" titer (275 units) and the mean titer in a group of patients with acute glomerulonephritis (1015 units) is much greater than the corresponding difference in ASO titers (Wannamaker, 1960).

An assay for streptokinase (a plasminogen activator) antibodies has been described as another indicator of recent infection. However, because it is technically difficult to perform, it is not used routinely.

These antibody determinations are used in patients suspected of having rheumatic fever or acute glomerulonephritis. The ASO titer is the single best test to document antecedent streptococcal infection, elevated titers being present in 80 per cent of patients with recent pharyngitis. To obtain a 90 per cent probability of documenting such infection, it is recommended that titers with two different tests be measured. Perhaps an additional 5 per cent are identified if a third different test is performed. The AH and anti-DNAse-B are the two most frequently used secondary procedures; however, the anti-DNAse-B would appear preferable because of its utility in patients with streptococcal pyoderma. Some patients may already have reached a plateau in titer rise when first examined, but it is more definitive to demonstrate a fourfold rise in titer in paired samples taken two to four weeks apart.

Streptozyme is a commercial reagent con-

5

sisting of formalin-treated sheep erythrocytes that are coated with group A streptococcal "extracellular products." Serum diluted 1:100 is mixed on a glass slide with a drop of this cell suspension, and the agglutination is observed macroscopically. A serial dilution scheme can be used and a titer determined. These cells are coated with multiple different streptococcal antigens, including those described above, and a significant elevation of antibody titer to one or a combination of antigens results in a positive test. The sensitivity of this procedure varies depending upon what it is compared with. In patients with known post-streptococcal glomerulonephritis, acute rheumatic fever, and proven streptococcal infection, it is better than any single antigen procedure and appears equal to combinations of three single antigen tests (Bisno, 1974). However, when the streptozyme test is compared with multiple single antigen tests without consideration of the clinical history, there are as many as 30 per cent "false" negative streptozyme tests in sera yielding slight elevations of a single titer. Thus, it appears that the streptozyme test may miss a borderline streptococcal antibody titer (Kholy, 1974). The rate of false positives varies, but it is generally between 3 and 5 per cent when compared with titers obtained with multiple tests of sera. The post-streptococcal conditions usually manifest considerable elevation in titer to single antigens, so that the streptozyme procedure would appear appropriate to study such cases.

Streptolysin O antigen coated on latex beads is available as a rapid screening test for ASO antibodies. This test generally becomes positive with sera containing titers of 150 Todd Units or greater.

There are other streptococcal antigens known to be important in the pathophysiology of group A streptococcal infections and their sequelae. The M- and T-proteins are antigenic cell wall proteins. Antibodies against the type-specific M-protein are important in type-specific immunity. The mucopeptide or peptidoglycan of the inner layer of the cell wall elicits antibodies in rabbits that appear to cross-react with rabbit hearts, suggesting a relationship between this antigen and the etiology of rheumatic fever. Humans do not, however, appear to develop significant antibody levels against the group-specific carbohydrates of the cell wall, which form the basis of the Lancefield serologic grouping of the streptococci.

FEBRILE AGGLUTININS

The group of serologic antigens that comprise the traditional febrile agglutinin panel (Salmonella, Proteus, Francisella, Tularensis, and Brucella) have been used for decades in screening patients with unexplained fever. Our understanding of these diseases and our abilities to isolate the causative organisms, as well as the development of other improved serologic methods, have altered this approach to the diagnosis of these diseases. In addition, the incidence of these diseases has significantly decreased, and there are other more common causes of fever. Thus, the blind use of this group of "traditional" antigens should be discouraged, and the selective use of serologic tests based on clinical impressions and epidemiologic consideration is recommended.

SALMONELLA

The Widal test was established early in this century for the demonstration of serum antibodies in typhoid fever. However, the incidence of infections due to *Salmonella typhi* has fallen off markedly in the United States, while the incidence of infections due to other members of the *Salmonella* group has in-

Table 54–1. THE O ANTIGEN GROUPS OF SALMONELLA USED COMMONLY

GROUP	EXAMPLES OF SALMONELLA SEROTYPES FOUND IN THE GROUP
A	Paratyphi A
B	Typhimurium Paratyphi B Derby San Diego
C	Paratyphi C *choleraesuis* Montevideo Newport
D	*typhi* Enteritidis Dublin Gallinarum Pullorum
E	Anatum Meleagridis Give Newington Illinois Senftenberg

creased. Thus, the selection of antigens has been expanded to represent the several bioserotypes commonly encountered. Indeed, each laboratory may want to limit the antigens it has available only to those serotypes that are most common in its geographic area. The hundreds of bioserotypes of *Salmonella* isolated from humans can be divided into 17 groups on the basis of O (somatic) antigens; however, 95 per cent of isolates from human infections fall into one of five O antigen groups designated A, B, C, D, and E. These five O antigen preparations are often used in testing (Table 54-1).

The H antigens are present on the flagella of the *Salmonella* and often elicit an antibody response in infected patients. These antigens exist in two distinct phases, and transformation from one phase to the other occurs in the living bacteria under cultured conditions. Occasionally, a given isolate of *Salmonella* may exhibit antigenicity of both phases simultaneously. These are designated as phase 1 and phase 2 H antigens. The phase 1 antigens are relatively specific for the bioserotype and are designated with lower case letters a through z. Phase 2 H antigens are shared by several different species of *Salmonella* and are referred to as group-specific H-antigens. These are designated with Arabic numerals and certain lower case letters. Commonly, four H antigen preparations are used (Table 54-2).

A third antigen, the Vi or envelope antigen, is not used in the diagnosis of infections. It has been suggested as a means of identifying typhoid carriers who often have negative O and H titers; however, its reactivity in this group appears variable.

The H-antigen preparations consist of formalin-killed suspensions of appropriate motile species of *Salmonella*. The O antigen is prepared in a similar manner from a 24-hour culture, with the exception that the organisms

Table 54-2. COMMONLY USED SALMONELLA H AGGLUTININ ANTIGENS

| | FLAGELLAR ANTIGENS | |
ORGANISM	phase 1	phase 2
S. enteritidis Paratyphi A	a	-
S. enteritidis Paratyphi B	b	1,2
S. enteritidis Paratyphi C and		
S. choleraesuis	c	1,5
S. typhi	d	-

are washed with alcohol to remove H-antigen activity. The antigens thus prepared are used in both a rapid macroscopic slide test and in a more dilute suspension in the macroscopic tube dilution procedure. Serum dilutions corresponding to 1:40 and 1:80 are recommended in the slide procedure as a screening test, and any positive reaction should be confirmed by determining titers in tube dilution tests. A hemagglutination procedure in which antigens eluted from bacteria are absorbed to human group O red cells has been described. This method gives higher numerical titers than the bacterial agglutination procedures (Neter, 1956).

Interpretation of *Salmonella* O agglutination titers must be done with caution and with the knowledge of the patient's typhoid immunization status and the possibility of recent infection with other members of the Enterobacteriaceae. A fourfold rise in paired serum samples must be considered presumptive evidence of infection. Generally, titers of O agglutinins become elevated in 50 per cent of *Salmonella* infections by the end of the first week and significantly elevated in 90 per cent of infected persons by the fourth week. Titers peak between the third and sixth weeks and then slowly fall to low or absent levels in six to 12 months. The titers of H agglutinins rise more slowly and may remain elevated for a few years. H agglutinins are not always demonstrable in *Salmonella* infections. Antibiotic therapy early in disease often blunts the serum agglutinin response.

Salmonellae are probably more widely present in our environment than we realize, and indeed we may suffer multiple episodes of undocumented *Salmonella* enteritis during our lifetime. This exposure, plus typhoid immunizations, create moderate agglutinin titers in many individuals. Indeed, titers of 1:40 or 1:80 of either O or H agglutinins are considered within the range of "normal." Other Enterobacteriaceae have cross-reacting antigens that may cause a rise in O agglutinin titers, but generally do not cause a rise in H agglutinins. It is recommended, therefore, that one not place great significance on a single titer, regardless of its level, and some authorities seriously question the use of the Widal test at all in clinical medicine (Rose, 1976). Certainly it is of no use in the diagnosis of *Salmonella* gastroenteritis, in which symptoms abate before antibody titers rise. The test is sometimes used in patients with immu-

5

nologic deficiency syndromes to determine if they can produce antibodies in response to typhoid immunization.

BRUCELLA

The isolation of brucellae from the blood or tissues of infected individuals is seldom achieved beyond the acute phase of infection; therefore, serology is often used to establish the diagnosis. The serum agglutinin titer is measured with either a formalin-killed or a phenolized heat-killed suspension of a smooth colonial variety of *Brucella abortus*. The three species (*B. abortus*, *B. suis*, and *B. melitensis*) share common surface antigens (designated A and M), and infection with any one elicits antibodies that react with this one antigen preparation.

The antigen is used in both a macroscopic slide test and a tube dilution procedure. The slide test should be used only as a screening test of serum diluted 1:40 and 1:80. Any positive reaction is followed by a tube dilution test. The serial tube dilution technique using doubling dilutions of serum in saline starts at a dilution of 1:20 and ranges up to 1:2560. The test is incubated at 37°C. for 48 hours and read macroscopically. A prozone phenomenon is occasionally observed but only rarely extends beyond a 1:320 dilution. Heat inactivation of the patient's serum for 15 minutes at 56°C. reduces the incidence of the prozone phenomenon. Also, centrifugation of the tubes just prior to reading the reaction increases the sensitivity of the test.

The titer starts to rise in acute brucellosis during the second week of disease and usually peaks between the third and sixth weeks. A titer of 1:320 is considered presumptive evidence of acute active disease, although peak titers are often in the 1:640 to 1:2560 range. Following recovery, patients usually maintain an elevated titer of at least 1:80 for five or more years. Persons living in highly endemic areas or working closely with animals may demonstrate significantly higher titers (1:320) without a history of clinically apparent acute disease.

The serologic diagnosis of chronic brucellosis is more difficult. The agglutinin titer may be low or even absent unless a Coombs' (antiglobulin) technique is employed to demonstrate human immunoglobulin reacting with the antigen preparation (Kerr, 1966). Immu-

nofluorescence and complement-fixation procedures do not seem to offer any advantages over the agglutinin and antiglobulin techniques. A skin test is no longer generally available; it does not increase case detection and may, in turn, induce serum agglutinins, usually in low titer. It is important to remember that the absence of *Brucella* agglutinins does *not* rule out the diagnosis of brucellosis.

Infections with *Francisella tularensis*, *Vibrio cholerae*, and *Yersinia enterocolitica* induce serum agglutinins that cross-react with the *Brucella* antigen. Occasionally, persons with healed brucellosis will experience a transient rise in agglutinin titer associated with a febrile disease. Such titers are reported to rise as high as 1:160 in a few days and then fall below 1:80 in a week or 10 days.

TULAREMIA

The bacterial agglutination titer is the most commonly used serologic test in the diagnosis of tularemia. The antigen, which is available commercially, consists of a formalin-killed suspension of a standard strain of *Francisella tularensis*. It has been used in a slide agglutination procedure, but is more commonly performed as a tube dilution procedure. In the latter, the serum dilutions are incubated with antigen suspensions for two hours at 56°C. or at 37°C. Following this period of incubation, the tubes are refrigerated overnight (4 to 6°C.) and then examined for evidence of agglutination. "Normals" may have titers as high as 1:40. In patients with tularemia, the titer usually rises during the second week of disease to 1:80 or higher and peaks between two and three months. Mean peak titers are 1:640; but may vary between 1:160 and 1:2560. Thereafter, serum titers fall off slowly to a level of approximately 1:80, where they remain for years or perhaps for life.

Cross-reactions occur with *Brucella* antigens in approximately 25 per cent of cases, but virtually always at a lower titer. *Proteus* OX-19 antigens also cross-react somewhat. The determination of simultaneous titers with these three antigens is suggested to aid in interpretation of results.

A variety of other methods have been used but have not gained much acceptance. A hemagglutination procedure using human O red cells coated with *F. tularensis* polysaccharide gives higher numerical titers, and a fourfold rise in titer is observed earlier (Charkes, 1959). A skin test antigen, known as Foshay antigen, has not become widely available and gave a moderate number of adverse reactions. Workers of the U.S. Public Health Service have developed a less toxic skin test antigen (Buchanan, 1971) which generates a positive reaction before the agglutinin titer rises in most patients and does not induce a positive agglutinin titer in uninfected persons. However, some persons with a pre-existing low agglutinin titer experience a rise in titer following skin testing.

Weil-Felix Reaction in Rickettsial Diseases

The classic serologic diagnosis of rickettsial disease has depended upon the cross-reactivity between some of the rickettsiae and certain strains of *Proteus* species. The so-called Weil-Felix reaction grew out of the demonstration of agglutinins in the serum of several patients with typhus, which reacted with a strain of *Proteus* isolated from one patient with typhus. The strain of *Proteus*, designated OX-19 or, when used in a battery with two other *Proteus* strains, OX-2 and OX-K, gives various patterns of reactions that are described in Chapter 52. These reactions are non-specific and can be considered only presumptive evidence of disease. It is best to confirm positive reactions with procedures using specific antigens for the infection being considered. Also, a rise in titer must be demonstrated for a definitive diagnosis to be made; this frequently occurs too late in the course of the disease to be helpful in deciding on therapy.

The *Proteus* antigens consist of formalin-killed saline suspensions of the bacteria that are used in both the rapid slide agglutinin and the macroscopic tube agglutination procedures. The former is often used as a screening procedure, while titers for diagnostic purposes are obtained from the tube procedure. Agglutinins may appear in these diseases as early as the fifth or sixth day of disease and generally by the twelfth day. Peak titers are reached in early convalescence and then fall to undetectable levels in several months. The absence of *Proteus* agglutinins does not rule out rickettsial disease. Rickettsialpox, trench fever, and Q fever fail to generate such agglutinins, and patients with Brill-Zinsser frequently do not either. Early treatment with antibiotics delays

and suppresses the agglutinin response. One must beware of false positive non-specific agglutination with outdated antigen. In addition, *Proteus* agglutinin reactions may be found in sera from patients with leptospirosis, borreliosis, severe liver disease, and *Proteus* infections, such as in the urinary tract.

GONOCOCCAL SEROLOGY

Infection with *Neisseria gonorrhoeae* is best diagnosed by culture and Gram's stain of the organism. There is a problem of compliance with this approach in females, especially those who are asymptomatic. Yet it is this group that represents a significant link in the epidemiology of gonorrhea and in whom a "blood test" would be highly desirable as a screening test. The frequency and the epidemiologic role of the asymptomatic male has not yet been worked out.

The complement fixation (CF) method, employed early in this century, used a heat-treated whole or disrupted organism as the antigen. However, interest in a serologic test dropped off when penicillin was introduced and temporarily reduced the public health problems associated with gonorrhea. With a resurgence of infections, the CF methods have been re-evaluated and have been found to be less sensitive than newer methods. CF positivity occurs in 50 per cent of culture-positive females (Rodas, 1974).

The indirect fluorescent antibody (IFA) technique has greater sensitivity. It is dependent on the use of a strain of *N. gonorrhoeae* that contains sufficient antigen common to the various antigenic types prevalent in the population. Antibody in patients' sera reacts with bacteria on a slide before the fluorescein-labeled anti-human gamma globulin is applied. This method has been reputed to be comparable to cervical culture in its rate of detection of asymptomatic females (O'Reilly, 1973; Gaafar, 1976a).

Attaching gonococcal antigens to various particles has also been reported. Latex particle agglutination, cholesterol-lecithin flocculation, hemagglutination, and charcoal particle agglutination have generally given similar levels of sensitivity (75 to 85 per cent), and have the advantage of requiring less sophisticated equipment. These methods and the IFA have similar rates of false-positives in that between

5 and 15 per cent of culture-negative females with negative clinical histories will have a positive or borderline result with present methods.

Dans (1977) has questioned the use of currently available serologic methods for screening the general population where the prevalence of gonorrhea is very low (2 per cent or less in clinically non-infected females in the young adult age group). In this group the predictive value of a positive serologic test would be less than 10 per cent, and it is questionable whether the high rate of false positives is acceptable in a disease with such a social stigma. The statistics are more favorable in patients seen in clinics for sexually transmitted disease, yet in this group a culture may still be a more efficient method of diagnosis.

Most individuals develop positive gonococcal serology well into the second week of infection. Such information would not be useful in males, who generally become symptomatic and seek treatment three to five days after being infected. In females, symptoms may develop later or not at all, and serology is generally positive in 80 per cent of those with positive cultures. Also individuals with gonococcal arthritis have a similar rate of positivity (Hess, 1965), and serology may be very useful here when cultures fail to produce an organism.

The high number of false positives is thought to result from antibodies developed in response to infections due to *N. meningitidis* or other *Neisseria* species that are common as indigenous bacterial flora, particularly in the upper respiratory tract. However, there are conflicting results in regard to this interpretation (O'Reilly, 1973). It appears, therefore, that the optimal gonococcal serologic test is not yet available.

OTHER BACTERIAL SEROLOGY

There are several bacterial infections in which serologic tests have been developed as diagnostic aids. However, the isolation of bacteria is still the preferred and more rapid method of diagnosis, and most of the serologic methods are available only through more specialized laboratories. (See p. 1579 for CIE.)

Teichoic acid antibodies in serious infections caused by *Staphylococcus aureus* have been shown to be helpful in assessing the significance of isolates from blood cultures. Teichoic acid is a constituent of the cell wall of this organism, and a crude sonicate of the organism has been used as an antigen preparation. Nagel (1975) suggests using counterimmunoelectrophoresis (CIE) to demonstrate the presence of antibodies, followed by a determination of the titer by double diffusion in agar. Patients with endocarditis usually have titers above 1:4, while patients with other localized staphylococcal infections have lower or absent titers; thus, an elevated titer may be helpful in interpreting the significance of an isolate of *S. aureus* from blood. Cross-reaction and positive titers in patients with infection due to some streptococcal species, *S. epidermidis*, *Haemophilus influenzae*, and diphtheroids have been reported (Tuazon, 1976).

The immune responses to several other bacterial infections are being studied extensively, not so much for diagnostic purposes, but in order to gain an understanding of "protective" antibodies that result from natural infection and to isolate the appropriate antigen to incorporate into a vaccine. The various serogroups of *Neisseria meningitidis* are being studied in this regard, and polysaccharide antigens are available for the induction of antibodies against the capsules of groups A and C. The group B capsular polysaccharide is a very poor antigen, and efforts to produce an effective vaccine against it are continuing. Hemagglutination procedures with the capsular polysaccharide coated onto human group O red blood cells and the indirect immunofluorescent antibody procedure are the most common methods used to identify antibody response to meningococci. It is interesting that the antibody titer in natural infections falls to undetectable levels in a few years, while the response to purified antigen injections is still demonstrable many years later. Also, young children respond very poorly to the vaccine, and it is not until the teen years and young adulthood that good responses are consistently obtained.

Considerable effort is also going into the development of vaccines against *Haemophilus influenzae*. The high incidence of cross-reacting antigens in staphylococci and *Escherichia coli* is being explored, with the potential of colonizing individuals with such strains to induce immunity. Definition of the protective antibody against *H. influenzae* remains a problem. Finally, a vaccine composed of capsular polysaccharides from prevalent types of pneumococci is available (p. 1598).

REFERENCES

Bisno, A. L., and Ofek, I.: Serologic diagnosis of streptococcal infection. Comparison of a rapid hemagglutination technique with conventional antibody tests Am. J. Dis. Child., *127*:676, 1974.

Bisno, A. L., and Stollerman, G. H.: Streptococcal antibodies in the diagnosis of rheumatic fever. *In* Cohen, A. S. (ed.) Laboratory Diagnostic Procedures in the Rheumatic Diseases, 2nd ed. Boston, Little, Brown & Company, 1975, p. 207.

Bodily, H. L., Updyke, E. L., and Mason, J. O. (eds.): Diagnostic Procedures for Bacterial, Mycotic and Parasitic Infections, 5th Ed. New York, American Public Health Association, 1970.

Bradstreet, C. M., Tannahill, A. J., Pollock, T. M., and Magford, H. E.: Intradermal test and serological tests in suspected brucella infection in man. Lancet, *2*:653, 1970.

Buchanan, C. S., and Haserick, J. R.: FTA-ABS test in pregnancy: A probable false positive reaction. Arch. Dermatol., *102*:322, 1970.

Buchanan, T. M., Brooks, G. F., and Brachman, P. S.: The tularemia skin test. Ann. Intern. Med., *74*:336, 1971.

Caloenescu, M., Clecner, B., Petrow, S., and Kasatiya, S. S.: Immunofluorescent antibody test for diagnosis of gonorrhea. J. Clin. Microbiol., *1*:143, 1975.

Charkes, N. D.: Hemaglutination test in tularemia. Results in 56 vaccinated persons with laboratory acquired infection. J. Immunol., *83*:213, 1959.

Dans, P., Rothenberg, R., and Holmes, K. K.: Gonococcal serology: How soon, how useful, and how much? J. Infect. Dis., *135*:330, 1977.

Edwards, J. M. B., Tannahill, A. J., and Bradstreet, C. M. P.: Comparison of the indirect fluorescent antibody test with agglutination, complement fixation and Coombs test for brucella antibody. J. Clin. Pathol., *23*:161, 1970.

Escobar, M. R., Dalton, H. P., and Allison, M. J.: Fluorescent antibody tests for syphilis using cerebrospinal fluid: Clinical correlation in 150 cases. Am. J. Clin. Pathol., *53*:886, 1970.

Gaafar, H. A.: Evaluation of the fluorescent gonococcal test—heated. J. Clin. Microbiol., *4*:423, 1976a.

Gaafar, H. A., and D'Arcangelis, D. C.: Fluorescent antibody test for the serological diagnosis of gonorrhea. J. Clin. Microbiol., *3*:438, 1976b.

Goldman, J. N., and Lantz, M. A.: FTA-ABS and VDRL slide test reactivity in a population of nuns. J.A.M.A., *217*:53, 1971.

Hess, E. V., Hunter, D. K., and Ziff, M.: Gonococcal antibodies in acute arthritis. J.A.M.A., *191*:531, 1965.

Hooshman, H., Escobar, M. R., and Kapf, S. W.: Neurosyphilis. A study of 241 patients. J.A.M.A., *219*:726, 1972.

Hunter, C. A., Burdorff, R., and Colbert, B.: Flocculation tests for tularemia. J. Lab. Clin. Med., *51*:134, 1958.

Jaffe, H. W.: The laboratory diagnosis of syphilis. New concepts. Ann. Intern. Med., *83*:846, 1975.

Kaplan, E. L., Anthony, B. F., Chapman, S. S., Ayoub, E. M., and Wannamaker, L. W.: The influence of the site of infection on the immune response to group A streptococci. J. Clin. Invest., *49*:1405, 1970.

Kaufman, R. E., Olansky, D. C., and Wiesner, P. J.: The FTA-ABS (IgM) test for neonatal congenital syphilis: A critical review. J. Am. Vener. Dis. Assoc., *1*:79, 1974.

Kerr, W. R., Coghlan, J. D., Payne, D. J. H., and Robertson, L.: The laboratory diagnosis of chronic brucellosis. Lancet, *2*:1181, 1966.

Kerr, W. R., Payne, D. J. H., Robertson, L., and Coombs, R. R. A.: Immunoglobulin class of brucella antibodies in human sera. Immunology, *13*:223, 1967.

Kholey, A. E., Hafez, K., and Krause, R. M.: Specificity and sensitivity of the Streptozyme test for the detection of streptococcal antibodies. Appl. Microbiol., *27*:748, 1974.

Makk, L., Christain, A. B., Showalter, D., and Skaggs, D. R.: A comparison of ART to VDRL slide test. Lab. Med., *2*:34, 1971.

McCormick, J. B., and Bennet, J. V.: Public health considerations in the management of meningococcal disease. Ann. Intern. Med., *83*:883, 1975.

McKenna, C. H., Schroeter, A. L., Kierland, R. R., Stillwell, G. G., and Pien, F. D.: The fluorescent treponemal antibody absorbed (FTA-ABS) test beading phenomenon in connective tissue diseases. Mayo Clin. Proc., *48*:545, 1973.

Nagel, J. G., Tuazon, C. U., Cardella, T. A., and Sheagren, J. M.: Teichoic acid serologic diagnosis of staphylococcal endocarditis. Ann. Intern. Med., *82*:13, 1975.

Neter, E., Gorzynski, E. A., Gino, R. M., Westphal, O., and Luderitz, O.: The enterobacterial hemagglutination test and its diagnostic potentialities. Can. J. Microbiol., *2*:232, 1956.

O'Reilly, R. J., Welch, B. G., and Kellogg, D. S.: An indirect fluorescent antibody technique for study of uncomplicated gonorrhea. II. Selection and characterization of the strain of Neisseria gonorrhea used as antigen. J. Infect. Dis., *127*:77, 1973.

Peter, G., and Smith, A. L.: Group A streptococcal infections of the skin and pharynx. N. Engl. J. Med., *297*:311, 1977.

Ravel, R.: Hemagglutination test for syphilis (MHA) as alternative to the FTA-ABS. Lab. Med., *7*:22, 1976.

Robertson, D. H. H., McMillan, A., Young, H. and Henricksen, C.: Clinical value of the treponemal pallidium hemagglutination test. Br. J. Vener. Dis., *51*:79, 1975.

Rodas, C. U., and Ronald A. R.: Comparison of three serological tests in gonococcal infection. Appl. Microbiol., *27*:695, 1974.

Rose, N. R., and Friedman, H. (eds.): Manual of Clinical Immunology, Washington, D.C. American Society for Microbiology, 1976.

Roy, S. B., Sturgis, G. P., and Massell, B. F.: Application of the antistreptolysin-O titer in the evaluation of joint pain and in the diagnosis of rheumatic fever. N. Engl. J. Med., *254*:95, 1956.

Schroeter, A. L., Lucas, J. B., Price, E. V., and Falcone, V. H.: Treatment for early syphilis and reactivity of serologic tests. J.A.M.A., *221*:471, 1972.

Sparling, P. F.: Diagnosis and treatment of syphilis N. Engl. J. Med., *284*:642, 1971.

Tuazon, C. U., and Sheagren, J. M.: Teichoic acid antibodies in the diagnosis of serious infections with Staphylococcus aureus. Ann. Intern. Med., *84*:543, 1976.

U. S. Public Health Service: Manual of tests for syphilis. P. H. S. Publication No. 411. Washington, D.C., U.S. Government Printing Office, 1969.

Wallace, A. L., and Norins, L. C.: Syphilis serology today. *In* Steffanini, M. (ed.): Progress in Clinical Pathology, vol II. New York, Grune and Stratton, Inc., 1970, p. 198.

Wannamaker, L. W., and Ayoub, E. M.: Antibody titers in acute rheumatic fever. Circulation, *21*:598, 1960.

Welch, B. G., and O'Reilly, R. J.: An indirect fluorescent antibody technique for study of uncomplicated gonorrhea. I. Methology. J. Infect. Dis., *127*:69, 1973.

Wilson, G. S., and Miles, A.: Topley and Wilson's Principles of Bacteriology, Virology, and Immunity, 6th ed. Baltimore, Williams and Wilkins Company, 1975.

Wright, J. T., Cremer, A. W., and Ridgway, G. L.: False positive FTA-ABS results in patient with genital herpes. Br. J. Vener. Dis., *51*:329, 1975.

5

55

BACTERIAL SUSCEPTIBILITY TESTING AND ASSAYS

John M. Matsen, M.D.

GENERAL PRINCIPLES AND CONSIDERATIONS

Historical perspectives

In the period antedating the development of the first agents of the modern era of antimicrobial therapy, namely the sulfonamides, medical scientists utilized the first forms of *in vitro* testing to determine the potency of antiseptic agents. Fleming (1924), the discoverer of penicillin, reported on a "slide cell," which he used to test the effects of various antiseptics on bacterial agents. Fleming (1938) also later described a similar technique for study-

ing the effect of various sulfonamide derivatives on *Streptococcus pneumoniae*.

Reddish (1929) described a diffusion susceptibility test for testing antiseptics, ointments, etc. At the same time, Fleming (1929) used a gutter cut into an agar plate, which he filled with the compound to be tested. Organisms were streaked at right angles to the gutter and susceptibility was determined by the distance of inhibition. The first susceptibility testing for systemically used antimicrobials was carried out with the sulfonamides in the 1930's. In 1939 Rose and Miller attempted to standardize the multiple testing variables present in the plate diffusion method by addressing the inoculum size, the composition of media, organisms tested, etc. Subsequently, various methods were described, first for the sulfonamides and penicillins and, later, for other agents as they were discovered, utilizing various broth dilution techniques or techniques incorporating antimicrobials in varying concentrations directly into agar media. The principle of the diffusion test was first described, as noted above, by Fleming (1929). By placing the agent to be tested in a "gutter" or well in an agar plate, he was then able to measure the margin of inhibition against the organism to be tested. Others subsequently modified this principle by filling cylinders placed on the surface of the agar, placing a drop of an antimicrobial on the surface of the agar, and applying absorbent paper discs as reservoirs of known amounts of antimicrobial agents on the surface of the agar plate, which was seeded with the test organism.

Subsequently, all of the above tests have been refined in order to obviate problems which initially affected the precision of the methodologies. It is the purpose of this chapter to define currently used techniques for antimicrobial susceptibility testing and assay, and to outline the advantages, difficulties, and comparison factors. Each of the methods thus described has historical precedents dating back 30 to 50 years. Even the automated methods are based upon principles related to conventional techniques that were modified from the ideas first explored many years ago.

Definition of terms

The vocabulary of antimicrobial susceptibility testing includes several terms with which the reader should become conversant.

Susceptibility. The level of antimicrobial at which the growth of a given strain or microorganism is inhibited or killed by an antimicrobial compound.

A Susceptible Organism. An organism which is inhibited or killed by the concentration of the antimicrobial usually achieved in the serum, other body fluids, and tissues of the patient who has been given the usual dose of the antimicrobial by the usual route of administration.

Resistance. An organism is resistant to an antimicrobial when its level of susceptibility is beyond that normally achieved in the human body by the usual dose given by the usual route of administration.

Intermediate Susceptibility. Sometimes referred to as indeterminate or equivocal susceptibility, this category includes strains that are not clearly resistant or susceptible to a given antimicrobial agent but for which an *in vivo* response is probable if the agent were given in high dosages (see Group II, p. 1905).

Minimal Inhibitory Concentration (M.I.C.). In simplest terms, the lowest concentration of antimicrobial at which no bacterial growth occurs for a given bacterial strain.

Minimum Lethal Concentration (M.L.C.) or Minimum Bactericidal Concentration (M.B.C.). The lowest concentration of antimicrobial at which no viable bacterial cells remain for a given strain.

Antimicrobial Assay. The determination of the concentration of an antimicrobial present in serum or other body fluid.

Serum Bactericidal Assay. The determination of the titer of serum which will, in combination with the antibiotic present in the serum, kill 99.9 per cent of the inoculum in the serum sample.

Which organisms should be tested for antimicrobial susceptibility?

Bacteria for which susceptibility testing should be performed are potential pathogens or those which are likely pathogens in unusual situations, such as in the compromised patient. Susceptibility testing should be avoided for organisms with predictable susceptibility patterns, as the chance of a laboratory error is greater than the potential presence of a resistant organism among some species. This point is demonstrated in susceptibility testing of Group A streptococci with penicillin. Any potential pathogen with a significant proportion of resistant strains will require appropriate susceptibility testing. Organisms that develop resistance rapidly on exposure to antimicrobial agents should be tested again if isolated during therapy, as should certain antimicrobial agents for which a propensity exists for the development of resistance during their clinical use. Organisms not usually considered to be pathogenic may be pathogenic in patients with immune deficiencies where the antibiotic must act alone, and, in that context, isolates in those clinical circumstances may well require susceptibility testing that would not otherwise be necessary. Caution should be exercised to avoid susceptibility testing of organisms representing normal flora that are not acting as pathogens in the clinical setting and of mixed organism cultures. In the latter instance, susceptibility testing should be delayed until the organisms have been separated on isolation plates.

Generally speaking, the following organism groups are currently tested:

Staphylococcus aureus

Staphylococcus epidermidis (when associated with clinical disease)

The Enterobacteriaceae

Pseudomonas species and other gram-negative non-fermentative bacilli

Haemophilus influenzae (ampicillin)

Neisseria gonorrhoeae (in treatment failure situations or where resistant organisms are endemic)

Other infrequently isolated organisms with unpredictable susceptibility

Antimicrobials to be tested

Recommendations of the National Committee for Clinical Laboratory Standards (1975) and recommendations promulgated by the Center for Disease Control (Thornsberry, 1977b) generally include the grouping of antimicrobials for susceptibility testing into those being used for gram-positive organisms and those being used for gram-negative organisms. A further subgrouping of the gram-negative organism panel into one for gram-negative infections and urinary tract isolates and one for the *Pseudomonas* and non-fermenter group of organisms may be desirable. It is this latter approach that will be outlined here for the reader's consideration (Table 55-1).

Use of susceptibility testing

Susceptibility tests, in the clinical setting, are justified in terms of the guidance that they provide for the physician. Where specific susceptibility testing results are not available, the physician, under ideal conditions, bases his or her approach to therapy upon accumulated knowledge regarding the organisms likely to be present in the specific disease entity, as well as the most likely susceptibility profile based upon past experience. Some organisms, such as Group A *Streptococcus*, are almost absolutely predictable with respect to their susceptibility to penicillin. Other organisms may have very little predictability of susceptibility. Such is the case with some of the gram-negative organisms, such as *Proteus rettgeri*. The majority of organisms with which the physician must deal in clinical settings have greater or lesser predictability depending upon the antibiotic being considered.

Susceptibility testing results, when available, should help the physician to select the most effective and preferred agent for the organism in question. In most instances, the physician will also have a number of other considerations to take into account when choosing the antimicrobial to be administered. Factors relating both to the antimicrobial and to the patient's underlying circumstances must be taken into consideration. The physi-

Table 55-1. PROPOSED ANTIMICROBIALS FOR ROUTINE TESTING

GRAM-POSITIVE ORGANISMS	ENTEROBACTERIACEAE	OTHER GRAM-NEGATIVE ORGANISMS
Amikacin	Amikacin	Amikacin
Ampicillin	Ampicillin	Carbenicillin
Cephalothin	Carbenicillin	Colistin (or polymyxin B)
Chloramphenicol	Cephalothin	Gentamicin
Clindamycin	Chloramphenicol	Tobramycin
Erythromycin	Colistin (or	Chloramphenicol‡
Gentamicin	polymyxin B)	Kanamycin‡
Methicillin, nafcillin	Gentamicin	Sulfonamide‡
or oxacillin	Tetracycline	Tetracycline‡
Penicillin	Tobramycin	
Tetracycline	Nitrofurantoin*	
Vancomycin	Sulfonamide*	
	Trimethoprim-	
	sulfamethoxazole*†	
	Kanamycin§	
	Nalidixic acid§	

*Reported for urinary tract isolates only.
†Trimethoprim-sulfamethoxazole may be effective against organisms isolated from other sites.
‡Reported for non-fermentative bacilli other than *Pseudomonas aeruginosa*.
§May be substituted for other agents, depending upon physician use and preference.

cian must also consider economic factors in administering antimicrobial agents, either in the hospital or in the office or clinic setting.

In many respects, the narrower the spectrum of the antimicrobial, the more preferred is its use when one knows specifically the organism being treated. However, the converse is true when one thinks in terms of approaching an unknown infection, where one may or may not know the susceptibility pattern. In that context, the broader spectrum antibiotics have great value. In gram-negative sepsis, the more common approach is to use an aminoglycoside antibiotic in conjunction with one of the cephalosporin or semisynthetic penicillin agents. This allows for the broad coverage necessitated by the unknown status of the organism's susceptibility.

In an ideal setting, susceptibility data should also provide some indication to the physician as to what level of antimicrobial is necessary. With the existing high content disk diffusion methodology, the values that have been established for the "susceptible" category take into consideration the usual dosage of antimicrobial, administered by the usual route, in systemic infections. For those agents for which toxicity is not a factor, an intermediate or indeterminate reading allows the physician to increase the dosage with some degree of confidence. However, for most antimicrobials the values reported for the disk diffusion method do not completely reflect the high concentration of antimicrobial in the urine owing to its excretion through the kidney. The level of susceptibility should ideally provide some correlation and provide some understanding as to the level of antimicrobial necessary to treat the specific infection effectively.

The degree of susceptibility of an organism at times can assist in determining the length of therapy. It has been suggested that viridans streptococci, in cases of endocarditis, inhibited by less than 0.2 μg/ml of penicillin, can be treated in one half to two thirds the time normally required for treatment of those organisms demonstrating a lesser degree of susceptibility. However, in most circumstances the degree of susceptibility of an organism is not the determining factor in the length of therapy. Rather, it is the specific clinical condition and the identity of the organism that provide the more appropriate guidelines for that decision.

In those settings where it is desirable to use a combination of antimicrobials, the classic approach to dilution or diffusion susceptibility testing will only infrequently provide assistance regarding the preferred antimicrobial combination. However, special testing can be performed, in which antimicrobials are tested in combination and in varying concentrations against the organism to be treated. These tests, however, can be rather expensive for the patient because of their complexity.

An age-old dilemma of the physician, that of receiving susceptibility results for a patient who is already receiving antimicrobial therapy, requires a decision as to whether or not susceptibility test results warrant a change in therapy. This dilemma is lessened when the patient is not doing well or when susceptibility results indicate resistance to the compound being used. However, in those instances in which susceptibility tests demonstrate susceptibility to the agent being used and to another agent or agents that are less expensive or less toxic, the physician will be required to exercise clinical judgment in determining the therapeutic approach. Our experience indicates that the physician will alter therapy in 20 to 30 per cent of such instances.

The need for assay information

The physician, for the support of antimicrobial therapy, often requires information relating to the pharmacokinetics of an antimicrobial agent in serum, urine, or other body fluids. Assays of antimicrobial levels may be helpful in predicting the likelihood of success of antimicrobial usage and as a means of attempting to prevent the potential toxicity which accompanies the use of a number of antimicrobial agents.

Both the estimation of therapeutic success and the prevention of toxicity may be important in the patient with normal excretory function but are of more frequent concern in the patient who has compromised renal function. One is much more likely to perform assays in patients in whom kidney or liver failure or dysfunction is present. Examples would include the use of an aminoglycoside antibiotic in a patient in whom the serum creatinine values were elevated, or the use of chloramphenicol in a newborn infant in whom the liver-conjugating enzymes are immature.

Another consideration in the use and the need for antimicrobial assays is whether or not the sample should be tested at the anticipated trough or peak level. To measure maximum effect, peak levels become an obvious

5

choice; however, there is evidence to indicate that the trough level of aminoglycoside antibiotics may assist in preventing both oto- and nephrotoxicity.

Antimicrobial assays may also be used to resolve quandaries relating to the failure of therapy where *in vitro* susceptibilities would have predicted response.

All in all, the assay of antimicrobial agents becomes an important part of most clinical microbiology laboratories. The methodology and specific approaches will be discussed later in this chapter.

Serum 'cidal assays, or serum bactericidal titers, have become increasingly important in many clinical microbiology laboratories. Another name for this test is the Schlichter (1947) test, which is used primarily in the management of endocarditis, osteomyelitis, or other serious bacterial infections. The methodology of this test will also be explained subsequently in this chapter. For introductory purposes, it is sufficient to explain that this test provides a quantitation of the combined effect of serum (or other body fluid) and the antibiotic which the patient is receiving. The assumption may be made, in the absence of an implanted prosthesis or other foreign material, that therapy can be anticipated to be successful if bactericidal activity has been demonstrated in a dilution of serum of 1:8 or 1:16 or greater. In staphylococcal endocarditis it is preferable to have activity of 1:32 or greater. Again, this test is used as a predictor of success in antimicrobial usage and also to monitor the appropriateness of therapy.

Timeliness of results

The potential exists for rapid answers in both susceptibility testing and antimicrobial assays. Currently, for example, instrumentation and other methodology exists which will allow for rapid susceptibility information within three to six hours following the isolation of an organism. In other circumstances, studies have demonstrated that with urine and other body fluids, where assessment by Gram stain has indicated the probable presence of a single organism, susceptibility results can be generated within a shorter time frame.

In part, the challenge to the pathologist is to coordinate susceptibility and culture information. A laboratory locked into set protocols at times is unresponsive to the individual cases in which this particular information becomes

very important to the physician. Certain kinds of cultures such as those of blood or cerebrospinal fluid, carry with them the greater likelihood that information received from the laboratory with regard to organism susceptibility may have an impact on patient care, on success of therapy, and on the length of hospital stay. In that context, one hopes that the clinical laboratory will be responsive to processing these cultures as rapidly as possible. Studies we have performed would indicate that there is a substantial impact on patient care when the susceptibility information is received simultaneously with preliminary culture information or within a short time after the beginning of therapy. The longer the result is in arriving, the less chance the physician will use the data in altering or modifying therapy.

The pressure for rapid susceptibility and assay testing results has its practical considerations, and if physicians know that rapid answers can be forthcoming, they will learn to expect this service and will plan their therapeutic decisions accordingly. In our own hospital, for example, where radioimmunoassay is currently used for gentamicin and bioassay for tobramycin, physicians indicate that they are much more likely to use gentamicin than tobramycin, largely on the basis of having access to the more rapid assay information provided by radioimmunoassay. They can determine trough levels and anticipate that within one hour they will know the dose they should provide the patient. In the case of peak levels, additional doses of antimicrobials can be given should these levels not be sufficient in terms of the current dosage, or the dosage can be reduced if these levels approach toxic ranges.

The clinical laboratory, along with providing rapid answers, should also pay attention to the details of result transmission and reporting. Just as the laboratory usually calls results of positive cultures of body fluids and tissues, it should also call results of priority susceptibility or assay tests, alterations in susceptibility or abnormal assay results, or in instances of resistance to an antimicrobial agent that is listed as therapy on the laboratory request slip.

In general, susceptibility results that do not become available until physicians have made their late afternoon rounds may have less impact on physicians' antimicrobial usage than if they are transmitted as quickly as possible for the physician to review on the same day that test results become available.

Regulating agencies, standardization, and "approved" methods

Valid and accurate results are more likely to be received from any clinical laboratory today than at any time previously. The regulation of antimicrobial susceptibility testing in the past has been very loose and has resulted in considerable variation in test methodology and test results. In 1966 Bauer et al. published their classic paper on the high content disc diffusion technique. This served as the basis for a number of recommendations for standardization and led to its recognition and promulgation by the Food and Drug Administration (Federal Register, 1972, 1973), to whom responsibility for antimicrobial susceptibility testing materials and methodology has been given. Other groups, such as the National Committee for Clinical Laboratory Standards (1975), have essentially agreed to this methodology and described it in greater detail. Textbooks and other manuals, such as the Manual of Clinical Microbiology for the American Society for Microbiology (Matsen, 1974), have also promulgated this methodology, adding emphasis to the desirability and necessity of uniform testing approaches.

It is anticipated that further standardization will occur for the alternative susceptibility methods, as has occurred with the diffusion method noted above and with the agar dilution methodology as advocated by the International Collaborative Study Group (Ericsson, 1971). It is of note that the latter group has achieved almost universal acceptance of this agar dilution methodology.

Quantitative vs. qualitative testing

Historically, clinical laboratories have been restrained in their ability to do quantitative susceptibility testing because of practicality and economics. Until a standardized agar dilution method was available, only a very few institutions, such as the Mayo Clinic, performed agar dilution susceptibilities on a routine basis (Washington, 1969). The advent of the Steers (1959) replicator and the practical approach, as developed by the Mayo Clinic (Washington, 1974a), has made this a very useful quantitative method for those institutions with high volumes of susceptibility tests. Broth dilution capability, while always available to the routine laboratory, was very prohibitive because of the cumbersome nature of the individual dilution sets for each antibiotic.

With the advent of microbroth dilution techniques, this approach has become convenient and economical (Gavan, 1970; Gavan, 1974; Gerlach, 1974, 1977; Goss, 1968; MacLowry, 1968, 1970; McMaster, 1978). In essence, microdilution costs are close enough to those of the disc diffusion test to make this method economically feasible. In addition, the advent of instrument-generated laboratory or commercially produced microbroth dilution plates, conveniently provided in bulk quantities, has made this a practical method as well (Tilton, 1973).

If a laboratory chooses to provide quantitative results to the physician, it is obliged to provide a ready reference for understanding the meaning and interpretation of the results being reported. In this context, it is important to determine whether the physician population one serves even desires to have quantitative data. Most commercial firms now producing the microdilution plates provide tables and reference data sufficient for appropriate physician education.

Disc diffusion testing, if carefully standardized, can provide quantitative information by extrapolating the MIC from zone diameters on the basis of previously derived regression plots. For an explanation of regression analysis and the uses to which it can be put, refer to page 1915.

In conjunction with the usage of the susceptible, intermediate, and resistant categories, it is pertinent to explain the four categories of susceptibility proposed by the International Collaborative Group (Ericsson, 1971). Group I includes high degrees of bacterial susceptibility, which would provide a strong likelihood of *in vivo* response if mild to moderately severe systemic infections were treated with the usual (orally administered where applicable) dosage of antibiotic. This group could be defined as "susceptible" without further qualifications.

Group II would include a level of susceptibility which would make the *in vivo* response probable in systemic infections if the antimicrobial were given in high dosage or up to the limits of toxicity. Group III would comprise that level of susceptibility which would make *in vivo* response probable in the treatment of localized infections at sites where the agent could be concentrated by the physiologic processes or by direct local application. Group IV, then, would include organisms of a degree of resistance which would make the *in vivo* response improbable. This group would be designated as resistant. The International Collaborative Group further advocated that the application of these categories would be antimicrobial-specific, with various modifications to fit each agent's unique pharmacokinetic features.

Susceptibility testing results usually reflect inhibition, rather than destruction or killing, of growth. This result can be of concern in certain types of infections, such as those due to staphylococci, where there may be a rather marked difference between the inhibitory and the killing or bactericidal concentration for several antibiotics, even with those which are ordinarily considered to be bactericidal in nature. For most infections, the inhibitory result is sufficient to direct the therapeutic choice of an antimicrobial agent. However, as indicated above, certain categories of infections may require determination of bactericidal concentrations.

One of the major problems in the use of susceptibility data is its relationship to anticipated urinary antimicrobial concentrations. It is generally acknowledged that urinary tract infections respond to the concentrations of antimicrobial in the urine which significantly exceed those generally present in the serum. The standardized disc diffusion method does not provide the physician with appropriate information regarding achievable urine levels. Unless the physician determines that the intermediate or indeterminate interpretive criteria are applicable to the urinary tract, the therapeutic approach may be far too conservative in terms of achievable antimicrobial levels in the urine, where they tend to be highly concentrated. In most instances, concentrations of antimicrobials tested by dilution methods range from those attainable in urine to those attainable in serum. Quantitative data, as provided by dilution testing, also has potential value, clinically, in the management of bacterial endocarditis, as well as in serious infections of compromised patients. Furthermore, it is becoming apparent that both quantitative inhibitory and bactericidal information can be of considerable help with staphylococcal infections, in which up to 40 per cent of the strains isolated from clinically significant infections may be termed "tolerant," with a considerable spread between the inhibitory and bactericidal concentrations (Sabath, 1977). Broth dilution testing allows determination of bactericidal endpoints.

Media: Type and content

One of the major problems in performing susceptibility tests is not only the variation among different formulations but also lot-to-lot and manufacturer-to-manufacturer variations of specific formulations. Whereas Mueller-Hinton medium has been chosen for standardized diffusion and dilution testing purposes because of its growth-potentiating properties for *Neisseria* and other fastidious organisms, it continues to be vulnerable to lot-to-lot and manufacturer-to-manufacturer variations. Our own experience would indicate that over the past three years there have been substantial problems in susceptibility testing media performance, and at almost all times one or more antibiotics will be outside the limits of quality control as established by regulating agencies and advisory committees. We have recently explored the susceptibility of one of the new cell wall active antimicrobials in six different media, and the MIC's varied by as much as tenfold with the same strain depending upon which medium was used. Some of this variation relates to cation differences and some relates to the digestion process necessary for the production of the protein components of the media. Much remains to be done in terms of providing a stoichiometrically precise medium which can be manufactured uniformly to provide a consistent end-product.

It is important, therefore, that the performance of media to be used by a laboratory be regularly assessed by appropriate quality control means. It is also hoped that media manufacturers will be placed under the constraints to adhere to performance standards of media in order to assure more uniform results in the clinical laboratories of this country.

DILUTION TESTING

GENERAL CONSIDERATIONS

Stock Solutions. The preparation of stock solutions necessitates obtaining standard preparation either from the manufacturer or from laboratory supply firms* which can provide the testing material. In most instances, antimicrobial preparations intended for clinical use are not acceptable as laboratory testing reagents, as they may be chemi-

---

*These compounds are also available from United States Pharmacopeia Convention, Inc., 12601 Twinbrook Parkway, Rockville, Md., 20852.

cally impure and inaccurate as to stated activity. Laboratory testing materials should:

1. Have a date of expiration clearly visible on the container.
2. Have a readily apparent statement of activity in μg or IU per mg or ml of preparation.
3. Be dated on arrival in the laboratory.
4. Be dated when opened.
5. Be stored in a desiccator after opening.
6. Be carefully weighed in an analytical balance or measured with pipettes of appropriate volumetric capacity.
7. Be sterilized by membrane filtration if necessary.
8. Be stored at $-20°$C. or colder.
9. Be dissolved or diluted in the appropriate solvent and diluent (see Table 55-2).

Inoculum Standardization. The use of a barium sulfate standard for standardization of inoculum has become routine for most susceptibility procedures. It should be stressed that this step is vulnerable to inefficient use of time, to errors in formulation and, therefore, determinations of turbidity, and to visual aberrations due to improper mixing. To ensure the maximum efficiency and accuracy, the following measures should be considered:

1. The turbidity standard is prepared by adding 0.5 ml of 0.048 M $BaCl_2$ (1.175 per cent, w/v, $BaCl_2 \cdot 2H_2O$) to 99.5 ml of 0.36 N H_2SO_4 (1 per cent, v/v). This is then equivalent to one half the density of a MacFarland No. 1 barium sulfate standard.
2. The standard should be placed in a sealed tube

Table 55–2. PREPARATION AND STORAGE OF ANTIMICROBIAL AGENTS*

The following table indicates the solvents and diluents to be used in the preparation of stock antibiotic solutions from antibiotic powder.

ANTIMICROBIAL	SOLVENT	DILUTION
Amikacin	[3]Water	Water
Amphotericin B	Dimethylsulfoxide	Water, adjust to pH 9.0 with NaOH
Ampicillin	[1]Phosphate buffer, pH 8.0, 0.1 M	Phosphate buffer, pH 6.0, 0.1 M
Carbenicillin	Water	Water
Cephalothin	Phosphate buffer, pH 6.0, 0.1 M	Water
Chloramphenicol	Ethanol	Water
Clindamycin	Water	Water
Cycloserine	Water	Water
Erythromycin	Ethanol	Water
Ethambutol	Water	Water
5-Fluorocytosine	Saline, 0.85%	Saline, 0.85%
Gentamicin	[3]Water	Water
Isoniazid	Water	Water
Kanamycin	[3]Water	Water
Nalidixic acid	1 N NaOH	Water
Nitrofurantoin	Dimethylformamide	Water
Oxacillin	Water	Water
Penicillin	Water	Water
Polymyxin B	Water	Water
Rifampin	Dimethylsulfoxide	Phosphate buffer, pH 7.0
Streptomycin	Water	Water
Sulfonamides	10% NaOH + hot water	Water
Tetracyclines	Water	Water
Tobramycin	Water	Water
Vancomycin	Water	Water

COMMENTS:
1. Phosphate buffers should be kept in the refrigerator for use as diluents.
2. Stock solutions are stored in the freezer at $-35°$C. At this temperature, stock solutions of most antibiotics (except penicillins, which should be replaced monthly) are stable for approximately six months.
3. The aminoglycoside antibiotics may also be dissolved in the phosphate buffer pH 8.0, 0.1 M.

*Modified from Washington (1974b).

to avoid fluid loss by evaporation (Washington, 1973).

3. The standard should be agitated with a vortex mixer prior to each use.

4. The actual process of inoculum standardization can be enhanced and time conserved by utilizing the modified Rh view box apparatus described by Stemper and Matsen (1970). This reference provides both a narrative descrip-

5. The use of a black on white background, either as a feature of the apparatus referred to above or separately, will also facilitate turbidity comparison.

Agar Dilution Susceptibility Testing

The agar dilution method, as described initially by the International Collaborative Study Group (Ericsson, 1971) and later in greater detail by Washington (1974b), has been used on a routine clinical basis primarily for research purposes and in larger clinical laboratories. To make this particular method economical on a day-to-day basis, at least 20 organisms should probably be tested daily. If the laboratory is performing more than 20 tests per day, then this method is the most economical of all of the susceptibility test methodologies.

Instrumentation. In order to achieve the economical advantage described above, this method requires an inoculum-replicating device, such as that of Steers (1959). Modifications of the instrumentation are possible by using a spring-loaded device which allows for more rapid and potentially more uniform application of the inoculum to the individual plates. In addition, the Steers device (Melrose Machine Shop, Woodlyn, Pa.) has been modified for use with a larger, square plate which provides for 36 inoculum implants. Though the seed plate and inoculating prongs can be made out of either aluminum or stainless steel, the aluminum construction is more vulnerable to erosion and pitting. The care of the instrumentation is important. Washington (1974a) advocates soaking the seed plate and inoculating prongs overnight in 70 per cent ethyl alcohol, after scrubbing them clean with a brush. They are then wrappd in a cloth towel and this pack is placed in a large glass Petri dish and autoclaved prior to use. Glass rings, called by some "Raschig"rings, can be placed around the inoculum of spreading *Proteus* strains in order to inhibit their dispersion across the agar test plate. These rings can be cleaned by boiling in water for 20 minutes and then soaking in 70 per cent ethyl alcohol prior to use.

Medium. Mueller-Hinton agar (MHA) or other agar media may be used for this method. One may also add whole, chocolatized, lysed, or peptic digest of blood, usually in a 5 per cent v/v amount for those organisms that require this enrichment.

Brain-heart infusion or Wilkins-Chalgren (1976) agar with 5 per cent sheep blood can be used for testing anaerobic organisms.

One should establish performance standards for each of the several antimicrobials to be used. It is important to note that cation differences can be substantial among the three media mentioned above, and in this context, performance, especially with the aminoglycoside antibiotics, can vary from lot to lot and from manufacturer to manufacturer, as well as from medium to medium (Reller, 1974; Washington, 1978).

Antimicrobial Preparations. Individual antimicrobials are prepared in sterile distilled water for later addition to the melted agar medium. The simplest approach to this task is to follow a systematized guide such as that presented in Table 55–3, as modified from Ericsson (1971). By preparing concentrations in this manner, 1.5 ml of antimicrobial solution can be added to 13.5 ml agar suspension or, alternatively, 2 ml of antimicrobial solution to 18 ml suspension for pouring into 100 mm plates.

Use of the scheme in Table 55–3 is made additionally practical in that only one pipette need be used for each series of three dilutions. Furthermore, this method is not as vulnerable to the cumulative error which can pose a serious problem in fixed and repetitive serial dilution methods.

The general approach, in the past, to tube dilution testing has been strictly in terms of twofold dilutions. Whereas this does provide considerable information with respect to the level of antimicrobial susceptibility, in actuality it provides more information than is needed in most clinical circumstances. Therefore, institutions such as the Mayo Clinic (Washington, 1974a) have developed an abbreviated set of concentrations to be used for agar dilution susceptibility testing. In most instances, this set includes only three or four concentrations. The determination of the concentrations of antimicrobial to be tested is based upon an assessment of the levels in serum likely to be attained in the treatment of systemic infection with the usual dose by the usual route of administration, and levels relating to expected urinary tract concentrations. This abbreviated scheme has obvious economic advantages over a ten- or twelve-level twofold dilution approach.

Preparation of Plates. The medium, once it has been prepared according to the manufacturer's directions, is allowed to cool to approximately 45° to 50°C. in an appropriately adjusted waterbath. The medium is usually prepared in screw-cap bottles, as these allow for ease of mixing.

Considerations in the preparation of plates include the ability to produce a plate which is level and uniform in consistency. In addition, the antimicrobials should be evenly distributed throughout the agar medium. Therefore, one should take care to add the antibiotic quickly in order that the agar medium not cool below 45°C. This prevents partial

---

*Available from Steuer Medical Inc., 1744 E. 3045 South, Salt Lake City, Utah 84106.

Table 55-3. MODIFIED GUIDE FOR DILUTION OF ANTIMICROBIALS IN AGAR

ANTIMICROBIAL SOLUTION		VOLUME OF STERILE WATER TO BE ADDED (IN ML)	CONCENTRATION AS ADDED TO MELTED AGAR 1:9 OR FOR FURTHER DILUTION ON LINES BELOW	FINAL CONCENTRATION IN AGAR	
μg or IU/ml	Stock vol. (in ml)		μg or IU/ml		LOG$_2$
2000	6.4	3.6	1280	128	7
1280	2	2	640	64	6
1280	1	3	320	32	5
1280	1	7	160	16	4
160	2	2	80	8	3
160	1	3	40	4	2
160	1	7	20	2	1
20	2	2	10	1	0
20	1	3	5	0.5	−1
20	1	7	2.5	0.25	−2

coalescence of the agar, which can result not only in uneven plates but also in non-uniform distribution of the antimicrobial. Similarly, adding an antimicrobial prior to cooling to 50°C. can be detrimental in that the increased temperature can have an adverse effect on the activity of some antimicrobials. In mixing the antimicrobial and agar, one should take care not to introduce bubbles by being too vigorous in the mixing process. Bubbles can result in an uneven surface, and the usual method of handling these bubbles, that of flaming the surface of the plate, can also have an adverse effect with respect to certain antimicrobials.

A separate plate of Mueller-Hinton agar without added antibiotics should also be poured for each dilution series in order to provide an appropriate growth control.

Once plates have been allowed to harden, they should be carefully marked as to the type and concentration of antimicrobial agent present. These plates can then be used within a short period of time or can be packaged in plastic bags and stored at 4°C. Studies by Ryan (1970) have shown that most antimicrobial agents in agar can be stored in this fashion for four weeks. The exceptions are the penicillins and nitrofurantoin. These should not be stored longer than one week. For reference work and other investigational studies, plates should be used within 24 hours of preparation.

Because of the need for uniformity and to obviate the possibility of inoculum spot coalescence on the agar, plates should be dried sufficiently to remove surface moisture before use.

A special note should be made at this point that blood products are usually added to the agar after the antimicrobial has been added and thoroughly mixed. Once the blood has been added, the plates should be poured immediately in order to avoid the possibility of coalescence of agar.

Inoculum is prepared as for other susceptibility tests. Between four and six morphologically identical colonies are touched with an inoculating loop or needle and suspended in 2 ml of an appropriate sterile medium. Either soybean-casein digest broth (e.g., Trypticase Soy Broth [TSB]) or Mueller-Hinton Broth (MHB) is usually used. One should be aware that streptococci do not generally grow well in MHB and that TSB should routinely be used for these organisms. There are several approaches to the standardization of the density of the inoculum (Ericsson, 1971; Washington, 1974a). A suitable approach is as follows: after inoculating 2 ml of sterile broth, the organisms are allowed to grow for 2 to 4 hours at 35°C. or are allowed to incubate overnight at the same temperature, and the turbidity of the broth culture is then adjusted to match that of the 0.5 MacFarland standard, by diluting the suspension with similar broth. A 1:200 dilution of the standardized organism suspension is made so that the final inoculum is in the range of 5×10^6 CFU/ml. An alternate approach to achieving this inoculum size is either to perform a 1:200 dilution of an overnight broth culture or to use a 0.5 ml broth culture that has been heavily inoculated and allowed to incubate for four hours.

Once the inoculum has been standardized, it should be transferred to the test medium without delay before organism replication occurs.

The whole process of inoculum preparation is facilitated if one uses a rack for the inoculated tubes with the same configuration as that of the replicator device's seed plate (Washington, 1974a). This will also facilitate the recording of specimen numbers onto a grid sheet marked in such a way that the location of each organism being tested can be easily noted.

Transfer of Inoculum. The first step in preparing for the transfer of inoculum from the standardized broth cultures into the seed plate wells should be to fill one well, usually in a corner, with India ink to define clearly the orientation of the organisms being tested. From the standardized broth tubes, an amount of inoculum approximately equivalent to one half to two thirds the potential volume of each well in the seed plate well is transferred to that well. Individual pipettes must be used for each organism; however, the amount to be transferred need only be approximate, so that less expensive Pasteur pipettes can be used. The head of the replicating device, containing the individual inoculation prongs corresponding with the wells in the seed plate, is then lowered into the seed plate, raised, and lowered onto the agar surface. The prongs are constructed so as to deliver approximately 0.001 to 0.003 ml or approximately 1×10^4 colony-forming units (CFU). The size of the inoculum spot on the agar surface is approximately 5 to 8 mm.

As one transfers the inoculum from a seed plate to the agar surface with any replicator device, one should be careful to use smooth hand movements to prevent splatter. One should avoid pressure on the agar surface with the inoculating head and should allow it to remain on the agar for 3 to 5 seconds prior to returning it to the seed plate. One should move from the least concentrated antimicrobial plate toward the most concentrated in the series in order to avoid the possibility of transfer of antimicrobial either to the seed plate or to subsequent dilutions in the series.

As has already been mentioned, 12×12 mm Raschig rings (Scientific Glass Apparatus, Bloomfield, N.J.) can be used to prevent spreading by *Proteus*. Once inoculation has taken place, these rings should be set on the agar. After the transfer of inocula has been completed, the plate is covered and allowed to stand until the inoculum droplets are absorbed into the agar; however, the surface of the agar should be carefully examined immediately after inoculum transfer in order to ensure that there is an inoculum droplet at each location where this transfer should have occurred. One can use a 0.001 ml calibrated loop for the transfer, on a single specimen basis, of inoculum from the appropriate seed plate well to the location on the agar surface where any droplets were not transferred.

Incubation. The plates are incubated at 35°C. in an inverted position for 16 to 20 hours. The atmosphere of incubation is usually ambient air, although, for those organisms requiring increased CO_2, incubation in CO_2 is possible as long as one tests appropriate controls in the same environment. In testing anaerobic organisms, these plates can be incubated in an anaerobic environment.

Results. According to the report of the International Collaborative Study (Ericsson, 1971), a barely visible haze of growth or a single colony is disregarded; if several colonies are found extending more than one dilution beyond an obvious endpoint, the purity of this strain is checked and the test repeated. The results are recorded on the grid which has been used to define the geographic location, both in the seed plate and on the agar surface, of the several specimens being tested.

HAEMOPHILUS INFLUENZAE. Because of the advent of ampicillin-resistant *H. influenzae*, the need has arisen for testing of this organism either by dilution or disc diffusion techniques or by determining beta-lactamase production. When several strains of *Haemophilus* are to be tested simultaneously, the agar dilution method facilitates this evaluation.

A stock antibiotic solution of ampicillin and the medium is prepared according to procedures already described. The test medium is Mueller-Hinton agar with added sterile horse blood or 1 per cent hemoglobin and IsoVitaleX (BioQuest, Cockeysville, Md.). The inoculum is prepared by scraping the growth from a pure culture (on chocolate or other suitable medium) of the *Haemophilus* with a sterile platinum loop into 4 ml of TSB to a density matching the 0.5 MacFarland turbidity standard (approximately 10^8 CFU/ml). This standardized suspension is then diluted 1:100. A suitable control (*Escherichia coli*, ATCC 25922) should be prepared and tested concurrently. If several strains are tested, the inoculating apparatus of Steers (1959) may be used; however, for few strains it is easier to spot inoculate the agar with a sterile 0.001 ml calibrated loop. It is suggested that an atmosphere with increased CO_2 should not be used unless it is required for the growth of a specific strain.

Results are determined in the same way as that described above for the agar dilution method. This procedure can be very helpful in those situations where there is equivocation about the results of disc diffusion testing. It can also be of value in those situations where ampicillin resistance is suspected despite the absence of beta-lactamase production. It should be stressed that some strains of *Haemophilus influenzae* that are resistant to ampicillin are not beta-lactamase producers.

Macrobroth dilution methods

The details of this procedure are described elsewhere (Ericsson, 1971; Washington, 1974b). Because of the necessity of preparing dilution series singly, macrobroth dilution methods are quite cumbersome and time-consuming.

Medium. The medium is usually Mueller-Hinton broth, although many other media have been used, including those resulting from soy digests, tryptose phosphate, nutrient, Eugon, brain-heart infusion, etc. Comparative studies have clearly indicated that the MIC and MBC values for test organisms can vary widely depending upon the type of media used, pH, osmolality, and electrical conductivity. Results can vary with certain antimicrobials by more than tenfold by employing different test media for determining the MIC in broth.

This variation should be of major consideration in attempting to provide data that can be of value to the physician and that can be compared among laboratories. It is the position of the author that, for the present time, media other than Mueller-Hinton should be used only when organisms fail to grow well in Mueller-Hinton medium.

Antimicrobial Preparation. The method of arriving at stock solutions for broth dilution testing has been previously described in this section. As for agar dilution, a table modified from the International Collaborative Study Report by Ericsson (1971) is included (Table 55-4) for use in the preparation of these dilutions.

Dilutions either can be twofold, with a wide or narrow range, or can be set at various predetermined levels in order to derive an appropriate analysis of high and low susceptibility. It has been our experience that when macrobroth dilution testing is done in the laboratory, it is often done for single organism determinations; however, it is still necessary to test control organisms concurrently.

Inoculum. The inoculum in the macrobroth method is in the range of 10^5 to 10^6 CFU/ml. One can use a 1:1000 or 1:2000 dilution of either an overnight broth culture, a 4 to 6 hour, 0.5 ml broth culture, or a 1:200 dilution of a broth culture adjusted to match the turbidity of a MacFarland 0.5 standard. It is customary to add 1 ml of standardized organism suspension to 1 ml of antibiotic solution in each tube. Tubes are incubated, with caps or plugs, in order to obviate evaporation and contamination, at 35°C.

Results. Since Mueller-Hinton broth has a slight turbidity, one must be careful to compare it with an uninoculated control. The MIC is determined as the least amount of antibiotic that results in complete inhibition of growth as judged by visual examination.

One advantage of this type of dilution test is that one can proceed to transfer aliquots from those tubes which demonstrate no visible growth to agar plate surfaces in order to determine the minimal bactericidal concentration, a concept discussed on page 1927.

Microbroth dilution testing

Microbroth dilution or microdilution technology has gained great acceptance over the past few years. Whereas microdilution trays, made of molded plastic, have been available for serologic determinations for a number of years, it is only in recent years that this methodology has taken hold for use with antimicrobial susceptibility testing. The method has some very real advantages in terms of the availability of commercially prepared trays containing prefrozen and diluted antimicrobials, and, for the larger clinical laboratories, instrumentation can be purchased for producing plates (Tilton, 1973).

The basic methodology, therefore, will vary, depending upon the amount of equipment available in that laboratory and whether or not the laboratory purchases the preprepared dilution trays. Although the description provided in this section includes the entire methodology, it should be recognized that one can step into this process at any step along the way.

Available Equipment. The basic unit of the microdilution system is the molded plastic tray or plate which contains 8 rows of 12 small, either flat bottomed or V-shaped cups to which can be delivered a small volume (usually 0.1 ml) of inoculum.

Table 55-4. MODIFIED GUIDE FOR DILUTION OF ANTIMICROBIALS IN BROTH

ANTIMICROBIAL SOLUTION		VOLUME OF BROTH DILUENT TO BE ADDED	CONCENTRATION AS ADDED TO CULTURE INOCULUM AT 1:2 OR FOR FURTHER DILUTION ON LINES BELOW	FINAL CONCENTRATION IN BROTH	
µg or IU/ml	Stock vol. (in ml)		µg or IU/ml		LOG₂
2000	2	13.62 ml	256	128	7
256	2	2 vols	128	64	6
256	1	3	64	32	5
256	1	7	32	16	4
32	2	2	16	8	3
32	1	3	8	4	2
32	1	7	4	2	1
4	2	2	2	1	0
4	1	3	1	0.5	−1
4	1	7	0.5	0.25	−2
0.5	2	2	0.25	0.125	−3
0.5	1	3	0.125	0.063	−4
0.5	1	7	0.063	0.031	−5

These trays can be purchased from several commercial manufacturers, and the author knows of no reason why one particular tray should be favored over another. Of consideration in the use of the trays is whether or not they can be reused. It should be pointed out that whereas it might be economically advantageous to wash and reuse trays, scratching of plastic surfaces, as will occur on the outer surface of the bottom of the individual wells, can interfere with the reading of broth dilution tests.

It is helpful, when performing microdilution tests, to have some way of dispensing the transparent tape for sealing the individual trays once the inoculum and the antimicrobial have been delivered; therefore, a small device for dispensing transparent tape may facilitate this procedure. In addition, one should also consider obtaining a reading rack with mirror to facilitate determination of the results.

Other factors to be considered are the specially calibrated loops that can be used for the dilution of antimicrobial solutions, and the specially constructed pipettes that can be used for the delivery of inoculum. Several levels of mechanization are available, including inoculating heads, much like those used for agar dilution testing, which can be used either manually or in a mechanized fashion for the delivery of inoculum into the antimicrobial-containing plates. It is not within the scope of this chapter to review all of the equipment available for the microdilution method; however, potential users should carefully consider the various alternatives in instrumentation that are available.

Media. The microdilution test can be performed with Mueller-Hinton broth; however, because of the deficiency of cations in formulations of this medium, it is suggested that it be supplemented with cation to assure appropriate susceptibility results (Thornsberry, 1977a). Reller (1974) recommends a final concentration of 50 mg of calcium and 25 mg of magnesium per liter of Mueller-Hinton broth to obviate this problem. This can be accomplished by preparing Mueller-Hinton broth, according to the manufacturer's directions, and adding the appropriate concentrations of calcium and magnesium with $CaCl_2$ and $MgCl_2$. As has been noted previously, the concentration of these divalent cations in Mueller-Hinton broth is so small that one can add these cations as though none were present originally.

Antimicrobials. Commercial firms have now developed the capacity for local distribution of prefrozen or lyophilized antimicrobial-containing trays for use in the clinical laboratory. The Food and Drug Administration has developed criteria for the quality control of these commercially prepared dilution sets, and the clinical laboratory can be assured that these trays will perform appropriately. The trays come individually or multiply packaged.

In preparing one's own trays, dilutions can be prepared by using the dilution schedule shown in Table 55-4, or one can use specially calibrated microdilution loops for serially diluting these trays. If one uses the fully instrumented approach to the preparation of trays, then the manufacturer's directions should be closely followed.

To be considered in the preparation of microdilution trays is the matter of using frozen stock solutions. Barry (1976) has suggested that allowing a stock solution to freeze, thawing it for preparing the dilutions, transferring these dilutions to the trays, and then refreezing them for storage, despite two freeze-thaw cycles, may be acceptable.

These trays, once prepared, can be frozen and stored in plastic bags for at least two weeks. If plates are purchased commercially, one should follow the manufacturer's outdate suggestions carefully.

Inoculation. The desired density of organisms is 5000 CFU per 0.1 ml of final volume in the tray wells. The inoculators deliver approximately 5 to 10 μl per prong or loop or 1 to 2 μl per pin. Therefore, the final inoculum delivered will depend upon the type of delivery system used. A final concentration in the well should be 10^5 CFU/ml. Another variable to be considered is that instruments deliver various volumes of antimicrobial solutions. Therefore, one must have a carefully defined protocol for delivery of the antimicrobial solutions into the trays and for diluting the inoculum. Once the inoculum has been delivered to the tray, it is sealed with transparent tape and incubated for 16 to 20 hours at 35°C.

Results. The MIC is defined as the lowest concentration without visible turbidity or a button of cells at the bottom of the well. Gerlach (1974) has demonstrated 95 per cent reproducibility in MIC determinations, a value which is consistent with the reproducibility of other susceptibility tests.

RAPID RESULTS. Preliminary information (Bartlett, 1976) indicates that the addition of tetrazolium can expedite determination of the MIC in microdilution tests; however, the reproducibility of this procedure remains to be established, and it appears that an adjustment in inoculum must be made to assure reproducibility. It would seem best to assume that the microdilution method requires a 16- to 20-hour incubation period until more studies become available regarding rapid techniques.

Special Considerations. It is tempting to stack microdilution trays in order to conserve incubator space; however, uniformity in temperatures of individual trays within an incubator depends on the circulation of air. Stacking trays, therefore, may well prevent trays from arriving at the appropriate temperature within the 16- to 20-hour incubation period. The longer the incubation time, the less impact this variable would have on the final result.

Thornsberry (1977a) has reported that some beta-lactamase-producing strains of *Staphylococ-*

cus aureus may give spuriously low penicillin or ampicillin MIC's in microdilution tests despite their production of beta-lactamase and probable resistance to penicillins in severe infections. It is suggested that all *Staphylococcus aureus* determined to be susceptible in the microdilution method be evaluated for the production of beta-lactamase.

NEWER AUTOMATED BROTH DILUTION ADAPTATIONS

Special Considerations in Automation. The advent of automation brings with it some very intriguing possibilities for clinical microbiology, but also presents potential problems. Because of automation, it is very likely that we will need to redefine certain performance guidelines. Yet, at the same time, the only meaningful way to evaluate these newer methods is to compare them with the reference or standard methods. Currently, therefore, newer methods may be compared with the agar dilution method, as described by the International Collaborative Study (Ericsson, 1971); however, it may be more meaningful, if the automated method procedurally resembles the broth dilution test, to equate performance to standard or reference broth dilution methods.

Any automated approach ought to have the same degree of precision or reproducibility that we expect from the other methods, and one would anticipate that these new techniques should approach 95 per cent reproducibility.

Cost should be taken into account in the overall evaluation of the practicality and use of instrumentation. Increased costs may be acceptable if precision, objectivity in determining results, convenience, uniformity, economy of time, and speed in obtaining results are enhanced and if there is a potential interface with a computer for both quality control and data processing. Automation does add another variable to quality control related to the maintenance and performance of instrumentation.

Instrumentation alone is difficult to justify, and it is to be hoped that automated, semiautomated, and mechanized procedures will be critically evaluated and the results reported to the profession to provide a reasonable basis for all of us to make a judgment regarding the incorporation of these innovations into our own clinical laboratories.

Devices

AUTOBAC I (PFIZER, INC.). Autobac I is a semiautomated system for measuring antimi-crobial susceptibilities of bacteria within a three- to five-hour time period. Although the basic system is adaptable to several aspects of clinical microbiology, the discussion here will be limited to its performance of susceptibility tests.

Instrumentation. The system comprises four separate components (McKie, 1974; Praglin, 1974). The central component of the system is a light-scattering photometer which also possesses the electronic capability to alter the evaluation mode and to be umbilicized to a free-standing computer unit that will become more important in future uses of this instrument (Matsen, 1977).

The second component is a cuvette comprising 12 individual test chambers and a thirteenth control chamber. This cuvette is molded so a broth inoculum tube can be firmly attached to it. It has a removable thick plastic manifold allowing access to the individual control chambers for the delivery of individual paper discs containing the antimicrobial substances.

The third component is a dispenser which delivers the antimicrobial discs to the individual chambers of the cuvette. The order of alignment of the antimicrobial substances is predetermined and cannot be randomly varied by the operator. The discs serve as the vehicles for delivering the antimicrobial agents by the principle of disc elution.

The fourth component is a dedicated, combined incubator and shaker. The internal housing within this incubator-shaker is designed to firmly hold the individual cuvettes.

An additional component of this system is a calibration wedge, by which the photometer is adjusted and can be checked. Finally, there is a multi-copy report form which is fed into the photometer housing for printing of results.

Susceptibility Testing Procedure. As the manufacturer provides complete testing procedures, the instructions will not be repeated here. Basically, the method involves selecting an organism from an initial isolation plate or directly from what appears to be a unimicrobially infected fluid specimen, and standardizing its inoculum density in saline with the light-scattering photometer. Newer models of the Autobac have the capacity for varying the meter reading in order that different inocula may be used. An aliquot of the standardized inoculum is then transferred into a tube of eugonic broth which is then screwed into the cuvette and firmly seated. The cuvette is then inverted on a level surface so that all the broth is distributed to a holding chamber situated at one end of the cuvette. Further manipulations of the cuvette are made so

5

as to distribute the broth evenly along the length of the cuvette. Thus, 1.5 ml aliquots are delivered into each of the individual chambers of the cuvette, which have been previously loaded with the antimicrobial discs by the disc dispenser.

The cuvette is then placed in the incubator-shaker for approximately three hours. The cuvette is then placed on a holding bar or carriage in the light-scattering photometer housing and the photometer lid is closed. A report form is inserted to record the result and the machine begins its computation. Sufficient growth must be obtained in the control chamber for the photometer to accept the report slip. If growth is insufficient, the cuvette is returned to the incubator-shaker for an additional period of time. If there is sufficient growth in the control chamber, a light-scatter index is calculated by means of a minicomputer within the photometer housing. This index is a numerical value between 0 and 1 with 0.01 subdivisions. An interpretation of susceptible, intermediate, or resistant is calculated for each antimicrobial agent in the control chamber and in each chamber containing antimicrobial (light-scatter index, or LSI). Modifications of the antimicrobial content of the discs and of the instrument's program can be made. For example, discs containing two or three amounts of each antimicrobial may be tested, and a result (MIC) formulated either from the absolute LSI derived from each chamber or by using a mathematical calculation based on a regression analysis of the LSI from the high and low antimicrobial discs used in the series.

Problem Areas. A seven-laboratory collaborative study evaluated the Autobac instrument and compared it to disc diffusion and the ICS agar dilution methods (Thornsberry, 1975). There was an overall agreement of about 90 per cent between the automated results and those of the other two methods. The principal difficulties were encountered with testing *Enterobacter* against ampicillin and cephalothin, and with *Pseudomonas aeruginosa* tested against chloramphenicol, tetracycline, and gentamicin. It has also been shown that the Autobac instrument is unlikely to detect methicillin- or nafcillin-resistant strains of *Staphylococcus;* therefore, it is suggested that when multiply resistant strains of staphylococci are encountered, they should be considered potentially resistant to the penicillinase-resistant semisynthetic penicillins and tested by another acceptable procedure (Cleary, 1978). Experience also demonstrates that ampicillin-resistant enterococci should be rechecked for susceptibility by a dilution or diffusion method. As with the disc diffusion method, one should also run a purity check on any specimen being tested in the Autobac.

Other Devices. Other forms of automation currently being marketed are limited to those used for the microdilution test. However, under evaluation are instruments manufac-

tured by the McDonnell Douglas Astronautics Company (AutoMicrobic System or AMS), Abbott Laboratories (MS-2), and Cathra (Repliscan). In addition, testing has been done of radiometric, laser-light scattering, and electrical impedance devices; however, none of these three systems is currently projected for marketing within the near future.

It is very likely that the Automicrobic, the MS-2, and the Repliscan devices will become available for susceptibility testing purposes in the near future. Since published results of clinical trials of these devices are not yet available, it seems premature to review their operation or instrumentation further.

DIFFUSION TESTING

PRINCIPLES

The observation that an antibiotic that diffused from antibiotic-impregnated material or from a reservoir cut in the surface of an agar plate inhibited the growth of a susceptible organism led ultimately to the development of a standardized antibiotic-impregnated paper disc diffusion method of susceptibility testing (Bauer, 1966). Historically many methods were employed, and a number are still in use or are being proposed for use in clinical laboratories. However, it is of major significance that the U.S. Food and Drug Administration, given the responsibility in this area by the United States Supreme Court, has recently recommended similar methodology for use in all laboratories (Federal Register, 1972, 1973). A subcommittee of the National Committee for Clinical Laboratory Standards (1975) has also recommended essentially the same method.

In brief, this method involves placing a known amount of antibiotic in a small, absorbent paper disc measuring 6 mm in diameter. The placement of this disc on an agar surface previously inoculated with the organism to be tested will result in a concentric zone of inhibited growth for susceptible organisms. The zone of inhibition for the great majority of antimicrobial agents has been shown to relate linearly to the minimal inhibitory concentration (MIC) of the antibiotic as measured by dilution susceptibility testing (Matsen, 1970; Ericsson, 1971).

This relationship is of great importance in understanding the principle of the disc diffusion susceptibility test and the genesis of the interpretive criteria. The relation between

MIC and zone diameter of inhibition can be expressed by regression analysis (Fig. 55-1). A sample of at least 100 to 150 organisms, representing the species of bacteria for which the antimicrobial agent might be used, is tested by both disc diffusion and agar or broth dilution. Organisms are selected to provide MIC values that are fairly evenly spread over the clinically relevant ranges of concentrations. Any values representing no zone of inhibition are excluded from the graphs and from the calculations of the regression lines. The ordinate or Y-axis denotes the MIC on a logarithmic scale, whereas the abscissa or X-axis represents zone diameters of inhibition on an arithmetic scale (Fig. 55-1). Since the distribution of plots with most antimicrobials is linear, application of the formula of least squares results in the mathematical computation of the "regression line" (line of best fit) shown in the figure. In those situations in which the relationship is not linear, this line has diminished significance. The calculated line is not, however, the "true" regression line. This is because, in the twofold dilution test, as used in this graph, the *average* true value of the MIC is one half of a twofold dilution lower than the observed value. Organism values, as derived from the dual test evaluation, are distributed on either side of these regression lines, and the pattern of organism scatter must be considered in arriving at susceptibility category breakpoints.

By defining the serum levels of the antibiotic achievable with the recommended dosages given by the usual routes of administration,

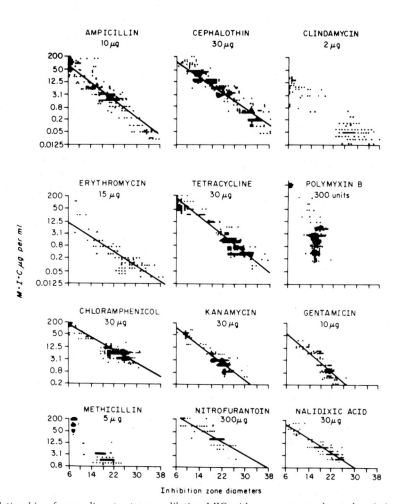

Figure 55-1. Relationship of zone diameter to agar dilution MIC with some commonly used antimicrobials. All except polymyxin and gentamicin show combined data from clinical laboratories of the Universities of Minnesota and Washington. The disc content is shown below each antimicrobial. Polymyxin MIC's are in units per milliliter. (From Matsen, 1974.)

one derives the MIC values in micrograms per ml (μg/ml) which would be expected to be inhibitory *in vivo*. The zone diameter interpretive criteria for susceptibility are then based on the zone of inhibition corresponding to this MIC value, while the criteria for defining intermediate susceptibility and resistance are based on considerations of toxicity and pharmacokinetics of the individual compounds, as well as the scatter of organisms on the histogram, as shown in Figure 55-1. The intermediate zone, in addition to providing an indication for maximum dosage if that particular antimicrobial is to be used, also serves as a buffer zone to minimize false susceptible or resistant interpretations related to the scatter of organisms.

DISC CONTENT SELECTION

The proper disc content for each antimicrobial should be based upon a number of experimentally derived factors, among which are the following:

1. Zone sizes of very susceptible organisms should preferably be in the range of 20 to 30 mm and no more than 35 mm. When larger zone sizes occur, reproducibility becomes increasingly difficult. Examples of large zone sizes are those occurring with susceptible staphylococci and the 10 unit penicillin disc.

2. Zone sizes should be large enough that the test maintains discriminating capability for organisms with intermediate levels of susceptibility, i.e., an intermediate-resistant zone diameter partition greater than 12 mm. There is an interesting corollary which holds true for certain antibiotics: the regression line usually crosses the Y-axis at a point where the MIC value is three to five times the stated content of the disc.

3. The stability of the antibiotic under routine storage conditions has a bearing on disc content. The smaller the disc content of unstable antimicrobial agents, the more crucial is the proportional deterioration of the antibiotic. The concept of the high content disc was an important feature of the standardized method originally proposed by Bauer (1966). The higher the disc content, the less likely is antimicrobial deterioration to be significant in the test.

4. Other considerations include the linearity and slope of the regression line and the standard deviation of organism plots about the line of regression. An error rate-bounded method for examining the relationship between zone diameter and MIC was described by Metzler (1974), who recommended limiting the rates of false susceptibles and false resistants obtained by the disc diffusion technique to 1 and 5 per cent, respectively.

The content of the discs is under the regulation of the Food and Drug Administration. Currently, the content of the discs must be not more than 150 per cent or less than 67 per cent of their stated content. Therefore, there is a possibility of considerable variation in content, and many large disc manufacturers aim for a modest overfill.

INDICATIONS AND LIMITATIONS

Indications for disc diffusion susceptibility testing are similar to the indications for susceptibility testing in general. In addition, it is important to understand that the standardized disc diffusion method should be used only for rapidly growing organisms for which an end-point can be determined within an 18- to 24-hour period. Continued incubation beyond that time interval may sufficiently alter the interaction between organism and antimicrobial to give erroneous results. Furthermore, certain organisms or antibiotics require special test conditions. *Haemophilus influenzae*, as has already been discussed, requires the addition of special nutrients to the medium. Streptococci grow poorly on Mueller-Hinton medium and require the addition of 5 per cent sheep blood. In testing sulfonamides or the combination of sulfamethoxazole and trimethoprim, blood additives cannot be used owing to the antagonistic effect of paraaminobenzoic acid present in blood. When sulfonamides are tested against *Neisseria meningitidis*, special factors must be considered. Disc diffusion susceptibility testing of penicillin is not standardized for *Neisseria meningitidis;* therefore, susceptibility testing of this antibiotic-organism pair should be carried out with agar dilution methods. Susceptibility testing should not be done with either methenamine mandelate or methenamine hippurate, as there is not sufficient analogy between the *in vivo* and *in vitro* conditions.

The disc diffusion method can be used for susceptibility testing of some anaerobic bacteria; however, the test procedures differ substantially from those used with rapidly growing aerobic and facultatively anaerobic bacteria (see p. 1923).

RECOMMENDED ANTIMICROBIALS

Currently, it is recommended that only one agent from each class of closely related antimicrobials be tested. Generally, this is the only agent available owing to Food and Drug Administration regulations. Although the class representative is usually sufficient for most testing situations, a few circumstances do exist wherein one cannot extrapolate susceptibility results to other agents within the class. Dilution testing is indicated in the unusual cases where this differentiation is clinically important. Two examples within the cephalosporin group illustrate this point. *Haemophilus influenzae* is usually susceptible to cephalothin, the class disc representative of the cephalosporin group, but is resistant to cephalexin. Therefore, one cannot extrapolate susceptibility to cephalexin from the cephalothin results in this instance. Cefazolin is usually more active *in vitro* than cephalothin against *Escherichia coli* and a zone diameter of 13 mm with the cephalothin disc can be used to indicate *E. coli* susceptibility to cefazolin. With few exceptions, however, the general guidelines in Table 55-1 should be used for selecting antimicrobials to be tested routinely against rapidly growing aerobic and facultatively anaerobic bacteria.

RECOMMENDED METHODS FOR DISC DIFFUSION TESTING

Agar diffusion surface-streak method

This method of susceptibility, as proposed in 1966 by Bauer, Kirby, Sherris, and Turck, is the basis for the methods recommended by the United States Food and Drug Administration (Federal Register, 1972, 1973) and the National Committee for Clinical Laboratory Standards (1975). The method described here is essentially that of the latter group and is given here because it encompasses the details of the method recommended by the Food and Drug Administration and emphasizes a few additional details which the author feels are important in the performance of the disc diffusion test. The method should be followed closely if accurate, reproducible results are to be anticipated.

Medium and Preparation of Plates. Mueller-Hinton medium is the recommended medium, and emphasis should be made that the interpretive chart (Table 55-5) is valid only when this medium is used in the prescribed manner. For justification of the use of Mueller-Hinton medium, the reader is referred to the report of the International Collaborative Study (Ericsson, 1971). Although Mueller-Hinton supports the growth of most organisms for which susceptibility testing will be done, 5 per cent defibrinated sheep, horse, or other animal blood should be added to ensure adequate growth of

streptococci and other fastidious organisms, and 5 per cent laked horse blood, Fildes digest, or other similar nutrient additive should be added for testing *Haemophilus*.

In general, it is advisable to use 150 mm Petri plates, although current recommendations do allow use of 100 mm plates instead. Agar depth should be in the range of 4 to 6 mm (Barry, 1973a) (20 to 25 ml of agar for the 100 mm plates and 79 to 80 ml for the 150 mm plates). After plates are prepared, they are best stored at 4°C. in cellophane wrapping, and should be used within a two-week period. Immediately prior to use plates should be "dried" in an incubator for 30 minutes to facilitate removal of excess surface moisture.

Preparation of Inoculum. An inoculating needle or loop is used to transfer portions of four or five colonies of the organism into 4 or 5 ml of a suitable broth medium (soybean-casein digest or tryptose phosphate broths are suggested) which is allowed to incubate at 35°C. until the turbidity of the culture compares to that of the recommended turbidity standard (see p. 1907). The standard is agitated on a vortex mixer immediately prior to use. Unless the standard is contained in heat-sealed glass tubes, it should probably be replaced every six months. If appropriately sealed, the standard may last indefinitely (Washington, 1973). The turbidity of the culture, if excessive, may be adjusted by the addition of sterile saline or broth or, if inadequate, by the addition of colonies, provided they are well isolated and are morphologically identical to those originally selected. The modified laboratory view box previously described (Stemper, 1970) enhances the process of handling the culture tubes and the standard during turbidity adjustment. The standardized inoculum suspension should be inoculated within 15 to 20 minutes.

Inoculation of Medium. A sterile cotton swab on a wooden applicator stick is dipped into the standardized inoculum suspension. Excess broth is expressed by pressing and rotating the swab against the inside of the suspension tube. The swab is then streaked evenly in three directions on the surface of the agar plate. A final sweep is made of the agar rim with the cotton swab. This inoculum is allowed to dry for three to five minutes and discs are then applied, either by a mechanical dispenser or by hand using sterile forceps. After placement, discs are pressed firmly but gently onto the agar surface. The spatial arrangement of the discs should preclude the development of overlapping zones of inhibition and, therefore, limits the number of discs that can be placed to 12 or 13 (9 in the outer ring) on a 150 mm plate.

Quality Assurance. Quality assurance should extend to all phases of the testing procedure. The Mueller-Hinton medium should be of proper depth (4 to 6 mm), should not be allowed to dry out excessively (store refrigerated, in cellophane wrapping, and use within two weeks), and should be checked

5

Table 55–5. ZONE DIAMETER INTERPRETIVE STANDARDS[1,2]

ANTIMICROBIAL AGENT		DISC POTENCY	ZONE DIAMETER (mm)			APPROXIMATE MIC CORRELATES	
			Resistant	Intermediate	Susceptible	Resistant	Susceptible
Amikacin[3,4]		30 μg	≤14	15–16	≥17	>16 μg/ml	≤8 μg/ml
Ampicillin[5]	Enterobacteriaceae & Enterococci	10 μg	≤11	12–13	≥14	≥32 μg/ml	≤8 μg/ml
	Staph/Pen susc. orgs.	10 μg	≤20	21–28	≥29	≥2.0 μg/ml penicillinase[6]	≤0.2 μg/ml
	Haemophilus	10 μg	≤19	—	≥20	—	≤2.0 μg/ml
Carbenicillin	*Proteus* & *E. coli*	100 μg	≤17	18–22	≥23	≥32 μg/ml	≤16 μg/ml
	P. aeruginosa[7]	100 μg	≤11	12–14	≥15	≥250 μg/ml	≤125 μg/ml
Cephalothin[8]		30 μg	≤14	15–17	≥18	≥32 μg/ml	≤10 μg/ml
Chloramphenicol		30 μg	≤12	13–17	≥18	≥25 μg/ml	≤12.5 μg/ml
Clindamycin[9]		2 μg	≤14	15–16	≥17	≥2 μg/ml	≤1 μg/ml
Colistin[10]		10 μg	≤8	9–10	≥11	—	—
Erythromycin		15 μg	≤13	14–17	≥18	≥8 μg/ml	≤2 μg/ml
Gentamicin		10 μg	≤12	13–14	≥15	≥6 μg/ml	≤6 μg/ml
Kanamycin		30 μg	≤13	14–17	≥18	≥25 μg/ml	≤6 μg/ml
Methicillin[11]		5 μg	≤9	10–13	≥14	—	≤3 μg/ml
Nafcillin[12]		1 μg	≤10	11–12	≥13	—	≤3 μg/ml
Nalidixic acid[13]		30 μg	≤13	14–18	≥19	≥32 μg/ml	≤12 μg/ml
Neomycin		30 μg	≤12	13–16	≥17	—	≤10 μg/ml
Nitrofurantoin[13]		300 μg	≤14	15–16	≥17	≥100 μg/ml	≤25 μg/ml
Penicillin G[14]	Staphylococci	10 units	≤20	21–28	≥29	penicillinase[6]	≤0.1 μg/ml
	Other organisms	10 units	≤11	12–21	≥22	≥32 μg/ml	≤1.5 μg/ml
Polymyxin B[10]		300 units	≤8	9–11	≥12	≥50 units/ml	
Streptomycin		10 μg	≤11	12–14	≥15	≥15 μg/ml	≤6 μg/ml
Sulfonamides	*N. mening.* only	250/300 μg			≥40		
	Other organisms[13]	250/300 μg	≤12	13–16	≥17	≥350 μg/ml	≤100 μg/ml
Tetracycline[15]		30 μg	≤14	15–18	≥19	≥12 μg/ml	≤4 μg/ml
Tobramycin		10 μg	≤12	13–14	≥15	≥6 μg/ml	≤6 μg/ml
Trimethoprim-sulfamethoxazole[13]		1.25 μg/23.75 μg	≤10	11–15	≥16	≥200 μg/ml	≤35 μg/ml
Vancomycin		30 μg	≤9	10–11	≥12	—	≤5 μg/ml

[1] Bauer (1966).

[2] NCCLS Subcommittee on Antimicrobial Susceptibility Testing (1975); Federal Register (1972, 1973).

[3] Tentative standards from Bristol Laboratories.

[4] Kelly, M.T., and Matsen, J.M.: In vitro activity, synergism, and testing parameters of amikacin, with comparisons to other aminoglycoside antibiotics. Antimicrob. Agents Chemother., *9*:440, 1975.

[5] Class disc for ampicillin, hetacillin, and amoxicillin.

[6] Resistant strains of *S. aureus* produce penicillinase. There are significant reports of ampicillin-resistant strains which produce penicillinase.

[7] Tentative standards from UUMC Clinical Microbiology Laboratory.

[8] Class disc for cephalothin, cephaloridine, cephalexin, cefazolin, cephacetrile, cephradrine, and cephapirin.

[9] The clindamycin disc is used to test susceptibility to both clindamycin and lincomycin. Owing to the greater activity of clindamycin, separate interpretive categories of zone diameters are recommended when reporting susceptibility to lincomycin as follows: ≤16 = R, 17–20 = I, ≥21 = S.

[10] Colistin and polymyxin B diffuse poorly in agar, and thus the accuracy of diffusion tests is less than that found with other antimicrobics, and MIC correlates cannot be calculated reliably from regression analysis.

[11] Class disc for penicillinase-resistant penicillins (i.e., methicillin, cloxacillin, dicloxacillin, oxacillin, and nafcillin).

[12] Class disc for penicillinase-resistant penicillins used at UUMC Clinical Microbiology Laboratory.

[13] Urinary tract infections only.

[14] Class disc for penicillin G, phenoxymethyl penicillin, and phenthicillin.

[15] Class disc for tetracyclines.

for appropriate pH. Discs should be stored frozen (−12° to −20°C.) and should be removed from the freezer as individual cartridges; the cartridge in use should be kept in a desiccated container at 4°C. and allowed to equilibrate to room temperature prior to use each day. Discs should be purchased through a local distributor whose storage conditions (4°C.) are known or directly from the manufacturer. The practice of receiving discs from pharmaceutical representatives is to be avoided because of the unknown storage conditions prior to receipt.

A representative disc from each cartridge should be tested with control bacterial strains (*Staphylococcus aureus* ATCC 25923 for antimicrobials to be tested against gram-positive organisms, *Escherichia coli* ATCC 25922, and *Pseudomonas aeruginosa* ATCC 27853 for agents to be tested against gram-negative bacilli) prior to the routine use of other discs from that cartridge. The control strains should be tested frequently and, ideally, each time a set of susceptibility tests is performed. An easily accessible, easily readable chart is recommended to facilitate recording and interpretation of quality assurance testing. Limits of excursion for the control *S. aureus*, *E. coli*, and *P. aeruginosa* are given in Table 55-6; however, it should be stressed that these limits are rather broad, and ideally each laboratory would establish its own, narrower limits of control.

A separate sheep blood agar plate should be streaked in quadrants, with the swab used for streaking the surface of each Mueller-Hinton plate to check for purity of inoculum.

Results. Zone diameters are measured under reflected light with a ruler or calipers on the undersurface of the Petri dish. If blood has been added to the Mueller-Hinton agar, the zones are measured from the surface of the agar after removing the cover. The end-point is complete inhibition of growth as determined visually, except in the case of sulfonamides, where organisms may grow through several generations before inhibition occurs. In this instance, slight growth (80 per cent or greater inhibition) is disregarded, and the margin of heavy growth is measured. The swarming of *Proteus* is also disregarded, and the margin of heavy growth which is usually clearly apparent is measured.

While preliminary readings may be obtained as soon as growth patterns become apparent (usually 6 to 8 hours), readings made at this time should be verified at 18 to 20 hours. Measurement of zones should include the entire diameter of the zone, including the disc. Should colonies be seen within the zone of inhibition, the purity check plate should be analyzed. If it is obvious that more than one organism is present, the test should be repeated. If the culture is pure, the colonies are regarded as significant and included in zone diameter measurement. Fortunately, this is not a frequent occurrence.

The zone diameter interpretive criteria, along with the MIC correlates, are shown in Table 55-5. This table contains a compilation of data from the Center for Disease Control (Thornsberry, 1977b) and from the National Committee for Clinical Laboratory Standards recommendations (1975).

Should a physician desire quantitative information, these MIC correlates can be referred to, as can the regression line plots such as that shown in Figure 55-1. One may give a range of MIC values for any given zone size based upon these regression line plots if one strictly adheres to the standard method.

Agar overlay diffusion method

An acceptable alternative method of inoculating disc diffusion test plates is the agar overlay method (Barry, 1970). This method is also applicable only to tests with commonly isolated, rapidly growing aerobic and facultatively anaerobic bacteria, such as *S.*

Table 55-6. SUSCEPTIBILITY OF CONTROL STRAINS*

ANTIBIOTIC	DISC POTENCY	ZONE DIAMETER OF INHIBITION (mm)		
		S. aureus (ATCC 25923)	*E. coli* (ATCC 25922)	*P. aeruginosa* (ATCC 27853)
Amikacin	10 μg	18–24	18–24	15–22
Ampicillin	10 μg	24–35	15–20	—
Bacitracin	10 U	17–22	—	—
Carbenicillin	100 μg	—	24–29	20–24
Cephalothin	30 μg	25–37	18–23	—
Chloramphenicol	30 μg	19–26	21–27	6
Clindamycin	2 μg	23–29	—	—
Colistin	10 μg	—	11–15	12–16
Erythromycin	15 μg	23–30	8–14	—
Gantrisin	250 or 300 μg	23–27	22–26	6
Gentamicin	10 μg	19–27	19–26	16–21
Kanamycin	30 μg	19–26	17–25	6
Methicillin	5 μg	17–22	—	—
Nalidixic acid	30 μg	—	21–25	—
Neomycin	30 μg	18–26	17–23	—
Nitrofurantoin	300 μg	—	20–24	—
Penicillin G	10 U	26–37	—	—
Polymyxin B	300 U	7–13	12–16	—
Streptomycin	10 μg	14–22	12–20	—
Tetracycline	30 μg	19–28	18–25	9–14
Trimethoprim-sulfamethoxazole	1.25 μg 23.75 μg	24–32	24–32	—
Tobramycin	10 μg	19–29	18–26	19–25
Vancomycin	30 μg	15–19	—	—

*From Thornsberry (1977b).

aureus, Enterobacteriaceae, *P. aeruginosa,* and other non-fermentative gram-negative bacilli.

Preparation of Plates. Mueller-Hinton agar is poured to a depth of 4 mm in 150 × 15 mm plastic Petri dishes.

Preparation and Incorporation of Inoculum. Four to five isolated colonies of the same morphologic type are selected from a primary isolation plate. A turbid suspension is prepared in 0.5 ml of brain-heart infusion broth in a 13 × 100 mm tube, which is then incubated in a 35 to 37°C. waterbath or heating block for four to eight hours. This suspension is well mixed after incubation, and a 0.001 loopful is transferred to a 9 ml aqueous solution of agar that has been held no longer than 8 hours in a 45° to 50°C. heating block (16 × 125 mm screw-capped tubes are routinely used). Tubes not used within this time interval are discarded. The melted agar, now inoculated with the test organism, is mixed by inverting several times before being poured over the surface of Mueller-Hinton agar in the 150 × 15 mm plastic Petri plate. The thin layer of melted agar will solidify too quickly on the Mueller-Hinton agar unless it is first brought to room temperature. Plates should be left for 3 to 5 minutes on a flat surface so that the agar overlay can harden properly before the discs are placed on the surface as described above.

Incubation. After the discs have been placed on the agar surface, the plates are inverted and incubated at 35°C. within 15 minutes for 16 to 18 hours.

Results. The plates are read in a manner similar to that employed with the surface streak disc diffusion method. The interpretive criteria are those listed in Table 55-5.

INTERPRETATION OF RESULTS

If the standard method is followed closely, results are reliable and reproducible. Interpretation is based upon the establishment, for each antimicrobial, of zone diameters which correlate with MIC values and which, in turn, relate to achievable levels of antimicrobial in body fluids and tissues. The categories of susceptible, intermediate, and resistant apply to systemic infections (except for nitrofurantoin, sulfonamides, and nalidixic acid). In situations where an antibiotic dose may be safely increased, concentrations far in excess of the levels considered in the establishment of these interpretive criteria may be reached. Similarly, the concentration of certain antimicrobials in the urine is many-fold higher than that considered as the upper limit of susceptibility in systemic infection. The interpretive criteria and MIC correlates presented in Table 55-5 are rough guidelines which provide, in most situations, a certain margin of safety

to cover biologic differences among organisms and differences in the human host's response to the organism and to the antibiotic. Furthermore, the disc producing the greatest zone of inhibition does not necessarily indicate that that particular agent is the agent of choice for a given pathogen.

REGRESSION INFORMATION FOR COMMONLY USED THERAPEUTICS

Each antibiotic varies somewhat or greatly from other agents in its regression analysis. For this reason, and because of the added information these analyses provide, regression lines for all of the currently commonly used antibiotics are helpful for reference purposes. While these regression plots can be used as already described elsewhere in this chapter, each laboratory desiring to use these plots in this manner should verify by control organism plots that these results are reproducible in their own laboratory. For further information on regression plots, the reader is referred to more detailed sources of information (Chabbert, 1949; Matsen, 1970, 1974).

COMMON ERRORS

Though the disc diffusion method is a fairly forgiving method, there are errors that occur which compromise accuracy and reliability, and one error can obviously compound another. Included below is a list of what might be considered "common errors" occurring in clinical microbiology laboratories.

1. Failure to use Mueller-Hinton medium.
2. Use of outdated medium or plates.
3. Failure to test the pH of Mueller-Hinton medium or committing other media preparation mistakes.
4. Failure to standardize the inoculum or to use proper density standardization procedures.
5. Use of an inaccurate turbidity reference standard (usually due to incorrect preparation, leakage, or evaporation).
6. Failure to express excess fluid from swab used for plate inoculation.
7. Excessive time lapse between inoculum standardization and plate inoculation.
8. Use of outdated or improperly stored discs.
9. Prolonged time lapse in applying discs after plates have been inoculated.
10. Delay in incubation following inocula-

tion and disc placement, thus allowing antibiotic "prediffusion" prior to optimal organism growth conditions.

11. Failure to use quality control strains or the use of improper quality control strains.
12. The testing of mixed cultures.
13. Transcription errors.
14. The testing of organisms which require anaerobic incubation, or which are so slow in their growth as to preclude a zone reading within an 18- to 24-hour time frame.

It is apparent that problems in each of these situations can be obviated by closely adhering to the prescribed methods.

INDICATIONS FOR DIRECT SUSCEPTIBILITY TESTING ON CLINICAL MATERIALS

While permissible in emergency situations in which cerebrospinal fluid or other body fluid specimens with gram-stained smears indicating that a pure culture may be expected, direct susceptibility testing of clinical material on a routine basis is to be avoided and discouraged. Mixtures of organisms, common in many specimens, may produce inaccurate interpretations (Shahidi, 1969). It may also be difficult to standardize the inoculum from direct clinical material (Ellner, 1976; Hollick, 1976; Wegner, 1976). The use of a purity check will be of great assistance in these emergency situations, as will an assessment of the nature of the "lawn" of inoculum on the susceptibility test plate. Results reported from such emergency tests should, unless a pure culture results and the appropriate inoculum has been achieved, be reported as preliminary or tentative and should be repeated and confirmed using one of the recommended methods (Barry, 1973b).

QUALITY CONTROL

As indicated in the preceding section, adherence to the prescribed methodology is important in the performance of the disc diffusion test. Attention to these detailed instructions is the best approach to quality control. The actual approach to quality assurance in the laboratory is geared to the various test materials (Mueller-Hinton medium, bar-

ium-sulfate turbidity standard, and antimicrobial discs), to the use of control organisms, and to the appropriate reading, interpretation, and transcription of zone sizes (Blazevic, 1972).

SPECIAL CONSIDERATIONS

Anaerobes. Because of the unusual features associated with the growth of anaerobic organisms, which include the requirements for an anaerobic environment, wide variations in replication times, as well as other organism-specific features, the susceptibility testing of anaerobic organisms poses special problems for the clinical microbiology laboratory. In this context, the methodologies that have been previously described do not have the same broad applicability for this group that they do for the aerobic or facultatively anaerobic and rapidly growing organisms. However, modifications of each of the susceptibility systems previously described have been worked out either for anaerobes in general or for specific groups of anaerobic organisms.

Problems with anaerobic susceptibility testing have been related to the polymicrobial nature of anaerobic infections, which also pose problems in the approach to therapy. In addition, delays in reporting anaerobic susceptibilities have led to less than optimal application of results to the therapy of the patient. Furthermore, the vast majority of anaerobic organisms are predictably susceptible to penicillin G, carbenicillin, and ticarcillin (*Bacteroides fragilis* and some *Bacteroides melaninogenicus* excepted) and chloramphenicol and clindamycin (*B. fragilis* and *B. melaninogenicus* included); and are variably susceptible to the tetracyclines and erythromycin. Newer cephalosporin-like antimicrobials, such as the cephamycins, are potentially useful in treating anaerobic infections, as may be newer agents now being investigated, e.g., piperacillin.

Anaerobic susceptibility testing, in our experience, has been of limited utility. We specifically inquire of the physician submitting any non-body fluid anaerobic isolate as to whether or not susceptibility testing is desired. In almost all instances, the physician elects to forego the susceptibility testing. This area, therefore, represents one of the most selective ones in all of clinical microbiology with respect to the need and clinical usefulness of susceptibility testing.

5

Physicians at times will order anaerobic susceptibility tests, and there is no question about their utility in certain specific clinical instances, especially those in which the clinical disease is still present after two or three days of therapy. It should, however, be realized that just as anaerobic infections can develop insidiously, they may be slow in demonstrating clinical and laboratory evidence of response to therapy.

Of considerable potential utility because of its simplicity in a wide spectrum of clinical laboratories is the broth-disc method of Wilkins (1973), which was carefully evaluated by Blazevic (1975) and found to be very reproducible and comparable to standard methodology. The test is based on the principle of disc elution; however, the discs are not specially prepared but rather are multiples of the discs used in the standard disc diffusion test. Therefore, the availability of discs presents, for most laboratories, no problem, and the quality control of the performance of the discs can be tied in with the quality control of the standard methodology.

MATERIALS. The medium is pre-reduced brain-heart infusion broth supplemented with 0.005 per cent hemin, 0.002 per cent menadione, and 0.05 per cent yeast extract (BHI-S). The amount of broth per tube is important, as one is dealing with a quantitative dilution of antimicrobial agents.

INOCULUM. The inoculum is one drop of a turbid 18- to 24-hour culture grown in pre-reduced chopped meat broth, chopped meat glucose broth, or peptone-yeast-extract-glucose broth.

PROCEDURE. The test is conducted in an anaerobic environment, either in a glovebox or in roll tubes inoculated with the Virginia Polytechnic Institute Cannula Apparatus. The appropriate number of antimicrobial discs is added to each tube of BHI-S (Table 55-7). When large numbers of discs are to be added they should be incubated anaerobically prior to addition to the broth (to avoid false sensitivities of strict anaerobes). In addition to the tubes containing antimicrobials, a tube without antimicrobials is inoculated as a growth control. One drop of inoculum is added to each tube, which is then sealed with a rubber stopper and incubated for 18 to 24 hours at 35°C. After incubation, a gram-stained smear should be made of the growth control to check for purity of the test suspension.

TEST INTERPRETATION. The interpretation of this particular susceptibility test differs from that used in the standard broth dilution test. In this particular test the end-point is determined by comparing the growth in each tube with that of the control. Susceptibility is defined by concentrations of antimicrobial yielding turbidity less than 50 per cent of that found in the growth control. Resistance is the presence of turbidity greater than 50 per cent of that in the growth control. Kurzynski (1976) has described a modification of this method in which the test is performed in thioglycollate broth incubated in air rather than anaerobically. This modification requires that the tubes be left at room temperature for two to three hours to ensure elution of the antimicrobial agent from the discs, since diffusion occurs more slowly because of the 0.05 per cent agar usually present in thioglycollate. The incubation time and determination of end-points are similar to those above, although with the more fastidious organisms 48 hours of incubation may be necessary.

Anaerobic Agar Dilution Testing. The basic principles of this test are the same as

Table 55-7. BROTH-DISC METHOD FOR ANAEROBIC SUSCEPTIBILITY TESTING

ANTIMICROBIAL	DISC CONTENT	NO. OF DISCS PER TUBE	FINAL CONCENTRATION (μg/ml)
Ampicillin	10 μg	2	4
Carbenicillin	100 μg	5	100
Cephalothin	30 μg	1	6
Chloramphenicol	30 μg	2	12
Clindamycin	2 μg	4	1.6
Clindamycin	4 μg	8	3.2
Doxycycline	5 μg	3	3
Erythromycin	15 μg	1	3
Gentamicin	10 μg	3	6
Penicillin G	10 units	1	2 units
Tetracycline	30 μg	1	6

those previously described for routine agar dilution testing. However, there are several modifications due to the unique nature of the anaerobic organisms.

MEDIUM. Brucella or brain-heart infusion agar with vitamin K_1, 10 µg/ml and 5 per cent whole or laked sheep blood, has been used by many investigators in the past; however, a subcommittee of the National Committee for Clinical Laboratory Standards, which has been developing a standard method for testing anaerobic bacteria, is recommending the Wilkins-Chalgren (1976) medium for this purpose.

The inoculum can be brought to desired density in thioglycollate-135 C without an indicator (Bio-Quest, Cockeysville, Md.) and enriched with hemin (0.005 per cent), menadione (0.002 per cent), and $NaHCO_3$ (1 mg/ml).

INOCULUM. A 24- to 48-hour incubation is required to bring organism turbidity to the equivalent of a MacFarland 0.5 standard. There is no further dilution of the broth suspension, and inoculation is made onto the agar as described previously. Incubation is at 35°C. for 48 hours in an anaerobic jar or chamber. The remaining test procedure is carried out as described for the ICS agar dilution methodology.

ANTIMICROBIALS. The antimicrobials usually tested are those listed in Table 55-7 for the broth-disc method. The plates should be prepared within 18 to 24 hours of use and should be stored at room temperature to delay absorption of oxygen, which occurs more rapidly at lower temperatures.

Whenever this test is performed, a plate containing no antibiotics should be inoculated and incubated simultaneously with the test plates, in the same environment.

The agar dilution method lends itself very readily to the testing of large numbers of organisms; hence, its principal uses in testing anaerobes are in the evaluation of new antimicrobial agents and in epidemiologic surveys of collections of strains to determine whether or not alterations in susceptibility have occurred.

Anaerobic Micro broth Dilution. The basic methodology, again, for testing anaerobes with the micro broth method is similar to that employed for regular aerobic organisms. The limitations of this method relate to the fact that the work should be performed, ideally, in an anaerobic chamber, which limits the ability of many laboratories to perform these tests.

MEDIUM. Brucella or brain-heart infusion broth supplemented with menadione (0.005 per cent) and hemin (0.001 per cent) or Schaedler broth should be used for both inoculum preparation and for dilution of antimicrobials.

Disc Diffusion Susceptibility Testing for Anaerobic Organisms. Sutter (1975) has provided guidelines for disc diffusion testing of anaerobes. Freshly prepared Brucella agar containing 5 per cent defibrinated sheep blood and 0.5 µg/ml menadione is used in 90 × 15 mm Petri dishes. The agar is poured to a depth of 5 to 6 mm, and not more than 4 antibiotic discs are applied to each plate. A few colonies or a 3 mm loopful from a broth culture of each strain to be tested is inoculated into a tube containing thioglycollate 135-C medium to which is added 5 mg/ml hemin prior to autoclaving and 1 µg/ml $NaHCO_3$ plus 0.5 µg/ml of filter-sterilized menadione after autoclaving. These tubes are incubated for 4 to 6 hours and then diluted to the density of a 0.5 MacFarland standard.

Streaking of the agar surface is done according to the method of Bauer (1966) with cotton swabs (Acme Cotton Company, Valley Stream, Long Island, N.Y.), and the plates are incubated at 37°C. in anaerobic incubators. Results are read after approximately 24 hours by measuring the diameter of the zone of inhibition around the antibiotic discs. Interpretation of results is made according to criteria published by Sutter (1975). An anaerobic control strain, selected for its susceptibility to penicillin, should be tested simultaneously with the test bacteria in order to demonstrate appropriate function of the test.

The Category Method for Anaerobic Bacteria. The category test (Thornsberry, 1977a) has been shown to be simple and reproducible and is another method which will be mentioned in order to give appropriate alternatives for anaerobic susceptibility testing. This method tests anaerobes with two or three concentrations of appropriate antimicrobials that have been selected to conform generally to the categories of susceptibility suggested by the International Collaborative Study (p. 1905).

MEDIUM. The concentrations of antimicrobial agents specified in Table 55-8 are prepared in prereduced Schaedler broth.

As with the broth-disc method of Wilkins (1973), the antimicrobial agents may also be added by means of paper discs; however, the authors (Thornsberry, 1977a) are careful to point out that it is impractical to use commercial discs, and advocate that discs of the proper concentrations can be easily prepared in the laboratory by adding the proper

Table 55–8. CONCENTRATIONS OF ANTIMICROBIAL AGENTS TO BE USED IN CATEGORY TEST

ANTIMICROBIAL AGENT	CONCENTRATION (µg/ml)
Penicillin G	0.25, 16, 128
Tetracycline	2, 8, 32
Clindamycin	2, 8, 64
Erythromycin	2, 4, 64
Chloramphenicol	1, 8

amount of antimicrobial to blank discs, drying them, and storing them with a desiccant at $-70°C$.

INOCULUM. The inoculum is prepared by removing an amount of overnight growth from a Schaedler agar plate and suspending it in Schaedler broth in order to adjust the turbidity to that of a 0.5 MacFarland standard. Alternatively, an overnight broth culture can be adjusted to the same turbidity.

TEST. PERFORMANCE. Antimicrobial solutions or discs are added to Schaedler broth so that the final concentrations are those listed in Table 55-8. A calibrated dropper is used to add 0.25 ml of the adjusted inoculum to each tube containing the antimicrobial and to a tube containing broth but no antimicrobial. The tubes are incubated anaerobically for 18 to 24 hours at $35°C$. The end-point is the lowest concentration without macroscopic growth, and one should be careful to ensure that there is adequate growth in the control broth. The results can be reported as MIC's or as categories of susceptibility. For all but chloramphenicol three concentrations are tested, which allows interpretation as shown in Table 55-9.

Susceptibility Testing of Haemophilus influenzae. Susceptibility testing with *Haemophilus influenzae* has assumed increased significance in that this organism has also demonstrated the capacity to produce beta-lactamase and manifest absolute resistance to the penicillin and semi-synthetic penicillin compounds. For most serious infections, such as meningitis, determination of the MIC is desirable. One can also test for the production of beta-lactamase and in most circumstances this information is sufficient. There are rare strains of *H. influenzae* that demonstrate resistance to penicillin by mechanisms other than beta-lactamase; therefore, susceptibility testing assumes increased significance with this particular organism. Agar dilution testing of *H. influenzae* has already been described in this chapter (see p. 1910).

BROTH DILUTION TESTING FOR HAEMOPHILUS INFLUENZAE. Schaedler's broth supplemented with 5 per cent Fildes reagent is used in either the microbroth or the macrobroth procedure (Thornsberry, 1977a), as has already been described. The inoculum can be prepared by suspending organisms taken from a chocolate agar plate, in Schaedler broth, to equal the density of a 0.5 MacFarland standard.

INTERPRETATION. Susceptible strains of *H. influenzae* are inhibited by 1 μg/ml or less of ampicillin. Ampicillin-resistant strains generally have MIC's of 8 μg/ml or higher, although occasional ones may have an MIC value of 4 μg/ml. Strains from patients with meningitis with MIC values of 2 μg/ml or greater should be considered ampicillin-resistant (Thornsberry, 1977a).

DISC DIFFUSION TESTING WITH HAEMOPHILUS INFLUENZAE. Mueller-Hinton agar (pH 7.2) should be supplemented with 1 per cent IsoVitaleX (BBL) and 1 per cent hemoglobin (Thornsberry, 1974). This preparation is superior to one with chocolatized sheep blood because the zones on chocolatized blood agar are very difficult to read. The disc diffusion test is carried out exactly as that described for the standard method, except that for ampicillin a zone diameter of 20 mm or greater defines susceptibility. Some ampicillin-resistant strains produce zone diameters close to 19 mm; however, there will almost always be varying numbers of colonies within this zone. Thornsberry (1977a) indicates that a 10-unit penicillin disc can also be used, as it discriminates between ampicillin-resistant and susceptible strains very well with the same zone diameter interpretive criteria as those described for ampicillin.

The susceptibility of *H. influenzae* to other antimicrobial agents can be determined by using the interpretive criteria listed in Table 55-5 (Thornsberry, 1977a).

Susceptibility Testing of Staphylococcus aureus. Problems associated with susceptibility testing of staphylococci fall into three main categories:

1. Detection of resistance to the semi-synthetic, penicillinase-resistant penicillins requires an incubation temperature of $35°C$. Alternatively, detection of this resistance can be enhanced by using a heavy inoculum, extending the incubation time to 48 hours, or adding 5 per cent NaCl to the testing medium. For all practical purposes, unless there is a specific epidemiologic problem requiring added surveillance, an incubation temperature of $35°C$. suffices.

2. Resistance to the semi-synthetic, penicillinase-resistant penicillins will not be reliably detected with cloxacillin or dicloxacillin (Drew, 1972). Susceptibility testing by the disc diffusion method should be done with methicillin, nafcillin, or oxacillin. Methicillin is probably the most widely used, but is also the least stable of the three compounds. Because resistance to methicillin is still uncommon in the United States, finding a resistant strain should prompt confirmation of its identity to be sure that it is *S. aureus* and repeat testing because of the possibility of reduced potency of the disc.

3. Staphylococci exist in which there is a large

Table 55-9. INTERPRETIVE GUIDELINES FOR CATEGORY METHOD OF SUSCEPTIBILITY TESTING

| | GROWTH IN FOUR TUBES | | | |
CATEGORY	Control	Low	Medium	High
I	+	−	−	−
II	+	+	−	−
III	+	+	+	−
IV	+	+	+	+

discrepancy between the MIC and MBC values when they are tested against the semi-synthetic penicillinase-resistant penicillins (Sabath, 1977). This phenomenon has been called "tolerance" and has led to a significant increase in the number of laboratory requests for both MBC and MIC determinations. It is estimated that as many as 40 per cent of the isolates of *Staphylococcus aureus* from clinically significant infections in hospital settings may demonstrate "tolerance." Both *Staphylococcus aureus* and enterococci may appear to be fully susceptible to a penicillin by MIC criteria, but they may be very resistant when one assesses the MBC of the penicillin or related compound.

Tolerance may be important in some patients and should be taken into account by the physician in the approach to the therapy of staphylococcal disease. It also has ramifications in the laboratory, not only in terms of additional requests for MBC testing, but also in the potential usage of combinations of antibiotics, i.e., an aminoglycoside and a semi-synthetic penicillinase-resistant penicillin, and the monitoring of therapy with aminoglycosides.

It should be noted at this point that *Staphylococcus epidermidis* is often resistant to the penicillinase-resistant, semi-synthetic penicillins (methicillin, nafcillin, and oxacillin).

Susceptibility Tests for Neisseria gonorrhoeae. Two types of resistance exist with *Neisseria gonorrhoeae*. One is a relative resistance which has been present for many years and seems to have reached a peak and remained stable over the recent years. This type of resistance has led to the current use of 4.8 million units of penicillin, in contrast to much lower dosages which at one time were uniformly effective in treating gonorrhea. A second type of resistance has manifested itself in recent years and is mediated through the production of penicillinase. Therefore, one can approach the assessment of susceptibility of *Neisseria gonorrhoeae* in two ways. One can test for its absolute susceptibility by means of the agar dilution test. Moreover, one can test for the production of beta-lactamase or penicillinase, as will be described in this section. A disc diffusion test was described by Ronald (1968) in which a zone diameter of 20 mm was equivalent to susceptibility of less than 1 unit of penicillin. This method did not gain wide acceptance; however, a modified disc diffusion test with the same zone diameter interpretive criterion has been shown to correlate with beta-lactamase production (Thornsberry, 1977a). In this test, an inoculum equivalent in density to a 0.5 MacFarland standard is applied, as for the standard disc diffusion method, to GC base agar supplemented with 1 per cent IsoVitaleX. A single 10 U penicillin disc is placed on the agar surface. Strains that produce beta-lactamase produce zone diameters of less than

19 mm. This method allows most laboratories to test for gonococcal susceptibility patterns and the likelihood of beta-lactamase production. Other than testing for beta-lactamase, there is seldom a need for susceptibility testing of *Neisseria gonorrhoeae*, except in instances of treatment failure, in epidemiologic investigations, or in studies of *in vitro* antibiotic susceptibility. In such instances, agar dilution studies can be performed. The growth from four or five colonies of the organism, grown on chocolate agar or modified Thayer-Martin medium, is suspended in TSB and adjusted to the appropriate density by comparison to a MacFarland 0.5 standard. A 1:20 dilution is made in broth and is streaked directly onto GC medium containing hemoglobin (1 g/100 ml), 1 per cent IsoVitaleX (BioQuest), or Supplement C (Difco) and the appropriate concentrations of antimicrobial. These plates should be used within 48 hours of preparation. They are incubated at 35°C. in an environment of increased CO_2 and are read at 24 hours if sufficient growth has occurred.

One should also test a control strain of *Neisseria gonorrhoeae* with known susceptibility, and it is recommended that *Sarcina lutea* be included to provide additional technical control. Barry (1976) stresses that the density of the inoculum is an important variable and suggests checking the adjusted cell suspension by diluting it by a factor of 50 and streaking it onto a chocolate agar plate with a 0.001 ml calibrated loop. If the inoculum is correct, from 10 to 100 colonies should grow on the agar.

Susceptibility Testing of Neisseria meningitidis. Susceptibility testing of *Neisseria meningitidis* is rarely required because beta-lactamase production by this species has not yet been demonstrated. Testing is usually carried out for research or epidemiologic purposes. However, since sulfonamides can prevent meningitis in close contacts of patients with meningococcal meningitis and because sulfonamide resistance is not uncommonly present in meningococci, susceptibility testing of sulfonamides may be necessary. A slight modification of the disc diffusion methodology, as described by Bennett (1968), is used with a zone diameter of 40 mm defining susceptibility. Susceptibility testing by the agar dilution method can also be carried out as described for *Neisseria gonorrhoeae*.

THE DETERMINATION OF BETA-LACTAMASE PRODUCTION

Beta-lactamase production is primarily determined with *H. influenzae*, *N. gonorrhoeae*, and *S. aureus*. Several methods exist that are applicable for testing these three organisms. Whereas the production of beta-lactamase is usually very rap-

5

idly demonstrated with *Haemophilus* and *Neisseria*, it can take longer to manifest itself with staphylococci, so that the tests should be allowed to incubate for at least one hour. Staphylococcal beta-lactamases are inducible, while the beta-lactamases of *H. influenzae* and *N. gonorrhoeae* are not.

Four tests will be described for the production of beta-lactamase. Each has its advantages and disadvantages (Thornsberry, 1977c). The reagents for each of the tests, with the exception of the chromogenic cephalosporin, are widely available and easy to prepare. For the purposes described above, the sensitivity and specificity of these tests are equivalent; however, the chromogenic cephalosporin test is more sensitive than the others for investigating the presence of beta-lactamases in other gram-negative bacilli, e.g., Enterobacteriaceae. Each of the tests can be performed rapidly and will provide results within minutes. The selection of one of these tests for routine purposes depends on various factors, including availability of reagents, stability of reagents, personal experience and expertise, ease of performance of the test, and clarity of end points.

Chromogenic cephalosporin test (O'Callaghan, 1972)

Reagents

Cephalosporin 87/312*
Dimethylsulfoxide (DMSO)
Phosphate buffer, pH 7

Monopotassium phosphate, M/15	39.2 ml
Disodium phosphate, M/15	60.8 ml

Dissolve cephalosporin in DMSO and mix in phosphate buffer to final concentration of 500 μg/ml.

Test

MICRODILUTION PLATE OR SMALL TUBE. Add 0.05 ml cephalosporin substrate to a well of a microdilution plate (or to a small tube). With a loop, remove the growth from several colonies of the test organism. Make a heavy turbid suspension in the cephalosporin solution. Mix for 1 minute. Observe for color change immediately, after 10 minutes, and after 1 hour. If the culture produces beta-lactamase, the color of the substrate will change from yellow to red. Beta-lactamase-producing *H. influenzae* or *N. gonorrhoeae* usually turn the solution red in less than 10 minutes, but staphylococci may require an hour. Run the test with a known beta-lactamase- and a non-beta-lactamase-producing strain of *N. gonorrhoeae*, *H. influenzae*, or *S. aureus*.

AGAR PLATE MODIFICATION. The agar plate should contain the organism in pure culture. Place

a drop (approximately 0.05 ml) of the cephalosporin reagent on an area of bacterial growth. Tilt the plate slightly to permit the drop to spread across the plate. If the organism produces beta-lactamase, the reagent will turn red along the streak; if it is beta-lactamase-negative, the reagent will be yellow along the streak. Because the red color is not as easily seen as in the test done in the microdilution well, the test should be repeated in a microdilution well or small tube if there is any doubt about the result. Usually a positive test can be read immediately, but the plate should be reexamined after 10 minutes. Experience with staphylococci in this test is very limited.

Precautions

1. Primary isolation media (e.g., modified Thayer-Martin medium) may contain beta-lactamase-producing bacteria in addition to those of interest (e.g., *N. gonorrhoeae*) and may cause a false-positive test.

2. Clinical specimens (e.g., urethral discharge, vaginal secretion) cannot be tested directly with the chromogenic cephalosporin test.

Rapid microtube iodometric test (Catlin, 1975)

Reagents

Penicillin G powder
Phosphate buffer, pH 6

Monopotassium phosphate, M/15	87.7 ml
Disodium phosphate, M/15	17.7 ml

Starch
Iodine
Potassium iodide

Solution. Add sodium or potassium penicillin G powder (most readily available as sodium or potassium penicillin G for intravenous human use) to freshly prepared pH 6.0 phosphate buffer to obtain a solution with a concentration of 6000 μg/ml. Small aliquots of the penicillin solution can be dispensed into vials that can be tightly sealed and frozen in non-frost-free freezers. Frost-free freezers are unsuitable because repeated thawing cycles cause deterioration of the penicillin. Aliquots can be thawed and used for up to one week or as long as correct results are obtained with control cultures of known reactivity.

STARCH SOLUTION. Add 1.0 g of soluble starch to 100 ml of distilled water. Place in boiling water bath until the starch goes into solution. Prepare fresh or store in refrigerator for no more than one week. Smaller volumes of this 1 per cent solution can be made because 10 ml is enough for over 100 tests. Starch designated for use in iodometric tests is commercially available.

IODINE. Dissolve 2.03 g of iodine and 53.2 g of potassium iodide in 100 ml of distilled water. Store at room temperature in brown glass bottle. Prepare fresh when the solution develops excessive precipi-

---

*Glaxo, Ltd., Greenford, Middlesex UB6 OHE England.

tate (usually several months). Run the test with known beta-lactamase-positive and beta-lactamase-negative strains of *N. gonorrhoeae, H. influenzae,* or *S. aureus.*

Test Procedure. Dispense 0.1 ml of the penicillin solution into a well of a microdilution plate or a small test tube. Remove several colonies of an 18- to 24-hour pure culture with a loop and make a *heavy* turbid suspension in the penicillin solution in the well. Stir for 30 seconds and *let the mixture stand for one hour at room temperature to allow time for the beta-lactamase to break down the penicillin to penicilloic acid.* *H. influenzae* and *N. gonorrhoeae* usually do not require an hour of incubation, but staphylococci may. Add 2 drops of starch solution to the suspension of bacteria and penicillin. Mix. Add 1 drop of iodine reagent. The solution will immediately turn blue because of the reaction of the iodine and the starch. If the iodine is added prematurely, the enzymatic reaction may stop and a false-negative test may result. Stir the mixture for one minute. Rapid decolorization indicates the production of beta-lactamase. If the solution remains blue for longer than 10 minutes, the organism did not produce the enzyme.

Precautions

1. Primary isolation medium (e.g., modified Thayer-Martin medium) may contain beta-lactamase-producing bacteria in addition to the bacteria of interest (e.g., *N. gonorrhoeae*) and cause a false-positive test.

2. Clinical specimens (e.g., urethral discharge, vaginal secretions) cannot be tested directly with the iodometric test.

Rapid slide iodometric test (Rosenblatt, 1978)

Penicillin Solution. Dissolve penicillin (Penicillin G, potassium, for injection U.S.P. [buffered], one million units per vial) in 1 ml sterile water and remove 0.15 ml aliquots for freezing at −20°C. (frozen vials may be used for as long as 30 days, but should be discarded after use, once thawed).

Iodine. Dissolve 1.5 g potassium iodine and 0.3 g iodine in 100 ml of 0.1 M phosphate buffer at pH 6.4. This buffer is prepared by the addition of 60 ml pH 6.0 buffer to 40 ml pH 7.0 buffer. The iodine solution is stored in a brown bottle at 4°C.

Starch Solution. Dissolve 0.4 g soluble starch (Difco) in 100 ml distilled water. Autoclave and store at 4°C.

A penicillin-iodine mixture is prepared by adding 1.1 ml of the iodine solution to a vial containing 0.5 ml of thawed penicillin G. Once this mixture has been prepared it should be used within one hour. A loopful of test organisms is removed from growth on the surface of an agar plate and emulsified in 1 drop of the penicillin-iodine mixture on an ordinary glass microscope slide. Immediately, one drop of starch solution is added. A negative test for

penicillinase is indicated by the development of a purple or lavender color which remains for 5 minutes.

A white color indicates a positive test. Most reactions will be complete by 30 seconds, with a final reading taken at 5 minutes for the detection of small amounts of penicillinase.

Rapid acidimetric test for beta-lactamase production in bacteria (Thornsberry, 1977c)

Reagents
Phenol red solution, 0.5%
Penicillin G
Sodium hydroxide, 1 M
Two ml of 0.5 per cent phenol red solution is added to 16.6 ml of sterile distilled water. This solution is then added to a vial containing 20 million units of potassium penicillin G (Pfizer). Sodium hydroxide (1 M) is added drop by drop until the test solution turns violet (pH 8.5). The test solution is either used immediately or divided into portions in screwcapped tubes and frozen at −60°C. for as long as one week.

Test Procedure. Dip a capillary tube (0.7 to 1.0 mm OD) into the test solution and allow liquid to flow by capillary action for a distance of 1 to 2 cm into the tube. The tip of the capillary tube is scraped lightly across several *H. influenzae* colonies from an agar plate (chocolate agar plus 1 per cent IsoVitaleX [BioQuest]) that has been incubated 24 hours, so that a plug of bacteria fills the bottom of the tube. Allow no air to be trapped between the test solution and the bacteria, since the two must be in contact. The filled capillary tubes are incubated at room temperature in a vertical position. This is achieved by sticking the empty end of the capillary tube into clay and letting it hang straight down. If the organism produces beta-lactamase, the test solution turns a bright yellow in 5 to 15 minutes. In the tests with organisms that do not produce beta-lactamase, the test solution either does not change color at all or changes to no more than a pale pink color. Include a penicillin-resistant *S. aureus* as a positive control and a penicillin-susceptible *S. aureus* as a negative control with each *Haemophilus* tested.

Special tests

Bactericidal Activity Testing. The majority of bacterial susceptibility testing is to determine inhibitory end-points. While antimicrobials may exert a killing effect in their action on bacteria and the concentration of antibiotic required for this lethal or bactericidal activity may, in fact, be very close to that of the inhibitory concentration, there may be situations, as with some staphylococci and enterococci, in which the inhibitory and bactericidal concentrations vary considerably. In addition, the assessment of an antimicrobial's bactericidal activity becomes all the more important in the patient whose immune defense mechanisms are compromised. In this circumstance an adjustment of antimicrobial therapy may well be warranted on the basis of the bactericidal test result.

Recently, the "minimal lethal concentration (MLC)" has been proposed for the effect previously known as the minimal bactericidal concentration (MBC). The reader should be aware that the terms are analogous.

In order to establish the MBC or MLC of an antimicrobial one begins by performing a standard broth dilution test, as for determining the MIC. For this test, however, it is necessary to quantitate the inoculum; this may be done by streaking 0.1 ml of 1:100 and 1:1000 dilutions of the inoculum over an agar surface. After the inhibitory phase of the test has been completed, a 0.01 ml calibrated loop is used to subculture from each tube to a quadrant of a blood agar plate. The plates are then incubated overnight, and the MBC or MLC is the lowest concentration (in μg/ml) of antimicrobial, subculture of which is lethal to 99.9 per cent of the original inoculum.

This method provides the greatest efficiency for the clinical laboratory. Were one to perform bactericidal testing for reference or investigational purposes, a more carefully defined and volumetrically determined procedure should be used.

Combination Testing.   Therapy in serious infections is very often approached with combinations of antimicrobials. In the compromised patient and in unusual clinical circumstances, testing of the combined action of antimicrobials may be warranted. There are several ways in which this testing can be accomplished, although what is described here is meant to be a practical method that can be used efficiently and economically in the clinical laboratory. An approach to testing combinations of three or more antimicrobials has been described by Berenbaum (1978).

Materials.   The test procedure outlined here requires two microdilution plates, a set of 15 μl pipette droppers, and 50 μl diluters. Mueller-Hinton broth is used, and the antimicrobials to be tested are made up in solutions so that they can be utilized alone and in various combinations. The inoculum density should be standardized with a 0.5 MacFarland standard and then diluted 1:100 in Mueller-Hinton broth.

Procedure.   Two microdilution plates are placed side by side, and the first four rows of the second plate are relabeled I through L. Only four rows are used in this second plate (Fig. 55-2). 50 μl of MHB are dispensed to all wells except A-1 with a 50 μl pipette dropper. The antibiotic solutions are labeled No. 1 and No. 2 and are diluted to contain concentrations equivalent to four times those finally desired. 100 μl of antibiotic solution No. 1 are added to well A-1, and 50 μl to the rest of the wells in column No. 1 (B through L) with the pipette dropper. The antibiotic in the first well (column 1) of each row is then serially diluted across the plates through column 11 (do not dilute into wells in column 12). With the 50 μl pipette dropper, dispense 50 μl of antibi-

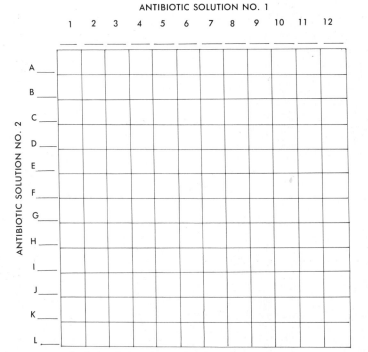

Figure 55-2. Arrangement of tubes and chart for results of combination study of two antimicrobial agents.

otic solution No. 2 into each well in row A (1 through 12). Again, with the 50 μl diluters, dilute serially down each column from each well in row A through wells in row K (do not dilute into wells in row L). Add 50 μl of the standardized inoculum to each of the 144 wells using a 50 μl pipette dropper. Cover the plate with a plastic tape and incubate. The MIC for antimicrobial No. 1 can be obtained from the wells in row L and the MIC for antimicrobial No. 2 from the wells in column 12. Well L-12 contains no antimicrobial and serves as the growth control. Results are recorded on a chart as shown in Figure 55-2. This chart serves as a laboratory work sheet and for plotting an isobologram. A straight line is drawn between the MIC values of each antimicrobial. A curve is constructed from the MIC of the combinations of the two antimicrobials. If the curve falls below the line that has been drawn between two MIC values of each antimicrobial, a synergistic effect has been demonstrated (Fig. 55-3). If the curve is outside this line, then antagonism has been demonstrated. A detailed discussion of the mathematical considerations involved in the determination of synergy can be found elsewhere (Berenbaum, 1978).

QUALITY CONTROL OF SUSCEPTIBILITY TESTING

Quality control is extremely important in antimicrobial susceptibility testing and for the other tests performed in the support of

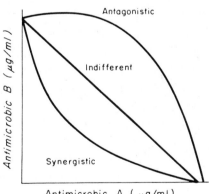

Figure 55-3. Isobologram portraying three possible results when two antimicrobics (A and B) are tested singly and in various combinations; either MIC or MLC endpoints may be plotted. A straight line joining the values obtained with each drug separately represents an isobol which indicates indifference. Antagonism is indicated by an isobol which bows upward away from the coordinates, and a bowing toward the coordinates indicates synergism. With permission from Barry, A. L., and Sabath, L. D.: Special tests: Bactericidal activity and activity of antimicrobics in combination. *In* Lennett, E. H., Spaulding, E. H., and Truant, J. P. (eds.): Manual of Clinical Microbiology, 2nd ed. Washington, D.C., American Society for Microbiology, 1974. p. 431.

antimicrobial therapy. All of the various parameters of each test should be regularly evaluated in order to ensure confidence in the performance of the test.

This section will outline an overall quality control program for the various tests that have been described.

Stock cultures

One should maintain a collection of all organisms needed for quality control of the media, the actual tests themselves, and any reagents that may be needed. Stock cultures of most organisms may be maintained on sealed agar deeps at 25°C. in the dark, at −70°C., or in a lyophilized state. Stock cultures of organisms with ATCC designation may be obtained from the American Type Culture Collection (12301 Parklawn Drive, Rockville, Md. 20852): *Staphylococcus aureus* ATCC 25923, *Escherichia coli* ATCC 25922, and *Pseudomonas aeruginosa* ATCC 27853 for disc diffusion susceptibility testing; *S. aureus* ATCC 29213 and *Streptococcus faecalis* ATCC 29212 for dilution susceptibility testing; *S. aureus* ATCC 25923, *P. aeruginosa* ATCC 27853, and *E. coli* ATCC 29194 for Autobac I; and *Bacillus subtilis* ATCC 6633, *Klebsiella pneumoniae* ATCC 27799, and *Clostridium perfringens* UUMC 9758 for antimicrobial assays.

Stock Culture Storage

GRAM-NEGATIVE BACILLI. These can be stored on small soybean-casein digest agar slants at room temperature in the dark and should be transferred weekly or twice monthly to new slants. Reference strains of these organisms should be kept in a lyophilized or frozen state in the event that the performance of the organisms on slants should change. Both the *E. coli* (ATCC 25922) and the *K. pneumoniae* (ATCC 27799) have proven to be extremely stable over many years. The *P. aeruginosa* (ATCC 27853) control strain, if subcultured daily, has a tendency to develop colonies resistant to carbenicillin. It is suggested that subculturing of this strain on a daily basis be limited to one week and that a fresh subculture be obtained from a lyophilized or frozen stock culture (Thornsberry, 1977a).

GRAM-POSITIVE COCCI. The *S. aureus* (ATCC 25923) and *S. faecalis* (ATCC 29212) are maintained on sheep blood agar at room temperature or transferred weekly or when new sheep blood plates are tested. Again, reference cultures are maintained in a lyophilized or frozen state in case questions arise about organism performance.

CLOSTRIDIUM PERFRINGENS. *Clostridium perfringens* can be maintained at room temperature in chopped meat medium and needs to be transferred to new chopped meat medium only every three months.

Media

Sterility. A sample of each lot of plated medium prepared in the clinical laboratory should be incubated to check for sterility. Plates containing media from commercial sources should also be checked for sterility.

Performance. Mueller-Hinton agar plates are tested with both *E. coli* (ATCC 25922) and *S. aureus* (ATCC 25923). These are incubated in an aerobic environment for 24 hours at 35°C. The pH of the medium should be 7.2 to 7.4 at 25°C., and the agar depth should be 4 to 5 mm. The surface of the agar should be even and the depth of the agar uniform. Mueller-Hinton broth is also tested with the same control organisms as the Mueller-Hinton agar plates.

Antimicrobial Discs and Stock Solutions. Stock antimicrobial solutions are frozen in readily usable aliquots. Once thawed they are not to be reused. Control organisms should be tested each time a new lot of antimicrobial is prepared or each time a new vial of antimicrobial discs is to be used. The vial of discs should be tested the day prior to its being used on a routine basis. All antimicrobial materials should be labeled as to the date of expiration, the date received in the laboratory, and the date opened. Unused lots of stock solutions should be discarded after the expiration date. Stock solutions can be stored at −20°C. or below for six months, with the exception of the penicillins and nitrofurantoin. All antimicrobial discs should be frozen at −20°C. in containers with desiccant. After removal from the freezer, discs should be allowed to equilibrate to room temperature before the containers are opened.

Procedural Checks. Each procedure has its own quality control checks. These are listed in the order that they have been presented in this chapter.

Dilution Testing. Dilution test series should be inoculated with the control strains listed above for dilution testing. At the Mayo Clinic, *E. coli* (ATCC 25922), *S. aureus* (ATCC 25923), and a strain of *P. aeruginosa* are used on a daily basis for quality control of agar dilution tests. The means and ranges of minimal inhibitory concentrations with these organisms are published elsewhere (Washington, 1974a). In agar dilution testing, it is important to inoculate an agar plate without antimicrobials in order to verify the viability of the test organism. In addition, each well of the seed plate should be subcultured to a quadrant of a blood agar plate in order to verify the purity of the inoculum. Dilution testing, in general, presents some special quality control problems. With all but the category or abbreviated methods of dilution testing, each dilution set will contain 8 to 12 twofold dilution steps. Control organisms should ideally provide a means of evaluating the performance of each antimicrobial agent by providing MIC values that are at least one twofold ($\log_2$) dilution from either end of the dilution scale for each antimicrobial being evaluated. Since the selection of the control strains for disc diffusion testing was made on the basis of

their susceptibility (vs. resistance) to various antimicrobials, it has been suggested that *S. aureus* ATCC 29213 and *S. faecalis* ATCC 29212 be used for quality control of dilution tests. These strains are more likely to yield MIC values above the lowest level of susceptibility tested (Thornsberry, 1977a). It should be noted that the only difference between *S. aureus* ATCC 25923 and *S. aureus* ATCC 29213 is that the former does not produce beta-lactamase, whereas the latter does and is, therefore, resistant to penicillin. Extensive data regarding the MIC values of various antimicrobials with these strains are not yet available.

The two control strains described above should be tested with each set of dilutions performed. Since most laboratories will perform susceptibility tests of a number of organisms each day, it is to be expected that, in order to control the performance of dilution tests, control organisms should be run with each group of organisms tested. This is especially important with broth dilution tests because of their vulnerability to inoculum size variations.

Since the 0.5 MacFarland turbidity standard is used for adjusting the inoculum of all antimicrobial susceptibility tests, it should be carefully maintained, as has already been described in this chapter.

Autobac I. Because discs are used as the source of antimicrobial and because of the number of test variables, including instrument function, control strains should be tested regularly in the Autobac. The manufacturer provides detailed quality control guidelines for those who purchase this instrument.

Disc Diffusion Testing. Considerable work has been done with the quality control of the disc diffusion methodology, and the performance of the three ATCC strains used for quality control has been carefully defined. The control limits for the zone diameters of inhibition of the control strains are listed in Tables 55-10 to 55-12. These are important tables for those using the disc diffusion method and should be maintained for reference purposes. Some antimicrobials are tested against two or three of the control strains. This overlap provides a double check on the performance of most antimicrobials and on the test itself.

The control strains should be tested daily or at least each time the test is conducted, and the zone diameters should be recorded on a quality control chart for easy visualization. Should the zone diameters fall outside the expected ranges, an investigation must be made to determine what has gone wrong.

Pretest monitoring of the performance of new vials of antimicrobial discs must be performed to detect any potential problems with the discs in this vial. This step is highly recommended, as it will obviate the necessity of having to repeat all of the susceptibility tests any time a disc from a new vial might perform poorly. At least in some instances, it

Table 55-10. CONTROL LIMITS FOR MONITORING PRECISION AND ACCURACY OF INHIBITORY ZONE DIAMETERS OBTAINED IN GROUPS OF FIVE SEPARATE OBSERVATIONS WITH ESCHERICHIA COLI ATCC 25922[*]

ANTIMICROBIAL AGENT	DISK CONTENT (μg)	INDIVIDUAL TEST CONTROL (zone diam. mm)	ACCURACY CONTROL (zone diam. mm)[a]	PRECISION CONTROL (RANGE OF FIVE VALUES[b]) Maximum	Average[c]
Ampicillin	10	15–20	15.8–19.2	6	2.9
Carbenicillin	100	24–29	25.0–28.0	7	3.5
Cephalothin	30	18–23	18.8–22.2	6	2.9
Chloramphenicol	30	21–27	22.0–26.0	7	3.5
Colistin	10	11–15	11.7–14.3	4	2.3
Erythromycin	15	8–14	9.0–13.0	7	3.5
Gentamicin	10	19–26	20.2–24.8	8	4.1
Kanamycin	30	17–25	18.3–23.7	9	4.7
Neomycin	30	17–23	18.0–22.0	6	3.5
Polymyxin B	300 U	12–16	12.7–15.3	4	2.3
Streptomycin	10	12–20	13.3–18.7	9	4.7
Tetracycline	30	18–25	19.2–23.8	8	4.1
Tobramycin	10	18–26			
Trimethoprim-sulfamethoxazole	1.25 23.75	24–32	25.3–30.7	9	4.7

[*]From Thornsberry (1977c).

[a]Mean of five values.

[b]Maximum value minus minimum value obtained in a series of five consecutive tests should not exceed the listed maximum limits, and the mean should fall within the range listed under "accuracy control."

[c]In a continuing series of ranges from consecutive groups of five tests each, the average range should approximate the listed value.

Table 55-11. CONTROL LIMITS FOR MONITORING PRECISION AND ACCURACY OF INHIBITORY ZONE DIAMETERS OBTAINED IN GROUPS OF FIVE SEPARATE OBSERVATIONS WITH STAPHYLOCOCCUS AUREUS ATCC 25923[*]

ANTIMICROBIAL AGENT	DISK CONTENT (μg)	INDIVIDUAL TEST CONTROL (zone diam. mm)	ACCURACY CONTROL (zone diam. mm)[a]	PRECISION CONTROL (RANGE[b] OF FIVE VALUES) Maximum	Average[c]
Ampicillin	10	24–35	25.8–33.2	13	6.4
Cephalothin	30	25–37	27.0–35.0	14	7.0
Chloramphenicol	30	19–26	20.2–24.8	8	4.1
Clindamycin	2	23–29	24.0–28.0	7	3.5
Erythromycin	15	23–30	23.3–28.7	9	4.7
Gentamicin	10	19–27	20.3–25.7	9	4.7
Kanamycin	30	19–26	20.2–24.8	8	4.1
Methicillin	5	17–22	17.8–21.2	6	2.9
Neomycin	30	18–26	19.3–24.7	9	4.7
Penicillin G	10 U	26–37	27.8–35.2	13	6.4
Polymyxin B	300 U	7–13			
Streptomycin	10	14–22	15.3–20.7	9	4.7
Tetracycline	30	19–28	20.5–26.5	11	5.2
Tobramycin	10	19–29			
Vancomycin	30	15–19	15.7–18.3	4	2.3
Trimethoprim-sulfamethoxazole	1.25 23.75	24–32	25.0–31.0	7	3.5

[*]From Thornsberry (1977c).

[a]See footnote a in Table 55-10.

[b]See footnote b in Table 55-10.

[c]See footnote c in Table 55-10.

Table 55-12. SUGGESTED QUALITY CONTROL
LIMITS FOR INHIBITORY ZONE DIAMETERS WHEN
TESTING WITH PSEUDOMONAS AERUGINOSA ATCC 27853*

ANTIMICROBIAL AGENT	DISK CONTENT (μg)	INDIVIDUAL TEST CONTROL ZONE DIAMETER (mm)
Carbenicillin	100	19–25
Gentamicin	10	16–22
Tobramycin	10	19–25
Polymyxin B	300 U	13–18
Colistin	10	11–15
Tetracycline	30	6–14
Chloramphenicol	30	6–12

*From Thornsberry (1977c).

will assist in making a decision as to whether or not to report susceptibility testing results if the zone diameters of the control strain(s) are not within the control limits on a particular day's run. If problems do occur, a log should be kept as to what they are and their disposition.

Other Susceptibility Testing. Currently, there are no established reference strains for control of susceptibility tests of anaerobic bacteria, haemophili, and neisseriae. Therefore, the laboratory should attempt to maintain stock cultures of each of these organisms for control purposes. *Neisseria* and *Haemophilus* species are very difficult to maintain in a clinical laboratory setting short of freezing at −70°C., and, even there, there is considerable risk of loss of viability, especially during the freezing and thawing processes themselves.

Proficiency Testing. Proficiency testing for clinical laboratories is an important part of monitoring of actual performance. It may be carried out with well-characterized internal unknowns or with external unknowns provided by the proficiency testing program conducted by the College of American Pathologists or by the Center for Disease Control.

ASSAYS OF ANTIMICROBIAL AGENTS

Indications for Assays. Basically, the assessment of the concentration of an antimicrobial in the serum or a body fluid of a patient is made in order to determine potential effect of that agent or the likelihood of toxicity. The circumstances in which antimicrobial assays are ordered, therefore, are those in which a low therapeutic-toxic ratio may exist, as in the case of the aminoglycosides or of chloramphenicol in newborn infants. A second circumstance would be in a patient in whom the anticipated clinical effect has not occurred, possibly owing to individual variations in the pharmacokinetics of the antimicrobial in the patient or to particular characteristics of the patient, organism, or antimicrobial that interfere with the activity of the antimicrobial. It is not the scope of this chapter to go

into all of the factors that can lead to the failure of antimicrobial therapy; however, it should be pointed out that these factors must be assessed because something can often be done to obviate their effects in the patient. A third circumstance in which antimicrobial assays become important is in the treatment of severe local infections, where fluid specimens may be available for assay, or in situations where the underlying disease of the patient is such that the antibiotic must do more of the job of eradicating the organism than would be the case in a normal patient with appropriately functioning host defense capabilities.

There are many methods for performing antimicrobial assays, including chemical, turbidimetric, agar diffusion, pH alteration and inhibition, enzymatic, radioimmunoassay, hemoglobin reduction, chromatographic, and many other techniques. Radioimmunoassay (RIA) and high pressure liquid chromatography (HPLC) have opened a new era in the assay of antimicrobials; however, not only is there a substantial investment in the equipment to perform these tests, but a certain level of expertise is required. These tests, nonetheless, will become more and more available in the future. In the interim and for those clinical laboratories where the availability of this instrumentation will continue to be a problem, there are several bioassay means that can be used very effectively to assay most antimicrobials. In addition, there are several innovations being used which will allow for greater ease in testing for antimicrobials in the presence of other agents being used in combination therapy. The three test organisms listed in Table 55-13 cover well over 90 per cent of the assay requests at the University of Utah Medical Center. Currently, for the high volume assay requests (for gentamicin) we use the radioimmunoassay (RIA) during the daytime hours and utilize the bioassay for single test requests in the evening and on

Table 55-13. ORGANISMS TO BE USED IN BIOASSAY OF ANTIBIOTICS IN SERUM AND BODY FLUIDS

ANTIMICROBIAL	TEST ORGANISM	ANTIMICROBIALS THAT DO NOT INTERFERE WITH TEST RESULTS
Ampicillin	*Clostridium perfringens*	Aminoglycosides
Amikacin	*Klebsiella pneumoniae* ATCC 27799	Ampicillin, carbenicillin, cephalothin, chloramphenicol, clindamycin, other penicillins
Carbenicillin	*C. perfringens*	Aminoglycosides
Cephalothin	*Bacillus subtilis* ATCC 6633	
Cephazolin	*B. subtilis* ATCC 6633	
Clindamycin	*C. perfringens*	Aminoglycosides
Chloramphenicol	*C. perfringens*	Aminoglycosides
Gentamicin	*K. pneumoniae* ATCC 27799	See amikacin above
Nafcillin	*B. subtilis* ATCC 6633	
Penicillin	*B. subtilis* ATCC 6633	
Tobramycin	*K. pneumoniae* ATCC 27799	See amikacin above
Vancomycin	*C. perfringens*	Aminoglycosides

weekends. For the less frequently used aminoglycosides, we continue to do the bioassay, as it is more economical. If more than three aminoglycoside assays can be done on a daily basis, RIA is cost-justifiable. The organisms used in the bioassay of antibiotic levels in serum and body fluids are listed in Table 55-13. It is not within the scope of this chapter to discuss the radioimmunoassay procedures in detail, as they are discussed elsewhere in this volume.

***Bacillus subtilis* Assay.** The *Bacillus subtilis* assay can be used for antimicrobials listed in Table 55-13 when no other antibiotics are present. It can also be used as a general method for assaying the aminoglycoside antibiotics in the presence of beta-lactam antibiotics if beta-lactamase is added to inactivate the cephalosporins and penicillins. Therefore, it has broad applicability and is presented here not only to provide an alternative for the testing of the aminoglycosides but also as a method for assaying antibiotics not covered by the other assay methods. The method outlined here is based on the description by Sabath (1974a).

PREPARATION OF ASSAY STRAIN. The assay organism is the spore form of *Bacillus subtilis* ATCC 6633, which can be used as a lyophilized preparation (Difco Laboratories, Detroit, Mich.) or prepared spores as described elsewhere (Sabath, 1974a).

PREPARATION AND STORAGE OF ASSAY PLATES. Plates for assay are prepared by adding 0.1 ml of the *B. subtilis* spore suspension to 100 ml of molten medium (Difco antibiotic assay medium No. 5 or Grove and Randall medium No. 5) at 48° to 65°C. and pouring 5 ml of the seeded agar into 100 mm plastic Petri dishes, which are allowed to remain on a level surface (check with spirit level) at room temperature until the agar has hardened. The plates can be used immediately, or they can be

stored at 4°C. in sealed plastic bags: plates stored for less than 2 weeks provide results after 2 hours of incubation, while those stored for 2 to 6 weeks require 4 to 5 hours of incubation before readings can be made.

PROCEDURE. The assay of a single serum sample requires two assay plates and 16 0.25 inch (0.6 cm) paper discs No. 740-E (Schleicher and Schuell Company, Keene, N.H.). The discs are arranged in four rows of four discs inside the lid of one of the assay plates, and 0.02 ml of the sample is placed on each of the four discs in the top row. Normal human sera (previously checked to be sure it does not contain antibacterial activity) are prepared with 12, 6, and 1.5 μg/ml for the gentamicin serum assay (suggested standards for other assays are streptomycin, 25, 12.5, and 3.1 μg/ml; vancomycin, 40, 20, and 10 μg/ml; kanamycin, 27, 9, and 3 μg/ml; and tobramycin and neomycin, 12, 6, 1.5 μg/ml), and 0.02 ml of each standard is placed on each of the four paper discs in the bottom row. A reference mark should be made on the bottom of each assay plate to designate the location of the 12-μg standard on the surface of the seeded agar. Discs with samples for assay are placed on the surface of the agar in a clockwise sequence. The duplicate discs containing samples are placed on the agar surface of the same plate so that pairs containing the same fluid are opposite each other. The other eight discs are placed in identical fashion to form a ring on the surface of the seeded agar in the second plate, and the two assay plates are placed on a level shelf at 37°C.

INCUBATION AND READING. Zone diameters of inhibition can be measured with a ruler or, for greater accuracy, with a vernier caliper after approximately four hours of incubation. The rapidity of formation of zones depends upon how long the plates have been stored.

CALCULATION. The results are calculated by plotting a dose response ("standard") curve (Fig. 55-4)

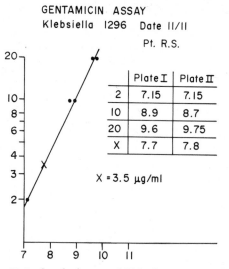

GENTAMICIN ASSAY
Klebsiella 1296   Date 11/11
Pt. R.S.

	Plate I	Plate II
2	7.15	7.15
10	8.9	8.7
20	9.6	9.75
X	7.7	7.8

X = 3.5 μg/ml

Figure 55-4. Standard curve of *Klebsiella pneumoniae* ATCC 27799 with gentamicin in bioassay.

Table 55-14. SUSCEPTIBILITY OF KLEBSIELLA ATCC 27799 TO 19 ANTIBIOTICS

ANTIBIOTIC	MIC*	ZONE SIZE†
Ampicillin	>1,000	6
Amikacin	0.8	
Carbenicillin	>2,000	6
Cephalothin	300	6
Chloramphenicol	>2,000	6
Clindamycin	500	6
Colistin	3.1	14
Erythromycin	800	8
Gentamicin	1.5	20
Kanamycin	>1,000	6
Methicillin	>1,000	6
Nalidixic acid	12.5	16
Nitrofurantoin	500	7
Penicillin G	>2,000	6
Polymyxin B	1.5	15
Streptomycin	>1,000	6
Tetracycline	>2,000	6
Tobramycin	0.2	
Vancomycin		6

*Minimum inhibitory concentration in μg/ml (U/ml for penicillin G and polymyxin B).
†Inhibition zone diameter in mm from disc diffusion method.

on semilogarithmic paper, relating the concentration (μg/ml) of antibiotic in the standard sera (log scale) to the zone diameter (mm) of inhibition. A separate curve is plotted for each of the two plates. Each point plotted represents the mean of the duplicate standards, as do diameters of the zones of inhibition around the two sample discs on each plate. The concentration in the unknown serum being assayed is extrapolated from the standard curve.

Assay of Samples Containing More Than One Antibiotic. The agar diffusion assay described above can be used to measure gentamicin or other aminoglycosides in the presence of any other penicillin or cephalosporin currently in use in the United States by simply adding 0.02 ml of beta-lactamase II (Whatman Biochemicals, Maidenhead, Surrey, England) to 0.1 ml of the serum for assay a few minutes before loading the discs (in calculating results, allow for dilution of sample by enzyme fluid by increasing "apparent" gentamicin value by 20 per cent). Alternatively, a beta-lactamase II may be prepared by simply growing *Bacillus cereus* 569 (ATCC 27348) at 37°C. for 18 hours in Difco brain-heart infusion broth containing 20 μg of cephalothin per ml and using the supernatant fluid as a crude beta-lactamase II. Should a non–beta-lactam antibiotic, such as tetracycline or clindamycin, be present, the assay should be performed with a test organism highly resistant to the interfering antibiotic.

Another bioassay, developed by Lund (1973), for the rapid measurement of aminoglycosides in blood and other body fluids, especially for those in which there are other antimicrobial agents, utilizes a multiply resistant *Klebsiella pneumoniae* (ATCC 27799) (Table 55-14). The basic principles of this test are the same as those described for the

B. subtilis assay; however, the advantages of using the *Klebsiella* are that non-beta-lactam antibiotics do not interfere with the bioassay of aminoglycosides. The reader should consult the description by Lund (1973) for details of performing this bioassay.

Assay for Antibiotics Other Than Aminoglycosides. There are numerous bioassay procedures described for antibiotics other than aminoglycosides; however, the presence of aminoglycosides in the fluid to be assayed usually interferes with reliable measurement of the non-aminoglycosidic antibiotic. In these instances, one may use *Clostridium perfringens* as the test organism for bioassays of penicillins (except nafcillin), clindamycin, chloramphenicol, and vancomycin (Sabath, 1974b), since *C. perfringens* is resistant to the aminoglycosides.

Interpretation of Assay Results. Interpretation of results of antimicrobial assays requires a knowledge of the pharmacokinetics of the agent in question, the timing of collection of the sample for assay, the status of the patient's renal and hepatic function, and the potential interactions of antimicrobial combinations. Anticipated peak serum and urine concentrations with moderate doses of antimicrobials are listed in Table 55-15.

SERUM BACTERICIDAL TESTING. The serum bactericidal or Schlichter test is often used to monitor the therapy of patients with endocarditis and osteomyelitis and for evaluating therapy in other serious infections (Jawetz, 1962; Klastersky, 1974; Pien,

Table 55–15.　ANTICIPATED PEAK ANTIBIOTIC SERUM LEVELS
(MODERATE DOSE)

ANTIMICROBIAL	SERUM CONCENTRATION (μg/ml)	URINE CONCENTRATION (μg/ml)
Amikacin (I.M.)	10–25	150–250
Amoxicillin (P.O.)	5–7	1000–1500
Ampicillin (P.O.)	2–4	100–600
(I.V.)	3–7	100–600
Carbenicillin (P.O.)	5–15	600–1200
(I.V.)	100–200	600–1500
Cefazolin (I.M.)	25–50	1500–3000
Cephalexin (P.O.)	6–20	800–2000
Cephalothin (I.V.)	10–60	1000–1500
Chloramphenicol (P.O.)	4–14	50–120
Clindamycin (P.O.)	2–5	8–25
(I.V.)	10–20	20–45
Colistimethate	4–8	50–250
Erythromycin (P.O.)	1–4	15–50
(I.V.)	5–15	50–200
Gentamicin (I.M.)	4–7	100–300
Kanamycin (I.M.)	12–30	150–300
Methicillin (I.V.)	10–20	50–120
Penicillin G (P.O.)	0.5	70–100
Polymyxin B (I.M.)	2–6	15
Tetracyclines (P.O.)	1–4	1200
(I.M.)	4–6	100–300
Tobramycin (I.M.)	4–7	100–300

1974; Schlichter, 1947). Much confusion about this test exists in the literature because of the lack of a standardized method for performing it (Pien, 1974). In fact, the original test described by Schlichter (1947) was a serum inhibitory titer at the anticipated nadir or trough antimicrobial level. In principle, it involves serial dilution of the patient's serum during antimicrobial therapy to determine the maximum dilution or titer of antimicrobial activity of the serum/antibiotic combination against the organism isolated from an infectious process in the patient being studied. The inoculum should be quantitated in order to give an indication of the sensitivity of the test and also to provide a means by which one may assess the reproducibility or precision of the test should repeat determinations be necessary. The interpretation of this test should not be generalized to all infections. One may anticipate that the effect achieved in the patient is adequate if a peak level of bactericidal activity has been demonstrated in a serum dilution of 1:8 or greater. In staphylococcal endocarditis, a titer of 1:32 or greater is desirable. Whereas this test may be extremely helpful in predicting the outcome of osteomyelitis and endocarditis, it has been our experience that the test is not as predictive of outcome when prosthetic devices are present. In certain kinds of infections, therefore, the serum bactericidal test is an indicator of therapeutic effect and a predictor of therapeutic success.

To perform the test, it is necessary to use the organism isolated from the patient's site of infection. If the patient has endocarditis, then the organism is taken from the blood. If the patient has osteomyelitis, then the organism is either a blood stream isolate or an isolate aspirated directly from the lesion. The organism is inoculated into 4 ml of Trypticase soy broth, which is incubated at 35°C. for four hours or until its turbidity matches that of an 0.5 MacFarland standard. It should be noted that endocarditis may be caused by slow-growing organisms, such as viridans streptococci, which may require the addition of 5 per cent horse serum to TSB and overnight incubation. Where serum has been added, as a facilitator of growth, it should be used throughout the entire test in order to enhance the growth of the organism.

A sample of blood is obtained from the patient, usually at the anticipated peak antimicrobial level. The serum is separated aseptically and stored at −20°C. until used. If the patient has a positive blood culture, the serum should be filtered prior to use.

Sterile TSB, 0.5 ml, is pipetted into each of 7 tubes. The patient's serum is thawed and mixed, and 0.5 ml is added to a tube without broth. This serves as an undiluted test tube. A half milliliter of serum is added to the first tube containing TSB; it is mixed and 0.5 ml is then serially diluted through all of the remaining tubes; 0.5 ml is discarded from tube 6, and tube 7 serves as the organism growth control and contains only broth.

The adjusted inoculum of the test organism is diluted 1:1000, and 0.5 ml of this dilution is added to each tube in the series, mixed, and incubated at 35°C. for 24 hours. With a 0.001 ml calibrated loop, duplicate blood agar plates are streaked with the inoculum and also incubated at 35°C. After 24 hours of incubation, the number of organisms present is determined and should approximate 10^5 CFU/ml (the actual number will vary from 5×10^4 to 5×10^5 CFU/ml). After 24 hours incubation, the test series of tubes are shaken and the results recorded as "growth" or "no-growth" for each tube. All tubes without visible growth are subcultured with a 0.01 ml calibrated loop on a quadrant of a sheep blood agar plate which is incubated overnight at 35°C. The next day the number of colonies subcultured from each tube is recorded, and the results reported as the highest dilution or titer of serum resulting in complete or 99.9 per cent killing of the original inoculum.

REFERENCES

Barry, A. L.: The Antimicrobic Susceptibility Test: Principles and Practices. Philadelphia, Lea and Febiger, 1976.

Barry, A. L., and Fay, G. D.: The amount of agar in antimicrobic disk susceptibility test plates. Am. J. Clin. Pathol., *59*:196, 1973a.

Barry, A. L., Garcia, F., and Thrupp, L. D.: An improved single-disk method for testing the antibiotic susceptibility of rapidly growing pathogens. Am. J. Clin. Pathol., *53*:149, 1970.

Barry, A. L., Joyce, L. J., Adams, A. P., and Benner, E. J.: Rapid determinations of antimicrobial susceptibility for urgent clinical situations. Am. J. Clin. Pathol., *59*:693, 1973b.

Bartlett, R. C., Mazens, M., and Greenfield, B.: Acceleration of tetrazolium reduction by bacteria. J. Clin. Microbiol., *3*:327, 1976.

Bauer, A. W., Kirby, W. M. M., Sherris, J. C., and Turck, M.: Antibiotic susceptibility testing by a standardized single disk method. Am. J. Clin. Pathol., *45*:493, 1966.

Bennett, J. V., Camp, H. M., and Eickhoff, T. C.: Rapid sulfonamide disc sensitivity test for meningococci. Appl. Microbiol., *16*:1056, 1968.

Berenbaum, M. C.: A method for testing for synergy with any number of agents. J. Infect. Dis., *137*:122, 1978.

Blazevic, D. J.: Evaluation of the modified broth-disk method for determining antibiotic susceptibilities of anaerobic bacteria. Antimicrob. Agents Chemother., *7*:721, 1975.

Blazevic, D. J., Koepcke, M. H., and Matsen, J. M.: Quality control testing with the disc antibiotic susceptibility test of Bauer-Kirby-Sherris-Turck. Am. J. Clin. Pathol., *57*:592, 1972.

Catlin, B. W.: Iodometric detection of *Haemophilus influenzae* beta-lactamase: Rapid, presumptive test for ampicillin resistance. Antimicrob. Agents Chemother., *7*:265, 1975.

Chabbert, Y.: Titrage de la sensibilite des germes aerobies aux antibiotiques par la methode de la cupule en gelose. Ann. Inst. Pasteur (Paris), *76*:68, 1949.

Cleary, T. J., and Maurer, D.: Methicillin-resistant *Staphylococcus aureus* susceptibility testing by an automated system. Autobac I. Antimicrob. Agents Chemother., *13*:837, 1978.

Drew, W. L., Barry, A. L., O'Toole, R., and Sherris, J. C.: Reliability of the Kirby-Bauer disc diffusion method for detecting methicillin-resistant strains of *Staphylococcus aureus*. Appl. Microbiol., *24*:240, 1972.

Ellner, P. D., and Johnson, E.: Unreliability of direct antibiotic susceptibility testing on wound exudates. Antimicrob. Agents Chemother., *9*:355, 1976.

Ericsson, H. M., and Sherris, J. C.: Antibiotic sensitivity testing. Report of an international collaborative study. Acta. Pathol. Microbiol. Scand., Sect. B., Suppl. 217, p. 1, 1971.

Federal Register, Rules and Regulations: Antibiotic susceptibility discs. *37*:20525, 1972.

Federal Register, Rules and Regulations: Antibiotic susceptibility discs: Correction. *38*:20076, 1973.

Fleming, A.: The antibacterial action *in vitro* of 2-(p-aminobenzenesulphonamido) pyridine on pneumococci and streptococci. Lancet, *2*:74, 1938.

Fleming, A.: A comparison of the activities of antiseptics on bacteria and on leukocytes. Proc. R. Soc. Lond. (Biol.), *96*:171, 1924.

Fleming, A.: On the antibacterial action of cultures of penicillium, with special reference to their use in the isolation of *B. influenzae*. Br. J. Exp. Pathol., *102*:226, 1929.

Gavan, T. L., and Butler, D. A.: An automated microdilution method for antimicrobial susceptibility testing. *In* Balows, A. (ed.): Current Techniques for Antibiotic Susceptibility Testing. Springfield, Ill., Charles C Thomas, Publisher, 1974, p. 88.

Gavan, T. L., and Town, M. A.: A microdilution method for antibiotic susceptibility testing: An evaluation. Am. J. Clin. Pathol., *53*:880, 1970.

Gerlach, E. H.: Dilution test procedures for susceptibility testing. *In* Bondi, H., Bartola, J. T., and Prier, J. E. (eds.): The Clinical Laboratory as an Aid in Chemotherapy of Infectious Diseases. Baltimore, University Park Press, 1977, p. 45.

Gerlach, E. H.: Microdilution I: A comparative study. *In* Balows, A. (ed.): Current Techniques for Antibiotic Susceptibility Testing. Springfield, Ill., Charles C Thomas, Publisher, 1974, p. 63.

Goss, W. A., and Cimijotti, E. B.: Evaluation of an automatic diluting device for microbiological applications. Appl. Microbiol., *16*:1414, 1968.

Hollick, G. E., and Washington, J. A., II: Comparison of direct and standardized disk diffusion susceptibility of testing urine cultures. Antimicrob. Agents Chemother., *9*:804, 1976.

Jawetz, E.: Assay of antibacterial activity in serum. Am. J. Dis. Child., *103*:113, 1962.

Klastersky, J., et al.: Antibacterial activity in serum and urine as a therapeutic guide in bacterial infections. J. Infec. Dis., *129*:187, 1974.

Kurzynski, T. A., Yrios, J. W., Helstad, A. G., and Field, C. R.: Aerobically incubated thioglycolate broth disk method for antibiotic susceptibility testing of anaerobes. Antimicrob. Agents Chemother., *10*:727, 1976.

Lund, M. E., Blazevic, D. J., and Matsen, J. M.: Rapid gentamicin bioassay using a multiple antibiotic-resistant strain of *Klebsiella pneumoniae*. Antimicrob. Agents Chemother., *4*:569, 1973.

MacLowry, J. D., Jaqua, M. J., and Selepak, S. T., Detailed methodology and implementation of a semiautomated serial dilution microtechnique for antimicrobial suscep- tibility testing. Appl. Microbiol., *20*:46, 1970.

MacLowry, J. D., and Marsh, H. H.: Semiautomatic microtechnique for serial dilution-antibiotic sensitivity testing in the clinical laboratory. J. Lab. Clin. Med., *72*:685, 1968.

Matsen, J. M., and Barry, A. L.: Susceptibility testing: Diffusion test procedures. *In* Lennette, E. H., Spauld- ing, E. H., and Truant, J. P. (eds.): Manual of Clinical Microbiology, 2nd ed. Washington, D.C., Am. Soc. Mi- crobiol., 1974, p. 418.

Matsen, J. M., Koepcke, M. J. H., and Quie, P. G.: Evalua- tion of the Bauer-Kirby-Sherris-Turck single-disc dif- fusion method of antibiotic susceptibility testing. Anti- microb. Agents Chemother., 1969. Am. Soc. Microbiol., Washington, D.C., p. 445, 1970.

Matsen, J. M., Sielaff, B. H., and Buck, G. E.: Rapid auto- mated bacterial identification with computerized pro- gramming of augmented Autobac I results. *In* Sharpe, A. N., and Clark, D. S. (eds.): Mechanizing Microbiology. Springfield, Ill., Charles C Thomas, Pub- lisher, 1977, p. 240.

McKie, J. E., Jr., Borovoy, R. J., Dooley, J. F., Evanega, G. R., Mendoza, G., Meyer, F., Moody, M., Packer, D. E., Praglin, J., and Smith, H.: Autobac 1-A 3-hour automated, antimicrobial susceptibility system: II. Microbiological studies, *In* Heden, C., and Illeni, T. (eds): Automation in Microbiology and Immunology. New York, John Wiley & Sons, Inc., 1974.

McMaster, P. R. B., Robertson, E. A., Witebsky, F. C., and MacLowry, J. D.: Evaluation of a dispensing instrument (Dynatec MIC-2000) for preparing microtiter antibiotic plates and testing their potency during storage. Anti- microb. Agents Chemother., *13*:842, 1978.

Metzler, C. M., and Dettaan, R. M.: Susceptibility tests of anaerobic bacteria: Statistical and clinical considera- tions. J. Infect. Dis., *130*:588, 1974.

National Committee for Clinical Laboratory Standards. Performance standards for antimicrobial disc suscepti- bility tests. Approved Standard ASM-2, Villanova, Pa., 1975.

O'Callaghan, C. H., Morris, A., Kirby, S. M., and Shingler, A. H.: Novel method for the detection of β-lactamases by using a chromogenic cephalosporin substrate. Anti- microb. Agents Chemother., *1*:283, 1972.

Pien, F. D., and Vosti, K. L.: Variation in performance of the serum bactericidal test. Antimicrob. Agents Chemother., *6*:330, 1974.

Praglin, J., Curtis, A. C., Longhenry, D. K., and McKie, J. E., Jr.: Autobac 1—A 3-hour automated anti- microbial susceptibility system: I. System description: *In* Heden, C., and Illeni, T. (eds.): Automation in Micro- biology and Immunology. New York, John Wiley & Sons, Inc., 1974.

Reddish, G. F.: Methods of testing antiseptics. J. Lab Clin. Med., *14*:649, 1929.

Reller, L. B., Schoenknecht, F. D., Kenny, M. A., and Sherris, J. C.: Antibiotic susceptibility testing of *Pseu- domonas aeruginosa:* Selection of a control strain and criteria for magnesium and calcium content in media. J. Infect. Dis., *130*:454, 1974.

Ronald, A. R., Eby, J., and Sherris, J. C.: Susceptibility of *Neisseria gonorrhoeae* to penicillin and tetracycline. Antimicrob. Agents Chemother., p. 431, 1968.

Rose, S. B., and Miller, R. E.: Studies with the agar cup- plate method I. A standardized agar cup-plate tech- nique. J. Bacteriol., *38*:525, 1939.

Rosenblatt, J. E., and Neuman, A. M.: Laboratory sugges- tions—A rapid slide test for penicillinase. Am. J. Clin. Pathol., *69*:351, 1978.

Ryan, K. J., Needham, G. M., Dunsmoor, C. L., and Sherris, J. C.: Stability of antibiotics and chemothera- peutics in agar plates. Appl. Microbiol., *20*:447, 1970.

Sabath, L. D., and Matsen, J. M.: Assay of antimicrobial agents (Antibiotic Section). *In* Lennette, E. H., Spaulding, E. H., and Truant, J. P. (eds.): Manual of Clinical Microbiology, 2nd ed. Washington, D.C., Am. Soc. Microbiol., 1974a.

Sabath, L. D., and Toftegaard, I.: Rapid microassays for clindamycin and gentamicin when present together and the effect of pH and of each on antibacterial activity of the other. Antimicrob. Agents Chemother., *6*:54, 1974b.

Sabath, L. D., Wheeler, N., Laverdiere, M., Blazevic, D., and Wilkinson, B. J.: A new type of penicillin resistance of *Staphylococcus aureus.* Lancet, *1*:443, 1977.

Schlichter, J. G., and Maclean, H. A.: A method of deter- mining effective therapeutic level in the treatment of subacute bacterial endocarditis with penicillin. Am. Heart J., *34*:209, 1947.

Shahidi, A., and Ellner, P. D.: Effect of mixed cultures on antibiotic susceptibility testing. Appl. Microbiol., *18*:766, 1969.

Steers, E., Foltz, E. L., and Graves, B. S.: An inocula replicating apparatus for routine testing of bacterial susceptibility to antibiotics. Antibiot. Chemother. (Basel), *9*:307, 1959.

Stemper, J. E., and Matsen, J. M.: Device for turbidity standardizing of cultures for antibiotic sensitivity test- ing. Appl. Microbiol., *19*:1015, 1970.

Sutter, V. L., Vargo, V. L., and Finegold, S. M.: Wads- worth Anaerobic Bacteriology Manual, 2nd ed. The Re- gents of the University of California, Los Angeles, 1975.

Thornsberry, C.: Rapid laboratory tests for β-lactamase production by bacteria. U.S. Dept. of Health, Education and Welfare, Public Health Service, Center for Disease Control, Atlanta, Ga., 1977c.

Thornsberry, C., Gavan, T., and Gerlach, E. H.: New de- velopments in antimicrobial agent susceptibility test- ing. *In* Sherris, J. C. (ed.): Cumitech 6. Am. Soc. Micro- biol., Washington, D.C., 1977a.

Thornsberry, C., Gavan, T. L., Sherris, J. C., Balows, A., Matsen, J. M., Sabath, L. D., Schoenknecht, F., Thrupp, L. D., and Washington, J. A., II.: Laboratory evaluation of a rapid, automated susceptibility testing system: Report of a collaborative study. Antimicrob. Agents Chemother., *7*:466, 1975.

Thornsberry, C., and Hawkins, T. M.: Agar disc diffusion susceptibility testing procedure. U.S. Dept. of Health, Education and Welfare, Publ. Health Serv., Center for Disease Control, Atlanta, Ga., 1977b.

Thornsberry, C., and Kirven, L. A.: Antimicrobial suscep- tibility of *Haemophilus influenzae.* Antimicrob. Agents Chemother., *6*:620, 1974.

Tilton, R. C., Lieberman, L., and Gerlach, E. H.: Micro- dilution antibiotic susceptibility testing: Examination of certain variables. Appl. Microbiol., *26*:658, 1973.

Washington, J. A., II.: Antimicrobial susceptibility of *Enterobacteriaceae* and nonfermenting gram-negative bacilli. Mayo Clin. Proc., *44*:811, 1969.

Washington, J. A., II, Snyder, R. J., Kohner, P. C., Wiltse, C. G., Ilstrup, D. M., and McCall, J. T.: Effect of cation content of agar on the activity of gentamicin, tobra- mycin and amikacin against *Pseudomonas aeruginosa.* J. Infect. Dis., *137*:103, 1978.

Washington, J. A., II., Warren, E., Dolan, C. T., and Karlson, A. G.: Antimicrobial susceptibility tests of bacteria. *In* Washington, J. A., II (ed.): Laboratory Procedures in Clinical Microbiology. Boston, Little, Brown and Company, 1974a, p. 286.

Washington, J. A., II, and Barry, A. L.: Dilution test procedures. *In* Lennette, E. H., Spaulding, E. H., and Truant, J. P. (eds.): Manual of Clinical Microbiology, 2nd ed. Washington, D.C., American Society for Microbiology, 1974b, p. 410.

Washington, J. A., II., Warren, E., and Karlson, A. G.: Stability of barium sulfate turbidity standards. Appl. Microbiol., *24*:1013, 1972.

Wegner, D. L., Mathis, C. R., and Neblett, T. R.: Direct method to determine the antibiotic susceptibility of rapidly growing blood pathogens. Antimicrob. Agents Chemother., *9*:861, 1976.

Wilkins, T. D., and Thiel, T.: Modified broth-disk method for testing the antibiotic susceptibility of anaerobic bacteria. Antimicrob. Agents Chemother., *3*:350, 1973.

Wilkins, T. D., and Chalgren, S.: Medium for use in antibiotic susceptibility testing of anaerobic bacteria. Antimicrob. Agents Chemother., *10*:926, 1976.

56

QUALITY CONTROL
IN MICROBIOLOGY

Thomas L. Gavan. M.D.

PERSONNEL

DOCUMENTATION OF PROCEDURES

SPECIFIC AREA OF QUALITY CONTROL
  Media
  Reagents
  Antisera

Antimicrobial Susceptibility Tests or
  Assays
Equipment
Stock Organisms, Source and Storage

PROFICIENCY TESTING

DOCUMENTATION OF QUALITY CONTROL

During the past 20 years quality control and quality assurance procedures have been increasingly emphasized. Procedures that provide information useful in the diagnosis of human disease are subject to variables that may lead to errors in test results and subsequently to diagnostic errors. Clinical chemistry and hematology lend themselves easily to well-established statistical quality control procedures because of the quantitative nature of many of the tests performed. In contrast, clinical microbiology is primarily a qualitative discipline, which, in addition, requires subjective interpretation. The variables of specimen collection and transport, selection and use of appropriate isolation media, incubating conditions, identification criteria, antimicrobial susceptibility testing, and reporting methods contribute to the list of possible sources of error that can lead to the production of irrelevant or (worse) misleading information (Dolan, 1977). Therefore, a quality assurance program in clinical microbiology must encompass all these aspects so that the limits of accuracy and reproducibility of microbiologic procedures can be determined and maintained at levels that can consistently and reliably provide at reasonable expense clinically relevant diagnostic information.

The degree of effort expended on a quality assurance program will vary widely, depending upon the size of the laboratory and the variety of procedures employed. However, the program instituted must encompass all procedures in use. In larger laboratories a specific technologist may be assigned responsibility for quality control on a full-time basis; in small laboratories this may be a part-time assignment.

The laboratory director should plan the quality assurance program, and if he or she does not take personal charge, should delegate responsibility and authority for its implementation. Quality control records must be reviewed at least monthly to assure that deficiencies noted are corrected.

The essential areas to be considered in implementing a comprehensive quality assurance program are as follows:
1. Personnel
2. Documentation of procedures
3. Specific areas of quality control
   a. Media
   b. Antimicrobial susceptibility tests
   c. Equipment
   d. Stock organisms, source and storage
4. Proficiency testing

PERSONNEL

Because of the high level of subjective interpretation required at nearly every step in processing specimens submitted for microbiologic evaluation, the qualifications, experience, and motivation of the personnel must be of the highest level. Individuals who aspire to perform a useful service in a microbiology laboratory must have not only a broad education in the basic fundamentals of the discipline, but also adequate training in practical laboratory work under the supervision of an experienced microbiologist. It has been shown that errors resulting in erroneous laboratory reports are closely related to the type of training, experience, and supervisory ability of the technologist immediately responsible for the microbiology section (Barry, 1968). New employees must be taught simple basic principles and continually supervised to discourage the all-too-common tendency of adopting more expedient but less effective methods.

Continuing education of the microbiology laboratory worker is essential if high levels of quality are to be maintained. This can take the form of seminars, journal clubs, and laboratory rounds where current developments can be presented and discussed. Because the handling of many microbiologic specimens may be dependent upon a particular clinical situation, microbiological-clinical correlations should be stressed. Personnel should be encouraged to attend meetings and seminars and to read current literature in clinical microbiology. Up-to-date reference books as well as appropriate journals should be available in the laboratory library.

DOCUMENTATION OF PROCEDURES

A detailed procedure manual is a necessary first step in developing a comprehensive quality control program. In such a manual are included all the policies which will guide the operation of the laboratory.

The organization of the laboratory should be outlined, with the responsibility and authority of all personnel at various levels clearly defined. Availability of services during regular working hours as well as evenings, nights, weekends, and holidays should be stated. Instructions for appropriate specimen collection, labeling, and transport to the laboratory, as well as criteria for the acceptability of these specimens, are especially important. The above information regarding availability of services, collection, labeling and transport of

specimens, and criteria for specimen acceptability should also be included in a manual for physicians and nurses and should be readily available to them to minimize the frequency of inappropriate specimens and to define clearly the laboratory's policy when such specimens are submitted.

For intralaboratory specimen handling, there should be instructions for appropriate accession procedures and internal laboratory communication for each specimen type (e.g., urine, blood, etc.). Worksheets, log books, and result reporting are included. For each category of specimen there should be an outline providing the technologist with instructions for processing. This includes specimen requirements, media to be inoculated, incubation conditions (temperature and atmosphere), criteria for initial culture review, criteria for the selection of colonies to be further isolated and identified, the extent to which identification should be carried out, and criteria for the reporting of test results (e.g., under what circumstances are immediate telephone reports required).

Laboratory safety should be a part of every procedure manual. This section should stress biologic, chemical, mechanical, and electrical hazards that may be encountered in the laboratory and how each employee is expected to handle situations involving these hazards. Special attention should be given to proper procedures for the safe disposal of contaminated materials.

The procedure manual should include a concise systematic description of all serologic procedures, biochemical tests, reagents, and media prepared in or used by the laboratory. This description should include the principles involved, source of materials, instructions for preparation and for use, significance of test results, and references where appropriate.

The quality control section should include a description of the program for monitoring equipment function, media, reagents, and stains, as well as the criteria for judging these items acceptable. The details of such a program are the subject of subsequent sections of this chapter. Finally, the procedure manual, once developed, must be reviewed at least annually to ensure that it is consistent with current operating procedures. As new procedures or changes in existing procedures are approved and introduced into the laboratory, appropriate entries must be made in the procedure manual. These should be initialed by the laboratory supervisor and/or the laboratory director. At the time of the annual review, a cover letter signed by the laboratory director should be included in the manual, indicating that the contents were reviewed and that they reflect the approved operating procedures of the laboratory.

SPECIFIC AREAS OF QUALITY CONTROL

MEDIA

Sterility and intended performance of all culture media must be established before use in the clinical laboratory. This applies both to media prepared in house from individual ingredients or dehydrated materials and to media received from commercial manufacturers already prepared and ready for use. The latter category must also include those commercially available "kit" products consisting of fixed batteries of media to be used in the identification of various groups of microorganisms. One can argue that commercially prepared media do not require the same degree of quality control as those that are prepared in the laboratory (Nagel, 1973). In recent years the Food and Drug Administration has established regulations for manufacturers of prepared media, which requires them to adhere to manufacturing, labeling, and quality control practices that yield a high quality finished product. These control measures insure that these products are satisfactory for the stated shelf life of the product when stored under stated conditions. The greatest variables in this situation can occur during transport of the product from manufacturer to consumer, at times due to storage for varying lengths of time by intermediaries. Although most manufacturers strive to provide appropriately insulated shipping containers, exposure to excessive heat or cold can damage a medium to the point that reliable results may not be obtained. It is prudent, therefore, to monitor sterility and performance of these media, at least in the case of those most sensitive to deterioration and at least concurrently with clinical use.

Laboratory Prepared Media. Media preparation should be scheduled so that all required quality control testing can be performed and evaluated prior to use. Raw materials should be dated upon receipt, and when the container is opened, the suppliers' recommendations for storage and expiration dates

should be rigidly followed. When a batch of medium is prepared, a production record should be kept. This will include the name of the medium, volume produced, formulation, manufacturer and lot numbers of ingredients, expiration date, and sterilization, dispensing, packaging, and labeling requirements. This information can be very useful for resolving problems that may occur. Sources of error in preparation of media from commercial dehydrated products include:

1. Improper storage
2. Outdated materials
3. Incorrect weighing
4. Incorrect measurement of water
5. Use of tap water, or use of water from a malfunctioning still
6. Use of glassware or stainless steel containers contaminated with detergents or chemicals
7. Incomplete mixing of ingredients or incomplete solution of ingredients
8. Overheating at any time during preparation or sterilization
9. Remelting solid media more than once
10. Improper determination of pH

Sterility Testing. Sterility testing must be applied to all batches of tubed or plated media, whether manufactured in-house or purchased ready for use. This is especially true with those media to which one or more sterile components are added after sterilization of the basal medium. It is obvious that the entire lot cannot be checked for sterility because of the possibility of deterioration. Therefore, a reasonable sample must be selected. When batches consist of 100 units or less, a 5 to 10 per cent sample should suffice. With batches of more than 100 units, 10 plates or tubes taken at random will usually detect batch contamination. Even though the batch has passed this sterility check, the technologist should be aware that random surface contamination can occur and should examine each plate at the time of inoculation for visible colonies. Growth of a specific colonial type beginning partway through the streaked area of a plate should alert the technologist to the possibility of contamination.

Special sterility problems can be seen with a selective medium. In this case the inhibiting properties of the medium may suppress growth of a contaminating organism to the extent that visible colonies are not produced, but at the same time viable organisms may make their appearance when isolated colonies are picked and transferred to a non-inhibiting medium. If aliquots of the finished medium are inoculated into 10 to 20 volumes of a non-inhibiting broth medium, contamination can be detected and subsequent problems eliminated.

In addition to sterility testing, all media prepared or received should be examined visually, and the color, clarity, and state of hydration determined. These characteristics also should be observed by technologists as part of their preinoculation inspection of all tubes and plates. Unless the medium contains some insoluble component (e.g., starch in Mueller-Hinton medium), the presence of turbidity or a precipitate indicates a defect on the medium. This may occur after storage. If the precipitate fails to disappear upon heating the medium to the temperature of incubation, the lot should be rejected. Media containing pH indicators provide a degree of built-in control. The color of each new lot should be compared with that of a previous satisfactory lot, and if the color differs, the pH should be rechecked. The pH of most media should fall ±0.2 unit of that specified by the manufacturer. The pH of all media should be determined electrometrically at room temperature. Media should not be tested when hot, because the pH tends to rise on cooling and the amount of change varies with the formulation.

To prevent dehydration of prepared or purchased media, proper storage conditions should be maintained. Problems should not occur with liquid or solid media stored in sealed, screw-capped containers. Dehydration of plated media cannot be prevented as completely, even when sealed in plastic bags. Media which show surface cracks or separation from the edge of the plate are not satisfactory for use and should be discarded.

Performance Tests of Media. The ability of isolation, selective, and differential media to perform as expected must be determined. Full scale performance testing of media prepared in house is essential. With commercially prepared media, which has been subjected to extensive quality control during manufacture, a modified system for performance testing may be satisfactory. It is recommended that before omitting pre-use performance testing, all media obtained ready for use be subjected to an extensive control program for at least several consecutive batches to ascertain reliability.

For purposes of this discussion, a quantity of medium prepared in the laboratory at one time is considered to be a batch. A "batch" of commercial medium is defined as a shipment of a common lot number received at one time. If a "batch" is not used in one month, the medium should be rechecked.

A collection of stable stock cultures with known characteristics is essential. Table 56-1 provides a list of quality control organisms for a wide variety of media and their expected reactions. These recommendations have been found useful in a large diagnostic laboratory, but may not be applicable to all laboratories, and some additional tests or media may be added to reflect local evaluation and identification practices. The source and storage of stock strains are discussed later.

Media intended for isolation should be tested using the most fastidious organism expected to be isolated. If more than one bacterial characteristic is to be demonstrated, multiple organisms may have to be used. For example, sheep blood agar plates are almost universally employed as a routine isolation medium. Both the ability to detect small numbers of fastidious organisms and the ability to demonstrate characteristic hemolysis must be manifest. This requires the use of several test organisms (Table 56-1). Furthermore, the inoculum chosen for testing isolation media must be light. Plates are inoculated with a 1:10 dilution in broth of a suspension of the test organism(s) adjusted to the density of a McFarland 0.5 standard. This provides a relatively standardized inoculum for obtaining isolated colonies. The colony counts, particularly on highly enriched isolation media, with or without inhibitors, can serve as a guide for evaluation of batch-to-batch reproducibility. In these mixtures a 1:1000 dilution (or one which yields 10^5 cfu/ml) of the McFarland adjusted suspension would be more appropriate. The inoculum and method of inoculation for biochemical or other differential tests should be that actually used in the laboratory.

Rapid identification "kit" systems should be controlled according to the recommendation of the manufacturer. In some laboratories highly specialized media, such as Bordet-Gengou, are made up and stored until the occasion for use when the basal medium is remelted, appropriate enrichments added, and plates poured. In these instances quality control prior to use may not be practical, but should be carried out concurrently with inoculation of clinical material. Similarly, media for the isolation of fungi

(*Text continued on p. 1946*)

Table 56-1. RECOMMENDED CHALLENGING ORGANISMS FOR USE IN PERFORMANCE TESTING OF PLATED AND TUBED CULTURE MEDIA

MEDIUM	POSITIVE CONTROL	EXPECTED RESULT	NEGATIVE CONTROL	EXPECTED RESULT	FREQUENCY TESTED
Bile-Esculin	Enterococcus	Growth; medium turns black	Group A streptococcus	No change in color of medium	Each lot
Bird seed agar	*Cryptococcus neoformans*	Colonies turn brown	*Candida albicans*	Colonies do not turn brown	Each lot
Chocolate agar	*Neisseria gonorrhoeae*	Enhanced growth	None		Each lot
	Neisseria meningitidis	Enhanced growth	None		Each lot
	Haemophilus influenzae	Enhanced growth	None		Each lot
Columbia blood agar	*Escherichia coli*	Growth and typical colonial morphology	None		Each lot
	Pseudomonas aeruginosa	Growth and typical colonial morphology	None		Each lot
	Acinetobacter calcoaceticus var. *antitratus*	Growth and typical colonial morphology	None		Each lot
	Group A streptococcus	Typical colonial morphology and growth, beta-hemolysis	None		Each lot
	Streptococcus pneumoniae	Typical colonial morphology and growth, alpha-hemolysis	None		Each lot
	Enterococcus	Growth and typical colonial morphology	None		Each lot
Corn meal agar	*Candida albicans*	Production of chlamydospores and pseudohyphae	*Cryptococcus neoformans*	No production of chlamydospores or pseudohyphae	Each lot
Citrate agar slant	*Enterobacter cloacae*	Growth—slant turns Prussian blue	*Escherichia coli*	No growth	Each lot
Cystine trypticase agar	*Escherichia coli* and dextrose disk	Growth, fermentation, acid (yellow) production	*Escherichia coli* (no dextrose disk)	Growth, no fermentation or acid production	Each lot
Decarboxylase broth	None		*Escherichia coli*	Growth is indicated by the yellow color of the broth	Each lot
Fletcher's medium	*Leptospira interrogans* ser. *icterohaemorrhagiae*	Growth	None		
Hippurate broth	Group B streptococcus (hemolytic and nonhemolytic strains)	Medium turns purple on addition of Ninhydrin	Group D streptococcus	Medium does *not* turn purple on addition of Ninhydrin	Each lot
Indole-nitrate-motility media	*Bacteroides fragilis* ssp. *thetaiotaomicron*	Indole produced	*Bacteroides fragilis* ssp. *fragilis*	No indole produced	Each lot
	Clostridium novyi Type A	Positive motility	*Bacteroides fragilis*	Negative motility	
Lysine-iron agar	*Edwardsiella tarda*	Alkaline/alkaline/(+)* H$_2$S	*Proteus rettgeri*	Red/alkaline/(−)H$_2$S*	
Lowenstein-Jensen agar	*Mycobacterium tuberculosis*	Characteristic growth	None		Each lot

(Table continued on following page)

5

Table 56-1. RECOMMENDED CHALLENGING ORGANISMS FOR USE IN PERFORMANCE
TESTING OF PLATING AND TUBED CULTURE MEDIA (continued)

MEDIUM	POSITIVE CONTROL	EXPECTED RESULT	NEGATIVE CONTROL	EXPECTED RESULT	FREQUENCY TESTED
Lowenstein-Jensen-Gruft	*Mycobacterium tuberculosis*	Characteristic growth	*Klebsiella pneumoniae*	No growth	Each lot
			Staphylococcus species	No growth	
Malonate broth	*Enterobacter aerogenes*	Prussian blue color change	*Escherichia coli*	No color change (stays green)	Each lot
Motility (BHI)	*Escherichia coli*	Growth out from stab	*Klebsiella pneumoniae*	No growth out from stab	Each lot
Methyl red broth	*Escherichia coli*	Color change from yellow to red with addition of reagent	*Enterobacter aerogenes*	No color change	Each lot and weekly
Mycobiotic agar	*Candida albicans*	Growth	*Cryptococcus neoformans*	Growth inhibition	Each lot
			Escherichia coli		
Phenyl-ethyl-alcohol agar	*Staphylococcus aureus*	Enhanced growth	*Proteus mirabilis* stab	Growth inhibition	Each lot
			Pseudomonas aeruginosa	Growth inhibition	
Sabouraud dextrose agar	*Candida albicans*	Growth	None		Each lot
	Cryptococcus neoformans	Growth			
Sabouraud dextrose agar w/gentamicin	*Candida albicans*	Growth	*Escherichia coli*	Growth inhibition	Each lot
	Cryptococcus neoformans	Growth	*Staphylococcus aureus*	Growth inhibition	
			Klebsiella pneumoniae	Growth inhibition	
Thayer-Martin agar	*Neisseria gonorrhoeae*	Growth	*Staphylococcus aureus*	Growth inhibition	
	Neisseria meningitidis	Growth	*Candida albicans*	Growth inhibition	Each lot
			Escherichia coli	Growth inhibition	
			Proteus mirabilis stab	Growth inhibition	
Tryptic soy agar	*Staphylococcus aureus*	Growth	None		Each lot
	Enterococcus	Growth			
Rabbit blood agar	*Haemophilus haemolyticus*	Beta-hemolysis and growth	*Haemophilus influenzae*	Growth and no hemolysis	Each lot
Xylose-lysine-desoxycholate agar	*Shigella sonnei*	Colorless colonies	*Staphylococcus aureus*	Growth inhibition	Each lot
	Salmonella typhi	Growth—H_2S production			
	Escherichia coli	Yellow colonies			
Brain-heart-infusion broth	*Staphylococcus aureus*	Growth	None		Each lot
	Escherichia coli	Growth			
Chocolate agar slants	*Haemophilus influenzae*	Growth	None		Each lot
	Neisseria gonorrhoeae	Growth			
Tryptic soy broth with 6.5% NaCl	Enterococcus	Turbid growth	Group B streptococcus	No growth	Each lot
Triple sugar iron agar	*Proteus vulgaris*	Acid/acid/+H_2S*	*Pseudomonas aeruginosa*	Alkaline/alkaline/−H_2S*	Each lot
Tryptic soy broth blood bottles	*Clostridium novyi* Group A	Growth	None		Each lot
	Bacteroides fragilis	Growth			
	Haemophilus influenzae				

(*Table continued on opposite page*)

Table 56–1. RECOMMENDED CHALLENGING ORGANISMS FOR USE IN PERFORMANCE TESTING OF PLATING AND TUBED CULTURE MEDIA (continued)

MEDIUM	POSITIVE CONTROL	EXPECTED RESULT	NEGATIVE CONTROL	EXPECTED RESULT	FREQUENCY TESTED
Urea agar slants	*Cryptococcus neoformans*	Medium changes to pink color	*Candida albicans*	No change to pink color in medium.	Each lot
Voges-Proskauer broth		Broth changes from yellow to red with addition of reagents	*Escherichia coli*	Broth remains yellow, i.e., no color change	
Nitrate agar slants	*Escherichia coli*	Red color when reagents are added	*Acinetobacter calcoaceticus* var. *anitratus*	No color change when reagents are added	Each lot
O-F dextrose	*Pseudomonas aeruginosa* (open)	Acid production (yellow)	*Pseudomonas aeruginosa* plus oil overlay	No acid production in fermentative tube	Each lot
	Klebsiella pneumoniae (open)	Acid production (yellow)	*Alcaligenes faecalis* plus oil overlay	No acid production in fermentative tube	
	Klebsiella pneumoniae plus oil overlay	Acid production (yellow)	*Alcaligenes faecalis* (open)	No acid production in oxidative tube	
O-F plain	*Pseudomonas aeruginosa* + dextrose disc	Acid production (yellow) oxidative positive	*Pseudomonas aeruginosa* + dextrose disc + oil	No acid production in fermentative tube	Each lot
			Pseudomonas aeruginosa	No acid production in oxidative tube	
			Pseudomonas aeruginosa + oil	No acid production in fermentative tube	
Phenylalanine deaminase agar slant	*Proteus mirabilis*	Reagent ferric chloride changes from yellow to green	*Escherichia coli*	Reagent ferric chloride stays yellow	New lot
Sorbitol phenol-red broth	*Enterobacter aerogenes*	Acid production (yellow)	*Proteus mirabilis*	No acid production, broth remains red in color	Each lot
Selenite F broth	*Shigella sonnei*	Enhanced growth	None		Each lot
	Salmonella typhi	Enhanced growth			
Thioglycollate broth	*Clostridium novyi* Type A	Growth	None		Each lot
	Enterococcus	Growth			
Todd-Hewitt broth	Group A streptococcus	Growth	None		Each lot
	Group B streptococcus	Growth			
	Group C streptococcus	Growth			
	Group D streptococcus	Growth			
	Group G streptococcus	Growth			
Colistin-nalidixic acid agar	Enterococcus	Enhanced growth	*Escherichia coli*	Growth inhibition	Each lot
	Staphylococcus aureus	Growth	*Pseudomonas aeruginosa*	Growth inhibition	
	Group A streptococcus	Enhanced growth			
Deoxyribonuclease agar	*Serratia marcescens*	Red colored zone around growth	*Escherichia coli*	No red colored zone around growth	Each lot
	Staphylococcus aureus	Red colored zone around growth	*Staphylococcus epidermidis*	No red colored zone around growth	

5

(*Table continued on following page*)

Table 56-1. RECOMMENDED CHALLENGING ORGANISMS FOR USE IN PERFORMANCE TESTING OF PLATING AND TUBED CULTURE MEDIA (continued)

MEDIUM	POSITIVE CONTROL	EXPECTED RESULT	NEGATIVE CONTROL	EXPECTED RESULT	FREQUENCY TESTED
Egg yolk agar	*Clostridium novyi* Type A	Lecithinase positive, i.e., zone of precipitation in agar around colony	*Bacteroides fragilis*	Lecithinase negative, i.e., no zone of precipitation	Each lot
		Lipase positive, i.e., formation of an iridescent "pearly" luster over and around the colony		Lipase negative, i.e., no iridescent "pearly" luster over or around the colony	
MacConkey agar	*Escherichia coli*	Lactose positive—pink colonies	*Proteus mirabilis* stab	Inhibition of swarming growth	Each lot
	Shigella sonnei	Lactose negative—colorless colonies	Enterococcus	Growth inhibition	
			Staphylococcus aureus	Growth inhibition	
Mueller-Hinton agar	*Escherichia coli* ATCC 25922	See Tables 56-6 and 56-8			Each lot, then daily
	Staphylococcus aureus ATCC 25923	See Tables 56-6 and 56-8			
	Pseudomonas aeruginosa ATCC 27853	See Table 56-7			

*The reactions are listed in the following order: slant/butt/H$_2$S production.

and mycobacteria may require concurrent testing. Tables 56-2 and 56-3 list recommendations for expiration dating of plated and tubed media prepared and stored in the laboratory.

Reagents

Reagents used in the microbiology laboratory include stains, chemicals, antimicrobials, impregnated paper discs or strips, and antisera. All must be monitored for effective performance. Stains and chemicals obtained from reputable sources should be labeled with lot number, dates of preparation or receipt, opening, and expiration. Freshness and stability can be assured if relatively small quantities are purchased or prepared at one time. Performance tests of each batch should be carried out prior to use and at appropriate intervals during the life time of the batch. These intervals are dependent upon the inherent stability of the reagent or stain and the frequency with which they are used. For example, Gram's stain may be checked on preparation and at weekly intervals, whereas less frequently used stains, such as flagella stain, should be tested concurrently with use with control organisms having known flagellar characteristics. Also, stable chemical reagents such as Kovacs' reagent for the indole test should be tested on preparation and at weekly intervals. Unstable reagents, such as hydrogen peroxide for the catalase test or tetramethyl-p-phenylenediamine dihydrochloride for the oxidase test, should be tested on each day of use. Table 56-4 lists recommended challenge organisms for use in the control of a variety of reagent materials and the maximum intervals for testing. These organisms provide both positive and negative reactions for each reagent.

Reagent-impregnated paper discs or strips obtained from reputable manufacturers should be stored with a desiccant (usually supplied with the original packaging) under the conditions described by the manufacturer. Suitable organisms for testing these items are listed in Table 56-4. Antimicrobial impreg-

Table 56–2. EXPIRATION DATING FOR PLATED MEDIA, CALCULATED FROM DATE OF PRODUCTION*

MEDIUM	EXPIRATION DATE
Bile-esculin agar	6 weeks
Bird seed agar	6 weeks
Brain-heart infusion agar	6 weeks
Brain-heart infusion w/blood	1 month
Brain-heart infusion w/gentamicin	6 weeks
Chocolate agar	1 month
Columbia blood agar	1 month
Columbia CNA agar	1 month
Corn meal agar w/Tween 80	6 weeks
DNase agar w/methyl green	6 weeks
DNase test agar w/toluidine blue	6 weeks
EMB agar	1 month
Hektoen agar	1 month
Mycobiotic agar	6 weeks
MacConkey agar	1 month
Phenylethyl alcohol agar w/blood	1 month
Potato dextrose agar	6 weeks
Rabbit blood agar	1 month
Sabouraud dextrose agar	6 weeks
Sabouraud dextrose agar w/gentamicin	6 weeks
Schaedler blood agar w/vitamin K	1 month
TB sensitivity plates	3 weeks
Thayer-Martin medium	1 month
Tryptic soy agar	6 weeks
XLD agar	1 month

*Stored in airtight wrappers at 2 to 8°C.

Table 56–3. EXPIRATION DATING OF TUBED MEDIA CALCULATED FROM DATE OF PRODUCTION*

MEDIUM	EXPIRATION DATE
Bordet-Gengou agar base	6 months
Biphasic fungal blood culture bottles	6 months
Brain-heart infusion broth	6 months
Brain-heart infusion agar	6 months
CTA medium plain	6 months
CTA medium w/carbohydrate	6 weeks
Fletcher's medium	3 months
Hippurate substrate (frozen at −20°C.)	3 months
Indole-nitrate broth	1 month
Indole-nitrate motility medium	1 month
KCN broth base	6 months
KCN broth w/KCN	2 weeks
Lysine iron agar	6 months
Malonate broth	6 months
Middlebrook 7H9 broth	3 months
Middlebrook 7H11S agar (Mitchison)	1 month
Motility GI medium	6 months
Mueller-Hinton broth bottles	6 weeks
MR-VP medium	6 months
Nitrate agar	6 months
Nutrient agar	6 months
Nutrient broth	6 months
OF medium plain	3 months
OF medium w/carbohydrate	6 weeks
Selenite broth	6 months
Sabouraud dextrose agar	6 months
SF broth	6 months
Simmons citrate agar	3 months
Thioglycollate broth	1 month
Todd-Hewitt broth	6 months
Tryptic soy broth w/6.5% NaCl	6 months
Trichophyton agars 1-7	6 months
Triple sugar iron agar	6 months
Urea agar	6 months

*Stored at 2 to 8°C. (except Hippurate substrate) with tubes tightly capped.

nated discs are covered under susceptibility testing control.

Antisera

Antisera for organism grouping and typing should be dated when received and when reconstituted. Storage at refrigerator temperatures is mandatory, with minimal exposure to room temperature at the time of use. Antisera must not be used beyond the manufacturer's expiration date and, when used, should be carefully inspected for turbidity or precipitate which may indicate contamination. Such sera must be discarded as unsatisfactory.

Each antiserum should be tested with organisms that produce a positive reaction and no reaction (negative). Table 56–5 lists suggested organisms that may be used with commonly used antisera. Each new vial of antiserum should be checked prior to initial use and at monthly intervals thereafter until the expiration date is reached. Saline should not be substituted for a negative control.

Antimicrobial susceptibility tests and assays

Since 1961, the FDA has certified the antibiotic content of all discs manufactured in the United States for antimicrobial susceptibility testing. This program enables users of these discs to rely on the labeled antibiotic content. However, the discs must be stored and used carefully after they are received in the laboratory. Discs must not be used beyond the manufacturer's expiration date. They must be stored with a desiccant at temperatures less than 8°C. If possible, all discs, but especially those of the penicillin family, should be stored at −14°C. or less with desiccation. When a working supply of discs is removed from stor-

5

Table 56–4. RECOMMENDED CHALLENGING ORGANISMS FOR USE IN PERFORMANCE TESTING OF REAGENTS, STRIPS, AND DISCS

MEDIUM	POSITIVE CONTROL	EXPECTED RESULT	NEGATIVE CONTROL	EXPECTED RESULT	FREQUENCY TESTED
Arginine decarboxylase	*Enterobacter cloacae*	Broth with arginine and test organism is purple; growth control is yellow	*Enterobacter aerogenes*	Broth with arginine and test organism is yellow; growth control is yellow	New lot, then weekly
Bacitracin disc	Group A streptococcus	Zone of inhibition measuring 10-18 mm around the disc	Group B streptococcus	No zone of inhibition around the disc	New lot, then weekly
Carbohydrate discs	Use appropriate positive controls	Acid production (yellow color)	Use appropriate negative controls	Acid production (yellow color)	New lot, then each test
Coagulase plasma	*Staphylococcus aureus*	Plasma clotted	*Staphylococcus epidermidis*	Plasma not clotted	New lot, then daily
Cytochrome oxidase strips	*Pseudomonas aeruginosa* ATCC 27853	Bacteria on strip turns blue-black	*Escherichia coli* ATCC 25922	No change in color of bacteria on strip	New lot, then daily
Ehrlich's reagent	*Escherichia coli*	A red ring will develop just below the xylene layer	*Enterobacter aerogenes*	Red ring does not develop	New lot, then weekly
Factor strips on tryptic soy agar plates "X"	*Haemophilus aphrophilus*	Growth around strip	*Haemophilus influenzae*	No growth around strip	New lot, then weekly
			Haemophilus parainfluenzae	No growth around strip	
"V"	*Haemophilus parainfluenzae*	Growth around strip	*Haemophilus influenzae*	No growth around strip	New lot, then weekly
"XV"	*Haemophilus influenzae*	Growth around strip	None		New lot, then weekly
	Haemophilus parainfluenzae	Growth around strip			New lot, then weekly
	Haemophilus aphrophilus	Growth around strip			
Ferric chloride	*Proteus mirabilis*	Slant of phenylalanine deaminase agar turns green	*Escherichia coli*	Slant of phenylalanine deaminase agar does not change color	New lot, then weekly
Gelatin strips	*Pseudomonas aeruginosa*	Organism liquefies the gelatin, leaving the clear blue supporting base, within 48 hours	*Pasteurella multocida*	Organism does *not* liquefy the gelatin revealing the clear blue supporting base	New lot, each test
Germ tube serum	*Candida albicans*	Germ tube production in 2 hours	*Candida tropicalis*	No germ tube production in 2 hours	New lot
			Candida parapsilosis		
Gram stain reagents	*Staphylococcus aureus* ATCC 25923	Purple organisms	*Escherichia coli* ATCC 25922	Red organisms	Daily
Hydrogen peroxide	*Staphylococcus aureus* ATCC 25923	Bacteria "bubbles" on glass slide	Group A streptococcus	No bubbles produced by bacteria on glass slide	Daily

(*Table continued on opposite page*)

Table 56–4. RECOMMENDED CHALLENGING ORGANISMS FOR USE IN PERFORMANCE
TESTING OF REAGENTS, STRIPS, AND DISCS (continued)

MEDIUM	POSITIVE CONTROL	EXPECTED RESULT	NEGATIVE CONTROL	EXPECTED RESULT	FREQUENCY TESTED
KCN broth base with potassium cyanide	*Proteus vulgaris*	Growth	*Shigella sonnei*	No growth	Each test
Kovacs	*Escherichia coli*	Tryptophane broth will turn a deep red color after the addition of 5 drops of reagent	*Enterobacter aerogenes*	Tryptophane broth will *not* change color after the addition of 5 drops of reagent	New lot, then weekly
Methyl red	*Escherichia coli*	Broth turns red	*Enterobacter aerogenes*	Broth remains yellow	New lot, then weekly
Ninhydrin	Group B streptococcus	1% aqueous sodium hippurate substrate turns purple with addition of reagent	Group A streptococcus	1% aqueous sodium hippurate substrate does *not* turn purple with addition of reagents, i.e., remains cloudy	New lot, then each test
Nitrate Nitrate I (0.8% sulfanilic acid) Nitrate II (0.5% N,N, dimethyl-1-naphthylamine)	*Escherichia coli*	Nitrate agar slant turns red on addition of reagents	*Acinetobacter calcoaceticus var. anitratus*	Nitrate agar slant produces *no* color change when reagents are added	New lot, then weekly
ONPG (beta-galactosidase) tablets	*Shigella sonnei*	Water around dissolved tablet turns yellow in 6 hours or less	*Salmonella typhi*	No color change in water around dissolved tablet	New lot, each test
Optochin disc	*Streptococcus pneumoniae*	Zone of inhibition measuring greater than 15 mm around the disc	Alpha hemolytic (viridans) streptococcus	No zone of inhibitor around the disc	New lot, then weekly
Ornithine decarboxylase	*Enterobacter hafniae*	Broth with ornithine and test organism is purple; growth control is yellow	*Proteus vulgaris*	Broth with ornithine and test organism is yellow; growth control is yellow	New lot, then weekly
Sodium desoxycholate	*Streptococcus pneumoniae*	Colonies on blood agar plate	Alpha hemolytic (viridans) streptococcus	Colonies remain unchanged	New lot, then weekly
Voges-Proskauer Voges-Proskauer I (alpha-napthol) Voges-Proskauer II (potassium hydroxide)	*Enterobacter aerogenes*	VP broth changes from yellow to red with addition of reagents	*Escherichia coli*	VP broth produces *no* color change with addition of reagents	New lot, then weekly

5

Table 56–5. CHALLENGE ORGANISMS FOR USE IN QUALITY CONTROL
OF DIAGNOSTIC ANTISERA

ANTISERUM	CHALLENGE ORGANISM	EXPECTED REACTION
Arizona	*Arizona hinshawii*	Agglutination
Alkalescens—dispar	Alkalescens—dispar	Agglutination
Arizona—mono	*Arizona hinshawii*	Agglutination
Bethesda—Ballerup	*Citrobacter freundii*	Agglutination
Escherichia coli	*Escherichia coli*	
Poly A	026:B_6	Agglutination
Poly B	086:B_7	Agglutination
Poly C	018:B_{21}	Agglutination
Haemophilus influenzae	*Haemophilus influenzae*	Capsular swelling (Quellung)
Herellea vaginicola*	*Herellea vaginicola*	Agglutination
Mima polymorpha**	*Mima polymorpha*	Agglutination
Neisseria meningitidis	*Neisseria meningitidis*	Agglutination
Salmonella		
Polyvalent	*Salmonella* sp.	Agglutination
Polyvalent H	*Salmonella paratyphi*	
Salmonella		
Group A	*Salmonella paratyphi* A	Agglutination
Group B	*S. typhimurium*	Agglutination
Group C_1	*S. thompson*	Agglutination
Group C_2	*S. virginia*	Agglutination
Group D	*S. enteriditis*	Agglutination
Group E	*S. newington*	Agglutination
Group Vi	*S. typhi*	Agglutination
Shigella		
A	*Shigella dysenteriae*	Agglutination
B	*S. flexneri*	Agglutination
C	*S. boydii*	Agglutination
D	*S. sonnei*	Agglutination
Streptococcus pneumoniae	*Streptococcus pneumoniae*	Capsular swelling (Quellung)

* Acinetobacter calcoaceticus var. anitratus.
**Acinetobacter calcoaceticus var. lwoffi.

age, the container should be allowed to warm to room temperature before opening to prevent condensation of moisture on the disc surfaces. Disc cartridges not used can be stored in the refrigerator at 2 to 8°C. Discs should be arranged on the plates to avoid overlapping of inhibitory zones or distortion of zones by synergistic or antagonistic drugs.

Discs used with the Autobac 1 system (Pfizer Diagnostics) are similarly subjected to FDA certification. In some instances these discs have a different antimicrobial content, as well as tighter tolerance limits than those manufactured for the diffusion test. In no instance should discs for diffusion testing be used with the Autobac 1 system or vice versa.

Antimicrobials to be used in dilution tests should be reference standard materials rather than preparations manufactured for clinical administration. Appropriate reference standards assayed for specific drug activity can be obtained from the drug manufacturer or purchased from the United States Pharmacopeia (USP-NF Reference Standards, 12601 Twinbrook Parkway, Rockville, Maryland 20852).

Unopened powder standards may be stored for several years at room temperature. Once opened they should be stored with a desiccant in an anhydrous jar. Synthetic penicillins and cephalosporins should be stored at 2 to 8°C. Solutions of aminoglycosides, tetracycline, erythromycin, and clindamycin are stable at room temperature. Synthetic penicillins and cephalosporins may be stored at −20°C. for up to one month.

Because of the large number of variables affecting all types of susceptibility tests, it is not practical to monitor each one. A program to monitor endpoint reproducibility and accuracy is sufficient to detect when significant changes have been introduced. When results depart significantly from the expected, then factors known to be sources of error, such as inoculum density, medium pH, disc storage, etc. can be considered individually to resolve the problem.

Table 56-6. EXPECTED RANGE OF INHIBITORY ZONE DIAMETERS FOR ANTIMICROBIAL SUSCEPTIBILITY TESTING DISCS TESTED WITH *S. aureus* ATCC 25923 AND *E. coli* ATCC 25922

ANTIMICROBIAL AGENT	DISC POTENCY	INHIBITORY ZONE DIAMETER RANGE (mm)	
		S. aureus ATCC 25923	*E. coli* ATCC 25922
Ampicillin	10 µg	24–35	15–20
Bacitracin	10 units	17–22	–
Carbenicillin	100 µg	–	24–29
Cephalothin	30 µg	25–37	18–23
Chloramphenicol	30 µg	19–26	21–27
Clindamycin	2 µg	23–29	–
Colistin	10 µg	–	11–15
Erythromycin	15 µg	22–30	8–14
Gentamicin	10 µg	19–27	19–26
Kanamycin	30 µg	19–26	17–25
Methicillin	5 µg	17–22	–
Nafcillin	1 µg	19–22	–
Neomycin	30 µg	18–26	17–23
Penicillin	10 units	26–37	–
Polymyxin B	300 units	7–13	12–16
Tetracycline	30 µg	19–28	18–25
Tobramycin	10 µg	19–29	18–26
Trimethoprim-sulfamethoxazole	1.25 µg/23.75 µg	24–32	24–32
Vancomycin	30 µg	15–19	–

Endpoint surveillance programs, regardless of the test method to be controlled, involve the repetitive testing of "standard" strains of bacteria. With the disc diffusion test, the following reference strains have been designated: *Staphylococcus aureus* ATCC 24923; *Escherichia coli* ATCC 25922; and *Pseudomonas aeruginosa* ATCC 27853. Expected inhibitory zone diameters have been determined for the *S. aureus* and *E. coli* through a collaborative study carried out by the FDA. The *P. aeruginosa* has only recently been recommended as a reference strain to monitor tests with gentamicin because the other reference cultures do not readily detect the effects of divalent cations in the medium on this antibiotic (Thornsberry, 1977).

Currently the best estimate of the true inhibitory zone diameters to be expected with the standard reference cultures of *S. aureus* and *E. coli* has been determined from a multilaboratory collaborative study conducted by the FDA. This determined the mean inhibitory zone diameters for the drug tests and also established tolerance limits for single observations. These data are the basis for the control limits listed in antimicrobial susceptibility testing disc package inserts and are summarized in Table 56-6. Table 56-7 lists suggested inhibitory zone diameters for use with *P. aeruginosa* ATCC 27853.

The National Committee for Clinical Laboratory Standards (1975) has recommended a simplified system for monitoring both precision and accuracy of zone diameters. The mean inhibitory zone is determined from a series of tests done on five consecutive days on which the test is performed. The range of these values is the difference between the largest and smallest values in the series of five measurements. These two parameters are compared with the limits listed in Table 56-8 under accuracy control and precision control. The observed mean and range for each antimicrobial tested would be expected to fall outside the maximum limits specified in no more than 1 of

Table 56-7. SUGGESTED QUALITY CONTROL LIMITS FOR INHIBITORY ZONE DIAMETERS WHEN TESTING WITH *P. aeruginosa* ATCC 27853

ANTIMICROBIAL	DISC POTENCY	INHIBITORY ZONE DIAMETER (mm)
Gentamicin	10 µg	16–22
Carbenicillin	100 µg	19–25
Chloramphenicol	30 µg	6–12
Tobramycin	10 µg	19–25
Polymyxin B	300 U	13–18
Colistin	10 µg	11–15
Tetracycline	30 µg	6–14

Table 56-8. CONTROL LIMITS FOR MONITORING PRECISION AND ACCURACY OF INHIBITORY ZONE DIAMETERS OBTAINED IN GROUPS OF FIVE SEPARATE OBSERVATIONS*

ANTIMICROBIAL AGENT	DISC POTENCY	*E. coli* ATCC (25922) ACCURACY CONTROL ZONE DIAMETER (mm) Mean of 5 Values	*E. coli* PRECISION CONTROL RANGE OF 5 VALUES (mm) Maximum	Average	*S. aureus* ATCC 25923 ACCURACY CONTROL ZONE DIAMETER (mm) Mean of 5 Values	*S. aureus* PRECISION CONTROL RANGE OF 5 VALUES (mm) Maximum	Average
Ampicillin	10 µg	15.8–19.2	6	2.9	25.8–33.2	13	6.4
Carbenicillin	100 µg	25.0–28.0	7	3.5	-	-	-
Cephalothin	30 µg	18.8–22.2	6	2.9	27.0–35.0	14	7.0
Chloramphenicol	30 µg	22.0–26.0	7	3.5	20.2–24.8	8	4.1
Clindamycin	2 µg	-	-	-	24.0–28.0	7	3.5
Colistin	10 µg	11.7–14.3	4	2.3	-	-	-
Erythromycin	15 µg	9.0–13.0	7	3.5	23.3–28.7	9	4.7
Gentamicin	10 µg	20.2–24.8	8	4.1	20.3–25.7	9	4.7
Kanamycin	30 µg	18.3–23.7	9	4.7	20.2–24.8	8	4.1
Methicillin	5 µg	-	-	-	17.8–21.2	6	2.9
Neomycin	30 µg	18.0–22.0	6	3.5	-	-	-
Penicillin G	10 units	-	-	-	27.8–35.2	13	6.4
Polymyxin B	300 units	12.7–15.3	4	2.3	-	-	-
Tetracycline	30 µg	19.2–23.8	8	4.1	20.5–26.5	11	5.2
Vancomycin	30 µg	-	-	-	15.7–18.3	4	2.3
Trimethoprim-sulfamethoxazole	1.25 µg/23.75 µg						

* Adapted from National Committee for Clinical Standards, Approved Standard ASM-2.

20 tests. Furthermore, the average range, over a period of time, should fall close to or less than the average range listed.

Standards for evaluating precision and accuracy of broth or agar dilution susceptibility testing procedures have not been developed to the extent that has been established for the disc diffusion test. Reproducibility of broth and agar dilution procedures is said to be on the order of $\pm\log_2$ dilution interval. In addition to the standard reference cultures of *S. aureus, E. coli,* and *P. aeruginosa,* other organisms must be used when monitoring dilution tests. Suitable reference cultures are listed in Table 56-9.

Reference standard cultures appropriate for monitoring each drug tested should be employed with each run of tests. The minimum inhibitory concentration (MIC) of the reference standard is then recorded and plotted. After 10 such tests have been made, a trend toward a median MIC value will be noted. Tests can be considered out of control if the MIC departs from the median by more than one $\log_2$ dilution.

Reference cultures recommended by the manufacturer for monitoring the Autobac 1 system are the same as those recommended for the disc diffusion test. The endpoints for these organisms fall, for the most part, at the extreme end of the instrument's light scatter-ing index scale (0.0 to 1.0) and not midway between where the test condition variations can be detected with greater sensitivity. Additional organisms having wider range light scattering indices should be sought for control purposes if this method is used.

Disc diffusion assay methods have widespread application in clinical laboratories for determining the levels in serum and other body fluids of potentially toxic antimicrobial agents and should be subjected to quality control. Serum assay procedures can be controlled by testing frozen aliquots of a pool of serum to which has been added the antimicrobial being tested in a concentration equivalent to the peak serum level obtained with normal doses. The serum pool should be tested for non-specific or antibiotic inhibition before antimicrobials are added. A blank control consisting of serum pool without antimicrobial should be run with each serum assay. Frozen aliquots of previously tested patient serum may also be retested.

Aliquots of the control serum must be kept frozen at $-20°$C. until used. Sera containing cephalosporins and penicillins should be stored at $-70°$C. Such pools should remain stable for six months if they are not thawed and refrozen.

One is often asked to assay one antimicrobial when a second antimicrobial is present. In some instances agents such as beta-lactamase or penicillinase, which inhibit the undesired drug but have no effect on the drug to be assayed, are added to the test system. In other situations, a test organism susceptible to the desired drug but resistant to the undesired drug may be used. In either case, the fact that the test conditions have actually suppressed the activity of the undesired drug should be demonstrated. This can be accomplished simply by placing an ordinary susceptibility testing disc containing the undesired drug on the test medium along with the standards, unknowns, and controls. Since each 6-mm assay disc will absorb 20 μl, the equivalent serum concentration in μg or units/ml represented by a susceptibility disc is 50 times the disc content. For example, if the test assay system successfully suppresses the inhibitory effect of a 10-unit penicillin disc, then one can assume the test system can suppress the equivalent of 500 units/ml of penicillin in the serum specimen. This can be reassuring when reporting levels of toxic agents.

Equipment

Properly functioning equipment is essential. A quality control program should include routine surveillance of all temperature-controlled mechanical and electrical apparatus. Preventive maintenance schedules should be established according to the recommendations of the equipment manufacturers. A maintenance manual listing the frequency and nature of the maintenance required should be attached to or located near each piece of equipment. These should be reviewed periodically to ascertain that the required maintenance has actually been performed and actions to correct defects noted. The maintenance manual should clearly define who is responsible for each maintenance item. In larger institutions these functions should be carried out by maintenance or engineering personnel.

Temperatures of incubators, refrigerators, freezers, water baths, heating blocks, and ovens should be recorded daily. Preferably, this should be done at the beginning and end of each day or on the day of use in the case of equipment used intermittently. It is good practice to make it a habit among personnel to check the temperature each time the equipment is used throughout the day. Recording these intermediate observations is not necessary. Thermometers vary widely in their calibration accuracy. All thermometers used should be calibrated against a National Bu-

Table 56–9. EXPECTED MINIMUM INHIBITORY CONCENTRATION (MIC) ENDPOINTS* FOR QUALITY CONTROL OF DILUTION ANTIMICROBIAL SUSCEPTIBILITY TESTS

ANTIMICROBIAL AGENT	MINIMUM INHIBITORY CONCENTRATION (μg/ml)			
	E. coli ATCC 25922	Enterococcus ATCC 29212	*S. aureus* ATCC 29213	*P. aeruginosa* ATCC 27853
Clindamycin	>16	8	≤0.25	>16
Erythromycin	>16	2	≤0.25	>16
Methicillin	>16	>16	1	>16
Nafcillin	>16	4	≤0.25	>16
Penicillin G	>4	2	0.5	>4
Ampicillin	2	1	0.5	>16
Cephalothin	8	32	≤1	>64
Tetracycline	1	16	0.5	8
Carbenicillin	≤8	32	≤8	32
Chloramphenicol	4	4	4	>32
Vancomycin	>64	2	1	>64
Kanamycin	2	32	≤1	>64
Gentamicin	0.5	8	≤0.25	0.5
Tobramycin	0.5	16	≤0.25	<0.25
Amikacin	1	>64	≤1	≤1
Nitrofurantoin	≤8	≤8	16	>512
Nalidixic Acid	≤2	>128	32	128
Trimethoprim-sulfamethoxazole	≤0.5/9.5	≤0.5/9.5	≤0.5/9.5	16/304

*Endpoints are based on broth microdilution test. Differences of one or two dilutions may be anticipated with broth macrotube dilution or agar dilution tests. Tests are considered in control if observed MIC is ± one dilution interval from the above listed mean.

reau of Standards thermometer, and the correction factor, if any, should be noted on a tag attached to the thermometer. Since thermometers in air can respond to transient temperature fluctuations when incubator or refrigerator doors are opened, the thermometer should be immersed in propylene glycol or water (if temperature range permits). A temperature log or graph should be attached in a prominent position to each piece of equipment for convenience in recording and as an obvious reminder to observe and record the temperature. The acceptable temperature range should be indicated and space should be provided to record the source of trouble and corrective action taken when temperatures fall outside the established limits. Temperature chart recorders and thermostatic devices that sound an alarm locally or at a remote location should be considered to prevent loss of cultures or materials due to excessively large temperature changes as a result of thermostat malfunction or electrical failure, particularly at night. Continuous monitoring is not practical or even desired for all pieces of temperature-controlled equipment. Commonly available high-low thermometers are relatively inexpensive and establish the range of temperature fluctuation that has occurred since the last reading and resetting.

The interiors of incubators, refrigerators, freezers, and water baths must be periodically cleaned. Freezers should be defrosted at appropriate intervals. The use of frost-free freezers in clinical laboratories is subject to question, since the temperature may rise above the melting point of some of the stored materials during the defrost cycle. Appropriate back-up storage facilities are required so that the above maintenance can be carried out.

Autoclaves should be equipped with temperature chart recorders so that the operation has evidence and documentation that appropriate temperatures were maintained during the entire sterilizing cycle. In addition, a suspension of or strips impregnated with spores of *Bacillus stearothermophilus* should be used regularly to monitor sterilization. Ampules or strips may be placed in a test pack. An indicator should be placed in the coolest part of the chamber, usually the front of the lowest shelf. In large autoclaves or ones with large loads, several locations should be checked to assure an even distribution of sterilizing conditions. These biologic checks should be made *at least monthly*. The use of tape with heat-sensitive dye markers is useful for monitoring each load, but does not supersede the biologic tests. It is essential that autoclave operators understand the principles of steam sterilization and follow standardized procedures.

The atmosphere in carbon dioxide incubators and anaerobic jars and chambers requires continued surveillance. Carbon dioxide can be accurately measured by trapping a sample in a syringe or balloon and measuring the CO_2 with the instruments used to measure expired CO_2 in a pulmonary function laboratory. This degree of accuracy is seldom required and a more practical method is to use a Fyrite (Scientific Products, No. G 1725) CO_2 measuring device. This apparatus, originally intended for measurement of furnace flue gases, is easy to use and provides measurements of CO_2 satisfactory for clinical laboratory purposes. These checks should be made daily. The concentration of CO_2 should not exceed 10 per cent after flushing the chamber and should not fall below 5 per cent overnight. When a new CO_2 incubator is put into service, frequent checks during the CO_2 cycling process should be made to determine the characteristics of the system. In addition to direct measurement of CO_2, biologic indicators such as a CO_2-dependent strain of *Neisseria gonorrhoeae* are recommended. This procedure should be controlled by a parallel culture incubated without CO_2 to verify CO_2 dependency.

Each time anaerobic jars are used, a freshly activated cold catalyst should be installed. Used catalyst can be reactivated by heating in an oven at 160°C. for one and a half to two hours. Reactivated catalyst should be stored in an air-tight container with a desiccant. Chemical indicators, such as methylene blue or resazurin, and/or biologic indicators (e.g., a culture of *Clostridium novyi*) should be included in each jar to confirm that anaerobic conditions were achieved. Similar controls and precautions with catalyst are required with anaerobic chambers.

Biologic safety cabinets are required, especially for handling specimens or cultures containing mycobacteria and pathogenic fungi. The air flow across the face of the hood should be checked periodically to determine that it meets the manufacturer's specifications. The air flow velocity should not be less than 100 feet per minute. Filters should be replaced after appropriate decontamination according to the manufacturer's instructions. A qualified technician should certify that it is free of leaks and that original specifications are met. Ul-traviolet lamps used in hoods or elsewhere in the laboratory for decontamination purposes must be checked for efficiency at three-month intervals or replaced according to the schedule provided by the lamp manufacturer. Ultraviolet lamps must be kept free of dust which markedly reduces their efficiency.

All balances, particularly analytical balances, must be protected against temperature variation, vibration, and humidity. Knife edges must be smooth and the pans scrupulously clean. National Bureau of Standards Class S weights should be available and used to check the accuracy of analytical balances monthly.

A regular schedule of cleaning and maintaining microscopes should be followed. All personnel must be instructed in the proper procedures for microscope alignment, usage, and cleaning. Without careful attention to these details, the finest microscope will give mediocre performance.

Glassware used in the laboratory must be inspected, and chipped or cracked pieces should be discarded. Glassware must be free of all detergents. Volumetric glassware, especially pipettes and pipettors, should be subjected to a routine checking procedure to verify their calibration accuracy.

Stock organisms, source and storage

As indicated previously, a collection of stable organisms with reliable morphologic, biochemical, physiologic, and serologic charac-teristics is essential to a quality control program. The desired characteristic(s) for each organism in the collection must be reproducible when maintained under proper conditions. Stock organisms can be obtained from a variety of sources, e.g., (1) The American Type Culture Collection, Rockville, Maryland; (2) Bactrol Discs, Difco Laboratories; (3) Bact-Chek Discs, Roche Diagnostics, Hoffman La Roche; (4) proficiency testing programs; (5) reference laboratories or public health laboratories; and (6) your own laboratory. Tables 56-1 and 56-4 list the kinds of organisms that should be included.

Three methods can be used to store stock cultures: (1) lyophilization (freeze drying); (2) ultra freezing; and (3) use of appropriate storage media at room temperature in the refrigerator or incubator. Lyophilization is the most reliable method but also the most elaborate. Most laboratories will lack the facilities for this process, although cultures may be obtained from outside sources in the lyophilized state.

Ultrafreezing may be used for aerobic and anaerobic organisms. A loop full of a log phase culture can be suspended in 0.5 to 1.0 ml of sterile defibrinated sheep blood in a screw cap vial. These vials can be quick frozen in a dry ice ethanol bath, in liquid nitrogen, or in an ultrafreezer and then stored at $-40°$C. or lower. Organisms can be recovered after thawing at $37°$C. in a water bath for several minutes. A modification of this method is to include sterile glass beads in the vial so that each bead is uniformly coated with the orga-

Table 56-10. RECOMMENDED MEDIA FOR STORAGE OF STOCK CULTURES

MEDIUM	ORGANISMS	STORAGE TIME*
Cystine-trypticase agar (CTA)	Enterobacteriaceae Non-fermenters Staphylococci Streptococci Pneumococci *Listeria*	2-3 months
Soybean casein digest agar (deeps or semisolid)	Enterobacteriaceae Staphylococci	1 year
Blood or chocolate agar slants	Fastidious organisms Pneumococci Streptococci *Haemophilus influenzae* *Neisseria gonorrhoeae* *Neisseria meningitidis*	variable
Cooked meat medium	Anaerobes Facultative anaerobes	2-3 months
Lowenstein-Jensen	Mycobacteria	3 months

*At 4 to 8°C.

nism blood suspension (Nagel, 1972). Individual beads can be quickly removed from the vial and placed in a tube of an appropriate broth medium for growth. The remaining unused beads are returned promptly to the freezer before they have a chance to thaw.

The simplest methods involve the use of solid, semisolid, or broth media for storage. These media should preserve the viability and stability of the organism without excessive growth or metabolic activity. Table 56-10 lists several suitable media and the organisms which can be stored.

PROFICIENCY TESTING

Proficiency testing, required by certain government and private accrediting or auditing agencies, provides a valuable adjunct to a laboratory's quality control program as a means of judging overall quality. Satisfactory performance indicates that all procedures, equipment, media, reagents, and personnel involved in the processing of these samples are working as expected. For optimal use as a quality control measure, these external unknowns should be introduced to the laboratory as clinical specimens and not identified as test samples. Similarly, internally fabricated specimens using organisms from the laboratory's own culture collection can be submitted as a "blind" to evaluate performance problems. These "blind" unknowns present several problems which must be overcome. The quality control technologist must introduce the samples in a form indistinguishable from routine clinical specimens. Care must be taken that reports are not included inadvertently in any real patient's record, and where organisms are used that will prompt a telephone call to the "requesting physician," he be notified in advance or the culture labeled as an autopsy. A mechanism should be worked out with the hospital business office so that there will be no confusion over laboratory charges.

Proficiency testing programs provided by external agencies (e.g., College of American Pathologists, Center for Disease Control, or state or local health departments) in general provide information which allows comparisons of the performance of the laboratory with that of all other participants in the program. In addition, these programs as a rule provide a considerable amount of timely educational material which addresses problems in evalua-

tion and identification procedures that may be encountered by participants when dealing with clinical specimens similar to the test sample. Some programs provide data regarding the results obtained by participants from the important differential tests used in identifying the test organism(s). This information can be valuable in several ways. It can verify that the test procedures used in the laboratory are adequate and that the individual test results are in agreement. When misidentification occurs, specific defective differential tests can be pinpointed. In addition, these data document the differential characteristics of the test organism(s), making it extremely valuable for future use as internal blind unknown organisms or as organisms to be implemented into the laboratory's media and reagent control program.

Results of internal and external testing programs should be reviewed on a regular basis and discussed with all personnel. These discussions should be an educational exercise with emphasis on laboratory and personnel improvement.

DOCUMENTATION OF QUALITY CONTROL

The quality control program should be completely described in the laboratory procedure manual. This should include a definition of the person or persons responsible for carrying out the program, as well as the mechanism whereby information obtained as a result of the program is communicated to the laboratory director. Each procedure, medium, reagent, item of equipment, etc. to be controlled should have the control methods defined, as well as the frequency of testing, limits for acceptability, and action to be taken when not acceptable. Appropriate work forms should be developed to assist persons making the control observations to record these results. For example, simple logs or graphs for daily temperature recordings of refrigerators and incubators can be attached to the unit. It is important to include in these records the limits of acceptability and to provide a place to record the reasons for the unacceptable result (if known), and the action taken to correct the defect.

These working records must be reviewed at least monthly by the person responsible for the quality control program, the laboratory director, or a supervisor. If the laboratory director does not personally inspect all control records, a summary report should be prepared which lists the item controlled, the number of control observations made, the number of times out of control, a summary of the reasons (if known), and the corrective actions taken.

All records should be signed or initialed by the person making the observation as well as by the supervisor reviewer. Bartlett (1974, 1975) describes and illustrates numerous forms and recording methods which provide excellent assistance in developing the documentation aspects of a control program.

REFERENCES

Barry, D. L., and Bernsohn, K. L.: The role of quality control in the clinical bacteriology laboratory. Am. J. Med. Tech., *34*:195, 1968.

Bartlett, R. C.: Functional quality control. *In* Prier, J. E., Bartola, J., and Friedman J. (eds.): Quality Control In Microbiology. Baltimore, University Park Press, 1975, p. 145.

Bartlett, R. C.: Medical Microbiology: Quality, Cost and Clinical Relevance. New York, Wiley-Interscience, 1974.

Blazevic, D. J., Hall, C. T., and Wilson, M. E.: Cumitech 3. Practical Quality Control Procedures for the Clinical Microbiology Laboratory, Washington, D.C., American Society for Microbiology, 1976.

Dolan, C. T., Gavan, T. L., King, J W., Marymont, J. H., Smith, J. W., and Sommers, H. M.: Clinical Relevance in Microbiology. Chicago, College of American Pathologists, 1977.

Lennette, E. H., Spaulding, E. H., and Truant, J. P. (eds.): Manual of Clinical Microbiology, 2nd ed., Washington, D.C., American Society for Microbiology, 1974.

Nagel, J. G., and Kunz, L. J.: Needless retesting of quality-assured, commercially prepared culture media. Appl. Microbiol., *26*:31, 1973.

Nagel, J. G., and Kunz, L. J.: Simplified storage and retrieval of stock cultures. Appl. Microbiol., *23*:837, 1972.

National Committee for Clinical Laboratory Standards. Approved Standard ASM-2. Performance Standards for Antimicrobial Disc Susceptibility Tests. Villanova, Pa., 1975.

Prier, J. E., Bartola, J. T., and Friedman, H. (eds.): Quality Control in Microbiology. Baltimore, University Park Press, 1975.

Russell, R. L.: Quality control in the microbiology laboratory. *In* Lennette, R. H., Spaulding E. H., and Truant, J. P. (eds.): Manual of Clinical Microbiology, 2nd ed. Washington, D.C., American Society for Microbiology, 1974, p. 862.

Russell, R. L., Yoshimori, R. S., Rhodes, T. F., Reynolds, J. W., and Jennings, E. R.: A quality control program for clinical microbiology. Tech. Bull. Reg. Med. Tech., *39*:195, 1969.

Thornsberry, C., Gavan, T. L., and Gerlach, E. A.: Cumitech 6. New Developments in Antimicrobial Agent Susceptibility Testing. Washington D.C., American Society for Microbiology, 1977.

Vera, H. D., and Dumoff, M.: Culture media. *In* Lennette, E. H., Spaulding, E. H., and Truant, J. P. (eds.): Manual of Clinical Microbiology, 2nd ed. Washington, D.C., American Society for Microbiology, 1974, p. 881.

5

57

HOSPITAL INFECTION CONTROL

Thomas F. Keys, M.D.

HISTORICAL PERSPECTIVE

The communicability of infectious diseases was clearly recognized four centuries ago by Fracastorius, an Italian, who wrote in his book *Contagion* that "there are, it seems, three fundamentally different types of contagion: the first infects by direct contact only; the second does the same, but in addition leaves fomes . . . ; thirdly, there is a kind of contagion which . . . also infects at a distance" (Fracastorius, 1930). Florence Nightingale uttered a prophetic statement 100 years ago in her classic text on the design, construction, and facilities of hospitals: "It may seem a strange principle to enunciate as the very first requirement in a hospital that it should do the sick no harm" (Nightingale, 1863).

In the nineteenth century, Ignaz Semmelweiss, a Hungarian physician, emerged as a tragic figure in the control of a serious hospital infection, puerperal sepsis (childbed fever). Semmelweiss conducted classic studies on the cause and prevention of childbed fever shortly after graduating from medical school in Vienna and then upon his return to Hungary several years later. Unfortunately, he did not publish his studies until 1861, several years before his death. Throughout his professional

career, Semmelweiss was opposed in his theories about this infectious disease. He died at the age of 47, ironically of streptococcal sepsis after performing an autopsy on a victim of the disease. Semmelweiss's bitterness was expressed in an open letter to one of his colleagues, Professor Scanzoni of Wurzburg, in 1862: "You have proved, Sir, that one can murder exceedingly well in your new and well-equipped maternity hospital, if one is properly qualified" (Antall, 1973).

With the advancement of techniques for surgical procedures and anesthesia, it was Joseph Lister, an Englishman who lived from 1827 to 1912, who stressed his concern about wound infections: "You must be able to see with your mental eye the septic ferments as one sees flies and other insects with the corporal eye. If you can, you will be properly on your guard against them" (Guthrie, 1949).

Lister was the first physician to use a phenol (carbolic acid) locally following repair of open compound fractures to prevent serious wound infections. He later extended this application to silk, catgut, and even to a carbolic steam spray for the operating room!

The genius of Louis Pasteur, his discovery of fermentation, and the germ theory prompted him to discuss avoidance of wound sepsis in a talk to Paris physicians in the late 1870's:

If I had the honor of being a surgeon, convinced as I am of the dangers caused by the germs of microbes scattered on the surface of every object, particularly in the hospitals, not only would I use absolutely clean instruments, but after cleansing my hands with the greatest care and putting them quickly through a flame, I would only make use of charpie, bandages and sponges which had previously been raised to a heat of 130 to 150 degrees centigrade.... All that is easy to practice, and, in that way, I should still have to fear the germs suspended in the atmosphere surrounding the patient; but observation shows us every day that the number of those germs is almost insignificant compared to that of those which lie scattered on the surface of objects or in the cleanest, ordinary water" (Vallery-Radot, 1916).

Pasteur's statements remain lucid and exceedingly to the point as one examines our approach to prevention of wound sepsis in today's hospitals.

SIGNIFICANCE

Hospital-associated infections have been estimated to occur in 3 to 13 per cent of all inpatients (Barrett-Connor, 1972). Lower rates are reported in patients residing in community hospitals, whereas higher rates are noted in major medical centers. In 1967 Altemeier estimated that over two million cases of wound infections had occurred in the United States alone. There is no reason to believe the problem has become less frequent in the intervening years. The financial burden of hospital infections is enormous. There is a direct expense borne by both patient and hospital estimated at six to nine thousand dollars per infection. In addition, there is loss of gainful employment as well as associated pain and discomfort from the infection. Mortality is high in patients with hospital-associated infections. Lorian (1972) has stated that excess mortality is either coincidental or an expression of the debility of this patient population. One must realize that patients with terminal disease may succumb to infection during hospitalization, often from bacteria in their own gastrointestinal tract. It is always difficult to "blame" the hospital for such an infection associated with a disease that has a hopeless prognosis.

Perhaps one of every three doctors in the United States is subjected to legal investigation related to possible malpractice. Unless negligence is proven on the part of the physician, other staff, and the hospital, most cases are not justified (Dornette, 1973). Successful legal action might occur if a newly operated patient is moved into a room shared by a patient with an obvious wound infection. Other examples might be not culturing a wound when pus is clearly present; not examining a wound when there is pain and fever; and not obtaining a chest x-ray if a patient is suspected of having pneumonia. Unfortunately, standards of hospital care are so high in the public mind that complications are simply not expected. Therefore, it is important that all individuals working in the hospital conform to procedures and practices that are currently acceptable and in keeping with professional standards of the community. In short, it is necessary that any conditions that might cause hospital infection be remedied by an active infection control program.

There are few objective data currently available to support a highly structured infection-control program. Nevertheless, some program must be adapted to the needs of the individual hospital. This must include a system for the recognition and control of infection hazards. Newly established guidelines by the Joint Commission on Accreditation of Hospitals (1975) clearly state that there must be an effective infection control program within the hospital. Unfortunately, the program by itself does not generate an income, and it is often difficult for administrators to justify this expense. In 1970 Edwards (1971) estimated the cost of a surveillance program for a 600-bed hospital in Chicago. The cost to the hospital was approximately $100,000 per year, which amounted to less than $3.00 per patient admission. Comparing this cost with an anticipated expense of six to nine thousand dollars for a serious hospital infection, a surveillance program appears justified. Or phrased another way, if such a program were available and might spare the possibility of a serious hospital infection, would you as a patient be willing to spend several dollars to maintain it? I doubt if many of us would decline to participate.

ORGANIZATION

The purpose of the infection control program is to develop and maintain effective measures for the recognition and prevention of hospital-associated (nosocomial) infections.

If the following goals or objectives are met, the program will be successful:

A practical surveillance system to detect nosocomial infections.

Written procedures for controlling all infection hazards to patients, employees, and visitors.

A strong employee health program, including orientation of new employees to the hazards of hospital infections.

An effective continuing education program for all staff.

THE HOSPITAL INFECTION COMMITTEE

According to the recent guidelines established by the Joint Commission on Accreditation of Hospitals (1975), the following criteria should be applied in staffing the hospital infection committee:

Responsibility for monitoring the infection control program shall be vested in a multidisciplinary committee. . . . Its membership shall include representation from the medical staff, administration, nursing services, and where available, the microbiology section of the laboratory. Any individual employed in a surveillance or epidemiologic capacity shall be a member of the committee.

The hospital infection committee must receive enthusiastic support from administration and all staff personnel. It is not a policeman, but it must have the authority to conduct epidemiologic investigations when appropriate, and it must be objective in making decisions and firm in implementing them. It is vital that the infection committee be well-represented by members of the medical and surgical staff. If the committe is heavy with administrators, nurses, and members of support facilities, it will have serious problems in initiating policies that affect professional activities of the medical and surgical staff. In addition to the chairperson and surveillance officer (who should also be the committee's secretary), other members should include:

Nursing service—two members: one responsible for inservice training; the other supervisory for general ward nursing.

Medical staff—one member, preferably involved in the care of immunologically compromised patients.

Surgical staff—two members: a general surgeon and either an orthopedic surgeon, a cardiac surgeon, or a neurosurgeon.

Pediatric staff—one member, preferably involved in the newborn nursery and neonatal intensive care unit.

Clinical laboratory—one member with knowledge of clinical microbiology (if not already the chairperson, surveillance officer, or environmental officer).

Employee health—one member, preferably nursing supervisor of the area.

Administration—one member, preferably knowledgeable about the nursing and support facilities for patient care.

The chairperson is the key to the success of the committee and to the entire infection control program. An individual whose "credentials document knowledge of and special interest or experience in infection control" is suited for the role (Joint Commission, 1975). Preferably, this might be a physician specializing in infectious diseases or a pathologist-microbiologist, or a surgeon. However, of greater importance is the personality of the individual and an ability to handle tactfully individuals engaged in medical, surgical, nursing, and support activities in the hospital. It is desirable that the chairperson remain in the position for at least five years and be remunerated financially for time and effort. Financial re-imbursement proportional to the time spent in infection-control activities should be provided by the hospital administration.

The committee should meet at least every one to two months and more frequently if necessary, depending on the complexities of the institution and the nature of the day-to-day problems. There is no point in meeting regularly without a well-conceived and prepared agenda, despite the attractiveness of having a fancy lunch in a quiet dining room for a change! It is important for the committee to seek advice and counsel from additional individuals representative of dietary, pharmacy, central supply, engineering, and housekeeping when the need arises. If a problem develops in a special area, the chairperson may designate a subcommittee or an *ad hoc* committee composed of individuals expert therein to review the situation in detail and present the problem and possible solutions to the entire committee at a later date.

The responsibilities of the hospital infection committee include:

1. To review nosocomial infections in regard to their management and epidemic potential.

2. To review and make recommendations regarding infection control procedures throughout all areas in the hospital, such as pharmacy, central supply, housekeeping, laundry, surgery, anesthesia, nursing, die-

tetics, engineering, surgical pathology, clinical pathology, radiology, respiratory therapy, physical medicine, and employee health.

3. To implement policies to control community epidemic problems as they might affect the hospital.
4. To review antibiotic usage as related to emergence of antibiotic-resistant bacteria.
5. To review and endorse ongoing educational programs in infection control for staff and hospital employees.
6. To review and endorse studies involving infection control.

The Infection Control Team

The team is composed of individuals who are regularly active on the hospital infection committee and includes the chairperson, individual(s) performing surveillance, and a member of the clinical laboratory. The team may expand with individuals expert in certain areas, as during an investigation of a possible outbreak or epidemic problem.

The infection control officer

Qualifications are the same as those for chairperson of the hospital infection committee. Responsibilities include:

a. Chairmanship of the hospital infection committee.
b. Effective communication among all professional and non-professional staff working in the hospital environment.
c. Regular review of recognized nosocomial infection cases and, as well, autopsy cases for possible unrecognized infection.
d. Information relay of potential epidemiologic significance from the laboratory to appropriate staff (for example, informing a ward nurse that a patient's sputum smear has just been reported as positive for acid-fast bacilli or that a patient's serum sample is positive for hepatitis B surface antigen).
e. Consultation with administration to discuss problems and policies of infection control, especially with new construction, remodeling, and purchase of any items that present infection hazards.
f. Evaluation of the effectiveness of other infection control team members.
g. Consultation with Employee Health Service as needed, especially with regard to potential communicable disease in employees.

h. Epidemiologic investigation and, if necessary, request for assistance from state and federal health authorities.
i. Educational programs on infection control for medical staff and other employee groups.
j. Clinical laboratory research to better understand the problems and improve the quality of infection control procedures.

The surveillance officer

This individual is usually a nurse or other qualified person who has a special interest, dedication, and training in practical matters of hospital infection control. Like the infection control officer, the surveillance officer must know the hospital and relate well to administration, staff, and patients at all levels. Responsibilities include:

a. Surveillance according to procedures approved by the hospital infection committee.
b. Instruction on practices and procedures of infection control to nursing service (including the operating room), dietetics, employee health, and other hospital departments (physical medicine, radiology, etc.)
c. Orientation of new employees on infection control, including personal hygiene and their attentiveness to the existing policies and procedures.
d. Written guidelines regarding isolation and care of patients with communicable diseases as recommended by the hospital infection committee.
e. Regular follow-up of patients with communicable diseases and recommendations for isolation procedures and other precautions as indicated.

It is obvious that more than one surveillance officer or infection control nurse will be required to discharge these responsibilities if the hospital is of significant size and complexity. Current recommendations are that one individual be employed full time for every 250 to 300 acute medical and surgical beds.

The environmental officer

This individual must be knowledgeable about the practical applications of microbiology to the infection control program. In general, a clinical microbiologist or laboratory technologist would be considered for this position. The responsibilities include:

a. Assistant to director in performance of duties and investigations.

b. Guidelines and instruction on infection control in hemodialysis, pharmacy, clinical pathology, central supply, housekeeping, and engineering. In conjunction with engineering, the environmental officer should provide guidelines and recommendations for the maintenance of adequate ventilation and waste disposal.

c. Collection and interpretation of environmental cultures as approved by the hospital infection committee.

Excellent training programs on hospital infection control are available at Center for Disease Control in Atlanta and at the University of Ottawa in Canada. I would strongly recommend these courses for any fledgling members on the Infection Control Team.

RESPONSIBILITIES OF THE INFECTION CONTROL TEAM

The responsibilities of the Infection Control Team include maintenance of approved isolation standards, surveillance of hospital-associated infections, collection and interpretation of environmental cultures, and investigation of a suspected outbreak or epidemic of hospital infection. Each one of these responsibilities is described in detail below.

Isolation procedures

Sir William Osler was once quoted as saying that "Soap and water and common sense are the best disinfectants" (Bean, 1930). This simple statement illustrates well the basic approach to handling patients admitted to the hospital or those who develop infections of a communicable nature while within the hospital. The purpose of isolation is to prevent access of infectious particles from air and contact to patients, sources recognized by Fracastorius in 1565 and Florence Nightingale in 1863. Unfortunately, well-designed controlled studies have not been possible to determine the beneficial aspects of certain isolation procedures. However, the theory is with us, and until our knowledge expands, the somewhat conservative isolation measures recommended by the American Hospital Association and Center for Disease Control should be adhered to. Despite the deficiencies in any plan for isolating patients with potentially communicable disease, it is critical that a program be simple and applicable to the day-to-day problems of a hospital. The standards must apply equally to physicians, nurses, visi-

tors, housekeepers, technicians, and so forth. On occasion, physicians will not adhere to established isolation procedures and a gentle reprimand by the chairperson of the infection committee is necessary. In a sense, physicians, like patients, are guests of the hospital and must abide by established guidelines for infection control. An invitation to attend an infection committee meeting sometimes is advisable so that the situation or problem may be aired more fully. Modification of an existing isolation policy can even be considered. It is important to realize that isolation procedures must not isolate the patient from the devotion, attention, evaluation, and therapy of health care providers. In addition, the need for isolation must be reviewed with the patient and with his family and other visitors not only by the nurse who is fulfilling the request by a physician, but by that physician as well. If the need arises, any member of the infection control team should be available for counsel.

We have used as a guide, "Isolation techniques for use in hospitals," developed by the Center for Disease Control (CDC), Atlanta, Georgia (CDC, 1975). A copy of this very valuable booklet is available directly from the Center. Modification of their isolation standards may be necessary, depending on the complexity and uniqueness of an individual hospital. Guidelines should be available at every nursing station for review on the wards. At our institution, physicians are provided with an abbreviated outline of isolation protocol that is conveniently carried in a pocket calendar notebook (Fig. 57-1). Guidelines for these categories are elaborated below:

Strict Isolation. This form of isolation is used principally for patients with severe burns, disseminated herpes infections, and well-documented staphylococcal pneumonia. A private room is required, with gown, mask, and gloves for direct patient contact. When the degree of contagiousness lessens, strict isolation is no longer necessary. For example, when a patient with staphylococcal pneumonia is responding clinically to appropriate antibiotic therapy and secretions can be adequately contained, strict isolation is no longer required. Similarly, after disseminated herpes lesions have resolved to the crusting and healing stages, the same principle holds.

Respiratory Isolation. Candidates for respiratory isolation include patients with suspected or culturally documented active pulmonary tuberculosis, influenza, and several

CATEGORIES	CRITERIA	PRECAUTIONS
STRICT ISOLATION (Yellow card)	Burns, extensive Staphylococcal pneumonia Diphtheria Chickenpox Disseminated herpes Congenital rubella Smallpox	Private room Gown Mask Gloves for patient contact Scrupulous handwashing Disinfection of patient-associated articles
RESPIRATORY ISOLATION (Red card)	Tuberculosis, pulmonary suspected or sputum-positive Influenza pneumonia Meningitis (meningococcal) Measles Pertussis Mumps Rubella	Private room Mask Scrupulous handwashing Disinfection of articles contaminated with secretions
ENTERIC PRECAUTIONS (Brown card)	Diarrhea, acute or until etiology established Salmonella Shigella	Private room Gown and gloves for contact with patient or articles likely contaminated with fecal material Scrupulous handwashing Disinfection of articles contaminated with feces
HEPATITIS PRECAUTIONS (Brown card with green *H* and *BLOOD* attached)	Hepatitis; viral (B or non-B)	Same as above plus special blood precautions
WOUND AND SKIN PRECAUTIONS (Green card)	Burns, moderate Pyogenic wound and skin infections where drainage cannot be contained in dressing Puerperal sepsis Eruptive herpes	Private room Gown Mask and gloves for direct wound contact Scrupulous handwashing Disinfection of contaminated articles
PROTECTIVE ISOLATION (Blue card)	Agranulocytosis Certain patients receiving immunosuppressive therapy Certain patients with lymphomas and leukemia	Private room Gown Mask Scrupulous handwashing Gloves at discretion of service

Figure 57–1. Hospital isolation procedures.

other acute respiratory infections. Although the justification for placing patients with meningitis in respiratory isolation is poorly documented, this is done until a preliminary diagnosis is established and the patient is on appropriate antimicrobial therapy, generally within 24 to 48 hours. On the other hand, it is important for patients admitted with measles to be in respiratory isolation because of viable viral particles in their respiratory secretions. Respiratory isolation should include a private room, preferably with ventilation exhausted to the outside. Although masks only trap large particulate matter and do not prevent entry of respiratory droplet nuclei, they heighten the awareness of staff for a patient's respiratory infection. For pulmonary tuberculosis, dura-

tion of isolation after therapy has commenced is not clear-cut. Communicability appears to be higher in patients with active open cavitary disease, as well as in those with tracheobronchial and vocal cord involvement. As a rule, therapy should be continued for at least 7 to 10 days before taking patients with pulmonary tuberculosis out of respiratory isolation, provided the patient is cooperative and capable of containing respiratory secretions.

Enteric Precautions. This isolation category applies principally to patients with acute diarrhea (often caused by *Salmonella*, *Shigella*, and parvoviruses) and viral hepatitis. For the patient with hepatitis B infection, additional precautions for collection and processing of blood specimens must be taken. The need for utilizing isolation for patients with asymptomatic hepatitis B infection is uncertain, but such isolation is practiced at our institution. Again, the most important precaution is careful handling of blood and tissue specimens from these patients. Duration of isolation for patients on enteric precautions depends to a great extent on the clinical illness and the infecting agent. Patients with gastrointestinal salmonellosis may remain with stool positivity for several weeks after they become asymptomatic, particularly if they have received antibiotic treatment. On the other hand, by the time patients are admitted to the hospital with acute hepatitis A infection, they no longer have viable virus in their feces. On a dialysis unit it is important to place HBsAg carriers on enteric precautions.

Wound and skin precautions. This isolation category generally applies to purulent postoperative wound infections with drainage that cannot be contained within a simple, dry dressing. The category is also useful for patients with local herpes infections until the lesions are in a final stage of healing. A private room is recommended, and patients are generally confined to their room until drainage is under control. When caring for a patient's wound, disposable gloves must be worn with scrupulous handwashing afterward. For patients with mild to moderate burn wounds, we have used a modified form of wound isolation. This allows a more liberal approach to ambulation and greater interaction with staff, other patients, family, and visitors. Such an approach reduces the incidence of deprivation problems, especially in pediatric burn wound cases after youngsters are on prolonged rigorous isolation.

Protective Isolation. Protective isolation has been intended for patients whose host defense mechanisms are highly compromised, such as for patients with leukocyte counts below 1000 cells/cu mm. For the average hospital not designed to care for highly compromised patients, this category is probably not necessary (Bodly, 1975). Laminar flow of ventilation, sterile food, and oral prophylactic antibiotics are provisions generally available only at a large referral cancer hospital. In most instances the general hospital can provide these patients with a private room close to a nursing station but distant from clinically infected cases.

Surveillance of hospital infections

Although arguments exist about the usefulness of surveillance for the regular detection of hospital-associated infections, I believe that collection of these data provides useful information for an infection control program. Surveillance allows the infection control team to appreciate the cause and origin of hospital infections. It provides a data base that can be readily reviewed if a potential epidemic or outbreak situation develops. Furthermore, surveillance stimulates a greater awareness of infection control problems and provides a format of continuing education of medical and nursing staff. In addition, if the surveillance system is comparable with that of other hospitals, causes and solutions to problems may be found simply by reviewing others' experience, either in the literature or by direct communication.

In order for surveillance of hospital infections to be useful, definitions of infection must be clear, and basic epidemiologic data must be collected, reviewed weekly, and disseminated regularly to the hospital infection committee. Detection of hospital infections involves assessment of both laboratory culture results and the patient's clinical condition. The infection control team is ideally suited for this task. In the past, physicians were asked to submit infection reports regularly as their patients acquired hospital infections. As one might anticipate, such data were rarely complete and in fact, detracted from the accuracy of a surveillance program. Occasionally a "prevalence survey" may be useful to determine the efficiency of a regular surveillance program. This involves an intensive search for hospital infection in all hospitalized patients during a particular day or portion of a week. Records, including charts and medication notes, are carefully scrutinized by trained personnel. Patients may even be interviewed and examined. If a regular surveillance program detects 70 per cent of hospital infections, it is satisfactory. If it detects a greater percentage, surveillance may be consuming time that could be spent in better ways by members of the infection control team.

A data collection card (epi-card) is ideal for recording basic surveillance information (Fig. 57-2). The card must be easy to use and carry. It is hardly necessary, in fact superfluous, to record a wealth of detail on the epi-card. Only

NAME _____   I.D. No. _____

AGE _____   TODAY'S DATE _____   ROOM NO. _____

ADM _____   DISM _____   SERVICE _____

DIAGNOSIS _____

SURGERY THIS ADMISSION:

Date   Procedure   Doctor   O.R.

PATHOGEN(S)

Site   Lab No.   Date   Organism   Antibiotic
                                                                                   Susceptibility

_____   _____   _____   _____   _____

_____   _____   _____   _____   _____

INFECTION SITE

☐ Surg Wound   ☐ Super   ☐ Deep   ☐ Clean   ☐ Clean-Contam

                    ☐ Foreign body   ☐ Prophy Antibiotics

☐ Urinary   ☐ Asx   ☐ Other ☐ Cath   Date _____ to _____

☐ Pneumonia   ☐ Trach   ☐ Intub ☐ IPPB   Date _____

☐ Skin   ☐ IV   ☐ Biopsy ☐ Angio ☐ Cardiac Cath   ☐ Other

☐ Bacteremia   ☐ Secondary ☐ Primary   ☐ Indeterm

☐ Other _____

☐ Hospital Infection   Ward _____   Room _____   ☐ Endogenous

                                                                                       ☐ Exogenous

Figure 57–2. Hospital infection surveillance card.

information necessary to document a hospital-associated infection is needed. By and large, most hospital-associated infections occur after a patient has been hospitalized for at least 48 to 72 hours. Although it is important to be aware of community-associated infections, it is not necessary to keep a record of these data on the epi-card. Our epi-card contains information necessary for reporting hospital infections and for reviewing problems when the possibility exists of an outbreak or epidemic. Bacteriologic data as reported by the clinical laboratory are entered on the central portion of the epi-card. On the top portion of the card, the patient's name, identification number, room number, admission date, service, and working diagnosis are recorded. The surveillance officer, working with laboratory and clinical clues, makes the diagnosis of hospital infection. Afterward, the remainder of the card is filled out with facts related to the infection site. Our definition of infection is in keeping with that established by the Center for Disease Control (Garner, 1970).

Wound Infection. A surgical wound with purulent drainage is infected. If it develops or extends below the fascial plane, it is considered a deep infection. If it is confined to the subcutaneous space, the infection is superficial. It is important in reporting wound infec-

---

Clean

Non-traumatic
No inflammation encountered
No break in technique
Respiratory, alimentary, genitourinary tracts not entered

Clean-contaminated

Gastrointestinal or respiratory tracts entered without significant spillage
Appendectomy
Oropharynx entered
Vagina entered
Genitourinary tract entered in absence of infected urine
Biliary tract entered in absence of infected bile
Minor break in technique

Contaminated

Major break in technique
Gross spillage from gastrointestinal tract
Traumatic wound, fresh
Entrance of genitourinary or biliary tracts in presence of infected urine or bile

Dirty and Infected

Acute bacterial inflammation encountered, without pus
Transection of "clean" tissue for the purpose of surgical access to a collection of pus
Perforated viscus encountered
Traumatic wound with retained devitalized tissue, foreign bodies, fecal contamination and/or delayed treatment, or from dirty source

---

Figure 57–3. Classification of operative wounds in relation to contamination and increasing risk of infection.

tions that they all be accurately classified at the time of surgery. Altemeier's categories of clean, clean-contaminated, contaminated, and dirty serve this purpose (Fig. 57-3). Most meaningful "attack rates" are derived by considering only the clean and clean-contaminated wound categories. Wound infections may not necessarily present during the same hospitalization as for surgery. Those following insertion of prosthetic devices, including cardiac valves and hip appliances, may not emerge until weeks, months, or sometimes years after operation.

Urinary Infection. Hospital-associated urinary tract infections most frequently occur following urologic instrumentation, usually with urethral catheters. Colony counts of 100,000 colonies of organisms or greater per ml of urine are generally diagnostic of significant infection. Most often catheter-associated bacteriuria is asymptomatic; nevertheless, it still represents a potential problem either later in the hospital or after the patient has left for home. Because urine cultures are not routinely done, it may be difficult to know if asymptomatic bacteriuria was present on admission. As a general rule, if the patient has a negative admission urinalysis but develops urinary symptoms 48 to 72 hours later, the infection should be classified as hospital-associated.

Pneumonia. Hospital-associated pneumonia is often exceedingly difficult to diagnose. Symptoms, signs, x-rays, and laboratory findings of pneumonia may be confused with those of pulmonary infarction, edema, atelectasis, and the shock lung syndrome. Ideally, diagnostic criteria should include a cough productive of purulent sputum, fever, and evidence of pneumonia on chest x-ray that was not present on admission.

Other infection sites include skin, as at the point of entry of an intravascular line or biopsy tool, burn wounds, gastroenteritis, meningitis, and endometritis.

Bloodstream. All bacteremias should be noted on the epi-cards. They may occur secondarily from wound, urinary, lung, and skin infections. Bacteremias cannot be taken lightly, since they carry significant morbidity and mortality for the hospitalized patient. When the source of bacteremia is uncertain, it may be designated as either indeterminate or primary if it may have resulted from direct inoculation of contaminated material into the bloodstream.

The reverse side of the epi-card may be used for recording other clinical information on the patient, such as fever, leukocytosis, pyuria, and chest x-ray findings. Certain risk factors that might predispose to infection may be recorded: obesity, age, antibiotic usage, cancer, alcoholism, and so forth. However, this is not necessary for routine surveillance. The reverse side may be better used by the surveillance officer for recording follow-up information on the case. Surveillance cards should be reviewed at least weekly by the infection control officer. In addition, the cards may be used for line-listing certain infections, such as wound infections, urinary infections, and bacteremias. While line-listings do not indicate attack rates of hospital infections, because they lack denominator data (number of cases at risk), they are still helpful if a trend toward a certain type of infection is developing in the hospital environment.

As noted previously, surveillance data must

fulfill a greater role than occupying the surveillance officer's filing cabinet. Data must be organized in such a fashion that they can be reviewed and understood by all members of the hospital infection committee. Such data must also be available for instant retrieval if review is necessary during investigation of a possible outbreak or epidemic of hospital infection.

Surveillance data gathered at our institution are routinely organized in several forms. First, a line-listing for all clean and clean-contaminated wound infections is prepared on a monthly basis for review by members of the hospital infection committee. To illustrate, the following heading is used to prepare the line-listing sheet of surgical wound infections:

Date (week, month)   **Hospital**
Organism/Surgeon/Procedure   *Date/ O.R./Date and Ward Cultured/Patient ID*

Secondly, the surveillance data are organized for a monthly nosocomial infection report, which provides a summary of cases with infections over cases at risk during the same period, usually by procedures or dismissals, for computation of hospital infection attack rates or "percentages" (Fig. 57-4). This basic report

1. *TOTALS*   Infections _____   Dismissals _____   Attack Rate _____ %

    Wounds _____   Skin _____

    Urinary _____   Other _____

    Pneumonia _____

2. *OPERATIVE WOUNDS* (Clean and Clean-Contaminated cases only)

Service	Infections	Total Cases	Attack Rate (%)
General Surgery	_____	_____	_____
Orthopedics	_____	_____	_____
Cardiac	_____	_____	_____
Etc.	_____	_____	_____

3. *NON-WOUNDS*

Service	Urinary	Pneumonia	Skin	Other	Total	Dism	Attack Rate (%)
Medicine	_____	_____	_____	____	____	____	_____
Surgery	_____	_____	_____	____	____	____	_____
Pediatrics	_____	_____	_____	____	____	____	_____
Obstetrics	_____	_____	_____	____	____	____	_____
Nursery	_____	_____	_____	____	____	____	_____
Etc.	_____	_____	_____	____	____	____	_____

4. *BACTEREMIAS*

Service	Ward	Date Cultured	Organism	Focus	Antibiotic Susceptibility
Hematology	____	_____	_____	____	_____
Nephrology	____	_____	_____	____	_____
Surgery	____	_____	_____	____	_____
Etc.	____	_____	_____	____	_____

Figure 57-4. Hospital-associated monthly infection report.

contains enough information for regular review by the hospital infection committee. If an increased number of certain infections is noted, it may be necessary to collect more denominator information before one can accurately assess the problem. For example, if during a reporting period an increased number of urinary tract infections was noted, one also must know how many patients during that same period underwent urologic instrumentation, especially urethral catheterization. Antibiotic susceptibility data are recorded on a monthly basis for all bacteremias, allowing for inspection of changing patterns of antibiotic susceptibility. This information may also be correlated with intrahospital antibiotic usage.

Although monthly surveillance reports are intended for review mainly by the hospital infection committee, they may also be useful for educating physicians, nurses, and other staff about principles and practices of infection control. It is possible to condense surveillance data to those applicable only on certain wards or in certain sections of the hospital. The ward or "unit" report can be forwarded to the nursing supervisor on a regular basis. This reporting system is best adapted for high-risk patient areas such as medical and surgical intensive care units. A regular review of the unit report by the infection control team to the medical and nursing staff not only makes them aware of potential epidemic problems but also provides them with essential inservice training.

Environmental cultures

Within the past several decades, many hospitals have dutifully collected a large variety and number of bacterial cultures from their environment. This labor has contributed greatly to the cost and, it is believed, to the effectiveness of an infection control program. Specimens have come from floors, sinks, walls, ceilings, staircases, air, water, and linen on a routine basis. These microbiologic data accumulate in hospital files and serve no useful purpose except perhaps to satisfy the requirements of certain regulatory agencies. In fact, when routine environmental cultures are examined with more than a passing glance and found to be positive, chaos occurs in the regular day-to-day operation of a hospital. On the other hand, negative cultures produce a feeling of contentment and complacency. It has only been within the past several years, with

support from the American Public Health and American Hospital Associations (1974, 1975), that the trend has reversed against routine environmental culturing. A change of heart has also been noted in a recent statement by the Joint Commission on Accreditation of Hospitals (1975). With few exceptions, environmental cultures should be employed only during an investigation of an outbreak or for research purposes. Routine environmental sampling for bacteria is still recommended for:

a. Hospital-prepared infant formula (weekly according to the American Academy of Pediatrics).
b. Hospital sterilizers, including steam, gas, and dry heat ovens (using spore strips).
c. Reusable inhalation therapy equipment and anesthesia equipment that cannot be sterilized (monthly according to Center for Disease Control).

While it is stated that routine culturing of the environment may serve as an educational device for nursing and housekeeping personnel, the time and expense might be better spent in teaching a basic course on microbiology and reviewing the writings of Semmelweiss, Lister, Pasteur, and Nightingale. To my way of thinking, it is nonsense to culture the environment merely to prove that germs exist!

Investigation of an outbreak

Emotions run high when word leaks out that a certain hospital has an epidemic. The term, defined by Webster as "common to, or affecting at the same time, many in a community," is usually misused and not truly representative of the problem at hand. Nevertheless, an investigation may be required, and this can only be done through the hospital infection committee with firm support by administration and staff. Occasionally, a complex problem, which may be scientific or political, may require outside resources for assistance. Public health authorities, beginning at the local level, should first be consulted. If necessary, state agencies may ask for assistance from the federal government through the Epidemiological Investigation Service, a branch of the CDC.

It is crucial to establish first whether or not a "problem" (avoid the word epidemic) really exists. As a rule, two or more cases of a clinical infection of identical cause or circumstance appearing within a limited time qualify for an investigation (Castle, 1977). The etiology must be determined as rapidly as possible by a competent clinical microbiology laboratory.

The next task is to identify all other clinical cases that have been recognized by routine surveillance within the past several months. Review of line-listing sheets, monthly surveillance reports, and details as recorded on the epi-cards is extremely helpful. In addition, it is desirable to locate additional cases that may not have been recognized by routine surveillance, since this usually reflects only 60 to 70 per cent of actual hospital infections. An intensified surveillance in areas where the index of suspicion is high may provide more cases. Even though they may not be definite, they should at least be examined to assess their epidemiologic significance. All suspected and confirmed cases are entered on a special line-listing sheet that is constructed to assess the clinical and epidemiologic features of the problem. For example, if there was concern about an increased incidence of operative wound infections, the following line listing might be used:

Culture results/Date/Ward
Operation/Date/Room/Team
Pre-op diagnosis/Patient identification

The next step in the investigation is to develop an attack rate for the recognized infections:

Attack rate (%) =
$$\frac{\text{number of infected cases}}{\text{number of cases at risk}} \times 100$$

Although it may not be completely accurate, the denominator figure in this formula usually represents the number of patients operated on, instrumented, or dismissed during the study period. Attack rates can be computed by the week, month, quarter, or year, depending on the nature of the investigation. A comparison of these data with those generated during a comparable period when there did not appear to be a problem is done using simple statistical analysis (Chi square) (Hill, 1971). If a significant difference in attack rates is documented, the investigation is continued. If there is not, the investigation is usually terminated. Often, however, review of the case material and epidemiologic features of the suspected outbreak generate significant concern among staff and administrators. Certain flaws and problems in existing infection control programs and policies can be recognized and hopefully remedied. On the other hand, if there is firm statistical support for an epidemic problem, the investigation must continue. A critical analysis of all procedures, including dates and locations of operations and use of catheters (urinary and vascular) and inhalation equipment, must take place. This information can also be line-listed and compared with those of a control population without infection but subjected to the same variables as the case population. After the data have been further refined, an hypothesis or tentative explanation of the problem is offered. It is extremely important to consult outside resources, including the literature, before formulating an hypothesis. Hypothesis testing may be done by instituting appropriate control measures for variables that the investigation has determined might have influenced the outcome of the population at risk. Once the hypothesis is verified, a corrective policy or procedure must be quickly drafted by the infection committee, approved by administration, and implemented. A strong educational program is essential to guarantee its effectiveness. Staff simply have to know about the problem before cooperation and adherance to a new policy will take place.

THE CLINICAL MICROBIOLOGY LABORATORY

The clinical microbiology laboratory provides vital objective data for routine surveillance and during the course of an investigation of a possible epidemic problem. Microbiologic data must be assessed regularly by the surveillance officer as to what is actually going on at the patient's bedside, where a clinical infection must be differentiated from colonization or contamination.

Problems in the collection and transportation of specimens must be avoided to prevent misinterpretation of culture results. The laboratory is required to accurately identify isolates and perform *in vitro* antibiotic susceptibility tests according to standardized techniques. Antibiotograms may be helpful in separating strains of similar species by noting a difference in susceptibility to antimicrobial agents. For example, an apparent "outbreak" of wound infections may appear to be due to a single strain of *Staphylococcus aureus*. If wound isolates show varied susceptibility to penicillin, this rules out the possibility that they are all caused by a peculiar strain of *Staphylococcus*. The antibiotogram may also be helpful when looking at infections due to aerobic gram-negative bacteria such as *Serratia marcescens, Pseudomonas, Proteus, Klebsiella, Enterobacter,* and *Providencia* species. Antimicrobials useful to survey these organisms include nitrofurantoin, chloramphenicol, trimethoprim-sulfamethoxazole, cephalothin, tetracycline, ampicillin, carbenicillin, kanamycin, gentamicin, tobramycin, amikacin, colistin, and nalidixic acid (Center for Disease Control, 1974).

For investigation of a suspected epidemic or outbreak, cultures of the environment, staff, and other patients may be necessary. They should be done only after approval by the infection control officer and preferably not until after the clinical impact of the suspected problem is appreciated. I recall a respected physician who, not very long ago, requested a culture of ice water because his patient had developed diarrhea. However, he failed to recognize that the onset of his patient's symptoms coincided with the administration of an antibiotic that commonly produces diarrhea as a side effect!

The clinical microbiology laboratory should suggest a method of culturing appropriate for the individual problem. Microbiologic sampling of prepacked, sterile, commercial products is not recommended. If contamination is suspected, the Center for Disease Control or the Federal Drug Administration should be contacted immediately. When culturing objects in the environment, such as equipment, soap dispensers, hand lotions, medicines, and food, a premoistened swab or immersion of the object in broth enriched with 0.5 per cent beef extract is recommended. To neutralize residual disinfectant, the broth should also contain 0.07 per cent lecithin and 0.5 per cent polysorbate-80. Fluid samples may be cultured by passing them through a 0.45 or 0.22 micron millipore filter and culturing the filters directly in broth or on an agar plate (Center for Disease Control, 1974). For air sampling, simple Rodac plates set on horizontal surfaces or specially designed and more sophisticated equipment may be used. However, often air sampling is not helpful during the investigation of an outbreak. The time and expense involved are great and interpretation of the data is difficult and may be misleading.

Isolates of unusual characteristics should be forwarded to the state health department or to other reference laboratories for special studies. All isolates of potential epidemiologic significance should be stored by the clinical laboratories, subject to final review by the infection control officer before discarding. Most hospital laboratories do not have facilities for bacteriophage typing of *Staphylococcus aureus* isolates. This may be performed by the Center for Disease Control when a hospital epidemic is identified and reported to the Epidemiological Investigation Service. For an alternative phage typing resource, it is suggested that the Directory of Rare Analyses (DORA) be consulted (Young, 1977). Isolates from patients with infections due to group A beta-hemolytic streptococci may be forwarded to state health or other reference laboratories for special typing procedures. Unfortunately, no simple, well-established uniform procedure is currently available for typing aerobic gram-negative bacteria.

ENVIRONMENTAL SERVICES (HOUSEKEEPING)

Hospital staff, particularly physicians, often fail to recognize the responsibility that housekeeping has in maintaining an effective infection control program. While it is obviously impossible to maintain a totally "germ-free" hospital environment, effective cleaning measures do greatly reduce the germ load to a susceptible patient population. Details of cleaning procedures are well-outlined in recent publications (Altemeier, 1976).

It is important for housekeeping personnel to understand the reasons behind the cleaning procedures and their key role in prevention of hospital infections. They will work harder with this knowledge if it is tactfully presented. Furthermore, employees must be cautioned regarding their exposure to potentially contaminated materials and wastes in the course of their duties. Of greatest concern at present is the possibility of hepatitis B infection after accidental inoculation from contaminated needles, syringes, and glassware in loose refuse. Such materials must be secured in a firm, clearly designated container to reduce this possibility. Needle sticks and other wounds should be promptly reported to the Employee Health Service for evaluation and follow-up.

The housekeeping department is frequently assaulted by detailmen who are in the business of selling items allegedly helpful in infection control. While it is important to be tactful and courteous, all such inquiries should be channeled through the hospital's purchasing service and administration prior to consideration by the infection control committee. For example, a variety of disinfectants are currently available for cleaning floors, but their over-all usefulness has not been well-established. It may be argued that germicidal cleaners are even not necessary in operating rooms and intensive care units because bacterial counts on floors rapidly increase within 20 to 30 minutes after application of germicides. Furthermore, certain germicides may prove so toxic to the housekeeping staff that their cleaning procedures become less effective. The plain fact is that the liberal application of a good detergent with generous amounts of water is the surest and most economical method for general cleaning. It is also important to realize that incompatibilities may exist between detergents and germicides, particularly with the quaternary ammonium compounds (QUATS). QUATS have themselves been associated with outbreaks of infections due to gram-negative bacteria, and they probably serve no useful purpose in a modern-day hospital (Dixon, 1976). A wet vacuum system with a mechanical pickup has been recommended for use on operating room floors. Our hospitals have not used this system, and to my knowledge, no problems with operative wound infections have occurred.

Last, the Housekeeping Department has the responsibility for maintaining adequate handwashing facilities for staff, patients, and visitors. The recent promotion of handwashing as a sound practice (Steere, 1975), which it certainly is, has resulted in the availability of many handwashing preparations. Soap products ranging from dispensable, impregnated dry soap leaves to foam compounds containing hexachlorophene, alcohol, and emolliants are now produced. Liquid soaps are often said to be superior to bar soaps, but there is no good scientific evidence to support this. In fact, contaminated liquid soap dispensers have been implicated in outbreaks of hospital infections. If bar soap is adequately maintained, it should be satisfactory in most areas of the hospital, provided that people know how to wash their hands. Plain soap without germicides does not promote the growth or transmission of bacteria (Bamran, 1965). For handwashing in the operating room theater and prior to performing other invasive procedures,

germicidal soaps are recommended. They may also be advisable for staff working in high-risk areas, such as intensive care units and the nursery, although sparse data are available on this subject.

EMPLOYEE HEALTH SERVICE

The hospital employee health service is integral to infection control. It protects employees from acquiring infections at work by offering immunization and surveillance for infections likely to occur in the susceptible population. It insures that other employees and patients are not exposed to potential communicable diseases by clearing employees with infections before they return to work. The infection control officer should be available for consultation and education to all employees. Common infections communicable to employees include tuberculosis and hepatitis B virus infection. In addition, pregnant women employees, depending on their immune status, may also be susceptible to rubella and perhaps to cytomegalovirus infections.

Tuberculosis is not nearly as prevalent now as it was 25 years ago. Even though the classic features of the disease may be present on admission, the diagnosis may not be suspected by a physician unfamiliar with the disease (Furrey, 1976; MacGregor, 1975). Such patients often reside on a general medical ward for several weeks before the diagnosis is considered. During this time, liberal exposure with infected respiratory droplet nuclei may occur to other patients and staff. Therefore, the health service must provide an active surveillance program for the early detection of tuberculosis for all their employees (Craven, 1975). Those who are tuberculin-negative should have tuberculin skin testing done annually. Employees with well-documented previous tuberculin positivity should have chest x-rays obtained annually to screen for reactivation of old pulmonary tuberculosis. Additional surveillance may be necessary after inadvertent heavy exposure from a highly contagious patient. Prior knowledge of an employee's recent tuberculin status always makes the job easier.

With the commercial availability of serologic tests, hepatitis B infection can now be recognized and differentiated from other types of diseases affecting the liver (Walsh, 1970). Employees working in certain hospital areas, such as the hemodialysis unit and clinical laboratory, are at significant risk of acquiring hepatitis B infection. Such "high-risk" employees should be initially tested, then monitored regularly for evidence of hepatitis B infection (Center for Disease Control, 1976; Melnick, 1976). Hepatitis B surface antibody should detect more subclinical cases of hepatitis B infection than does surface antigen, since the latter's persistence in the blood is uncommon. Hiring employees with positive hepatitis B surface antigen to work in "high-risk" areas in the hospital is controversial (Blumberg, 1976). The ideal candidate for such a job would be antigen-negative but antibody-positive, and thus presumably protected from reinfection.

Employees must be knowledgeable about infections that they may bring into the hospital. These include skin and acute respiratory infections and diarrhea. The health service must be consulted promptly to assess the significance of these problems. Active skin lesions due to *Staphylococcus aureus*, *Streptococcus pyogenes*, and *Herpes simplex* will restrict employees from working in patient care areas until healing has occurred. Similarly, employees with streptococcal pharyngitis must not work around patients until they have received effective treatment for this disease. Influenza is a highly contagious respiratory infection; employees should always be reminded about this at the beginning of every "flu" season; they also should be encouraged to participate in annual influenza vaccination. While most cases of gastroenteritis are nonspecific, they may be due to communicable pathogens such as *Salmonella*, *Shigella*, and parvovirus-like agents (for example, Norwalk agent) (Flewett, 1975). It would be neither wise nor prudent for an employee to return to work until after gastrointestinal symptoms have subsided.

The employee health program should provide active vaccines against influenza, rubella, measles, mumps, and poliomyelitis viruses, as well as against diphtheria and tetanus. BCG vaccine for tuberculosis and smallpox vaccine are generally not indicated for the average community or medical center hospital unless there is a good possibility of exposure to these diseases because of their location and population served.

Gamma globulin prophylaxis should be considered for employees exposed to patients with viral hepatitis and, if possible, given within several days after exposure. For sig-

nificant exposure to non-B viral hepatitis, 0.03 ml/kg is given intramuscularly. For documented exposure to contamination by hepatitis B surface antigen, a commerical preparation of hepatitis B immune globulin has recently become available. Although the long-term benefit of this preparation is not yet well-documented (Grady, 1975), the following conditions warrant consideration for its use: accidental needle stick, direct mucous membrane contact, and oral ingestion. All potential recipients should be proven hepatitis B antigen-and antibody-negative before receiving this preparation. The standard dosage is 0.06 ml/kg, given intramuscularly.

Antibiotic prophylaxis has been advised to employees, usually physicians or nurses, that have had significant exposure to patients with acute meningococcal meningitis (McCormick, 1975). Indication should include only intimate contact with potentially infected respiratory secretions, as might occur during mouth-to-mouth resuscitation. Rifampin, 300 mg by mouth twice daily for two days, is the antibiotic currently recommended unless the organism is known to be susceptible to sulfa drugs (Pickering, 1976).

CONCLUSION

In conclusion, the fundamental principles of infection control are not difficult to understand. As our knowledge of hospital-associated infections advances, new methods of prevention must be devised. Concern is currently directed at controlling spread of infection from the animate and inanimate environment of the hospital. Reasonably sound practices have been established for the care of operative wounds (Subcommittee on Aseptic Methods, 1968; Cruse, 1973), urinary catheters (Stamm, 1975), inhalation equipment (Pierce, 1973), and intravascular devices (Maki, 1973). However, many infections in hospitalized patients arise from their own endogenous flora. More knowledge about patient host defenses is required before a solution to this problem can be found. Polyvalent vaccines against aerobic gram-negative bacteria have been proposed to protect the susceptible hospitalized patient (Hewitt, 1974). Replacement of host flora with less virulent and yet protective organisms has also been suggested (Feingold, 1970).

For the present time there is much we can do to educate ourselves and colleagues about the merits of already established practices and procedures of infection control. Special presentations to employees working in housekeeping and dietetics are necessary because they are not as knowledgeable about medical topics as are physicians and nurses. Of the latter, it is unfortunate but true that some physicians are less inclined to follow established infection control practices, simply because they fail to realize their importance and significance. An occasional stimulating, clinically oriented presentation to the medical and surgical staff about the hazards of hospital infections can be quite helpful in this regard. Although physicians are rarely incriminated outside of the operating room as a source of hospital infection, they are objects of scrutiny by all other hospital employees, as well as by patients and visitors. Physicians' words, and actions can do much to improve rather than detract from a hospital infection control program.

REFERENCES

Altemeier, W. A., Burke, J. F., Pruitt, B. A., et al.: Manual on Control of Infection in Surgical Patients. Philadelphia, J. B. Lippincott, 1976.

American Hospital Association, Committee on Infections Within Hospitals: Statement on microbiologic sampling in the hospital. Hospitals, *48*:125, 1974.

American Public Health Association, Committee on Microbial Contamination of Surfaces: Environmental microbiologic sampling in the hospital. Health Lab. Sci., *12*:234, 1975.

Antall, J., and Szebelledy, G.: Pictures from the History of Medicine: The Semmelweis Medical Historical Museum. Budapest, Corvina Press, 1973, p. 15.

Bamran, E. A., et al.: Bacteriologic studies relating to handwashing. I. The inability of soap bars to transmit bacteria. Am. J. Publ. Health, *55*:915, 1965.

Barrett-Connor, E.: Control and prevention of hospital-acquired infection. Prevent. Med., *1*:195, 1972.

Bean, W. B.: Sir William Osler: Aphorisms from his bedside teachings and writings collected by Robert Bennett Bean. New York, Henry Schuman, 1930, p. 130.

Blumberg, B. S.: Bioethical questions related to hepatitis B antigen. Am. J. Clin. Pathol., *65*:848, 1976.

Bodey, G. P.: Isolation for the compromised host. J.A.M.A., *233*:543, 1975.

Castle, M., and Mallison, G. F.: Effective investigations of nosocomial outbreaks. Assoc. Prac. Infec. Control, *5*:13, 1977.

Center for Disease Control, Committee on Viral Hepatitis: Perspectives on the control of viral hepatitis, type B. Morbid. Mortal. Rep. (Suppl), *25*:3, 1976.

Center for Disease Control: Isolation Techniques for Use in Hospitals. Washington, U.S. Government Printing Office, 1975.

Center for Disease Control: Laboratory aspects in the control of nosocomial infections. National Nosocomial Infection Study Report, Annual Summary 1974, p. 27.

Craven, R. B., Wenzel, R. P., and Atuk, N. O.: Minimizing tuberculosis risk to hospital personnel and students exposed to unsuspected disease. Ann. Intern. Med., *82*:628, 1975.

Cruse, P. J. E., and Foord, R.: A 5 year prospective study of 23,649 surgical wounds. Arch. Surg., *107*:206, 1973.

Dixon, R. E., Kaslow, R. A., Mackel, D. C., et al.: Aqueous quarternary ammonium antiseptics and disinfectants. J.A.M.A., *236*:2415, 1976.

Dornette, W. H. L.: Legal aspects of hospital-acquired infection. J. Legal Med., p. 37, 1973.

Edwards, L. D., Levin, S., and Lepper, M. H.: Descriptive epidemiology. Environ. San., *45*:75, 1971.

Feingold, D. S.: Hospital-acquired infections. N. Engl. J. Med., *283*:1384, 1970.

Flewett, T. H., Bryden, A. S., Davies, H., et al.: Epidemic viral enteritis in a long-stay children's ward. Lancet, *1*:4, 1975.

Fracastorius, H.: Contagion—History of Medicine Series II. New York, G. P. Putnam's Sons, 1930, p. 7.

Furey, W. W., and Stefancic, M. F.: Tuberculosis in a community hospital. J.A.M.A., *235*:168, 1976.

Garner, J. S., Bennett, J. V., Scheckler, W. E., et al.: Surveillance of nosocomial infection. Proceedings of the International Conference on Nosocomial Infections, Atlanta, 1970, p. 277.

Grady, G. F., and Lee, V. A.: Hepatitis B immune globulin—prevention of hepatitis from accidental exposure among medical personnel. N. Engl. J. Med., *293*:1067, 1975.

Guthrie, D.: Lord Lister, His Life and Doctrine. Edinburgh, E. S. Livingstone, 1949, p. 55.

Hewitt, W. L., and Sanford, J. P.: Workshop on hospital-associated infections. J. Infect. Dis., *130*:680, 1974.

Hill, A. B.: Principles of Medical Statistics. New York, Oxford University, 1971.

Joint Commission on Accreditation of Hospitals: Infection Control—Standards Adopted by Board of Commissioners, December, 1975.

Lorian, V., and Topf, B.: Microbiology of nosocomial infections. Arch. Intern. Med., *130*:104, 1972.

MacGregor, R. R.: A year's experience with tuberculosis in a private urban teaching hospital in the post sanatorium era. Am. J. Med., *58*:221, 1975.

Maki, D. G., Goldmann, D. A., and Rhame F. S.: Infection control in intravenous therapy. Ann. Intern. Med., *79*:867, 1973.

McCormick, J. B., and Bennett, J. V.: Public health considerations in the management of meningococcal disease. Ann. Intern. Med., *83*:883, 1975.

Melnick, J. L., Dreesman, G. R., and Hollinger, F. B.: Approaching the control of viral hepatitis, type B. J. Infect. Dis., *133*:210, 1976.

Nightingale, F.: Notes on Hospitals. London, Longman, Green, Longman, Roberts and Green, 1863, preface p. iii.

Pickering, L. K.: Chemoprophylaxis against *Neisseria meningitidis*. J.A.M.A., *236*:1882, 1976.

Pierce, A. K., and Sanford, J. P.: Bacterial contamination of aerosols. Arch. Intern. Med., *131*:156, 1973.

Stamm, W. E.: Guidelines for prevention of catheter-associated urinary tract infections. Ann. Intern. Med., *82*:386, 1975.

Steere, A. C., and Mallison, G. F.: Handwashing practices for the prevention of nosocomial infections. Ann. Intern. Med., *83*:683, 1975.

Subcommittee on Aseptic Methods in Operating Theatres:

Preparation of the patient and performance of the operation. Lancet, *1*:834, 1968.

Vallery-Radot, R.: The Life of Pasteur. New York, Garden City, 1916, p. 274.

Walsh, J. H., Yalow, R., and Benson, S. A.: Detection of Australia antigen and antibody by means of radioimmunoassay techniques. J. Infect. Dis., *121*:550, 1970.

Young, D. S., Hicks, J. M., and Pestaner, L. C.: Directory of rare analyses. Clin. Chem., *23*:323, 1977.

Part 6

ADMINISTRATION OF THE CLINICAL LABORATORY

*Edited by William W. McLendon, M.D.,
and John Bernard Henry, M.D.*

58

ORGANIZATION AND MANAGEMENT OF THE CLINICAL LABORATORY

William W. McLendon, M.D. and
Michael D. Reich

The efficient operation of a clinical laboratory and the effective delivery of medical laboratory services to clinicians and their patients require a complex interdigitation of expertise in medical, scientific, and technical areas; resources in the form of personnel, equipment, supplies, and facilities; and skills in organization, management, and communication. Laboratory directors today and in the future must also be aware of the many accreditation standards and governmental regulations which apply to laboratory practice and must assure quality laboratory performance. The spiralling costs of medical care mandate that those in clinical laboratories and their clinical colleagues be concerned as well with the effective utilization of laboratory services in medical care.

Although the medical, scientific, and technical expertise covered in preceding sections of this text are an essential prerequisite for the provision of medical laboratory services, success in applying these techniques to benefit patient care is vitally dependent on the management and communication skills of laboratory directors, supervisors, and technologists.

The relationship of these aspects of laboratory practice to science and medicine can be best understood in reference to Figure 58-1. The discipline of laboratory medicine can be viewed as a bridging endeavor linking the basic medical, biologic, and physical sciences with the applied medical sciences. Those working in clinical laboratories have the exciting opportunity and challenge to apply advances in the sciences to assist their clinical colleagues in making diagnostic, therapeutic, and prognostic decisions. In this role the laboratorian serves as a clinical consultant to the clinician and the patient. Most persons in laboratory medicine also serve roles as research or developmental scientists and as educators.

As shown in the same illustration, however, this purely scientific and clinical approach to laboratory medicine is no longer sufficient. The bridge between the basic sciences and the clinical services is now buttressed by essential support derived from computer science, management techniques, technology, and industry. In the future this entire activity will be guided, and to an ever greater extent restricted, by the proliferation of accreditation

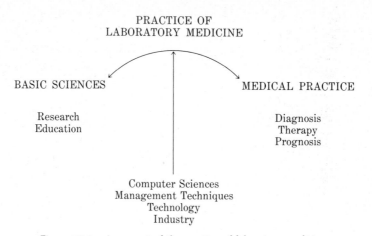

PRACTICE OF
LABORATORY MEDICINE

BASIC SCIENCES   MEDICAL PRACTICE

Research   Diagnosis
Education   Therapy
                                  Prognosis

Computer Sciences
Management Techniques
Technology
Industry

Figure 58–1. A concept of the practice of laboratory medicine.

standards, governmental regulations, and financial constraints.

An overview of the multiple functions performed by those in laboratory medicine is seen schematically in Table 58–1.

To be successful today, persons in laboratory medicine must be aware of all these functions and all those external influences affecting the practice of laboratory medicine and must assume other roles as well—those of managers and executives. Managers are those who manage the work of others, while executives are all those knowledge workers in a modern organization who, by virtue of position and knowledge, are responsible for contributions that significantly affect the capacity of the organization to perform and obtain results (Drucker, 1967). By this definition, all the key persons in a modern clinical laboratory are executives; that is, laboratory directors, managers, supervisors, and technologists.

Dorsey (1969) has summarized the most prominent indicators of a lack of management and communications skills on the part of clinical laboratory executives:

1. Inability to maintain an adequate staff. The deficiency may be due to an insufficient number of trained workers or inefficient use of the personnel available.

2. Recurring or persistent misunderstandings with the hospital administration.

3. Frequent or recurrent confusion concerning requisitions or reports of laboratory work. It makes little difference how accurately a technologist performs a test if the report doesn't reach the doctor until 48 hours later, or if the result is reported on the wrong chart.

Table 58–1. SCHEMATIC OUTLINE OF ACTIVITIES IN LABORATORY MEDICINE

MANAGEMENT					
Planning	Fiscal	Facilities	Materials	Personnel	Licensure and accreditation
PATIENT CARE SERVICE					
Indications and selection of procedures		Technology and generation of data	Data evaluation, interpretation, and communication	Quality assurance	Effective utilization of the laboratory
TEACHING					
Medical technologists	Residents and fellows in laboratory medicine (clinical pathology)	Medical students	Clinical house staff	Attending staff	Other medical and health related professionals
RESEARCH					
Basic		Methodological			Clinical

4. Frequent "rush" orders for supplies.

5. Low morale in the laboratory.

6. Requests for deserved pay raises by competent workers [when funds are available].

7. Excessive cost of operation.

8. Ignorance of the cost of operation.

9. Expenditure of much of the director's time in making minor decisions.

10. Inability to do one or more tests when a key individual has a day off.

Success as an executive in a clinical laboratory is dependent upon the acquisition of management knowledge and skills as well as the development of certain personal characteristics. Scheer provides five such characteristics essential to success for an executive, whether one is in business or in laboratory medicine (Dorsey, 1969):

1. *Motivation.* The executive's value is in direct proportion to his ability to motivate himself and his workers.

2. *Vision.* Every executive is a supervisor. The word supervisor carries the connotation of someone possessed with "super" vision; hence, one capable of seeing over and beyond the obvious.

3. *Decision-making ability.* The man who cannot make decisions must yield authority to one who can.

4. *Good health.* In this case good health embodies more than physical fitness. It means living a balanced life physically, emotionally, and spiritually as the best antidote to the tensions, frustrations, strain, and effort which are the lot of the executive.

5. *Humility.* This implies the recognition that we each have shortcomings, that we are not self-sufficient, and that we need the help of our subordinates just as much as they need our help.

It is our purpose to provide guidelines for operation of laboratories with consideration of the organization and management of clinical laboratories in this chapter; fiscal management in Chapter 59; communications and data processing in Chapter 60; legal aspects of laboratory medicine in Chapter 61; effective utilization of laboratory services in Chapter 62; and monitoring quality of laboratory measurements in Chapter 63. Space limitations preclude a thorough coverage of these topics, and readers are referred to the works cited in the References of each chapter, as well as those general references and sources listed at the end of this chapter. The recent volumes on clinical laboratory management, as well as the more general works on management, particularly those of Peter Drucker, are highly recommended. *The Effective Executive* by Drucker is a readable introduction to the problems and challenges of being an executive with practical suggestions for becoming a more effective executive. The *Achievement Planning Calendar* (source listed at the end of this chapter) provides a valuable tool for setting individual goals and objectives on a five-year, one-year, and monthly basis. The format of the calendar encourages systematic planning for the year and month with the opportunity to review what has, and has not, been accomplished at the end of each month and year. Every laboratory director and supervisor should also be familiar with the regulations of the Joint Committee on Accreditation of Hospitals (JCAH) in regard to pathology services and the applicable local, state, and federal governmental regulations. The *Laboratory Regulation Manual,* a publication of the Health Law Center with quarterly supplements and newsletter, provides detailed current information on laboratory regulations at the local, state, and federal level. The *Standards for Accreditation of Medical Laboratories,* the *Inspection Checklists,* and the *Inspection and Accreditation Newsletter,* all available from the College of American Pathologists, are particularly valuable, since they provide a distillation of laboratory regulations from a variety of sources.

SETTING GOALS AND OBJECTIVES

The first step in a systematic approach to the organization and management of the clinical laboratory begins with the establishment of general goals and specific objectives by the laboratory staff. The use of such objectives for purposes of management is known as management by objectives or MBO (Bennington, 1977). In order to achieve these objectives, the clinical laboratory must have adequate facilities, equipment and supplies, and an adequate number of qualified personnel; each of these three areas is briefly considered in the succeeding sections of this chapter.

As used here, *goals* are those general and qualitative statements of overall philosophy of the organization. An example of a goal is: "a commitment by the laboratories to be a vital component of a hospital whose goal is to provide a patient care environment of excellence, to serve the community, and to serve as the primary setting for clinical teaching and research for the medical school." *Objectives* are

6

the statements of the more specific and quantifiable steps taken to achieve the organizational goals (Bennington, 1977). An example of an objective is: "to evaluate the available methods and to introduce into regular use an LDH isoenzyme procedure by January."

The goals should be consistent with the organizational structure, the management style of the laboratory director, and the available resources. In turn, such goals should influence the future programs of the laboratory and the activities of the director and the laboratory staff.

The types of goals set for a laboratory will vary greatly. For instance, the goals for the operation of an office laboratory with two physicians are vastly different from those of a reference laboratory serving thousands of physicians and patients in a large geographic area. Almost as great a difference in goals may exist for laboratories in similar sized hospitals, depending upon the types of patients served, the nature of the hospital (acute care versus chronic care; secondary versus tertiary care), and the nature of the educational and research commitments.

A useful exercise for a new laboratory, or periodically for an existing laboratory, is to put into writing the *overall goals* of the laboratory after discussions with the appropriate persons in the organization. Such written goals may be organized as follows:

1. A statement of the primary external goals of the laboratory. Most laboratories exist within the framework of some other institution such as a hospital, clinic, practice, or corporation. The goals of the laboratory should thus be a subset of the overall goals of that organization or institution. As pointed out by Drucker (1967), "what happens inside any organization is only effort and cost while the results of those efforts and costs are on the outside." Specifically, a hospital or laboratory has results only with respect to the patient, who is not a member of the hospital or laboratory organization. Without a stated primary commitment to the patient, Lundberg (1975) has commented that "in a complicated health-care organization the patients' true needs are often lost in the clamor of special interests."

2. A statement of the primary internal goal of the laboratory in reference to service, research, and education.

3. A statement as to the secondary and tertiary goals of the laboratory in reference to service, research, and education.

4. A statement in reference to the management philosophy and need for cost effectiveness.

5. A statement as to what kind of environment is desired in the laboratory with respect to interpersonal relationships, working conditions, and attitudes toward teaching and scholarly activities.

Such overall goals, once established, like laboratory procedure manuals and policies, should be reviewed every year and appropriate modifications made. If the goals have been thoughtfully composed, such modifications should be minimal unless a major change has been made in the parent organization or in the leadership of the laboratory. Such a review can most productively be done at the time of the year when the current year's accomplishments are being reviewed and the goals for the next budget year are being established.

In contrast to the more general goals mentioned above, objectives should be quantifiable statements of aims which are achievable in a designated time frame. They should be formulated as part of planning for the next year's budget and as part of a multi-year long-range planning effort (See Chap. 59). Experience indicates that success in attaining objectives is enhanced when the affected personnel have input into formulating the objectives, as contrasted with the objectives being decreed from above. Priority ranking of objectives based on organizational goals is useful, since resources may limit the ability to implement all objectives within a designated planning period. They should be designed to measure specific results in the organization rather than simply stating philosophical goals. Management by objectives, to be effective, should lead to specific results which can be quantitatively monitored over time to see if the objectives are achieved as scheduled.

LABORATORY FACILITIES AND ORGANIZATION

This discussion of laboratory design is intended as an outline of the considerations necessary in preparing a functional design for a clinical laboratory. A *Manual for Laboratory Planning and Design* should be consulted for details, specific suggestions, examples of laboratories, and an excellent bibliography (Thomas, 1977).

The successful design of a functional clinical laboratory, either new or renovated, requires the close cooperation of several groups of professionals. First, the laboratory director and the entire laboratory staff need to be intimately and continually involved with the process. The laboratory director should have a clear understanding with the appropriate administrative personnel concerning the right to final review of all plans and any changes. In order to prevent misunderstandings, all recommendations and changes must be documented in writing. Second, outside consultants or designers of laboratories may be utilized, although this is not an essential feature. Third, an architect or architectural firm is essential to prepare the various drawings and specifications, the final approved copies of which will be used in the bidding process and by the contractor for construction. Fourth, a contractor is needed to construct the facility.

FUNCTIONAL CONSIDERATIONS IN LABORATORY DESIGN

The laboratory director having the opportunity to design a new laboratory or make major renovations in an older laboratory should think in functional terms about the laboratory operation and its facility needs.

Traditionally laboratories have been organized in relationship to techniques or historical accident rather than in relationship to clinical problems, disease orientation, or functional efficiency. It has been pointed out that traditional laboratories have a mixture of approaches: for example, clinical chemistry is technique oriented; clinical microbiology is technique and disease oriented; urinalysis is specimen oriented; hematology is specimen and organ system oriented; and blood bank is product oriented. Such an organizational approach may continue to be of value in the future, but the following functional approaches should also be considered.

TAT Laboratories. In an effort to make laboratories more responsive to the needs of the using physician, the concept of laboratory organization based on turn-around time (TAT) has evolved (Lundberg, 1975). In this approach, laboratories are organized on the basis of turn-around time, that is, the elapsed time from arrival of the specimen in the laboratory to the availability of the result in the laboratory. No STAT requests are accepted. The one-hour-or-less TAT laboratory operates 24 hours a day, 7 days a week and manually performs those procedures such as electrolytes, amylase, and blood gases needed for immediate patient care. The four-hour-or-less TAT laboratory also operates around the clock but uses predominantly automated equipment to meet the bulk of on-going patient care requirements. The 24-hour-or-less TAT laboratory operates one or more shifts 7 days a week with predominately automated equipment to provide the less urgent routine procedures. The greater than 24-hour TAT laboratory may operate one shift 5 days a week and provides the more sophisticated, low-volume procedures. This approach to the organization of laboratories is analogous to recent trends in hospitals to organize patient care in a progression of levels of care, such as critical care, routine, and ambulatory care units.

Disease- or Problem-Oriented Laboratories. Another approach to functional organization of the laboratory includes the development of disease- or problem-oriented laboratories. In some medical centers these may be satellite laboratories devoted to areas such as birth defects, immunology, or rheumatology, but such laboratories are best developed as components of centralized laboratories. An approach not requiring complete functional reorganization of the central laboratories is to offer panels of procedures for the specific disease or problem-oriented situation. The individual tests composing the panels (Henry, 1977) can be performed in the traditional laboratories with data correlation done manually or automated. The development of computer systems for handling all of the laboratory data allows sorting of data into meaningful and appropriate test groupings on reports, thus permitting a disease- or problem-oriented approach within a traditional laboratory organization.

Automated Laboratories. Still another functional approach to the organization of laboratories has been proposed by Reece (1974). He believes that the automated laboratory of the future should use production-line techniques and statistical methods to produce clinician-oriented results. This will be accomplished by reorganizing laboratories into three major divisions:

THE RECEIVING DIVISION. This area would be charged with receiving the specimen, re-

6

cording the requisition and patient data, and preparing the specimen for analysis. All information affecting the subsequent interpretation of the results (e.g., drugs, pregnancy, lipemia) would be entered in the computer here.

THE PROCESSING DIVISION. This division would consist of the laboratory where procedures are performed and data generated.

THE TRANSMITTING DIVISION. This division would process the data output from the laboratory and then transmit the results in comprehensive, readable, problem-oriented reports to the requesting physician. It also would provide the means for the monitoring of the data by the laboratory directors and supervisors.

SPATIAL CONSIDERATIONS IN LABORATORY DESIGN

Spatial Relationships Within the Institution. If the laboratory director has the opportunity to design a laboratory for an entirely new building or hospital, or to relocate a laboratory in an existing hospital or building, it is critical that the location of the laboratory be studied in relationship to the other hospital services, to traffic, and to supporting services and users. For example, the blood bank and the stat laboratory procedures should be readily accessible to the emergency room, operating rooms, and intensive care unit. The location of the blood bank should allow rapid access and egress of donors and adequate parking for donors. The blood drawing areas and specimen collection areas need to be planned in relationship to the ambulatory care facilities. The relationship to the central supply and other supporting areas needs to be considered. If the laboratory is serving an inpatient population, the accessibility to corridors and elevators providing access to the main patient care units is essential.

Intralaboratory Relationships. The relationship of various laboratories to each other and to supporting areas such as blood drawing, data processing, glass washing, and storage should be taken into account. An ideal arrangement is to have a receiving, data processing, and reporting center serve as the hub of the laboratory. Radiating from this could be the various laboratories. The stat laboratories and large volume laboratories such as hematology and chemistry might be most closely related to these central areas, while the labo-

ratories with greater turn-around time and/or less volume, such as clinical microbiology and radioassay laboratories, might be located at a somewhat greater distance from the central areas.

A systematic approach to determining the optimal internal layout of laboratories is available (Gonzales-Menocal, 1973). The same system may be used when designing a hospital to determine the best location for a laboratory in relationship to other hospital services.

Traffic Flow. It is very important to plan the traffic flow so that intralaboratory traffic is separated from outside traffic. Provisions should be made for ambulatory patients and blood bank donors coming into the laboratory. The flow of specimens can be coordinated through a central receiving area which is readily accessible to those bringing specimens to the laboratory. If possible, this function may be coordinated with the ambulatory blood drawing area. The hub concept of a central receiving and processing area is a useful one, with requisitions flowing into the laboratory and data for reporting flowing back to this center. All inquiries can be directed to this central area; only those for procedures which are in process would have to be referred to individual laboratories.

SPECIFIC DESIGN CONSIDERATIONS

Square Footage. The gross square footage of laboratory space can be calculated by using the outside dimensions of laboratory sections or of an entire laboratory to determine the square footage. A more important consideration, however, is the net square footage. This represents the gross square footage less the square footage occupied by halls, stairways, walls, chases, elevators, restrooms, and other common spaces. The net square footage thus gives one an indication of the actual square footage available for laboratory use. Depending on the design of the laboratory, the net square footage in modern clinical laboratories varies from approximately 65 per cent to 90 per cent of the gross square footage, according to a recent survey (Thomas, 1977).

Mechanical Services. Proper planning of mechanical services is essential for any laboratory. Special attention should be paid to temperature control and air handling, especially in reference to staff comfort and safety.

Noise control is also of vital importance for the morale and productivity of the laboratory staff.

Casework and Interior Design. One of the most important decisions the laboratory director has to make in regard to a new or renovated laboratory is the nature of the casework (laboratory benches and cabinets) which will be used in the laboratory. In a small laboratory it is usually appropriate simply to design the casework as part of the internal planning for the laboratory and to have this built in by the contractor. In the larger laboratory with multiple laboratory sections, however, it is generally preferable to obtain standard casework from some reputable manufacturer. Because it is impossible to anticipate completely the future needs of the laboratory, many manufacturers are offering modular designs for laboratory casework. This approach may provide utilities along the outer walls of the laboratory with some flexibility in the cabinet components which can be attached to supporting framework. Such a system allows the laboratory to make future changes in one or more laboratory sections by exchanging component parts or obtaining additional component parts from the manufacturer. It also tends to minimize the amount of plumbing and carpentry work which is necessary as changes are made. Such cabinet work generally adds a higher cost initially; hence, this must be weighed against the likelihood that this flexibility will be required in the future.

On a larger scale, the laboratory director should also investigate the desirability of a modular approach to interior walls within the laboratory. Such a system has to be carefully designed by the architect to coordinate with a modular or grid system in the ceiling and floor utilities. This can be very expensive, but may be worthwhile if the laboratory anticipates major changes. Another approach is to have the laboratory built with rigid outside walls and the interior divided by partial or complete modular walls as part of the casework.

Communications. By the nature of its activity, a clinical laboratory has as one of its primary functions the process of communication of information, both within the laboratory and between the laboratory and the physician users (See also Chap. 60). In the one- or two-room laboratory, a telephone with one or two extensions and one or two incoming lines may suffice. The problem is much more complex in the multi-section laboratory. Here a decision must be made as to whether there will be a central answering service with the ability to transfer calls to the individual sections or whether each section will have its own line or lines. The use of consultants from the local telephone company in the planning stage can be very helpful to the laboratory director in making these plans.

Intercom systems usually are essential within larger laboratories and may be of two types. One is the hands-on, private communication which is a part of the telephone system. This has the advantages that additional equipment is not needed, telephone conversations can be private, and switching from the intercom to telephone lines is convenient. For laboratory areas where persons are performing tests and may not be able to answer a telephone, a public address type of intercom system may be desirable. This has the disadvantage of contributing significantly to the noise level of the laboratory environment, but the trade-off in terms of efficiency of operation may be necessary.

Since most larger laboratories today, or in the not-too-distant future, will have automated data processing, planning should include consideration of the installation and location of conduits and terminal boxes for data processing equipment. Even if a system does not exist in the laboratory, advice can be obtained concerning the nature of conduits and the location of terminal boxes for future systems. If one is planning to build an entire institution, of which the laboratories are a part, consideration should also be given to the necessity for conduits connecting the laboratory and hospital computer systems with nursing stations and other hospital areas. A computer located within the laboratory may require special attention to air conditioning and humidity.

Safety. During the planning stage the laboratory director should become thoroughly familiar with the federal Occupational Health and Safety Act regulations as well as state and local regulations. The current checklists of the College of American Pathologists Inspection and Accreditation Program offer a convenient guide to safety requirements, since they are designed to highlight the major safety requirements of the laboratory. The Joint Commission on Accreditation of Hospitals also offers a useful self-evaluation form on Safety and Sanitation.

The fire safety measures will be determined

6

to a large extent by local regulations. Biologic, toxic, and radioactive hazards also have to be considered. Design of hoods and ventilation systems should be based on the anticipated use of toxic or biologic hazards in the various laboratory areas.

General Laboratory Support Functions.
The following are some of the general laboratory support functions which are frequently neglected in laboratory planning.

STOREROOMS. It should be determined whether the major storage will be handled outside of the laboratory or whether a central laboratory storeroom will be needed. Regardless of this decision, sufficient storage should be available within each laboratory to handle several days to several weeks supply of critical material. Modular storage cabinets which can be filled in a central storeroom and then transported to the laboratory areas should be investigated. Special consideration should be given to the storage of flammables and compressed gases.

GLASSWARE WASHING. Although at one time it seemed that most of the glassware being used in laboratories would be replaced by disposables, the need to conserve energy has forced laboratories to reconsider recycling many items. Washroom and appropriate sterilization facilities should be included in any laboratory design. Media and reagent preparation facilities may also be needed.

LOUNGES AND TOILETS. These are essential for the comfort and morale of the employees and must be included in any plans. Local building codes generally will specify the minimum facilities of this type which must be made available.

BLOOD COLLECTING AREA AND EXAMINING ROOMS. If the laboratory provides blood collection for ambulatory patients, adequate facilities including waiting rooms and restrooms for patients should be designed. Many laboratories are finding that this can be most effectively planned as part of a central receiving and processing area. Data processing terminals should be available in this area for entry of patient test requisitions and for preparation of blood collection labels.

LIBRARY AND CONFERENCE ROOMS. These facilities are essential both for teaching programs and for continuing education.

SPACE FOR RESEARCH AND DEVELOPMENT. Depending upon the goals and needs of the laboratory, space may be allotted for research and development work.

STAGES IN LABORATORY DESIGN AND BUILDING

Preparation of a Functional Program.
The functional program is defined as a written document giving the purposes of the laboratory, the functions which are necessary to achieve these purposes, and the various interrelationships of functions within the laboratory. The program should not include square footage estimates as such, but should include detailed information concerning the current and proposed figures for the number of patients to be served and specimens to be processed; the number of technical, clerical, and supervisory personnel; and the number of clinical scientists and pathologists. A detailed listing of bench space required per technologist is desirable as well as a detailed listing of the present and anticipated bench top and freestanding equipment. If teaching programs exist, the number of students to be housed in the laboratory for both lecture and bench type instruction should be taken into consideration.

During the development of the functional program, the temptation to sketch out the laboratory design should be resisted and saved for the architect at a later stage. It is essential, however, to generate functional flow diagrams of the processes proposed for the laboratory; this is invaluable to the architect.

One should also avoid the temptation to adopt some standardized square footage figure or to copy some other laboratory. It is, however, useful to visit other laboratories, especially recently constructed or renovated laboratories, to profit by their successes and failures. The Manual cited (p. 1980) provides information on a number of recently constructed clinical laboratories (Thomas, 1977), while the Veterans Administration Manual on Planning Criteria for Medical Facilities (Veterans Administration, 1974) gives guidelines on square footage for various laboratories; both of these sources may be consulted after the determination of needed square footage is made to detect omissions or other errors.

In the preparation of the functional program, general statements about flexibility and the potential need for expansion in the future are essential. In terms of flexibility, one might consider modular laboratory furniture and perhaps modular wall systems. In view of the continuing growth of laboratory services, one must also plan for future expansion.

If a specific budget exists for the construction, this amount should be made known to the architects at this stage to assist in their planning.

Schematic Design Drawing. In this stage the laboratory personnel responsible for planning the new or renovated laboratory should meet with the architects to help them develop an understanding of the relationships of one laboratory to another and of the laboratories to other services in the institution. The architect will use the functional program narrative at this point to translate the specific functional requirements into an architectural program which assigns space to the functions. From this point simple line drawings are developed to show the possible arrangements of laboratories and their divisions with suggested corridors, stairways, elevators, lounges, and other common areas.

Design Development Drawing. These drawings represent the next stage of architectural design and provide the detailed location of doors, windows, partitions, fixed and movable equipment, bench space, seats, furniture, and associated support facilities. They also include details of the proposed mechanical, electrical, and plumbing needs. At this point it is extremely important for the laboratory to furnish the architect with a complete list of present and proposed equipment, including specific electrical requirements, size, and estimated BTU output. The latter is of extreme importance, since too often air conditioning systems are designed for the number of personnel in an area, neglecting the much greater output of heat by modern automated laboratory equipment.

Working Drawings and Specifications. These drawings represent the final or contract documents and give the detailed information necessary for construction of the proposed laboratory. Architectural drawings of the structure are supplemented by detailed drawings of the plumbing, electrical, and mechanical services. A set of specifications is also prepared to document the quality of materials, as contrasted to the working drawings which delineate the location of materials.

Period of Construction. After bids are let and the contractor is chosen, the laboratory director will have to deal through the owner's representative or the architect. It is important that the progress of the building be monitored and that problems be called to the attention of the appropriate person. Change orders must be in writing and must go through the archi-

tect or owner's representative to the contractor. The director should be aware of the fact that change orders may be very expensive and should be avoided except where absolutely necessary. The more comprehensive the planning prior to construction, the less the need for change orders during construction.

At the conclusion of the construction, the owner or person responsible makes a final inspection, with documentation of those items which must be corrected before the building is accepted. The laboratory director or a designee should be involved in this process.

PURCHASING

Clinical laboratories, as a business, require raw materials for successful operation. Whereas equipment idled by breakdowns or lack of supplies is an economic loss for business, the same situation in the clinical laboratory can seriously interfere with the delivery of patient care.

Responsible people must decide what supplies they need, when they need them, and in what quantities. Much time can be wasted in the purchasing procedure unless a workable procurement system is developed. In the larger medical centers, the purchasing process may involve many people and elaborate systems for obtaining bids, for quantity buying, and for sharing purchasing power with other institutions. In contrast, in the physician's office laboratory, the entire process may be handled by the technologist dealing directly with the vendors.

Whatever the environment, two essential components are common to most purchasing systems. Product research and well-developed specifications help assure adequate quality of purchases, while inventory control helps assure adequate quantity of materials for the laboratory operation.

PRODUCT SPECIFICATIONS

Since the basis for any purchasing process is the need to procure goods to meet specific needs, time must be spent on product research leading to the development of product specifications. The medical laboratory supply market is very competitive, with many similar items available for each need; only through product investigation can the best product for the available funds be determined.

This process can be accomplished by comparative evaluations within the laboratory, by consultation with other users, or by reference to publications offering comparative studies of equipment and supplies. Product specifications prepared after such a study help assure adequate quality of purchased reagents and supplies.

A similar process of evaluation and product specification is necessary prior to purchase of major equipment. In addition, the following considerations are important:

1. Written specifications must include a detailed description of the required equipment; specifications should never be made by verbal agreement.
2. On-site visits to see equipment operating in other laboratories is encouraged. More valuable is the trial installation of the equipment within the laboratory. This allows operation of the equipment under the particular conditions of the laboratory; equally importantly, it gives personnel an opportunity to test the equipment and have input into the purchase decision.
3. An environment necessary to accommodate the equipment must be prepared in advance. Such special requirements as high amperage, special gases, controlled humidity, unusual weight loads, or high BTU output are but a few of the considerations. Not infrequently laboratories receive much-needed equipment which then lies idle for weeks or months while an adequate area is belatedly prepared.
4. A more complicated decision, but one that must be made, is whether to lease, rent, or buy major equipment. See Chapter 59 for discussion of this issue.
5. In the United States, approval by a Health Systems Agency under Public Law 93-641 may be necessary for major equipment (see Chap. 59). This process can usually be accomplished in parallel with the product evaluation and specifications.
6. Complete instruction manuals should be obtained with the instrument and preventive maintenance schedules established (Hamlin, 1974).

PURCHASING OF SUPPLIES

Orders should be placed only by authorized staff members who are familiar with the quality of service and reliability of the suppliers. Delivery schedules are a major factor in determining whether a purchasing system is in or out of control. High-use items should be delivered frequently. Release orders and standing orders are excellent methods of doing this and can save the laboratory time and money. Release orders are annual contracts in which the vendor agrees to deliver goods at a predetermined price as notified by the laboratory. The standing order is an annual contract in which the vendor agrees to deliver goods at a predetermined price and on an established schedule.

RECEIVING AND ACCOUNTS PAYABLE

Goods should be unpacked and inspected as soon as possible to insure that everything is delivered or that some acknowledgement of back-ordered items is made. Damaged or defective goods should be identified early in order to assure replacement or credit.

Three pieces of information must agree before the vendor's bill will be paid by most accounts payable systems: the purchase request must agree with the invoice, the invoice must agree with the packing slip, and they all must agree with the final bill from the vendor. Any non-agreement between the figures results in payment to the vendor being withheld.

RECORDS AND INVENTORY CONTROL

Much has been written about inventory control, and there are elaborate formulas for deciding inventory size and reordering time, but for most laboratories simpler methods will serve as well. One of these methods is through the use of an inventory system using stock record cards, as shown in Figure 58-2.

In an inventory system levels are set at low and high points. The low level is that point at which on-hand supplies are sufficient to carry the laboratory through until goods on order are received. The upper limit is that level which will meet the laboratories requirements for a longer period of time, such as several months to a year. The primary factors determining these limits are the anticipated delivery time for each item, the available storage space, the shelf life of the item, and the anticipated rate of usage.

An effective inventory control system requires excellent communications between all sections of the laboratory and the person(s) responsible for purchasing. The latter must be made aware of anticipated increases or de-

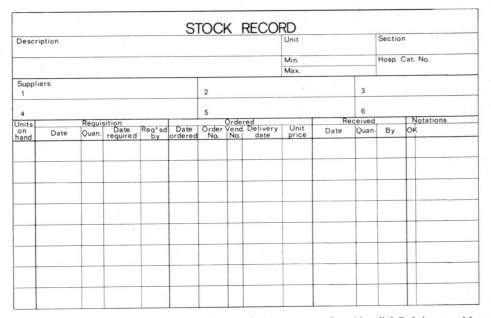

Figure 58–2. Stock record card for inventory system. (Reprinted with permission from Newell, J. E.: Laboratory Management. Boston, Little, Brown and Company, 1972, p. 144.)

creases in requirements for all items and must closely monitor delivery times and vendor performance.

PERSONNEL

A clinical laboratory should have goals and objectives and must have facilities, supplies, and equipment. The most essential component in any health care activity, however, is people. In addition, salaries and related benefits comprise 60 to 70 per cent of most laboratory expense budgets. The responsible laboratory director thus should be concerned with developing this human resource to its optimal level, as management has been defined as "getting things done through the efforts of other people." This requires an understanding of those factors affecting motivation and those techniques available for personnel management.

MOTIVATION

The day-to-day operation of a laboratory and the motivation of the persons in that laboratory will be determined to a large extent by the management style of those responsible for directing the institution, the laboratory, and the various laboratory sections. Such manage-

ment styles are determined by a person's personality and previous experience, but can be modified if a conscious effort is made.

Current understanding of the influence of leadership and management styles on the operation of organizations and the motivation of personnel has been derived from the work of a number of persons, particularly Maslow (1954), McGregor (1960), and Herzberg (1968).

Maslow developed a theory of human motivation based on the fact that man is a wanting animal, that his behavior is determined by unsatisfied needs, and that these needs form an internal hierarchy. He identified five needs and arranged them in a hierarchy of importance from the most fundamental to the ones providing the most satisfaction. These are as follows: bodily needs such as food, clothing, and shelter; the need to feel secure; the need to feel loved or wanted; the ego need to feel important; and the self-actualization need, or the need to feel that one is doing well and is developing in one's ability. For those who have a job with a reasonable salary and working conditions, the first three levels of internal needs are usually reasonably well satisfied. It is the satisfaction of their needs at the fourth and fifth levels which determine how well persons perform on a job and how well they are motivated.

6

Based on the work of Maslow, McGregor (1960) has described two extreme management styles: Theory X style, which unfortunately still exists in many medical care settings, is a model patterned after Caesar's legions and the medieval church. Such a management style is based on the assumption that people hate work; that they have to be driven, threatened, and punished to achieve organizational goals (such as "good patient care"); and that they lack ambition and want only security. Such an approach worked reasonably well in a time when the average soldier or worker was uneducated and dependent on orders from an authority who had almost unlimited power over a person's life. In today's medical care institutions, where well-educated and highly motivated staff are essential for medical care, such a management style can be disastrous.

At an opposite pole is McGregor's Theory Y management style. This is based on the following assumptions, which he argues are more valid in present-day organizations: work is as natural as rest or play; people don't have to be forced or threatened to work; they will commit themselves to the external organization only to the extent that they can see ways of satisfying their own internal ego and developmental needs; and people want responsiblity and will seek out such responsiblity in the proper environment when given the opportunity.

The degree of delegation of authority and sharing of responsibility will be a reflection both of the size of the laboratory and of the management style of the persons in charge. A Theory X organization will have little delegation of authority and sharing of responsibility. A Theory Y organization, however, is characterized by a decentralized type of organization with greater delegation of authority and sharing of responsibility. As the laboratory organization becomes larger, the need for more delegation should be apparent; failure to ac-

knowledge this will generally lead to major organizational problems. One of the most common management failures in clinical laboratories is the reluctance to share responsibility, thus resulting in the underutilization of talented persons.

The need for delegated authority and shared responsibility is related to the concept of *span of control:* that is, how many persons or operations can one person effectively direct? It is usually felt that one person can direct the activities of some four to eight other persons or groups, although exceptions obviously exist. A laboratory with many individual sections or persons reporting to one director will usually be much less well-managed than a laboratory in which the individuals are consolidated into approximately four or five larger laboratory sections, each of which reports to the laboratory director (Figs. 58-3 and 58-4). The latter laboratory organization provides a well-defined vertical communication structure and also illustrates the difference in line and staff positions. *Line positions* are filled by directors, supervisors, and technologists who are primarily responsible for the delivery of clinical laboratory services and are in a direct line from the director of laboratories, while the *staff positions* are filled by persons who provide a supportive or administrative service for the organization. This distinction is carried over from military organizations, in which the commanding officer, company commander, and platoon leader are line officers, whereas the executive officer is a staff officer.

Other more recent writers on management have recognized many gradations of management styles between the two extremes described by Theory X and Theory Y. It is important to remember that no one style is appropriate in all situations in any one laboratory or organization; the director or supervisor must be able to use the appropriate style for

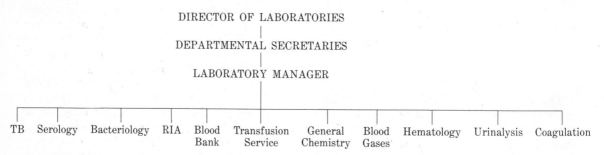

Figure 58-3. A clinical laboratory table of organization showing an extended span of control for the director of laboratories and no recognition of line and staff functions.

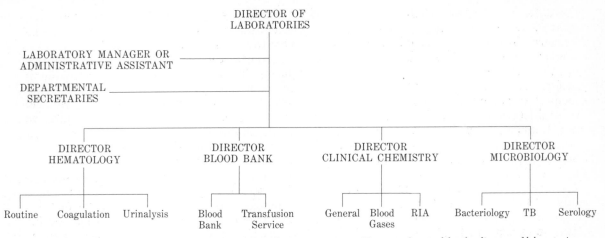

Figure 58-4. A clinical laboratory table of organization illustrating a reasonable span of control for the director of laboratories and delineating the laboratory manager and departmental secretaries as staff functions.

the situation or person with which one is dealing at the moment. Proper understanding and use of these observations on human motivation, however, can lead to better motivated and more productive personnel in the laboratory. In our experience the most effective way to accomplish this is to begin with a mutual commitment by all those in the clinical laboratories to create a working environment in which there is concern for each patient served, mutual respect for each co-worker, and enthusiasm for teaching and advancement of the field of laboratory medicine.

PERSONNEL MANAGEMENT

The more tangible aspects of dealing with personnel in the clinical laboratory setting are addressed in the discussion of personnel management. Personnel policies, procedures, and records are vital to the smooth operation of any laboratory and are necessary to meet accreditation and legal requirements.

Policy Manual. All laboratories should have readily available administrative policy manuals which state the laboratory and institutional policy for the guidance of those working in the laboratory. Recurrent crises concerning the same problems are symptomatic of a laboratory that has no clearly understood and documented policies.

The policy should reflect the philosophy and overall goals of the larger organization as well as those of the laboratory. They should be written in consultation with the persons involved and reviewed by the appropriate per-

sons in the institution (e.g., the personnel department) to be certain they are consistent with institutional policy. Like the laboratory procedure manuals, policies should be dated and approved by the laboratory director. Because of the rapidly changing nature of most laboratory operations they should be reviewed and updated at least annually, with a signature or initials and a date to document this review.

Job Description. A job description is a summary of all the important or significant facts about a particular job. It is a useful tool in classifying positions, determining pay grades, recruitment, orientation of new employees, and setting employee performance standards.

A properly prepared job description answers the following questions:
1. *What* are the duties and responsibilities (including percentages of time spent at the various tasks)?
2. *How, where, and when* are the duties and responsibilities performed?
3. *What* qualifications are required; that is, the knowledge, skills, and abilities needed to do the work?
4. *Why* is the job necessary; that is, what is the purpose of the job?
5. *How* does the job relate to other jobs in the organization?

Each point should be written in a concise, clear way so that anyone can identify the job from the description.

Position Classification. In most organizations, a method for position classification has been developed. This involves determining the different kinds or "classes" of positions existing in the institution. The duties and responsibilities of the positions (job descriptions) are the basis upon which the individual positions are assigned to the appropriate class.

Each class consists of all positions (e.g., medical technologists), regardless of departmental location, that are sufficiently alike in duties and responsibilities to have the same descriptive title, to have the same pay scale, and to require substantially the same qualifications. Within each class, such as Medical Technologist I, a number of pay steps are established. This provides a means to compensate the experienced employee at job entry. The steps also facilitate annual and merit raises, when available.

Recruitment and Selection of Employees. The recruitment and selection of new employees is one of the most crucial management tasks performed in the laboratory, since each person added to the staff influences positively or negatively the future of the laboratory.

The first step in the selection process is the initial screening. Minimum criteria should be defined for each position, and all applicants should be compared to these criteria. The criteria should include such things as minimum education and experience and any required licensure or certification. This initial screening can be accomplished by the personnel department; only those candidates meeting the minimum qualifications should be referred to the laboratory for interviewing. Although the laboratory director may elect to delegate the selection of the personnel to supervisors or others, the final responsibility for the choice rests with the director.

It is much easier to insure that important considerations are not overlooked if the interviewer uses an informal list of established criteria based upon the job description. In the case of a supervisory position these criteria may be qualitative. Such things as problem solving aptitude, ability to communicate, creativity, and innovation may be more important and harder to define than the applicant's technical expertise. This approach also insures that all candidates are compared equitably.

As the selection process narrows to serious contenders, it is appropriate to check the candidates' past employment records. It is helpful to structure questions to past employers around those criteria used in the interview. This gives excellent comparison between the candidates' responses and proven work habits.

Through such a standardized screening and interviewing process, the laboratory should be able to recruit quality personnel.

Orientation. The important step of introducing the employee to his or her new environment comes after the selection and hiring process. An orientation program is probably one of the most overlooked tools available to the manager.

Each laboratory should have a program of orientation for new employees to make them aware of the policies and procedures used in the particular laboratory. Even though a new employee may be a registered technologist, his or her experience with the particular procedures in use in a new environment may be limited. During this orientation it should be emphasized that suggestions for changing procedures or methods are welcome and will be given due consideration, but that each employee must follow the laboratory method and procedure exactly as prescribed. Individual initiative in modifying laboratory determinations without consultation and proper documentation should not be tolerated.

Done correctly, orientation can establish early in the employee's career an understanding of the philosophy of the laboratory and the institution. It can correct those misunderstandings that are so often present with new employees and can establish in the beginning an open channel of communcation between the supervisor and the new employee.

Although there are numerous formats for accomplishing orientation, the following is a minimum list of items that should be covered:

Location of policy manuals and their contents

The job description—the duties and responsibilities

The overall objectives of the laboratory and the employee's role in meeting these objectives

The employee evaluation form and how it is used

The departmental organization and the "key" personnel

The location of the procedure manuals and their contents

Time sheets and how they are handled

What to do if the employee has a job-related accident

Laboratory policies relative to meal times, breaks, vacations, and holiday scheduling

The department's and employee's role in the fire and disaster plans

Employee's Health Service

In-Service Continuing Education. Because of the rapidly changing nature of laboratory medicine, it is also desirable to have regular continuing education sessions for laboratory staff. These can be developed and presented by the laboratory staff and directors, with outside participants as needed. In addition, the staff should be given the time, and encouraged to attend, appropriate medical staff meetings in the institution as well as continuing education programs in laboratory medicine elsewhere. Documentation of attendance at such meetings, as well as topics covered, should be maintained to meet accreditation requirements.

Intralaboratory Staff Meetings. Intralaboratory communications are enhanced and crises minimized when regularly scheduled meetings of laboratory directors, associates, supervisors, and staff are held. Meetings of the supervisors and laboratory director are usually held weekly to discuss administrative, professional, and technical problems. Periodic full laboratory staff meetings are also useful as a forum for discussing problems, new policies and procedures, and for planning. Such meetings, if properly organized and directed, tend to promote teamwork in the laboratory and to bring problems to light before they become crises.

Personnel Records. All institutions maintain some personnel records on employees, but the laboratory may wish to keep a duplicate set of records for their use. If so, consideration should be given to what information should be, and legally can be, kept in these records.

The question of employee privacy has become a much-discussed issue recently, and court cases have been brought relative to this question. Since laws pertaining to this are changing rapidly, the reader is encouraged to determine what current organizational or federal guidelines exist relative to this matter. Before duplicating existing personnel records, thought should be given to the implications and responsibilities related to such an act, and counsel with appropriate personnel authorities is advised.

Evaluations. An important part of employee development is feedback, whether negative or positive. This can be accomplished through random meetings, memoranda to the file, or through a structured evaluation system. The latter offers the opportunity for the employee and supervisor to take time to review past performance, as well as to project future expectations. It provides both parties the framework within which constructive criticism can be given and provides the vehicle by which relationships can be redefined.

As with other management tools, the format of the evaluation forms can vary according to preference. For fairness and uniformity, the same form should be used for all employees. The form need not be complex, and the most frequently measured areas are the following:

ADAPTABILITY. The employee's ability to change behavior, attitude, and work methods to meet demands of the situation.

ATTENDANCE. Faithfulness in coming to work and conforming to work schedule.

JOB KNOWLEDGE AND SKILLS. The employee's use of his training and experience in performing the assigned job duties.

QUALITY OF WORK. Accuracy, thoroughness, and precision of work performed.

QUANTITY OF WORK. Amount of work performed in comparison with normal amount expected.

WORK RELATIONSHIPS. Quality of relationships with co-workers, supervisory staff, patients, and the public.

INITIATIVE. Extra effort.

RESPONSIVENESS. How quickly an individual accomplishes an assignment.

Each employee should be evaluated at regular intervals. In most laboratories this is done on a yearly basis, usually on the anniversary of the employee's hiring date. The evaluation should be reviewed with the employee and signed by the employee before it is placed in the personnel file.

Discipline and Dismissal. Some employees will fall short of expected standards. When this situation arises decisive action is imperative. "No action" is not an acceptable approach; how much action to take will depend upon the type of infraction and the circumstances surrounding it.

Most employee infractions fall into two general categories: those relating to performance of duties and those relating to personal conduct.

Some examples of failures of performance of duties requiring disciplinary action are:

1. Inefficiency or incompetency in the performance of duties.

2. Negligence in the performance of duties.

3. Physical or mental incapability for performing duties.

6

4. Habitual improper use of sick leave privileges.

5. Failure to maintain satisfactory and harmonious working relationships with the public and fellow employees.

All of these have in common the failure of the employee to meet standards related to the quality and/or quantity of work.

When a disciplinary action becomes necessary because of failure of performance of duties the following steps are usually considered essential:

1. An oral warning (memorandum for record maintained by the department).

2. A second oral warning with a follow-up letter to the employee. A re-evaluation of the employee's performance should be made in a specified period of time, not to exceed a maximum of six months. This evaluation serves as a method to rescind the previous action (by written notice to the employee) or, if warranted, to move the disciplinary action to the next step.

3. A written final warning to the employee. An evaluation of the employee's performance should again be made prior to a maximum of six months. At this time the decision is made to rescind the previous actions or to proceed with disciplinary action, which may include dismissal.

4. The notice of dismissal should be in writing and should inform the employee of the reason for dismissal and the method of appeal, if applicable.

Some examples of job-related personal conduct requiring disciplinary action are:

1. Conviction of a felony.

2. Falsified job information to secure a position.

3. Willful damage, destruction, or theft of property.

4. Possession of unauthorized fire arms or lethal weapons on the job.

5. Insubordination.

6. Reporting to work under the influence of alcohol or non-prescribed drugs, or partaking of such on the job.

Because of the seriousness of such acts, the laboratory director or supervisor may elect to recommend dismissal of the employee immediately rather than following the sequences noted above. In most hospitals, however, the procedure for such dismissals would include consultation with the personnel department.

Success in handling disciplinary problems comes with consistency of approach, promptness, and equity in dealing with all personnel. The importance of thorough documentation of personnel problems and resulting actions cannot be overemphasized. With proper employee recruitment, selection, orientation, and motivation, disciplinary problems should be minimized.

REFERENCES

Bennington, J. L.: Management by objectives. *In* Bennington, J. L. et al. (eds.): Management and Cost Control Techniques for the Clinical Laboratory. Baltimore, University Park Press, 1977.

Dorsey, D. B., et al. (eds.): Administration in the Pathology Laboratory, rev. ed. Skokie, Ill. College of American Pathologists, 1969.

Drucker, P. F.: The Effective Executive. New York, Harper & Row, 1967.

Gonzales-Menocal, P., et al.: A quantitative approach to the solution of laboratory layout problems. Lab. Med., vol. 4, no. 11, p. 17, 1973.

Hamlin, W. B., et al. (ed.): Laboratory instrument maintenance and function verification. Skokie, Ill., College of American Pathologists, 1974.

Henry, J. B.: Introduction to organ panels. *In* Henry, J. B., and Giegel, J. L. (eds.): Quality Control in Laboratory Medicine. New York, Masson Publishing USA, Inc., 1977.

Herzberg, F.: One more time: How do you motivate employees? Harvard Business Review, January-February, 1968.

Joint Commission on Accreditation of Hospitals: Pathology services. *In* Accreditation Manual for Hospitals. Chicago, 1976.

Lundberg, G. D.: Managing the patient-focused laboratory. Oradell, N. J., Medical Economics Company, 1975.

Maslow, A. H.: Motivation and Personality. New York, Harper & Row, Publishers, Inc., 1954.

McGregor, D.: The human side of enterprise. New York, McGraw-Hill Book Co., Inc., 1960.

Reece, R. L.: The screening laboratory of 1980. Perspect. Biol. Med., *17*:227, 1974.

Thomas, R. G. (ed.): Manual for laboratory planning and design, rev. ed. Skokie, Ill., College of American Pathologists, 1977.

Veterans Administration, Department of Medicine and Surgery: Chapter 240, Laboratory Services. *In* Planning Criteria for Medical Facilities, Manual M-7. Washington, D.C., U.S. Government Printing Office, 1974.

MANAGEMENT, GENERAL

Books

Drucker, P. F.: The Effective Executive. New York, Harper & Row, Publishers, Inc., 1967.

Drucker, P. F.: Management: Tasks, Responsibilities, Practices. New York, Harper & Row, Publishers, Inc., 1974.

Levey, S., and Loomba, N. P. (eds.): Health Care Administration: A Managerial Perspective. Philadelphia, J. B. Lippincott Company, 1973.

Organizations

The American Management Associates, 135 West 50th Street, New York, N.Y. 10020, offer courses and publications for members and non-members.

Personal time management

Achievement Planning Calendar. May be purchased from Achievement Resources, Inc., P.O. Box 2120, Ann Arbor, Michigan 48106.

MANAGEMENT, CLINICAL LABORATORY

Books

Bennington, L., et al. (eds.): Management and Cost Control Techniques for the Clinical Laboratory. Baltimore, University Park Press, 1977.

Dorsey, D. B., et al. (eds.): Administration in the Pathology Laboratory, rev. ed. Skokie, Ill., College of American Pathologists, 1969.

Lundberg, G. D.: Managing the Patient-focused Laboratory. Oradell, N. J., Medical Economics Company, 1975.

Newell, J. E.: Laboratory Management. Boston, Little, Brown & Co., 1972.

Periodicals

Laboratory Management. A monthly publication of the Medical Division of United Business Publications, Inc., 750 Third Avenue, New York, New York 10017.

Laboratory Medicine. A monthly publication of the American Society of Clinical Pathologists. Published by J. B. Lippincott Company, East Washington Square, Philadelphia, Pennsylvania 19105.

Pathologist. A monthly publication of the College of American Pathologists, 7400 N. Skokie Boulevard, Skokie, Illinois 60076.

Workshops

The College of American Pathologists, in cooperation with the American Management Association, presents workshops in management for laboratory personnel at various sites in the United States. For further information, contact the College of American Pathologists, 7400 N. Skokie Boulevard, Skokie, Illinois 60076.

LABORATORY DESIGN AND SAFETY

JCAH Hospital Staff-Evaluation Survey, Safety and Sanitation, 1976. May be obtained from the Joint Commission on Accreditation of Hospitals, 875 North Michigan Avenue, Chicago, Illinois 60611.

Thomas, G. (ed.): Manual for Laboratory Planning and Design, rev. ed. Skokie, Ill., College of American Pathologists, 1977.

Veterans Administration, Department of Medicine and Surgery: Chapter 240, Laboratory services. In Planning Criteria for Medical Facilities, Manual M-7. Washington, D.C., U.S. Government Printing Office, 1974.

REGIONALIZATION OF LABORATORY SERVICES

The American Hospital Association, 840 North Lake Shore Drive, Chicago, Illinois, 60611, offers assistance to health care institutions interested in multi-institutional or regional approaches to delivery of health services.

COMMUNICATIONS AND DATA PROCESSING

Books

Enlander, D. (ed.): Computers in Laboratory Medicine. New York, Academic Press, Inc., 1975.

Grams, R. R.: Problem solving, Systems Analysis and Medicine. Springfield, Ill., Charles C Thomas, Publisher, 1972.

J. Lloyd Johnson Associates: Achieving the Optimum Information System for the Laboratory. Northbrook, Ill., J. Lloyd Johnson Associates, 1975.

J. Lloyd Johnson Associates: Achieving the Optimum Information System for the Laboratory, Update, 1976. Northfield, Ill., J. Lloyd Johnson Associates, 1976.

Payne, L. C., and Brown, P. T. S.: An Introduction to Medical Automation, 2nd ed. Philadelphia, J. B. Lippincott Co., 1975.

Organizations

Society for Computer Medicine, 5100 Edina Industrial Boulevard, Suite 231 F, Edina, Minnesota 55435.

Periodicals

Computers and Medicine. A bi-monthly publication of the American Medical Association, 535 N. Dearborn St., Chicago, Illinois 60610.

Datamation. A monthly publication by Technical Publishing Company, 1301 South Grove Avenue, Barrington, Illinois 60010.

Infosystems. A monthly publication by Hitchcock Publishing Company, Hitchcock Building, Wheaton, Illinois 60187.

Issue on Electronics, Science, *195*:1085, 1977.

Issue on Microelectronics, Scientific American, *237*:62, 1977.

Journal of Medical Systems. A quarterly publication by

6

Plenum Publishing Corporation, 227 West 17th Street, New York, N.Y. 10011.

CONTINUING EDUCATION

The American Society of Clinical Pathologists, 2100 W. Harrison Street, Chicago, Illinois 60612, provides a broad range of A-V materials, workshops, and publications for continuing education in laboratory medicine.

LABORATORY ACCREDITATION AND REGULATIONS

Books

Feegel, J. R.: Legal Aspects of Laboratory Medicine. Boston, Little, Brown & Co., 1973.

Laboratory Regulation Manual. Health Law Center, Aspen Systems Corporation, 20010 Century Boulevard, Germantown, Maryland 20767. Loose-leaf manual of laboratory regulations with quarterly Newsletter and Supplements.

Accrediting agencies

Commission on Inspection and Accreditation, College of American Pathologists, 7400 N. Skokie Boulevard, Skokie, Illinois 60076. This is a voluntary program of laboratory improvement and accreditation which can serve in many instances in lieu of state or federal programs.

Joint Commissions on Accreditation of Hospitals, 875 N. Michigan Avenue, Chicago, Illinois 60611. Laboratories and pathology services are inspected and accredited as part of hospital inspection and accreditation by the JCAH.

Licensure and Proficiency Testing Division, Bureau of Laboratories, Center for Disease Control, Atlanta, Georgia 30333. Provides licensure for interstate laboratories covered under the Clinical Laboratory Improvement Act of 1967. Laboratories not covered by this or other acts may voluntarily elect to be inspected.

The American Association of Blood Banks, 1828 L Street, N.W., Washington, D.C. 20036, publishes Standards for Blood Banks and Transfusion Services and sponsors a voluntary inspection and accreditation program for blood banks.

PROFICIENCY TESTING

CDC Proficiency Testing. U.S. Department of Health, Education and Welfare, Public Health Service, Center for Disease Control, Atlanta, Georgia 30333. U.S. federal government program of clinical laboratory proficiency testing.

College of American Pathologists Survey. College of American Pathologists, 7400 N. Skokie Boulevard, Skokie, Illinois 60076. Provides proficiency testing for most laboratory areas. Approved by most states for Medicare and State licensure and are equal to or more stringent than the requirements for the current governmental requirements under CLIA 1967.

Proficiency Test Service. Institute for Clinical Science, 1833 Delancey Place, Philadelphia, Pennsylvania 19103. Monthly evaluation service, primarily in clinical chemistry.

59

FISCAL MANAGEMENT

Michael D. Reich and
William W. McLendon, M.D.

The ability of the laboratory to meet the goals and objectives as discussed in Chapter 58 (p. 1979) depends on the availability and management of fiscal resources to provide facilities, equipment, supplies, and personnel. In this chapter we will address external factors which influence fiscal decisions, tools which are available for fiscal decision-making, and techniques available for developing and monitoring laboratory budgets utilizing the concept of responsibility budgeting.

FACTORS INFLUENCING
FISCAL DECISIONS

Government. As the government has become more involved with financing medical care in the United States with the passage of the various federal health legislative acts, the degree of external control over hospital and laboratory fiscal decisions has increased tremendously. Although we will not attempt to review these influences in detail, the laboratory director and his associates should be familiar with such programs and the restrictions which they bring to the financing of hospital and laboratory services. The federal legislation establishing health system agencies is an outgrowth of earlier, more voluntary efforts to review on a regional basis health care planning and expenditures. Under the National Health Planning and Resources Development Act of 1974 (PL 93-641), the Department of Health, Education and Welfare (HEW) was instructed to divide each state into health service areas. A health systems agency (HSA) is designated for each area and is charged with the development and review of short- and long-range health care plans for the area. In addition, the HSA must give prior approval to all changes in hospital bed size and to all program changes or capital requests exceeding a dollar amount (e.g., $100,000).

In addition, laboratory directors in institutions financed by cities, counties, states, or other governmental entities should also be aware of the financial constraints imposed by such entities.

Non-governmental Third-Party Payors. Since the 1930's an extensive system of private health care financing has also developed in the United States. This is generally of two types. One is the non-profit health and hospital insurance plans such as the Blue Cross and Blue Shield Insurance, which are available in every state and which now pay for some 20 to 25 per cent of the health and medical care costs in the United States. The second type is the commercial health insurance companies, which pay for less than 5 per cent. By contrast, the federal government is now paying half or

6

more of health and medical care costs in the United States, with the balance being paid by individuals.

Both private insurance companies and other agencies concerned with rising costs of health care have established means of reviewing charges for laboratory and hospital services and the expenditure of health and medical care funds. Recently an increasing amount of influence is also being exerted by industry, labor, and consumer groups. Such reviewing authorities and interest groups will influence the laboratory director's program and fiscal planning and should be considered in making such plans.

Regionalization and Shared Services. Because of concern with cost containment, increasing pressure will be placed upon laboratories to prevent duplication and provide regionalization of services, particularly in the area of the specialized and non-emergency laboratory services. A system of regional laboratories has already been established in the United Kingdom under the National Health Service, and pressure to establish a similar pattern of services in the United States is already being exerted.

Numerous voluntary efforts are being made to curb the rising costs of providing medical care by preventing unnecessary duplication of efforts or facilities. These multi-institutional efforts take many forms, ranging from simple sharing of joint services to the merging of institutions or the formation of consortia.

The decision as to what laboratory procedures should be done locally and what might be done in a regional laboratory or on a shared basis may be made according to the criteria advanced by Hain (1972). Although he was concerned with those procedures which should be done in a physician's office and those which could be done in a centralized laboratory facility, the criteria could be useful in a more general context:

The procedures which can be done more reliably or at less cost centrally and for which the turn-around time from collection of the specimen to reporting of results to the attending physician will not impede the immediate effective care of the patient should be done in the community core laboratory [regional or shared laboratory]. All others would be done in the peripheral facility [hospital or office laboratory].

In theory this approach is attractive, but in actual practice it may break down, since different measurements can become critical, depending on the patient rather than some other criteria. As a result, laboratories may still maintain back-up capability for a wide range of measurements and defeat the purpose of centralization.

Brown (1975) provides practical guidelines for those considering regional or shared laboratory services, with a checklist of questions to be considered in the planning stages of such a venture.

TOOLS FOR FISCAL DECISION-MAKING

An accepted premise in management states that one cannot manage that which one cannot measure. The laboratory director thus needs certain quantitative management tools in order rationally to approach the development of budgets, the monitoring of budgets, and the utilization of fiscal resources.

LABORATORY WORKLOAD RECORDING METHOD

Until relatively recently clinical laboratories had no standard method of workload measurement related to the time expended by laboratory technologists in performing laboratory measurements and examinations. Utilizing the experience of the workload system developed by the Canadian Association of Pathologists, and working in conjunction with the Veterans Administration and other groups, the College of American Pathologists (CAP) has developed a standardized workload recording method for clinical laboratories (CAP, 1978). This method is now recognized as a means of recording laboratory workload by the American Hospital Association and other organizations.

A laboratory utilizing this method makes a *raw count*, which is a simple tally of all procedures performed. The CAP workload recording method provides each determination or procedure with a *unit value*, weighted according to the methodology used and to the degree of automation involved. As a result, the system is applicable to both the large, highly automated laboratory and the small laboratory using manual procedures. The official unit value for each procedure is derived after performance of time studied in sufficient laboratories to provide a statistically meaningful data base. Temporary unit values may be assigned to new or infrequent procedures after a standardized time study is performed by the laboratory and submitted to CAP.

Each *unit* in the workload recording method represents one minute of technical, clerical, and aide time. The *unit value* of a particular procedure includes the time for specimen processing and testing; clerical work including logging and recording of results; and supportive activities such as solution preparation and glassware washing. It does not include the interpretation of results by pathologists, or their assistance to clinical colleagues in terms of what to order and in what order to request it; nor does it include the time for specimen collection, quality control samples, or reports. Quality control determinations, standards, and repeat measurements are given the same unit value as the patient specimen and considered as additional procedures. When specimen collection is performed by the laboratory, additional units of work are credited to the laboratory. Monthly totals of the raw counts of procedures are collected by the laboratory and then multiplied by the appropriate unit value of each procedure to produce the total unit value or total workload in minutes.

Although the system may be used locally by an individual laboratory, the greatest value and ease of operation are provided when the monthly figures are submitted to the CAP Computer Assisted Workload Program on standardized workload reporting forms (Fig. 59-1). In addition to workload figures, the laboratory submits the number of worked and paid man hours of technical, clerical, and aide time during the month. The *worked man hours* are defined as the actual number of hours employees worked in the laboratory during the month, whereas *paid man hours* reflect the total number of paid hours and include holiday, sick leave, and vacation hours. Utilizing these monthly inputs, the computer program then provides reports (Fig. 59-2) giving the laboratory workload in raw count and total units by sections, along with the listing of paid and worked hours plus a calculated productivity figure. The *paid productivity* is calculated by dividing the total number of workload units for the month by the number of paid man hours, while the *worked productivity* is similarly calculated utilizing the number of worked man hours. Since the workload unit was defined as one minute of technical, clerical, and aide time, in an ideal situation there should be a productivity of 60

workload units (that is, 60 minutes of productive work) for each hour of worked time. In actual practice, the average workload productivity in most laboratories is in the range of 30 to 60 workload units per hour. Because of the many variables that enter into the calculation of this figure, one should not interpret it as an absolute indication of productivity. On the other hand, it can be of great value in comparing current with previous productivity, in comparing sections within a laboratory, and in comparing one laboratory with other comparable laboratories (such data are provided by the CAP computerized service). If a laboratory section consistently has a workload productivity in the range of 20 to 30, for example,

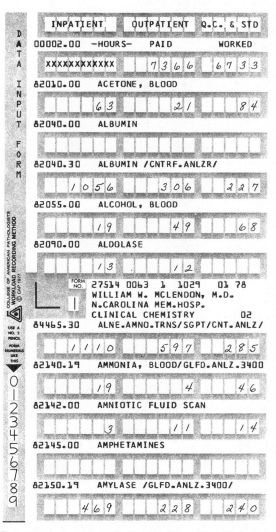

Figure 59–1. Input form for Workload Recording Method of the College of American Pathologists.

02/03/78   PAGE   1

COLLEGE OF AMERICAN PATHOLOGISTS
WORKLOAD - COMPUTER ASSISTED PROGRAM
MONTHLY COMPARATIVE ANALYSIS REPORT

MONTH ENDING DEC. 1977

LAB. NO. 27514-0063

SECTION INFORMATION			TOTAL RAW COUNT	TOTAL UNIT VAL.	WORKED MAN HRS.	WORKED PROD.	PAID MAN HRS.	PAID MAN-HOUR PRODUCTIVITY				
YOUR NO.	CAP. NO.	NAME						LAST 6 MON.	LAST 12 MON.	CURR. MONTH	YOUR GP. SIZE	ALL LAB. GROUPS
05	***	IMMUNOLOGY	2631	65742	113	581.7	348	370.3	247.0	188.9*		
08	***	RADIOISOTOPES	0	0	0	.0	0	.0	.0	.0*		
30	***	SPECIAL HEMATOLOGY	520	11360	480	23.6	480	37.4	36.6	23.6*		
31	***	PCC LAB	0	0	0	.0	0	.0	.0	.0*		
65	***	VIROLOGY	214	1941	302	6.4	415	.0	.0	4.6*		
73	***	HYPERTENSION LAB	0	0	0	.0	0	.0	.0	.0*		
74	***	UROLOGY LAB	0	0	0	.0	0	.0	.0	.0*		
01	01	BLOOD BANK	18708	132758	4,344	30.5	4,969	27.9	27.9	26.7		
STANDARD		BLOOD BANK	18708	132758	4,344		4,969			26.7	38.4	37.7
02	02	CLINICAL CHEMISTRY	105324	392893	6,733	58.3	7,366	59.2	58.2	53.3		
20	02	ENDOCRINOLOGY	8478	113260	1,968	57.5	2,326	49.4	48.1	48.6		
71	02	BLOOD GASES	38061	315145	1,467	214.8	1,702	200.6	189.9	185.1		
STANDARD		CHEMISTRY	151863	821298	10,168		11,394	72.0	72.0		47.1	52.5
03	03	HEMATOLOGY	30530	183506	3,086	59.4	4,181	36.5	35.8	43.8		
72	03	CLINICAL COAGULATION	5732	62642	1,639	38.2	2,006	37.1	37.1	31.2		
STANDARD		HEMATOLOGY	36262	246148	4,725		6,187			39.7	40.7	42.9
STD..04		HISTOLOGY									40.9	38.7
64	05	SEROLOGY	3039	20549	304	67.5	338	65.3	60.4	60.7		
STANDARD		IMMUNOLOGY	3039	20549	304		338			60.7	48.3	44.6
06	06	MICROBIOLOGY	89032	203694	4,218	48.2	5,080	35.5	32.3	40.0		
61	06	AFB	3456	21941	339	64.7	389	61.6	47.7	56.4		
62	06	MYCOLOGY	5464	18725	339	55.2	389	49.1	42.9	48.1		
63	06	PARASITOLOGY	456	3010	340	8.8	372	13.5	12.0	8.0		
STANDARD		MICROBIOLOGY	98408	247369	5,236		6,230			39.7	46.6	47.0
STD..07		MISCELLANEOUS								.0	.0	40.5
STD..08		RADIOISOTOPES								.0	.0	21.1
09	09	LAB CENTRAL	7639	62024	3,179	19.5	3,652	22.5	25.1	16.9		
STANDARD		SPECIMEN PROCUREMENT	7639	62024	3,179		3,652			16.9**	35.1	39.1
10	10	URINALYSIS	5057	30960	320	96.7	320	103.1	93.1	96.7		
STANDARD		URINE AND FECES	5057	30960	320		320			96.7**	39.0	34.3
MONTHLY TOTALS - ALL SECTIONS			324341	1640149	29,171		34,333					

Figure 59-2. Example of one of the monthly reports from the Computer Assisted Workload Program of the College of American Pathologists.

then one must assume a low productivity for this laboratory, probably implying an over-staffing of the laboratory. On the other hand, if a laboratory's productivity consistently runs over 60, then the laboratory may well be understaffed and need additional personnel support. Both of these judgments assume that the workload units are reasonable for the laboratory's methods and that input errors are excluded.

The utilization of this tool provides a well-standardized and relatively flexible approach to documenting workload and determining productivity. Laboratories are encouraged to utilize this tool, since it provides useful information for budget forecasting and determining future staffing levels.

In projecting workload figures for purposes of future planning, one should take into account two types of growth. One is the *intrinsic growth* in the utilization of laboratory services resulting from improvements in the available laboratory services and from physicians' greater utilization of these services. Such intrinsic growth in recent years has been as much as 15 per cent for areas such as clinical chemistry, with an overall growth of clinical laboratory procedures averaging about 5 to 10 per cent per year. Such growth is in addition to the *growth due to increased volume;* that is, growth related to new beds or different types of beds (e.g., intensive care), expanded outpatient or other services (e.g., transplantation, oncology, burn unit). Both the intrinsic growth and the growth due to new services are obviously influenced by many factors. Thus a laboratory should not base planning on growth figures such as those cited above, but must utilize realistic figures from its own experience and projections for the future. Tools available for workload forecasting are presented in much greater detail by Westlake (1977).

COST FINDING

Cost finding is the means by which a laboratory documents its costs for performing a particular procedure and then establishes its charges based on the involved direct and indirect costs. This approach is in contrast to the frequently used approach in the past of telephoning a few other hospitals and laboratories in the region to request their charges and setting charges or fees based on such a survey.

Ideally, cost finding should be done by laboratory personnel in consultation with the fiscal staff in the hospital. This combination is necessary, since laboratory staff can analyze steps involved in performing procedures, while fiscal personnel are needed to provide the indirect (or overhead) expenses and to assist in preparing the data for submission to the hospital administration, board of trustees, and third party payors for approval.

Direct vs. Indirect Costs. Two general types of costs are involved in the operation of a laboratory or in costing any single procedure. The first of these is *direct costs*, which are the costs of materials, supplies, and personnel time directly attributable to the specific measurement or examination. Equipment depreciation may be included as part of direct or of indirect costs, depending upon the accounting method in use. Equipment leasing is generally considered a direct cost. *Indirect costs* are those costs necessary to operate a laboratory that are not directly attributable to specific measurements or examinations. Such costs include allocated portion of utilities, laboratory and institutional administrative expenses, building depreciation, and janitorial service. The allocation of the costs to the laboratory may be done by various approaches. One (known as step down allocation method) is to take the cost of operating the non–revenue-producing services in a hospital and then allocate this cost to the revenue-producing department on the basis of some formula, such as the number of personnel employed by the area (in the case of the personnel department expense) or the number of square feet in an area (in the case of the janitorial services). Another approach is to determine total expenses for the non–revenue-producing departments as a percentage of the total expenses for operating the hospital or institution. This percentage, representing the indirect expenses, would then be added to the direct expenses for any test procedure to determine the total charge.

In many states cost allocation has been directed by third party agencies through reimbursement based on a step down procedure.

Fixed vs. Variable Costs. The concept of fixed and variable costs is useful in analyzing the effects of changing volumes of determinations on expenses and revenue. The *fixed costs* in a laboratory are constant over time regardless of volume of determinations. Depreciation, supervisor salaries, and rental charges are examples. The laboratory will incur these charges at a fixed rate that should not vary with reasonable changes in work volume. On the other hand, *variable costs* are those costs (for items such as supplies and reagents) which will vary in a linear relationship to the volume of determinations. Fixed costs are much larger costs, since personnel costs usually amount to about 60 to 70 per cent of the total budget of most hospitals. In general, therefore, the greater the workload performed by the laboratory, the less the per unit cost.

Revenue is also dependent on volume, so that the *break-even point* for a laboratory is attained at the time revenue exceeds total expenses (that is, the sum of the fixed expenses and the variable expenses). This is graphically shown in Figure 59-3. By use of such a diagram with the current and historical data from a laboratory, one may predict the effect of changing total volume, increasing or decreasing charges, or changing the fixed expenses by adding personnel or equipment (Louvau, 1977). This approach is not applicable to all hospitals, however, since revenue may be dependent upon state regulations on reimbursements rather than upon those variables.

Development of Charges. The development of charges is a necessary part of most laboratory operations, if the patient or a third-party payor is to be billed for laboratory determinations on an individual basis. Although in the past charges for pharmacy, lab-

oratory, and other diagnostic or therapeutic services were often excessive in order to cover losses in other hospital areas, this practice is being challenged by those third-party payors who reimburse actual costs rather than charges. In addition, laboratories outside of hospitals have demonstrated that laboratory services can be offered at a lesser charge if the laboratory is not saddled with expenses of many other operating divisions of the hospital. When comparing charges from a non-hospital laboratory with those from a hospital laboratory, however, one should be aware of increased overall costs necessary to operate a "full service" laboratory in a large community hospital or a medical center with its requirements for emergency services, specialized services, and training programs.

The method of development of charges will vary from institution to institution depending on the fiscal structure of the institution. Figure 59-4 shows a form used in one institution for the development of charges. In modified fashion this can serve for other institutions.

COST-EFFECTIVENESS AND COST-BENEFIT ANALYSES

The ever-increasing emphasis on costs of health and medical care has led to the development of tools for the evaluation of the effectiveness or benefits of proposed courses of action in relationship to the costs to be incurred. Although the terms "cost-effectiveness" and "cost-benefit" are sometimes used interchangeably, Smith (1973) distinguishes the two as follows:

In *cost-benefit analysis*, the monetary cost of a program is normally compared with its expected benefits, and normally those benefits are expressed in dollars. . . . In a cost-benefit analysis of alternate programs, we compare the expected benefits to determine what is the best investment . . . both costs and benefits are usually expressed in dollars to permit ready comparison.

Cost-effectiveness analysis differs from cost-benefit analysis in that costs are calculated and alternate ways are compared for achieving a specific set of results. Our objective is not just how to use funds most wisely; it also includes the constraint that a specific output must be achieved. Very often this output is not expressed in dollars.

Cost-benefit analysis is a useful tool for making decisions such as the purchase of new instrumentation, the addition or deletion of measurements and examinations in a labora-

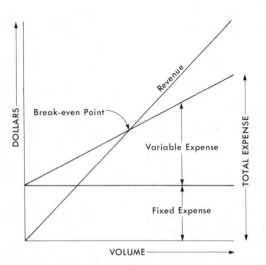

Figure 59-3. Relationships of expenses and revenues to the break-even point. (Modified from Bennington, J. L., et al. (eds.): Management and Cost Control Techniques for the Clinical Laboratory. Baltimore, University Park Press, 1977.)

LABORATORY: T.B./Mycology
NAME OF PROCEDURE: Fungus Culture

A. <u>SALARIES:</u>

	Employee 1	Employee 2
Employee Classification	MT II	MT III
Work Time per Unit	15 min.	15 min.
Rate per Hour	4.67	5.57
	$ 1.16	$ 1.39
TOTAL		$ 2.55

B. <u>REAGENTS AND SUPPLIES</u>

Include the cost of supplies consumed in performing the procedures. Do not include such things as equipment depreciation, housekeeping expense, lights, and water; these will be accounted for in the indirect expenses.

Media .30/tube × 2 = .60	
Media .20/tube × 2 = .40	
Misc. .25	
TOTAL	$ 1.25

C. <u>SPECIMEN COLLECTION</u>

Employee Classification		
Time per Unit		
Rate per Hour		
TOTAL	$	

D. <u>SPECIALIZED REPORTING</u>

Employee Classification	MT III	
Time per Unit	10 min.	
Rate per Unit	.92	
TOTAL	$ .92	
TOTAL DIRECT COSTS	$ 4.72	
DEPT. INDIRECT COSTS (including professional)	$ 3.14	
TOTAL COST	$ 7.86	
SUGGESTED CHARGE	$ 8.00	

Figure 59-4. An approach to charge development.

tory, or whether a measurement is to be sent to an outside laboratory or performed locally. Böer (1977) provides more details on this type of analysis and gives examples of the use of this technique in clinical laboratory decisions.

Cost-effectiveness analysis is useful when various approaches are being investigated to ascertain the most effective way to achieve a desired result, for example, to determine the best program to train 10 medical technologists per year or to determine the best instrumentation to perform blood gases on a 100-μl sample. Smith (1973) provides other examples and advice on avoiding errors in using cost-effectiveness and cost-benefit analysis.

RESPONSIBILITY BUDGETING

A budget is an itemized statement of estimated income and expenses which is prepared as a financial plan for the coming year. Once prepared, it is then used as a guideline for fiscal management and cost control on an ongoing basis. In order to do this one must have a means of comparing on a regular basis the projected budget with the actual expenses and making adjustments where necessary during the year.

In the past most budgets have been formulated on the basis of negotiating for additional funds for growth and expansion with little attention directed to the base (or continuing) budget from the previous year. *Zero-base budgeting*, in contrast, is founded on the assumption that no base budget is carried forward to the next year and that existing as well as proposed expenditures must be justified. It should be observed, however, that a zero-base budget approach is time-consuming and expensive to institute properly and that alternate ways exist to achieve the same goal. The discussion which follows will be applicable to either the usual budget procedure or the zero-base budget procedure.

Responsibility budgeting follows the philosophy of placing the accountability for the budget at the lowest level of management possible. It is generally recognized that in order for this approach to be successful, five concepts basic to this form of budgeting must be followed (Bennington, 1977):

1. Planned and actual expenses are to be charged to the lowest level of the organization which can cause their being incurred.
2. No expense item is to be charged to a department unless the department can exercise control of that expense item.
3. All departments included in the budget must be headed by someone who can be held responsible for the cost of that department.
4. Every item of expense can be controlled by someone in the total organization.
5. The department head must participate in the budget formulation process and agree that the planned expenditure of his or her organizational unit is realistic.

BUDGET DEVELOPMENT

Table of Organization and Chart of Accounts.   Before a laboratory can introduce the concept of responsibility budgeting, an organizational chart which accurately reflects the actual budgetary responsibility centers in the laboratory must be developed. The financial or *budgetary organizational chart* (Fig. 59-5) does not necessarily have to agree with the administrative organizational chart, but it must recognize all areas within the laboratory which incur expenses, which generate income, and for which a separate budget is developed. In most accounting systems each area will be given a unique cost center and a unique revenue code. It is also important to clearly identify the person responsible for the budget in each of these areas.

The *chart of accounts* is developed for each budget center by listing the expense items for that center broken down into the usual categories such as salaries, fringe benefits, overtime, supplies, reagents, and equipment repairs (Fig. 59-6).

The design of such an organizational chart and the development of a chart of accounts thus gives the laboratory the information necessary to monitor trends in expenses and revenues by budgetary responsibility centers within the laboratory and to project such expenses and revenues for budget preparation.

The actual budget process should allow adequate time to review past performance compared with planned performance; to establish plans for the next year; and to convert these plans into quantitative financial data for review and approval of the next year's budget. The steps to accomplish this process are outlined in the following section.

Objectives.   As noted in Chapter 58, objectives should be made annually for each section having responsibility for development of the budget, as well as for the entire laboratory. Such objectives should be achievable, quantifiable, and consistent with the institutional philosophy. They should include projections of growth and new programs and reflect needs for personnel and capital equipment. We have

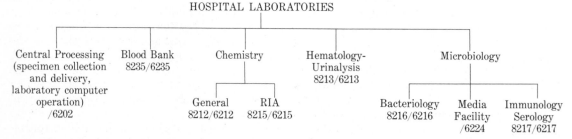

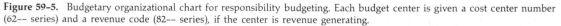

Figure 59-5. Budgetary organizational chart for responsibility budgeting. Each budget center is given a cost center number (62-- series) and a revenue code (82-- series), if the center is revenue generating.

CHART OF ACCOUNTS

120—SALARIES & WAGES—SPA

1210   Salaries—SPA. Compensation for services of employees regularly employed on a permanent basis (permanent full time and permanent part time) and subject to the State Personnel Act.

1211   Shift Differential. Additional compensation to employees who work on the evening or night shift.

1213   On-Call Pay. Additional compensation paid to those employees who stand by and remain ready to perform their normal duties on a specific pre-determined date when called upon.

1220   Salaries—Overtime. Additional compensation paid to those employees who are subject to the Fair Labor Standards Act whenever those employees work in excess of 40 hours during the hospital's work week.

1250   Holiday Premium Pay. Additional compensation paid to SPA employees who are required to work on days designated as "Holiday Premium" days.

1255   Longevity Pay. Additional compensation recognizes the long term service of Permanent Full Time Staff employees who have at least fifteen years of Aggregate State Service.

1260   Employees on Loan. Compensation paid to Hospital employees on loan to other State Agencies.

1290   Workmen's Compensation. Wage continuation payments to those employees who sustain job-related illness or accidents.

Figure 59-6. Portion of a typical chart of accounts.

found that objectives can be best developed as a response to observed needs and can be best evaluated when coupled with a strategy for implementation (Fig. 59-7).

Expense Projections. When a decision is first made to implement responsibility budgeting in the laboratory, it may be difficult to find detailed fiscal information on expenses for preceding years in the records of either the laboratory or the accounting department. After the chart of accounts has been established for a year or so, such records will become available and will be useful tools for future budget preparation.

The projection of expenses for the coming year is ordinarily based on at least six to nine months of actual expense data, which are then annualized to serve as a baseline for the preparation of the next year's budget. The projected expenses for the next 12 months are then arrived at from the annualized current data, taking into account anticipated changes in the following areas: inflation, workload, inpatient census, outpatient visits, and new or deleted hospital programs which would affect the laboratories. In addition, input should be obtained from the various laboratories concerning addition of new services, deletion of obsolete measurements, introduction of automated equipment, and anticipated changes in vendor's prices to the laboratories.

Revenue Projections. Revenue projections are best made by projecting the number of procedures to be performed during the budget year and calculating the revenue based on the current charges. Whereas the cost of purchased supplies and other items will change without direct control from the laboratory or hospital, any necessary changes in the charge structure must be initiated by the laboratory and hospital administration. Part of the budget process usually consists of determining whether the proposed expense budget will be covered by the revenues to be generated at the current level of charges. If this appears unlikely, and if the expenses cannot be trimmed further without compromising patient care, then part of the budget recommendation may be that certain or all charges are increased. On the other hand, if new services and equipment significantly reduce the cost of certain measurements, the budget planning may lead to recommendations that selected charges be reduced. In either case, the projection of new charges as anticipated revenue must be made and incorporated into the budget. Unfortunately, this approach is not universally applicable, since certain states penalize any hospital with revenue over a predetermined amount and all additional revenue is lost. It is likely that such regulations will be applied nationally in the near future.

6

HOSPITAL LABORATORIES
PLANNING STATEMENTS

NEED STATEMENT	OBJECTIVES	STRATEGY STATEMENTS	
1. Currently, delays exist in data input into the computer for the Chemistry and Coagulation Laboratories, and no computerized reportings exist for Urinalysis, Hematology, and Blood Bank.	1. Develop an on-line laboratory information system for all laboratories by the end of the fiscal year. The Blood Bank program at this stage would include only reporting of transfusions to appear on the cumulative reports.	a. Renovation of existing Lab Central, to accommodate Data Acquisition Computer (DAC)	April
		b. Complete Systems design of Lab Information Systems (LIS)	June
		c. Purchase first DAC	June
		d. Testing DAC	June–Oct.
		e. Programming and testing of LIS	June–Oct.
		f. Obtain funding and purchase second (back-up) DAC	Oct.
		g. Obtain funding for 24-hour Lab Central coverage	July
		h. Establish Lab Central positions, recruit, and train	Oct.
		i. Training lab and hospital staffs	Oct.–Dec.
		j. Parallel testing of LIS	Dec.–Jan.
		k. Implementation	Feb.

Figure 59-7. Planning statements developed as a part of budget preparation.

Capital Equipment Budget. In most institutions a capital equipment budget is prepared in parallel with the operating budget, but it is a separate budget. Capital budget requests are obviously closely related to the short- and long-range goals of the institution and the laboratories.

The decision of whether major capital equipment should be purchased outright or financed through leasing or rental must be made. The trend today is toward lease or rental of such equipment. The principal advantages of leasing are the low capital outlay and the ability to surrender the equipment when it becomes obsolete. The decision, however, is a complex one involving not only institutional fiscal policy but also outside influences. Böer (1977) provides a more detailed discussion.

If equipment is to be purchased, then the operating budget must show the anticipated annual depreciation of this equipment, as either a direct cost or an indirect cost, depending upon the accounting procedure used by the particular institution. If the equipment is to be leased or rented, then the annual lease or rental amount for the equipment must be shown in the appropriate line as operating expense for the year.

A justification for new equipment generally is based on one or more reasons. Replacement equipment is best justified by thorough documentation of the extent of the down time and cost of repairs of current equipment. This can be done by maintaining a log listing the type and duration of such problems; most current accreditation standards require such documentation.

A second type of justification for capital equipment is based on the projection that the new equipment will provide labor savings and greater efficiency for the laboratory and possi-

Year:_____   LABORATORY SECTION:___**Bacteriology**___   Cost #__6216__   Revenue #__8216__

		PREVIOUS YEAR ACTUAL	JULY	AUG	SEPT	MAY	JUNE	CURRENT YEAR BUDGETED
HOSPITAL	Average Daily Census	507.7	508.3	547.1	531.6	525		498
	Admissions	18,568	1723	1660	1649	1718		20,127
	Outpatient Visits, Total	228,426	17,517	18,746	17,591	18,250		215,415
	Emergency Room Visits	21,773	2109	1934	1836	1912		23,515
PERSONNEL	FP (full, perm.) Positions	33	35	35		35		35
	FP (full, perm.) Employees		31	31		35		
	PP (part, perm.) Positions	1						
	PP (part, perm.) Employees		12	14		0		
	FT & PT (temporary) Employees							
CAP WORKLOAD	Raw Count of Tests (Incl. Std., QC)	299,312	71,057	61,931	67,554	102,452		
	Total Units (Incl. Std., QC)	2,331,643	181,204	194,788	209,693	227,412		
	Worked Manhours	58,584	5062	5110	5116	5146		
	Worked Productivity	39.8	35.7	38.1	40.9	44.1		
TREND REPORTS	Revenue: Inpatient — Actual (A)	700,551	59,037	125,921	191,553	702,361		695,249
	Budgeted (B)		64,686	131,981	186,738	684,706		
	Outpatient — Actual (A)	238,003	17,093	34,400	54,862	201,161		240,087
	Budgeted (B)		19,792	41,304	62,090	227,663		
	Total Direct Expenses (A)	584,619	44,385	81,649	122,920	450,706		540,882
	(B)		39,948	87,432	132,998	487,629		
	Subtotal: Payroll & Benefits (A)	327,909	35,516	63,367	95,380	349,726		407,016
	(B)		32,083	66,968	101,755	373,101		
	Overtime (A)	7,778	167	1005	1509	5533		8125
	(B)		725	1450	2175	7975		
	Subtotal: Supplies & Materials (A)	45,180	7330	10,018	13,736	49,173		52,499
	(B)		3579	7158	10,737	40,735		
	Subtotal: Miscellaneous Obligations (A)	10,137	62	837	1528	9215		10,940
	(B)		1408	2321	3234	9825		
	Subtotal: Fixed Charges (A)	8000	101	250	350	7500		8300
	(B)		693	1252	1811	7780		
	Capital Equipment Purchases (A)	23,428	1285	1879	5320	8175		9472
	(B)		9472	9472	9472	9472		

Figure 59-8. Example of a budget monitoring report.

6

bly greater revenue. A cost-benefit analysis as previously described will help document this justification. If the laboratory is not willing to give up positions in trade for such equipment, then the laboratory director must be prepared to justify with workload statistics the fact that the personnel are currently overworked and/or document that the persons freed from one task will be assigned to other needed tasks.

Capital expenses also may be justified on the basis of new or improved services. Such justification usually is based on the medical necessity to improve the quality or efficiency of services or the variety and complexity of measurements and examinations offered. Again, a cost-benefit analysis is useful in justifying such a request.

BUDGET MONITORING

No budgeting system is complete without consistent financial feedback during the budget year. This is usually accomplished through the use of some type of accounting report. Such reports come in many different formats but have as their basic goal the presentation of current monthly and year-to-date data on revenue, expenses, and statistics as compared with the previously projected budget figures. An example of a simple format to accomplish this monitoring is shown in Figure 59-8.

These reports are most useful when they are monitored on a monthly basis by meetings of persons from each responsibility center with the laboratory director. At such meetings the data can be checked for accuracy, and unexpected variances from the budgeted projections can be investigated to determine the cause and to implement corrective action.

In summary, responsibility budgeting provides laboratory directors and supervisors with a way to have meaningful input into fiscal decisions being made on their behalf and a mechanism to monitor and control the fiscal operation of the laboratory. The process requires a plan, as outlined previously, as well as careful monitoring of the results at least monthly during the budget year. With each succeeding month and year of the use of this system, the preparation of budgets and accurate projection of income and revenue should become less difficult and more accurate. Furthermore, sound fiscal management of the laboratory contributes to improved and expanded patient care services within the confines of inevitable financial constraints.

REFERENCES

Bennington, J. L.: Responsibility budgeting. *In* Bennington, J. L., Boer, G. B., Louvau, G. E., and Westlake, G. E. (eds.): Management and Cost Control Techniques for Clinical Laboratory. Baltimore, University Park Press, 1977.

Böer, G. B.: Cost analysis. *In* Bennington, J. L., et al. (eds.): Management and Cost Control Techniques for Clinical Laboratory. Baltimore, University Park Press, 1977.

Brown, M., McCool, B., Matti, L., and Shipley, L.: Shared laboratory services? What to consider. Hospitals, *49*:48, 1975.

CAP: Laboratory Workload Recording Method. Skokie, Ill., College of American Pathologists, 1978.

Hain, R. F.: The community core laboratory: The laboratory of the future. South. Med. J., *65*:379, 1972.

Louvau, G. E.: Break-even and bivariate linear regression analysis. *In* Bennington, J. L., Boer, G. B., Louvau, G. E., and Westlake, G. E. (eds.): Management and Cost Control Techniques for Clinical Laboratory. Baltimore, University Park Press, 1977.

Smith, W. F.: Cost-effectiveness and cost-budget analyses for public health programs. *In* Levey, S., and Loomba, N. P. (eds): Health Care Administration. Philadelphia, J. B. Lippincott Company, 1973.

Westlake, G. E.: Forecasting and test volume projection. *In* Bennington, J. L., Boer, G. B., Louvau, G. E., and Westlake, G. E. (eds.): Management and Cost Control Techniques for Clinical Laboratory. Baltimore, University Park Press, 1977.

60

COMMUNICATIONS AND DATA PROCESSING

William W. McLendon, M.D.

Communications, both written and verbal, are a major component of all medical care. The essence of laboratory medicine or clinical pathology is the acquisition of data by analytical procedures performed on patient specimens, the determination of the validity of those data by laboratory professionals, and the communication of those data with appropriate interpretation to the patient's physician to assist the physician in diagnostic, therapeutic, and prognostic decisions.

The typical cycle of communications necessary to completely process a request for laboratory procedures is shown in Figure 60-1. In a physician's office laboratory only the patient, the physician, and the laboratory technologist may be involved in the cycle. In a large medical center, however, as many as 30 or more persons and steps may be involved in carrying out this cycle. With each additional step or person involved, an additional potential source of error, confusion, or delay is introduced. In order to contribute effectively to medical care, the modern clinical laboratory must concern itself with the ramifications of this entire cycle rather than confining its interest only to the traditional area of data acquisition.

The first step in the cycle of physician-laboratory communications is the encounter between the patient and the physician, resulting in a decision on the part of the physician that a laboratory examination or measurement is necessary to assist in making a specific diagnosis, in providing a prognostic judgment, or in monitoring the results of therapy. The physician's decision is translated into a written order, which in turn is recorded, usually by a physician, nurse, or clerk, through a written requisition for laboratory measurements or examinations. The requisition includes the requested determinations as well as basic demographic information about the patient derived from the ADT (admission, discharge, transfer) function. Either it is accompanied by a specimen or laboratory personnel collect the specimen. When both the completed requisition and the appropriately labeled specimen are available in the laboratory, the requested

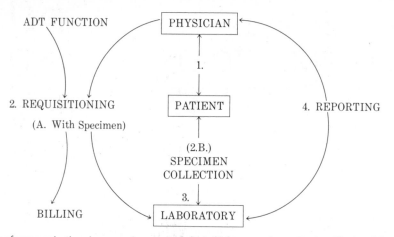

Figure 60-1. Cycle of communications in processing a typical clinical laboratory determination. The intralaboratory component of this cycle comprises only step 3 (the data acquisition from performance of the requested determination) plus step 2.B., when the laboratory performs the specimen collection. All the other essential components (patient-physician encounter, requisitioning, and reporting) are extralaboratory activities. The ADT function provides the admission, discharge, and transfer information necessary for the requisitioning process, while the billing function is usually a by-product of the requisitioning process.

measurements and/or examinations are performed, the resulting data are processed and checked for validity, and a report is returned to the physician.

Although this simplified cycle highlights the essential communication function involving a clinical laboratory, many other intralaboratory and extralaboratory communications are necessary, especially in the larger laboratories. Some of these functions are reviewed subsequently.

In settings such as the physician's office laboratory, the intralaboratory and extralaboratory communications are essentially the same. In a large institution the requirements for both intralaboratory and extralaboratory communications increase greatly, frequently resulting in significant increases in response time to the physician's request for laboratory support in caring for the patient. In a biologic analogy, Drucker (1967) has pointed out that an organization, like an animal, has to devote an ever greater portion of its resources to internal tasks of circulation and information transfer as the mass of the organization grows. Whereas all of the single cell animal, such as an amoeba, is in constant direct contact with its environment and all its energies can

be devoted directly to the task of survival and procreation, much of the resources of a higher animal have to be devoted to the internal task of circulation and communication. The speed and effectiveness with which this internal communication is accomplished may be a significant factor in the survival of the organism. This same problem occurs as laboratories and medical institutions grow. Not infrequently, so much effort is put into data acquisition that the staff becomes concerned only with the specimen and requisition orders which are received in one window and the report which goes out another. Contrariwise, the physician may conceive of the laboratory as only a "black box" into which a specimen and requisition are inserted, and from which a report usually is generated. Such a situation denotes a failure on the part of both the laboratory and the clinician to recognize the essential components of patient-physician-laboratory communication as outlined in Figure 60-1.

In this chapter I will outline the various essential steps in communications both inside and outside the laboratory and comment on some of the tools that are available to the clinical laboratory to assist in data acquisition, data processing, and telecommunications.

COMMUNICATIONS

Standard III of the College of American Pathologists (CAP) Standards for Accreditation of Medical Laboratories (CAP, 1974) states that, "channels of communications within the laboratory as well as with all other closely affiliated sections of services in the hospital and the medical staff shall be appropriate to the size and complexity of the organization."

INTRALABORATORY COMMUNICATIONS

Policy Manual. All laboratories should have administrative policy manuals which state the laboratory and institutional policy for the guidance of those working in the laboratory. Recurrent crises concerning the same problems are symptomatic of a laboratory that has no clearly understood and documented policies.

The policy should reflect the philosophy and overall goals of the larger organization as well as those of the laboratory. They should be written in consultation with the persons involved and reviewed by the appropriate persons in the institution (e.g., the personnel department) to be certain they are consistent with institutional policy. Like the laboratory procedure manuals, policies should be dated and approved by the laboratory director. Because of the rapidly changing nature of most laboratory operations, they should be reviewed and updated at least annually with a signature or initials and a date to document this review.

Policy manuals should be readily available to all laboratory employees and the orientation of new employees should include an introduction to the laboratory policies.

Procedure Manual. Standard IV of the College of American Pathologists (CAP) Commission on Laboratory Inspection and Accreditation (CAP, 1974) states that "quality control systems for laboratories should be designed to assure the medical reliability of the laboratory data." In the explanatory notes, the following statement is made concerning procedure manuals:

All laboratory methods in current use must be recorded in notebooks, card files, or sets of flow charts available at all times in the immediate bench area where the tests are performed. Each method description must be complete, including reagent brands, source and content of standards, calibration procedures, any special precautions, anticipated reactions, and pertinent literature references. Each method must be dated and initialed by the director, or responsible supervisor, initially and at least annually.

Similar requirements exist in most state and federal regulations concerning clinical laboratory practice. Thus good laboratory practice, as well as law, requires a well-documented laboratory procedure manual.

Orientation and Continuing In-service Education. Each laboratory should have a program of orientation for new employees to make them aware of the laboratory policies and the procedures used in the particular laboratory. Even though a new employee may be a registered technologist, his or her experience with particular procedures in use in a new environment may be limited. During this orientation it should be emphasized that suggestions for changing procedures or methods are welcome and will be given due consideration, but that each employee must follow the laboratory method and procedures exactly as prescribed. Individual initiative in modifying laboratory determinations without consultation and proper documentation should not be tolerated.

Because of the rapidly changing nature of laboratory medicine, it is also desirable to have regular continuing education sessions for laboratory staff. These can be developed and presented by the laboratory staff and directors with outside participants as needed. In addition, the staff should be given the time, and encouraged to attend, appropriate medical staff meetings in the institution as well as continuing education programs in laboratory medicine elsewhere. Documentation of attendance at such meetings, as well as topics covered, should be maintained to meet accreditation requirements.

Intralaboratory Staff Meetings. Intralaboratory communications are enhanced and crises minimized when regularly scheduled meetings of laboratory directors, associates, supervisors, and staff are held. Meetings of the supervisors and laboratory director are usually held weekly to discuss administrative, professional, and technical problems. Periodic full laboratory staff meetings are also useful as a forum for discussing problems, new policies, and procedures and for planning. Such meetings, if properly organized and directed, tend

6

to promote teamwork in the laboratory and to bring problems to light before they become crises.

EXTRALABORATORY COMMUNICATIONS

Manual of Procedures and Collection Instructions. The CAP Standards insist that "the laboratory must maintain a complete and detailed book of instructions covering the ordering of tests, precautions for special procedures, the proper method for preservation of specimens, and pertinent standard procedures of the laboratory. The procedures used for collection of all specimens, their proper identification, their storage and their preservation must be clearly described in writing and available to those collecting specimens. All procedures shall be such as to insure satisfactory specimens for procedures to be performed" (CAP, 1974).

At a minimum, such manuals should be available at every patient unit, both inpatient and outpatient. A loose-leaf format with each page dated allows sections to be updated without having to reprint the entire volume. A list of locations of all notebooks should be maintained by the laboratory and one person designated to update the manuals as changes are made. Where it is available, a computerized list in alphabetical order of all determinations performed by the laboratory is very useful. If the data are stored on computer tape or disc, updating and printing of dated, revised procedure lists are facilitated (Fig. 60-2).

Laboratory Users' Manual. In addition to the manual of laboratory procedures and collection instructions in notebooks located at each patient unit, many laboratories find it useful to produce a pocket-sized manual for the attending and the house staffs. This is particularly useful in teaching institutions where there is a large and frequently changing group of attending physicians, house officers, and students who need ready access to information about laboratory services. A users' manual of two sections has been found to be most useful. The first section contains a directory of the laboratory sections (e.g., hematology, chemistry) with listings of the key staff, the laboratory location, telephone numbers, operating hours, and special instructions (Fig. 60-3). The second half of the manual consists of an alphabetical computer listing of laboratory measurements and examinations.

This contains the same information as shown in Figure 60-2 but is reduced in printing to the appropriate size for the laboratory users' manual.

Laboratory Bulletins. Periodic laboratory bulletins, newsletters, or measurements of the month, circulated to the medical staff, are a useful means of communicating information about new laboratory services or policies. These are generally most effective when a standard format has been devised and when they are issued on a regular basis. Because of the information explosion with which the clinician must deal daily, these should be concisely written, carefully edited discussions of topics of current interest. Many problems can be avoided if a draft copy of a proposed bulletin is reviewed prior to distribution by those physicians most knowledgeable or most affected by the topic being discussed. An effective approach is to use a one-page or multiple-page issue on one major topic with brief general announcements at the end.

Other Extralaboratory Communications. One of the most important functions of laboratory directors is to be available and responsive to written or verbal communication from the clinician users of the laboratory. It is by such extralaboratory communications that the laboratory staff becomes aware of its failure or success in meeting the needs of the users, for, as emphasized by Drucker (1967): "There are no results within the organization. All the results are on the outside . . . a hospital has results on a respective patient."

If the laboratory director or staff have a negative or defensive attitude about constructive criticism or other extralaboratory communications, they will soon discover that these communications have greatly diminished or ceased. This will result in the unrealistic impression that no problems exist; it will become apparent that communications have failed only when a major crisis arises.

Such informal communications can be enhanced by making the physician welcome in the laboratory. Some laboratories have a physicians' lounge with coffee available for the attending physicians. The laboratory director can also promote this sort of exchange by regular attendance at general medical staff meetings as well as specialty service meetings, by eating in the doctors' dining room, and by occasionally joining the physicians in the operating room or medical staff lounges for an informal conversation.

```
                    NORTH CAROLINA MEMORIAL HOSPITAL
              INSTRUCTIONS FOR COLLECTION OF LABORATORY SPECIMENS
                                 05/11/77

    PROCEDURE              LABORATORY    SPECIMEN REQUIREMENT       REFERENCE INTERVALS

    ABO GROUP & RH TYPE    BLOOD BANK    2 ML BLOOD,RED TOP (2)     NA
                                            MICRO: 1 POLY TUBE

    ABSOLUTE EOS COUNT     HEMATOLOGY    3 ML BLOOD,LAV TOP         100-300/CUMM

    ACETAMINOPHEN          CHEMISTRY     7 ML BLOOD,RED TOP         THERAP 10-25 UG/ML
                                                                   TOXIC 100-250 UG/ML

    ACETEST (KETONES)      CHEMISTRY     3 ML BLOOD,RED TOP (1)     NEGATIVE

    ACETONE                CHEMISTRY     SEE ALCOHOL SCREEN (1)     MIN DETECT: 20 MG/DL

    ACID HEMOLYSINS        HEMATOLOGY    BLOOD,1 BLUE TOP           NO HEMOLYSIS

    ACID PHOSPHATASE       CHEMISTRY     2 ML BLOOD,RED TOP         0-12 U/LITER

    ACID PTASE PROSTAT.    CHEMISTRY     2 ML BLOOD,RED TOP         0-4 U/LITER

    ACTH                   RIA-ENDO      20 ML BLOOD,GREEN TOP      C.02-0.10 NG/ML A.M.

    ADENOVIRUSES           VIROLOGY      3 ML BLOOD,YELLOW TOP      PAIRED SERA 4X INCRS

    ADMISSION PANEL        CHEMISTRY     21 ML BLOOD,RED TOP          SEE INDIVIDUAL TESTS
                                            INCLUDES NA,K,CL,CO2,BUN,CREATININE,ALK
                                            P'TASE,ALT,AST,LDH,TOTAL PROTEIN,ALBUMIN
                                            URIC ACID,TOTAL BILIRUBIN & CALCIUM

    ADRENOCORTCOTROP HOR   RIA-ENDO      SEE ACTH                   0.02-0.10 NG/ML A.M.

    AGAROSE ELECT SCRN     CHEMISTRY     SEE SERUM PROTEIN PROFILE INTERPRETATION

    AGBM                   IMMUNOLOGY    SEE GLOMERUL BASE MEM AB   NEGATIVE

    ALANINE AMINOTRANS     CHEMISTRY     1 ML BLOOD,RED TOP (2)     8-60 UNITS/ML
                                            MICRO: 150 MICROLITERS WHOLE BLOOD
                                            MICRO: 1 POLY TUBE

    ALBUMIN,CSF            CHEMISTRY     .5 ML CSF                  5-50 MG/DL

    ALBUMIN,SERUM          CHEMISTRY     1 ML BLOOD,RED TOP (3)     3.5-5.0 G/DL
                                            MICRO: 50 MICROLITERS WHOLE BLOOD

    ALBUMIN,URINE          CHEMISTRY     24 HR URINE REFRIGERATE    9-22 MG/24 HRS
                                            OBTAIN CONTAINER "A" FROM CHEM LAB

    ALCOHOL,ETHYL          CHEMISTRY     SEE ALCOHOL SCREEN (1)     >300 MG/DL TOXIC
                                                                   MIN DETECT: 20 MG/DL

    ALCOHOL,ISOPROPYL      CHEMISTRY     SEE ALCOHOL SCREEN (1)     >350 MG/DL TOXIC
                                                                   MIN DETECT: 1C MG/DL

    ALCOHOL,METHYL         CHEMISTRY     SEE ALCOHOL SCREEN (1)     >80 MG/DL TOXIC
                                                                   MIN DETECT: 5 MG/DL

    ALCOHOL SCREEN         CHEMISTRY     7 ML BLOOD,RED TOP (1)       SEE INDIVID TESTS
                                            INCLUDES ACETONE,ETHYL ALCOHOL,METHYL
                                            ALCOHOL & ISOPROPYL ALCOHOL
                                            DO NOT PREP PATIENT WITH ALCOHOL

    ALDOLASE               CHEMISTRY     1 ML BLOOD,RED TOP         3-8 UNITS/ML

    ALDOSTERONE,SERUM      RIA-ENDO      28 ML BLOOD,RED TOP          SEE POCKET MANUAL

    ALDOSTERONE,URINE      RIA-ENDO      100 ML OF 24 HR COLLECTN   2-16 UG/24 HR
                                            ADD 20 ML 33% ACETIC ACID TO CONTAINER
                                            AT START OF COLLECTION

    ALKALINE PHOSPHATASE   CHEMISTRY     1 ML BLOOD RED TOP (2)     ADULT 2-6 UNITS
                                                                   CHILD 6-12 UNITS
                                            MICRO: 150 MICROLITERS WHOLE BLOOD

    ALK PTASE ISOENZYME    CHEMISTRY     CONTACT LABORATORY         NA
```

Figure 60-2. Computer-generated listing of procedures, specimen requirements, and reference intervals.

6

The importance of open communications and mutual respect between the laboratory staff and the nursing and clerical staffs throughout the hospital is frequently overlooked. The work of these persons in collecting specimens, transmitting orders, completing requisitions, and charting laboratory reports have a direct impact on the laboratory's ability to perform its function. As a result, orientation programs and in-service education by laboratory staff covering these subjects can promote good will and minimize misunderstandings between these various groups in the hospital.

HEMATOLOGY LABORATORY

Location: 1st Floor, Ambulatory Patient Care Facility, Room 1258

Extensions: 64087 (Hematology and Urinalysis)
64661 (Special Hematology)
Note: If no answer in hematology between midnight and 7:00 AM, call beeper #5567

Staff
Director: John A. Johnson, M.D.
Associate Director: Eugene Patterson, M.D.
Supervisor: Jane A. Smith, MT(ASCP)
Assistant Supervisors:
  Routine Hematology: Anne Gillis, MT(ASCP)
  Special Hematology: Langley Arlington, MT(ASCP)
  Evening & Mornings: Charles A. Johnston, MT(ASCP)
  Urinalysis: David R. Charles, MT(ASCP)

Hours of Operation
Hematology and Urinalysis: 24 hours a day, 7 days a week
Special Hematology: 8:00 AM–5:00 PM, Monday through Friday

Resident On-Call: A Laboratory Medicine Resident is on-call during holidays, nights, and weekends for problems arising in the laboratory. The resident on call may be contacted through the Hospital Operator.

General Guidelines
1. A Complete Blood Count (CBC) includes the following determinations done on the Coulter S: Hemoglobin, Hematocrit, RBC, Indices, and WBC. If one or more components of a CBC are ordered, all are done since the charge to the patient is the same.
2. The following procedures are offered between 10:00 PM and 8:00 AM: CBC, WBC differential, platelet count, fluid cell count, and urinalysis. Other determinations must be approved by the Laboratory Medicine Resident On-Call.
3. All urine specimen containers (not lids) must be labeled with the full name and unit number of the patient. Urine specimens must be received in the laboratory within 2 hours of collection.
4. Bone marrows should be scheduled with the Special Hematology Section at extension 64661.
5. Consult the Procedures Directory for a complete list of available determinations and examinations.

Figure 60-3. Page from first section (Laboratory Directory) of laboratory users manual. The second section (Procedures Directory) is shown in Figure 60-2.

REQUISITIONING AND REPORTING

REQUISITIONING

Proper requisitioning procedures assure adequate identification of the patient and the specimen, indicate the measurements or examinations desired, and facilitate reporting of the results. An additional important function is the provision of administrative and billing data.

Both the Joint Commission on Accreditation of Hospitals (JCAH, 1976) and the CAP Standards for Accreditation of Medical Laboratories (CAP, 1974) recognize the key role of requisitioning. The explanatory notes for CAP Standard III (CAP, 1974) state:

All requests for clinical laboratory tests must be made in writing. A time stamp should be used to establish the date and hour that the request was received by the laboratory . . . these requests and reports shall identify the patient with certainty. Minimum identification data shall include at least

the full name of the patient, hospital number, room number or address, age, sex and attending physician. Requisitions should clearly specify the tests to be performed and the kind of service required (routine, pre-op, STAT, etc.) and, where appropriate, should specify the time when the specimen was collected.

The JCAH also requires the following record in the laboratory (JCAH, 1976, Standard II, Interpretation):

A record should be maintained of the daily accession of specimens, each of which should be numbered, or otherwise appropriately identified. This record should contain at least the following information:
  Laboratory procedure number or other identification
  Identification of the patient
  Name of the practitioner
  Date and time the specimen was collected
  Date and time the specimen was received
  Date, time, and by whom the specimen was examined
  Condition of any unsatisfactory specimen
  Type of test or procedure performed
  Results and date of reporting

The format of laboratory requisitions will vary considerably from hospital to hospital, although all have a basic similarity. Although many sizes of requisitions have been used in the past, most requisitions today are either the size of a Hollerith computer card ($3\frac{1}{4}$ by $7\frac{3}{8}$ inches or 8.3 by 18.7 cm.) or medical record size ($9\frac{1}{2}$ by 11 inches or 21.5 by 28 cm.). The former are generally multipart forms, one of which is usually a computer card for the business office. The top sheet is used as the report copy, with other sheets used as laboratory and physician copies.

The larger, medical-record size requisitions (Fig. 60–4) can be used for both the physician's order and the requisition, thus preventing transcription errors in ordering. The original is sent to the laboratory as a requisition and the second copy is left in the chart as a record of the order. In general these types of requisitions are used with computerized systems where reports will be given on other forms. Such a requisition, however, can also serve as a manual back-up report for an automated reporting system.

In order to facilitate the use of requisitions by nursing, clerical, and laboratory personnel, the design should be such that each requisition has specific areas for the following types of information: (1) Patient identification, usually in the upper right hand corner. Provisions should be made for either hand-written or imprinted information. (2) The date and time of specimen collection and identification of the person who collected the specimen. (3) The measurement or examination requested. When the same requisition is to be used for reporting, appropriate space for the results should be included in the same area. (4) Date and time of reporting and the initials of the technologist performing the determination. (5) The identification of the laboratory. It is also desirable to have imprinted on the form the name of the director of laboratories and/or the associate director of the laboratory section in which the requisition is used. If the procedure is performed by another laboratory, that laboratory's name must also be shown on the report.

If the laboratory has different requisitions for different sections, it is essential that the general layout of the forms be the same in order not to confuse clerical and nursing personnel who will be completing the requests. The requisition itself should be black ink on white paper for best results if medical records containing these reports are later to be micro-filmed; the requisitions for different sections can be color coded for quick identification on the tab or in other areas without data.

PATIENT AND SPECIMEN IDENTIFICATION

At this time no completely reliable, generally acceptable, and cost-effective system of total patient and specimen identification is available. This area thus remains one of the greatest unsolved problems in the clinical laboratories, since reliable patient and specimen identification is an essential feature of any accurate laboratory testing and reporting system. Progress has been reported by the Committee for Commonality in Blood Banking Automation in applying the bar-coded label technique used in grocery stores and other businesses to the area of blood banking (ABC, 1977).

It is anticipated that in the next decade reliable and cost-effective methods of patient and specimen identification will be more readily available. If a laboratory is considering such an approach, however, it should be planned in conjunction with a total hospital approach to this problem, since any identification system being used for laboratory purposes should be the same as that being used for admitting, nursing, pharmacy, radiology, and other services. Otherwise the expense will be prohibitive and great confusion may result.

Until such time as a more reliable automated identification system is available, laboratory professionals must take utmost care with the manual system and insist on proper identification of patients and specimens. Most hospitals apply an armband on inpatients at admission, and laboratory personnel should check this armband with the requisition. A useful additional check is to ask the patient for his or her name and birthdate and to check this against the data available on the armband and the requisition. If the patient is not lucid or if the proper identification is not on the patient (identification on the bed or in the room is not acceptable, since patients are moved without changing such identification), laboratory personnel should be instructed to seek positive identification by other persons who know the patient. Such identification should be documented on the requisition. Each specimen should be labeled immediately by the person collecting the specimen with the patient's full name (correctly spelled), hospital numbers, and date. Blood specimens for

6

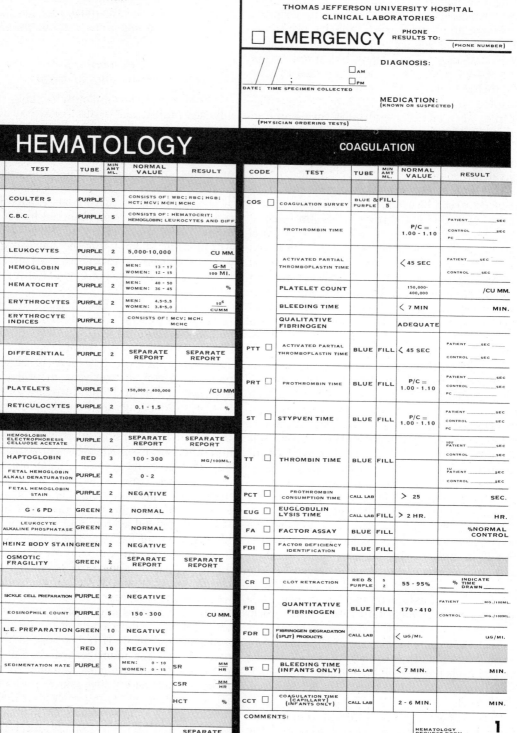

Figure 60-4. A requisition form which can be used as an order sheet (the second copy remaining in the chart). This form is used with a computerized reporting system, but is designed to serve also as a temporary report form on a back-up basis.

cross-matching should also show on the label the name of the phlebotomist. When specimens are collected by other than laboratory personnel, these data should be verified; improperly labeled or unlabeled specimens should not be accepted by the laboratory.

REPORTS

Written reports

Both the Joint Commission on Accreditation of Hospitals and the College of American Pathologists state that the laboratory director is responsible for all laboratory reports and that "authenticated and dated reports of clinical pathology tests should be filed promptly with the patient's record and duplicate copies kept in the laboratory" (CAP, 1974). The CAP Standards further state:

Each report should be time stamped to record the date and hour the procedure was completed. Each request and report should identify the patient with certainty . . . whenever feasible, reports should all be signed or initialed by the technologist responsible for performing this procedure or by the pathologist.

When computerized laboratory reports are used the presence of technologist's initial or numbers on the report can be confused with patient data by the clinician; in such instances it is generally accepted that documentation of the technologist performing the determination in the laboratory log or on worksheets is sufficient.

General Qualities of a Laboratory Report. A subcommittee of the College of American Pathologists reported in 1974 on general qualities of a good laboratory report (Burns, 1974). These considerations are of value in designing either a manual or a computer-generated reporting system. They are as follows:

1. Compactness
2. Consistency of terminology, format, and usage of abbreviations and symbols
3. Clear understandability
4. Logical and accessible location in medical chart
5. Statement of date and time of collection
6. Gross description and source of specimen when pertinent
7. Sharp differentiation of reference or normal and abnormal values
8. Sequential order of multiple results on single specimen
9. Identification of patient, patient location, and physician
10. Assurance of accuracy of transcription of request
11. Ease of preparation
12. Administrative and record-keeping value

Verbal Reports. Verbal reports constitute a major problem for most laboratories. It is essential that verbal or telephone reports be given in order to facilitate medical care, particularly in an emergency situation. On the other hand, this is a major potential source of errors and medical liability. At a minimum, the laboratory should require proper identification of the person receiving the report and of the patient. The person giving the report should repeat the patient's name, identification number, and location along with the results in order to further confirm the identification.

As an alternate to verbal reports, many laboratories are using various transmission devices from the laboratory to key areas such as the emergency room and intensive care unit which require immediate reports. One type allows a hand-written result on either blank paper or a preprinted form to be transmitted electronically and generated in a similar form at the receiving end. This has the advantage of being reliable and relatively inexpensive, but it is subject to transcription errors. A newer approach is facsimile transmission, a process similar to photocopying a document, but done electronically to a remote output device. This has the advantage of giving an exact facsimile of the original test report, but has the disadvantage of being more expensive, generally slower, and in some cases less reliable. Such devices as these provide a rapid, on-line report for immediate patient care; a permanent report from the laboratory in the usual format would follow for medicolegal and medical record purposes.

MANUAL SYSTEMS FOR TEST REQUISITIONING AND REPORTING

Although automated data processing is increasingly being used for laboratory requisitioning and reporting, manual means for doing this same task will undoubtedly be used in many laboratories and in many situations for years to come. A properly designed manual system can provide many beneficial features of a computerized system without the investments necessary for a computerized system. A

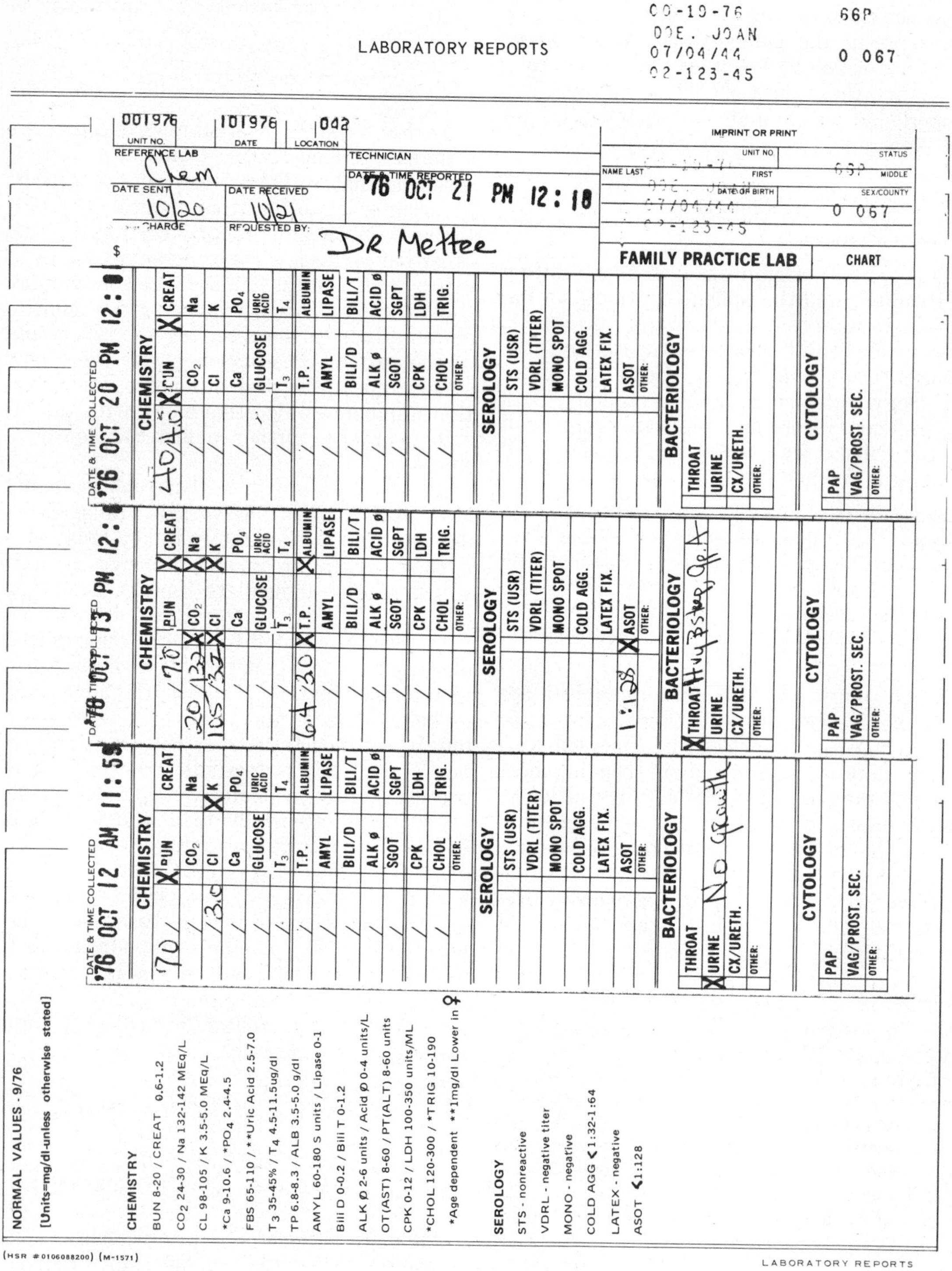

LABORATORY REPORTS

CO-19-76   66P
DOE, JOAN
07/04/44   0 067
02-123-45

Figure 60–5. Use of carrier sheet in chart with reporting slips designed to provide a manual cumulative report.

poorly designed manual system, however, can be a major hindrance for a laboratory operation, and, more importantly, for the medical care of the patients served by the laboratory. Furthermore, experience has shown that computerization of a laboratory with a poorly or-

ganized manual system leads only to more chaos, rather than solving any problems. As the volume increases for manual systems, the point will be reached where automated data processing is essential. The laboratory director should try to anticipate this development by implementing an effective manual system and planning ahead to an automated data processing system before a crisis situation is reached.

Most manual systems are based on combined test requisitioning and reporting forms, usually in the size of a Hollerith card, as noted previously.

Although a requisitioning and reporting system may meet the needs of the laboratory, it is important that the laboratory director be aware of the needs of the clinician for a concise, readable, and chronologic presentation of related laboratory data. Traditionally this has been performed by shingling the laboratory reports in the patient record. If these reports are color coded by originating laboratory and the reports from a single laboratory are put together on a carrier page, this can provide a chronologic reporting system. This can be facilitated by using reports designed in a vertical format so that the date and time of collection are seen across the top and the results are written vertically (Fig. 60-5).

An alternative method exists for providing a chronologically oriented type of report that simulates a computerized cumulative report. (Henry, 1964) (Fig. 60-6). The laboratory has an 8½ by 11 inch or larger master card (cumulative report card or CRC) on which the patient's demographic data are written or imprinted at the time of admission or of first laboratory activity. A simple disposable requisition is used to request testing (and for billing purposes, if necessary). After the determinations are performed in the laboratory, the results are written in the proper position on the master card (CRC) in the laboratory along with the date and time of collection at the head of the column. If the laboratory is large and organized in sections, each section may have a separate CRC for its data. After the laboratory data are placed on the CRC, a dated photocopy is made; this copy is sent to the physician or chart as the report. As subsequent data are added to the card and copies made, the earlier copies in the chart are removed and replaced by the updated photocopy of the CRC. This system has the advantage of providing a cumulative report to both the physician and the laboratory and of allowing the laboratory to make "delta checks" on the data before releasing new data (that is, checking the current data against the previous data to determine if the results are reasonable). It can be used either as a totally manual system or as a temporary manual back-up approach for a computerized reporting system. The disad-

vantages of the system relate to the investment of clerical time and photocopying, as well as the possibility of transcription errors. Also, if the patient volume is high, the cost of filing and retrieving the master cards can be considerable.

AUTOMATED DATA PROCESSING AND TELECOMMUNICATIONS

Although automated data processing has been used in routine clinical laboratories for only little over a decade, the concept of using machine-readable information is almost two centuries old. The Jacquard Loom, which was invented about 1800 in France, utilized punched paper cards to control automatically the pattern woven by the loom. Even earlier, rolls of punched paper had been used to program automatically some musical instruments. The first major practical use of automated data processing equipment occurred at the end of the nineteenth century when Hermann Hollerith used punched cards (the size of the old U.S. dollar bill) and automated data sorters for tabulating the 1890 census in the United States. His work and his tabulating card company later led to the founding of the International Business Machine Company in the early part of the twentieth century and to the rapid expansion of the use of keypunched data and tabulating machines. World War II led to the development of electronic data processing units for military purposes, followed in the postwar years by a rapid expansion of their use in commercial and other ventures. In the 1950's and 1960's three "generations" of large commercial computers were developed and marketed. Each succeeding generation was marked by increased reliability and speed, coupled with decreases in costs and size, as computer technology shifted from vacuum tubes to transitors and then to large scale integrated circuits.

The rapid advances being made in microelectronics during the 1960's led to the introduction of the minicomputers beginning with the PDP5 and PDP8 introduced in 1963 and 1965 by the Digital Equipment Corporation. Although these were minicomputers in terms of their size (approximately the size of a one- or two-drawer file cabinet) they were in many respects as powerful as the much larger, more costly, and less flexible traditional computers then available.

The further development of microelectron-

6

STATE UNIVERSITY HOSPITAL

Upstate Medical Center

CLINICAL PATHOLOGY — MICROSCOPY

Last Reporting Date: _____

	Normal Values	Date:							LEGEND
Appearance									A. Laboratory Accident
Color									B. Confirmed
Sample-Type									E. Recollect Specimen
Volume-ml.									F. Unit notified
Specific Gravity									G. Specimens not rec'd
PH									H. Hemolysis
Protein-(qualitative)	0.6								J. Xanthochromic
(quanitative)									K. Marked (over 100/hpf)
Glucose-(qualitative)(quan.)	0-0.18								L. Lactescence
Bilirubin	0								M. Minimum (less than 0-1/hpf)
Acetone	0								N. Not done-See Schedule
Hemoglobin	0								Q. Quantity not sufficient
Reducing Substances (quan.)									T. Improperly labeled
Phenylpyruvic Acid	0								U. Test cancelled by physician
Cystine	0								W. Improper specimen
MICROSCOPIC EXAM.									X. Report to follow
Cells RBC/hpf	0-2								Y. Obscured by dye
Cells WBC/hpf	0-3								
Cells epith									REMARKS:
Casts									
Other:									
Bacteria									
Mucus									
CSF CELL CT RBC/mm3									
WBC/mm3									
poly									
mono									
HCG									
Microscopy Accession No.									
Technologist									

SPECIAL MICROSCOPY	Date:							
ANALYSIS	Normal Values							
17 OH	M 7-15 / F 4-8 MG/TV							
17 Ketosteroids	M 10-20 / F 5-15 MG/TV							
Ketogenic Steroids	M 5-23 / F 3-15 MG/TV							
Urine Na	75-200mEq/L							
Urine K	26-123mEq/L							
Urine Creatinine	1.0-1.8gm/24o							
Creatinine Clearance	M 123± 16 / F 97±10 ml./min							
V M A	Up to 7.0 mg/24o							
Serum Creatinine	mg/100ml.							
Total Volume								
Accession No.								
Technologist								

40410

M.D. ⑪

Clinical Pathologist

Figure 60-6. Example of a Cumulative Report Card (CRC) for one laboratory section.

ics has led to the production in the 1970's of the microprocessor and microcomputer (Noyce, 1977). These are programmable computers with the entire central processing unit in one or more silicone chips measuring only a fraction of an inch each. Although micro-computers are somewhat slower than mini-computers and do not yet have available as versatile computer languages, they will undoubtedly revolutionize the application of computers in laboratories and elsewhere in the next decade. The same microelectronic technology has already made available to laboratories during the last decade very powerful programmable calculators as well as the small, relatively inexpensive calculators for ordinary problem solving in the laboratory. This technology has also resulted in the use of microprocessors in many clinical laboratory instruments for preprocessing of data and generation of digital outputs and printed reports.

The pioneering work in the application of computers to practical problems in the clinical laboratory occurred in the early 1960's with the work of Arthur Rappoport, George Williams, and others utilizing larger, commercially available computers applied to clinical laboratory problems. Pioneering work in the application of the minicomputer to the clinical laboratory was done by Phillip Hicks, utilizing first the LINC computer and later the PDP series of computers produced by Digital Equipment Corporation.

The enthusiasm engendered by these pioneer efforts in clinical laboratory computerization resulted in an explosion of interest both by clinical laboratory directors and computer vendors during the next decade. Such enthusiasm was frequently uncritical, leading to many failures and much wasted effort and money. By the mid-1970's, however, a number of successful laboratory information systems utilizing various approaches existed.

SCOPE OF CLINICAL LABORATORY DATA PROCESSING

Planning for the data processing and communication needs of clinical laboratories, especially those in a hospital setting, involves a consideration of much more than just the laboratory. As shown in Figure 60-1, many of the most essential components of a data communication system for a clinical laboratory are outside the walls of the laboratory. Furthermore, the laboratory in the hospital setting is dependent upon others to gather the basic administrative and medical data about the patient and to assign a unique medical record or unit number. The recognition of the interrelationship of various hospital activities has led to the development of Hospital Information Systems.

Ball (1973) has represented a Hospital Information System (HIS) as a pyramid with three levels of activity (Fig. 60-7). The administrative and financial level serves as the base

for the clinical subsystems such as the laboratories; all these functions are coordinated by a system of data collection, storage, retrieval, and communications.

Other medical computer systems have evolved with an emphasis on the medical record and are known as Medical Information Systems. Shannon and Ball (1976) have recently classified the various types of patient-oriented data processing systems as follows:

Class A. Individual, stand-alone systems, usually serving one speciality area or department such as the clinical laboratories or admitting.

Class B. The typical Hospital Information System (HIS), as shown in Figure 60-7. This is usually an institutionally oriented, interdepartmental system centering on communications.

Class C. Medical Records or Medical Information System (MIS), as shown in Figure 60-8. These systems have many features in common with the HIS but are oriented to patients, diseases, and medical records rather than to departments and the institution.

Although the ideal laboratory system today and in the future will address all the laboratory's communication problems, most laboratory systems in hospitals to date have approached the intra- and extralaboratory aspects in one sequence or another. Where the initial efforts at computerization have been made in the laboratory, the intralaboratory data processing and communication problems have been solved first with a Class A system. In other hospitals the initial computerization effort has been made on a hospital-wide basis (Class B or C system), so that extralaboratory communication needs (admission, discharge, and transfer functions, test requisitions, and sometimes reporting) have been met first. In such hospitals, the laboratory has then had to develop an intralaboratory system later as a dedicated system interfaced to the larger system or as a component of the larger system. In some hospitals components of both systems are available; for example, a laboratory-based computer system with terminals in the admitting office providing the ADT (admission, discharge, and transfer) function for the laboratory and perhaps other hospital areas. Other laboratory-based systems have terminals at the patient

6

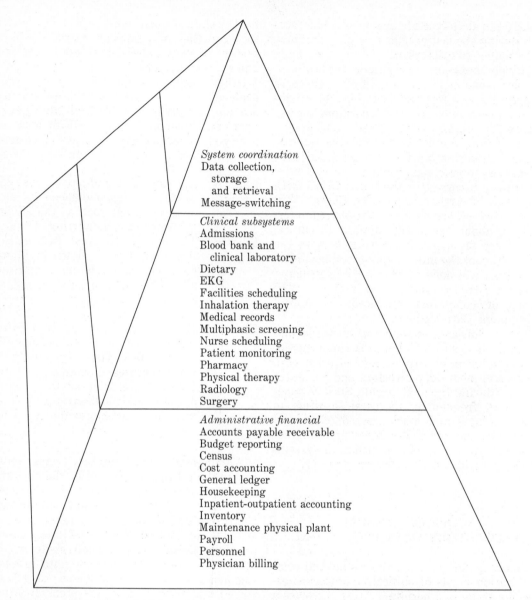

System coordination
Data collection,
   storage
   and retrieval
Message-switching

Clinical subsystems
Admissions
Blood bank and
   clinical laboratory
Dietary
EKG
Facilities scheduling
Inhalation therapy
Medical records
Multiphasic screening
Nurse scheduling
Patient monitoring
Pharmacy
Physical therapy
Radiology
Surgery

Administrative financial
Accounts payable receivable
Budget reporting
Census
Cost accounting
General ledger
Housekeeping
Inpatient-outpatient accounting
Inventory
Maintenance physical plant
Payroll
Personnel
Physician billing

Figure 60–7. Structure of a hospital information system (HIS, Class B). (Used with permission from Ball, M. J.: How to Select a Computerized Hospital Information System. Basel, S. Karger, 1973.)

units for laboratory requisitioning and reporting; this may be difficult to cost-justify, however, when compared with HIS or MIS terminals at the patient units serving multiple uses.

Ideally a laboratory information system (LIS) in a hospital will include both the intralaboratory and extralaboratory functions. Because of available resources and priorities, however, it may be necessary to develop one area prior to the other. In such a case, it is essential that all involved recognize the total needs of the laboratory and the hospital for data processing and develop the components in a way that will allow them to be used as modules for a total system to be developed later.

The intralaboratory approach to a laboratory information system provides the means for data acquisition in the laboratory and the generation of reports for internal use and reports for manual external distribution to

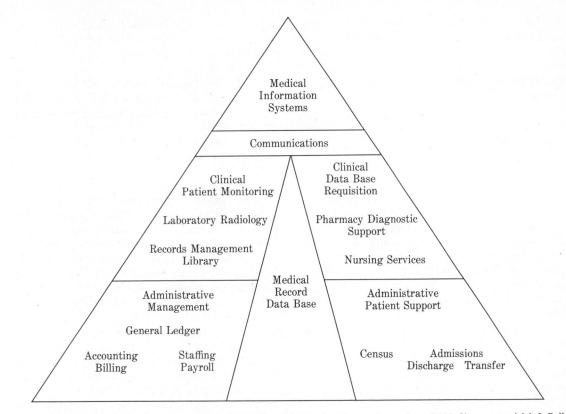

Figure 60–8. The medical information system (MIS, Class C). (Used with permission from R. H. Shannon and M. J. Ball, Bioscience Communications, 2:282, 1976.)

clinicians and to medical records. In a stand-alone laboratory system (Class A system) requisitions are generally received at the laboratory in the traditional fashion and entered in the computer by card readers or cathode ray tubes (CRT's). Admission, discharge, and transfer data (ADT) may have to be entered in a similar manner as information is received manually from the admitting office. The laboratory computer system may produce billing reports, or this information may be transmitted to an on-site or off-site hospital business computer by manual or electronic means.

The extralaboratory approach to a laboratory information system generally is a part of a larger Hospital Information System. Such systems are usually oriented to the patient units with on-line input of physicians' orders into the computer terminals and with feedback to the unit of confirmations, instructions, and reports. An essential feature of such a system is an on-line ADT function from the admitting office in order that the system know the current location and status of each patient.

Hospital charges are captured automatically by the system at the time requests are made at the nursing station. The various professional supporting services such as the clinical laboratory, radiology, and pharmacy are notified of orders, usually by printers located in these areas. In some systems, programs exist to permit the immediate print-out of emergency or timed requests to be collected by the laboratory, while storing the routine requests to be printed in the form of a collection list at the time the blood drawing team makes the next collection.

In considering a laboratory computer system it is thus essential for the planners to realize the distinction between these two approaches and to determine if both are to be done simultaneously or if they are to be phased in one sequence or another. Whereas the first approach (a Class A system) may be successfully accomplished primarily as a laboratory venture, the second approach (Class B or C system) involves the planning and cooperation of almost the entire institution. Even though a stand-alone laboratory system may be the only computerization contemplated in the near future, an institution-wide approach to its planning and implementation is still highly recommended for the reasons discussed previously.

DEFINITION OF TERMS AND CONCEPTS

The laboratory director involved in automated data processing or considering this for the clinical laboratory should have a knowledge of the basic principles and concepts of data processing in order to communicate the laboratory's needs to computer specialists and possible vendors. In order to avoid the excesses of the past, the computer should be looked upon as another tool, rather than as an end in itself. Like other tools, it is an extension or amplification of man's ability to solve a problem. Because it is an extension of man's mind, it is a very powerful tool. Like other powerful tools available in medicine (chemotherapy, surgery, radiation), it has potential for great benefits but also the potential for great harm. Harmful effects can be avoided by a critical approach to the field and by a basic understanding of the general principles involved.

A few basic definitions and concepts are given in the discussion to follow, and the reader seeking greater detail is directed to the works cited in the references for this chapter and Chapter 58. The reports on clinical laboratory computerization by J. Lloyd Johnson Associates are particularly recommended (Johnson, 1975; 1976).

In very simple terms a computer goes through the same steps to solve a problem as does a human being. To solve a problem such as "2 + 2," a person must have an input device (ears or eyes), a memory to provide processing instructions and to store the intermediate and final answers, a brain to process the problem, and some way to produce the answer (in writing or by voice). The computer uses input devices such as card readers or cathode ray tubes (CRT or TV tubes) to receive the instructions, problem, and data. The central processing unit (CPU) of the computer uses a program stored in its memory for instructions. Certain simple problems may be solved directly by the arithmetic portion of the computer, whereas more complicated problems may be directed step by step by the computer program, utilizing in

sequence multiple simple logic circuits. Once the problem is solved, the computer then stores the answer for later output in various forms. Most commonly the output is in the form of some type of printing, either in hardcopy by a printer or on a CRT. Many other forms of computer output are available, including punched cards and even a vocal output utilizing prerecorded numbers and words assembled by the computer to give a verbal answer.

A *computer system* has two essential components for complete operation. The *hardware* is the physical structure of the computer. This includes the central processing unit with its associated control units, arithmetic (logic) circuits, and timing devices. It also includes the peripheral memory storage devices (usually in the form of magnetic tape or magnetic discs) and the various input and output devices (known as I/O devices). In order for the computer to accept information, solve problems, and properly produce the solutions to the problems, the computer must also have a program of instructions known as *software*. In the human analogy the hardware and software are comparable to structure and function (or anatomy and physiology).

Human beings are accustomed to thinking and solving problems utilizing a *decimal system of numbers* (such as ones, tens, and hundreds), and characters (such as A, B, C) linked together in words of variable length. For example, we might say, "The hematocrit is 39 per cent." The computer can handle similar data but must encode it into a much simpler common denominator. Otherwise the computer designers would be faced with an impossible task of being able to electronically represent ten different levels of numbers (0 to 9), 26 English characters (A to Z), and a multitude of words of variable length.

The modern computer is thus based on the *binary number system;* all decimal numbers and natural language inputs are encoded into this system by the computer input devices. All computer processing and storage occurs in a binary form, which is then decoded into the decimal and natural language form for the output devices.

The basic building block of computer languages is the *bit* (abbreviation of *bi*nary dig*it*). This is expressed as either a zero or a one. This binary expression of information gives the computer designer multiple options for expressing mechanically or electronically binary information. These include the presence or absence of a punched hole in a computer card; the presence or absence of a pencil mark on an optically sensed document; the rotational direction of a magnetic charge on a magnetic core; or the presence or absence of an electrical charge in an electronic circuit.

Alphabetical characters of information can be coded in the binary system by groups of 8 bits, based on a standardized scheme. The term *byte* (or *character*) is used to refer to a group of 8 bits when one is speaking of the size of computer storage. Computers also use *computer words*. These are generally fixed length words in multiples of four bits, (for example, a 4 bit word, 8 bit word, 16 bit word, or 32 bit word). Current microcomputers generally use the shorter word lengths (4 to 16 bits), while most minicomputers use 8 to 32 bit computer words. The longer computer words permit more efficient handling of large numbers and more efficient use of large computer memories.

The computer programmer instructs the computer by means of a *computer language*. Although the computer itself is run by instructions in zeros and ones, this approach is awkward, time consuming, and error prone for the human. *Assembly languages* permit the programmer to write the list of instructions in mnemonics. These are then translated by a computer program known as an *assembler* on a one-to-one basis into the machine language instructions which will be used by the computer. Assembly languages are specific for each type of computer.

In an effort to further simplify computer programming and increase the productivity of programmers, various *higher level programming languages* have been developed. With slight modifications the same language can be used in different computers. They are organized in a way to reflect human thought. For example, COBOL (*Common Business Oriented Language*) has been designed for business oriented computer programming, while FORTRAN (*Formula Translation*) is designed for scientific use and permits the programmer to write programs in essentially the same way one would state a problem in a formula. The higher level languages require a *compiler program* to translate the instructions into machine instructions for use by the computer. The higher level languages are much easier to use for the programmer but are not as efficient in terms of required memory in the computer

as is assembly language. Now that computer hardware is more compact and much less expensive, however, the size of the computer memory is no longer the critical determinant, as it once was in the smaller laboratory computers.

The laboratory director planning a computer system will not need to know the detailed internal processing of the computer but should be familiar with the various hardware components, since these may influence greatly the performance of the computer. The central portion of the computer hardware is known as the *central processing unit* (CPU). This consists of the computer memory as well as arithmetic (logic) and control circuits. Until recently most CPU memory was composed of small magnetic cores threaded by several tiny wires, and thus were known as *core memory*. The bits of information were stored as zeros and ones based on the rotational direction of the magnetic charge. The core memory is now being replaced by solid state semiconductor memory. Memory size is indicated by the number of K of computer words which can be stored in the core memory. One K represents roughly 1000 computer words, or more specifically 2^{10} or 1024 computer words. A sixteen K computer thus has a core storage of 16×2^{10} or 16,384 separate words. The actual number of bits being stored would depend on the computer word length (for instance, 8 bit or 16 bit). In general, the larger the computer memory, the more powerful the computer. This is not a direct relationship, however, since the type of language used for programming, the size of the computer word, and the nature of the hardware all determine the requirements for memory.

The laboratory director also needs to be concerned with the peripheral devices, since these will also have a major effect on the operation of a laboratory computer system. The peripheral memory devices such as discs must be of sufficient speed to handle all of the anticipated transactions and must be of sufficient size to store all of the required data for the desired period of time. At a minimum the system speed should allow response times on the terminals of no more than several seconds and the storage capacity should permit active, on-line files for all inpatients, for discharged patients for 30 to 60 days, and for outpatients for 30 to 60 days after the last activity. The growth of the laboratory volume should also be taken into account; if possible, the initial sys-

TABLE 60–1. COMMON INPUT AND OUTPUT (I/O) TECHNIQUES USED
IN LABORATORY INFORMATION SYSTEMS

	TECHNIQUES	APPROXIMATE SPEED OF INPUT OR OUTPUT	COMMENTS
Key punch	Holes punched in 80 column Hollerith card using card punch and verifier; computer input by card reader	An experienced key punch operator can input approximately 130 characters per minute. Card reader: 300-1200 cards/min.	Noisy and slow; requires handling large volume of cards. Machine and human readable. Not commonly used for output.
Mark sense	Preprinted card marked with a pencil to indicate data for computer entry; computer input by card reader.	Card readers: 300 cards/min.	May have significant error rate. Machine and human readable. Not used for output.
Paper tape	Holes punched into paper tape.	Punched at 50 characters/second; read at 300 characters/second.	Messy; problems if tape torn or wet. Machine readable only. May be useful for instrument output (e.g., gamma counters) with later input into computer through paper tape reader.
Cathode ray tube (CRT) with keyboard	Typewriter-like keyboard for data entry with verification on screen.	Speed variable by function but can be enhanced using formatted screens. Speed usually figured in transactions per minute or hour.	Relatively rapid. Quiet. Coded or free text entry. Requires typing skills for rapid input. Useful for input or output.
Cathode ray tube (CRT) with light pen	Formulated data on screen; data or requests indicated by light pen pointed to appropriate place.	Quite rapid for fixed entry functions but drops off when free text data also entered.	Relatively rapid and easy to learn. Quiet. Useful for input or output.
Printing terminal or teletype	Data entered by typing on the keyboard; verified on printed page. Output printed a character at a time.	Input speed depends on function and can be enhanced using coded entries. Output usually 30 characters per second.	Requires typing skills for rapid input. Noisy. Human readable hard copy for documentation of input. Useful for input or output.
Line printer	Prints one line at a time of data on continuous paper (hard copy).	Output of 200 to 1200 lines/min.	Hard copy output only. Noisy. Rapid method for large volume output (cumulative reports, etc.)
Computer-outputted microfilm or microfiche (COM)	Computer formulates reports or tabulation of data which is transferred to tape, then to microfilm or microfiche.	Very rapid; usually at tape reading and writing speed.	Useful for storage of large quantities of data not needed immediately. May access through microfilm or microfiche readers. COM usually done off-site by special equipment not a part of an LIS.

tem should be able to handle at least a doubling of volume without degradation of these standards. The I/O devices are also of great importance. These should be sufficient in number to prevent bottlenecks in the laboratory operation. They should also be of size and design to permit efficient use by technologists and clerical personnel. The common types of peripheral memory devices and I/O devices used in laboratory information systems are listed in Tables 60-1 and 60-2.

Practically all computers being used in clinical laboratories and in most commerical operations are *digital computers*, since they are based on the concept of dealing with discrete digits or pieces of information. Certain machine outputs, such as an electrocardiogram or the single channel AutoAnalyzer, generate an *analog* or continuous signal. Data in analog form must be converted to digital form either by the instrument or by the computer in order to be processed in a digital computer. This is known as *A to D* (Analog to Digital) *Conversion*. In the original laboratory computer sys-

Table 60–2. AUXILIARY STORAGE DEVICES COMMONLY USED IN LABORATORY INFORMATION SYSTEMS

	PHYSICAL MEDIUM FOR STORAGE OF DATA	SPEED AND CAPACITY	COMMENTS
Magnetic Tape			Unlimited off-line storage; removable. Relatively slow access
Cassette	Magnetic tape in plastic cassette	90,000 characters/reel	Convenient
DEC tape	Magnetic tape on reels	295,000 characters/reel	Slow access time
Industry-compatible	Magnetic tape on reels; 1600 bytes per inch	38,000,000 characters/reel	Large volume storage but mainly useful for sequential processing
Disks			Fast access when on-line. Efficient bulk storage
Floppy disk	Flexible plastic magnetic disk	125,000 words	Inexpensive storage, slower access than others
Disk cartridge	Firm magnetic disk in a plastic cover	1.2 million words	Widely used in LIS. Intermediate access time
Disk pack	Multiple plastic magnetic disks	44 million words	Rapid access time; removable medium; unlimited off-line storage

tems, this was an important and very useful function of the computer itself. More recently, many of the automated instruments are equipped, as a standard or optional feature, with preprocessors which perform this function and which provide digital outputs to printers, displays, or interfaced computers.

Telecommunications refers to the transmission of data over a distance. The most common example of this process is, of course, the telephone. The laboratory may use non-computer means of telecommunication or may develop a computer system with telecommunication capability as noted previously.

FEATURES OF A LABORATORY COMPUTER SYSTEM

The features of an automated data processing system can be divided into two categories.

Those features which are essential for the operation of a basic laboratory system include (1) Method for requisition of test requested, either preceded by or with the concurrent entry of patient administrative data such as name, identification number, age, sex, physician, and location. (2) The preparation of lists, generally in the form of gummed labels, for the blood drawing team use. (3) Preparation of worklists. (4) Manual and on-line methods for entry of laboratory data with procedures for verification of the data entry and hard copy print-outs of check lists. (5) The generation of reports for the physicians' use. At a minimum

these should include location reports, with the data sorted by all patients for a particular location (i.e., clinic or floor), and patient interim and cumulative reports. (6) Billing data should be available for either manual or on-line transmission to the hospital billing computer. (7) Feedback to laboratory management as to performance of the system, probably in the form of a discrepancy report. Feedback is required to assure stable operation of the system.

Other features which are desirable but may not be essential in the first stage of development include the following. Many of these are by-products of the data base provided by the essential features noted above. (1) Detailed quality control reports. (2) Workload reports, preferably in the format of the College of American Pathologists standardized workload reporting system. (3) Other statistical reports, tailored for the needs of the specific laboratory. (4) Other management reports. (5) More sophisticated billing either by the laboratory computer or by on-line transmission of data to the hospital computer. (6) Epidemiologic reports as a by-product of the clinical microbiology laboratory system. (7) Ability to retrieve laboratory data for educational or research purposes (for example "all patients with a hematocrit of 20 per cent or less" or "all patients having a positive blood culture with a *Staphylococcus aureus* for the previous six months"). (8) Telecommunications capabilities to remote locations served by the laboratories. (9) Instructions to nursing personnel in regard to collection of specimens and preparation of patients. (10) Graphic display or reporting of data. (11) Interpretative reporting of data with suggested follow-up laboratory studies. (12) Reports on physician utilization of laboratory services.

APPROACHES TO LABORATORY COMPUTERIZATION

The practical use of computer techniques in the routine clinical laboratory began in earnest in the mid-1960's and has shown a great burst of activity during the 1970's. In the first decade of this development, the laboratory director planning a laboratory information system generally had one of two major approaches to consider: the first was a "do-it-yourself" approach, generally utilizing the personnel and equipment resources of the hospital data processing department (unfortunately, usually a business-oriented department with little or no experience in on-line data acquisition). The second was the purchase of a "turnkey" computer system developed by a commercial vendor in one or more developmental laboratories and then marketed more generally. To a limited extent the director might have had an alternative approach utilizing terminals from a remote computer system in a shared approach. The latter approach was generally restricted to more specific programs and applications rather than providing a complete laboratory information system. Programmable calculators have also been widely used to solve specific data acquisition and reporting needs in the laboratory (Westlake, 1975), although again these generally are not suitable for a total laboratory information system.

In more recent years the rapid development of the hardware and software for minicomputers and the introduction of microcomputers has offered the laboratory a third major approach. This can be considered a combined approach, since it utilizes commerically available hardware and software packages for on-line data acquisition and preprocessing of laboratory data interfaced with a larger hospital or business computer for large scale data processing, report generation, storage of a data base, and communications. This approach is also known as *distributed data processing*, since two or more computers are distributed within an institution or organization to perform specialized tasks and are joined together by a communication network.

Before describing the several approaches and their advantages and disadvantages, it is important to emphasize that no one approach is ideal for all laboratories. The laboratory director considering computerization of the clinical laboratory should examine all approaches. Special local needs and resources should be considered before making a decision.

Many observers of the laboratory computing field have seen examples of successful approaches under much less than ideal conditions, while at the same time approaches which seem to be ideal have failed. In both instances the difference between success and failure was the degree of determination and dedication of the laboratory director and other people involved with the computer development.

These three major approaches will be reviewed briefly with comments on the advantages and disadvantages of each.

In-House Development of a Laboratory Computer System

The development of a laboratory information system utilizing personnel and hardware of an existing hospital business computer system is frequently the first suggestion of the hospital administrator or member of the hospital board when approached about laboratory computerization. This is a result of a belief on the part of business-oriented persons that a computer system which can serve the business needs of a bank, hospital, or industrial concern certainly should be able to handle the data processing needs of a clinical laboratory. In addition, such an approach *seems* to be most cost effective, since it would make use of computer equipment, programs, and expertise already present in the hospital computer department. Unfortunately, far more failures than successes have resulted to date from such an approach (Johnson, 1975). The failures can be attributed in part to the great differences in needs between the simultaneous on-line processing of multiple automated instruments and the production of various laboratory reports on demand versus the batch processing of payrolls and patient billing. Such an approach also overlooks the fact that software development now may account for up to 90 per cent of the costs of a computer system. A reason frequently cited for a laboratory undertaking to develop its own laboratory information system is that "its needs are unique and cannot be met by a more standard approach." Johnson (1975) has documented the failure of so many of these unique in-house developments and answers this rationale for their development as follows:

The laboratory with so called unique requirements—which, consequently *must* develop its own automated information system, is a laboratory with a director who is incapable of defining correct objectives and/or who is on a ego trip. "Unique requirements" and "maximum flexibility because the laboratory needs are changing" is the last refuge of the incompetent. Those unique requirements are the very tip of the iceberg. With regards to the changing needs of the laboratory which no one can anticipate, it is said in the *Rubaiyat*, "If you don't know where you're going, any road will take you there."

Successful examples of in-house developed systems do exist where the resources and talent were available to see the task to completion. In most cases these have been stand-alone systems developed in the laboratory environment.

TURNKEY LABORATORY COMPUTER SYSTEMS

An alternative and increasingly popular approach to laboratory computerization is the purchase or lease by the laboratory or hospital of a vendor-developed system of hardware and software specifically designed for use in the clinical laboratory environment (Fig. 60–9). Such systems have been called a "turnkey system," since at least in theory one can purchase the entire computer package, have it installed, and simply "turn the key" to have it operational. The laboratory director should be aware, however, that the director and laboratory staff will be required to make many decisions about their operation and about the design of the computer system before it is actually installed. Also there will be a period of parallel testing and the necessity for many adjustments in both the computer and the laboratory operation in order to achieve a successful installation.

The advantages to this approach are many, and it is highly recommended for most hospital and clinical laboratory settings. The extremely high cost of development of a computer system can be distributed among many users rather than being borne entirely by one

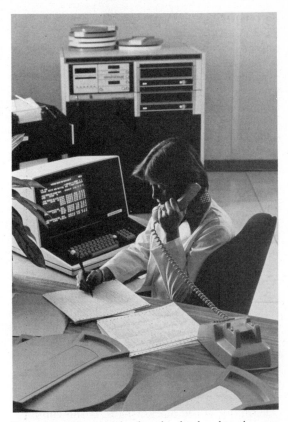

Figure 60–9. An example of vendor-developed turnkey system of hardware and software for the clinical laboratory. (Photograph courtesy of B-D Spear Medical Systems.)

user, thus lowering the initial and the operating costs. Furthermore, if the company remains in business and has a continuing commitment to the laboratory system, then the user has the added and continuing advantage of obtaining corrections for "bugs" in the program, improvements in programs, and new programs which are developed by the vendor for new users. Although some costs may be associated with such updates and additions (either a one-time cost or a monthly payment for software maintenance), the cost should be less than one would experience in having such modifications done on a cost basis for each individual system. Most vendors of dedicated laboratory systems also have a users group which provides suggestions for future development to the vendor and which helps advise the vendor about improvements in programs or programs for new laboratory areas. Users in such groups also serve a valuable function in sharing their experiences and solutions to problems. The availability of local or conven-

6

ient hardware and software support should be an important determinant in decisions regarding a turnkey system or a particular turnkey vendor.

The disadvantages of a "turnkey" system are real, however, and must be weighed against the advantages. Foremost in most laboratory directors' minds is the apparent disadvantage of the lack of "flexibility" to meet individual laboratory needs. This was a real problem in the earlier systems in the 1960's which required reprogramming to make even minor changes in the system, such as the addition or deletion of determinations. The modern systems, however, have modular programs and are table driven so that changes in the program can be simply made on-site by the users. Such programs allow the user to add or delete procedures as well as reorganize reporting formats in a matter of a few minutes.

A more real potential disadvantage of a dedicated laboratory system is the fact that the laboratory having such a system is "married" to the company for the period of time the system is in use. It is thus important that a prospective purchaser thoroughly evaluate the company's track record and prospect for continuing in the marketplace. If the vendor's system uses standard computer hardware from one of the reputable hardware manufac-

turers, then service for the hardware would be available elsewhere even if the vendor went out of business. By the same token the more modern programs allow the laboratory so much flexibility that the laboratory is not so dependent upon the vendor as with older versions. In order to protect oneself, however, the laboratory might wish to require complete documentation of the system as part of the purchase contract. This would then allow the laboratory to maintain the system and to train programmers in the unlikely event that the vendor would not be able to do it in the future.

DISTRIBUTED PROCESSING

Many larger laboratories are now taking a third approach which is based on the following premises: first, many of the problems faced by those taking option one above (total in-house development of a system) have been in the area of the on-line monitoring of the automated instruments and the initial processing of such data (that is, data acquisition and preprocessing or reduction of data). Programmable calculators and mini- and microcomputers with the appropriate software for data acquisition for clinical laboratory instruments and preprocessing of that data are now commerically available and can be purchased or

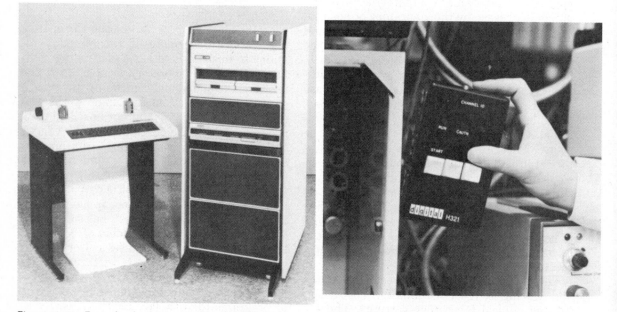

Figure 60–10. Example of a data acquisition computer for use in a distributed processing approach to a LIS. At left is a I/O terminal and minicomputer, which is capable of interfacing with as many as 15 laboratory instruments. At right is the local operator's console, which permits the technologist to communicate directly with the computer when starting or stopping a run. (Programmable Data Logger, courtesy of Digital Equipment Corporation.)

leased to accomplish this vital function in the laboratory (Fig. 60-10). Second, many of the problems faced by those taking the second option above (the purchase or lease of the "turnkey" laboratory system) concern the limited storage, computing, printing, and telecommunication capability of some of the smaller computers and peripheral equipment used in these systems. By use of an in-laboratory data acquisition and preprocessing computer (which may be a modified turnkey laboratory system), coupled with a larger host computer system for preparation of reports, storage of data, and telecommunications, the laboratory can theoretically overcome both of these problems. In such a system the hospital computer would generally already have available the admission, discharge, and transfer function as well as the billing function. In many situations, telecommunications to patient units would also be available so that the use of the data acquisition computer(s) in the laboratory would complete the total cycle, as described previously in Figure 60-1. Such a system provides considerable flexibility to the laboratory, but at the same time this requires considerable in-house expertise and commitment.

Because of these rapid advances in computer technology in recent years, the question for many laboratory directors is now "which computers shall we use?" rather than "which computer shall we use?" Integrated laboratory systems with several computers are already in use (Williams, 1975; Seligson, 1975) and more are being developed. This distributed processing approach has many advantages over the previous approach of either a large computer *or* a minicomputer for laboratory data processing. With the advances in hardware, software, and telecommunications the laboratory director now has the option of putting together computers in a system to meet the specific laboratory and institutional needs.

PLANNING FOR A LABORATORY COMPUTER: SYSTEMS ANALYSIS

One of the most common errors of laboratory directors in regard to data processing for their laboratories has been the assumption that the introduction of a computerized system to the laboratory will automatically solve all of their organizational, workload, and workflow problems. Experience has shown to the contrary that the introduction of a computer system into a poorly organized and chaotic laboratory situation only increases the degree of chaos.

The technique of systems analysis can be utilized in order to avoid this problem (Grams, 1972). By this technique a systematic study of the present system, a review of available systems to solve the laboratory's problems, and a proposal for a new system for the laboratory can be made. As part of this process a manual back-up system for the proposed computer system can be designed and implemented prior to the actual implementation of the computerized system. In many instances, the process of systems analysis, with the resulting improvement of the current operating system and the establishment of a manual back-up system for the computer, provides benefits to the laboratory's operations almost equal to those provided by the ultimate installation of the computer system.

The laboratory director may receive professional assistance from systems analysts, although analysis itself should be done by the laboratory staff along with guidance from available materials. The steps to be undertaken can be briefly summarized as follows (Grams, 1972):

1. *The Descriptive Phase.* In the first step of this phase, the exact *definition of the problem* to be solved is stated in a single statement with qualifiers to define in order of importance the various components of the major problem statement. An example of such a problem statement for a laboratory computer system might be: "How to create a system of hardware and software within the hospital laboratories, with appropriate interfaces to the hospital computer system, to provide the necessary manual and on-line acquisition and processing of patient laboratory data, to provide physicians with prompt and accurate reporting of laboratory results, to provide data retrieval for educational, research and management purposes; and to be cost justifiable to the hospital administration and third parties as a result of increased productivity, expanding laboratory services, and improved quality and availability of laboratory data." As pointed out by Grams, such a problem statement is a preliminary statement and should be re-evaluated and reconfirmed after each successive stage in the systems analysis.

A second and very important step in the descriptive phase of systems analysis is a *de-*

6

BLOOD DRAWING TEAM (BDT) OPERATION

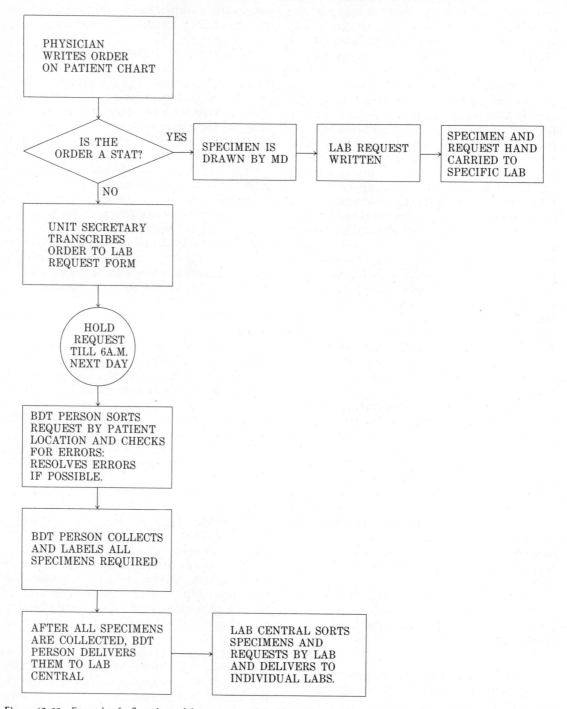

Figure 60–11. Example of a flow chart of the operation of the Blood Drawing Team (BDT) in a hospital laboratory prepared as part of a systems analysis.

scription of the operational system, that is, a description of the current approach to the flow of specimens and data within the laboratory and institution. In this description, as with the others to follow, the use of flow charts com-posed of standardized symbols will greatly facilitate the process (Fig. 60–11). At the end of the operational systems description, the problem statement should be reconfirmed and modified as necessary.

2. *The Investigative Phase* (Research). At this phase the laboratory director and the project team research the current literature, consult vendors, make personal contacts, and make on-site visits to determine the *relevant existing systems* which might be available to solve the laboratory's problems. The material included in this section will generally consist of a description of more than one system, but an attempt should be made to describe only those systems which have been successful or have great promise for success in the near future. The systems described also should not be unique ones confined to one institution. The description should be limited to those systems which are readily available and may likely be able to be utilized in part or in whole in solving the current problem. At the end of this phase, the initial problem statement should again be reconfirmed and modified if necessary.

3. *Creative Phase*. After study and documentation of the present system and of relevant existing systems elsewhere, the laboratory director and his team are now ready to describe the proposed system for the laboratory. The *proposed system description* is done in a similar fashion to the description of the existing system and the relevant outside systems. In addition, however, one must list ways in which the proposed system could be evaluated once it is implemented and reasons justifying the proposed system versus other systems.

4. *Implementation Phase*. A description of the planned implementation schedule for the proposed system is developed (see below).

5. *Evaluation Phase*. A description of the evaluation of the proposed system is developed in order to determine if the system as installed is meeting the previously developed functional specifications.

IMPLEMENTATION AND EVALUATION

Although actual implementation of a clinical laboratory computer system may take only a few weeks or at the most several months, planning for successful implementation should begin months earlier at the time the initial decision is made concerning a computer system.

The following are examples of the multiple plans which must be made in order finally to implement a laboratory computer system. This assumes that a systems analysis has been made, that necessary corrections have been made in the operation of the laboratory, and that a decision has been made concerning the approach to be used for computerization. Some of the considerations leading to successful implementation are as follows:

1. Remodeling, if necessary, of space for the computer, with considerations of humidity, air conditioning, etc.

2. Many laboratories find it useful to combine the computer operation function with a reorganization of the laboratory to provide a central receiving and information area (Lab Central for short) or a Central Processing Area (CPA). With such a concept a single physical location serves well for the laboratory computer system operation and for a central receiving area. With proper telephone equipment this can serve as a central information area for the entire laboratory with only those calls for determinations actually in progress being referred to individual sections. The blood drawing team operation may also be successfully operated out of this area.

3. The necessary personnel for step 2 should be funded, recruited, and trained.

4. New requisition forms and report forms should be designed and purchased. All other computer supplies should be purchased and a sufficient stock kept on hand. Storage cabinets for discs and other computer materials should be available.

5. A back-up manual system should be designed and tested prior to implementation of the computer system.

6. A program of in-service education should be started. This first should involve the laboratory personnel who will be most intimately involved with the computer. Ideally they should be involved with the entire planning process and should have input their needs in the system design. If such is the case then the actual in-service training will consist of familiarizing them with the details of the operating system. Much of this can be accomplished during the parallel operation before final implementation of the computer system. In-service training will also have to be provided for the hospital clerical personnel and staff physicians, for both of whom the system will have a major impact. In addition, many laboratories have found that a centrally located display, showing the key steps in the computer operation and the samples of the types of reports, is useful as a training aid for new personnel and staff and to explain to visitors the operation of the system.

Because of the large number of items to be coordinated, all of which must be done in a certain time frame in order to successfully accomplish the implementation, the use of a PERT (*Program Evaluation* and *Review Technique*) chart is of value.

Once the computer is installed the laboratory will go through a period of parallel operation as the various programs are tested internally in the laboratory. This can be a difficult period for laboratory personnel, since they may be doing twice as much work but not receiving many advantages from the system. On the other hand, if it is handled well and planned for in advance, the excitement of using the new system will make up for any added burden during the time. It is essential during this period of time to thoroughly test the system and to work with the vendor or local systems people to make any necessary corrections in the system.

If one is dealing with a very large institution, the implementation of the reporting system for physicians may be staged, that is, shifting from the manual to the computer reporting system on a few locations at a time in sequence. This allows the computer and laboratory staff to concentrate on the problems in a few areas rather than being overwhelmed with a transition accomplished all at one time. On the other hand, if the planning and in-service education have been thoroughly performed, the switch-over may be achieved throughout the institution at a specific date.

During both the implementation phase and the early operational phase, a continuing evaluation of the computer function should be performed and documented. The evaluation should be based on the functional specifications and on the evaluation procedure developed during the systems analysis.

REFERENCES

ABC (American Blood Commission) CCBBA Simplified Uniform Blood Bag Labels. June 17, 1977. American Blood Commission, 1901 North Ft. Myer Drive, Suite 300, Arlington, VA 22209.

Ball, M. J.: The need for a hospital information system. *In* Ball, M. J. (ed.): How to Select a Computerized Hospital Information System. Basel, S. Karger, 1973.

Burns, E. L., Hanson, D. J., Schoen, I., Barnett, R. N., Minckler, T., and Winter, S.: Communication of laboratory data to the clinician. Am. J. Clin. Pathol., *61*:900, 1974.

CAP Standards for accreditation of medical laboratories. Skokie, Ill., College of American Pathologists, 1974.

Drucker, P. F.: The Effective Executive. New York, Harper & Row, Publishers, Inc., 1967.

Grams, R. R.: Problem solving, systems analysis and medicine. Springfield, Ill., Charles C Thomas, Publisher, 1972.

Henry, J. B., and Pruitt, C. T.: This report system reduces lab errors. Mod. Hosp., *104*:118, 1964.

JCAH Accreditation Manual for Hospitals. Chicago, Ill., Joint Commission on Accreditation of Hospitals, 1976.

Johnson, J. L.: Achieving the Optimum Information System for the Laboratory. Northbrook, Ill., J. Lloyd Johnson Associates, 1975.

Noyce, R. N.: Microelectronics. Sci. Am., *237*:63, 1977.

Seligson, D.: Current trends in laboratory automation and computerization. *In* Enlander, E. (ed): Computers in Laboratory Medicine. New York, Academic Press, Inc., 1975.

Shannon, R. H., and Ball, M. J.: A patient-oriented classification of medical data: An aid to systems analysis and design. Biosci. Comm., *2*:282, 1976.

Westlake, G.: Microprocessors, programmable calculators and minicomputers in the clinical laboratory. *In* Enlander, E. (ed.): Computers in Laboratory Medicine. New York, Academic Press, Inc., 1975.

Williams, G. Z.: New directions in clinical laboratory computerization. *In* Enlander, E. (ed): Computers in Laboratory Medicine. New York, Academic Press, Inc., 1975.

Note: See also general references at the end of Chapter 58.

61

LEGAL ASPECTS OF LABORATORY MEDICINE

John R. Feegel, M.D., J.D.

While the practice of laboratory medicine is not free from liability, it does carry a lower risk for malpractice suits among the medical specialties. Improper identification of specimens or reports leading to erroneous diagnoses, negligent blood banking, misdiagnoses on frozen sections, and autopsies performed without valid consents are the areas which generate the majority of liability suits against pathologists.

But malpractice suits are not the only legal problems which the pathologist may face. Contractual problems with hospitals, associates, and technologists; performance on hospital committees; retention of records; release of information; government rules and regulations; and the occasional duty as medical examiner or coroner may generate an additional spectrum of legal challenges for the laboratory physician.

No brief discussion can substitute for competent legal advice. Local and state laws vary, making a self-protective review mandatory whenever a pathologist accepts a new hospital contract. A competent attorney on whom the pathologist can personally rely should be among the items he considers indispensable for the practice of laboratory medicine. The attorney who represents the hospital may often be a friend and advisor, but he cannot ethically represent both the pathologist and the administration when a dispute arises between them, or when a suit by an unhappy patient forces them to be adversaries in court.

CONTRACTS

The pathologist has traditionally been an independent contractor rather than a hospital employee. The test has historically been a matter of "control." Recent cases have held that when the hospital provides the hospital-based physician with virtually everything he needs for his practice, pays his salary, and retains the power to fire him at will, he is in effect an employee, regardless of the wording of his contract. As an employee, liability for his poor performance may be passed on to the hospital, thereby involving them both. As an independent contractor, the pathologist would be liable for his own acts, while the hospital

6

would be responsible only for those of its employees. The laboratory technologists are usually considered employees of the hospital rather than of the pathologist. If the pathologist hires and fires the laboratory staff, paying their salaries and exercising "control," they may be found to be *his* employees, freeing the hospital from responsibility.

The chief pathologist may contract with the hospital, or several hospitals, for performance of professional duties which need not be specifically listed. As chief, he may then contract with associate pathologists to perform specific duties, but always with the approval of the hospital staffs concerned. Professional duties may be delegated to a competent associate without sharing liability for malpractice, but not to an associate who is known to be incompetent or untrained.

A pathologist considering a professional contract with a hospital or with associates should contact the College of American Pathologists, Skokie, Illinois, for advice on the business and ethical problems involved (College of American Pathologists, 1977). CAP supports more than one type of compensation. Under normal circumstances, a salary is not the preferred arrangement for him. A fee for service is considered better, although government positions and certain charitable institutions do not permit this and are acceptable exceptions. Recently, federal legislation has been suggested to limit hospital-based physicians to formula salaries or to other limitations, particularly when the fees are generated from large volume Medicare-Medicaid practices. A pathologist who hires professional personnel and others to perform duties in his laboratory should be aware of Civil Rights requirements, Workmen's Compensation regulations, and the licensure regulations for the state and the federal government before contracts are offered.

LICENSES AND REGULATIONS

As a physician, every pathologist must conform to the laws of his state applicable to the practice of medicine. Certain positions in state or federal institutions may be exempt from medical license requirements.

In addition, many states have passed laws to regulate the practice of laboratory medicine. These may apply to practices within as well as those separate from hospital laboratories. The state laws must be complied with by the pathologist-laboratory director as well as by the technical staff. These laws may describe the educational requirements of designated laboratory positions and require examinations to demonstrate competency. Such licenses may require annual renewal. Violations of these rules may result in the closure of the laboratory or may put the hospital and the pathologist in an untenable position for collection of bills from various governmental and health insurance agencies.

Additional regulations are applicable to laboratories participating in Medicare or Medicaid. These rules are complex, voluminous, and constantly changing. An alert pathologist will not only read the official guidelines available from the U.S. Department of Health, Education and Welfare, but will confer frequently with appropriate hospital representatives to make sure that the regulations are being met. The outline below is no substitute for personal effort.

Under federal regulations (CFR—Code of Federal Regulations), a laboratory is ". . . a facility for the biological, microbiological, serological, chemical, immunohematological, biophysical, cytological, pathological or other examination of material derived from the human body for the purposes of providing information for the diagnosis, prevention, or treatment of any disease or impairment or the assessment of the health of man." In addition, the regulations may vary depending on whether the laboratory is hospital-based or independent. A hospital laboratory which is reimbursed by Medicare must meet the Medicare conditions of participation or the Joint Commission (JCAH) Standards. If the laboratory is in interstate commerce by its shipment of specimens across state lines, or if it offers services to a health maintenance organization (HMO), further conditions may have to be met. These should be specifically investigated. The medical conditions of participation are given in the Code of Federal Regulations, Title 20, Sec. 405.1028.

The standards of the Joint Commission on Accreditation of Hospitals (JCAH) are found in a booklet published by that organization.*

---

* New manual with section for Pathology revised, effective after January, 1979.

The JCAH standards for pathology (I-VIII) require that the pathology service be directed by a physician qualified to assume the professional and administrative responsibilities for the services rendered, adequate space, equipment, and supplies, appropriate channels of communication within the hospital, quality control systems, proper labeling and delivery of specimens from surgery, proper space and equipment for autopsies, adequate blood banking facilities or services, and filing of all laboratory reports. The JCAH standards also require sufficient qualified personnel to perform the technical procedures and to comply with all local, state, and federal licensing rules. The standards offer guidelines for the proper storage of slides, blocks, and bone marrow aspirate, although strict time limits are not given. A pathologist who supervises a laboratory which has not complied with the JCAH standards may have difficulty defending himself against a subsequent liability suit. It would be embarrassing for any pathologist to learn of these standards in court while he is the defendant.

Regulations under the Clinical Laboratory Improvement Act of 1967 (CLIA) require a federal license if the laboratory accepts more than 100 specimens per year from outside the state wherein it normally operates. This regulation usually applies only to independent laboratories, since hospital laboratories seldom solicit specimens outside the state. However, laboratory participants under the Medicare program must meet the demands of the Medicare standards.

Under current federal regulations, inspection and accreditation by the College of American Pathologists program is equivalent to federal inspection and accreditation, since the standards of the CAP program are equal to, or more stringent than, the federal regulations. Whether accredited by the federal or CAP program, the licensed laboratory must be a regular participant in an approved proficiency testing service and maintain an acceptable level of performance on the surveys.

OFFICE LABORATORIES

In general, most laboratories operated within and solely for the benefit of a physician's private practice are not regulated by the specific state or federal regulations. This exemption will probably not survive much longer, since many of these procedures are billed to Medicare and Medicaid, thereby generating government interest in their performance. Small independent laboratories may also claim certain exceptions to selected regulations if they receive less than 100 specimens per year from other physicians. Obviously, these regulations should be investigated by the physician directly concerned.

OTHER REGULATIONS

Laboratory physicians should be aware that tax-free alcohol is regulated by the Alcohol, Tobacco and Firearms Bureau of the United States Treasury Department. Accurate records, inventory, and proper storage of alcohol is required. Local and state fire regulations may control the storage and transportation of many volatile liquids commonly used in the clinical laboratory or in tissue preparation. Radioactive materials must be stored and disposed of according to federal regulations (Atomic Energy Act, 1954). The shipment of some biologic specimens across state lines or in the United States mail is regulated to some extent. In short, there are many specific laboratory functions which require investigation of other local, state, or federal regulations that are not primarily health oriented.

CONSENTS

The consent for autopsy is regulated in each state by a statute which should be known by every pathologist in that state. In general, the spouse is the consenting party. Where there is no surviving spouse, the next-of-kin may consent. Some autopsy consent forms provide permission to investigate only the cause of death, while others allow the pathologist to retain specific organs or parts of organs, disposing of them later. The more liberal wording is to be appreciated by the hospital pathologist.

Selected specialized procedures such as needle biopsies or special bone marrow aspirations should have written consent from the patient or guardian added to the chart. Every consent should be an "informed consent." That is to say, the consenting party should have a clear idea of what he is agreeing to, what may go wrong, and what will probably result if all goes well. Minors, by special legislation in many states, can consent to therapy for venereal disease without notification of their parents. Some states permit minors to consent to a blood donation but not to the sale of blood. Persons who have been declared mentally incompetent may have consent granted for them by a guardian or by a court. In cases where a consent is lacking, and a medical procedure is appropriate for a minor, the physician should ask a local judge for assistance. Often a telephone call to a judge will suffice. The *Uniform Anatomical Gift Act* allows persons to donate parts of their bodies after death without conforming to the details of the statutes on wills and probate. Such gifts may be rescinded by the surviving next-of-kin after the donor's death.

PRIVACY

A patient retains his rights to reasonable privacy. Photographs, however interesting medically, should not be taken without permission. Photographs of specimens or tissues in which the patient is not named may be taken and published without specific permission unless the specimen is sufficiently unique as to embarrass or identify the patient. Anonymous photographs of tissues may be published in scientific journals without specific permission of the patient under the same reasoning.

RECORDS

The laboratory reports, slides, blocks, and other materials relating to a patient's treatment in the hospital laboratory are the property of the hospital, although the patient has a right to the information. The patient may also demand that the material be surrendered to another physician or hospital for the consultation of another physician. The pathologist should cooperate pleasantly with this request. Such slides and records should be stored for extended periods of time, often dictated by

the biologic activity of the disease or by the statute of limitations for liability suits. In any event, storage for several years should be minimum for most materials.

SUBPOENAS

A subpoena issued by a court or an attorney has the force of law behind it and should be complied with fully. Failure to conform may result in a contempt-of-court citation and embarrassment. A *Subpoena Duces Tecum* requires the production of all records, specimens, slides, or other materials specifically mentioned in the document.

The pathologist has no legal right to refuse to supply the material requested nor to insist that the identity of the consultant, if any, be disclosed before surrender.

In court, the pathologist should be a cooperative and objective witness, replying reasonably to all questions, and being an advocate for neither side. He should not allow himself to be angered by an attorney's technique of cross examination, nor supply information not asked for. As a professional person temporarily distracted from his practice, he may submit a bill for his time and anticipate full payment. When he is not paid his reasonable fee, the pathologist may contact the local Bar Association or the judge in the case to complain.

FORENSIC PATHOLOGY— POLICE CASES

Many hospital laboratories are asked to cooperate with selected police investigations, although these laboratories and their personnel have no official appointments to do so. Such cooperation is praiseworthy. Hospital laboratories should not refuse to draw or accept blood alcohols or to examine material obtained in assault or rape cases. Many communities have no other sources of scientific information available to them in times of great need. Hence, it is necessary for the laboratory personnel to be familiar with the state's blood alcohol law as supplied in the motor vehicle statutes. A patient who is not under arrest should not be forced to give blood against his will. When the test is properly requested by the police, the results should be given to them.

A specimen produced in a rape examination should be examined by a cooperative laboratory technologist without objection. Tests for vaginal acid phosphatase can be performed in hospital laboratories with a reasonable degree of accuracy using appropriate dilutions. A smear, wet or dried, should be viewed under a microscope by a laboratory technologist without hesitation, and the presence or absence of sperm reported when requested. Specific forensic training is not required to disclose whether sperm is recognized on the slide. Statements regarding probable source, longevity, or other sexual characteristics may require forensic training to be accurate.

A hospital pathologist is competent to perform blood typing for paternity disputes and to express an opinion on the possibility or impossibility of parentage. However, his lack of experience beyond the basic blood group systems may compromise his testimony in an area of often tricky serology. A prudent pathologist will seek help. (See Chapter 44.)

QUALITY CONTROL PROGRAMS

Quality control programs have been offered commercially for some time and are now an integral part of the inspection system for state and federal approval. The backbone of the quality control program is records. The supervising pathologist should insure that the quality control is organized for periodic review of every major portion of the clinical laboratory, and that the program can be documented for the inspector. The ability to prove that the various laboratory tests are accurate and that they have been repeatedly checked is a stout defensive tool in a lawsuit. Log books demonstrating the efficiency of the quality control program should be stored indefinitely.

RETIREMENT PROGRAMS

Many pathologists have chosen to defer payment to themselves from collectable fees, design retirement programs for themselves and their employees, and to provide group disability insurance or hospitalization plans for associates and employees. Space does not permit a comprehensive discussion of the business and tax aspects of these problems. However, before any pathologist launches into an extensive financial plan, he should seek competent advice from his CPA or from an attorney specializing in tax and estate planning. The effects may be adverse and create long-range problems which an otherwise intelligent pathologist may not anticipate.

GENERAL

The hospital-based pathologist and his colleagues in the independent laboratory are not immune from law suits, nor are they free to practice their specialties without regulations. The wider the scope of the practice, and often the larger the laboratory, the more likely the need for competent legal advice. Few attorneys are pathologists and therefore the regulations regarding laboratories may not be immediately available. However, a discussion with a personal lawyer will be a valuable investment for any pathologist. Somehow, pathologists find time to study diseases that, in all probability, they will never see in a lifetime of practice. Surely a few hours with a competent legal advisor is worth as much.

6

REFERENCES

Accreditation Manual for Hospitals, 1976. Joint Commissions on Accreditation of Hospitals, 645 N. Michigan Avenue, Chicago, Ill. 60611.

Atomic Energy Act of 1954, U.S.C. 73, Stat 689, Sec. 274.

Clinical Laboratories Improvement Act of 1967, U.S.C. 42, Sec. 263 (a).

Code of Federal Regulations: Distribution and Use of Tax-free Alcohol. Title 26, Pt. 213, Pub. No. 444. Washington, D.C., U.S. Government Printing Office.

Code of Federal Regulations: Federal Health Insurance for the Aged. Title 20, Ch. III, Pt. 405. HIR-10 (6/67). Washington, D.C., U.S. Department of Health, Education and Welfare, Social Security Administration.

College of American Pathologists: Guidelines for Pathologists: Professional Practices. Skokie, Ill., College of American Pathologists, 1977.

Death Investigation: An Analysis of the Laws and Policies of the United States. Washington, D.C., U.S. Department of Health, Education and Welfare Pub. No. (HSA) 78-5252.

Feegel, J. R.: Legal Aspects of Laboratory Medicine. Boston, Little, Brown and Company, 1973.

Hospital Laboratories—Fire Safety. National Fire Protection Association Bulletin No. NFPA 56C. Boston, Mass.

62

EFFECTIVE UTILIZATION OF CLINICAL LABORATORIES

John Bernard Henry, M.D., and
John Murphy, M.D.

To use clinical laboratory resources effectively, pertinent laboratory data must be generated in an appropriate and expeditious time interval as well as in the most logical and economical manner for optimal patient care (Table 62–1 and Table 58–1). Ideally this is a goal which all clinicians and pathologists strive to achieve. In practice, it is a difficult goal to attain. Based on imprecise criteria and ill-defined standards, many instances of charges of "underutilization," "overutilization," or "malutilization" of clinical laboratory services have appeared in both the medical and non-medical press.

Underutilization of clinical laboratories occurs when pertinent laboratory data are not sought or are not obtained (Table 62–2). Both of these situations fortunately are rare today.

Overutilization and/or *malutilization* results whenever superfluous or repetitious data are obtained, when pertinent data are obtained at inappropriate times, or in random or illogic sequences, or when the obtained data are ignored or obtained at excessive cost of time, effort, or money.

Optimal service or benefit to the patient is difficult to define by truly objective or statistical terms. There is conflicting evidence either to support or to refute charges of widespread *ineffective laboratory utilization*. Griner (1971) showed that the length of hospitalization of patients with ketoacidosis, whose diagnosis and management in large part are laboratory determined, was not correlated with the use of laboratory services (i.e., the number of laboratory tests ordered did not correlate with shortened hospitalization). Ashley (1972) has shown similar findings among patients with common medical and surgical illnesses. Furthermore, he found a marked variation in patterns of laboratory utilization among different hospitals. Carmalt (1971) concluded that there was no improvement in hospital care or a shortening of hospitalization with the introduction of chemical batteries or profiles for inpatients. This is in contrast to our favorable experience with "organ panels," which tend to suggest cost effectiveness and provide most pertinent laboratory data for medical problem solving as part of a problem-oriented medical record (POMR) (Hurst, 1972; Henry, 1970 and 1979).

The problem is complicated by the fact that

Table 62–1. SCHEMATIC OUTLINE OF ACTIVITIES IN CLINICAL LABORATORIES

ADMINISTRATION		
PATIENT CARE SERVICE		
Indications and Selection	Technology and Generation	Interpretation and Translation
TEACHING		
RESEARCH		

Table 62–2. INDICATIONS OR REASONS FOR ORDERING LABORATORY MEASUREMENTS AND/OR EXAMINATIONS

1. To confirm a clinical impression or establish a diagnosis.
2. To rule out a diagnosis.
3. To monitor therapy (management guide).
4. To establish prognosis.
5. To screen for or detect disease.

the increased use of laboratory measurements has been temporally associated with advances in cardiovascular, orthopedic, and transplantation surgery, and in the treatment of patients with various malignancies, to mention only a few. In most instances, the length of hospitalization has been shortened. At the University Hospital of the Upstate Medical Center, Syracuse, New York, the average duration of hospitalization was 9.0 days in 1977, compared with 12.9 days in 1967. Although there are many factors responsible, it appears that increased utilization of the diagnostic clinical laboratory has contributed to the success of modern medical advances and made possible greater patient turnover.

Compounding, intensifying, and focusing attention on the alleged problem of non-effective use of laboratories is the expense of this expanded testing to the patient in this age of economic instability and inflation. At the Upstate Medical Center the 1977 average cost per patient day in non-acute units is $240 and in acute treatment units is $825. This is an increase of 180 per cent since 1972. During this same time, the average laboratory expense per patient admission increased from $185 to $361. This is an increase of approximately 95 per cent. It is not unusual for laboratory charges to comprise 5 to 25 per cent of the entire hospital bill. These figures are not unique to University Hospitals like Upstate; similar figures have also been demonstrated in private, federal (V.A.), and HMO clinics and hospitals (Freeborn, 1972) in the United States and in government-directed hospitals in the United Kingdom (Ashley, 1972; Carmalt, 1971).

In order for the exponential increase in laboratory testing, which is of the order of 10 per cent per year, and the cost escalation to be controlled and in order for the patient to gain maximal benefit from laboratory services, the many interrelated factors that can contribute to utilization and thus malutilization must be recognized and appropriate and reasonable solutions found. If this is not accomplished in a systematic manner and if all who are involved do not join in to alleviate such overutilization and/or malutilization as may exist, it is probable, if not almost certain, that externally imposed and artificial constraints will be placed on physicians and institutions. This in turn will certainly result in underutilization at best, perhaps rationing at worst.

Some of the contributing causes have been identified and remedies proposed or introduced, but these examples have been most singular and fragmentary. Much more has to be accomplished and on a more universal scale.

Each clinical laboratory has to examine its internal operations to assess economy. The vast majority of laboratories in the United States exist to provide reliable measurements and examinations to patients through their physicians. In order to insure accurate and precise data, it is necessary that the laboratory have an *internal quality control program*, consisting of daily testing of pooled specimens, the results of which are statistically analyzed. Equally important is the development of an *external quality control program*, such as that of the College of American Pathologists or the Center for Disease Control. Since the introduction of these programs, interlaboratory comparability in the United States has been markedly improved. If these programs are well organized, the resulting extra time, effort, and cost of operation becomes minimal compared with the benefit to the patient. If reliable data are generated and if reference intervals are established for the population served (by statistical methods), the need for confirmatory testing of earlier laboratory data can be considerably reduced. In addition, a well-organized and thorough preventive maintenance program will increase the usefulness, operational time, and longevity of instrumentation.

To improve service, clinical laboratories are constantly evaluating new methods and measurements. It is important that the clinical relevance of a new or improved test (i.e., precision, specificity, sensitivity, etc.) be considered, as well as the cost impact; only if these considerations are found favorable should the new tests or methods be instituted and older tests discarded.

In order for the laboratory to function efficiently and economically, it is necessary that the pathologist, in addition to pursuing his other professional and scientific endeavors, assume an active medical-managerial role and become intimately involved in the actual day-to-day running of each area, with the intent of streamlining the work force and eliminating waste. Only a physician can function effectively in this role when direct and indirect patient care decisions are constantly required. He or she should be not only *visible* but also *accessible* to the laboratory staff while educating them about laboratory expenses and efficiency.

Besides internal self assessment, the laboratory director and staff should evaluate the external effectiveness of the laboratory, or its relationship to the clinical staff which makes use of the laboratory services. The clinical laboratory aids the physician by providing measurements and examinations for reasons noted in Table 62-2. The majority of tests (60 per cent) performed at Upstate Medical Center, with a heavy emphasis on tertiary care, is for the purpose of monitoring therapy (i.e., management).

Many of the recent developments in laboratory medicine have been in the area of enzymology, immunopathology, and therapeutic drug monitoring, which emphasize determinations valuable for following the progression of disease states and their responses to various therapeutic regimens. The introduction and use of these measurements and examinations are justified if used judiciously.

An area of significantly increased laboratory usage is the performance of measurements or groups of measurements on those who do not have clinical disease. The goal of these *"screening"* measurements is to detect biochemical disease states that can be corrected and/or reduced as well as to prevent or lessen eventual medical care and hospitalization with its resultant costs and at the same time increase the general health of the population. In order to detect the relatively few patients within the screened population with incipient or preclinical disease, amenable to alteration or amelioration, it is necessary to do comprehensive studies to determine cost effectiveness or cost-benefit ratio in various diseases that are routinely screened, determining the predictive value and efficiency of each measurement. A predictive method, taking into consideration the sensitivity and specificity of measurements and the prevalence of detected disease(s) in the population, has been emphasized by Galen (1975). Although these concerns are often stated, they have thus far been resistant to scientific study, leading to consensus conclusions.

In examining the relationship between the clinical staff and the laboratory, areas of undue "iatrogenic" enhancement have to be identified and controlled (Henry, 1976). Basic to the excessive use of the laboratory by some is their lack of knowledge concerning details of laboratory organization, test methods, including limitations, and most importantly, costs. This is directly related to the non-emphasis on laboratory medicine in some of the curricula during undergraduate medical education and the lack of involvement of medical students and clinical residents in the laboratory. All departments, from statistics to internal medicine, are trying to obtain more teaching time in the preclinical years of undergraduate medical education, but the increasing importance of the clinical laboratory and its influence on cost mandate that a strong clinical pathology course be incorporated into the curriculum. Ward (1976) at the University of Minnesota developed a course in interpretive aspects of laboratory medicine and subsequently found that students who took this course had greater competence in laboratory utilization than those students who did not take this course. One of the most direct and effective means of education during the clinical years is for rotation of medical students and house officers through the laboratory, combined with the active participation of pathologists "on rounds" and in clinical conferences. It is here that cost factors of the laboratory can be discussed, along with what measurements should be requested and in what order and how to get the most out of the laboratory in a cost effective, efficient manner. Pathologists should hear and see first-hand the logic or "why" of clinical colleagues' demand for increasingly varied or highly specialized laboratory services. At the same time, pathologists can become familiar with problems unique to the clinics and wards as they relate to the laboratory and the cost of testing. Schroeder (1973) at the George Washington University Medical Center demonstrated a 30 per cent reduction in laboratory utilization on selected medical outpatients when a cost audit of laboratory procedures was performed and made available to clinicians ordering the measurements and examinations. This concept is attractive, but its widespread extrapolation to other settings, including hospital inpatients, should be undertaken with extreme caution.

Other pertinent topics for discussion are physiologic variations of hormones and other organic molecules, variations in methods, and the random variations inherent in test methods (expressed as S.D. or C.V.) described in Chapter 1. Patient preparation, proper specimen collection, and the interferences of anticoagulants, drugs, and foods on test measurements can be stressed. If there is a better understanding of these variables and inter-

STATE UNIVERSITY HOSPITAL
UPSTATE MEDICAL CENTER

CLINICAL PATHOLOGY – ORGAN PANEL A

Last Reporting Date: _____

GENERAL HEALTH (Fasting)				
Creatinine mg/dl	0.6–1.2			
Urea Nitrogen (BUN) mg/dl	8–18			
SGO Transaminase (AST) IU/L	1 – 39			
Uric Acid mg/dl	Female 2.0–6.4 Male 2.1–7.8			
Chloride mEq/L	98–109			
CO₂ Content mM/L	24–30			
Sodium mEq/L	135–145			
Potassium mEq/L	4.0–4.8			
Calcium mEq/L	4.5–5.4			
Lactic Dehydrogenase IU/L	71–207			
Glucose mg/dl	65–115			
Cholesterol mg/dl	Age 20–30 130–230			
Triglyceride mg/dl	10–160			
CBC	See Hematology Report Sheet			
Urinalysis	See Microscopy Report Sheet			
PARATHYROID				
Calcium Total mEq/L	4.5–5.4			
Alkaline Phosphatase IU/L	Adult 4–13 Child 13–20			
Inorganic Phosphorus mg/dl	Adult 2.0–5.2 Child 4.0–7.0			

PROSTATIC				
Acid Phosphatase IU/L	0–0.8			
Creatinine ng/dl	0.6–1.2			
Calcium meq/L	4.5–5.4			
Alkaline Phosphatase IU/L	Adult 4–13			
Phosphorous mg/dl	Adult 2.0–5.2			

PANCREATIC				
Amylase, Serum Somogyi Units/dl	50–150			
Amylase Urinary units/min.	1–5			
Lipase, Serum units/ml	0.5–1.8			
Calcium mEq/L	4.5–5.4			
Creatinine Serum mg/dl	0.6–1.2			
Urine Creatinine mg/dl				
Amylase/Creatinine Clearance %	1–3.5			

THYROID				
T₄–RIA ug/dl	5.5–12.3			
Free Thyroxine ng/dl	0.9–2.3			
T₃–RIA mg/dl	92–217			
TSH–RIA µIU/L	Less than 10			

Figure 62–1. Cumulative report form of five organ panels.

ferences, what represents a change in the laboratory versus a change in the patient can be appreciated and laboratory measurements ordered and interpreted in a more logical and accurate fashion. At the Upstate Medical Center, written elaboration of these topics, which are called *Measurement of the Month,* are distributed to the medical staff, wards, and clinics. These topics can be further stressed and defined by the interaction of pathologists and clinicians both in the laboratory and in clinical settings.

Organ panels evolved and are expanded and updated at the Upstate Medical Center in response to this type of interaction with clinical colleagues (Figs. 62-1 to 62-3 and Table 62-3) (Henry, 1979). In the course of ordering measurements or examinations for the purpose of diagnosis or management, some physicians may request standing or routine (i.e., hourly, daily, etc.) laboratory orders without evaluating whether the patient needs these tests so often or without actually using the laboratory data for decision making. Edwards (1973) studied physician response to urine culture results and found that there was no consistent, logical approach to using bacteriologic culture results; but that in a significant percentage of cases, therapy was not changed when culture results indicated that it should have been changed.

Measurements may be ordered by some to "completely" work up the patient and to show fellow physicians or attending physicians that all possibilities have been considered. Models for this approach are present in case presentations of patients in medical journals, in which extensive laboratory data are prescribed in block form and the rationale or cost of ordering is not emphasized in the discussion.

There appears to be an undue concern over missed, occult, or unsuspected diagnoses,

STATE UNIVERSITY HOSPITAL
UPSTATE MEDICAL CENTER

CLINICAL PATHOLOGY -- ORGAN PANEL **B**

Last Reporting Date: _____

HYPOPITUITARISM PANEL (Insulin Tolerance)

Time	Glucose mg/dl	Cortisol RIA mcg/dl	Growth Hormone ng/ml
Control 1			
Control 2			
15 Min.			
30 Min.			
45 Min.			
60 Min.			
90 Min.			
120 Min.			

MICROCYTIC ANEMIA

Serum Iron µg/dl	50-150		
TI BC µg/dl	250-450		
Ferritin	M 10-273, F 5-99, Children (6 mos-15 yrs) 7-142 ng/ml		
Hemoglobin Electrophoresis	See Hematology Report Sheet		
CBC	See Hematology Report Sheet		

PULMONARY

Blood pH units	Art. 7.38–7.44 Ven. 7.36–7.41		
Blood PCO₂ mmHg	Art. 35–40 Ven. 40–45		
Blood PO₂ mmHg	Art. 95–100		
Oxygen Saturation Percent	Art. 94–100 Ven. 60–85		
CO₂ Content mM/L	24–30		
Sodium mEq/L	135–145		
Potassium mEq/L	4.0–4.8		
Chloride mmol/L	98–109		
Urea Nitrogen (BUN) mg/dl	8–18		
Glucose mg/dl	65–115		
CBC	See Hematology Report Form		

MUSCLE

Creatine Phosphokinase (CPK) IU/L	Male 55-170 Female 30-135		
Lactic Dehydrogenase IU/L	71-207		
T₄-RIA ug/dl	5.5-12.3		
Creatine Phosphokinase Isoenzymes	See Special Report		
Aldolase (S-L) units	3-8		

MALABSORPTION

Fecal Fat gm/day	2-5			
Xylose Tolerance Urine gm/5hr	5.3-7.7			
Calcium Total mEq/L	4.5-5.4			
Carotene ug/dl	50-360			
Albumin gm/dl	Age 15-35 3.44-5.64 Age 35-55 3.22-5.10			
Total Proteins gm/dl	6.78-8.3			
Folic Acid ng/ml	5-21			
Electrophoresis	See Chemistry Report Form			

METABOLIC

Glucose mg/dl	65-115			
Uric Acid mg/dl	Female 2.0-6.4 Male 2.1-7.8			
Cholesterol mg/dl	Age 20-30 130-230			
Triglycerides mg/dl	10-160			
T₄-RIA ug/dl	5.5-12.3			
Creatinine mg/dl	0.6-1.2			
Calcium mEq/L	4.5-5.4			
Alkaline Phosphatase IU/L	Adult 4-13 Child 13-20			
SGO Transaminase IU/L	1-39			
Lactic Dehydrogenase IU/L	71-207			
Phosphorous mg/dl	Adult 2.0-5.2 Child 4.0-7.0			

LEGEND

A. Laboratory Accident
B. Confirmed
C. Clotted
D. Moderate
E. Recollect Specimen
F. Unit Notified
G. Specimen not received
H. Hemolysis
J. Xanthochromic
K. Marked (Over 100/hpf)
L. Lactescence
M. Minimum (Less than 0-1/hpf)

N. Not done – see schedule
P. Patient not available
Q. Quantity not sufficient
R. Patient uncooperative
T. Improperly labeled
U. Test cancelled by physician
W. Improper specimen
X. Report to follow
Y. Obscured by dye

_____ M. D.
Clinical Pathologist

Figure 62-2. Cumulative report form of six organ panels.

STATE UNIVERSITY HOSPITAL
UPSTATE MEDICAL CENTER

CLINICAL PATHOLOGY -- ORGAN PANEL C

Last Reporting Date: _____

CARDIAC INJURY I

Creatine Phosphokinase (CPK) IU/L	Male 55-170 Female 30-135		
Lactic Dehydrogenase IU/L	71-207		

CARDIAC INJURY II

Lactic Dehydrogenase Isoenzymes	See Special Report		
Creatine Phosphokinase Isoenzymes	See Special Report		

CARDIAC EVALUATION

Cholesterol mg/dl	Age 20-30 130-230		
Triglyceride mg/dl	10-160		
T₄-RIA μg/dl	5.5-12.3		
Glucose mg/dl	65-115		
Uric Acid mg/dl	Male 2.1-7.8 Female 2.0-6.4		

HYPERTENSION

Creatinine mg/dl	0.6-1.2		
Creatinine Clearance ml/min.	80-120		
Urinary Free Cortisol mcg/24 hr	75-410		
Metanephrines μgm/mg creatinine	Less than 1.82		
Chloride mEq/L	98-109		
CO₂ Content mM/L	24-30		
Sodium mEq/L	135-145		
Potassium mEq/L	4.0-4.8		
Glucose mg/dl	65-115		

ARTHRITIS

%.S.R. %	40-54		
C-Reactive Protein	Negative		
Antinuclear Antibody Titer	Under 1:20		
Rheumatoid Factor Slide Latex Test			
Rheumatoid Factor Tube Latex Test			
Titer @ 56°C	1:20		
Titer @ 4°C	1:80		
Uric Acid mg/dl	Female 2.0-6.4 Male 2.1-7.8		
Total Proteins gm/dl	6.7-8.3		

TRANSITION PANEL

Alkaline Phosphatase IU/L	Adult 4-13 Child 11-20		
Lactic Dehydrogenase IU/L	71-207		
Uric Acid mg/dl	Female 2.0-6.4 Male 2.1-7.8		
Gamma Glutamyl Traspeptidase IU/L	Female 3-55 Male 15-85		
Serum Calcium meq/L	4.5-5.4		
CBC c̄ Differential	See Hematology Report Form		

HEPATIC

SGO Transaminase IU/L	1-39		
Alkaline Phosphatase IU/L	Adult 4-13 Child 11-20		
Bilirubin Total mg/dl	0.1-1.2		
Bilirubin Direct mg/dl	0.0-0.2		
Prothrombin time Seconds	9.2-11.2		
Gamma Glutamyl Traspeptidase IU/L	Female 3-55 Male 15-85		
Partial Thromboplastic time sec.	15-38		
Total Proteins gm/dl	6.7-8.3		
Albumin gm/dl	3.7-4.9		

RENAL

Urea Nitrogen (BUN) mg/dl	8-18		
Creatinine mg/dl	0.6-1.2		
Creatinine Clearance ml/min.	80-120		
Total Osmolality Serum mOsm/Kg	285-295		
Osmolality Urine mOsm/Kg	300-1000		
Osmolal Clearance ml/min			
Free Water Clearance ml/min			
Sodium mEq/L	135-145		
Potassium mEq/L	4.0-4.8		
Chloride mEq/L	98-109		
CO₂ Content mM/L	24-30		
Inorganic Phosphorus mg/dl	Adult 2.0-5.2 Child 4.0-7.0		
Calcium mEq/L	4.5-5.4		
Glucose mg/dl	65-115		
Uric Acid mg/dl	Female 2.0-6.4 Male 2.1-7.8		
Albumin gm/dl	Age 15-35 3.44-5.64 Age 35-55 3.22-5.10		
Total Proteins gm/dl	6.7-8.3		
Urinalysis	See Microscopy Report Sheet		
Urine Culture & Colony Count	See Bacteriology Report Sheet		

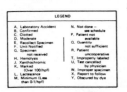

LEGEND	
A. Laboratory Accident	N. Not done — see schedule
B. Confirmed	P. Patient not available
C. Clotted	
D. Moderate	Q. Quantity not sufficient
E. Recollect Specimen	R. Patient uncooperative
F. Unit Notified	
G. Specimen not received	T. Improperly labeled
H. Hemolysis	U. Test cancelled by physician
J. Xanthochromic	W. Improper specimen
K. Marked (Over 100/hpf)	X. Report to follow
L. Lactescence	Y. Obscured by dye
M. Minimum (Less than 0-1/hpf)	

_____ M.D.
Clinical Pathologist

Figure 62–3. Cumulative report form of seven organ panels.

Table 62-3. LIST OF ORGAN PANELS CURRENTLY AVAILABLE AT SUNY UPSTATE MEDICAL CENTER

Arthritis	Metabolic
Cardiac evaluation	Microcytic anemia
Cardiac injury I	Muscle
Cardiac injury II	Pancreatic
General health	Parathyroid
Hepatic	Prostatic
Hypertension—Cardiovascular	Pulmonary
Hypopituitarism panel	Renal
(insulin tolerance)	Thyroid
Malabsorption	Transition panel

which has recently been intensified by large medical legal settlements and resultant increased liability insurance or defensive utilization of the laboratory. This cause of overutilization of laboratories will continue to escalate unless reasonable limits are placed on settlements and the public is educated about the seriousness and expense of these problems.

Direct and effective means of communication have to exist between laboratory technical staff, pathologists, and clinical staff in order that patient data generated by the laboratory be received by the physician. Tables of critical levels should exist in the laboratory and the importance of promptly relating critical data to the physician should be understood by all in the laboratory (Table 62-4). Reasonable turn-around times for all determinations should be decided on jointly by the various clinical departments and pathology staff (Table 62-5). Written protocols regarding the availabilities of test parameters can be posted in appropriate wards and clinics. This can reduce or eliminate the repeat ordering of tests in those situations in which the data are needed for immediate patient care.

Another area that can be explored is the feasibility of sharing reagents and instrumentation between laboratories. Problems of transportation of specimens, prolonged turn-around times, and communication between laboratory and ordering physicians have to be considered. In those instances in which the requested determinations are not urgent, sharing may be plausible and may eliminate the need for duplication of expensive instrumentation and laboratory personnel. This is particularly feasible for hormone determinations and drug assays. The possibility exists, however, that sharing will cause increased turn-around time, inflicting medical risks and perhaps extending hospitalizations.

If the goal of optimal patient care is to be achieved from a laboratory viewpoint, it will be necessary for all involved to become cognizant of the many subtle, inbuilt, and interrelating problems that can contribute to malutilization of laboratories and to develop and implement more efficient ordering and testing patterns. An example of this approach has been the implementation at the Upstate Medical Center of new crossmatch or blood ordering guidelines for elective surgical hemotherapy (Mintz, 1976). Surgical procedures were identified for which much more blood was routinely crossmatched preoperatively than utilized and others identified for which blood was rarely transfused. The pathologist in charge of the blood bank monitors preoperative crossmatch ordering and actively interacts with and educates his clinical colleagues. The average preoperative crossmatch orders for patients undergoing routine elective operative procedures requiring hemotherapy have been significantly reduced (Mintz, 1978) (Table 62-6). For those procedures during which blood was rarely transfused, preoperative crossmatching is not done, in lieu of ABO-Rh typing and irregular antibody screening. Boral (1977) has shown that such antibody detection virtually assures complete transfusion safety; therefore, in those instances in which blood is needed, transfusion need not be delayed while crossmatching is being done. The director of the blood bank assumes full responsibility for this action. The use of the "type and screen" together with adherence to crossmatch guidelines and realistic blood ordering for elective surgery has resulted in substantial monetary savings, increased effective blood utilization (reduced blood outdating), and a better use of technologist time (Henry, 1977). An alternative strategy for ordering blood has evolved.

It should be considered carefully that while many of the areas reviewed address the development of more appropriate utilization of the clinical laboratory, this will *not* necessarily reduce costs. Some evidence exists that a considerable increase in laboratory utilization could and would occur. If appropriate, this is not necessarily bad, but must be appreciated.

In conclusion, it is only through awareness and cooperation (i.e., technical inservice conferences), a strong clinical pathology curricu-

Table 62-4. CLINICAL PATHOLOGY STANDARD OPERATING PROCEDURE FOR
ABNORMAL RESULTS

HEMATOLOGY

Technologist will call patient's physician immediately for the following:

Hematocrit	<25 or >55
Hemoglobin	<7.5 or >18 g/dl
WBC (leukocyte count)	$<2 \times 10^3/\mu l$ or $>20 \times 10^3/\mu l$
Platelet count	$<50 \times 10^3/\mu l$ or $>1,000 \times 10^3/\mu l$
Prothrombin time	>60 sec (also make out "abnormal coag"
Thrombin time	>60 sec card for the resident)
Partial thromboplastin time (Activated)	>90 sec
Prothrombin time	>11 sec

Unexpected differential findings, including blasts in a new patient or a leukemic patient presumed to be in remission.

Notify Clinical Pathology Resident or Attending Pathologist for:

Partial thromboplastin time (Activated)	>32 sec	Make out "abnormal coagula-
Thrombin time	>29 sec	tion studies card" for the res-
Bleeding time	>7 min.	ident. The resident must
		check these cards at least
		once in the morning and once
		in the afternoon and notify ·
		the physician and determine
		if the patient is on anticoag-
		ulants.

BLOOD BANK

The Pathology Resident calls immediately either the patient's attending physician or appropriate house staff for the following:
  Transfusion reaction results
  Problems in compatibility testing
  Deviations from guidelines for ordering blood
The Pathology Resident and/or Attending Pathologist should be notified before reporting the following:
  Positive direct Coomb's test (antiglobulin test)
  Antibody identification and titer
  Positive indirect Coomb's (antiglobulin test)
  Isohemagglutinin titers
  Renal transplantation HLA typings and match as well as results of all HLA typing.

CHEMISTRY

Technologist calls patient's physician promptly for the following:
  Glucose under 50 mg/dl or over 500 mg/dl
  Calcium under 4 mEq/l or over 5.9 mEq/l
  Magnesium under 1 mEq/l or over 3 mEq/l
  Sodium under 125 mmol/l or over 150 mmol/l
  Potassium under 2.7 mmol/l or over 5.9 mmol/l
  CO_2 under 15 mmol/l or over 50 mmol/l
  All abnormal blood gas results not previously identified
  Positive screens for barbiturates
  Lactic acid greater than 3 mmol/l
  CO values greater than 20%
  Acetone greater than 30 mg/dl
Notify the Pathology Resident or attending for the following:
  Digoxin greater than 3.5 ng/ml
  Digitoxin greater than 35 ng/ml
  Lithium greater than 3 mmol/l
  Phenytoin greater than 50 μg/ml
  Ethosuximide greater than 150 μg/ml
  Phenobarbital greater than 75 μg/ml
  Primidone greater than 18 μg/ml
  Quinidine greater than 10 μg/l
  Cortisol less than 5 μg/dl or greater than 50 μg/dl
  All abnormally high values for catecholamines, metanephrines or VMA
  17 OH steroids less than 2 mg/24 hr or greater than 25 mg/24 hr
  17 ketosteroids less then 3 mg/24 hr
  24 hour urine volumes less than 500 ml for steroid measurements
  Procainamide greater than 15 μg/l

Table 62–5. AVAILABLE EMERGENCY CLINICAL PATHOLOGY PROCEDURES

BLOOD BANK

1. Whole blood crossmatched
2. Packed red blood cells crossmatched
3. Frozen, washed red cells
4. Albumin 25% (salt poor 100 ml)
   Albumin 25% (salt poor 50 ml)
5. Fresh frozen plasma
6. Group, Rh, and antiglobulin test
7. Platelet concentrates
8. Transfusion reaction evaluation
9. Process and collect blood from donors
10. Leukocyte-poor packed cells
11. Platelet-rich plasma
12. Cryoprecipitate
13. Factor VIII or AHF (antihemophilia factor) concentrate
14. Factor IX complex concentrate
15. Plasma protein fraction concentrate
16. Leukapheresis
17. Plateletpheresis
18. RhoGam
19. Antibody identification

CHEMISTRY

1. Blood ammonia
2. Blood amylase
3. Blood total bilirubin
4. Blood bromide level
5. Blood carbon dioxide
6. Blood chloride
7. Blood glucose
8. Blood pH, Pco_2, Po_2, & O_2 sat.
9. Blood potassium
10. Blood salicylate
11. Blood sodium
12. Blood urea nitrogen
13. Cerebrospinal fluid glucose
14. Cerebrospinal fluid protein
15. CSF glutamine
16. Creatine phosphokinase
17. R.B.C. potassium
18. Barbiturate screening
19. Blood calcium
20. Cardiac injury panel
21. Blood acetone
22. Creatinine
23. Blood alcohol
24. Lactate dehydrogenase
25. Lactic acid
26. Albumin
27. Alkaline phosphatase
28. Pseudocholinesterase
29. Transaminase (SGOT or ALT)
30. Total protein
31. Phenobarbital
32. Phenytoin
33. Digoxin
34. Theophylline

HEMATOLOGY

1. Hematocrit
2. White cell count
3. Differential count (including platelet estimate & RBC morphology)
4. CBC (WBC, RBC, Hgb, Hct, MCV, MCH, MCHC) scan for RBC morphology, platelet estimate, abnormal WBC's. Differential done only if ordered or if abnormal WBC count or abnormal cells seen in scan.
5. Prothrombin time
6. Partial thromboplastin time
7. Thrombin time
8. Platelet count
9. Fibrinogen
10. Fibrin split products (FSP) screen

MICROBIOLOGY

1. Specimens cultured
2. Gram stain, India ink prep.
3. Acid-fast stain
4. Counterimmunoelectropheresis

SEROLOGY AND IMMUNOLOGY

1. Monospot
2. Cryptococcal antigen (CSF)

MICROSCOPY

1. Urinalysis
2. Pregnancy (HCG) test
3. Osmolality
4. CSF cell count
5. Urine sodium and potassium

Performance of emergency procedures other than those listed above requires prior approval of the director of Clinical Pathology or attending pathologist. We invite consultations at any time concerning these and other problems.

6

Table 62–6. STATE UNIVERSITY OF NEW YORK UPSTATE MEDICAL CENTER BLOOD BANK WORKLOAD FROM 1972 TO 1976 REFLECTING IMPACT OF TYPE AND SCREEN INSTITUTED IN 1974

	NUMBER OF UNITS WHOLE BLOOD AND PACKED RED CELLS CROSSMATCHED	NUMBER OF UNITS WHOLE BLOOD AND PACKED RED CELLS TRANSFUSED	CROSSMATCH/TRANSFUSION (C/T) RATIO
1972	21,744	7688	2.82
1973	29,448*	9689*	3.03*
1974	28,236	9931	2.84
1975	24,078	9789	2.45
1976	21,528	10,942	1.96

*A decrease in crossmatches of approximately 8000 or ⅓ (33 per cent) from 1973 through 1976 with an increase in transfusions of 1300 (12 per cent); C/T ratio decreased from 3.03 to 1.96 during this interval.

lum in undergraduate medical education, and involvement of the pathologist in clinical situations on a universal scale that malutilization can be reduced in conjunction with optimal patient care and cost containment. More studies reflecting clinical outcome in terms of impact of laboratory testing need to be accomplished so that ideal or optimal laboratory utilization may be defined. The problems are urgent and if solutions are not found, artificial and external restrictions will be imposed which will create additional problems, i.e., increasing underutilization and restrictive use of laboratory services.

REFERENCES

Ashley, J. S. A., Parker, P., and Beresford, T. C.: How much clinical investigation? Lancet, *1*:890, 1972.

Boral L., and Henry, J. B.: The type and screen: A safe alternative and supplement in selected surgical procedures. Transfusion, *17*:165, 1977.

Carmalt, M. H. B., and Whitehead, T. P.: Biochemical profiles and length of hospital stay. Proc. Roy. Soc. Med., *64*:257, 1971.

Edwards, L. D., Levin, S., Balogtas, R., Lowe, P., Landon, W., and Lepper, M. H.: Ordering patterns and utilization of bacteriological culture reports. Arch. Intern. Med., *132*:678, 1973.

Freeborn, D. K., Baer, D., Greenlick, R. R., and Bailey, J. W.: Determinants of medical care utilization: Physicians use of laboratory services. Am. J. Publ. Health, *62*:846, 1972.

Galen, R. S., and Gambino, S. R.: Beyond Normality, the Predictive Value and Efficiency of Medical Diagnoses. New York, John Wiley and Sons, Inc., 1975.

Griner, P. F., and Liptzin, B.: Use of the laboratory in a teaching hospital. Ann. Intern. Med., *75*:157, 1971.

Henry, J. B., and Arras, M. J.: An innovation in delivery of health care: Organ panels. South. Med. J., *63*:907, 1970.

Henry, J. B., and Howanitz, P. J.: Organ panels and relationship of laboratory to the physician. *In* Clinician and Chemist: The Relationship of the Laboratory to the Physician. D. S. Young, M.D. (ed.). American Association of Clinical Chemistry, 1725 K Street, Washington, D.C. 20006, 1979.

Henry, J. B.: Principles of quality control. *In* Quality Control in Clinical Laboratory. Transactions of the 2nd International Symposium on Quality Control. Osaka, Japan, Daiwa Relief Art Printing Co. Ltd., 1976.

Henry, J. B., and Mintz, P. D.: Hemotherapy in elective surgery: Revised and realistic blood ordering. Joint Commission on Accreditation of Hospitals, Quality Review Bulletin, 1977.

Hurst, J. W., and Walker, H. K.: The Problem Oriented System. New York, Medcom Press, 1972.

Mintz, P. D., Lauenstein, K., Hume, J., and Henry, J. B.: Expected hemotherapy in elective surgery: A follow up. J.A.M.A., *239*:623, 1978.

Mintz, P. D., Nordine, R. B., Henry, J. B., et al.: Expected hemotherapy in elective surgery, N.Y. State J. Med., *76*:532, 1976.

Schroeder, S. A., Kenders, K., Cooper, J. K., and Piemme, T. E.: Use of laboratory tests and pharmaceuticals. J.A.M.A., *225*:969, 1973.

Ward, P. C. J., Harris, I. B., Burke, M. D., and Hurwitz, C.: Systematic instruction in interpretive aspects of laboratory medicine. J. Med. Ed., *51*:648, 1976.

63

MONITORING THE QUALITY OF LABORATORY MEASUREMENTS

George F. Grannis, Ph.D., and
Bernard E. Statland, M.D., Ph.D.

OVERVIEW

Clinical laboratories perform qualitative, semiquantitative, and quantitative tests on a variety of biologic specimens. Qualitative tests, in which a particular characteristic of the specimen is determined to be either present or absent, are called binary discrete variates (see Chap. 16). Examples of such tests are blood grouping or the identification of microbiologic organisms present in a specimen. The results of such tests are in the nature of "yes" or "no," or "positive" or "negative" answers. That is, the examination shows what particular characteristics are present or absent in the specimen. Semiquantitative tests are those in which the degree of positivity or negativity is roughly estimated, usually by visual observation. An example of such a test is the dipstick test for urinary glucose, in which the degree of reaction is visually estimated and indicated as negative, weakly positive, moderately positive, or strongly positive, or more simply as 0, +, ++, or +++. In the last example, we are

6

dealing with a discrete variate having four possible values. Quantitative tests are those in which the amount of a particular substance, or property, is measured by some instrument and the result is expressed numerically. Examples of quantitative measurements are the determination of the number of red or white cells in a blood specimen, the number of organisms found in a microbiologic culture, or the concentration of some analyte in a specimen of blood or urine. In the last example, we are dealing with a continuous variate (see Chap. 16). In this chapter we will be concerned with the techniques for monitoring and assessing the reliability of *quantitative* laboratory measurements (continuous variates) in laboratory medicine.

The basic principles of industrial quality control were set forth by Shewhart in 1931. Measurements were made of items produced by a machine or sequence of machines, and the average value and range of values of the measurements were determined. Tolerance limits that would result in an acceptable product then were established, and product uniformity could be assured by continual surveillance of these critical measurements to detect deterioration of machine performance and by correction of the problems as they became evident. The ways in which these basic principles have been extended to develop systems of quality assurance in clinical chemistry have been reviewed by Grannis (1977).

Most quantitative analytical procedures involve several operations, or steps, and each operation is subject to some degree of inaccuracy or imprecision or to the possibility of a mistake. The immediate aim of quality control is to assure that the end-products—the analytical values regularly produced by a clinical laboratory—are sufficiently reliable for their intended use. A broader objective is to assure that all laboratories produce analytical values that meet acceptable standards of precision and accuracy at all times. The attainment of these intra- and inter-laboratory aims requires that all laboratory personnel—technologists, supervisors, and directors—be knowledgeable of the causes of analytical inaccuracies and of the techniques that are available for their detection, correction, and control. In addition, knowledge is required of the degree of the inaccuracy and imprecision allowed if analytical values are to be clinically useful.

Quality control in laboratory medicine has been defined as the study of those errors which are the responsibility of the laboratory, and the procedures used to recognize and minimize them. An alternative term "quality assurance" has been used to represent the techniques available to insure with a specified degree of confidence that the result reported by the laboratory is correct. In order to have such confidence, the laboratory director must be assured that there is both "precision control" and "accuracy control" performed in the laboratory.

In this chapter we will consider some of the general principles of quality assurance of clinical laboratory data and some of the specific systems that have been developed for monitoring and improving the quality of clinical laboratory performance. However, before we consider these specific details, it will be helpful to review some basic concepts concerning quantitative measurements.

THE NATURE OF ANALYTICAL BIASES AND RANDOM VARIABILITY

In Chapter 1, two types of analytical bias—constant bias and proportional bias—were presented (see Fig. 1-5). We will refer to these types of biases again before introducing the major techniques of quality control.

ANALYTICAL BIAS

It is a basic premise of quality control that the analytical values actually reported by the laboratory ideally should correspond to the correct or expected values. Let us assume that we do have some specimens for which we know the *true* concentration (expected value) of an analyte. In the optimum case when those specimens are analyzed by the laboratory, the reported values should correspond exactly to the expected values. That is, the reported values should fall along a line of slope 1.00 when graphed as shown in Figure 63-1A (see Chap. 1). However, all analytical procedures are subject to a variety of analytical inaccuracies, or biases. Figure 63-1B illustrates the effects of a proportional bias in which the reported values are higher than the expected values. The bias is called proportional because the amount of bias increases in direct proportion to the concentration of analyte in the specimen. Figure 63-1C illustrates the effect

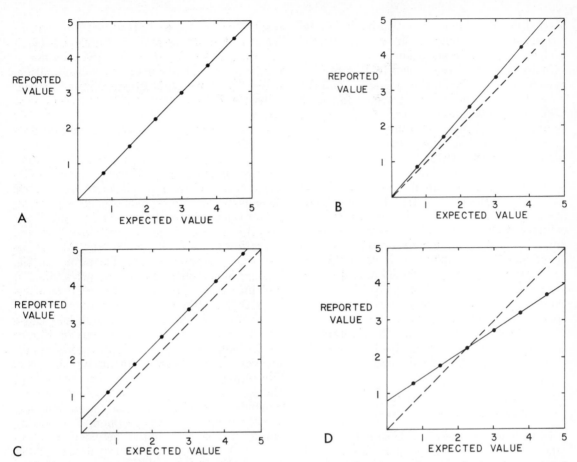

Figure 63–1. Illustration of the concept of the "operational line." When the laboratory's reported values for a series of specimens are plotted against the known, or expected, values, the data should fall along the straight line of slope 1.0, as shown in *A. B, C,* and *D* respectively illustrate the results observed when proportional, constant, or combined biases are present. The dashed lines in *B, C,* and *D* represent the case of no proportional bias and no constant bias. Every laboratory, in every analytical procedure, produces results that fall along some operational line, and one objective of quality control is to determine and optimize the laboratory's operational lines.

of a constant bias, in which the reported values are each higher than the expected values by a constant amount, at all concentrations of analyte.

The biases shown in Figures 63–1*B* and *C* are positive biases, because the reported values are greater than the expected values. Of course, negative biases may also occur; furthermore, the reported values may fall along a curve rather than a straight line. Nevertheless, Figures 63–1*B* and *C* illustrate the two major classes of biases that affect the accuracy of clinical analyses. Many analytical procedures are subject to either constant or proportional biases, or to both. Figure 63–1*D* illustrates how combined constant and proportional biases may affect the correlation of reported

and expected values. It is worth noting that when combined biases are present, there is frequently one concentration at which the reported value does correspond exactly to the expected value. This phenomenon—that the reported value at some analyte concentration is the same as the expected value while they disagree at all other concentrations—is commonly observed and must be considered when interpreting quality control data. The phenomenon is sometimes used to advantage to minimize analytical bias. For example, when a particular method is found to have a constant positive bias, that bias may be partially compensated by deliberately introducing a negative proportional bias. This principle, of introducing compensatory biases to minimize total bias, although widely employed in some analytical systems, may result in unexpected problems in certain situations.

Charts such as those shown in Figure 63-1 have been called "operational charts," and the lines on which the reported values fall have been called "operational lines," because every laboratory does produce results that tend to fall along some line when graphed as in Figure 63-1 (Grannis, 1972). That is, each laboratory for each analytical procedure customarily operates with a certain degree of bias that causes its results to be distributed along some operational line, as shown in the figures. One primary objective of quality assurance procedures is to determine a laboratory's operational line for each analytical method. Ideally, of course, all laboratories should have an operational line of slope 1.00 (Fig. 63-1A), so that their reported values are unbiased and correspond exactly to the known values. But if this ideal cannot be attained, then the laboratory's customary operational line should at least be maintained in a reproducible manner.

RANDOM ANALYTICAL VARIABILITY

In addition to analytical biases, laboratory analyses are also subject to imprecision, or random variability. The effects of random variation on analyses are illustrated in Figures 63-2A and B, which show how a laboratory's results may, on the average, fall along some operational line even though the individual results are distributed about the line, within certain limits of variability. Figure 63-2A illustrates limits of variability that increase in proportion to the mean analyte concentration, while Figure 63-2B illustrates limits of variability that are constant at all concentrations of analyte.

Knowledge of the kinds of bias and random variability that affect an analytical system is helpful in identifying their causes. For example, proportional limits of variability are commonly caused by imprecision in volumetric dispensing of the sample. An automatic pipettor is a mechanical device and as such there may be a certain amount of "play" in the operation of its parts, which may increase as the parts become worn. Variation in the amount of sample measured by such a pipettor will introduce variation in the analytical results that is proportional to the analyte concentration of the specimen, and will cause proportional variability as shown in Figure 63-2A. Similarly, constant limits of variability are commonly observed in analytical procedures that are influenced by the turbidity of the specimen. Sample turbidity is usually independent of analyte concentration, but may vary from specimen to specimen, thus causing results to be distributed between constant limits, as shown in Figure 63-2B. Thus, knowledge of how various sources of analytical bias and variability affect the accuracy and precision of the operational line can be most helpful in identifying and in correcting analytical problems as they arise.

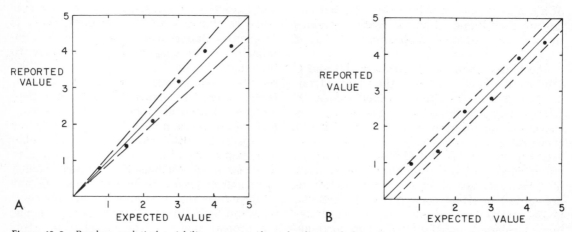

Figure 63-2. Random analytical variability causes results to be dispersed about the operational line, and may increase in proportion to analyte concentration (*A*) or may be constant at all concentrations (*B*).

Mistakes

In addition to analytical factors that introduce bias and random variability into the analytical procedure, laboratory analyses are also subject to "mistakes." It is sometimes difficult to determine whether an erroneous result was due to an analytical factor or to a mistake, but the differentiation is of some importance if the cause of a problem is to be identified and corrected. Analytical errors are usually systematic in nature. That is, they are caused by some factor in the analytical system which can affect a series of analyses. For example, an erroneously calibrated pipettor might cause a systematic proportional bias, while a pipettor that operates imprecisely will cause random variability of analyses. Mistakes occur rather seldom, however, and usually affect only a few analyses. The pipettor might be used to measure a sample into the wrong tube, or the analytical result might be assigned to the wrong specimen, or the numbers in the analytical value might be transposed. These kinds of incidents are due to human mistakes rather than to deficiencies in the analytical system. Table 63-1 lists further examples of mistakes in the laboratory.

Several studies have indicated that as many as 2 per cent of all clinical chemistry analyses may be erroneous due to mistakes (Grannis, 1972; Whitehurst, 1975; Ladenson, 1975). There are a multitude of steps involved in the processing of a specimen; thus, there are numerous points where a mistake may occur. Even when the probability of a mistake occurring is low at any one point, the probability that at least one error occurs can be quite high.

One important aspect of quality control is to identify those steps in the analytical process where the likelihood of mistakes is high, and to consider ways to minimize that likelihood.

Quality Control Specimens Used in Monitoring Analytical Bias and Variability

The use of samples obtained from the same pool for the comparison of laboratory analyses was introduced nearly three decades ago and is still the most direct and widely applied quality assurance technique (Henry, 1952; Henry, 1959). In a number of studies (Belk,

Table 63-1. SOME TYPES OF LABORATORY MISTAKES

1. Obtaining the specimen from the wrong patient
2. Specimen mix-up
   a. Specimens labeled with wrong accession numbers
   b. Sera transferred to mislabeled tubes
   c. An improper cup number was recorded when a specimen was removed from the AutoAnalyzer sampler wheel to insert an emergency specimen, and all specimens on the wheel were assigned false values.
   d. Analytical tubes interchanged during pipetting of specimens
3. Incorrect chart readings
   a. Incorrect reading of AutoAnalyzer peak.
   b. Incorrect read-off from standard curve.
   c. Read-off from standard curve assigned to wrong specimen.
   d. Read-off from wrong standard curve.
4. Dilution and calculation errors
   a. Analyst forgot to correct results for dilution.
   b. Samples diluted by first-shift technologist were analyzed by a second-shift technologist who was not informed of the prior dilution.
   c. A newly employed analyst thought a "1 to 2" dilution meant 1 volume of serum and 2 volumes of diluent rather than 1 volume of each.
5. Reagent and standard solutions
   a. Distilled water rather than buffer was used to prepare a reagent.
   b. pH meter standardized with wrong buffer.
   c. Reagent contaminated.
   d. New reagent used without checking against old reagent.
6. Instrument problems
   a. Slow clock used for a timed reaction.
   b. Recorder not properly warmed up; blank reading unstable.
   c. Broken balance used to weigh out standards.
7. Other
   a. Specimens left at room temperature by first-shift technologist to be analyzed by second-shift technologist; second-shift technologist did not report for work, and specimens were not analyzed until the next day.
   b. Analyst calculated results mentally rather than drawing a standard curve or calculating a factor; the results were grossly incorrect.
   c. Initial computer print-out was incorrect, and subsequent corrected print-out was ignored.

Modified from Grannis, G. F., Gruemer, H. D., Lott, J. A., Edison, J. A., and McCabe, W. C.; Clin. Chem., *18*:222, 1972.

1947; Shuey, 1949; Wootton, 1953) samples (assumed to be identical) of aqueous solutions of analytes, or of liquid serum or urine, were distributed to several laboratories for analysis. The results revealed clear evidence of substantial systematic differences among the laboratories. Similarly, when samples of the same serum pool were analyzed in a single laboratory over a period of time, variability in the measured values could be documented (Levey, 1950). These early studies established the important principle that a laboratory's analyses could be compared with those of other laboratories, or with its own prior analyses, simply by periodically analyzing samples that had been reserved from a large serum pool. The studies of Belk led directly to the establishment of interlaboratory comparison programs (Dorsey, 1975), and the studies of Levey led to the establishment of intralaboratory quality control programs.

However, the development of these programs was not without difficulty. In order to be effective the samples had to be essentially equivalent one to the other, the analytes in the sample had to be stable in storage over a substantial period of time, and the material had to be available in sufficient quantity to be used by many laboratories or by a single laboratory for a long period of time. It is beyond the scope of this chapter to consider the technical development of samples suitable for use in quality control. Suffice it to say that most samples used today are lyophilized products prepared from large pools of serum. As the interpretation of quality control data requires some appreciation of the limitations of these control specimens, it is worthwhile to consider some of the characteristics of such specimens.

The larger manufacturers of quality control specimens maintain blood plasma collection stations, and the fresh plasma is frozen for transport to a manufacturing plant. When a batch of control serum is to be prepared, as much as 2000 liters of plasma is thawed, pooled, defibrinated, supplemented with various analytes to achieve the desired concentrations in the final product, mixed thoroughly, filtered, and dispensed into vials. The vials are then lyophilized and capped under nitrogen. The steps in this manufacturing process which are most critical for assuring that the final specimens will contain essentially the identical quantities of the analyte(s) of interest are the dispensing and lyophilization procedures. In addition, the entire process must be completed expeditiously, to prevent deterioration of the pool. The dispensers used are precision instruments that deliver pre-set volumes with a coefficient of variation (CV) of less than 1 per cent, and can dispense 2000 liters in about 10 hours. The serum is processed at cold room temperatures to minimize deterioration. Lyophilization is carried out to a residual mois-

ture content of less than 2 per cent water to assure stability in transport and storage. In general, the final samples are found to have a vial-to-vial variability of about 1 per cent. Except for occasional loss of glucose due to bacterial contamination and occasional changes in enzyme activities, the lyophilized products are generally stable. Some preparations are found to have greater turbidity than is customarily seen with clinical specimens. However, currently available specimens are generally satisfactory for most quality control programs, and we may expect continuing product improvements as manufacturing technology is further developed. In practice, the laboratory should purchase a supply of commercial lyophilized serum pool sufficient to last one year. Unassayed material is less expensive and avoids the pitfalls of erroneous assay values or assay values which show methodology bias. Such unassayed material will be useful for "precision control"; however, it should not be considered adequate for "accuracy control."

INTRODUCTION TO QUALITY CONTROL TECHNIQUES

Quality control can be divided into two major types: internal quality control (intralaboratory quality control) and external quality control (interlaboratory quality control). Intralaboratory quality control can be based either on the results of control specimens or on the results of patient specimens.

INTRALABORATORY QUALITY CONTROL (INTERNAL QUALITY CONTROL) BASED ON USE OF CONTROL SPECIMENS

Quality control within the clinical chemistry laboratory should be thought of as a *system* for assuring the quality of total laboratory performance. The purpose of the control program is to assess realistically the laboratory's usual performance in relation to that of other laboratories, to identify significant problems as they arise, and to document that the problems are solved. This endeavor requires the involvement of all laboratory personnel and is most effectively coordinated by one individual who has the assigned responsibility of maintaining and reviewing the laboratory's quality control records and of making regular reports to the laboratory staff. A coordinated system of quality control provides a mechanism for the open discussion of current laboratory problems and for developing uniform standards of performance throughout the laboratory.

An effective system of quality control, developed by Sax (1967), modified by Allen (1969), and further refined by Grannis (1972) is illustrated in Figure 63–3. In this system each analyst in the chemistry laboratory routinely includes known quality control specimens in each analytical run. The expected values for these specimens are known to the analyst, and the purpose of these control specimens is to aid the analyst, who is responsible for a particular procedure, in deciding whether the analytical system is producing analytically reliable results for that particular analyte. Other quality control specimens, which may be duplicate patient specimens, commercial control specimens, or specimens with known additives, are prepared by the "Quality Control Laboratory" and interspersed randomly among the clinical specimens. The fact that these specimens are control specimens is unknown to the analysts in the laboratory. The purpose of the latter specimens is to obtain an independent assessment of all of the procedures performed in the laboratory. The data from both types of specimens are assessed on a daily basis, and the Quality Control Laboratory prepares a monthly statistical summary and a review of apparent problems. This summary is a permanent agenda item for the regular meeting of the laboratory supervisors and director.

The quality control laboratory also receives and distributes specimens from various interlaboratory surveys and maintains records of the survey reports. Thus, this system provides a mechanism for acquiring a variety of information about laboratory performance, for identifying and resolving problems, and for developing realistic standards of performance.

Although the system just described may appear suitable only for the larger clinical laboratories, the basic concept of having a regular review and discussion of quality control data, whether acquired with known or unknown samples, is applicable to all laboratories. In the following paragraphs we will consider some details in setting up and maintaining the system illustrated in Figure 63–3, but these details should be generally applicable to other systems as well.

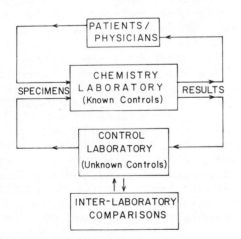

Figure 63–3. A system for intralaboratory monitoring of measurements. Analysts in the chemistry laboratory employ known control materials with each set of clinical analyses. The control laboratory obtains an independent assessment of overall laboratory performance by interspersing unknown specimens with the regular clinical specimens and evaluating the reported results. The control laboratory also processes samples from interlaboratory comparison programs. The control laboratory is responsible for reviewing all quality control data and for making regular reports to the laboratory's supervisorial staff.

SELECTION OF QUALITY CONTROL SPECIMENS

The commercial suppliers of control sera customarily provide "normal" (or "level 1") and "abnormal" (or "level 2") specimens, and for each analyte one or the other of these specimens usually provides values near the principal "clinical decision concentration." It is good laboratory practice to include both a "normal" and an "abnormal" control specimen in each analytical run. The unknown control specimens should not be identical to the known controls, and together the known and unknown controls should encompass the significant portion of the analytical range for each analyte. With judicious selection of control materials, the "operational lines" of the laboratory (see Fig. 63–1) may be monitored rather closely on a daily basis.

PREPARATION OF CONTROL SPECIMENS

Because an effective quality control program depends on having control specimens that are highly reproducible, it is absolutely essential that the lyophilized samples be reconstituted and handled with good quantitative technique. That is, the reconstitution fluid should be measured with a volumetric pipet or a well-calibrated dilutor; the proteinaceous material must be allowed to dissolve completely; and, as the specimens will be used over the course of several hours, they should be protected from deterioration due to bacterial action (glucose), exposure to light (bilirubin), evaporation (all analytes), or loss of CO_2. The preparation of the daily control specimens is a specialized task, and this task should be included in the laboratory's regular schedule of personnel rotation or assigned to one individual. If precautions such as these are not taken, then each questionable result may be "explained" as an erroneous control sample and real analytical problems may remain undetected.

FORMS AND CHARTS

Quality control programs quickly generate large amounts of data, and several forms and charts are most helpful in organizing the data in a useful format.

Results from Known Controls, By Analyte. The results from known control specimens should be tabulated on a standard form for each analyte. The form should have columns for each control specimen, and the successive analytical results are recorded in the appropriate column as they are acquired. After 20 or more values have been recorded, the mean and standard deviation of the values are calculated for each column. (See Chapter 1 for computing the mean and standard deviation.) As the form is intended for use at the bench to monitor the analytical procedure, the range of acceptable values should be listed for each control specimen.

An alternative and more effective way of monitoring the analytical procedure is to plot the control results serially as illustrated in Figure 63-4. This graph is similar to that introduced by Levey and Jennings and shows the expected mean value and the range of acceptable values. The determined values should fall within the indicated limits with a certain probability. Here, the use of "prediction intervals" would be appropriate (see Chap. 2). This chart is very useful at the bench because it provides an immediate visual comparison of the current analyses with prior analyses and aids in the detection of emergent problems.

By example, Figure 63-5 illustrates three types of changes that are commonly observed in quality control data. *Dispersion* of the data occurs when there is increased variability, or imprecision, in the analytical system. A *trend* in the data—i.e., a progressive drift of the determined values from the expected value—occurs when the analytical system becomes increasingly biased. An abrupt change from the expected value is called a *shift* and is indicative of the sudden appearance of bias.

The changes in control data illustrated in Figure 63-5 are indications that the analytical system has changed, and the analyst should determine what caused the change. This task is sometimes facilitated by remembering that a single control specimen allows one to evaluate a single point along the laboratory's operational line (see Fig. 63-1). If data from two or more control specimens are available, then additional points along the operational line are obtained. By observing how the analyses of the control specimens have changed, one can infer how the operational line has changed, and identify the kind of analytical problem that has occurred.

Results from Unknown Controls, All Analytes. It is convenient to record the daily results from unknown controls on a form that lists all of the tests being monitored and the range of acceptable values for each test. The recorded results are then compared with the ranges, outlying values are identified, and significant problems investigated. This form serves to organize the data in a format that is convenient for entry into a computer for statistical calculations, and the form also serves as a record of the frequency with which outly-

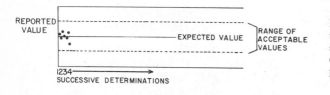

Figure 63-4. A modified Levey-Jennings quality control graph. Control data are graphed as acquired and should fall within the established limits. Values exceeding the limits are indicative of a possible analytical problem or of a mistake.

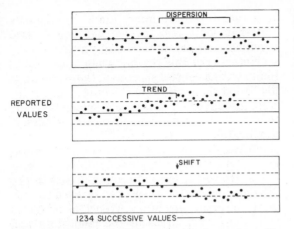

Figure 63-5. Examples of three common changes in quality control data. *Dispersion* is seen when there is an increased frequency of both high and low outliers. A progressive drift of the reported values from the prior mean value is called a *trend*. A *shift* occurs when there is an abrupt change from the established mean value.

ing values are observed in various portions of the laboratory.

The Monthly Report Form. The monthly report form simply lists the mean, standard deviation, and coefficient of variation (CV) for the various controls and the expected mean value and acceptable CV for each procedure. The data are listed in columns, and a new column is added each month, so that prior and current values may be easily compared. It is convenient to arrange the test procedures by supervisory areas of responsibility. The monthly report is accompanied by a summary of apparent problems to be discussed at the supervisors' meeting.

Long-Term Records. The setting of ranges for evaluating the acceptability of the quality control results is a critical aspect of the quality control program. Gooszen (1960) has noted that when the ranges are too narrow there will be frequent out-of-range results, tests will appear to be frequently "out-of-control," and concerned laboratory personnel may

spend an inordinate amount of time and effort pursuing insignificant problems. On the other hand, if the ranges are too wide, few out-of-range results will be observed, the test will appear always to be "in-control," and significant problems may go unnoticed. For these reasons, it is customary to define two limits for evaluating results: "warning limits" representing ± 2 standard deviation intervals from the expected value of a control specimen, and "action limits" representing ± 3 standard deviation intervals (Henry, 1959). On a statistical basis, about 19 of every 20 values should be expected to fall within the warning limits, and values exceeding the action limits should rarely be observed unless a real analytical change has occurred (Copeland, 1978b).

The data accumulated on successive monthly reports are an important source of information for setting practical ranges for acceptability of control results. For example, the monthly coefficients of variation may be graphed as in Figure 63-6 to provide an ongoing, long-term record of the analytical variability of each procedure. The figure shows that for a 12-month period during 1970 the CV of a glucose procedure, at a concentration of about 5.0 mmol/liter, was about 3.7 per cent. This CV was relatively low compared with prior values, and it was stable from month to month. The stability occurred because of some improvements that had been made in the analytical system. Thus, the laboratory demonstrated, over a 12-month period of time, that it could consistently produce reasonably precise analyses. Having documented this fact, laboratory staff should be expected to maintain at least this level of performance or to improve further. Assurance that this level of performance will be maintained may be gained by establishing a *laboratory policy* that (a) the ranges for acceptability of results will be based on the coefficients of variation observed during extended periods of good performance (i.e., low and stable CV's), (b) that the established ranges will be reviewed annually, and

6

Figure 63-6. Example of a long-term record of monthly coefficients of variation for serum glucose values. The mean concentration of serum glucose is approximately 5.0 mmol/l. See text for discussion of how this type of record may be used to establish optimum limits for control charts, to detect analytical problems, and to evaluate a new method.

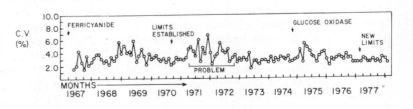

(c) that the established ranges may be narrowed when better performance is documented, but may not be widened.

This policy, when applied to all procedures performed by the laboratory, assures that the established ranges will be realistic, that frequent out-of-range values will be indicative of real problems that merit attention, and that the laboratory's standards for performance must remain constant, or improve, but may not be relaxed.

Figure 63-6 also shows how this policy may be used effectively. During 1971 and 1972, the CV's of the glucose procedure were increased and erratic. There were frequent out-of-range values over an extended period of time. These values could have been obscured simply by relaxing the established ranges, but, by maintaining the established ranges, the laboratory personnel were alerted to the fact that all was not well with the procedure. Eventually, the imprecision was found to be due to the use of reagents that were of variable quality (Lott, 1973). When new lots of reagents were evaluated more carefully before being placed in use and poor quality lots were rejected, the monthly CV's returned to their prior values.

Figure 63-6 also illustrates the value of long-term records when a new procedure is introduced. In 1974, the glucose procedure was changed from a ferricyanide method to a glucose oxidase method. The figure shows that the CV was reduced from 3.7 to 3.0 per cent. The ranges for acceptable results were narrowed accordingly. Thus, Figure 63-6 illustrates how long-term quality control data may be used to establish practical limits for the acceptability of results, to establish laboratory policies that will assure the detection and correction of analytical problems, and to assure the progressive improvement of laboratory performance.

Events and Action Records (Mistakes). If it is accepted that quality control specimens can be reproducibly prepared and that practical limits for analytical variability can be established, then it must be accepted that reported values which exceed these limits are exceptional and noteworthy. It is helpful to record the occurrence of these events and, whenever possible, to investigate their causes, and to record the corrective action that was taken. Such investigations will reveal that many of these out-of-range values are due to mistakes. From Table 63-1, it will be appreciated that there are many kinds of mistakes and that some will involve but one or two specimens, while others will involve many specimens. For this reason, when a mistake is found with a control specimen, there is a good likelihood that one or more clinical specimens were also involved, and efforts should be made to identify the specimens involved and correct the mistake. Control specimens make up a small fraction of the laboratory's total workload, and they cannot possibly detect all mistakes. However, the data accumulated in the "Events and Action Book" can be used to estimate the *frequency* of occurrence of mistakes in various work areas of the laboratory and can serve as a reminder to laboratory personnel to be alert to the probability of mistakes. The data of the Events and Action Book should be reviewed periodically and included with the quality control report.

USE OF CUMULATIVE SUM (CUSUM) TECHNIQUES

Woodard (1964) introduced a new approach to plotting the results obtained on control material, namely the computation of the cumulative sum of the differences of the measured values from the "assigned value" (the assumed correct value). The procedure is straightforward in that one merely subtracts the assigned value from the daily observed values and then notes the accumulated difference. The use of the cusum technique is illustrated by the following example. Table 63-2 presents the 20 daily observed values on control material for serum chloride, the differences from the assigned value, and the cumulative sums. The assigned value is 100 mmol/liter, i.e.; we assume that the correct value is 100 mmol/liter. In practice both the daily observed values and the daily cusums are plotted. The benefit of the cusum graph is that often changes which are not obvious in the conventional control charts (Figure 63-5) will be more apparent in the cusum plot. When interpreting the cusum graph, one is interested in the slope of the graph. Assuming that there is no appreciable change from day to day and assuming that the mean of the observed values is close to the assigned value, the slope should approximate zero, i.e., the cusum values should be parallel to the horizontal axis. This is essentially the case for the first eight days in our illustrative example (see Table 63-2). When

Table 63–2. CALCULATION OF CUMULATIVE SUMS FOR DAILY OBSERVED VALUES IN CONTROL SPECIMENS OF SERUM CHLORIDE

DAY NO.	SERUM CHLORIDE (MMOL/LITER)	ASSIGNED VALUE	DAILY DIFFERENCE	CUSUM
1	100	100	0	0
2	98	100	−2	−2
3	102	100	+2	0
4	99	100	−1	−1
5	101	100	+1	0
6	100	100	0	0
7	98	100	−2	−2
8	101	100	+1	−1
9	97	100	−3	−4
10	99	100	−1	−5
11	98	100	−2	−7
12	101	100	+1	−6
13	100	100	0	−6
14	99	100	−1	−7
15	99	100	−1	−8
16	101	100	+1	−7
17	97	100	−3	−10
18	100	100	0	−10
19	101	100	+1	−9
20	99	100	−1	−10

the material during the pre-instrumental phase of the analysis, eg., the reactivation of alkaline phosphatase activity with time (see Chap. 1). For the above reasons, the calculated variance of daily control values might overestimate the day-to-day analytical variance due to instrumental sources. Analytical variance alone, however, can theoretically be computed using multiple control specimens. The analysis of variance model permits one to partition the variance due to "analytical sources" from the variance due to "control specimens." In practice with each run of specimens at least two separate control pools are assayed in replicate. The results are analyzed using a two-way analysis of variance (ANOVA) model with the factors being "control material used" and "run number" (Winkel, 1976). This approach has been applied in the clinical setting, and the analysis of the results has been automated using a laboratory-based computer and the ANOVA program (Riddick, 1972).

the slope deviates markedly from zero, i.e., either an upward or a downward slope, we consider two possible explanations: (1) the assigned value is not the correct value, or (2) there is a bias (inaccuracy) in the measurements. In our example, we note a downward trend beginning on Day No. 9 and continuing through Day No. 17. Had we relied on the conventional control charts only, we might not have identified the shift in the observed values (Whitehead, 1977; Westgard, 1977). Of course, statistically significant deviation may not necessarily be "medically significant."

USE OF MULTIPLE CONTROL SPECIMENS

The basic assumption underlying the use of control specimen results to monitor the analytical variation is that the variation among samples obtained from the same control pool is an accurate reflection of the analytical variation. There are reasons to believe that the above assumption is not always correct: first, there may be additional variation in the control material results due to instability of the control material during storage, due to the variation in the initial aliquoting of the material and/or in the reconstituting of lyophilized material, and due to inconsistent handling of

INTRALABORATORY QUALITY CONTROL (INTERNAL QUALITY CONTROL) BASED ON PATIENT SPECIMENS

The reference sample approach to quality control (i.e., the use of identical samples over a long period of time) is widely used because it provides the laboratory with a rather constant frame of reference for the evaluation of its performance. However, commercial control specimens do not exactly simulate genuine clinical specimens, and occasionally changes in the control specimen (e.g., a loss of glucose) may incorrectly lead the laboratory personnel to believe that their analytical method is "out of control." In addition, the analytical biases observed with clinical specimens may not be identical to those observed with control specimens.

In the case of patient specimens, one must take into account the pre-instrumental sources of variation, including specimen collection, specimen transport, and specimen preparation. These same sources of variation are not present in the case of control material. For these reasons, a number of approaches of quality control (quality assurance) using the results observed on patient specimens have been proposed. They include determining the daily mean of certain patient results, using

6

one or more arithmetic checks on multiple results obtained on the same specimen, comparing the "present result" with any previous results from the same patient, noting apparently absurd results and "alert values," evaluating the combination of multiple results for unusual patterns, and assaying randomized duplicate patient specimens. Each of these approaches will be presented.

The Daily Mean

Waid (1955) and Hoffmann (1965) have postulated that if a significant analytical change occurs in a test procedure, that change should be reflected in the clinical data. They proposed several techniques (average of all values, average of values in the reference interval, number of values greater than the mode) for detecting changes in the frequency distribution of the clinical assay values. Although these procedures are basically attractive because they deal with clinical specimens, they have not been widely adopted. Several studies have shown the methods to be relatively insensitive to changes in analytical bias (Henry, 1959; Van Pennen, 1965; Frankel, 1967; Kilgariff, 1968; Amador, 1968). The reason these methods are insensitive may be understood by considering that for many analytes, the clinical assays include values both above and below the reference interval. When either constant or proportional biases are introduced (see Fig. 63–1), some clinical assays will move into the reference interval while others will move out, and the number of values within the central portion of the distribution curve will tend to remain constant (Kilgariff, 1968). In addition, many analytical systems employ the technique known as "single-point calibration." This technique is subject to combined constant and proportional systematic biases, and the "operational line" may pivot about the calibration value (see Fig. 63–1D). As the calibration point is often near the mean value of the clinical specimens, most clinical assays will be relatively unchanged even when the method is clearly biased at other concentrations. It is quite possible that in the routine operation of the clinical laboratory, a subtle combination of compensatory biases affects the clinical assays, making the detection of the biases from examination of the clinical data quite difficult. Nevertheless, a number of authors have reported successful application of the techniques, particularly when large biases were present (Dixon, 1970; Begtrup, 1971; Berry, 1973).

Arithmetic Check

Examination of clinical assays does have much value in the detection of mistakes. Whitehurst (1975) has described a computer-assisted program in which the clinical assay results are examined in several ways to detect questionable values. The arithmetic check compares two or more results from the same specimen that are related. For example, the difference between the major anions and cations of serum (i.e., the anion gap) was found most commonly to have a value between 10 and 21 mmol/liter.

Let us take the situation where S-sodium = 140 mmol/l, S-potassium = 5 mmol/l, S-bicarbonate = 26 mmol/l, and S-chloride = 100 mmol/l. In such a case the anion gap would be 145 minus 126, or 19 mmol/l.

The analysis as described by Whitehurst (1975) is automated using a computer program. According to the program, differences of less than 10.0 mmol/l or greater than 21 mmol/l are written into the discrepancy file for eventual computer printout. For checking acid-base calculation, actual bicarbonate and total CO_2 are calculated from pH and Pco_2 values by means of the Henderson-Hasselbalch equation (see Chap. 5), and the calculated values are compared with the observed values. In an analogous manner, when one knows the concentration values of serum sodium, urea, and glucose, one can compute a calculated osmolality and compare this value with the observed serum osmolality. The presence of significant discrepancies may not always be an indicator of analytical error; however, they should be cause for concern and further investigation.

Previous Value Check

The previous value check compares the result obtained for one specimen with the previous result(s) obtained for the same patient. Limits for the usual differences between specimens are entered into the computer program, and specimens having differences greater than these limits are listed for review by laboratory personnel. Here knowledge of the magnitude of the total (physiologic and analytical) intraindividual variation under various conditions is critical (see Chap. 2). The limits can be based solely on a statistical model and the width of the interval is dependent upon the probability value which one is using to decide if a measurement is outside the limits. Of course, finding such a result will not necessarily be associated with an analytical error. In fact, most often it is associated with a change in the disease course or a change in therapy. Some workers have used the term "delta check" to refer to this type of evaluation (Ladenson, 1975).

ALERT CHECK AND ABSURD VALUES

The alert check is designed to detect large errors or very unlikely values. For example, serum urea values less than 1.0 mmol/liter or greater than 18.0 mmol/liter are listed by the computer for review by laboratory personnel. Absurd values must also be recognized; e.g., a serum potassium of 40.0 mmol/l may represent a value in which the decimal point had been misplaced.

PATTERN RECOGNITION

Lindberg (1965, 1966) has described the use of pattern recognition techniques to detect unlikely combinations of values. As examples, (1) urea, creatinine, and uric acid values; or (2) sodium, potassium, chloride, and bicarbonate values are found to occur in clinical specimens in distinctive combinations, and the frequency of these various combinations can be calculated. The laboratory director should be aware of unusual combinations, e.g., grossly elevated serum alanine aminotransferase in association with a "normal" serum aspartate aminotransferase. An additional example is the situation when the results of the visual inspection of erythrocytes in a blood smear do not correspond to the values of red blood cell indices (see Chap. 29). When such unusual combinations occur, the possibility of laboratory error should be considered.

In all the cases presented, the laboratory-based computer could be programmed to detect unusual combinations of laboratory values. These various data analysis procedures are basically systems for checking and cross-checking the clinical assays for known internal consistencies, and for identifying unusual val-

ues. Whitehurst (1975) found that with his system, 8.4 per cent of all clinical assays were listed by the computer for review, 1.9 per cent of the specimens were re-analyzed, and 0.83 per cent were judged to be erroneous.

RANDOMIZED DUPLICATE SPECIMENS

An additional technique, which is useful for *occasional* checks of the reproducibility of a laboratory's analyses, is the use of randomized duplicate specimens (Bokelund, 1974). This technique is applied to serum analytes as follows: (1) Two blood specimens are obtained per venipuncture. (2) Each specimen is uniquely labeled and uniquely processed. (3) All specimens in a batch are placed in a randomized order. (4) The technologist is not informed as to which two samples are members of a duplicate pair. (5) The specimens are assayed for the analyte(s) of interest and the results are recorded. (6) The within-batch random analytical variation is computed on the basis of the "difference of duplicates" approach. (7) Whenever the absolute difference in duplicate values for any particular pair of results is greater than a predefined limit, both specimens are reassayed. The limit is based on the calculated standard deviation. (8) If the difference of the reassayed duplicates is still greater than the limit, the cause for the "apparent discrepancy" is sought. (9) If the difference is within the limit, the average of two replicates is computed and the resultant mean value is sent out to the requesting physician.

The use of randomized duplicates for monitoring within-batch quality assurance has certain advantages. Randomization of the specimens within a batch (as compared to the case where one replicate specimen follows the other) should overcome any possible correlation between "time of assay" and the "order of the specimen"; i.e., any general analytic drift occurring during the assaying of the batch of specimens will be included. In addition, the use of duplicates obtained at venipuncture allows estimation of the *total* (pre-instrumental and instrumental) within-batch analytical variation. Thus, this approach provides a realistic assessment of total variability in the entire analytical process and should give a greater degree of confidence in the quality of each particular measurement reported from the laboratory. Of course, the cost-benefit of this approach may be questioned; however, the availability of laboratory-based computers and analyzers with very high throughputs might make this method cost effective.

INTERLABORATORY COMPARISON PROGRAMS (EXTERNAL QUALITY CONTROL)

At present there are two principal types of programs in which laboratories may compare their analytical results. There are *survey programs* (proficiency testing) in which large numbers of laboratories analyze the same specimens several times each year, and there are *regional quality control programs* in which a group of laboratories in a geographical region use the same lots of quality control specimens on a daily basis for their internal quality control programs. The first of the survey programs was initiated in the late 1940's by Sunderman, and the most successful of these (The College of American Pathologists Survey Program) has grown to include more than 9000 of the approximately 13,000 clinical laboratories in the United States as well as several hundred laboratories in other countries (Gilbert, 1975a). The first regional quality control program was started by Preston in 1967 (Lawson, 1976). There are now many such regional programs, and by 1975 nearly 50 per cent of all laboratories in the United States participated in these programs. Thus, both regional quality control programs and survey programs are widely used by clinical laboratories to facilitate interlaboratory comparisons of analyses.

REGIONAL QUALITY CONTROL PROGRAMS

These programs are available from the major manufacturers of quality control specimens, as well as from various professional societies. In a typical program each participant receives a stock of quality control serum that is to be analyzed on a daily basis over a period of about one year. The analytical results are sent weekly or monthly to the supplier of the program for entry into a computer, and the participant receives a monthly report that compares the mean value and standard deviation of his analyses with those of peer laboratories—i.e., laboratories that use a comparable analytical method. Most of these

programs also supply computer-generated Levey-Jennings graphs of the data with ample room for the laboratory personnel to manually plot current results. This type of program is very useful to smaller laboratories that lack the personnel or computer facilities to perform the statistical calculations or to prepare the graphs that are necessary to maintain their internal quality control program.

Regional quality control programs are necessarily limited in size because of limitations in the volume of serum that can be processed to prepare the control specimens. However, some of these regional quality control programs have been integrated through the College of American Pathologists (CAP) Computer Center. That is, the data from various regional programs are processed by the CAP computer center. In this way the data from the various programs, even though based on the use of several different serum pools, may be combined for detailed statistical analyses. For example, Ross (1976) estimated the average median analytical variation obtained for 14 analytes at various analyte concentrations by both manual and automated methods. A condensed summary of some of these data is given in Table 63-3. These estimates are based

Table 63-3. ESTIMATES OF THE AVERAGE MEDIAN DAY-TO-DAY COEFFICIENT OF VARIATION OF MANUAL AND AUTOMATED ANALYSES, FOR EACH OF 14 ANALYTES, AT THE INDICATED CONCENTRATION OF ANALYTE

ANALYTE	CONCENTRATION	ESTIMATED AVERAGE MEDIAN COEFFICIENT OF VARIATION	
		Manual	Automated
Albumin	35 g/liter	5.6	3.8
Bilirubin	17 μmol/liter	13.4	10.2
Calcium	2.75 mmol/liter	3.4	2.6
Chloride	110 mmol/liter	1.9	1.6
Cholesterol	6.5 mmol/liter	4.5	4.6
Creatinine	440 μmol/liter	5.2	3.2
Glucose	6.7 mmol/liter	4.4	3.4
Phosphorus	1.5 mmol/liter	5.1	3.9
Potassium	6.0 mmol/liter	2.4	1.7
Protein	70 g/liter	2.8	2.1
Sodium	150 mmol/liter	1.3	1.3
Triglyceride	1.5 mmol/liter	7.5	5.5
Urea	10 mmol/liter	7.1	3.8
Uric acid	350 μmol/liter	5.3	3.0

Adapted from Ross, J. W., and Fraser, M. D.: Am. J. Clin. Pathol., *66*:203, 1976.

on hundreds of thousands of analyses performed on a daily basis in more than a thousand laboratories. These data may be used by the individual laboratories in evaluating their acceptable limits for quality control specimens in their internal control program as well as being an indicator of the current level of performance of laboratories throughout the country.

SURVEY PROGRAMS

Although there are many clinical chemistry survey programs available to laboratories through governmental, private, and professional agencies, the program developed by the College of American Pathologists is the largest in scope and is probably the most sophisticated at the present time. Participants in the program receive several specimens several times each year for analysis, and return their results to the CAP Computer Center. Shortly thereafter each participant receives a report that compares this reported value with the mean and standard deviation obtained by peer laboratories, the number of peer laboratories, and the "SDI" of the reported value. (The SDI is the *Standard Deviation Interval*, i.e., the difference between the reported value and mean value, divided by the standard deviation. An SDI of -0.4 means that the reported value is 0.4 standard deviation unit below the group mean value.) Reported values that differ excessively from the mean value are flagged to alert the participant to the possibility of an analytical error. In addition to this statistical summary, each participant receives a concise summary of the performance of all methods for each analyte covered in the survey. The summary lists results according to all method/instrument combinations that were used by 20 or more laboratories. The complete participant report includes data for each of more than 20 analytes. This kind of report provides an overview of the field at the time of each survey and is valuable to participants because it indicates the popularity of various methods and the relative bias and variability of the various methods as they are actually used in the field. As such summaries are provided with each survey, the popularity and performance characteristics of each method over a period of time are continuously documented.

In addition to the regular participant report

and method summaries, an annual report (called Survey Data) is also prepared for the participants. The specimens used in the CAP Survey Program are sometimes prepared to have subtle inter-relationships. The survey specimens are mailed during the year in various combinations that may include duplicate specimens, inter-related specimens, or unrelated specimens. It is possible to statistically analyze the data from such specimens to obtain estimates of the intra- and inter-laboratory variability of analyses, as well as the relative bias between analytical methods as a function of analyte concentration. This kind of data is most valuable to laboratories and to instrument/reagent manufacturers in comparing the analytical performance of various methods.

There are two other aspects of the CAP Survey Program that have important bearing on quality assurance. First, the specimens used in the survey program are manufactured in excess of survey needs, and after each survey is completed the excess serum is made available as a survey-validated reference material (SVRM). Thus, this reference serum is continuously renewed with each survey, is nationally available, and has consensus mean values assigned for more than 20 analytes and for all methods used by 20 or more laboratories. This reference serum has many practical uses for trouble-shooting analytical problems, comparing methods, or checking analytic values assigned to other reference, calibration, or quality control products. The consensus mean values attached to these reference sera have been evaluated for reliability (Gilbert, 1976; Grannis, 1976) and some specimens have been analyzed by the National Bureau of Standards using definitive (absolute) methods for some constituents (Gilbert, 1978). Second, laboratories that participate in the CAP Inspection and Accreditation Program receive a quarterly report that lists those tests for which the laboratory's reported results differed significantly from the consensus mean value. The report lists all such results for the preceding three years, unless satisfactory results were obtained in four successive surveys. This report serves to alert the laboratory to possible problem areas. As the inspection and accreditation procedure includes a review of such tests, an effective mechanism is established for assuring that these apparent problem areas will receive attention.

6

YOUDEN PLOTS

Youden (1960) presented a novel approach in plotting the results obtained from each of two control specimens sent out to various laboratories. The range of possible results of the one specimen, e.g., the "lower level," is marked on the abscissa (x-axis) and the range of the possible results of the second specimen, e.g., the "higher level," is marked on the ordinate (y-axis). The results from many laboratories are plotted on the same graph. The interlaboratory means and standard deviations are computed. The two scales are adjusted so that the actual measured distances of the standard deviations are the same for the two specimens.

Assuming that the mean values of the results represent a reasonable estimate of the "true values," one can determine how his laboratory performed as compared with other laboratories. Furthermore, one can verify the possibility of a consistent positive bias (right upper quadrant of the Youden plot) or of a consistent negative bias (left lower quadrant of the Youden plot). The relationship of the Youden plot to various kinds of operational lines (Figures 63-1A to D) has been described (Grannis, 1977).

ACCURACY CONTROL

The maintenance of analytical accuracy (i.e., reproducible method calibration) over extended periods of time is important. Each new analytical method introduced into the laboratory must undergo strict reliability checks (see Chap. 1) before it is used clinically. After being placed into use, a method may become inaccurate (biased) for many reasons, and it is helpful to monitor and occasionally confirm the method's "operational line." This may be done by plotting the difference between the laboratory's monthly mean and the expected value, for each control material (Grannis, 1977). The difference should, of course, be zero. Accuracy problems sometimes arise owing to the widespread use of secondary serum calibrators for some analytical systems. It may be found that the assigned values for some lots of such calibrators are not consistent with those of other lots. When this occurs, the appropriate calibrator value may be determined by concomitant analysis with the prior lot of calibrator, as well as with CAP Survey Serum or other well-assayed serum products. Method calibration may also be checked for some analytes by dilution of such well-assayed sera with diluents having weighed-in concentrations of analytes (Grannis, 1978). Using this technique the method calibration may be checked for correspondence to peer laboratories that established the mean value of the Survey Serum, as well as for ability to recover known amounts of added analyte. In addition, well-defined reference methodologies are becoming available, and these should be useful in providing a reliable reference base from which to determine appropriate calibrator values.

Changes in method calibration may occur when any part of the analytical system is altered, as, for example, by the replacement of instrument parts or the introduction of new reagents or standards. Whenever these kinds of changes are made they should be documented in a log book and the quality control results must be examined critically for the appearance of method bias. In addition, it is good laboratory practice to determine reference values on a defined population of apparently healthy subjects at least annually (Copeland, 1974).

AN INTEGRATED APPROACH TO QUALITY ASSURANCE

We have presented a variety of quality assurance techniques that are available to laboratories. The extent of usage of these techniques in any one laboratory will depend on the size and scope of that laboratory's services. However, regardless of the actual techniques used, all quality control programs should include a regular critical review of laboratory performance. The laboratory director, quality control coordinator, chief technologist, and section supervisors should meet regularly to evaluate the quality of measurements produced by the laboratory. On a monthly basis this group should have available various indicators of performance such as the statistical summaries of various control specimens, the control charts for those procedures in which significant change has occurred, and records of results obtained in proficiency survey programs. The possible causes of particular problems are discussed and corrective actions proposed. As was illustrated in Figure 63-6, analytical problems cannot always be resolved immediately. First, it must be recognized that a problem exists, then the nature of the problem must be clarified, and finally specific remedial action must be developed. When there are inconsistencies in results on performance using control specimens versus patient specimens, these may be explained on the basis of the obvious differences in the preinstrumental sources of variation for the two types of specimens.

The regular review of quality control data by the senior laboratory staff serves to focus attention on significant laboratory problems and to assure that the problems will be addressed. In the course of such meetings, as the resolution of problems is documented, and various laboratory policies are evolved, a confidence in the quality of the laboratory's performance develops. This confidence, which is based on documented, objective data, is necessary for making the many decisions that must be made in the daily operation of the laboratory. The most critical decisions involve whether to release particular batches of results to the requesting physicians. These decisions are aided by full knowledge of the usual analytical performance of the laboratory. Quality control programs provide the objective data base from which these decisions may be made with confidence. And it is through making the correct decisions that the physician-user is assured of the quality of the laboratory result. It should be emphasized that the laboratorian must be sensitive to feedback from the clinics and wards, i.e., is the laboratory result of the patient's specimen consistent with the clinical findings?

ANALYTICAL GOALS IN CLINICAL CHEMISTRY

From an idealistic viewpoint, quantitative clinical laboratory measurements should be highly accurate and precise. But it is a practical reality that the methods and techniques in common usage have various degrees of analytical bias and variability. Intra- and interlaboratory quality control programs provide a means for assessing the magnitude of bias and variability of various methods and for documenting changes in quality of performance, but they do not indicate whether laboratory results are in fact sufficiently accurate and precise for maximum clinical usefulness. The basic question we will now consider is "How accurate and precise must clinical laboratory measurements be in order to provide the most clinically useful results?"

ACCURACY GOALS

Few workers in the clinical laboratory field have attempted to define goals for analytical accuracy. Rather, mechanisms have evolved that assure that analytical biases will, in the course of time, become minimal. For example, the College of American Pathologists' Survey Program provides an excellent assessment of the relative bias among various methods. Table 63-4 compares the average bias found in calcium analyses by the major methods in use, relative to the atomic absorption procedure. The determination of calcium by atomic absorption spectrophotometry is considered to be a reference method, i.e., a method that is known to be specific for calcium, is believed to provide a good estimate of the true calcium concentration, and is quite easily applied in laboratories that have appropriate instrumentation.

Some samples of the CAP Survey Serum were analyzed for calcium by the National Bureau of Standards, and the consensus mean values obtained by hundreds of laboratories using atomic absorption were found to agree very well with the values obtained by the National Bureau of Standards. Thus, the method comparisons shown in Table 63-4 serve to relate all the methods commonly used by clinical laboratories to a definitive analysis. Similar studies have been made for sodium, potassium, chloride, lithium, magnesium, and iron, with quite similar results (Gilbert, 1978).

As reliable knowledge of the magnitude of analytical bias of various methods becomes known, we may expect the clinical laboratory field to voluntarily adopt such methods that show the least bias and are most cost-effective. Interlaboratory programs provide the data which document these changes in the field and such data provide abundant evidence that inferior methods are readily abandoned as improved methods become available (Gilbert, 1977).

PRECISION GOALS

The question of how precise clinical analyses should be was addressed at a recent conference (Elevitch, 1977). Clinical analyses are used in various medical situations, but the

Table 63–4. ANNUAL SUMMARY OF RANDOM ANALYTICAL VARIABILITY OF CALCIUM ANALYSES*

METHOD/INSTRUMENT		RANDOM ANALYTICAL CV				ANALYTICAL BIAS† (RELATIVE TO MANUAL ATOMIC ABSORPTION) PER CENT VARIATION
		No. Labs	Within Day	Within Lab	Among Labs	
Cresolphthalein	A.A. 2	105	1.2	2.5	3.1	−1.1
Cresolphthalein	12/30	45	1.2	2.7	2.9	−.4
Dupont ACA		273	1.3	3.1	3.6	1.3
Corning Titrator		81	1.9	2.4	3.2	−1.3
Cresolphthalein	A.A. 1	105	1.7	3.2	3.6	1.8
Cresolphthalein	12/60	1,108	1.5	2.5	2.8	−1.2
Atomic Absorption	Manual	216	2.0	3.0	3.8	Comparative Method
Cresolphthalein	Mark X	71	2.0	3.4	3.3	0.0
Cresolphthalein	ABA 100/50	53	2.0	4.6	5.5	−1.4
Cresolphthalein	Other Automat.	256	2.1	4.2	4.6	.8
Methyl Thymol Blue	Manual	93	2.7	4.3	5.2	−2.2
EDTA Titration Other	Manual	249	2.9	4.5	5.6	0.0
Calcein	Oxford	212	2.9	4.9	5.6	−1.7
Calcein, Fluorimetric	Manual	167	3.1	5.2	5.7	−1.5
Cresolphthalein	Manual	722	3.4	5.5	6.2	−1.7
Emission Flame Photometry	Manual	147	3.4	6.6	7.9	−1.4
Other, Not Listed	Manual	103	3.4	5.8	6.7	−2.3
HPE/Monitor	Manual	279	3.4	5.5	5.9	−1.6
Chloranilate Precipitation	Manual	126	3.5	6.2	6.4	−1.2
Calchrome	Oxford	125	3.7	6.1	6.7	−1.4
Clinicard		308	4.1	5.5	5.9	2.1
Cresolphthalein	Mark 17	101	2.2	3.7	3.9	1.3
ALL RESULTS		5,194	2.8	4.3	5.2	−.7

*The data are based on analyses by more than 5000 laboratories of 12 survey specimens that had calcium concentrations ranging from 2.37 to 3.03 mmol/liter. Similar summaries are available for other analytes included in the CAP survey program. Adapted from: Survey Data '75, p. 9, College of American Pathologists, Skokie, Illinois, 1976.

$$†\text{Analytical Bias} = \left(\frac{\text{Result of candidate method} - \text{Result of manual atomic absorption method}}{\text{Result of manual atomic absorption method}} \right) \times 100$$

most precise analyses are required when an individual's present value is to be compared with his prior value and a decision must be made as to whether a real change has occurred. Quite clearly, in this situation the laboratory's analytical variability must be less than the intraindividual physiologic variability. The conference recommended the goal that analytical variance ultimately should not exceed one fourth of the physiologic variance. The magnitude of physiologic variability for many analytes has been determined (see Chap. 2), and consequently the maximum desired analytical variability can be calculated. Table 63-5 compares the average coefficient of variation observed in a recent CAP survey with the coefficient of variation desired for maximum clinical usefulness, and it is apparent that for most analytes the average analytical variation at present is somewhat larger than required for maximum clinical utility, at least when following a patient's results sequentially (Elevitch, 1977).

An alternative approach, used to set performance goals for the analytical variation, is to survey clinicians in terms of asking, "At a defined, narrow concentration range, what do you consider to be the minimum change in the concentration of the analyte which would precipitate a change in your treatment/diagnostic plan?" Barnett (1977), Skendzel (1978), and Elion-Gerritzen (1978) have conducted investigations with practicing physicians to determine what levels of precision are utilized. The results of their studies, combined with the results of the regional quality control values throughout the USA compiled by Ross (1977), Gilbert (1975b), Kurtz, (1977), and Copeland (1978a), yield the major conclusions: that for the most frequently used assays—serum glucose, creatinine, urea, nitrogen, sodium, potassium—the physician's need for precision is easily met by the laboratory; cholesterol and triglyceride measurements meet the requirements, but calcium measurements do not meet the desired precision goals.

Table 63–5. COMPARISON OF AVERAGE COEFFICIENTS OF
VARIATION (CV) OBSERVED IN THE 1975 CAP SURVEY
PROGRAM WITH THE DESIRED ANALYTICAL COEFFICIENT
OF VARIATION

ANALYTE IN SERUM	ANALYTE CONCENTRATION	OBSERVED ANALYTICAL CV	DESIRED ANALYTICAL CV*
Calcium	2.75 mmol/liter	4.2	0.9
Chloride	110 mmol/liter	2.5	1.1
Cholesterol	6.5 mmol/liter	5.9	2.4
Creatinine	180 μmol/liter	11.7	2.2
Glucose	5.5 mmol/liter	5.4	2.2
Phosphate	1.5 mmol/liter	6.6	2.9
Potassium	3.0 mmol/liter	2.8	2.2
Sodium	130 mmol/liter	1.6	0.4
Protein, total	70 g/liter	3.6	1.5
Urea	10 mmol/liter	9.2	6.2
Urate	350 μmol/liter	6.6	3.7

Adapted from Elevitch, F. (ed.): Analytical Goals in Clinical Chemistry. Skokie, Ill. College of American Pathologists, 1977.

*Based on the intra-individual day-to-day physiologic variation; that is, the "desired analytical coefficient of variation" is computed as one-half the mean physiologic coefficient of variation (see Chap. 1).

SUMMARY

Powerful techniques for monitoring, assessing, and improving the quality of quantitative laboratory measurements have been developed and are widely used by clinical laboratories. Through their participation in interlaboratory comparison programs, the laboratories collectively generate a massive data base that provides information about the analytical bias and variability of the various methods that are in common use. With these data individual laboratories and manufacturers of analytical systems may make informed decisions as to which instrument and method they prefer to use. Through their participation the laboratories also collectively create well-assayed sera that are continually renewed and have well-characterized target values for all of the common analytes. These sera have use in aiding the solution of various problems brought to light in intralaboratory quality control programs, and as reference materials for checking the validity of target values assigned to other reference, calibration, or control materials. As intra- and interlaboratory monitoring programs are on-going endeavors, they serve continuously to document development of the clinical laboratory field as it evolves toward the goal of fully reliable laboratory measurements.

REFERENCES

Allen, J. R., Earp, R., Farrell, C. E., and Gruemer, H. D.: Analytical bias in a quality control scheme. Clin. Chem., 15:1039, 1969.

Amador, E.: Quality control by the reference sample method. Am. J. Clin. Pathol., 50:360, 1968.

Barnett, R. N.: Analytical goals in clinical chemistry. Pathologist, 31:319, 1977.

Begtrup, H., Leroy, S., Thyregod, P., and Wallow-Hansen, P.: Average of normals' used as control of accuracy, and a comparison with other controls. Scand. J. Clin. Lab. Invest., 27:247, 1971.

Belk, W. P., and Sunderman, F. W.: A survey on the accuracy of chemical analysis in clinical laboratories. Am. J. Clin. Pathol., 17:854, 1947.

Berry, A. J., Lott, J. A., and Grannis, G. F.: NADH preparations as they affect reliability of serum lactate dehydrogenase determinations. Clin. Chem., 19:1255, 1973.

Bokelund, H., Winkel, P., and Statland, B. E.: Factors contributing to intraindividual variation of serum consitutents: 3. Use of randomized duplicates to evaluate sources of analytic error. Clin. Chem., 20:1507, 1974.

Copeland, B. E., Day, K., Shruhan, C., and Doherty, A.: Long term human reference values in a specific age range: Report of five years' experience. J. Clin. Chem. Clin. Biochem., 5:252, 1974.

Copeland, B. E.: 1978—An evaluation of the state of the art of the precision of clinical chemistry measurements compared with the state of the art of medical decision making. Panel on Laboratory of the Council on Scientific Affairs. Chicago, American Medical Association, 1978a.

Copeland, B. E., Rosvoll, R. V., and Casella, J. M.: Quality control in clinical chemistry, 3rd ed. Chicago, Commission on Continuing Education. American Society of Clinical Pathologists, 1978b.

Dixon, K., and Northam, B. E.: Quality control using the daily mean. Clin. Chim. Acta, 30:453, 1970.

Dorsey, D. B.: The evolution of proficiency testing in the U.S.A., In Proceedings of the Second National Conference on Proficiency Testing. Bethesda, Md., Information Services, 1975.

Elevitch, F. (ed.): Proceedings of the 1976 Aspen Conference on Analytical Goals in Clinical Chemistry. Skokie, Ill., College of American Pathologists, 1977.

Elion-Gerritzen, W. E.: Medical significance of laboratory results in relation to analytical performance. Thesis. Rotterdam, Eramus University, 1978.

Frankel, S., and Ahrlen, R. C.: An evaluation of the number plus method of quality control. Am. J. Clin. Pathol., 37:248, 1967.

Gilbert, R. K.: The perspective (on proficiency testing) of the College of American Pathologists. In Proceedings of the Second National Conference on Proficiency Testing. Bethesda, Md., Information Services, 1975, p. 15.

Gilbert, R. K.: A comparison of participant mean values of duplicate specimens in the CAP chemistry survey program. Am. J. Clin. Pathol., 66:184, 1976.

Gilbert, R. K.: CAP interlaboratory survey data and analytic goals. In Elevitch, F. (ed.): Analytical Goals in Clinical Chemistry. Skokie, Ill., College of American Pathologists, 1977, p. 63.

Gilbert, R. K.: The accuracy of clinical laboratory study by comparison with definitive methods. Am. J. Clin. Pathol., 70:450, 1978.

Gooszen, J. A. H.: The use of control charts in the clinical laboratory. Clin. Chim. Acta, 5:431, 1960.

Grannis, G. F., Gruemer, H. D., Lott, J. A., Edison, J. A., and McCabe, W. C.: Proficiency evaluation of clinical chemistry laboratories. Clin. Chem., 18:222, 1972.

Grannis, G. F.: Studies of the reliability of constituent target values established in a large inter-laboratory survey. Clin. Chem., 22:1035, 1976.

Grannis, G. F., and Caragher, T. E.: Quality control programs in clinical chemistry. CRC Critical Reviews in Clinical Laboratory Sciences, 7:327, 1977.

Grannis, G. F.: Use of survey validated reference materials to establish target values of quality control pools. Pathologist, 32:96, 1978.

Henry, R. J., and Segalove, M.: The running of standards in clinical chemistry and the use of the control chart. J. Clin. Pathol., 5:305, 1952.

Henry, R. J.: Use of the control chart in clinical chemistry. Clin. Chem., 5:309, 1959.

Hoffman, R. G., and Waid, M. E.: The "average of normals" method of quality control. Am. J. Clin. Pathol., 43:134, 1965.

Kilgariff, M., and Owen, J. A.: An assessment of the "average of normals" quality control method. Clin. Chim. Acta, 19:175, 1968.

Kurtz, S., Copeland, B. E., and Straumfjord, J. J.: Guidelines for clinical chemistry quality control based on the long term experience of sixty-one university and tertiary care referral hospitals. Am. J. Clin. Pathol., 68:463, 1977.

Ladenson, J. H.: Patients as their own controls: Use of the computer to identify "laboratory error." Clin. Chem., 21:1648, 1975.

Lawson, N. S., and Haven, G. T.: The role of regional quality control programs in the practice of laboratory medicine in the United States. Am. J. Clin. Pathol., 66:286, 1976.

Levey, S., and Jennings, E. R.: The use of control charts in the clinical laboratory. Am. J. Clin. Pathol., 20:1059, 1950.

Lindberg, D. A., Van Peenen, H. J., and Couch, R.: Patterns in clinical chemistry. Am. J. Clin. Pathol., 44:315, 1965.

Lindberg, D. A., and Van Peenen, H. J.: The meaning of quality control with multiple chemical analysis. In Skeggs, L. T., Jr. (ed.): Automation in Analytical Chemistry. New York, Mediad, 1966, p. 433.

Lott, J. A., Mercier, J. E., and Durham, B. W.: Solution of a vexing problem with the automated alkaline ferricyanide method for glucose. Clin. Chem., 19:670, 1973.

Riddick, J. H., Flora, R., and Van Meter, Q. L.: Computerized prepration of two-way analysis of variance control charts for clinical chemistry. Clin. Chem., 18:250, 1972.

Ross, J. W., and Fraser, M. D.: The effect of analyte and analyte concentration upon precision estimates in clinical chemistry. Am. J. Clin. Pathol., 66:193, 1976.

Sax, S. M., Dorman, L., Lebenson, D. D., and Moore, J. J.: Design and operation of an expanded system of quality control. Clin. Chem., 13:825, 1967.

Shewhart, W. A.: Economic Control of Quality of Manufactured Products. New York, D. Van Nostrand Co., 1931.

Shuey, H. E., and Cebel, J.: Bull. U.S. Army Med. Dept., 9:799, 1949.

Skendzel, L. P.: How physicians use laboratory tests. J.A.M.A., 239:1077, 1978.

Sunderman, F. W., and Boerner, F.: Normal values in clinical medicine. Philadelphia, W. B. Saunders Company, 1949.

Survey Data 1975, R. K. Gilbert (ed.). Skokie, Ill., College of American pathologists, 1976.

Van Peenen, H. J., and Lindberg, D. A. B.: The limitations of laboratory quality control with reference to the "number plus" method. Am. J. Clin. Pathol., 44:322, 1965.

Waid, M. E., and Hoffman, R. G.: The quality control of laboratory precision. Am. J. Clin. Pathol., 25:585, 1955.

Westgaard, J. O., Groth, T., Aronsson, T., and de Verdier, C-H: Combined Shewhart-cusum control chart for improved quality control in clinical chemistry. Clin. Chem., 23:1881, 1977.

Whitehead, T. P.: Quality Control in the Clinical Laboratory. New York, John Wiley and Sons, Inc., 1977.

Whitehurst, P., DiSilvio, T. V., and Boyadjian, G.: Evaluation of discrepancies in patients' results—An aspect of computer-assisted quality control. Clin. Chem., 21:87, 1975.

Winkel, P., and Statland, B. E.: Two novel approaches combined for quality assurance in the routine clinical chemistry laboratory. Clin. Chem., 22:1216, 1976.

Woodard, R. H., and Goldsmith, P. L.: Cumulative Sum Techniques. ICi Monograph No. 3. Edinburgh, Oliver and Boyd, 1964.

Wooton, I. D. P., and King, E. J.: Normal values for blood constituents: Inter-hospital differences. Lancet, 1:470, 1953.

Youden, W. I.: The sample, the procedure and the laboratory. Anal. Chem., 32:23A, 1960.

PHYSIOLOGIC SOLUTIONS, BUFFERS, ACID-BASE INDICATORS, STANDARD REFERENCE MATERIALS, AND TEMPERATURE CONVERSIONS

PHYSIOLOGIC SOLUTIONS

A physiologic solution is one that contains various salts in concentrations that closely approximate the composition of fluids in the human body. The simplest of these is physiologic saline, which has the same osmotic pressure as the blood. There are more elaborate solutions, for example, to maintain tissues in a metabolically active state for longer periods of time. The table below gives formulas of solutions that are isotonic with respect to blood.

PHYSIOLOGIC SOLUTIONS

	SALINE	LOCKE'S SOLUTION	RINGER'S* SOLUTION	TYRODE'S SOLUTION
Sodium chloride	0.85 g	0.9 g	0.7 g	0.8 g
Calcium chloride		0.024 g	0.0026 g	0.02 g
Potassium chloride		0.042 g	0.035 g	0.02 g
Sodium bicarbonate		0.01–0.03 g		0.1 g
D-Glucose		0.1–0.25 g		0.1 g
Magnesium chloride				0.01 g
Monosodium phosphate				0.005 g
Distilled water	100 ml	100 ml	100 ml	100 ml

*Porter modification.

BUFFERS†

Buffers have the ability to resist changes in pH. Buffers usually consist of a weak acid and its salt or a weak base and its salt. The Henderson-Hasselbalch equation is useful in calculating the acid (or base) to salt ratio required to

---

†For a comprehensive discussion, including preparation of buffer solutions of a definite ionic strength, consult Roger G. Bates, Determination of pH—Theory and Practice, 2nd ed. New York, John Wiley & Sons, Inc., 1973.

establish a desired pH from a buffer system. For example, if 1 liter of 0.1 M acetic acid buffer (total molarity of acetate ion plus acetic acid) at pH 4.90 is desired, use the expression

(1) $pH = pK + \log \dfrac{[A^-]}{[HA]}$ (Henderson-Hasselbalch equation)

Substituting for pH = 4.90 and pK = 4.76 (for acetic acid),

(2) $4.90 = 4.76 + \log \dfrac{[acetate]}{[acetic\ acid]}$,

(3) $\log \dfrac{[acetate]}{[acetic\ acid]} = 0.14$,

(4) $\dfrac{[acetate]}{[acetic\ acid]} = 1.38$.

(5) $[acetate] + [acetic\ acid] = 0.1\ M$

(6)   and $\dfrac{[acetate]}{[acetic\ acid]} = 1.38$

(7)   or $[acetate] = 1.38\ [acetic\ acid]$

(8) $1.38\ [acetic\ acid] + [acetic\ acid] = 0.1\ M$

(9) $[acetic\ acid] = 0.042\ M = 2.52\ g$ acetic acid/liter

(10) $[acetate] = 0.058\ M = 4.76\ g$ sodium acetate/liter

Similarly, if 648 ml of 0.025 molar diethylbarbituric acid and 10 ml of 0.5 molar sodium diethylbarbiturate are mixed and diluted to 1 liter, the approximate pH of the solution is calculated, knowing that the pK for diethylbarbituric acid = 7.98.

(1)   Molar concentration $= \dfrac{moles}{liter}$

(2) $liters \left(\dfrac{moles}{liter}\right) = moles$

For diethylbarbituric acid

(3) $(0.648)(0.025) = 0.0162$ mole

(4)   which diluted to 1 liter $= 0.0162$ mole/liter

For sodium diethylbarbiturate

(5) $(0.010)(0.5) = 0.005$ mole

(6)   which, diluted to 1 liter $= 0.005$ mole/liter

(7) $pH = pK + \log \dfrac{[salt]}{[acid]} = pK - \log \dfrac{[acid]}{[salt]}$

(8) $= 7.98 - \log \dfrac{0.0162}{0.005}$

(9) $= 7.98 - \log 3.24$

(10) $= 7.98 - 0.51$

(11) $\therefore pH = 7.47$

The maximum buffering capacity is at the pK value of the weak acid or base. For instance, for acetic acid with a pH value of 4.76, more acid will be required to change the pH of an acetate buffer from 4.76 to 4.66 than from 4.20 to 4.10. Efficient buffering capacity covers a pH range of about 1 unit on either side of the pK value of the weak acid or base. For acetic acid, this would be from about pH 3.8 to 5.8.

SORENSEN'S PHOSPHATE BUFFERS

These buffer solutions are generally useful, since the range of the mixtures is from pH 5 to 8.

Fifteenth Molar Monobasic Potassium Phosphate Solution (KH_2PO_4). Weigh 9.0727 g of monobasic potassium phosphate. Dissolve it in distilled water and dilute to exactly 1 liter with distilled water. The solution must be absolutely clear and should yield no test for chloride or sulfates. Phosphate salt solutions should be kept in the refrigerator.

Fifteenth Molar Dibasic Sodium Phosphate Solution (Na_2HPO_4). Expose dibasic sodium phosphate containing 12 moles of water of crystallization to ordinary atmosphere for two weeks. It should then contain 2 moles of water of crystallization. Dissolve 11.867 g of disodium phosphate duohydrate in distilled water and dilute to exactly 1 liter with distilled water. The solution must be absolutely clear and should yield no test for chloride or sulfates.

SORENSEN'S TABLE OF BUFFER MIXTURES

Na_2HPO_4 SOLUTION (ml)	KH_2PO_4 SOLUTION (ml)	pH
0.25	9.75	5.288
0.5	9.5	5.589
1.0	9.0	5.906
2.0	8.0	6.239
3.0	7.0	6.468
4.0	6.0	6.643
5.0	5.0	6.813
6.0	4.0	6.979
7.0	3.0	7.168
8.0	2.0	7.381
9.0	1.0	7.731
9.5	0.5	8.043

TRIS(HYDROXYMETHYL)AMINOMETHANE BUFFER[*]

Tris(hydroxymethyl)aminomethane buffer can be used for a pH range between 7.0 and 9.0, but its best buffer capacity is between 7.5 and 8.5. It is practically ineffective below pH 7.0 and above pH 9.0. One advantage of the buffer is its excellent stability. The buffer can be prepared by weighing the desired amount of tris(hydroxymethyl)aminomethane, dissolving it in water and adjusting the pH to the desired value with HCl. For example, if 100 ml of 0.05 M buffer is desired, place 0.6057 g of tris(hydroxymethyl)aminomethane into a 100 ml volumetric flask. This is dissolved in approximately 50 ml of distilled water. Add 0.1 N HCl, as indicated in the table, and fill up to the mark with distilled water. The table shows the pH values obtained when 0.6057 g of tris(hydroxymethyl)aminomethane dissolved in water is mixed with the indicated amounts of 0.1 N HCl and diluted to 100 ml.

ACID-BASE INDICATORS[†]

An acid-base indicator is a weak acid or a weak base, the undissociated form of which has a color and constitution other than the iogenic form. Color change takes place over a certain narrow range of hydrogen ion concentrations. This range is called the color change interval and is expressed in terms of pH (the negative logarithm of the hydrogen ion concentration). A great number of

---

[*] If buffers of a higher molarity are desired, the 0.1 N HCl may have to be replaced by a 1.0 N HCl.

[†] Based on Lange, N. A.: Handbook of Chemistry. Revised 11th ed. New York, McGraw-Hill Book Company, Inc., 1973.

ML 0.1 N HCl ADDED	RESULTING pH AT 23°C.	RESULTING pH AT 37°C.
5.0	9.10	8.95
7.5	8.92	8.78
10.0	8.74	8.60
12.5	8.62	8.48
15.0	8.50	8.37
17.5	8.40	8.27
20.0	8.32	8.18
22.5	8.23	8.10
25.0	8.14	8.00
27.5	8.05	7.90
30.0	7.96	7.82
32.5	7.87	7.73
35.0	7.77	7.63
37.5	7.66	7.52
40.0	7.54	7.40
42.5	7.36	7.22
45.0	7.20	7.05

ACID-BASE INDICATORS

INDICATOR	pH RANGE	QUANTITY OF INDICATOR PER 10 ML	COLOR Acid	Alkaline
Thymol blue (A)*†	1.2–2.8	1–2 drops 0.1% soln. in aq.	red	yellow
Methyl orange (B)	3.1–4.4	1 drop 0.1% soln. in aq.	red	orange
Bromphenol blue (A)†	3.0–4.6	1 drop 0.1% soln. in aq.	yellow	blue-violet
Bromcresol green (A)†	4.0–5.6	1 drop 0.1% soln. in aq.	yellow	blue
Methyl red (A)†	4.4–6.2	1 drop 0.1% soln. in aq.	red	yellow
Bromcresol purple (A)†	5.2–6.8	1 drop 0.1% soln. in aq.	yellow	purple
Bromthymol blue (A)†	6.2–7.6	1 drop 0.1% soln. in aq.	yellow	blue
Phenol red (A)†	6.4–8.0	1 drop 0.1% soln. in aq.	yellow	red
Neutral red (B)	6.8–8.0	1 drop 0.1% soln. in 70% alc.	red	yellow
Thymol blue (A)†‡	8.0–9.6	1–5 drops 0.1% soln. in aq.	yellow	blue
Phenolphthalein (A)	8.0–10.0	1–5 drops 0.1% soln. in 70% alc.	colorless	red
Thymolphthalein (A)	9.4–10.6	1 drop 0.1% soln. in 90% alc.	colorless	blue

The letters A or B following the name of the indicator signify, respectively, that the compound is an indicator *acid* or *base*.
* For the acid range.
† Sodium salt.
‡ For the alkaline range.

COMMONLY USED ACIDS AND ALKALIES*

SOLUTION	MOL. WEIGHT	SPEC. GRAVITY†	GM. PER LITER†	MOLARITY†	NORMALITY†	APPROX. NUMBER OF ML REQUIRED TO MAKE 1000 ML OF 1 N SOLUTION
Conc. HCl	36.46	1.19	440	12	12	83
Conc. H_2SO_4	98.08	1.84	1730	18	36	28
Conc. HNO_3	63.02	1.42	990	16	16	64
Conc. lactic acid	90.08	1.21	1030	11	11	87
Glacial acetic acid	60.08	1.06	1060	17.5	17.5	57
Conc. NH_4OH	35.05	0.90	250	15	15	67

* Commercially available.
† Figures may vary slightly according to the lot or manufacturer.

STANDARD REFERENCE MATERIALS FOR CLINICAL MEASUREMENTS*†

SRM NO.	NAME	PURITY (%)	PROPERTY CERTIFIED	AMOUNT (gm.)	DATE ISSUED
40h	Sodium oxalate	99.95	Reductometric standard	60	April 24, 1969
83c	Arsenic trioxide	99.99	Reductometric standard	75	April 16, 1970
84h	Acid potassium phthalate	99.993	Acidimetric standard	60	July 9, 1969
136c	Potassium dichromate	99.98	Oxidation standard	60	March 24, 1970
186Ic	Potassium dihydrogen phosphate	99.9	pH	30	Sept. 1, 1970
186IIc	Disodium hydrogen phosphate	99.9	pH	30	Sept. 1, 1970
350	Benzoic acid	99.98	Acidimetric standard	30	April 15, 1958
911a	Cholesterol	99.4	Identity and purity	2.0	June 6, 1974
912	Urea	99.7	Identity and purity	25	Sept. 24, 1968
913	Uric acid	99.7	Identity and purity	10	Sept. 24, 1968
914	Creatinine	99.8	Identity and purity	10	Sept. 24, 1968
915	Calcium carbonate	99.9	Identity and purity	20	March 4, 1969
916	Bilirubin	99	Identity and purity	0.1	March 10, 1971
917	D-Glucose	99.9	Identity and purity	25	Nov. 18, 1970
918	Potassium chloride	99.9	Identity and purity	20	Jan. 22, 1971
922	tris(Hydroxymethyl)amino-methane	99.9	pH	25	Dec. 13, 1973
923	tris(Hydroxymethyl)amino-methane hydrochloride	99.7	pH	35	Dec. 13, 1973
930b	Glass filters for spectrophotom-etry		Absorbance	3 filters	Feb. 24, 1975
933	Clinical laboratory thermometers		Temperature	Set of 3	August 23, 1974
937	Iron metal	99.9		50	Summer, 1978
1571	Orchard leaves		Major and trace constituents	75	Oct. 1, 1971
2201	NaCl	99.9	pNa pCl	120	Feb. 22, 1971
2202	KCl	99.9	pK pCl	160	Feb. 22, 1971

*Orders and requests for information about these SRM's should be directed to the Office of Standard Reference Materials, Institute for Materials Research, National Bureau of Standards, Washington, D.C. 20234.
†NBS Spec. Publ. 260, Catalog of NBS Standard Reference Materials, 1975-1976 edition.

substances show indicator properties, although relatively few of them are practically applied for neutralization reactions and pH determinations. In general, weak acids should be titrated in the presence of indicators that change in slightly alkaline solutions. Weak bases should be titrated in the presence of indicators that change in slightly acid solutions.

The availability of precision pH meters allows titration to a selected end-point (pH) and may replace use of indicators for several applications.

TEMPERATURE CONVERSIONS

CENTIGRADE	FAHRENHEIT	CENTIGRADE	FAHRENHEIT
110°	230°	42°	107.6°
100	212	41	105.8
95	203	40.5	104.9
90	194	40	104
85	185	39.5	103.1
80	176	39	102.2
75	167	38.5	101.3
70	158	38	100.4
65	149	37.5	99.5
60	140	37	98.6
55	131	36.5	97.7
50	122	36	96.8
45	113	35.5	95.9
44	111.2	35	95
43	109.4	34	93.2

6

TEMPERATURE CONVERSIONS (*Continued*)

CENTIGRADE		FAHRENHEIT	CENTIGRADE		FAHRENHEIT
33°	....	91.4°	10°	....	50°
32	....	89.6	+5	....	41
31	....	87.8	0	....	32
30	....	86	−5	....	23
25	....	77	−10	....	14
20	....	68	−15	....	+5
15	....	59	−20	....	−4

$$0.54°C \quad = \quad 1°F$$
$$1°C \quad = \quad 1.8°F$$

To convert Fahrenheit into Centigrade, subtract 32 and multiply by 0.555.
To convert Centigrade into Fahrenheit, multiply by 1.8 and add 32.

REFERENCES

Lange, N. A., and Dean, I. A. (eds.): Handbook of Chemistry, 11th ed. New York, McGraw-Hill Book Company, 1973.

Long, C. (ed.): Biochemists' Handbook. Princeton, N.J., D. Van Nostrand Co., Inc., 1961.

Meinke, W. W.: Standard Reference Materials for Clinical Measurements. Anal. Chem., *43*:31A, 1971.

The Merck Index; an Encyclopedia of Chemicals and Drugs, 9th ed. Rahway, N.J., Merck & Co., Inc., 1976.

APPENDIX 2
DESIRABLE WEIGHTS AND BODY SURFACE AREA

DESIRABLE WEIGHTS FOR MEN AND WOMEN*
According to Height and Frame. Ages 25 and Over

HEIGHT (IN SHOES)	WEIGHT IN POUNDS (IN INDOOR CLOTHING)		
	Small Frame	Medium Frame	Large Frame
	MEN		
5' 2"	112–120	118–129	126–141
3"	115–123	121–133	129–144
4"	118–126	124–136	132–148
5"	121–129	127–139	135–152
6"	124–133	130–143	138–156
7"	128–137	134–147	142–161
8"	132–141	138–152	147–166
9"	136–145	142–156	151–170
10"	140–150	146–160	155–174
11"	144–154	150–165	159–179
6' 0"	148–158	154–170	164–184
1"	152–162	158–175	168–189
2"	156–167	162–180	173–194
3"	160–171	167–185	178–199
4"	164–175	172–190	182–204
	WOMEN		
4' 10"	92– 98	96–107	104–119
11"	94–101	98–110	106–122
5' 0"	96–104	101–113	109–125
1"	99–107	104–116	112–128
2"	102–110	107–119	115–131
3"	105–113	110–122	118–134
4"	108–116	113–126	121–138
5"	111–119	116–130	125–142
6"	114–123	120–135	129–146
7"	118–127	124–139	133–150
8"	122–131	128–143	137–154
9"	126–135	132–147	141–158
10"	130–140	136–151	145–163
11"	134–144	140–155	149–168
6' 0"	138–148	144–159	153–173

*Prepared by the Metropolitan Life Insurance Company. Derived primarily from data of the *Build and Blood Pressure Study, 1959*, Society of Actuaries. Reproduced with permission.

6

NOMOGRAM FOR THE DETERMINATION OF BODY
SURFACE AREA OF CHILDREN AND ADULTS*

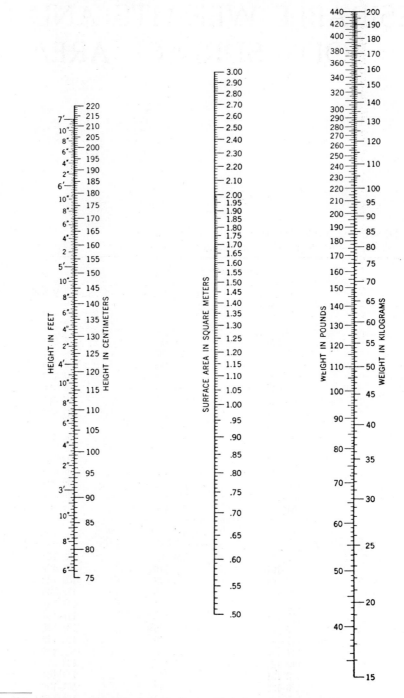

*From Boothby, W. M., and Sandiford, R. B.: Boston Med. Surg. J., *185*:337, 1921.

NOMOGRAM FOR THE DETERMINATION OF
BODY SURFACE AREA OF CHILDREN*

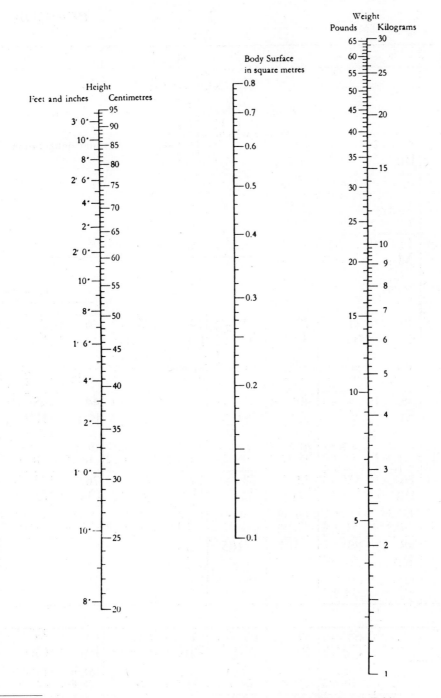

---

*From DuBois, E. F.: Basal Metabolism in Health and Disease. Philadelphia, Lea & Febiger, 1936.

APPENDIX 3

PERIODIC TABLE

KEY TO CHART

Atomic Number → **50** +2
Symbol → **Sn** +4 ← Oxidation States
Atomic Weight → 118.69
−18−18−4 ← Electron Configuration

Transition Elements — Group 8

1a	2a	3b	4b	5b	6b	7b	8		
1 H +1 −1 1.0080 1									
3 Li +1 6.94_1 2−1	**4** Be +2 9.01218 2−2								
11 Na +1 22.9898 2−8−1	**12** Mg +2 24.305 2−8−2								
19 K +1 39.102 −8−8−1	**20** Ca +2 40.08 −8−8−2	**21** Sc +3 44.9559 −8−9−2	**22** Ti +2,+3,+4 47.90 8−10−2	**23** V +2,+3,+4,+5 50.941_4 −8−11−2	**24** Cr +2,+3,+6 51.996 −8−13−1	**25** Mn +2,+3,+4,+7 54.9380 −8−13−2	**26** Fe +2,+3 55.847 −8−14 2	**27** Co +2,+3 58.9332 8−15−2	**28** Ni +2,+3 58.71 −8−16−2
37 Rb +1 85.467_8 −18−8−1	**38** Sr +2 87.62 −18−8−2	**39** Y +3 88.9059 18−9−2	**40** Zr +4 91.22 −18−10−2	**41** Nb +3,+5 92.9064 −18−12−1	**42** Mo +6 95.94 −18−13−1	**43** Tc +4,+6,+7 98.9062 −18−13−2	**44** Ru +3 101.07 −18−15−1	**45** Rh +3 102.9055 −18−16−1	**46** Pd +2,+4 106.4 −18−18−0
55 Cs +1 132.9055 −18−8−1	**56** Ba +2 137.34 −18−8−2	**57*** La +3 138.9055 −18−9−2	**72** Hf +4 178.49 −32−10−2	**73** Ta +5 180.947_9 −32−11−2	**74** W +6 183.85 −32−12−2	**75** Re +4,+6,+7 186.2 −32−13−2	**76** Os +3,+4 190.2 −32−14−2	**77** Ir +3,+4 192.22 −32−15−2	**78** Pt +2,+4 195.09 −32−16−2
87 Fr +1 (223) −18−8−1	**88** Ra +2 (226) −18−8−2	**89**** Ac +3 (227) −18−9−2	**104** — −32−10−2	**105** —					

*Lanthanides

58 Ce +3,+4 140.12 −20−8−2	**59** Pr +3 140.9077 −21−8−2	**60** Nd +3 144.24 −22−8−2	**61** Pm +3 (145) −23−8−2	**62** Sm +2,+3 150.4 −24−8−2	**63** Eu +2,+3 151.96 −25−8−2	**64** Gd +3 157.25 −25−9−2	**65** Tb +3 158.9254 −27−8−2

**Actinides

90 Th +4 232.0381 −18−10−2	**91** Pa +5,+4 231.0359 −20−9−2	**92** U +3,+4,+5,+6 238.029 −21−9−2	**93** Np +3,+4,+5,+6 237.0482 −22−9−2	**94** Pu +3,+4,+5,+6 (244) −24−8−2	**95** Am +3,+4,+5,+6 (243) −25−8−2	**96** Cm +3 (247) −25−9−2	**97** Bk +3,+4 (247) −27−8−2

Numbers in parentheses are mass numbers of most stable isotope of that element.

From Weast, R. C. (ed.): Handbook of Chemistry and Physics. 54th ed. Cleveland, Ohio, Chemical Rubber Co., 1973-1974.

OF THE ELEMENTS

1b	2b	3a	4a	5a	6a	7a	0	Orbit
							2 0 He 4.00260 2	– K
		5 +3 B 10.81 2-3	**6** +2 C +4 −4 12.011 2-4	**7** +1 N +2 +3 +4 +5 −1 14.0067 −2 2-5 −3	**8** −2 O 15.9994 2-6	**9** −1 F 18.9984 2-7	**10** 0 Ne 20.17₉ 2-8	– K–L
Transition Elements		**13** +3 Al 26.9815 2-8-3	**14** +2 Si +4 −4 28.086 2-8-4	**15** +3 P +5 −3 30.9738 2-8-5	**16** +4 S +6 −2 32.06 2-8-6	**17** +1 Cl +5 +7 −1 35.453 2-8-7	**18** 0 Ar 39.948 2-8-8	–K–L–M
29 +1 Cu +2 63.546 −8–18–1	**30** +2 Zn 65.38 −8–18–2	**31** +3 Ga 69.72 −8–18–3	**32** +2 Ge +4 72.59 −8–18–4	**33** +3 As +5 −3 74.9216 −8–18–5	**34** +4 Se +6 −2 78.96 −8–18–6	**35** +1 Br +5 −1 79.904 −8–18–7	**36** 0 Kr 83.80 −8–18–8	–L–M–N
47 +1 Ag 107.868 −18–18–1	**48** +2 Cd 112.40 −18–18–2	**49** +3 In 114.82 −18–18–3	**50** +2 Sn +4 118.69 −18–18–4	**51** +3 Sb +5 −3 121.75 −18–18–5	**52** +4 Te +6 −2 127.60 −18–18–6	**53** +1 I +5 +7 −1 126.9045 −18–18–7	**54** 0 Xe 131.30 −18–18–8	–M–N–O
79 +1 Au +3 196.9665 −32–18–1	**80** +1 Hg +2 200.59 −32–18–2	**81** +1 Tl +3 204.37 −32–18–3	**82** +2 Pb +4 207.2 −32–18–4	**83** +3 Bi +5 208.9806 −32–18–5	**84** +2 Po +4 (209) −32–18–6	**85** At (210) −32–18–7	**86** 0 Rn (222) −32–18–8	–N–O–P
								–O–P–Q

						Orbit
66 +3 Dy 162.50 −28–8–2	**67** +3 Ho 164.9303 −29–8–2	**68** +3 Er 167.26 −30–8–2	**69** +3 Tm 168.9342 −31–8–2	**70** +2 Yb +3 173.04 −32–8–2	**71** +3 Lu 174.97 −32–9–2	–N–O–P
98 +3 Cf (251) −28–8–2	**99** Es (254) −29–8–2	**100** Fm (257) −30–8–2	**101** Md (256) −31–8–2	**102** No (254) −32–8–2	**103** Lr −32–9–2	–O–P–Q

PERIODIC TABLE OF THE ELEMENTS

6

SEQUENCE OF CHEMICAL ANALYSIS OF CALCULI

CHEMICAL GROUP	REAGENTS AND TREATMENT	POSITIVE RESULTS AND INTERPRETATIONS
1. Carbonates	Relatively large sample of pulverized stone in test tube. 10-15 drops 10% HCl.	Foaming effervescence

CO_2 is displaced by HCl from the carbonates.

$$Na_2CO_3 + 2HCl \longrightarrow 2NaCl + H_2CO_3 \longrightarrow H_2O + CO_2\uparrow$$

If carbonates present, allow effervescence to cease. Save most of the supernatant for determinations 5, 6, and 7. Either pour off or take off the acid extract in an aspirating pipette, the tip of which has been lightly plugged with cotton. Remove the cotton by seizing the projecting wisp and divide the "filtrate" into three aliquots for 5, 6, and 7. The original test tube containing the pulverized stone and a few drops of HCl is then used for determination 2.

2. Oxalates	Test tube from determination 1. Add a pinch of MnO_2; do not mix or shake the tube. It may be necessary to warm the contents of the tube very slightly to obtain reaction of trace quantities.	Effervescence or tiny bubbles of CO_2 popping upward from the sediment of the tube.

MnO_2 acts as an oxidizing agent in the production of CO_2.
$$2CaC_2O_4 + 2HCl + MnO_2 \longrightarrow 2CaCO_3 + MnCl_2 + CO_2\uparrow$$

3. Phosphates	Pulverized stone in test tube. 1 drop 10% HCl 2 drops $H_2SO_4^-$ molybdate reagent 1 drop amino-naphtholsulfonic acid	Blue color develops. If present in trace quantities, this occurs upon standing in a few minutes.

The blue color is due to reduced oxides of molybdenum.

4. Urates and uric acid	Pulverized stone in test tube. 1 drop 20% Na_2CO_3 2 drops uric acid reagent	Prompt *deep* blue color. Pale blue color is negative.

Uric acid reduces orthophosphoric acid, producing a blue color.

5. Calcium	Acid extract on microscopic slide. 2-3 drops saturated $(NH_4)_2C_2O_4$	White precipitate or film. The film reaction is most noticeable if slide is held over a dark background.

Calcium ions in the presence of ammonium oxalate produce a white precipitate of calcium oxalate.

6. Magnesium	Acid extract in test tube 2-3 drops 20% NaOH 2-3 drops "Mg" reagent	Reddish purple reagent slowly becomes a definite (corn-flower) blue and precipitate forms.

By rendering the acid extract alkaline, $Mg(OH)_3$ is formed. The azo dye is absorbed by the $Mg(OH)_3$ in alkaline solution. The sensitivity is very dependent upon the OH-ion concentration.

7. NH_4 group	Acid extract in test tube 2-3 drops 20% NaOH 2-3 drops Nessler's reagent	Orange-brown (rusty) precipitate. Positive test differentiates NH_4-urates from uric acid. Positive test indicates triple phosphates vs. Ca or Mg phosphates.

Ammonia, produced from the NH_4 group in alkaline solution reacts with the double iodide in Nessler's reagent to form dimercuric ammonium iodide (the orange-brown precipitate)

8. Cystine	Pulverized stone in test tube 1 drop 10% NH_4OH 1 drop 5% NaCN (wait 5 min.) 2-3 drops sodium nitroprusside solution	*Beet-red* color is a positive reaction which may fade to orange-red upon standing.

Nitroprusside reaction: Proteins with a free SH (cysteine) group yield a reddish color with sodium nitroprusside in an ammoniacal solution. The cystine -S-S- groups in protein may be reduced to -SH groups by reducing agents such as NaCN, after which they give the nitroprusside reaction.

SEQUENCE OF CHEMICAL ANALYSIS OF CALCULI (*Continued*)

RARE STONES	REAGENTS AND TREATMENT	POSITIVE RESULTS AND INTERPRETATIONS
1. Sulfonamides	Pulverized stone in test tube 2 drops 10% HCl (wait 30 min.) 2 drops 0.1% $NaNO_2$ (wait 30-60 min.) 2 drops 0.5% NH_4-sulfamate 2-3 drops sulfa dye reagent	Magenta color is a positive reaction.

The presence of any sulfonamide derivative is determined by the diazotization of a free amino group. Excess $NaNO_2$ is destroyed by ammonium sulfamate and the purplish red azo dye is formed by the coupling of the diazotized sulfanilamide with N-(1-naphthyl) ethylenediamine dihydrochloride.

2. Cholesterol	Pulverized stone in test tube. Add 1 ml chloroform, mix, heat over steam bath. Allow to stand until the insoluble material settles out. Decant into test tube. To this add 3 drops acetic anhydride and 1 drop concentrated H_2SO_4.	Test solution becomes red, then blue, and finally blue-green in color.

Liebermann-Burchard reaction: Transient colors are probably due to halochromic salts of either the unsaturated sterol or a product of it further dehydrated.

3. Xanthine	Xanthine is difficult to separate from uric acid, so that the x-ray diffraction method is probably better for identification. Pulverized stone in evaporating dish, add 2 drops concentrated HNO_3, and evaporate to complete dryness over steam bath. Cool slightly. Add 1 drop 20% NaOH. Warm again.	Residue left after evaporation is yellow. After addition of NaOH, an orange color develops, which becomes red upon warming.

Xanthoproteic reaction: This is due to the nitration of the phenyl rings present in tyrosine, phenylalanine, and tryptophane to give yellow nitro substitution products, which become orange upon the addition of alkali (salt formation).

In doing the qualitative test for xanthine, colored reactions will also be obtained from uric acid. The dried residue after evaporation is lemon yellow with xanthine, but is orange with uric acid. After addition of NaOH, an orange color develops, becoming red with warming when xanthine is present; if uric acid is present, a cherry red to purple color develops immediately after addition of NaOH.

6

% TRANSMISSION–ABSORBANCE CONVERSION CHART*

% T	A	% T	A	% T	A	% T	A
1	2.000	1.5	1.824	51	.2924	51.5	.2882
2	1.699	2.5	1.602	52	.2840	52.5	.2798
3	1.523	3.5	1.456	53	.2756	53.5	.2716
4	1.398	4.5	1.347	54	.2676	54.5	.2636
5	1.301	5.5	1.260	55	.2596	55.5	.2557
6	1.222	6.5	1.187	56	.2518	56.5	.2480
7	1.155	7.5	1.126	57	.2441	57.5	.2403
8	1.097	8.5	1.071	58	.2366	58.5	.2328
9	1.046	9.5	1.022	59	.2291	59.5	.2255
10	1.000	10.5	.979	60	.2218	60.5	.2182
11	.959	11.5	.939	61	.2147	61.5	.2111
12	.921	12.5	.903	62	.2076	62.5	.2041
13	.886	13.5	.870	63	.2007	63.5	.1973
14	.854	14.5	.838	64	.1939	64.5	.1905
15	.824	15.5	.810	65	.1871	65.5	.1838
16	.796	16.5	.782	66	.1805	66.5	.1772
17	.770	17.5	.757	67	.1739	67.5	.1707
18	.745	18.5	.733	68	.1675	68.5	.1643
19	.721	19.5	.710	69	.1612	69.5	.1580
20	.699	20.5	.688	70	.1549	70.5	.1518
21	.678	21.5	.668	71	.1487	71.5	.1457
22	.658	22.5	.648	72	.1427	72.5	.1397
23	.638	23.5	.629	73	.1367	73.5	.1337
24	.620	24.5	.611	74	.1308	74.5	.1278
25	.602	25.5	.594	75	.1249	75.5	.1221
26	.585	26.5	.577	76	.1192	76.5	.1163
27	.569	27.5	.561	77	.1135	77.5	.1107
28	.553	28.5	.545	78	.1079	78.5	.1051
29	.538	29.5	.530	79	.1024	79.5	.0996
30	.523	30.5	.516	80	.0969	80.5	.0942
31	.509	31.5	.502	81	.0915	81.5	.0888
32	.495	32.5	.488	82	.0862	82.5	.0835
33	.482	33.5	.475	83	.0809	83.5	.0783
34	.469	34.5	.462	84	.0757	84.5	.0731
35	.456	35.5	.450	85	.0706	85.5	.0680
36	.444	36.5	.438	86	.0655	86.5	.0630
37	.432	37.5	.426	87	.0605	87.5	.0580
38	.420	38.5	.414	88	.0555	88.5	.0531
39	.409	39.5	.403	89	.0505	89.5	.0482
40	.398	40.5	.392	90	.0458	90.5	.0434
41	.387	41.5	.382	91	.0410	91.5	.0386
42	.377	42.5	.372	92	.0362	92.5	.0339
43	.367	43.5	.362	93	.0315	93.5	.0292
44	.357	44.5	.352	94	.0269	94.5	.0246
45	.347	45.5	.342	95	.0223	95.5	.0200
46	.337	46.5	.332	96	.0177	96.5	.0155
47	.328	47.5	.323	97	.0132	97.5	.0110
48	.319	48.5	.314	98	.0088	98.5	.0066
49	.310	49.5	.305	99	.0044	99.5	.0022
50	.301	50.5	.297	100	.0000		

*From Tietz, N. W.: Fundamentals of Clinical Chemistry. Philadelphia, W. B. Saunders Company, 1976.

APPENDIX 4

*John Bernard Henry, M.D., and
H. Peter Lehmann, Ph.D.*

SI UNITS

Recommendations for the standardized presentation of clinical laboratory data based on SI units were proposed by the Commission on Clinical Chemistry of the International Union of Pure and Applied Chemistry and the International Federation of Clinical Chemistry in 1967 (Dybkaer and Jørgensen, 1967). Revisions of the original recommendations were published as final proposals, Recommendations 1973, in 1974 (International Union of Pure and Applied Chemistry, 1974). Support for these proposals came from the International Committee for Standardization in Hematology and the World Association of (Anatomic and Clinical) Pathology Societies, in addition to the International Federation of Clinical Chemistry, who agreed to recommend to all concerned with health services throughout the world that, with regard to units of measurements for medical laboratory results, the International System of Units (SI) be accepted in its broad application (International Committee for Standardization in Hematology et al., 1973). The World Health Organization at the 30th World Health Assembly in 1977 recommended the adoption of the SI by the entire scientific community, and particularly the medical community throughout the world (World Health Organization, 1977). Thus, it is apparent that there is a movement toward the use of SI units in medicine and, therefore, that the system will be universally adopted over the next few years for reporting clinical laboratory data. The feasibility of rigid adoption of the SI to all clinical laboratory measurements has been discussed in a number of editorials (Beeler, 1973 and 1976; Conn, 1977; Copeland, 1976; Editorial, British Medical Journal, 1974; Ingelfinger, 1975) and articles (Baron et al., 1974; Dybkaer, 1967; Lehmann, 1976; Young, 1974 and 1975; Council on Scientific Affairs, 1978) in the medical literature.

The SI consists of 7 base units which are dimensionally independent. The base units are listed in Table 1, along with the symbols to be used to denote these quantities. Table 2 lists derived units of the SI that are used in the clinical laboratory. There are two kinds of derived units: coherent units, which are derived directly from the base units without the use of conversion factors, and non-coherent units, which are constructed from the base units and contain a numerical factor in order to make the numbers more convenient to use. The approved prefixes to denote fractions or multiples of basic and derived SI units are given in Table 3.

In making the conversion to SI units (Tables 4 to 12), the following guidelines were followed, based on the editorial policy of the American Journal of Clinical Pathology, whose guidelines were used for conversion to SI units throughout this book (see Chapter 1).

1. All normal ranges or reference intervals have been converted to SI units except in cases where the measurements are not quantitative.

Table 1 BASIC UNITS

QUANTITY	NAME	SYMBOL
Amount of substance	mole	mol
Mass	kilogram	kg
Length	meter	m
Time	second	s
Thermodynamic temperature	kelvin	K
Electric current	ampere	A
Luminous intensity	candela	cd

2. Chemical names have not been changed; e.g., urea is retained instead of changing to carbamide.

3. Factors were calculated on the basis of relative masses for atoms corrected to conform to the 1967 (amended 1973) values of the Commission on Atomic Weights of the International Union of Pure and Applied Chemistry.

4. Factors were calculated to the base unit for volume of one liter in accordance with Recommendation 1973.

5. The orders of magnitude of the factors were calculated to make the normal values in SI units convenient numbers, i.e., with prefixes, a number not greater than 1000 or smaller than 0.001.

6. The number "in SI Units" is equal to the number "in Conventional Units" times the "Factor."

7. For compounds where relative molecular masses are not definitely known, e.g., proteins, normal ranges or reference intervals are converted to mass amounts per liter.

8. For mixtures of indeterminate composition, e.g., 17-ketosteroids, reference intervals are converted to mass amounts per liter.

9. Quantities of a relative nature which are usually expressed as percentages, e.g., fractions of LDH isoenzymes, are given as fractions of the total.

10. Enzyme units are given as the International Unit per liter (U/l). Although the coherent SI unit for catalysts (including enzymes), the katal, has been defined as the number of moles of substrate converted per second under defined conditions, it has not yet been adopted for use with the SI.

11. The pH scale is retained for measurement of hydrogen ion concentrations.

12. The milliosmole per liter (mOsm/l) is retained for osmolality measurements instead of the SI unit, degree Celsius (1 Osm/l = 1.86°C.).

Table 2 DERIVED UNITS

QUANTITY	UNIT NAME	UNIT SYMBOL
Area	square meter[a]	m^2
Clearance	liter/second[b]	l/s
Concentration		
Mass	kilogram/liter[b]	kg/l
Substance	mole/liter[b]	mol/l
Density	kilogram/liter[b]	kg/l
Electric potential	volt[a]	$V = kg\ m^2/s^3A$
Energy	Joule[a]	$J = kg\ m^2/s^2$
Force	Newton[a]	$N = kg\ m/s^2$
Frequency	Hertz[a]	Hz = 1 cycle/s
Pressure	Pascal[a]	$Pa = kg/m\ s^2$
Temperature	degree Celsius[a]	$°C = °K - 273.15$
Volume	cubic meter[a]	m^3
	liter[b]	$1 = dm^3$

[a] Derived coherent unit.
[b] Derived non-coherent unit.

Table 3 PREFIXES

PREFIX	PREFIX SYMBOL	FACTOR
tera	T	10^{12}
giga	G	10^{9}
mega	M	10^{6}
kilo	k	10^{3}
hecto	h	10^{2}
deca	da	10^{1}
deci	d	10^{-1}
centi	c	10^{-2}
milli	m	10^{-3}
micro	μ	10^{-6}
nano	n	10^{-9}
pico	p	10^{-12}
femto	f	10^{-15}
atto	a	10^{-18}

REFERENCES

Baron, D. N.: SI units. Br. Med. J., *4*:509, 1974.

Baron, D. N., Broughton, P. M. G., Cohen, M., Langsley, T. S., Lewis, S. M., and Shinton, N. K.: The use of SI units in reporting results obtained in hospital laboratories. J. Clin. Pathol., *27*:590, 1974.

Beeler, M. F., Copeland, B. E., Gambino, S. R., and Powsner, E. R.: Editorial—The metric system and clinical chemistry. Am. J. Clin. Pathol., *59*:277, 1973.

Beeler, M. F.: Metrication from crawl to walk. Am. J. Clin. Pathol., *65*:19, 1976.

Conn, R. B.: Statement of the American Society of Clinical Pathology on the adoption of the International System of Units (SI). Am. J. Clin. Pathol., *67*:108, 1977.

Copeland, B. E.: SI units—a classification. Am. J. Clin. Pathol., *65*:20, 1976.

Council on Scientific Affairs: Adoption of International System of Units for Clinical Chemistry. J.A.M.A., *240*:2664, 1978.

Dybkaer, R., and Jørgensen, K.: Quantities and Units in Clinical Chemistry, Including Recommendation 1966 of the Commission on Clinical Chemistry of the International Union of Pure and Applied Chemistry and of the International Federation of Clinical Chemistry. Copenhagen, Munksgaard, 1967.

Dybkaer, R.: International recommendation for nomenclature of quantities and units in clinical chemistry. Am. J. Clin. Pathol., *52*:637, 1969.

Editorial: SI units. Br. Med. J., *4*:490, 1974.

Ingelfinger, F. J.: Metrication on the crawl. N. Engl. J. Med., *292*:805, 1975.

International Committee for Standardization in Hematology, International Federation of Clinical Chemistry, and World Association of (Anatomic and Clinical) Pathology Societies: Recommendations for use of SI units in clinical laboratory measurements. Br. J. Haematol., *23*:787, 1972, and Clin. Chem., *19*:135, 1973.

International Union of Pure and Applied Chemistry and International Federation of Clinical Chemistry: Quantities and Units in Clinical Chemistry Recommendation 1973. Pure Appl. Chem., *37*:519, 1974.

International Union of Pure and Applied Chemistry and International Federation of Clinical Chemistry: List of Quantities in Clinical Chemistry Recommendation 1973. Pure Appl. Chem., *37*:549, 1974.

Lehmann, H. P.: Metrication of clinical laboratory data in SI units. Am. J. Clin. Pathol., *65*:2, 1976.

World Health Organization: Use of SI units in medicine. WHO Official Records No. 240, 1977.

Young, D. S.: Standardized reporting of laboratory data: The desirability of using SI units. N. Engl. J. Med., *290*:368, 1974.

Young, D. S.: Normal laboratory values (case records of the Massachusetts General Hospital) in SI units. N. Engl. J. Med., *292*:795, 1975.

6

Table 4 WHOLE BLOOD, SERUM, AND PLASMA CHEMISTRY

TYPICAL REFERENCE INTERVALS

COMPONENT	SYSTEM	In Conventional Units	Factor*	In SI Units†
Acetoacetic acid:				
qualitative	Serum	Negative		Negative
quantitative	Serum	0.2–1.0 mg/dl	98	19.6–98.0 µmol/l
Acetone:				
qualitative	Serum	Negative		Negative
quantitative	Serum	0.3–2.0 mg/dl	172	51.6–344.0 µmol/l
Albumin:				
quantitative	Serum	3.2–4.5 g/dl (salt fractionation)	10	32–45 g/l
		3.2–5.6 g/dl (electrophoresis)	10	32–56 g/l
		3.8–5.0 g/dl (dye binding)	10	38–50 g/l
Alcohol, ethyl	Serum or whole blood	Negative—but presented as mg/dl	0.22	Negative—but presented as mmol/l
Aldolase	Serum:			
	adults	3–8 Sibley-Lehninger U/dl at 37°C.	7.4	22–59 mU/l at 37°C.
	children	Approximately 2 times adult levels		Approximately 2 times adult levels
	newborn	Approximately 4 times adult levels		Approximately 4 times adult levels
Alpha-amino acid nitrogen	Serum	3.6–7.0 mg/dl	0.714	2.6–5.0 mmol/l
δ-Aminolevulinic acid	Serum	0.01–0.03 mg/dl	76.3	0.76–2.29 µmol/l
Ammonia	Plasma	20–120 µg/dl (diffusion)	0.554	11.1–67.0 µmol/l
		40–80 µg/dl (enzymatic method)	0.554	22.2–44.3 µmol/l
		12–48 µg/dl (resin method)	0.554	6.7–26.6 µmol/l
Amylase	Serum	60–160 Somogyi units/dl	1.85	111–296 U/l
Argininosuccinic lyase	Serum	0–4 U/dl	10	0–40 U/l
Arsenic‡	Whole blood	<7 µg/dl	0.13	<0.91 µmol/l
Ascorbic acid (vitamin C)	Plasma	0.6–1.6 mg/dl	56.8	34–91 µmol/l
	Whole blood	0.7–2.0 mg/dl	56.8	40–114 µmol/l
Barbiturates	Serum, plasma, or whole blood	Negative	—	Negative
Base excess	Whole blood:			
	male	−3.3 to +1.2 mEq/l	1	−3.3 to +1.2 mmol/l
	female	−2.4 to +2.3 mEq/l	1	−2.4 to +2.3 mmol/l
Base, total	Serum	145–160 mEq/l	1	145–160 mmol/l
Bicarbonate	Plasma	21–28 mM	1	21–28 mmol/l
Bile acids	Serum	0.3–3.0 mg/dl	10	3.0–30.0 mg/l
Bilirubin:	Serum			
direct (conjugated)		Up to 0.3 mg/dl	17.1	Up to 5.1 µmol/l
indirect (unconjugated)		0.1–1.0 mg/dl	17.1	1.7–17.1 µmol/l
total		0.1–1.2 mg/dl	17.1	1.7–20.5 µmol/l
newborns total		1–12 mg/dl	17.1	17.1–205.0 µmol/l
Blood gases: (Chapter 5)	Whole blood			
pH		7.38–7.44 (arterial)	1	7.38–7.44
		7.36–7.41 (venous)	1	7.36–7.41

2086

Determination	Specimen	Conventional value	Factor	SI value
Pco$_2$	Whole blood	35-40 mm Hg (arterial)	0.133	4.66-5.32 kPa[a]
	Whole blood	40-45 mm Hg (venous)	0.133	5.32-5.99 kPa[a]
Po$_2$	Serum	95-100 mm Hg (arterial)	0.133	12.64-13.30 kPa[a]
Bromide	Serum	0-5 mg/dl	0.125	0-0.63 mmol/l
BSP (Bromosulphalein) (5 mg/kg)	Serum	less than 6% retention 45 min. after injection	0.01[b]	less than 0.06 retention 45 min after injection
Calcium: ionized	Serum	4-4.8 mg/dl	0.25	1.0-1.2
		2.0-2.4 mEq/l	0.5	1.0-1.2 mmol/l
total		30-58% of total	0.01[b]	0.30-0.58 of total
		9.2-11.0 mg/dl	0.25	2.3-2.8 mmol/l
		4.6-5.5 mEq/l	0.5	23-28 mmol/l
Carbon dioxide (CO$_2$ content)	Whole blood (arterial)	19-24 mM	1	19-24 mmol/l
	Plasma or serum (arterial)	21-28 mM	1	21-28 mmol/l
Carbon dioxide	Whole blood (venous)	22-26 mM	1	22-26 mmol/l
	Plasma or serum (venous)	24-30 mM	1	24-30 mmol/l
CO$_2$ combining power	Plasma or serum (venous)	24-30 mM	1	24-30 mmol/l
CO$_2$ partial pressure (Pco$_2$)	Whole blood (arterial)	35-40 mm Hg	0.133	4.66-5.32 kPa[a]
	Whole blood (venous)	40-45 mm Hg	0.133	5.32-5.99 kPa[a]
Carbonic acid (H$_2$CO$_3$)	Whole blood (arterial)	1.05-1.45 mM	1	1.05-1.45 mmol/l
	Whole blood (venous)	1.15-1.50 mM	1	1.15-1.50 mmol/l
	Plasma (venous)	1.02-1.38 mM	1	1.02-1.38 mmol/l
Carboxyhemoglobin (carbon monoxide hemoglobin)	Whole blood: suburban nonsmokers	<1.5% saturation of hemoglobin	0.01[b]	<0.015 saturation of hemoglobin
	smokers	1.5-5.0% saturation	0.01	0.015-0.050 saturation
	heavy smokers	5.0-9.0% saturation	0.01	0.050-0.090 saturation
Carotene, beta	Serum	40-200 µg/dl	0.0186	0.74-3.72 µmol/l
Ceruloplasmin	Serum	23-50 mg/dl	10	230-500 mg/l
Chloride	Serum	95-103 mEq/l	1	95-103 mmol/l
Cholesterol total (Chapter 8)	Serum	150-250 mg/dl (varies with diet, sex, and age)	0.026	3.90-6.50 mmol/l
esters	Serum	65-75% of total cholesterol	0.01[b]	0.65-0.75 of total cholesterol
Cholinesterase (Pseudocholinesterase)	Erythrocytes	0.65-1.3 pH units	1	0.65-1.3 units[c]
	Plasma	0.5-1.3 pH units	1	0.5-1.3 units
	Plasma	8-18 IU/l at 37°C.	1	8-18 U/l at 37°C.
Citrate	Serum or plasma	1.7-3.0 mg/dl	52	88-156 µmol/l
Copper	Serum, plasma: male	70-140 µg/dl	0.157	11.0-22.0 µmol/l
	female	80-155 µg/dl	0.157	12.6-24.3 µmol/l
Cortisol	Plasma: 8 a.m.-10 a.m.	5-23 µg/dl	27.6	188-635 nmol/l
	4 p.m.-6 p.m.	3-13 µg/dl	27.6	83-359 nmol/l

6

Table 4 WHOLE BLOOD, SERUM, AND PLASMA CHEMISTRY (*Continued*)

| | | TYPICAL REFERENCE INTERVALS | | |
COMPONENT	SYSTEM	In Conventional Units	Factor*	In SI Units†
Creatine as creatinine	Serum or plasma:			
male		.1-.4 mg/dl	76.3	7.6-30.5 μmol/l
female		.2-.7 mg/dl	76.3	15.3-53.4 μmol/l
Creatine kinase (CK)	Serum:			
male		55-170 U/l at 37°C.	1	55-170 U/l at 37°C.
female		30-135 U/l at 37°C.	1	30-135 U/l at 37°C.
Creatinine (Chapter 10)	Serum or plasma	0.6-1.2 mg/dl (adult)	88.4	53-106 μmol/l
		0.3-0.6 mg/dl (children < 2 yr.)	88.4	27-54 μmol/l
Creatinine clearance (endogenous) (Chapter 6)	Serum or plasma and urine:			
male		107-139 ml/min.	0.0167	1.78-2.32 ml/s
female		87-107 ml/min	0.0167	1.45-1.79 ml/s
Cryoglobulins	Serum	Negative	—	Negative
Electrophoresis, protein (Chapter 9)	Serum	per cent:		
Albumin		52-65% of total protein	0.01b	0.52-0.65 of total protein
Alpha-1		2.5-5.0% of total protein	0.01	0.025-0.05 of total protein
Alpha-2		7.0-13.0% of total protein	0.01	0.07-0.13 of total protein
Beta		8.0-14.0% of total protein	0.01	0.08-0.14 of total protein
Gamma		12.0-22.0% of total protein	0.01	0.12-0.22 of total protein
	Serum	Concentration		
Albumin		3.2-5.6 gm/dl	10	32-56 g/l
Alpha-1		0.1-0.4 gm/dl		1-4 g/l
Alpha-2		0.4-1.2 gm/dl		4-12 g/l
Beta		0.5-1.1 gm/dl		5-11 g/l
Gamma		0.5-1.6 gm/dl		5-16 g/l
Fats, neutral (see Triglycerides)				
Fatty acids:				
total (free and esterified)	Serum	9-15 mM	1	9-15 mmol/l
free (non-esterified)	Plasma	300-480 μEq/l	1	300-480 μmol/l
Fibrinogen	Plasma	200-400 mg/dl	0.01	2.00-4.00 g/l
Fluoride	Whole blood	<0.05 mg/dl	0.53	<0.027 mmol/l
Folate	Serum	5-25 ng/ml (bioassay)	2.27	11-56 nmol/l
		>2.3 ng/ml (radioassay)	2.27	>5.2 nmol/l
	Erythrocytes	166-640 ng/ml (bioassay)	2.27	376-1452 nmol/l
		>140 ng/ml (radioassay)	2.27	>318 nmol/l
Galactose	Whole blood:			
adults		none	0.055	none
children		<20 mg/dl	0.055	<1.1 mmol/l
Gamma globulin	Serum	0.5-1.6 gm/dl	10	5-16 g/l
Globulins, total	Serum	2.3-3.5 gm/dl	10	23-35 g/l
Glucose, fasting	Serum or plasma	70-110 mg/dl	0.055	3.85-6.05 mmol/l
	Whole blood	60-100 mg/dl	0.055	3.30-5.50 mmol/l

Test	Specimen	Conventional units	Factor	SI units
Glucose tolerance oral (See Table 7-4, p. 167, for criteria employed)	Serum or plasma:			
	fasting	70–110 mg/dl	0.055	3.85–6.05 mmol/l
	30 min.	30–60 mg/dl above fasting	0.055	1.65–3.30 mmol/l above fasting
	60 min.	20–50 mg/dl above fasting	0.055	1.10–2.75 mmol/l above fasting
	120 min.	5–15 mg/dl above fasting	0.055	0.28–0.83 mmol/l above fasting
	180 min.	Fasting level or below	0.055	Fasting level or below
intravenous	Serum or plasma:			
	fasting	70–110 mg/dl	0.055	3.85–6.05 mmol/l
	5 min.	Maximum of 250 mg/dl	0.055	Maximum of 13.75 mmol/l
	60 min.	Significant decrease	0.055	Significant decrease
	120 min.	Below 120 mg/dl	0.055	Below 6.60 mmol/l
	180 min.	Fasting level	0.055	Fasting level
Glucose 6-phosphate dehydrogenase (G6PD)	Erythrocytes	250–500 units/10⁶ cells	1	250–500 units/10^6 cells
		1200–2000 mIU/ml packed erythrocytes	1	1200–2000 U/l packed erythrocytes
γ-Glutamyl transferase	Serum	5–40 IU/l	1	5–40 U/l at 37°C.
Glutathione	Whole blood	24–37 mg/dl	0.032	0.77–1.18 mmol/l
Growth hormone	Serum	<10 ng/ml	1	<10 µg/l
Guanase	Serum	<3 nM/ml/min	1	<3 U/l at 37°C.
Haptoglobin	Serum	60–270 mg/dl	.01	0.6–2.7 g/l
Hemoglobin	Serum or plasma:			
	qualitative	Negative	10	Negative
	quantitative	0.5–5.0 mg/dl	10	5–50 mg/l
	Whole blood:			
	female	12.0–16.0 g/dl	10	1.86–2.48 mmol/l
	male	13.5–18.0 g/dl	10	2.09–2.79 mmol/l
α-Hydroxybutyrate dehydrogenase	Serum	140–350 U/ml	1	140–350 kU/l
17-Hydroxycorticosteroids	Plasma:			
	male	7–19 µg/dl	10	70–190 µg/l
	female	9–21 µg/dl	10	9–21 µg/l
	after 24 USP units of ACTH I.M.			
	Serum	35–55 µg/dl	10	350–550 µg/l
Immunoglobulins:	Serum			
IgG		800–1801 mg/dl	0.01	8.0–18.0 g/l
IgA		113–563 mg/dl	0.01	1.1–5.6 g/l
IgM		54–222 mg/dl	0.01	0.54–2.2 g/l
IgD		0.5–3.0 mg/dl	10	5.0–30 mg/l
IgE		0.01–0.04 mg/dl	10	0.1–0.4 mg/l
Insulin	Plasma:			
	bioassay	11–240 µIU/ml[d]	0.0417	0.46–10.00 µg/l
	radioimmunoassay	4–24 µIU/ml	0.0417	0.17–1.00 µg/l
Insulin tolerance (0.1 unit/kg) (See Fig. 14-6, p. 409)	Serum:			
	fasting	Glucose of 70–110 mg/dl	0.055	Glucose of 3.85–6.05 mmol/l
	30 min.	Fall to 50% of fasting level	0.01[b]	Fall to 0.5 of fasting level
	90 min.	Fasting level		Fasting level

6

Table 4 WHOLE BLOOD, SERUM, AND PLASMA CHEMISTRY (*Continued*)

COMPONENT	SYSTEM	TYPICAL REFERENCE INTERVALS		
		In Conventional Units	Factor*	In SI Units†
Iodine:				
butanol-extraction (BEI)	Serum	3.5–6.5 μg/dl	0.079	0.28–0.51 μmol/l
protein bound (PBI)	Serum	4.0–8.0 μg/dl		0.32–0.63 μmol/l
Iron, total	Serum	60–150 μg/dl	0.179	11–27 μmol/l
Iron binding capacity	Serum	300–360 μg/dl	0.179	54–64 μmol/l
Iron saturation	Serum	20–55%	0.01[b]	0.20–0.55 of total iron binding capacity
Isocitric dehydrogenase	Serum	50–240 units/ml at 25°C. (Wolfson-Williams Ashman units)	0.0167	0.83–4.18 U/l at 25°C.
Ketone bodies	Serum	Negative	—	Negative
17-Ketosteroids	Plasma	25–125 μg/dl	0.01	0.25–1.25 mg/l
Lactic acid (as lactate)	Whole blood:			
	venous	5–20 mg/dl	0.111	0.6–2.2 mmol/l
	arterial	3–7 mg/dl		0.3–0.8 mmol/l
Lactate dehydrogenase (LDH)	Serum	80–120 units at 30°C. (lactate → pyruvate)	0.48	38–62 U/l at 30°C. (lactate → pyruvate)
		185–640 units at 30°C. (pyruvate → lactate)	0.48	90–310 U/l at 30°C. (pyruvate → lactate)
		100–190 U/l at 37°C. (lactate → pyruvate)	1	100–190 U/l at 37°C. (lactate → pyruvate)
Lactate dehydrogenase isoenzymes:	Serum			
LDH$_1$ (anode)		17–27%	0.01[b]	0.17–0.27 of total LDH
LDH$_2$		27–37%		0.27–0.37 of total LDH
LDH$_3$		18–25%		0.18–0.25 of total LDH
LDH$_4$		3–8%		0.03–0.08 of total LDH
LDH$_5$ (cathode)		0–5%		0.00–0.05 of total LDH
Lactate dehydrogenase (heat stable)	Serum	30–60% of total	0.01[b]	0.3–0.6 of total LDH
Lactose tolerance	Serum	Serum glucose changes similar to glucose tolerance test	—	Serum glucose changes similar to glucose tolerance test
Lead	Whole blood	0–50 μg/dl	0.048	0–2.4 μmol/l
Leucine aminopeptidase (LAP)	Serum:			
	male	80–200 U/ml (Goldbarg-Rutenberg)	0.24	19.2–48.0 U/l
	female	75–185 U/ml (Goldbarg-Rutenberg)	0.24	18.0–44.4 U/l
Lipase	Serum	0–1.5 U/ml (Cherry-Crandall)	278	0–417 U/l
		14–280 mIU/ml	1	14–280 U/l
Lipids, total	Serum	400–800 mg/dl	0.01	4.00–8.00 g/l
cholesterol (see Chap. 8)		150–250 mg/dl	0.026	3.9–6.5 mmol/l
triglycerides (see Chap. 8)		10–190 mg/dl	0.109	1.09–20.71 mmol/l
phospholipids		150–380 mg/dl	0.01	1.50–380 g/l
fatty acids (free)		9.0–15.0 mM/l	1	9.0–15.0 mmol/l
		300–480 μEq/l	1	300–480 μmol/l
phospholipid phosphorous		8.0–11.0 mg/dl	0.323	2.58–3.55 mmol/l
Lithium	Serum	Negative	—	Negative
Therapeutic interval		0.5–1.4 mEq/l	1	0.5–1.4 mmol/l

Test	Specimen	Conventional	Factor	SI
Long-acting thyroid-stimulating hormone (LATS)	Serum	None	—	None
Lutenizing hormone (LH)	Serum:			
male		6-30 mIU/ml	0.23	1.4-6.9 mg/l
female		Mid cycle peak: 3 times baseline value	0.23	Mid cycle peak: 3 times baseline value
		Premenopausal <30 mIU/ml	0.23	Premenopausal <5 times baseline value
		Postmenopausal >35 mIU/ml		Postmenopausal >5 times baseline value
Macroglobulins, total	Serum	70-430 mg/dl	0.01	0.7-4.3 g/l
Magnesium	Serum	1.3-2.1 mEq/l	0.5	0.7-1.1 mmol/l
		1.8-3.0 mg/dl	0.41	0.7-1.1 mmol/l
Methemoglobin	Whole blood	0-0.24 g/dl	10	0.0-2.4 g/l
		<30% of total hemoglobin	0.01[b]	<.03 of total hemoglobin
Mucoprotein	Serum	80-200 mg/dl	0.01	0.8-2.0 g/l
Non-protein nitrogen (NPN)	Serum or plasma	20-35 mg/dl	0.714	14.3-25.0 mmol/l
	Whole blood	25-50 mg/dl	0.714	17.9-35.7 mmol/l
5'Nucleotidase	Serum	0-1.6 units at 37°C.	1	0-1.6 units at 37°C.
Ornithine carbamyl transferase	Serum	8-20 mIU/ml at 37°C.	1	8-20 U/l at 37°C.
Osmolality	Serum	280-295 mOsm/kg	1	280-295 mOsm/l
Oxygen: (Chapter 5)				
pressure (PO_2)	Whole blood (arterial)	95-100 mm Hg	0.133	12.64-13.30 kPa[a]
content	Whole blood (arterial)	15-23 volume %	0.01[b]	0.15-0.23 of volume
saturation	Whole blood (arterial)	94-100%	0.01[b]	0.94-1.00 of total
pH	Whole blood (arterial)	7.38-7.44	1	7.38-7.44
	Whole blood (venous)	7.36-7.41	1	7.36-7.41
	Serum or plasma (venous)	7.35-7.45	1	7.35-7.45
Phenylalanine	Serum: adults	<3.0 mg/dl	0.061	<0.18 mmol/l
	newborns (term)	1.2-3.5 mg/dl	0.061	0.07-0.21 mmol/l
Phosphatase				
acid phosphatase	Serum	0.13-0.63 U/l at 37°C. (paranitrophenyl phosphate)	16.67	2.2-10.5 U/l at 37°C. (p-nitrophenylphosphate)
				0.0-0.8 U/l at 37°C.
alkaline phosphatase	Serum	20-90 IU/l at 30°C. (paranitrophenylphosphate in AMP buffer)	1	20-90 U/l at 30°C. (p-nitrophenylphosphate)
				25-97 U/l at 37°C. (p-nitrophenylphosphate)
Phospholipid phosphorus	Serum	8-11 mg/dl	0.323	2.6-3.6 mmol/l
Phospholipids	Serum	150-380 mg/dl	0.01	1.50-3.80 g/l
Phosphorus, inorganic	Serum: adults	2.3-4.7 mg/dl	0.323	0.78-1.52 mmol/l
	children	4.0-7.0 mg/dl	0.323	1.29-2.26 mmol/l
Potassium	Plasma	3.8-5.0 mEq/l	1	3.8-5.0 mmol/l
Prolactin		1-25 ng/ml (females)		
		1-20 ng/ml (males)		
Proteins: (Chapter 9)	Serum			
total		6.0-7.8 g/dl	10	60-78 g/l
albumin		3.2-4.5 g/dl	10	32-45 g/l
globulin		2.3-3.5 g/dl	10	23-35 g/l

6

Table 4   WHOLE BLOOD, SERUM, AND PLASMA CHEMISTRY (*Continued*)

TYPICAL REFERENCE INTERVALS

COMPONENT	SYSTEM	In Conventional Units	Factor*	In SI Units†
Protein fractionation		See electrophoresis		See electrophoresis
Protoporphyrin	Erythrocytes	15–50 μg/dl	0.018	0.27–0.90 μmol/l
Pyruvate	Whole blood	0.3–0.9 mg/dl	114	34–103 μmol/l
Salicylates	Serum	Negative	—	Negative
therapeutic interval		15–30 mg/dl	0.072	1.44–1.80 mmol/l
		150–300 μg/ml	0.0072	1.08–2.16 mmol/l
Sodium	Plasma	136–142 mEq/l	1	136–142 mmol/l
Sulfate, inorganic	Serum	0.2–1.3 mEq/l	0.5	0.10–0.65 mmol/l
		0.9–6.0 mg/dl as SO_4^{--}	0.104	0.09–0.62 mmol/l as SO_4^{--}
Sulfhemoglobin	Whole blood	Negative	—	Negative
Sulfonamides	Serum or whole blood	Negative	—	Negative
Testosterone	Serum or plasma:			
male		300–1200 ng/dl	0.035	10.0–42.0 nmol/l
female		30–95 ng/dl	0.035	1.1–3.3 nmol/l
Thiocyanate	Serum	Negative	—	Negative
Thymol flocculation	Serum	0–5 units^f	1	0–5 units
Thyroid hormone tests: (Chapter 14)	Serum			
a) Expressed as thyroxine:				
T$_4$ by column		5.0–11.0 μg/dl	13.0	65–143 nmol/l
T$_4$ by competitive binding—Murphy-Pattee		6.0–11.8 μg/dl	13.0	78–153 nmol/l
T$_4$ RIA		5.5–12.5 mEq/dl	13.0	72–163 nmol/l
free T$_4$		0.9–2.3 ng/dl	13.0	12–30 pmol/l
b) Expressed as iodine:				
T$_4$ by column		3.2–7.2 μg/dl	79.0	253–569 nmol/l
T$_4$ by competitive binding—Murphy-Pattee		3.9–7.7 μg/dl	79.0	308–608 nmol/l
free T$_4$		0.6–1.5 ng/dl	79.0	47–119 pmol/l
T$_3$ resin uptake	Serum	25–38 relative % uptake	0.01^b	0.25–0.38 relative uptake
Thyroxine-binding globulin (TBG)	Serum	10–26 μg/dl	10	100–260 μg/l
TSH	Serum	<10 μU/ml	1	<10^{-3} IU/l
Transferases				
aspartate amino transferase (AST or SGOT)	Serum	10–40 U/ml (Karmen) at 25°C. 16–60 U/ml (Karmen) at 30°C.	0.48	8–29 U/l at 30°C. 8–33 U/l at 37°C.
alanine amino transferase (ALT or SGPT)	Serum	10–30 U/ml (Karmen) at 25°C. 8–50 U/ml (Karmen) at 30°C.	0.48	4–24 U/l at 30°C. 4–36 U/l at 37°C.
gamma glutamyl transferase (GGT)		5–40 IU/l at 37°C.	1	5–40 U/l at 37°C.
Triglycerides (Chapter 8)	Serum	10–190 mg/dl	0.011^e	0.11–2.09 mmol/l
Urea nitrogen	Serum	8–23 mg/dl	0.357	2.9–8.2 mmol/l

Test	Specimen	Conventional value	Factor	SI units
Urea clearance:	Serum and Urine			
maximum clearance		64–99 ml/min, or more than 75% of normal clearance	0.0167	1.07–1.65 ml/s
standard clearance		41–65 ml/min, or more than 75% of normal clearance	0.0167	0.68–1.09 ml/s or more than 0.75 of normal clearance
Uric acid	Serum:			
male		4.0–8.5 mg/dl	0.059	0.24–0.5 mmol/l
female		2.7–7.3 mg/dl	0.059	0.16–0.43 mmol/l
Vitamin A	Serum	15–60 µg/dl	0.035	0.53–2.10 µmol/l
Vitamin A tolerance	Serum: fasting 3 hr. or 6 hr. after 5000 units vitamin A/kg 24 hrs.	15–60 µg/dl	0.035	0.53–2.10 µmol/l
		200–600 µg/dl Fasting values or slightly above		7.00–21.00 µmol/l Fasting values or slightly above
Vitamin B$_{12}$	Serum	160–950 pg/ml	0.74	118–703 pmol/l
Unsaturated vitamin B$_{12}$ binding capacity	Serum	1000–2000 pg/ml	0.74	740–1480 pmol/l
Vitamin C	Plasma	0.6–1.6 mg/dl	56.8	34–91 µmol/l
Xylose absorption	Serum:			
normal		25–40 mg/dl between 1 and 2 hr.	0.067	1.68–2.68 mmol/l between 1 and 2 h
in malabsorption		Maximum approximately 10 mg/dl		Maximum approximately 0.67 mmol/l
Dose: adult		25 g D-xylose	0.067	0.167 mol D-xylose
children		0.5 g/kg D-xylose		3.33 mmol/kg D-xylose
Zinc	Serum	50–150 µg/dl	0.153	7.65–22.95 µmol/l

*Factor = Number factor (note that units are not presented).

†Value in SI units = Value in conventional units × factor.

‡Usually not measured in blood (preferred specimen is urine, hair, or nails except in acute cases where gastric contents are used).

6

Table 5 URINE

COMPONENT	TYPE OF URINE SPECIMEN	In Conventional Units	TYPICAL REFERENCE INTERVALS	
			Factor	In SI Units
Acetoacetic acid	Random	Negative	—	Negative
Acetone	Random	Negative	—	Negative
Addis count	12 hr. collection	WBC and epithelial cells: 1,800,000/12 hr.	1	1.8×10^6/12 h
		RBC 500,000/12 hr.	1	0.5×10^6/12 h
		Hyaline casts: 0–5000/12 hr.	1	5.0×10^3/12 h
Albumin:				
qualitative	Random	Negative	—	Negative
quantitative	24 hr.	15–150 mg/24 hr.	1	0.015–0.150 g/24 h
Aldosterone	24 hr.	2–26 μg/24 hr.	2.77	5.5–72.0 nmol/24 h
Alkapton bodies	Random	Negative	—	Negative
Alpha-amino acid nitrogen	24 hr.	100–290 mg/24 hr.	0.0714	7.14–20.71 mmol/24 h
δ-Aminolevulinic acid	Random:			
adult		0.1–0.6 mg/dl	76.3	7.6–45.8 μmol/l
children		<0.5 mg/dl	76.3	<38.1 μmol/l
	24 hr.	1.5–7.5 mg/24 hr.	7.63	11.15–57.2 μmol/24 h
Ammonia nitrogen	24 hr.	500–1200 mg/24 hr.	0.071	35.5–85.2 mmol/24 h
Amylase	2 hr.	35–260 Somogyi units/hr.	0.185	6.5–48.1 U/h
Arsenic	24 hr.	<50 μg/l	0.013	<0.65 μmol/l
Ascorbic acid	Random	1–7 mg/dl	0.057	0.06–0.40 mmol/l
	24 hr.	>50 mg/24 hr.	0.0057	>0.29 mmol/24 h
Bence Jones protein	Random	Negative	—	Negative
Beryllium	24 hr.	<0.05 μg/24 hr.	111	<5.55 nmol/24 h
Bilirubin, qualitative	Random	Negative	—	Negative
Blood, occult	Random	Negative	—	Negative
Borate	24 hr.	<2 mg/l	16	<32 μmol/l
Calcium:				
qualitative (Sulkowitch)	Random	1+ turbidity	1	1+ turbidity
quantitative	24 hr.:			
average diet		100–240 mg/24 hr.	0.025	2.50–6.25 mmol/24 h
low calcium diet		<150 mg/24 hr.	0.025	<3.75 mmol/24 h
high calcium diet		240–300 mg/24 hr.	0.025	6.25–7.50 mmol/24 h
Catecholamines	Random	0–14 μg/dl	0.059	0–0.83 μmol/l
	24 hr.	<100 μg/24 hr. (varies with activity)	0.0059	<0.59 μmol/24 h
Epinephrine		<10 ng/24 hr.	5.46	<55 nmol/24 h
Norepinephrine		<100 ng/24 hr.	5.91	<590 nmol/24 h
Total free catecholamines		4–126 mcg./24 hr.	5.91	24–745 nmol/24 h
Total metanephrines		0.1–1.6 mg./24 hr.	5.07	0.5–8.1 μmol/24 h
Chloride	24 hr.	140–250 mEq/24 hr.	1	140–250 mmol/24 h
Concentration test (Fishberg):	Random—after fluid restriction			

Specific gravity		>1.025	1	>1.025
Osmolality	24 hr.	>850 mOsm/24 hr.	1	>850 mOsm/l
Copper	Random: adult	0-50 µg/24 hr.	0.016	0-0.48 µmol/24 h
Coproporphyrin	24 hr.: adult	3-20 µg/dl	0.015	0.045-0.30 µmol/l
Creatine	24 hr.: adult	50-160 µg/24 hr.	0.0015	0.075-0.24 µmol/24 h
	children	0-80 µg/24 hr.	0.0015	0.00-0.12 µmol/24 h
Creatinine	24 hr.: male	0-40 mg/24 hr.	0.0076	0-0.30 mmol/24 h
	female	0-100 mg/24 hr.	0.0076	0-0.76 mmol/24 h
		Higher in children and during pregnancy	0.0076	Higher in children and during pregnancy
	24 hr.: male	20-26 mg/kg/24 hr.	0.0088	0.18-0.23 mmol/kg/24 h
		1.0-2.0 g/24 hr.	8.8	8.8-17.6 mmol/24 h
	female	14-22 mg/kg/24 hr.	0.0088	0.12-0.19 mmol/kg/24 h
		0.8-1.8 g/24 hr.	8.8	7.0-15.8 mmol/24 h
Cystine, qualitative	Random	Negative	—	Negative
Cystine and cysteine	24 hr.	10-100 mg/24 hr.	.0083[h]	0.08-0.83 mmol/24 h
Diacetic acid	Random	Negative	—	Negative
Epinephrine	24 hr.	0-20 µg/24 hr.	0.0055	0.00-0.11 µmol/24 h
Estrogens total	24 hr.: male	5-18 µg/24 hr.	1	5-18 µg/24 h
	female: ovulation	28-100 µg/24 hr.	1	28-80 µg/24 h
	luteal peak	22-80 µg/24 hr.	1	22-105 µg/24 h
	at menses	4-25 µg/24 hr.	1	4-25 µg/24 h
	pregnancy	Up to 45,000 µg/24 hr.	1	Up to 45,000 µg/24 h
	postmenopausal	Up to 10 µg/24 hr.	1	Up to 10 µg/24 h
fractionated	24 hr., non-pregnant, midcycle			
Estrone (E¹)	—	2-25 µg/24 hr.	3.7	7-93 nmol/24 h
Estradiol (E²)	—	0-10 µg/24 hr.	3.7	0-37 nmol/24 h
Estriol (E³)		2-30 µg/24 hr.	3.5	7-105 nmol/24 h
Fat, qualitative	Random	Negative	—	Negative
FIGLU (N-formiminoglutamic acid)	24 hr.	<3 mg/24 hr.	5.7	<17.0 µmol/24 h
	after 15 g of L-histidine	4 mg/8 hr.	5.7	23.0 µmol/8 h
Fluoride	24 hr.	<1 mg/24 hr.	0.053	0.053 mmol/24 h
Follicle-stimulating hormone (FSH)	24 hr.: adult	4-25 mIu/ml	1	6-50 Mouse uterine units (MUU)/24 h
	prepubertal	4-30 mIu/ml	1	<10 MUU/24 h
	postmenopausal	40-50 mIu/ml	1	>50 MUU/24 h
	midcycle	2+ baseline		
Fructose	24 hr.	30-65 mg/24 hr.	0.0056	0.17-0.36 mmol/24 h

6

Table 5 URINE (*Continued*)

COMPONENT	TYPE OF URINE SPECIMEN	TYPICAL REFERENCE INTERVALS		
		In Conventional Units	Factor	In SI Units
Glucose:				
qualitative	Random	Negative	—	Negative
quantitative:	24 hr.	0.5-1.5 g/24 hr.	1	0.5-1.5 g/24 h
copper-reducing substances		average 250 mg/24 hr.	1	average 250 mg/24 h
total sugars		average 130 mg/24 hr.	0.0056	average 0.73 mmol/24 h
glucose	24 hr.			
Gonadotropins, pituitary (FSH and LH)	24 hr.	10-50 MUU/24 hr.	1	10-50 MUU/24 h
Etiocholanolone	24 hr.:			
male		1.4-5.0 mg/24 hr.	3.44	4.8-17.2 μmol/24 h
female		0.8-4.0 mg/24 hr.	3.44	2.8-13.8 μmol/24 h
Dehydroepiandrosterone	24 hr.:			
male		0.2-2.0 mg/24 hr.	3.46	0.7-6.9 μmol/24 h
female		0.2-1.8 mg/24 hr.	3.46	0.7-6.2 μmol/24 h
11-Ketoandrosterone	24 hr.:			
male		0.2-1.0 mg/24 hr.	3.28	0.7-3.3 μmol/24 h
female		0.2-0.8 mg/24 hr.	3.28	0.7-2.6 μmol/24 h
11-Ketoetiocholanolone	24 hr.:			
male		0.2-1.0 mg/24 hr.	3.28	0.7-3.3 μmol/24 h
female		0.2-0.8 mg/24 hr.	3.28	0.7-2.6 μmol/24 h
11-Hydroxyandrosterone	24 hr.:			
male		0.1-0.8 mg/24 hr.	3.26	0.3-2.6 μmol/24 h
female		0.0-0.5 mg/24 hr.	3.26	0.0-1.6 μmol/24 h
11-Hydroxyetiocholanolone	24 hr.:			
male		0.2-0.6 mg/24 hr.	3.26	0.7-2.0 μmol/24 h
female		0.1-1.1 mg/24 hr.	3.26	0.3-3.6 μmol/24 h
Lactose	24 hr.	14-40 mg/24 hr.	2.9	41-116 μmol/24 h
Lead	24 hr.	<100 μg/24 hr.	0.0048	<0.48 μmol/24 h
Magnesium	24 hr.	6.0-8.5 mEq/24 hr.	0.5	3.0-4.3 mmol/24 h
Melanin, qualitative	Random	Negative	—	Negative
3-Methoxy-4-hydroxymandelic acid (VMA)	24 hr.:			
adults		1.5-7.5 mg/24 hr.	5.05	7.6-37.9 μmol/24 h
infants		83 μg/kg/24 hr.	0.0051	0.4 μmol/kg/24 h
Mucin	24 hr.	100-150 mg/24 hr.	1	100-150 mg/24 h
Myoglobin				
qualitative	Random	Negative	—	Negative
quantitative	24 hr.	<4 mg/l	1	<4 mg/l
Osmolality	Random	500-800 mOsm/kg water	1	500-800 mOsm/kg water
Pentoses	24 hr.	2-5 mg/kg/24 hr.	1	2-5 mg/kg/24 h
pH	Random	4.6-8.0	1	4.6-8.0

Phenosulfonphthalein (PSP)	Urine timed after 6 mg PSP IV			
	15 min.	20–50% dye excreted	0.01[b]	0.2–0.5 dye excreted
	30 min.	16–24% dye excreted	0.01	0.16–0.24 dye excreted
	60 min.	9–17% dye excreted	0.01	0.09–0.17 dye excreted
	120 min.	3–10% dye excreted	0.01	0.03–0.10 dye excreted
Phenylpyruvic acid, qualitative	Random	Negative	—	Negative
Phosphorus	Random	0.9–1.3 g/24 hr.	32	29–42 mmol/24 h
Porphobilinogen:				
qualitative	Random	Negative	—	Negative
quantitative	24 hr.	0–1.0 mg/24 hr.	4.42	0–4.4 μmol/24 h
Potassium	24 hr.	40–80 mEq/24 hr.	1	40–80 mmol/24 h
Pregnancy tests	Concentrated morning specimen	Positive in normal pregnancies or with tumors producing chorionic gonadotropin	—	Positive in normal pregnancies or with tumors producing chorionic gonadotropin
Pregnanediol	24 hr.:			
	male	0–1.5 mg/24 hr.	3.12	0–4.7 μmol/24 h
	female	1–8 mg/24 hr.	3.12	3–25 μmol/24 h
	peak pregnancy	1 week after ovulation	3.12	1 week after ovulation
	children	<50 mg/24 hr.	3.12	156 μmol/24 h
Pregnanetriol	24 hr.:	Negative		Negative
	male	0.4–2.4 mg/24 hr.	2.97	1.2–7.1 μmol/24 h
	female	0.5–2.0 mg/24 hr.	2.97	1.5–5.9 μmol/24 h
	children	Up to 1 mg/24 hr.	2.97	Up to 3 μmol/24 h
Protein, qualitative	Random	Negative	—	Negative
	24 hr.	40–150 mg/24 hr.	1	40–150 mg/24 h
Reducing substances, total	24 hr.	0.5–1.5 mg/24 hr.	1	0.5–1.5 mg/24 h
Sodium	24 hr.	75–200 mEq/24 hr.	1	75–200 mmol/24 h
Solids, total	24 hr.	55–70 g/24 hr.	1	55–70 g/24 h
		Decreases with age to 30 gm/24 hr.	—	Decreases with age to 30 g/24 h
Specific gravity	Random	1.016–1.022 (normal fluid intake)	1	Relative Density (U 20°C./water 20°C.)
		1.001–1.035 (range)		1.016–1.022 (normal fluid intake)
				1.001–1.034 (range)
Sugars (excluding glucose)	Random	Negative	—	Negative
Titratable acidity	24 hr.	20–50 mEq/24 hr.	1	20–50 mmol/24 h
Urea nitrogen	24 hr.	6–17 g/24 hr.	0.0357	0.21–0.60 mol/24 h
Uric acid	24 hr.	250–750 mg/24 hr.	0.0059	1.48–4.43 mmol/24 h
Urobilinogen	2 hr.	0.3–1.0 Ehrlich Units	—	
	24 hr.	0.05–2.5 mg/24 hr. or 0.5–4.0 Ehrlich units/24 hr.	1.69	0.09–4.23 μmol/24 h
Uropepsin	Random	15–45 units/hr. (Anson)	7.37	111–332 U/h
	24 hr.	1500–5000 units/24 hr. (Anson)	7.37	11–37 kU/h
Uroporphyrins:				
qualitative	Random	Negative	—	Negative
quantitative	24 hr.	10–30 μg/24 hr.	0.0012	0.012–0.037 μmol/24 h
Vanillylmandelic acid (VMA)	24 hr.	1.5–7.5 mg/24 hr.	5.05	7.6–37.9 μmol/24 h
Volume, total	24 hr.	600–1600 ml/24 hr.	0.001	0.6–1.61/24 h
Zinc	24 hr.	0.15–1.2 mg/24 hr.	15.3	2.3–18.4 μmol/24 h

6

Table 6   SYNOVIAL FLUID

COMPONENT	TYPICAL REFERENCE INTERVALS		
	In Conventional Units	Factor	In SI Units
Blood-serum-synovial fluid glucose difference	<10 mg/dl	0.055	<0.55 mmol/l
Differential cell count	Granulocytes < 25% of nucleated cells	0.01[b]	Granulocytes < 0.25 of nucleated cells
Fibrin clot	Absent	—	Absent
Mucin clot	Abundant	—	Abundant
Nucleated cell count	<200 cells/μl	10^6	<2 × 10^8 cells/l
Viscosity	High	—	High
Volume	<3.5 ml	0.001	<0.0035 l

Table 7   SEMINAL FLUID

COMPONENT	TYPICAL REFERENCE INTERVALS		
	In Conventional Units	Factor	In SI Units
Liquefaction	within 20 min.	1	within 20 min
Sperm morphology	>70% normal, mature spermatozoa	0.01[b]	>0.7 normal, mature spermatozoa
Sperm motility	>60%	0.01[b]	>0.6
pH	>7.0 (average 7.7)	1	>7.0 (average 7.7)
Sperm count	60–150 million/ml	10^3	60–150 × 10^9/l
Volume	1.5–5.0 ml	0.001	0.0015–0.005/l

Table 8   GASTRIC FLUID

COMPONENT	TYPICAL REFERENCE INTERVALS		
	In Conventional Units	Factor	In SI Units
Fasting residual volume	20–100 ml	0.001	0.02–0.10/l
pH	<2.0	1	<2.0
Basal acid output (BAO)	0–6 mEq/hr.	1	0–6 mmol/h
Maximum acid output (MAO) (after histamine stimulation)	5–40 mEq/hr.	1	5–40 mmol/h
BAO/MAO ratio	<0.4	1	<0.4

Table 9 HEMATOLOGY

COMPONENT	TYPICAL REFERENCE INTERVALS			
	In Conventional Units	Factor	In SI Units	
Red cell volume:				
male	25–35 ml/kg body weight	0.001	0.025–0.035 l/kg body weight	
female	20–30 ml/kg body weight	—	0.020–0.030 l/kg body weight	
Plasma volume:				
male	40–50 ml/kg body weight	0.001	0.040–0.050 l/kg body weight	
female	40–50 ml/kg body weight	—	0.040–0.050 l/kg body weight	
Coagulation tests:				
Bleeding time (Ivy)	1–6 minutes	1	1–6 min	
Bleeding time (Duke)	1–3 minutes	1	1–3 min	
Clot retraction	½ the original mass in 2 hr.	1	0.5 the original mass in 2 h	
Dilute blood clot lysis time	Clot lysis between 6 and 10 hr at 37°C.	1	Clot lysis between 6 and 10 h at 37°C.	
Euglobin clot lysis time	Clot lysis between 2 and 6 hr. at 37°C.	1	Clot lysis between 2 and 6 h at 37°C.	
Partial thromboplastin time	60–70 seconds	1	60–70 s	
Kaolin activated	35–50 seconds	1	35–50 s	
Prothrombin time	12–14 seconds	1	12–14 s	
Venous clotting time:				
3 tubes	5–15 minutes	1	5–15 min	
2 tubes	5–18 minutes	—	5–8 min	
Whole blood clot lysis time	None in 24 hr.	—	None in 24 h	
Complete blood count (CBC)				
Hematocrit:				
male	40–54%	0.01[b]	0.40–0.54	
female	38–47%	—	0.38–0.47	
Hemoglobin:				
male	13.5–18.0 g/dl	0.155	2.09–2.79 mmol/l	
female	12.0–16.0 g/dl	—	1.86–2.48 mmol/l	
Red Cell Count:				
male	$4.6–6.2 \times 10^6/\mu l$	0.155	$4.6–6.2 \times 10^{12}/l$	
female	$4.2–5.4 \times 10^6/\mu l$	—	$4.2–5.4 \times 10^{12}/l$	
White Cell Count	$4.5–11.0 \times 10^3/\mu l$	10^6	$4.5–11.0 \times 10^9/l$	
Erythrocyte indices:				
Mean corpuscular volume (MCV)	80–96 cu. microns	1	80–96 fl	
Mean corpuscular hemoglobin (MCH)	27–31 pg	1	27–31 pg	
Mean corpuscular hemoglobin concentration (MCHC)	32–36%	0.01[b]	0.32–0.36	

White blood cell differential (adult):	Mean per cent	Range of absolute counts		Mean fraction*	Range of absolute count
Segmented neutrophils	56%	1800–7000/μl	10^6	0.56	$1.8–7.0 \times 10^9/l$
Bands	3%	0–700/μl	10^6	0.03	$0–0.70 \times 10^9/l$
Eosinophils	2.7%	0–450/μl	10^6	0.027	$0–0.45 \times 10^9/l$
Basophils	0.3%	0–200/μl	10^6	0.003	$0–0.20 \times 10^9/l$
Lymphocytes	34%	1000–4800/μl	10^6	0.34	$1.0–4.8 \times 10^9/l$
Monocytes	4%	0–800/μl	10^6	0.04	$0–0.80 \times 10^9/l$
Hemoglobin A_2	1.5–3.5% of total hemoglobin		0.01[b]	0.015–0.035 of total hemoglobin	
Hemoglobin F	<2%		0.01[b]	<0.02	

6

Table 9   HEMATOLOGY (*Continued*)

	TYPICAL REFERENCE INTERVALS					
COMPONENT	In Conventional Units			Factor	In SI Units	
Osmotic fragility	% NaCl	% Lysis		% NaCl—171 % Lysis—0.01[b]	NaCl mmol/l	Fractional Lysis
		Fresh	24 hr. at 37°C.			Fresh	24 h at 37°C
	0.2	—	95–100		34.2	—	0.95–1.00
	0.3	97–100	85–100		51.3	0.97–1.00	0.85–1.00
	0.35	90–99	75–100		59.8	0.90–0.99	0.75–1.00
	0.4	50–95	65–100		68.4	0.50–0.95	0.65–1.00
	0.45	5–45	55–95		77.0	0.05–0.45	0.55–0.95
	0.5	0–6	40–85		85.5	0–0.06	0.40–0.85
	0.55	0	15–70		94.1	0	0.15–0.70
	0.6	—	0–40		102.6	—	0–0.40
	0.65	—	0–10		111.2	—	0–0.10
	0.7	—	0–5		119.7	—	0–0.05
	0.75	—	0		128.3	—	0
Platelet count	150,000–400,000/μl			10^6	0.15–0.4 × 10^{12}/l	
Reticulocyte count	0.5–1.5%			0.01[b]	0.005–0.015	
	25,000–75,000 cells/μl			10^6	25–75 × 10^9/l	
Sedimentation rate (ESR) (Westergren)						
Men under 50 yrs.	<15 mm/hr			1	<15 mm/h	
Men over 50 yrs.	<20 mm/hr			1	<20 mm/h	
Women under 50 yrs.	<20 mm/hr			1	<20 mm/h	
Women over 50 yrs.	<30 mm/hr			1	<30 mm/h	
Viscosity	1.4–1.8 times water			1	1.4–1.8 times water	
Zeta sedimentation ratio	41–54%			0.01	0.41–0.54	

* All percentages are multiplied by 0.01[b] to give mean fraction.

Table 10   AMNIOTIC FLUID

| | TYPICAL REFERENCE INTERVALS | | |
COMPONENT	In Conventional Units	Factor	In SI Units
Appearance:			
early gestation	Clear	—	Clear
term	Clear or slightly opalescent	—	Clear or slightly opalescent
Albumin:			
early gestation	0.39 g/dl	147	57.3 μmol/l
term	0.19 g/dl	147	27.9 μmol/l
Bilirubin:			
early gestation	<0.075 mg/dl	17.1	<1.28 μmol/l
term	<0.025 mg/dl	17.1	<0.43 μmol/l
Chloride:			
early gestation	Approximately equal to serum chloride	—	Approximately equal to serum chloride
term	Generally 1-3 mEq/l lower than serum chloride	1	Generally 1-3 mmol/l lower than serum chloride
Creatinine:			
early gestation	0.8-1.1 mg/dl	88.4	70.7-97.2 μmol/l
term	1.8-4.0 mg/dl (generally > 2 mg/dl)	88.4	159.1-353.6 μmol/l (generally > 176.8 μmol/l)
Estriol:			
early gestation	<10 μg/dl	0.035	<0.35 μmol/l
term	>60 μg/dl	0.035	>2.1 μmol/l
Lecithin/sphingomyelin		1	
Early (immature)	<1:1	1	<1:1
Term (mature)	>2:1	1	>2:1
Osmolality:			
early gestation	Approximately equal to serum osmolality	1	Approximately equal to serum osmolality
term	230-270 mOsm/l	1	<230-270 mOsm/l
Pco$_2$:			
early gestation	33-55 mm Hg	0.133	4.39-7.32 kPa[a]
term	42-55 mm Hg (increases toward term)	0.133	5.59-7.32 kPa[a] (increases toward term)
pH:			
early gestation	7.12-7.38	1	7.12-7.38
term	6.91-7.43 (decreases toward term)	1	6.91-7.43
Protein, total:			
early gestation	0.60 ± 0.24 g/dl	10	6.0 ± 2.4 g/l
term	0.26 ± 0.19 g/dl	10	2.6 ± 1.9 g/l
Sodium:			
early gestation	Approximately equal to serum sodium	1	Approximately equal to serum sodium
term	7-10 mEq/l lower than serum sodium	1	7-10 mmol/l lower than serum sodium
Staining, cytologic:			
Oil red O:			
early gestation	<10%	0.01[b]	<0.1
term	>50%	0.01	>0.5
Nile blue sulfate:			
early gestation	0	0.01[b]	0
term	>20%	0.01	>0.2
Urea:			
early gestation	18.0 ± 5.9 mg/dl	0.166	2.99 ± 0.98 mmol/l
term	30.3 ± 11.4 mg/dl	0.166	5.03 ± 1.89 mmol/l
Uric acid:			
early gestation	3.72 ± 0.96 mg/dl	0.059	0.22 ± 0.06 mmol/l
term	9.90 ± 2.23 mg/dl	0.059	0.58 ± 0.13 mmol/l
Volume:			
early gestation	450-1200 ml	0.001	0.45-1.2 l
term	500-1400 ml (increases toward term)	0.001	0.5-1.4 l (increases toward term)

6

Table 11   CEREBROSPINAL FLUID

| COMPONENT | TYPICAL REFERENCE INTERVALS | | |
	In Conventional Units	Factor	In SI Units
Albumin	10–30 mg/dl	10	100–300 mg/l
Calcium	2.1–2.7 mEq/l	0.5	1.05–1.35 mmol/l
Cell count	0–5 cells/μl	10^6	$0\text{–}5 \times 10^6/l$
Chloride:			
adult	118–132 mEq/l	1	118–132 mmol/l
Colloidal gold curve	0001111000	—	0001111000
Glucose	50–80 mg/dl	0.055	2.75–4.40 mmol/l
Lactate dehydrogenase (LDH)	Approximately 10% of serum level	—	Approximately 0.1 of serum level
Protein:			
total CSF	15–45 mg/dl	10	150–450 mg/l
ventricular fluid	5–15 mg/dl	10	50–150 mg/l
Protein Electrophoresis:			
Prealbumin	2–7%	0.01[b]	0.02–0.07
Albumin	56–76%	0.01	0.56–0.76
Alpha-1 globulin	2–7%	0.01	0.02–0.07
Alpha-2 globulin	4–12%	0.01	0.04–0.12
Beta globulin	8–18%	0.01	0.08–0.18
Gamma globulin	3–12%	0.01	0.03–0.12
Xanthochromia	Negative	—	Negative

Table 12   MISCELLANEOUS

| COMPONENT | SPECIMEN | TYPICAL REFERENCE INTERVALS | | |
		In Conventional Units	Factor	In SI Units
Bile, qualitative	Random stool	Negative in adults	—	Negative in adults
		Positive in children	—	Positive in children
Chloride	Sweat	4–60 mEq/l	1	4–60 mmol/l
Clearances:	Serum and urine (timed)			
creatinine, endogenous		115 ± 20 ml/min	0.0167	1.92 ± 0.33 ml/l
Diodrast		600–720 ml/min.	0.0167	10.02–12.02 ml/s
inulin		100–150 ml/min.	0.0167	1.67–2.51 ml/s
PAH		600–750 ml/min.	0.0167	10.02–12.53 ml/s
Diagnex blue (tubeless gastric analysis)	Urine	Free acid present	—	Free acid present
Fat:	Stool, 72 hr.			
total fat		<5 g/24 hr.	0.01[b]	<5 g/24 h
		10–25% of dry matter	0.01	0.1–0.24 of dry matter
neutral fat		1–5% of dry matter	0.01	0.01–0.05 of dry matter
free fatty acids		5–13% of dry matter	0.01	0.05–0.13 of dry matter
combined fatty acids		5–15% of dry matter	0.01	0.05–0.15 of dry matter
Nitrogen, total	Stool, 24 hr.	10% of intake	%—0.01[b]	0.1 of intake
		1–2 g/24 hr.	g/24 hr—0.071	0.071–0.142 mol/24 h
Sodium	Sweat	10–80 mEq/l	1	10–80 mmol/l
Trypsin activity	Random, fresh stool	Positive (2+ to 4+)	—	Positive (2+ to 4+)
Thyroid ^{131}I uptake		7.5–25% in 6 hr.	0.01[b]	0.075–0.25 in 6 h
Urobilinogen:				
qualitative	Random stool	Positive	—	Positive
quantitative	Stool, 24 hr	40–200 mg/24 hr.	0.00169	0.068–0.34 mmol/24 h
		80–280 Ehrlich units/24 hr.		

NOTES TO TABLES 4 THROUGH 12

a. It is recommended (World Health Organization, 1977) that the units mm Hg be retained for pressures (Pco_2, Po_2) at the present time.

b. Percentages are expressed as number fractions in the SI, where a number fraction is dimensionless quantity given by: the number of defined particles constituting a specified component divided by the total number of defined particles in the system.

c. Unit based on hydrogen ion concentration.

d. One (1) International Unit of insulin corresponds to 0.04167 mg of the 4th International Standard (a mixture of 52% beef insulin and 48% pig insulin).

e. Factor based on relative molecular mass of triolein (885.4)

f. One (1) International Unit of lutenizing hormone corresponds to 0.2296 mg of 2nd reference preparation (1964).

g. One (1) is equivalent to the turbidity of a solution containing 0.65 mmol/l of $BaSO_4$.

h. Factor based on the relative molecular mass of cysteine, 121.16.

6

SELECTED PEDIATRIC REFERENCE VALUES*

S†-Acid phosphatase

Newborn: 7.4–19.4 U/l
2–13 yrs: 6.4–15.2 U/l

S-Aldolase

Newborn: to 4 × adult value
Child: to 2 × adult value

S-Alkaline phosphatase

Newborn: 40–300 U/l
Child: 60–270 U/l

S-Alpha fetoprotein:

Newborn: up to 100 mg/l
2 weeks: undetectable

S-Amylase

Newborn: little, if any, amylase activity
1 year: adult values

S-Aspartate aminotransferase

Newborn: 16–74 U/l
1–3 yrs: 6–30 U/l

S-Bilirubin

Newborn:

	PRE-TERM	FULL-TERM
24 h	17.1–102.8 μmol/l (10–60 mg/l)	34.2–102.8 μmol/l (20–60 mg/l)
48 h	102.8–137.0 μmol/l (60–80 mg/l)	102.8–119.9 μmol/l (60–70 mg/l)
3–5 d	171.0–266.5 μmol/l (100–150 mg/l)	68.6–205.2 μmol/l (40–120 mg/l)

S-Calcium

Pre-term, first week: 1.5–2.5 mmol/l (60–100 mg/l)
Full-term, first week: 1.75–3.00 mmol/l (70–120 mg/l)
1–2 yrs: 2.5–3.0 mmol/l (100–120 mg/l)
2–16 yrs: 2.25–2.88 mmol/l (90–115 mg/l)

U†-Catecholamines

	NOREPINEPHRINE	EPINEPHRINE
1 yr:	29.5–86.8 nmol/d (5.4–15.9 μg/d)	0.6–25.4 nmol/d (0.1–4.3 μg/d)
1–5 yrs:	44.2–168.1 nmol/d (8.1–30.8 μg/d)	4.7–53.8 nmol/d (0.8–9.1 μg/d)
6–15 yrs:	103.7–388.1 nmol/d (19.0–71.1 μg/d)	7.7–62.1 nmol/d (1.3–10.5 μg/d)
>15 yrs:	188.8–474.8 nmol/d (34.4–87.0 μg/d)	20.7–78.0 nmol/d (3.5–13.2 μg/d)

U-Chloride

Infant: 1.7–8.5 mmol/d
Child: 17–34 mmol/d

S-Cholesterol

Cord blood: 1.2–2.5 mmol/l (460–980 mg/l)
1–2 yrs: 1.8–4.9 mmol/l (700–1900 mg/l)
2–16 yrs: 3.5–6.5 mmol/l (1350–2500 mg/l)

U-Cortisol (free)

4 mos–10 yrs: 2–27 μg/d
11–20 yrs: 0.7–55 μg/d

---

*Information based on: Meites, S. (ed.): Pediatric Clinical Chemistry. Washington, D.C., American Association for Clinical Chemistry, 1977.
†S = serum; U = urine

S-Creatine kinase

Newborn:	$3 \times$ adult values
3 wks–3 mos:	$1.5 \times$ adult values
>1 yr:	at adult values

S-Creatinine

Upper reference value:

Up to 5 yrs:	44 μmol/l (5.0 mg/l)
Up to 6 yrs:	53 μmol/l (6.0 mg/l)
Up to 7 yrs:	62 μmol/l (7.0 mg/l)
Up to 8 yrs:	70 μmol/l (8.0 mg/l)
Up to 9 yrs:	79 μmol/l (9.0 mg/l)
Up to 10 yrs:	88 μmol/l (10.0 mg/l)
>10 yrs:	106 μmol/l (12.0 mg/l)

S-Estradiol

0–2 yrs:	0–7 pg/ml
2–4 yrs:	0–7 pg/ml
4–6 yrs:	0–14 pg/ml
6–8 yrs:	0–10 pg/ml
8–10 yrs:	0–100 pg/ml
10–12 yrs:	0–100 pg/ml
12–14 yrs:	0–100 pg/ml
14–16 yrs:	7–105 pg/ml
16–25 yrs:	7–320 pg/ml

Fecal Fat:

Pre-term newborn:	up to 40% excreted
Full-term newborn:	up to 20% excreted
3 mos–1 yr:	up to 15% excreted
1 yr:	up to 8.5% excreted

P-Nonesterified fatty acids

Newborn:	0–1845 mmol/l
4 mos–10 yrs:	300–1100 mmol/l

S-Glucose

Pre-term newborn:	1.2–3.6 mmol/l (200–656 mg/l)
Full-term newborn:	1.1–6.0 mmol/l (200–1100 mg/l)
Child:	3.3–5.8 mmol/l (600–1050 mg/l)

S-γ-Glutamyltransferase

Premature newborn:	56–233 U/l
Newborn–3 wks:	10–103 U/l
3 wks–3 mos:	4–111 U/l
1–5 yrs:	2–23 U/l
6–15 yrs:	2–23 U/l
16 yrs–adult:	2–35 U/l

6

S-Haptoglobin

Newborn:	detectable haptoglobin in only 10–20%
1 yr and older:	at adult values

S-Immunoglobulin IgG

0–5 wks:	7500–15,000 mg/l
6 mos:	1500–7000 mg/l
1 yr:	1400–10,300 mg/l
5 yrs:	3700–15,000 mg/l
10 yrs:	4400–15,500 mg/l

S-Immunoglobulin IgA

0-5 wks:	none
6 mos:	200-1300 mg/l
1 yr:	200-1300 mg/l
5 yrs:	300-2000 mg/l
10 yrs:	500-2300 mg/l

S-Immunoglobulin IgM

0-5 wks:	less than 200 mg/l
6 mos:	300-600 mg/l
1 yr:	300-1600 mg/l
5 yrs:	200-2200 mg/l
10 yrs:	300-1700 mg/l

Inulin clearance

<1 mo:	29-88 ml/min per 1.73 m^2 of body surface
1-6 mos:	40-112 ml/min per 1.73 m^2 of body surface
6-12 mos:	62-121 ml/min per 1.73 m^2 of body surface
>1 yr:	78-164 ml/min per 1.73 m^2 of body surface

U-17-Ketosteroids

0-3 days:		0-0.5 mg/d
1-3 yrs:		<2.0 mg/d
3-6 yrs:		0.5-3.0 mg/d
6-9 yrs:		0.8-4.0 mg/d
10-12 yrs:	male:	0.7-6.0 mg/d
	female:	0.7-5.0 mg/d
Adolescent:	male:	3-15 mg/d
	female:	3-12 mg/d

S-Lactate dehydrogenase

1-3 days: up to 2 × adult values

S-Phosphorus (inorganic)

	PRE-TERM	FULL-TERM
Newborn:	1.8-2.6 mmol/l (56.0-80.0 mg/l)	1.6-2.5 mmol/l (50.0-78.0 mg/l)
6-10 days:	2.0-3.8 mmol/l (61-117 mg/l)	1.6-2.9 mmol/l (49-89 mg/l)

4 mos:	1.6-2.6 mmol/l (48-81 mg/l)
1 yr:	1.25-2.1 mmol/l (39-60 mg/l)
2-16 yrs:	0.9-1.5 mmol/l (26-50 mg/l)

S-Potassium

Pre-term newborn:	4.5-7.2 mmol/l
Full-term newborn:	5.0-7.7 mmol/l
2 d-2 wks:	4.0-6.4 mmol/l
2 wks-3 mos:	4.0-6.2 mmol/l
3 mos-1 yr:	3.7-5.6 mmol/l
1-16 yrs:	3.6-5.2 mmol/l

S-Testosterone

AGE	MALE	FEMALE
0-2 yrs:	40-370 ng/l	70-180 ng/l
2-4 yrs:	50-160 ng/l	70-200 ng/l
4-6 yrs:	80-400 ng/l	100-200 ng/l
6-8 yrs:	60-280 ng/l	150-300 ng/l
8-10 yrs:	90-500 ng/l	200-400 ng/l
10-12 yrs:	80-2900 ng/l	200-500 ng/l
12-14 yrs:	50-7600 ng/l	300-700 ng/l
14-16 yrs:	900-5600 ng/l	350-950 ng/l
16-18 yrs:	2600-7300 ng/l	400-950 ng/l
18-20 yrs:	4000-7200 ng/l	400-950 ng/l
20-25 yrs:	3400-11,200 ng/l	400-950 ng/l

S-Thyroxine

1–3 days:	142–296 nmol/l (11–23 μg/dl)
1 wk–1 mo:	116–232 nmol/l (9–18 μg/dl)
1–4 mos:	97–212 nmol/l (7.5–16.5 μg/dl)
4–12 mos:	71–187 nmol/l (5.5–14.5 μg/dl)
1–6 yrs:	71–174 nmol/l (5.5–13.5 μg/dl)
6–10 yrs:	64–161 nmol/l (5.0–12.5 μg/dl)

6

INDEX

SUBJECT INDEX

i

GUIDELINES FOR ORDERING BLOOD FOR ELECTIVE SURGERY

These guidelines have been developed and are used at the State University of New York, Upstate Medical Center University Hospital (1978). Each institution is urged to generate its own guidelines, as described in the references. Variations to fit individual patient requirements are recognized and orders modified accordingly.

General Surgery

Amputation A/K, B/K	T&S*
Cholecystectomy and CD exploration	T&S
Gastrectomy with/without vagotomy:	
Subtotal	3
Total	3
Splenectomy	1
Sympathectomy	T&S
†Exploratory laparotomy	T&S
Esophageal resection	2–4
Breast biopsy	T&S
Mastectomy:	
Simple	T&S
Radical	1
Pancreatectomy:	
Partial	4
Radical (Whipple)	4
Thyroidectomy:	
Partial	T&S
Total	T&S
Parathyroidectomy	T&S
Parotidectomy	T&S
Colon Resection:	
Total large colon	2
Hemicolectomy	2
Sigmoidectomy	2
Anterior resection	2
Abdominal-perineal resection	3
Small bowel segment resection	1
Colostomy, Gastrostomy	T&S
Hemorrhoidectomy	T&S
Pilonidal cyst	T&S
Hernias:	
Inguinal	T&S
Incisional	T&S
Umbilical	T&S
Ventral	T&S
Hiatal	T&S
Vein stripping	T&S
Aneurysm resection	6
Femoropopliteal bypass	3
Portocaval shunt	4
Hepatectomy	6

Cardiopulmonary

Coronary vein graft:	
Single	3
Double	3
Triple	3
With other procedure	8(3)
Valve replacement:	
Aortic	6(3)
Mitral	6(3)
Double valve	8(3)
Valve replacement plus single vein grafts	10(3)
Atrial septal defect repair	4(2)
Ventricular septal defect repair	4(2)
Tetralogy of Fallot correction	8(3)
Mitral commissurotomy	6(2)
Pulmonary valvulotomy	4(2)
Coarctation of the aorta correction	4
Aortic valvulotomy or annuloplasty	6
Pericardectomy	8
Thoracotomy:	
Pneumonectomy	2
Wedge resection, pulmonary	2
Esophagectomy	2
Bronchopleural fistula	2
Pectus excavatum	1
Tracheostomy	T&S
Embolectomy	2
Patent ductus arteriosus	4
Vascular tumors	4
Thoracic aneurysm	10(3)

Neurosurgery

Carpal tunnel procedures	T&S
Cranioplasty	1
†Craniotomy:	
Aneurysm	4–6
Subdural, epidural hematoma	2
Tumor	4–8
Cordotomy	T&S
†Laminectomy	T&S
Nerve repair	T&S
Hypophysectomy	T&S
Scalp and skull lesions (no intracranial communications)	T&S
Transphenoidal hypophysectomy	T&S
Ulnar nerve relocation	T&S
Ventricular peritoneal shunt	T&S

Otolaryngology

Branchial cleft cyst	T&S
Glossectomy	2
Laryngectomy	2
with radical neck dissection	4
Mandibulectomy	2
Ethmoidectomy	T&S
Caldwell-Luc operation	T&S
Orbital exploration	1
Mastoidectomy	2
Septoplasty	T&S
Tumor of palate	T&S
Maxillectomy	2
Jaw, neck, tongue dissection	4
Temporal bone resection	6